D1758826

DIAGNOSTIC IMAGING
BREAST

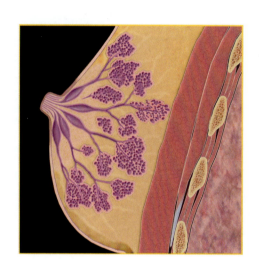

DIAGNOSTIC IMAGING
BREAST

Wendie A. Berg, MD, PhD, FACR

Breast Imaging Consultant
Study Chair ACRIN 6666
American Radiology Services,
Johns Hopkins Green Spring
Lutherville, Maryland

Robyn L. Birdwell, MD

Section Head, Division of Breast Imaging
Brigham and Women's Hospital
Associate Professor of Radiology
Harvard Medical School
Boston, Massachusetts

Eva C. Gombos, MD

Instructor in Radiology
Brigham and Women's Hospital
Dana-Farber Cancer Institute
Harvard Medical School
Boston, Massachusetts

Shih-chang Wang, BSc(Med), MBBS, FRANZCR, FAMS

Associate Professor in Diagnostic Radiology,
Yong Loo Lin School of Medicine
National University Hospital of Singapore
Singapore

Brett T. Parkinson, MD

Imaging Director Breast Care Services
Intermountain Healthcare
Adjunct Assistant Professor of Radiology
University of Utah School of Medicine
Salt Lake City, Utah

Sughra Raza, MD

Associate Director, Division of Breast Imaging
Brigham and Women's Hospital
Assistant Professor
Harvard Medical School
Boston, Massachusetts

Gretchen E. Green, MD, MMS

Clinical Fellow in Women's Imaging
Brigham and Women's Hospital
Harvard Medical School
Boston, Massachusetts
Present Address: Greensboro Radiology
Greensboro, North Carolina

Anne Kennedy, MD

Director of Women's Imaging
Associate Professor of Radiology
Adjunct Associate Professor of Obstetrics and Gynecology
University of Utah School of Medicine
Salt Lake City, Utah

Mark D. Kettler, MD

Director of Breast Imaging
Oregon Health & Science University
Portland, Oregon

AMIRSYS®
Names you know, content you trust®

AMIRSYS®

Names you know, content you trust®

First Edition

Text - Copyright Wendie A. Berg, MD, PhD, FACR 2006

Drawings - Copyright Amirsys Inc 2006

Compilation - Copyright Amirsys Inc 2006

All rights reserved. No part of this publication may be reproduced, stored in a retrieval system, or transmitted, in any form or media or by any means, electronic, mechanical, photocopying, recording, or otherwise, without prior written permission from Amirsys Inc.

Composition by Amirsys Inc, Salt Lake City, Utah

Printed in Canada by Friesens, Altona, Manitoba, Canada

ISBN-13: 978-1-4160-3337-0
ISBN-10: 1-4160-3337-8
ISBN-13: 978-0-8089-2380-0 (International English Edition)
ISBN-10: 0-8089-2380-3 (International English Edition)

Notice and Disclaimer

The information in this product ("Product") is provided as a reference for use by licensed medical professionals and no others. It does not and should not be construed as any form of medical diagnosis or professional medical advice on any matter. Receipt or use of this Product, in whole or in part, does not constitute or create a doctor-patient, therapist-patient, or other healthcare professional relationship between Amirsys Inc. ("Amirsys") and any recipient. This Product may not reflect the most current medical developments, and Amirsys makes no claims, promises, or guarantees about accuracy, completeness, or adequacy of the information contained in or linked to the Product. The Product is not a substitute for or replacement of professional medical judgment. Amirsys and its affiliates, authors, contributors, partners, and sponsors disclaim all liability or responsibility for any injury and/or damage to persons or property in respect to actions taken or not taken based on any and all Product information.

In the cases where drugs or other chemicals are prescribed, readers are advised to check the Product information currently provided by the manufacturer of each drug to be administered to verify the recommended dose, the method and duration of administration, and contraindications. It is the responsibility of the treating physician relying on experience and knowledge of the patient to determine dosages and the best treatment for the patient.

To the maximum extent permitted by applicable law, Amirsys provides the Product AS IS AND WITH ALL FAULTS, AND HEREBY DISCLAIMS ALL WARRANTIES AND CONDITIONS, WHETHER EXPRESS, IMPLIED OR STATUTORY, INCLUDING BUT NOT LIMITED TO, ANY (IF ANY) IMPLIED WARRANTIES OR CONDITIONS OF MERCHANTABILITY, OF FITNESS FOR A PARTICULAR PURPOSE, OF LACK OF VIRUSES, OR ACCURACY OR COMPLETENESS OF RESPONSES, OR RESULTS, AND OF LACK OF NEGLIGENCE OR LACK OF WORKMANLIKE EFFORT. ALSO, THERE IS NO WARRANTY OR CONDITION OF TITLE, QUIET ENJOYMENT, QUIET POSSESSION, CORRESPONDENCE TO DESCRIPTION OR NON-INFRINGEMENT, WITH REGARD TO THE PRODUCT. THE ENTIRE RISK AS TO THE QUALITY OF OR ARISING OUT OF USE OR PERFORMANCE OF THE PRODUCT REMAINS WITH THE READER.

Amirsys disclaims all warranties of any kind if the Product was customized, repackaged or altered in any way by any third party.

Library of Congress Cataloging-in-Publication Data

Diagnostic imaging. Breast / Wendie A. Berg ... [et al.]. — 1st ed.
    p. ; cm.
  Includes bibliographical references and index.
  ISBN-13: 978-1-4160-3337-0
  ISBN-10: 1-4160-3337-8
  ISBN-13: 978-0-8089-2380-0 (international English ed.)
  ISBN-10: 0-8089-2380-3 (international English ed.)
  1. Breast—Imaging—Handbooks, manuals, etc. 2. Breast—Cancer
—Diagnosis—Handbooks, manuals, etc.   I. Berg, Wendie A.
II. Title: Breast.
  [DNLM: 1. Breast Neoplasms—diagnosis—Handbooks. 2. Diag-
nostic Imaging—methods—Handbooks. 3. Mammography—Hand-
books.   WP 39 D536 2006]
RC280.B8D534 2006
618.1'90754—dc22

                               2006030829

This book would not have been possible without the ongoing support of our families, who not only tolerate our passion for our field, but encourage it. We thank our colleagues for alerting us to interesting case material and believing in this project. Lastly, and perhaps most importantly, we dedicate this book to our patients. We have learned a great deal from them, and we have a great deal still to learn.

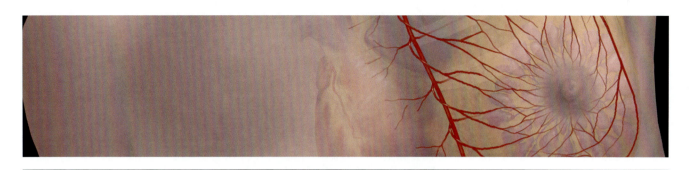

CONTRIBUTORS

Contributing Authors

Laura Amodei, MD
Instructor, Division of Breast Imaging
Department of Radiology
Johns Hopkins Hospital
Johns Hopkins University School of Medicine
Baltimore, Maryland

Gauri C. Bedi, MD, FACS
Breast Surgeon
The Hoffberger Breast Center at Mercy
Mercy Medical Center
Baltimore, Maryland

Jennifer R. Bellon, MD
Assistant Professor
Department of Radiation Oncology
Brigham and Women's Hospital
Dana-Farber Cancer Institute
Harvard Medical School
Boston, Massachusetts

Eric Berns, PhD
Research Assistant Professor
Department of Radiology
Northwestern University, Feinberg School of Medicine
Chicago, Illinois

Roger L. Christian, MD
Clinical Director Comprehensive Breast Health Center
Assistant Professor of Surgery
Brigham and Women's Hospital
Harvard Medical School
Boston, Massachusetts

Arthur J. Elman, MD, FACR
Instructor, Department of Radiation Oncology
Massachusetts General Hospital
Harvard Medical School
Boston, Massachusetts

Dianne Georgian-Smith, MD
Associate Professor of Radiology
Massachusetts General Hospital
Harvard Medical School
Boston, Massachusetts

Juan Godinez, MD
Instructor, Department of Radiation Oncology
Brigham and Women's Hospital
Dana-Farber Cancer Institute
Harvard Medical School
Boston, Massachusetts

R. Edward Hendrick, PhD, FACR
Research Professor and Director, Breast Imaging Research
Northwestern University, Feinberg School of Medicine
and Northwestern Memorial Hospital
Chicago, Illinois

Daniel F. Kacher, MS
Senior Engineer, Image-Guided Therapy Program
Brigham and Women's Hospital
Harvard Medical School
Boston, Massachusetts

Michael N. Linver, MD, FACR
Director of Mammography
X-Ray Associates of New Mexico, P.C.
Clinical Professor of Radiology
University of New Mexico School of Medicine
Albuquerque, New Mexico

M. Raquel Oliva, MD
Women's Imaging Fellow
Department of Radiology
Brigham and Women's Hospital
Harvard Medical School
Boston, Massachusetts

Ann H. Partridge, MD, MPH
Assistant Professor of Medicine
Brigham and Women's Hospital
Dana-Farber Cancer Institute
Harvard Medical School
Boston, Massachusetts

Cheryl A. Sadow, MD
Instructor of Radiology
Division of Abdominal Imaging and Intervention
Brigham and Women's Hospital
Boston, Massachusetts

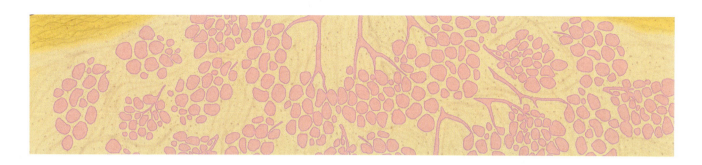

DIAGNOSTIC IMAGING: BREAST

We at Amirsys are proud to present **Diagnostic Imaging: Breast**, the ninth volume in our acclaimed *Diagnostic Imaging (DI)* series. We began this precedent-setting, image- and graphic-rich series with David Stoller's <u>Diagnostic Imaging: Orthopaedics</u>. The next volumes, <u>DI: Brain</u>, <u>DI: Head and Neck</u>, <u>DI: Abdomen</u>, <u>DI: Spine</u>, <u>DI: Pediatrics</u>, <u>DI: Obstetrics</u> and <u>DI: Chest</u>, are now joined by Wendie Berg & Robyn Birdwell's fabulous new textbook, **<u>DI: Breast</u>**.

In **<u>Diagnostic Imaging: Breast</u>**, all breast diagnoses with any form of imaging finding are included. As expected, mammographic images and BI-RADS® definitions are highlighted in this text. Breast MR and ultrasound along with clinical photographs & color graphics make this textbook into a feast for the radiologist's eyes. In addition, exhaustive coverage of clinical issues surrounding breast diagnoses including staging and therapeutic options can be found. Breast anatomy and procedures each have their own section in this textbook. Consequently, this image-rich offering covers all areas of breast imaging needed by the practicing radiologist.

The unique bulleted format of the DI series allows our authors to present approximately twice the information and four times the number of images per diagnosis compared to an old-fashioned traditional prose textbook. All the DI books follow the same format, which means that our many readers find the same information in the same place—every time! And in every body part! The innovative visual differential diagnosis "thumbnail" that provides you with an at-a-glance look at entities that can mimic the diagnosis in question has been highly popular (and much copied). "Key Facts" boxes provide a succinct summary for quick, easy review.

In summary, **<u>Diagnostic Imaging: Breast</u>** is a product designed with you, the reader, in mind. Today's typical practice settings demand efficiency in both image interpretation and learning. We think you'll find this new volume a highly efficient and wonderfully rich resource that will significantly enhance your practice—and find a welcome place on your bookshelf. Enjoy!

Anne G. Osborn, MD
Executive Vice President & Editor-in-Chief, Amirsys, Inc.

H. Ric Harnsberger, MD
CEO & Chairman, Amirsys, Inc.

Paula J. Woodward, MD
Senior Vice President & Medical Director, Amirsys, Inc.

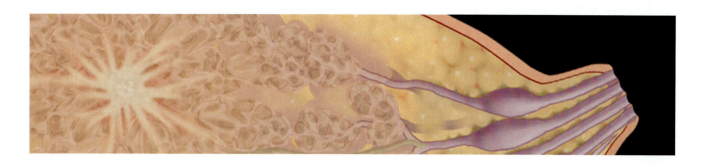

FOREWORD

The breast is an emblem of women. It has become a political organ and its symbolism is deeply rooted in our culture. Breast cancer, now out in the open, has become a target for conquest by very influential advocacy groups. Millions of women undergo annual screening mammography as part of their health maintenance programs. The widespread use of mammography, federal regulation of its quality, and frequent media coverage have introduced the public to radiology and radiologists. Mammography, combined with other imaging modalities in problem-solving, and image-guided percutaneous biopsies performed by radiologists to replace open surgical procedures for diagnosis, have brought radiologists into the clinical realm of direct patient management, while physician-patient relationships remain uncommon in other areas of radiology. Drs. Wendie Berg and Robyn Birdwell have created an outstanding, complete and comprehensive reference that places breast imaging in clinical context, is up-to-the-minute in detection, diagnosis, therapy and management of breast cancer, and is liberally and beautifully illustrated with correlative mammography, ultrasound, and MRI images and superb color graphics.

Diagnostic Imaging: Breast speaks in the language of the future to the broadened scope, greater clinical involvement, and rapidly advancing multimodality imaging and interventional technology of breast imaging. This comprehensive reference is an outstanding addition to a series of authoritative and attractive subspecialty imaging texts earning recognition for their completeness, economy of verbiage, illustrative richness, and clinical relevance. With the elimination of verbal fillers, there is space within the bulleted phrases that comprise the text to include additional detail, and space on the pages for more images. The formatting allows the reader using the book as a reference to scan quickly through the table of contents and/or index and to go immediately to the section that can provide an answer to a question or problem.

As utilization of mammography, breast ultrasound, and now MRI continues to grow, so does the need to manage the patient and to improve mammographic interpretation. This reference will prove invaluable to radiology residents during their three (or more) dedicated months of breast imaging, to breast imaging fellows, to radiology faculty members, to general radiologists, and to other breast physicians. The comprehensiveness, balance, and clinical practicality of this text will require that a copy be chained to the counter in the reading room for reference many times a day. For example, a gynecologist notes a dimple and swelling beneath the left breast of a pregnant patient and sends the patient for evaluation. What is the swelling? How can it be imaged or does it need to be? For a start, look in the embryology section with its lovely illustration of an embryo's two mammalian milk lines. Another example: APBI? The senior member of a group, who remembers ABPA (allergic bronchopulmonary aspergillosis), is perplexed but quickly discovers that the acronym stands for *accelerated partial breast irradiation* for breast cancer patients. APBI is a current area of research and clinical trials with newly developed devices. The method is defined and illustrated and clinical details are provided: eligibility criteria are outlined, methods of delivery shown, and follow-up mammography is illustrated. A third example: when silicone implants rupture, what is the ultrasound physical principle that accounts for the "snowstorm" or echogenic noise signature? Throughout the text, technical factors are discussed for each modality enabling the reader to appreciate the interdependence of interpretation and image quality.

Diagnostic Imaging: Breast will be the standard, authoritative reference for breast imaging. Its numerous, well-chosen images have been obtained with excellent up-to-date technique and equipment and include many digital mammograms, high resolution sonograms, and high-field-strength MR images. The book will be required reading for our residents and fellows, clinicians will find it to be of great value, and my colleagues and I will refer to it frequently. It's a great read, and Drs. Berg and Birdwell have our thanks for this monumental, fabulous effort.

Ellen B. Mendelson, MD

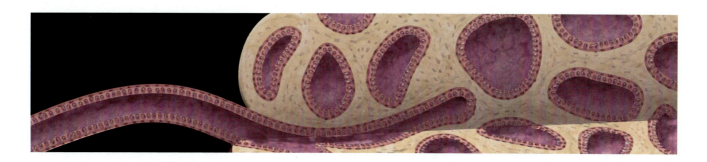

PREFACE

"You can see a lot by just looking."   *(Yogi Berra)*

Breast imaging is an exciting and challenging field. Each and every patient is concerned that she may be the next one we diagnose with cancer. The ability to "see" breast cancers by mammography has dramatically affected many women and has been proven to save lives. For mammography to be of maximal benefit, technique and positioning are critical. The radiologist must have the skills to distinguish normal variations from suspicious findings. Appropriate use of computer-assisted detection (CAD), ultrasound, and magnetic resonance imaging (MRI) can further improve the diagnostic yield of breast imaging.

The skills of the breast imager are largely developed through experience. Participating in the diagnostic workup of screen-detected abnormalities provides important feedback. There is no substitute for examining clinical abnormalities and correlating palpable findings directly with ultrasound while scanning. Learning occurs especially when we find out the results of our recommended biopsies. Core biopsy allows exquisite correlation of imaging and histopathologic findings. Understanding the histopathologic appearance of breast lesions facilitates recognition of specific entities on imaging. The more cancers one has seen, the more likely one will recognize their often subtle features.

We have put together our best images, experience, and an excellent multidisciplinary team in preparing this text. We hope we have developed a resource to improve recognition, understanding, and management of problems encountered in breast imaging. The bulleted text provides a concise summary of pertinent facts. The image galleries are extensive and cross modalities in breast imaging. Mammographic, sonographic, and MRI findings are all richly illustrated and discussed. We have incorporated early results in nuclear medicine imaging of breast cancer. Prognostic and treatment information is detailed for malignant and high-risk lesions, as is the natural history of benign conditions.

So roll up your sleeves, examine those clinical findings, lay your hands on the transducer, take time to look at prior exams, and don't be afraid to ask when you don't know. Perhaps you will find some answers in this book.

We welcome feedback, and encourage further studies to add to the science of what is fundamentally an art. Here's to the journey and the responsibility we all share.

"It's not too far, it just seems like it is."   *(Yogi Berra)*

Wendie A. Berg, MD, PhD, FACR and Robyn L. Birdwell, MD

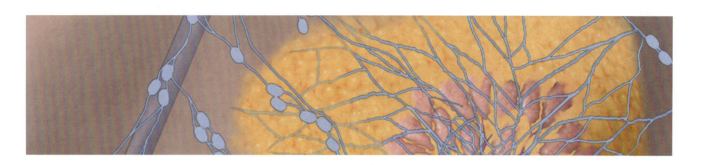

ACKNOWLEDGMENTS

Illustrations

Richard Coombs, MS
Lane R. Bennion, MS
James A. Cooper, MD

Image/Text Editing

Douglas Grant Jackson
Amanda Hurtado
Melanie Hall

Medical Text Editing

Gregory L. Johnson, MD

Case Management

Roth LaFleur
Christopher Odekirk

Case Contributors

(ALP) Amy L.M. Pang, FRCR
(DAL) Daniel A. Lehrer, MD
(DNS) Darrell N. Smith, MD
(DWM) Diana Weedman Molavi, MD
(EAM) Elizabeth A. Morris, MD
(EAR) Elizabeth A. Rafferty, MD
(EBM) Ellen B. Mendelson, MD
(FMD) Fred M. Dirbas, MD
(GMT) Gary M. Tse, FRCPC
(HKG) Harmindar K. Gill, MD
(JAW) Judith A. Wolfman, MD
(JJP) Julian J. Pribaz, MD, FRCS, FRACS
(KK) Katalin Kelemen, MD, PhD
(LG) Lorena Gutierrez, MD
(LPA) Lee P. Alder, MD via Naviscan PET Systems, Inc.
(LT) Lorraine Tafra, MD via Naviscan PET Systems, Inc.
(LWB) Lawrence W. Bassett, MD
(MP) Mayur Patel, MD
(MY) Martin Yaffe, MD
(OBI) Olga B. Ioffe, MD
(RAC) Ronald A. Castellino, MD
(RHH) Ralph H. Hruban, MD
(SJS) Stuart J. Schnitt, MD, PhD
(WLB) William L. Boren, MD via Dilon Technologies, LLC

Project Leads

Melissa A. Hoopes
Kaerli Main

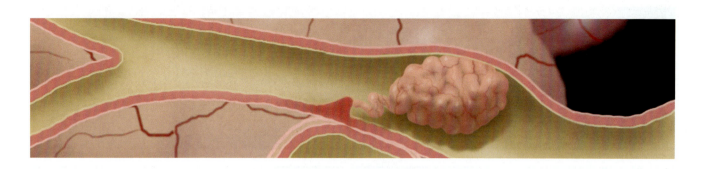

SECTIONS

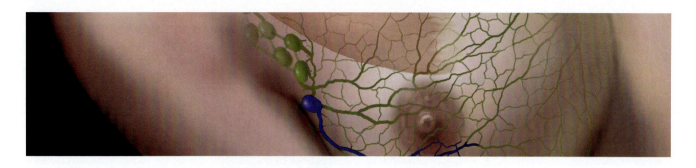

TABLE OF CONTENTS

MR Enhancement Patterns

SECTION 2
Histopathologic Diagnoses

Benign Lesions

Risk Lesions

Locally Aggressive Lesions

Malignant Lesions

SECTION 3
Anatomic Considerations

Nipple

Skin

Axilla

Chest Wall

Vascular Entities

SECTION 4
Post-Operative Imaging Findings

Results of Benign Intervention

Results Following Treatment for Malignancies

SECTION 5
Special Topics

Hormonal Changes

Pregnancy

SECTION 3
Procedures, Surgical

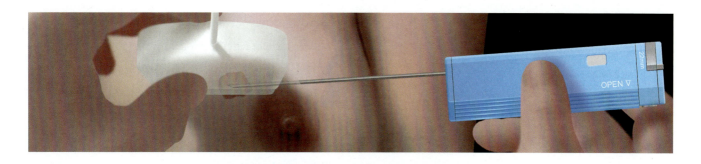

ABBREVIATIONS

AAPM: American Association of Physicists in Medicine

ACC: adenoid cystic carcinoma

ACR: American College of Radiology

ACS: American Cancer Society

ADH: atypical ductal hyperplasia

AEC: automatic exposure control

AI: aromatase inhibitor

AJCC: American Joint Committee on Cancer

ALH: atypical lobular hyperplasia

ALND: axillary lymph node dissection

AM: apocrine metaplasia

AP: anteroposterior

APBI: accelerated partial breast irradiation

BB: bee-bee (radiopaque marker)

BC: breast cancer

BCT: breast conservation therapy

BI-RADS: Breast Imaging Reporting and Data System® (registered trademark of the American College of Radiology)

Bq: becquerel, with 1 Bq = 1 disintegration per second

BSGI: breast-specific gamma imaging

bx: biopsy

c/w: consistent with

Ca++: calcifications or microcalcifications

CAD: computer-aided detection or computer-assisted detection

CALGB: Cancer and Leukemia Group B

CAPSS: columnar alteration with apical snouts and secretions

CBC: contralateral breast cancer

CBE: clinical breast examination

CC: craniocaudal

CCC: columnar cell change

CCFB: CC view from below (caudal-cranial)

CCH: columnar cell hyperplasia

CCL: columnar cell lesions

cCR: clinical complete response

CCRL: CC view with the top of the breast rolled laterally

CCRM: CC view with the top of the breast rolled medially

CDR: cancer detection rate

CECT: contrast-enhanced computed tomography

CI: confidence interval

CNB: core needle biopsy

CR: complete response

CR-FFDM: computed radiography full-field digital mammography

CSL: complex sclerosing lesion

dB: decibels

DCIS: ductal carcinoma in situ

DDFS: distant disease-free survival

DFS: disease-free survival

DIEP: deep inferior epigastric perforator

Dmax: maximum optical density in film

DVT: deep-vein thrombosis

EGF: epidermal growth factor

EGFR: epidermal growth factor (EGF) receptor

EIC: extensive intraductal component

ER: estrogen receptor

FA: fibroadenoma

FAC: fibroadenomatoid change

FAH: fibroadenomatoid hyperplasia

FAL: fibroadenolipoma

FCC: fibrocystic changes

FDA: Food and Drug Administration (United States)

FDG: 18F-fluorodeoxyglucose

FEA: flat epithelial atypia

FFDM: full-field digital mammography

FISH: fluorescence in situ hybridization

FN: false negative

FNA: fine needle aspiration

FNAB: fine needle aspiration biopsy

FOV: field of view

FP: false positive

FUS: focused ultrasound surgery

GCDFP: gross cystic disease fluid protein

GCSF: granulocyte colony stimulating factor

GCT: granular cell tumor

Gd-contrast: gadolinium-based contrast agent

H&E: haematoxylin and eosin

HCG: human chorionic gonadotropin

HIP: Health Insurance Plan of New York

HIV: human immunodeficiency virus

HRT: hormone replacement therapy

IBC: inflammatory breast cancer

ID: implant-displaced

IDC: infiltrating (invasive) ductal carcinoma

IDH: usual intraductal hyperplasia

IEA: inferior epigastric artery

I-GAP: inferior gluteal artery perforator

IHC: immunohistochemistry

ILC: infiltrating (invasive) lobular carcinoma

IMA: internal mammary artery

IMF: inframammary fold

IMLN: intramammary lymph node

IMN: internal mammary node

IMPC: invasive micropapillary carcinoma

IORT: intraoperative radiation therapy

ITC: isolated tumor cells

kVp: kilovoltage peak

LABC: locally advanced breast cancer

LCIS: lobular carcinoma in situ

LDM: latissimus dorsi myocutaneous

LIQ: lower inner quadrant

LITT: laser interstitial thermal therapy

LM: lateromedial view

LN: lobular neoplasia

LOH: loss of heterozygosity

LOQ: lower outer quadrant

lt: left

LVI: lymphovascular invasion

mAs: milliampere seconds

MB: megabyte

MBBC: metachronous bilateral breast cancer

mCi: millicurie

MDP: Tc-99m-methylene diphosphonate

MGA: microglandular adenosis

MIBI: Tc-99m-sestamibi

MIP: maximum intensity pixel

MLL: mucocele-like lesions

MLO: mediolateral oblique

MQSA: Mammography Quality Standards Act

MRI: magnetic resonance imaging

MRM: modified radical mastectomy

MRS: magnetic resonance spectroscopy

MRVAB: magnetic resonance imaging-guided vacuum-assisted biopsy

ML: mediolateral view

NAT: neoadjuvant chemotherapy

NHL: non-Hodgkin lymphoma

NOS: not otherwise specified

NPV: negative predictive value

NSABP: National Surgical Adjuvant Breast and Bowel Project

NST: no special type, no specific type

OR: odds ratio

OS: overall survival

PAAG: polyacrylamide gel

PACS: picture archiving and communications system

PASH: pseudoangiomatous stromal hyperplasia

pCR: pathologic complete response

PE: pulmonary embolism

PEM: positron emission mammography

PLB: primary lymphoma of breast

PLC: pleomorphic lobular carcinoma

PNL: posterior nipple line

PPV: positive predictive value

PR: progesterone receptor

PT: phyllodes tumor

QA: quality assurance

QC: quality control

RA: rheumatoid arthritis

RCTs: randomized controlled trials

RFA: radiofrequency ablation

RM: radical mastectomy

ROI: region of interest

RR: relative risk

RSL: radial sclerosing lesion

rt: right

RT-PCR: reverse transcriptase-polymerase chain reaction

SA: sclerosing adenosis

SBBC: simultaneous bilateral primary breast cancer

SC: Tc-99m-sulfur colloid

SEA: superior epigastric artery

SERM: selective estrogen receptor modulator

SFM: screen-film mammography

S-GAP: superior gluteal artery perforator

SI: signal intensity

SIEA: superficial inferior epigastric artery

SLN: sentinel lymph node

SMM-HC: smooth muscle myosin heavy chain

SMOLD: squamous metaplasia of lactiferous ducts

SMPTE: Society of Motion Picture and Television Engineers

SNB: sentinel lymph node biopsy

SNR: signal-to-noise ratio

SPECT: single photon emission computed tomography

SPGR: spoiled-gradient echo

STIR: short tau inversion recovery

STIR WS: short tau inversion recovery with water suppression

SUV: standardized uptake value

SVAB: stereotactic vacuum-assisted biopsy

T1WI: T1-weighted imaging

T2WI: T2-weighted imaging

T2WI FS: T2-weighted imaging with fat suppression

TAM: Tamoxifen

TB: tuberculosis

TDLU: terminal duct lobular unit

TGC: time gain compensation curve

TM: total mastectomy

TN: true negative

TNM: tumor, node, metastasis

TP: true positive

TRAM: transverse rectus abdominus myocutaneous

TSH: thyroid stimulating hormone

UBC: unilateral breast cancer

UIQ: upper inner quadrant

UK NHS: United Kingdom National Health Service

UOQ: upper outer quadrant

US: ultrasound

USA: United States of America

USCNB: ultrasound-guided core needle biopsy

USPSTF: United States Preventive Services Task Force

US-VAB or US-DVB: ultrasound-guided directional vacuum-assisted breast biopsy

VAB: vacuum-assisted biopsy

WBI: whole breast irradiation

WL: window level

WW: window width

XCCL: laterally exaggerated CC view

XCCM: medially exaggerated CC view

DIAGNOSTIC IMAGING
BREAST

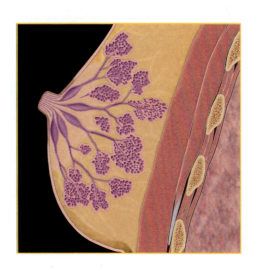

PART I

Anatomy

Breast Overview

Embryology and Normal Development

Nipple Areolar Complex & Skin

Segmental Anatomy

Chest Wall and Axilla

Neurovascular Supply

Lymph Nodes and Lymphatics

BREAST OVERVIEW

Terminology

Abbreviations
- Terminal ductal lobular unit (TDLU)
- Anterior mammary fascia (AMF)
- Posterior mammary fascia (PMF)
- Anterior suspensory ligament (ASL)
- Posterior suspensory ligament (PSL)

General Breast Anatomy

Overview
- Conical, round or hemispherical shape
- Comprised of 15-20 lobes, each encased in fascial sheath defined by AMF & PMF
- Extends from 2nd or 3rd intercostal space to 6th or 7th intercostal space
- Extends laterally to anterior axillary fold and medially to lateral sternum
- Relationship to chest wall
  - Superior two-thirds overlies pectoralis major muscle
  - Lateral portions overly serratus anterior muscle
  - Inferior-most margin overlies upper abdominal oblique muscles
- Axillary tail of Spence: Extension of normal breast tissue toward axilla
- Average breast size: Diameter 10-12 cm; thickness 5-7 cm; median 5 cm thick with mammographic compression
- Support and mobility relate to fascial attachments to skin and chest wall

Glandular Elements

Contents
- Extralobular ducts
- TDLUs
- Extralobular ducts and TDLUs contain two cell layers: Outer myoepithelial cell layer and inner epithelial cell layer

Stroma/Connective Tissue

Contents
- Fat
- Connective tissue
- ASLs (Cooper) and PSLs
- Nerves, blood vessels and lymphatics

Interlobular Tissue
- High in collagen content
- Relatively lower in cellular elements and hyaluronic acid

Intralobular Tissue
- Relatively lower collagen content
- Higher in cellular elements and hyaluronic acid

Zonal Anatomy

Premammary (Subcutaneous) Zone
- Most superficial zone
- Anterior margin defined by skin, posterior margin defined by AMF
- Contains subcutaneous fat, blood vessels, anterior suspensory (Cooper) ligaments
- May contain ectopic ducts and TDLUs
- ASLs (Cooper ligaments)
  - Formed from two leaflets of AMF inserting into dermis
  - Provide support for breast
  - Usually visible on mammograms and sonograms

Mammary Zone
- Defined anteriorly by AMF and posteriorly by PMF
- Contains majority of ducts/TDLUs, stromal fat and stromal connective tissue
- Subdivided haphazardly by interspersed ASLs

Retromammary Zone
- Most posterior of three zones
- Defined anteriorly by PMF and posteriorly by chest wall
- Contains fat and PSLs which attach PMF to chest wall

Imaging Principles

Mammography
- Overall breast density reflects ratio between glandular elements (higher density) and fat (lower density); usually symmetric between breasts but wide range of normal
- Fatty involution typically begins in lower-outer quadrant; progresses with age to upper-outer quadrant
- American College of Radiology Breast Imaging and Reporting and Database System (BI-RADS) density categories
  - 1: Almost entirely fat
  - 2: Scattered fibroglandular densities
  - 3: Heterogeneously dense
  - 4: Extremely dense

Ultrasound
- Thin echogenic skin line
- ASLs usually visible in subcutaneous zone
- Interlobular stroma and glandular elements usually hyperechoic relative to fat
- Pectoral muscles and ribs visible as hypoechoic posterior structures

MR
- Fibroglandular tissue/muscle often show physiologic enhancement
- Density and enhancement features of parenchyma vary with patient age and phase of menstrual cycle
- Ideally performed day 7-14 of menstrual cycle: Less dense stroma and lower breast water content
- Fibrocystic change may enhance/obscure pathology

BREAST OVERVIEW

Premammary zone

Mammary zone

Retromammary zone

Premammary zone

Mammary zone

Retromammary zone

Premammary zone

Mammary zone

Retromammary zone

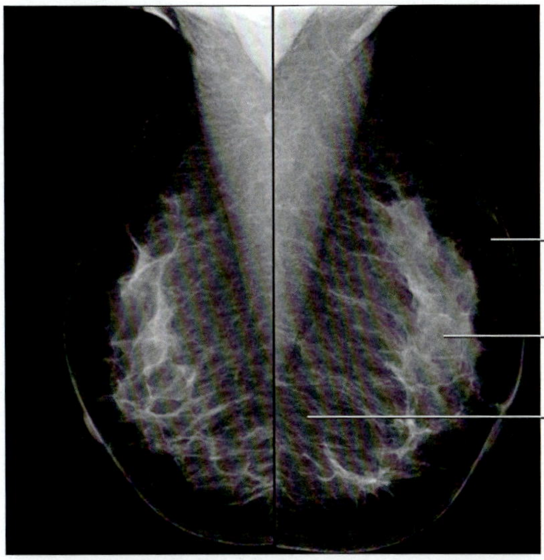

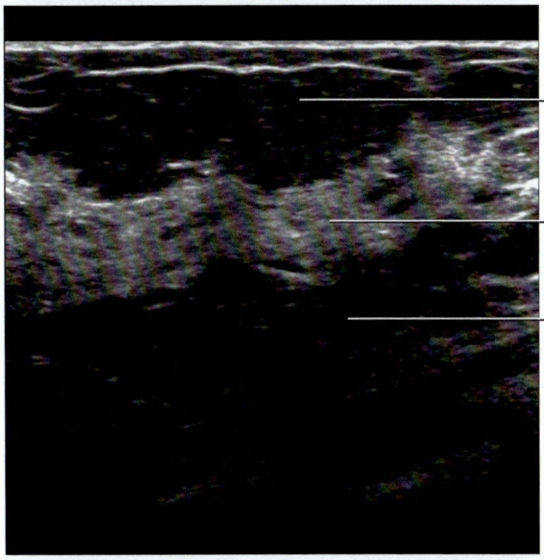

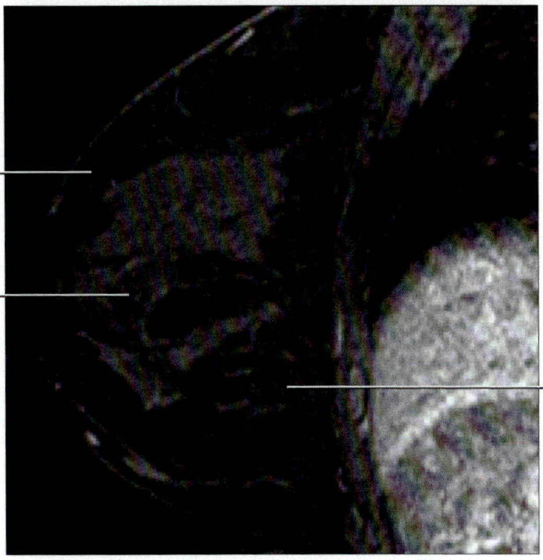

(Top) Bilateral MLO digital mammograms demonstrate the subcutaneous, premammary zone defined anteriorly by the skin and posteriorly by the anterior mammary fascia, the mammary zone defined anteriorly by the anterior mammary fascia and posteriorly by the posterior mammary fascia and the retromammary zone defined anteriorly by the posterior mammary fascia and posteriorly by the chest wall. (Middle) Breast ultrasound demonstrating zonal anatomy. (Bottom) Sagittal T1 C+ SPGR breast MR demonstrating zonal anatomy.

BREAST OVERVIEW

ANTERIOR SUSPENSORY (COOPER) LIGAMENTS

Premammary fat

Glandular elements

Retromammary fat

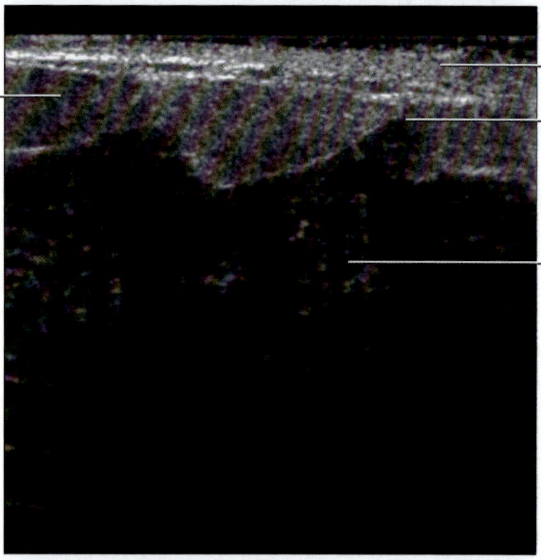

Anterior suspensory (Cooper) ligaments

Premammary fat

Skin

Anterior suspensory (Cooper) ligament

Fibroglandular elements

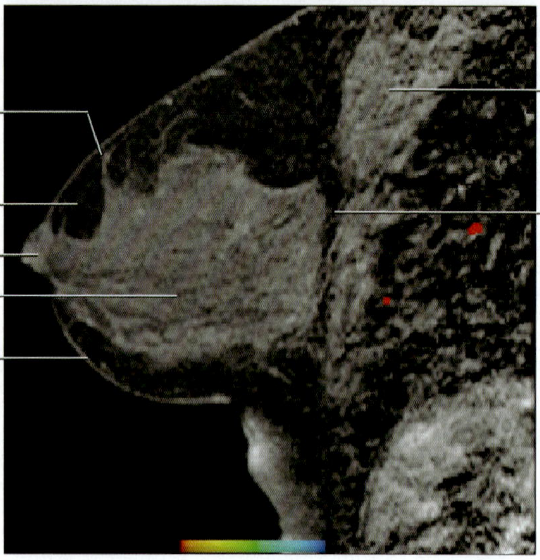

Anterior suspensory (Cooper) ligament

Premammary fat

Physiologic nipple enhancement

Dense glandular elements

Skin

Pectoralis major muscle

Retromammary fat

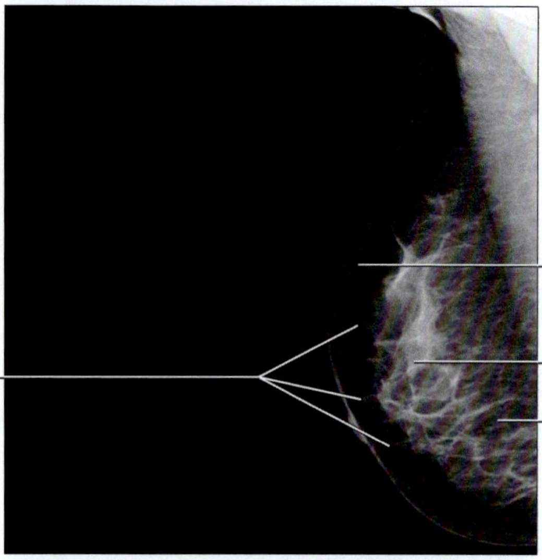

(Top) Right MLO digital mammogram with abundant fat in the subcutaneous (premammary) and retromammary zones and glandular elements and stroma in the mammary zone. Anterior suspensory (Cooper) ligaments are formed from leaflets of the anterior mammary fascia and insert into the dermis to stabilize the breast. **(Middle)** Breast ultrasound nicely demonstrates leaflets of anterior mammary fascia converging to form anterior suspensory (Cooper) ligaments. **(Bottom)** Sagittal T1 C+ FS MR in a pre-menopausal woman showing a few anterior suspensory (Cooper) ligaments, with mild physiologic enhancement of normal glandular elements and nipple.

BREAST OVERVIEW

BI-RADS BREAST COMPOSITION

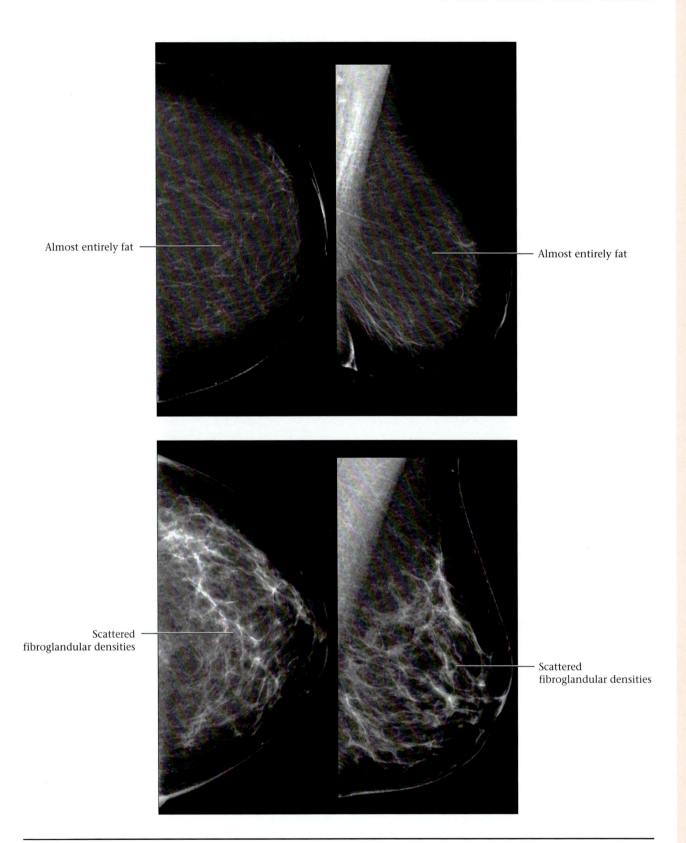

Almost entirely fat

Almost entirely fat

Scattered fibroglandular densities

Scattered fibroglandular densities

(Top) The American College of Radiology Breast Imaging and Reporting Database System (BI-RADS) divides breast composition into four categories: 1) almost entirely fat, 2) scattered fibroglandular densities (approximately 25-50% glandular), 3) heterogeneously dense (51-75% glandular), 4) extremely dense (greater than 75% glandular). These CC/MLO digital mammograms show almost entirely fat composition. **(Bottom)** These CC/MLO digital mammograms show a pattern of scattered fibroglandular density.

BREAST OVERVIEW

BI-RADS BREAST COMPOSITION

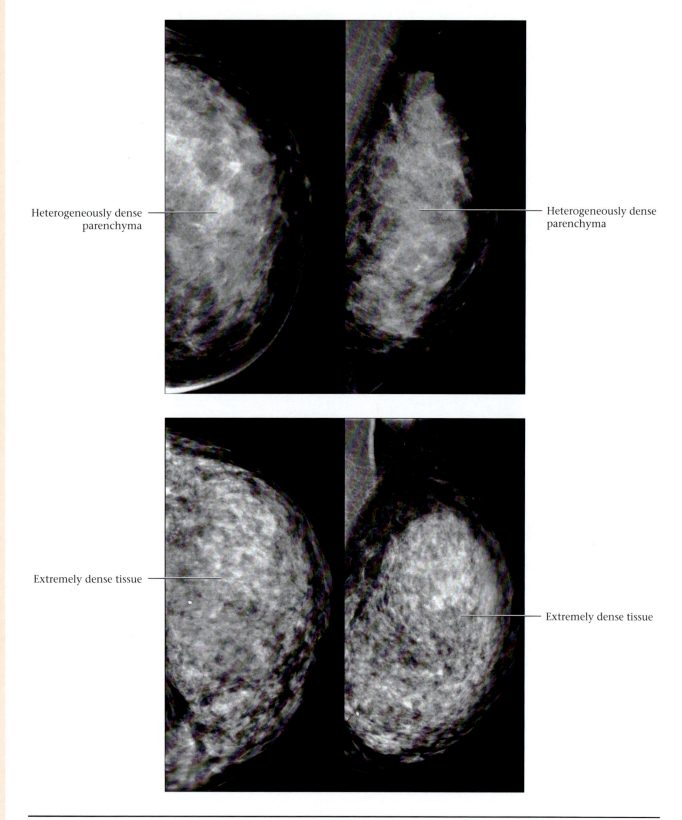

Heterogeneously dense parenchyma — — Heterogeneously dense parenchyma

Extremely dense tissue — — Extremely dense tissue

(Top) These CC/MLO digital mammograms show heterogeneously dense parenchyma, which could obscure detection of small masses. **(Bottom)** These CC/MLO digital mammograms show an extremely dense breast tissue composition, which lowers the sensitivity of mammography.

BREAST OVERVIEW

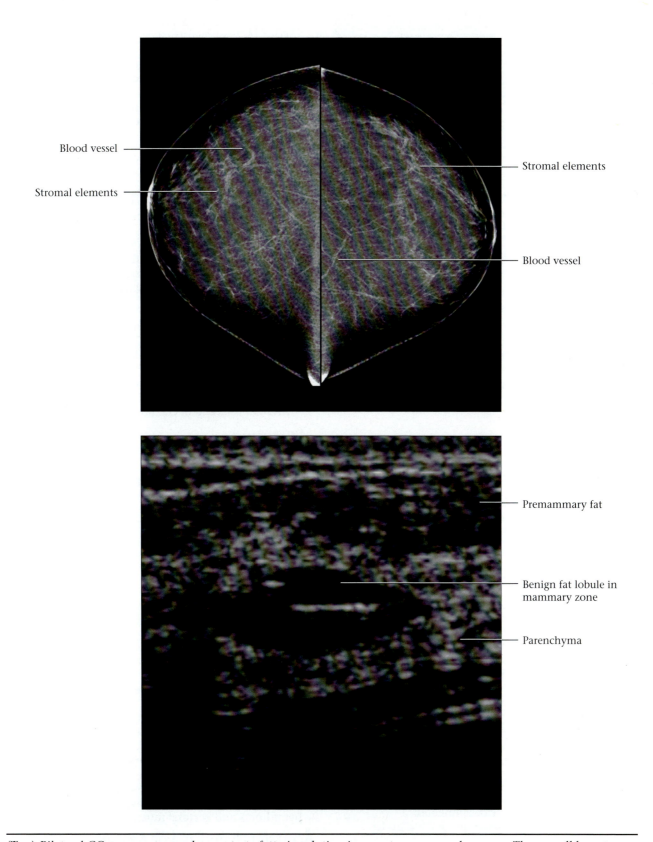

Blood vessel

Stromal elements

Stromal elements

Blood vessel

Premammary fat

Benign fat lobule in mammary zone

Parenchyma

(Top) Bilateral CC mammograms demonstrate fatty involution in a post-menopausal woman. The overall breast density is low, reflecting fatty replacement of most glandular elements. Residual scattered linear densities are stromal elements including connective tissue, blood vessels, and lymphatics. **(Bottom)** Breast ultrasound shows fat in the premammary zone and a classic benign fat lobule in the mammary zone. Fat lobules are circumscribed, isoechoic to subcutaneous fat, usually compressible, and often demonstrate linear echo(es) parallel to their long axis as seen in this example. This is a benign finding and does not require tissue sampling or excision. Surrounding parenchyma is hyperechoic to fat.

EMBRYOLOGY AND NORMAL DEVELOPMENT

Embryology

Embryologic Events
- Weeks 4-6
  - Ectodermal streaks develop from fetal axilla to groin
  - Mammary ridges develop in thoracic region
- Weeks 6-8
  - Mammary ridges involute
  - Invagination of chest wall mesenchyme
- Weeks 12-16
  - Differentiation of smooth muscle of nipple and areola
  - Development of epithelial buds and bud branching
- Weeks 16-20
  - Development of hair follicles, apocrine glands and glands of Montgomery
  - Appearance of primitive elements of breast parenchyma
- 3rd trimester
  - Epidermis depresses into shallow mammary pit
  - Nipple-areolar complex enlarges and develops pigmentation
  - Main ducts canalize
  - Lobules begin differentiation

Breast Development

Neonatal
- Connective tissue proliferates causing nipple to become erect
- Hormonally stimulated lobular tissue may secrete colostrum

Childhood and Puberty
- Main ducts branch; give rise to terminal buds, precursors of terminal ductal lobular units (TDLUs)
- Adipose cells proliferate, enlarge and extend into subcutaneous tissue
- Periductal tissues (stroma) increase; blood vessels proliferate
- Tanner phases of pubertal breast development
  - I: Nipple elevation but no palpable glandular elements
  - II: Nipple and breast project as mound from chest wall with palpable tissue in subareolar region
  - III: Increased glandular tissue/increased areolar size and pigmentation
  - IV: Development of separate nipple-areolar complex as secondary mound anterior to breast
  - V: Final adolescent development with smooth breast contour

Menarche
- Proliferative phase (follicular phase of ovary)
  - Days 3-14 of menstrual cycle
  - Overall regression of breast epithelium
  - Increase in ovarian estrogen production under pituitary control
  - Stroma becomes less dense
  - Duct lumens expand with increased epithelial cell activity
  - Lowest breast volume and water content

- Secretory phase (luteal phase of ovary)
  - Days 15-28 of menstrual cycle
  - Stromal density increases
  - Ductal epithelium proliferates
  - Water content of breast increases
  - Clinical symptoms relate to
    - Increased interlobular fluid
    - Generalized lobular proliferation

Pregnancy
- Marked ductal and lobular proliferation in early weeks of pregnancy
- Weeks 5-9
  - Generalized breast enlargement
  - Progressive increase in nipple-areolar complex pigmentation
- Second half of pregnancy
  - Progressive lobular proliferation
  - Stromal and fat elements increase
  - Colostrum accumulates in alveoli

Lactation
- Immediate post-partum enlargement due to colostrum accumulation
- Milk secreted into alveoli 3-7 days post partum
- Post-lactational changes
  - Periductal and perivascular stromal connective tissue increases
  - Alveolar cells and ductal branches regress

Menopause
- Generalized fatty replacement/atrophy of epithelium and stroma
- Hormone replacement therapy (HRT) stimulates residual elements; may ↑ mammographic density

Developmental Anomalies

Congenital
- Polymastia
  - Accessory tissue; incomplete involution of mammary ridge
  - Usually enlarges during pregnancy/lactation
- Polythelia
  - Accessory nipples
  - Most common congenital anomaly
- Amastia
  - Absence of breast development
- Amazia
  - Nipple present but no breast development
- Hyperplasia: Unilateral or bilateral
- Hypoplasia: Unilateral or bilateral
- Congential inversion of nipple
  - Incidence: 3% of live births
  - Association: Duct ectasia, periductal mastitis
- Poland syndrome: Unilateral hypoplasia of breast, hemithorax and pectoral muscle

Acquired Hypoplasia or Amastia
- Inadvertent biopsy of breast bud during childhood
- Trauma
- Chest wall radiation during childhood

EMBRYOLOGY AND NORMAL DEVELOPMENT

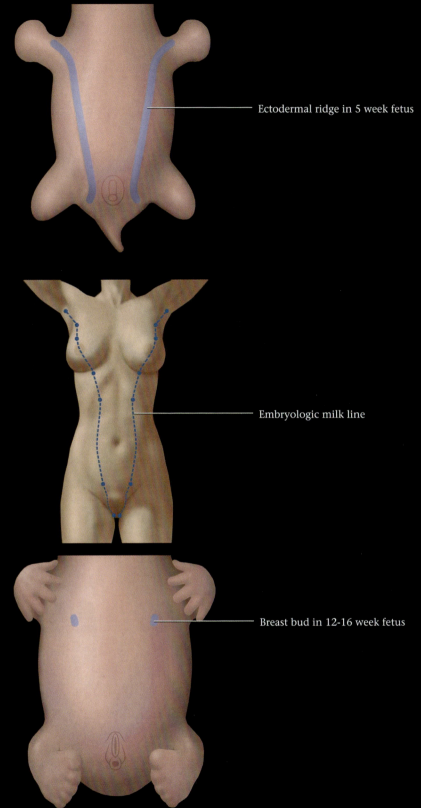

Ectodermal ridge in 5 week fetus

Embryologic milk line

Breast bud in 12-16 week fetus

(Top) The ectodermal milk streaks develop between the axillae and the inguinal regions during the 5th week of fetal growth and evolve into the mammary ridges in the thoracic region, the progenitor tissue of normal breasts. Incomplete involution of the ectodermal streaks produces accessory breast, nipple and areolar tissue which can present anywhere between the axillae and groin. **(Middle)** Schematic diagram demonstrates potential foci for accessory breast tissue in the adult woman. Accessory tissue may become clinically evident during pregnancy, lactation or hormone replacement therapy. **(Bottom)** The epithelial breast buds develop between weeks 12 and 16 of fetal growth. Breast buds may simulate cutaneous masses in infancy and childhood. Inadvertent biopsy of breast buds can cause acquired breast hypoplasia/amastia.

EMBRYOLOGY AND NORMAL DEVELOPMENT

PUBERTAL BREAST DEVELOPMENT

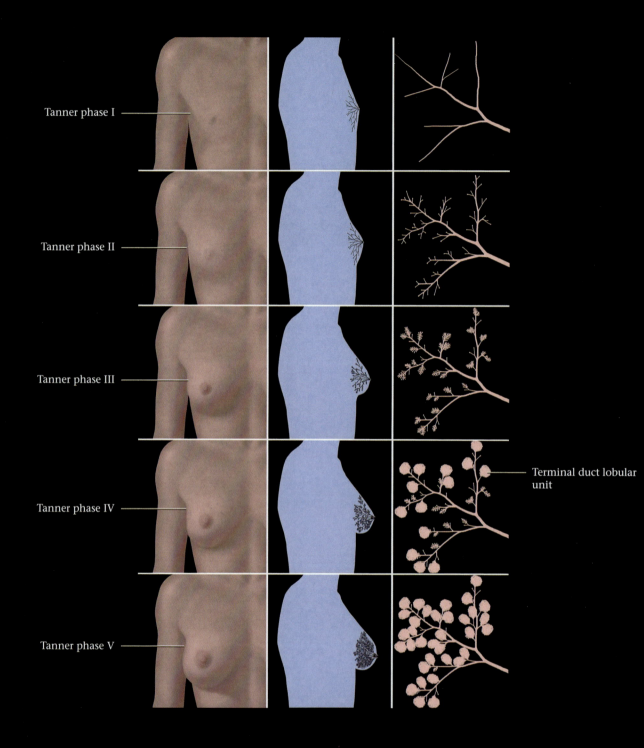

Tanner phase I

Tanner phase II

Tanner phase III

Tanner phase IV

Tanner phase V

Terminal duct lobular unit

During childhood, main ducts branch and give rise to terminal buds, the precursors of TDLUs. The diagram demonstrates the five Tanner phases of breast development with the left-hand column showing progressive changes in breast appearance as viewed from the front, the middle column representing glandular changes as viewed from the side and the right-hand column depicting corresponding changes in the ducts and TDLUs. I: Nipple elevation but no palpable glandular elements and minimal duct branching. II: Projection of nipple and breast as mound with small terminal buds projecting from ductal branches. III: Increased glandular and areolar tissue with primitive TDLUs. IV: Separate nipple-areolar complex as secondary mound, complete TDLUs. V: Final development with smooth breast and areolar contour and proliferation of TDLUs.

EMBRYOLOGY AND NORMAL DEVELOPMENT

No visible pectoral muscle — Normal left pectoral muscle

Right breast — Left breast

Fatty replacement — Fatty replacement

Normal lymph nodes

Right breast — Left breast

Stimulated glandular tissue

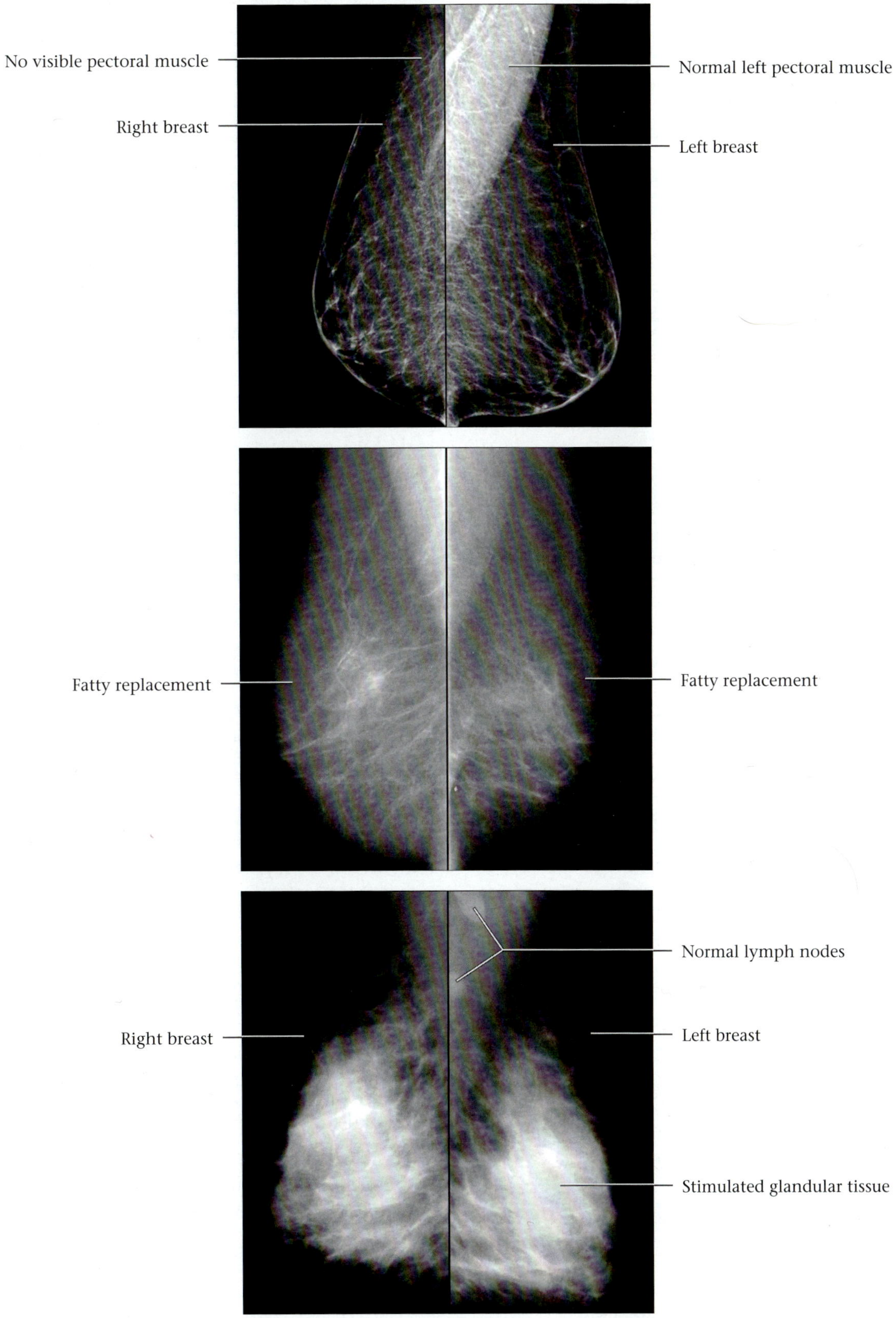

(Top) Bilateral MLO digital mammograms show characteristic appearance of Poland syndrome affecting the right breast. This is a congenital condition characterized by unilateral hypoplasia of the breast, hemithorax and pectoral muscle. (Middle) Bilateral MLO digital mammograms show generalized atrophy of epithelial and stromal elements with diffuse fatty replacement typical of post-menopausal change. (Bottom) Bilateral digital MLO mammograms show dramatic effects of HRT causing marked increase in overall breast density (same patient as prior image). Note normal lymph nodes in the left axilla.

NIPPLE AREOLAR COMPLEX & SKIN

Gross Anatomy

Overview
- Upper and medial aspect
  - Skin surface smoothly transitions to chest wall
- Inferior aspect
  - Skin surface smoothly transitions to upper abdominal skin
- Lateral aspect
  - Margin of breast clearly defined from chest wall and axillary tissues

Skin

Overview
- Average thickness 0.5-2 mm
- Contents
  - Sweat glands
  - Sebaceous glands
  - Hair follicles

Innervation
- Lateral cutaneous branches of 2nd-6th intercostal nerves

Arterial Supply
- Medial breast surface
  - Anterior intercostal artery branches
- Lateral breast surface
  - Lateral thoracic artery branches
  - Posterior intercostal artery branches

Venous Drainage
- Medial breast surface
  - Veins accompanying anterior intercostal artery branches
- Lateral breast surface
  - Veins accompanying
    - Lateral thoracic artery branches
    - Posterior intercostal artery branches

Lymphatic Drainage
- Breast tissue drainage
  - Dermal lymphatics
  - Periareolar lymphatics
- Periareolar lymphatic drainage
  - Axillary lymphatics
  - Internal mammary lymphatics
- Cutaneous anastomotic lymph channels are potential pathways for spread of contralateral breast cancer

Nipple-Areolar Complex

Overview
- Highly pigmented
- Covered by stratified squamous epithelium
- Long dermal papillae expedite capillary flow
- Subareolar smooth muscle arranged radially and circumferentially
  - Expedites nipple erection during nursing
- Increases in pigmentation and size during puberty

- Further increases in size and pigmentation during pregnancy

Nipple

Overview
- Projects at level of 4th intercostal space in non-pendulous breast
- Conical shape with average height of 10-12 mm
- 8-12 major duct orifices at bases of crevices on nipple surface
- Sensory nerve endings and sebaceous glands present but no fat, hair or sudoriferous (sweat) glands
- Subdermal smooth muscle present to facilitate nipple function during nursing

Areola

Overview
- Circular and pigmented, measuring 15-60 mm in diameter
- Contents
  - Apocrine sweat glands
  - Sebaceous glands
  - Hair follicles
  - Accessory areolar glands (of Montgomery)
- Areolar dermis contains smooth muscle in contiguity with nipple smooth muscle
- Lymphatic drainage pattern from subareolar (Sappey) plexus to axillary and internal mammary lymph nodes
  - Physiologic basis for sentinel node mapping

Imaging Principles

Mammography/Ductography
- Normal skin thickness is usually ≤ 2 mm
- Dermal papillae often visible as grooves in nipple
- Nipple usually everted
  - Nipples congenitally inverted in 3% of live births
- Should be seen in profile on at least one of two standard mammographic views
- New nipple inversion requires diligent search for subareolar pathology, esp. if unilateral
  - Can be caused by periductal mastitis, esp. bilateral
- Keratin plugs may form in duct orifices
  - Cleansing with alcohol facilitates duct cannulation

Ultrasound
- Normal breast bud in children may simulate mass
- Nipple is hypoechoic and may simulate subareolar mass
- Physiologic subareolar hypervascularity secondary to rich vascular/ductal network
- Scanning with warm acoustic gel minimizes periareolar smooth muscle contraction

MR
- Normal skin and mature scars do not enhance
- Nipple-areolar complex may enhance intensely
- Folliculitis/inflamed sebaceous cysts simulate neoplasm

NIPPLE AREOLAR COMPLEX & SKIN

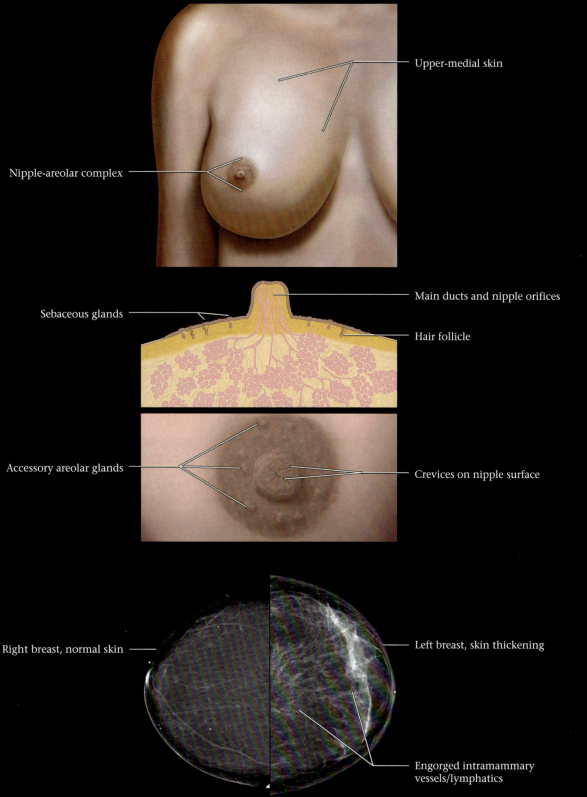

Upper-medial skin

Nipple-areolar complex

Sebaceous glands

Main ducts and nipple orifices

Hair follicle

Accessory areolar glands

Crevices on nipple surface

Right breast, normal skin

Left breast, skin thickening

Engorged intramammary vessels/lymphatics

(Top) Frontal view of the breast demonstrates a normal nipple-areolar complex projecting at the level of the fourth intercostal space. Note the smooth transition of the upper and medial breast to the chest wall. (Middle) Cross-sectional and frontal view schematics of the nipple-areolar complex. The 8-12 main ducts terminate as duct orifices on the surface of the nipple. The areola contains apocrine sweat glands, sebaceous glands, hair follicles and raised, visible accessory areolar glands (of Montgomery). (Bottom) Right and left digital CC views of different patients show a normal, fatty-replaced right breast with normal skin generally not more than 2 mm thick (though inframammary fold skin can be slightly thicker). The mammogram of the left breast shows markedly thickened skin and prominence of the intramammary vessels and lymphatics due to severe congestive heart failure.

NIPPLE AREOLAR COMPLEX & SKIN

MAMMOGRAPHY, NIPPLE-AREOLAR COMPLEX

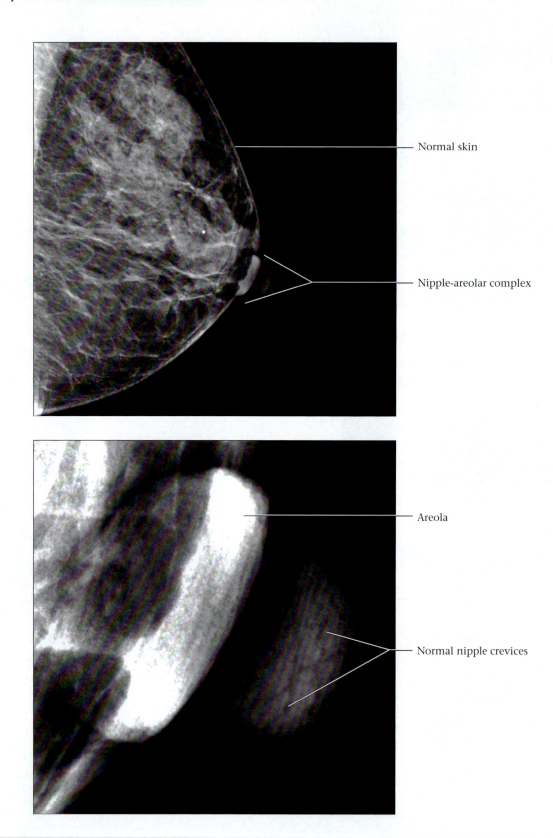

Normal skin

Nipple-areolar complex

Areola

Normal nipple crevices

(Top) MLO digital mammogram demonstrates normal breast skin measuring ≤ 2 mm in thickness and a normal everted nipple-areolar complex which should measure 15-60 mm in diameter. **(Bottom)** Magnification view of the nipple-areolar complex in profile demonstrates normal crevices in the nipple.

NIPPLE AREOLAR COMPLEX & SKIN

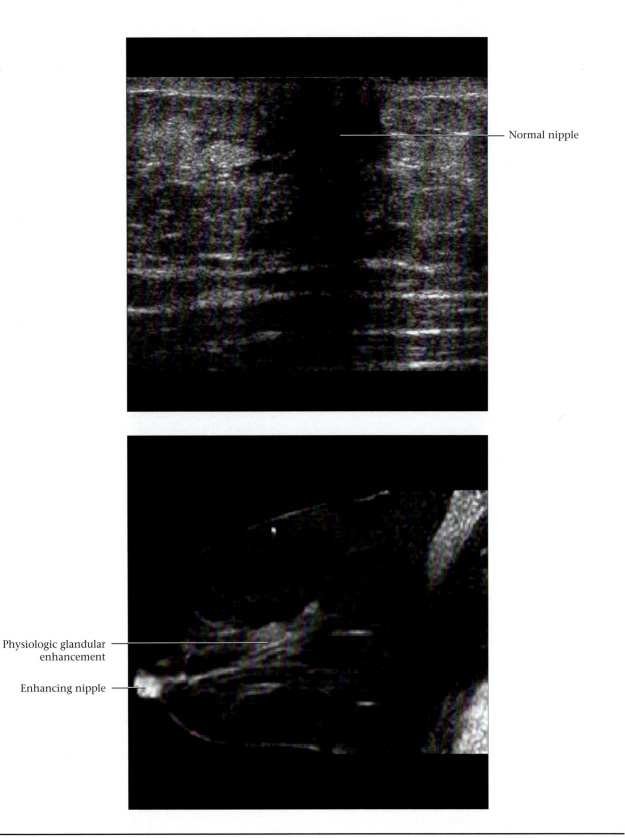

Normal nipple

Physiologic glandular enhancement

Enhancing nipple

(Top) Ultrasound of the nipple-areolar complex shows a typically hypoechoic nipple artificially flattened by the ultrasound transducer. This normal finding may simulate a subareolar mass. (Bottom) Sagittal enhanced T1 SPGR breast MR shows intense but physiologic enhancement of the nipple.

SEGMENTAL ANATOMY

Terminology

Definitions
- Lobe (segment): Drainage territory defined by each major duct
- Terminal duct: Final branch of segmental duct
  - Has two parts: Extralobular terminal duct (ELTD) and intralobular terminal duct (ILTD)
- Lobule: Composed of ILTD and complex system of tiny ducts terminating in blind-ending acini (alveoli)
- Terminal ductal lobular unit (TDLU): Lobule + ELTD

Clinical Implications

Clinical Importance
- Most invasive cancers arise from TDLU
- Ductal carcinoma in situ (DCIS) may extend into segmental and main ducts
- Papillomas and duct ectasia arise from ductal elements
- Duct orifices and subareolar ducts avenues for mastitis

Lobe/Segment

Composition
- Major ducts and branches → ELTDs → ILTDs → acini

Clinical Considerations
- Average of 15-20 lobes per breast
- Lobar volume and anatomy variable
- No discrete histologic or anatomic lobar boundaries
- Most, but not all, lobes drain to corresponding nipple duct orifice (some share common ducts)

Ductal System

Histology
- Inner lining of epithelial cells
  - Cell of origin of ductal carcinoma in situ, invasive ductal and invasive lobular carcinoma
- Outer discontinuous layer of myoepithelial cells
  - Function in milk expression during suckling
  - Cell of origin of adenomyoepitheliomas, other rare tumors
  - 'Biphasic' tumors are proliferations of both epithelial and myoepithelial elements: Papilloma, fibroadenoma, phyllodes, other
- Basement membrane between ducts and stroma
- Surrounded by fibroelastic stromal tissue less dense than interlobular breast stromal tissue

Duct Orifices
- Usually 8-12 per nipple
- Arranged radially in nipple crevices
- Some major ducts merge deep to nipple surface
- Quadrant of duct orifice on nipple surface does not always correspond to quadrant of lobe

Lactiferous Sinus (Ampullary Segment)
- Widened duct segment just deep to nipple orifice
- Average diameter = 4-5 mm

Major Ducts
- Average diameter = 1 mm
- Arborize into segmental and subsegmental branches of variable length and number
- Branches may extend into multiple breast quadrants
- Segmental and subsegmental branches give rise to terminal ducts
- Drain 20-40 lobules each containing 10-100 acini

Terminal Duct Lobular Unit (TDLU)

Overview
- Functional, glandular unit of breast
- May arise directly from major ducts or lactiferous sinuses
  - Possible explanation for subareolar invasive malignancies
- Multiple rows of TDLUs arise from distal segmental/subsegmental ducts
  - More numerous anterior rows have longer ELTDs
  - Less numerous posterior rows have shorter ELTDs
- Composition
  - ELTD is extralobar segment of terminal duct
  - ILTD is terminal intralobular segment of terminal duct
  - 10-100 acini drain into each ILTD
  - Loose stromal matrix of collagen and reticular fibers less dense than interlobular stroma

TDLU Proliferation
- Late adolescence
- Pregnancy and lactation
- Exogenous hormones: Birth control pills and hormone replacement therapy (HRT)
- Post-ovulatory (secretory) phase of menstrual cycle

TDLU Regression
- Postpartum and menopause
- May be nonuniform between breasts causing mammographic asymmetries

Imaging Issues

Mammography
- TDLUs ordinarily not visibile
- Dilated ducts often visible in subareolar region
- Isolated peripheral dilated ducts merit further evaluation for possible obstructing mass

Ultrasound
- Ducts frequently visible as linear, branching hypo- to isoechoic channels
- Physiologic duct dilatation occurs in menopause and pregnancy
- TDLUs occasionally visible

MR
- Benign ducts rarely enhance
- Fluid-filled, ectatic ducts appear as hyperintense tubular structures on more heavily T2-weighted scans

SEGMENTAL ANATOMY

TERMINAL DUCT LOBULAR UNIT

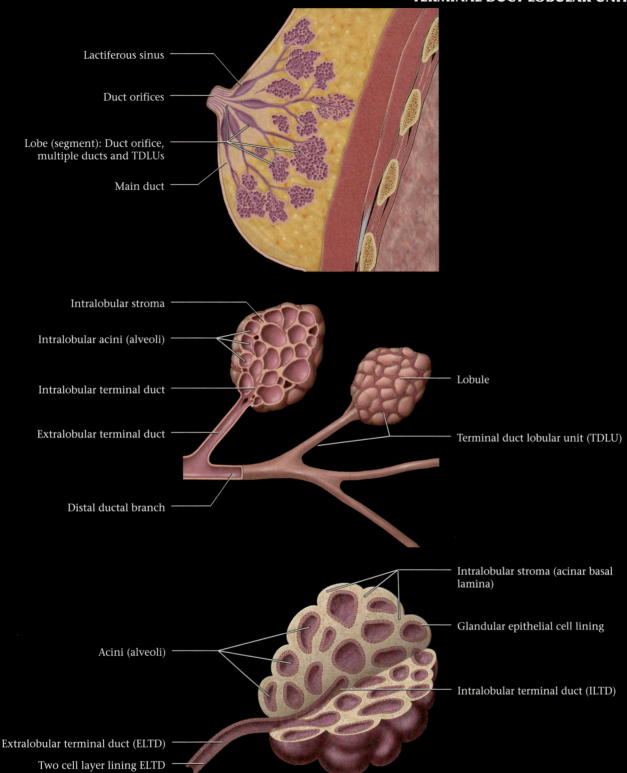

Lactiferous sinus

Duct orifices

Lobe (segment): Duct orifice, multiple ducts and TDLUs

Main duct

Intralobular stroma

Intralobular acini (alveoli)

Intralobular terminal duct

Extralobular terminal duct

Lobule

Terminal duct lobular unit (TDLU)

Distal ductal branch

Intralobular stroma (acinar basal lamina)

Glandular epithelial cell lining

Acini (alveoli)

Intralobular terminal duct (ILTD)

Extralobular terminal duct (ELTD)

Two cell layer lining ELTD

(Top) Sagittal schematic shows components of a lobe/segment from the duct orifice on the nipple surface to the TDLUs. Breasts average 15-20 lobes, draining into 8-12 duct orifices. (Middle) The TDLU arises from branches of distal subsegmental ducts and is composed of the extralobular terminal duct (ELTD), the intralobular terminal duct (ILTD) and multiple acini arranged around the ILTD. The TDLU on the left has been sectioned to demonstrate the relationship between acini and the ILTD. 10-100 acini drain into each ILTD. The intralobular stroma is composed of collagen and reticular fibers. (Bottom) Magnified schematic diagram of a sectioned TDLU. The ELTDs and ILTDs have an inner cellular layer of epithelial cells and an outer layer of myoepithelial cells enveloped by a basement membrane. The acini are lined by glandular epithelial cells.

SEGMENTAL ANATOMY

LOBAR ANATOMY

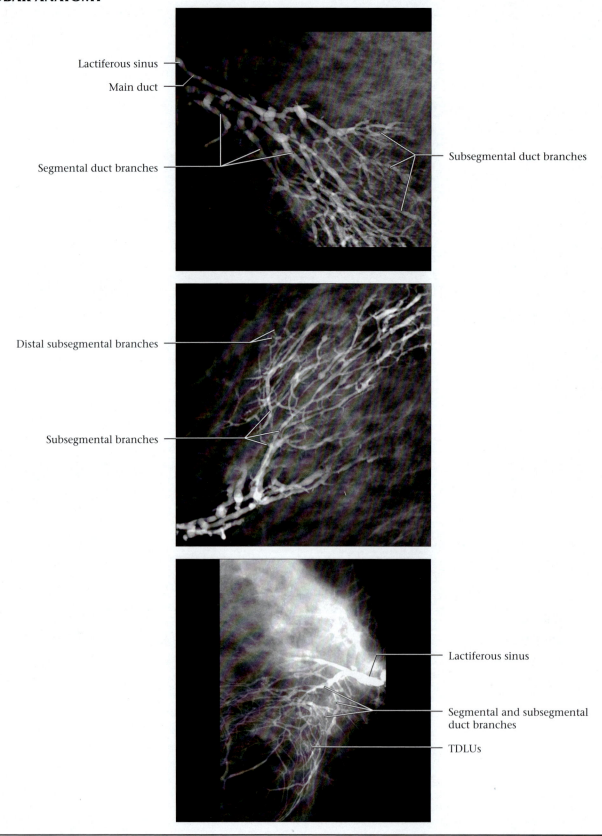

Lactiferous sinus

Main duct

Segmental duct branches

Subsegmental duct branches

Distal subsegmental branches

Subsegmental branches

Lactiferous sinus

Segmental and subsegmental duct branches

TDLUs

(Top) First of two magnification views in following ductography. This CC view shows the extensive branching pattern of ducts within a lobe. Occasionally, dilated TDLUs may be opacified with contrast. **(Middle)** ML view from the same case shows the distal subsegmental duct branches. The TDLUs arise from these distal subsegmental branches. **(Bottom)** This left breast ductogram nicely demonstrates the lactiferous sinus, the most proximal aspect of the main duct. The main duct has been sufficiently distended with contrast to opacify some TDLUs.

PHYSIOLOGIC DUCT DILATION

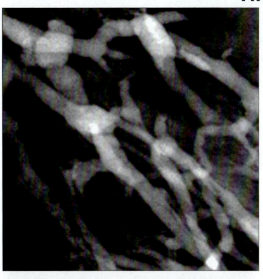

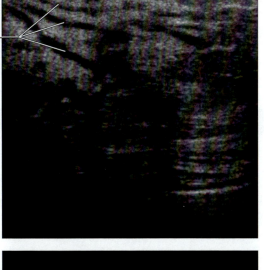

Subcutaneous fat

Multiple mildly ectatic ducts

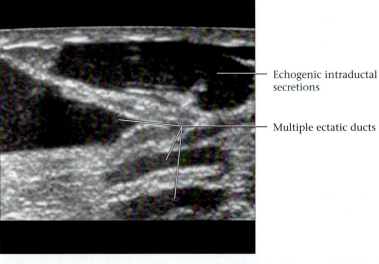

Echogenic intraductal secretions

Multiple ectatic ducts

(Top) Magnified image from a ductogram shows ectatic segmental ducts. Duct ectasia is more common in older patients but may develop at an earlier age in patients with congenitally inverted nipples. Dilated ducts are also seen in pregnant and lactating women. Dilated ducts are usually central. Isolated peripheral dilated ducts may signify obstruction as from a papilloma or other cause and merit further evaluation. (Middle) Breast ultrasound demonstrates mild physiologic ectasia of ducts in a pregnant patient. Note the branching, avascular channels in the anterior third of the breast. (Bottom) This breast ultrasound shows severely ectatic ducts containing echogenic secretions in this patient with chronic duct ectasia. Compression of the ducts with the transducer during real-time scanning may help distinguish benign secretions/debris from intraductal neoplasm.

SEGMENTAL ANATOMY

TERMINAL DUCTAL LOBULAR UNIT

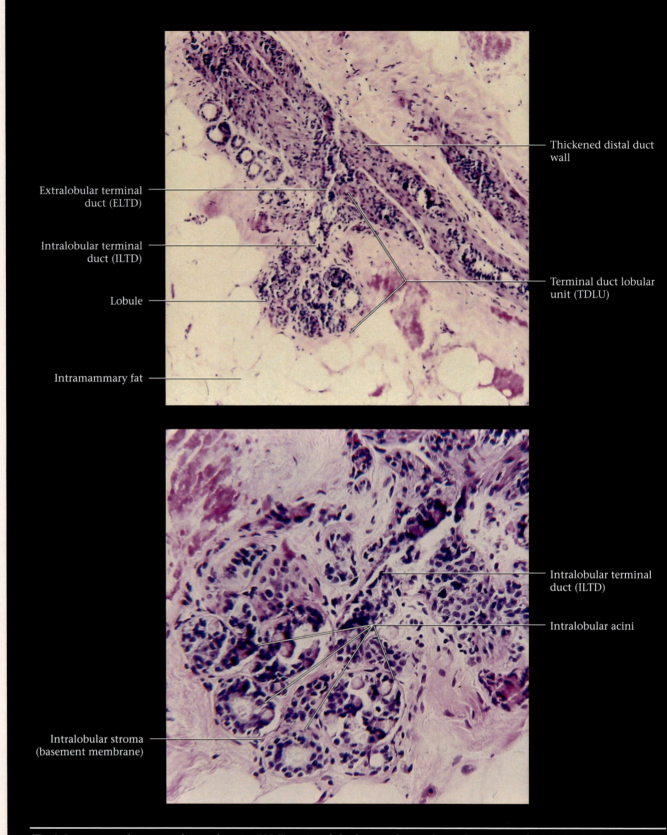

Thickened distal duct wall

Extralobular terminal duct (ELTD)

Intralobular terminal duct (ILTD)

Lobule

Intramammary fat

Terminal duct lobular unit (TDLU)

Intralobular terminal duct (ILTD)

Intralobular acini

Intralobular stroma (basement membrane)

(Top) Low-power hematoxylin and eosin (H&E) stain of the breast shows the architecture of a TDLU. An ELTD is seen emerging obliquely from a thickened distal duct. The ELTD continues as the ILTD as the duct enters the lobule. The TDLU includes the ELTD, ILTD and acini, and is the functional glandular unit of the breast. **(Bottom)** Medium-power H&E stain of the TDLU shows the clusters of intralobular acini. These acini are surrounded by a basement membrane, the integrity of which is used to distinguish in situ from invasive ductal carcinoma. Each lobule typically has 10-100 acini. The acini drain to the ILTD → ELTD → subsegmental duct → segmental duct → main duct.

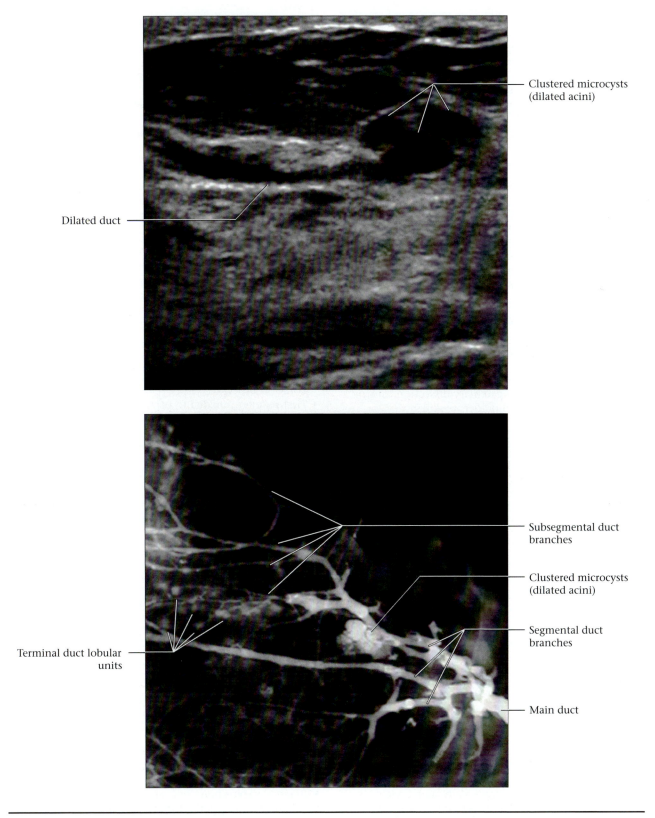

Clustered microcysts (dilated acini)

Dilated duct

Subsegmental duct branches

Clustered microcysts (dilated acini)

Segmental duct branches

Terminal duct lobular units

Main duct

(Top) Radial ultrasound shows a dilated duct terminating in a cluster of microcysts. These microcysts represent dilated acini within a TDLU. **(Bottom)** CC magnification view following ductography shows the extensive branching pattern of the ducts. The ducts become progressively smaller and eventually terminate as small, nodular tufts which are the TDLUs.

CHEST WALL AND AXILLA

Musculature

Pectoralis Major
- Immediately deep to superior 2/3 of breast tissue
- Smaller clavicular division originates from medial half of clavicle
- Larger costosternal division originates from sternum and 2nd-6th costal cartilages
- Inserts into greater tuberosity of humerus
- Innervated by medial and lateral pectoral nerves from brachial plexus
- Cephalic vein separates lateral border from deltoid muscle

Pectoralis Minor
- Located deep to the pectoralis major
- Origin from 2nd-5th ribs
- Inserts into coracoid process of scapula
- Innervated by medial pectoral nerve arising from medial division of brachial plexus
- Important landmark for zonal lymph node pathology

Serratus Anterior
- Immediately deep to lower breast tissue
- Origin from external surfaces of lateral upper eight ribs
- Inserts into medial border of scapula
- Innervated by long thoracic nerve (of Bell) arising from posterior C5, C6, & C7 brachial plexus roots
  - May be damaged during axillary dissection causing scapular "winging" & shoulder weakness

Latissimus Dorsi
- Largest muscle in human body: Can be used for myocutaneous flaps for breast reconstruction
- Origin from lowest 6 thoracic spinous processes, supraspinous ligaments of lower thoracic fascia and iliac crest
- Inserts into intertubercular groove of humerus via narrow tendon forming posterior axillary fold
- Innervated by thoracodorsal nerve from posterior brachial plexus & associated with scapular lymph node group

Subclavius
- Origin from first rib and costochondral cartilage
- Defines apex of axilla
- Inserts on inferior surface of mid clavicle
- Innervated by nerve to subclavius from C5 and C6 brachial plexus roots
- Terminates as costocoracoid ligament at entry of axillary vessels into chest

Congenital Muscular Abnormalities
- Absence of sternocostal division of pectoralis major (Poland syndrome)
- Sternalis muscle between sternal insertion of sternocleidomastoid muscle and rectus abdominus
  - May be visible mammographically on CC view
- Insertion of pectoralis muscle into both coracoid process and humeral head

Submuscular Chest Wall Structures
- Intercostal muscles, intercostal vessels and nerves, costal cartilage, parietal pleura

Axilla

Anatomic Boundaries
- Anterior wall: Formed by pectoralis major/pectoralis minor muscles and fascia
- Posterior wall: Formed by subscapularis, latissimus dorsi and teres major muscles and associated tendons
- Medial wall: Formed by serratus anterior muscle covering medial thoracic wall
- Lateral wall: Formed by bicipital (intertubercular) groove of humerus

Contents
- Fat, lymph nodes, arteries, veins and nerves
- Dense connective tissue (axillary sheath) surrounds nerves and vessels traversing axilla

Fascia
- Superficial layer (pectoral fascia composed of fascia from pectoralis major and minor muscles)
- Deep layer (clavipectoral or costocoracoid fascia) extending from clavicle to floor of axilla
  - Upper portion, the costocoracoid membrane, pierced by lateral pectoral nerve, cephalic vein & axillary artery branches

Axillary Artery
- Enters axilla posterior to pectoralis minor muscle near coracoid process
- First segment, medial to pectoralis minor muscle, supplies thoracic wall and first and second intercostal spaces
- Second segment, posterior to pectoralis minor muscle, has two major branches
  - Thoracoacromial trunk supplies pectoralis major and minor muscles and must be identified during axillary dissection
  - Lateral thoracic artery supplies parts of lateral breast tissue
- Third segment, lateral to pectoralis minor muscle; three major branches
  - Anterior humeral artery and posterior circumflex humeral artery supply arm and shoulder region
  - Subscapular artery is largest axillary arterial branch
    - Supplies latissimus dorsi, serratus anterior and subscapularis muscles
    - Closely associated with central and subscapular lymph nodal groups

Axillary Vein
- Projects medial and inferior to axillary artery
- Venous branches roughly parallel arterial branches

Nerves
- Medial, lateral and posterior cords of brachial plexus associated with and named for relationship to axillary artery
- Brachial plexus branches
  - Long thoracic nerve/intercostobrachial nerve
  - Prone to injury during axillary dissection

CHEST MUSCULATURE OVERVIEW

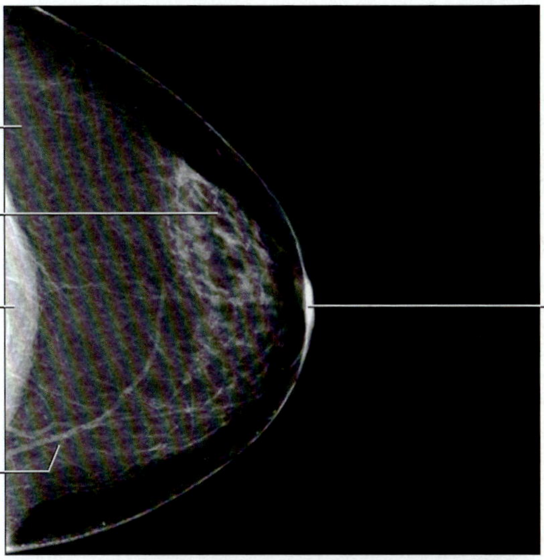

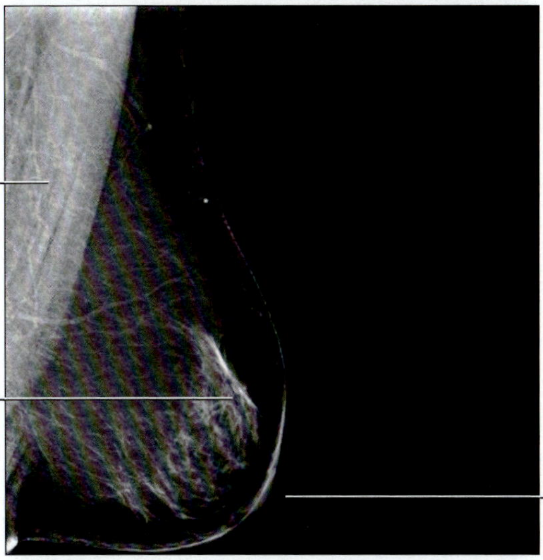

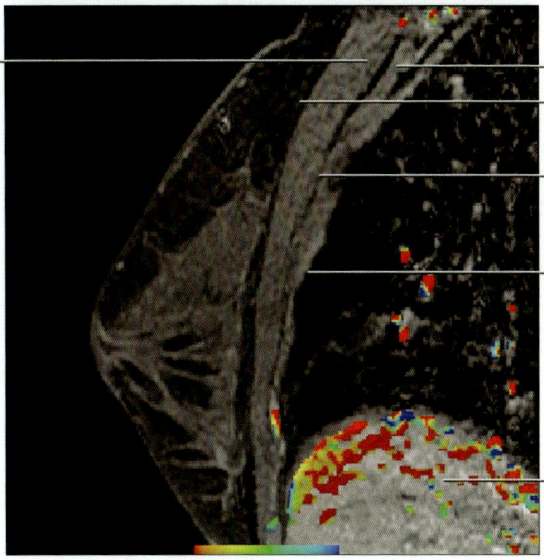

Posterior breast tissue
Fibroglandular elements
Pectoralis major muscle
Vessel
Nipple-areolar complex

Pectoralis major muscle
Residual fibroglandular elements
Nipple-areolar complex

Pectoralis major muscle
Pectoralis minor muscle
Anterior pectoralis major fascia
Anterior fascia of pectoralis minor muscle
Parietal pleura
Liver

(Top) CC view from a well-positioned digital mammogram demonstrates the posterior breast tissues and the pectoralis major muscle. (Middle) MLO projection of the same patient demonstrates satisfactory positioning and excellent depiction of the pectoralis musculature. (Bottom) Sagittal T1 SPGR contrast-enhanced MR toward the axillary aspect of the right breast depicts the anatomic relationship of the pectoralis minor muscle deep to the pectoralis major muscle. The pectoralis minor muscle is an important landmark for determining surgical levels of axillary lymph nodes.

CHEST WALL AND AXILLA

COMPUTED TOMOGRAPHY

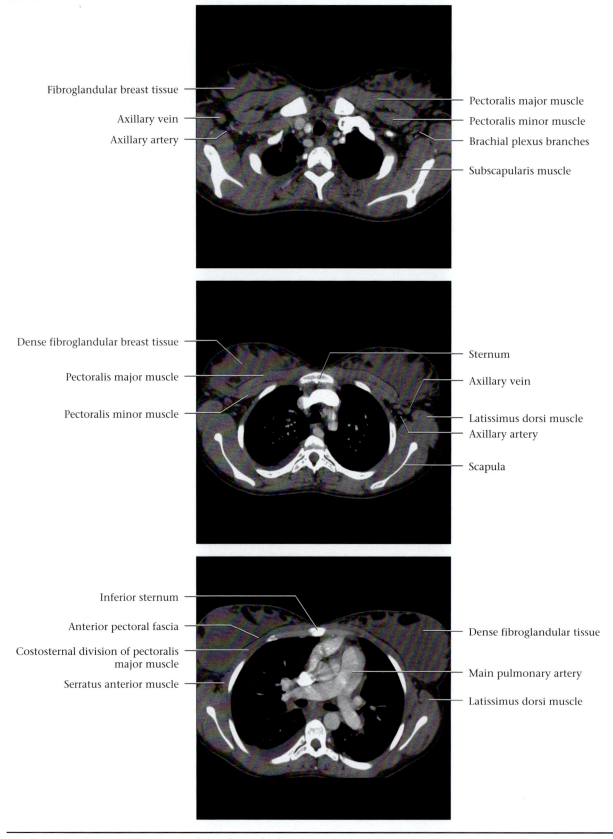

Fibroglandular breast tissue

Axillary vein

Axillary artery

Pectoralis major muscle

Pectoralis minor muscle

Brachial plexus branches

Subscapularis muscle

Dense fibroglandular breast tissue

Pectoralis major muscle

Pectoralis minor muscle

Sternum

Axillary vein

Latissimus dorsi muscle

Axillary artery

Scapula

Inferior sternum

Anterior pectoral fascia

Costosternal division of pectoralis major muscle

Serratus anterior muscle

Dense fibroglandular tissue

Main pulmonary artery

Latissimus dorsi muscle

(Top) Axial enhanced CT at level of the clavicular heads. Note the relationship between the pectoralis major and pectoralis minor muscles and the contents of the axilla. **(Middle)** Axial enhanced CT at mid-sternal level. The latissimus dorsi muscle can be used for myocutaneous flaps for breast reconstruction. **(Bottom)** Enhanced axial CT at level of pulmonary artery. The serratus anterior muscle projects at the inferior/posterior aspect of the breast.

CHEST WALL AND AXILLA

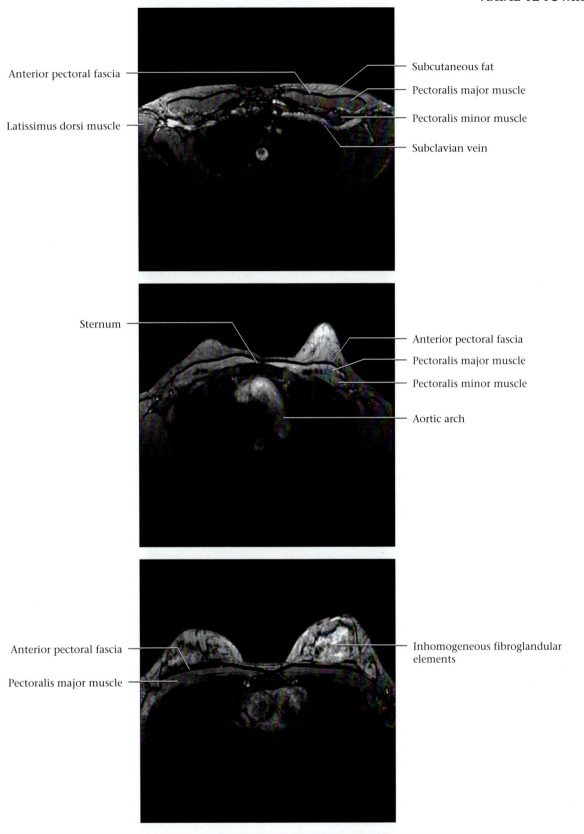

Anterior pectoral fascia

Latissimus dorsi muscle

Subcutaneous fat

Pectoralis major muscle

Pectoralis minor muscle

Subclavian vein

Sternum

Anterior pectoral fascia

Pectoralis major muscle

Pectoralis minor muscle

Aortic arch

Anterior pectoral fascia

Pectoralis major muscle

Inhomogeneous fibroglandular elements

(Top) Axial T2WI FS MR at level of subclavian veins. **(Middle)** Axial T2WI FS MR at level of aortic arch. With posterior breast neoplasms, MR is particularly sensitive for assessing invasion of the pectoral fascia and pectoral musculature as evidenced by contrast-enhancement of the musculature. **(Bottom)** Axial T2WI FS MR at level of heart. Note the normal thickness of the anterior fascia of the pectoralis muscle.

NEUROVASCULAR SUPPLY

Innervation

Innervation Overview
- Specialized fibers for nipple, areola and breast
  - Facilitate nipple erection
  - Allow flow of milk during suckling
- Sympathetic fibers to skin and breast tissue
  - Modulate blood flow
  - Affect apocrine function
- Three major groups innervate breast and converge on nipple-areolar complex
  - Supraclavicular nerves via cervical plexus
  - Thoracic nerve branches via brachial plexus
  - Intercostal nerves

Superior Breast Innervation
- Cutaneous branches of 2nd and 3rd intercostal nerves
- Anterior and medial branches of supraclavicular nerve via cervical plexus

Lateral Breast Innervation
- Lateral cutaneous branches of 4th and 5th intercostal nerves
  - Perforate chest wall in mid-axillary line
  - Posterior branches innervate lateral chest wall
  - Anterior branches provide perforating branches to glandular elements and nipple-areolar complex

Medial Breast Innervation
- Anterior branches of 2nd-5th intercostal nerves passing through intercostal spaces near sternum
  - Medial branches innervate chest wall
  - Lateral branches become medial mammary nerves

Arterial Supply

Overview
- Vessels enter via superolateral, superomedial and deep aspects of breast
- Multiple small perforating branches and intramammary anastomoses

Internal Mammary (Thoracic) Artery
- Supplies approximately 60% of breast medially and centrally
- Originates from subclavian artery
- Descends along lateral surface of sternum
- Anterior perforating branches pass through 2nd-4th intercostal spaces and become medial mammary arteries

Lateral Thoracic Artery
- Supplies approximately 30% of breast, primarily upper outer quadrant
- Origin
  - Most commonly arises from axillary artery
  - Less commonly arises from thoracoacromial or subscapular artery
  - Descends along axillary border of pectoralis minor muscle
- Provides multiple lateral mammary branches

Remainder of Breast Variable (10%)
- 3rd, 4th, and 5th posterior intercostal arteries
  - Lateral mammary branches of lateral cutaneous branches
- Pectoral branch of thoracoacromial artery
- Subscapular artery
- Thoracodorsal artery

Venous Drainage

Overview
- Multiple potential pathways for hematogenous metastases from breast cancer
- Lymphatic drainage pathways may parallel venous drainage

Superficial Systems
- Usually do not accompany arteries
- Form anastomotic circle near nipple-areolar complex (circulus venosus)
- Drain to periphery of breast and join deep venous system

Deep Systems
- May provide direct pathways for metastatic disease to lung
- Generally accompany arteries supplying region of breast
- Three principal routes of deep venous drainage
  - Posterior intercostal vein branches
  - Axillary vein branches
  - Internal mammary vein branches

Vertebral Plexus (Batson Plexus)
- Composed of valveless venous channels
- Surrounds vertebral column extending from skull to sacrum
- In contiguity with posterior intercostal vessels
- Potential route for hematogenous metastases from breast cancer to spine, ribs and brain

Imaging Issues

Mammography
- Physiologic calcification of arterial media often seen in post-menopausal population
- Arterial calcification in pre-menopausal population: Consider diabetes or other vasculopathy

Ultrasound
- Doppler assessment: Confirm vascular channel
  - Separate arteries from veins by direction of flow, pulsatility, etc.

MR
- Normal vessels identified by viewing course over contiguous images
- Maximum intensity projections (MIP): 3D display including vasculature
- Often see preferential physiologic enhancement in upper outer quadrant, periphery
- Increased vascularity in breast(s) with cancer

ARTERIAL/VENOUS/NEUROLOGIC ANATOMY

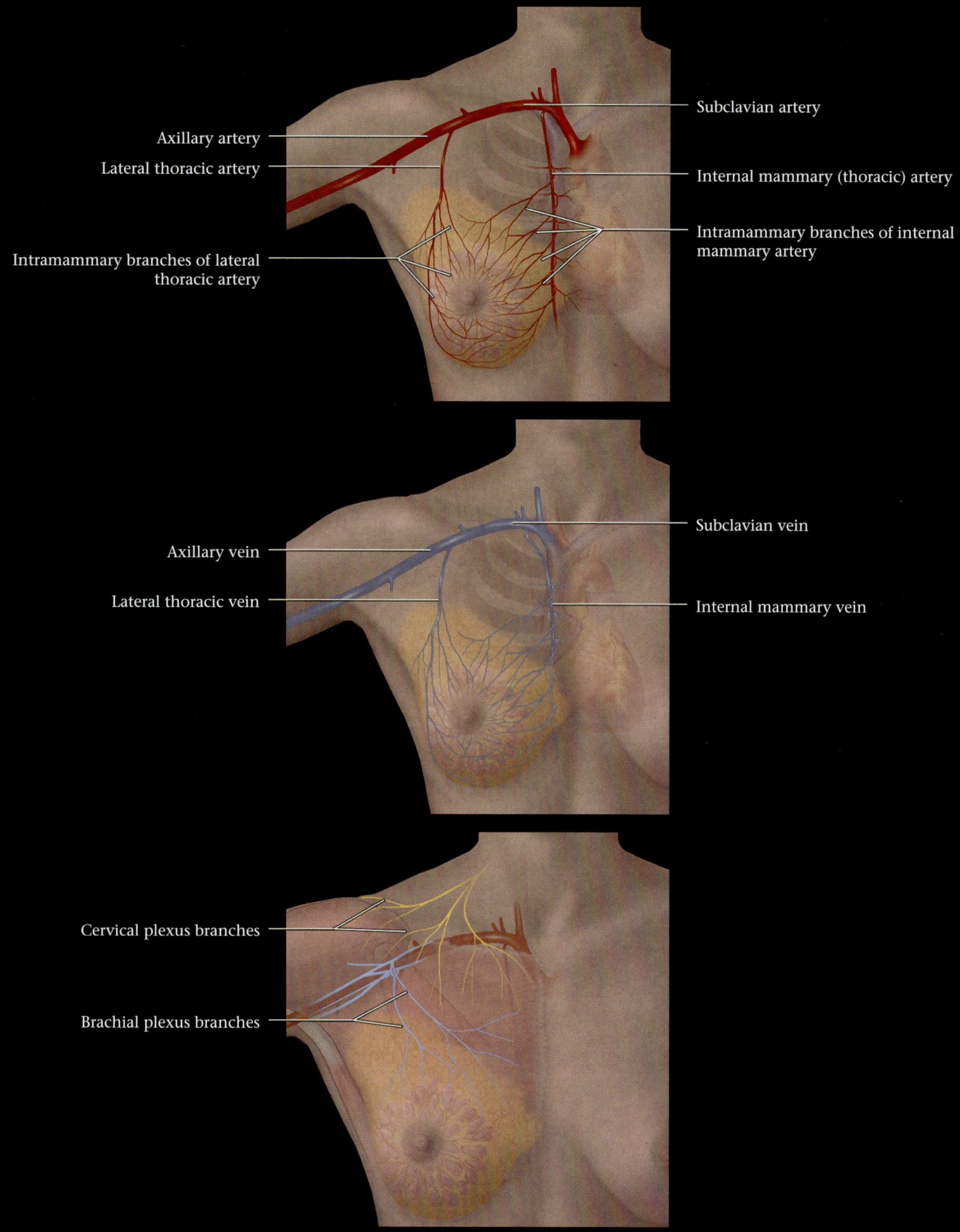

Axillary artery

Lateral thoracic artery

Intramammary branches of lateral thoracic artery

Subclavian artery

Internal mammary (thoracic) artery

Intramammary branches of internal mammary artery

Axillary vein

Lateral thoracic vein

Subclavian vein

Internal mammary vein

Cervical plexus branches

Brachial plexus branches

(Top) Vessels enter via the superolateral, superomedial and deep aspects of the breast. The internal mammary artery supplies 60% of the breast medially/centrally and the lateral thoracic artery supplies about 30% of the breast in the upper-outer quadrant. The remainder of the vascular supply to the breast is variable via posterior intercostal arteries, the pectoral branch of the thoracoacromial artery, the subscapular artery and the thoracodorsal artery. (Middle) The deep venous drainage of the breast parallels the arterial supply with the three principal routes via the internal mammary veins into the subclavian vein, the lateral thoracic veins into the axillary vein and the posterior intercostal vein branches into the vertebral plexus. (Bottom) The superior breast is innervated by branches from the cervical plexus and the remainder of the breast by intercostal branches from the brachial plexus.

VASCULAR STRUCTURES

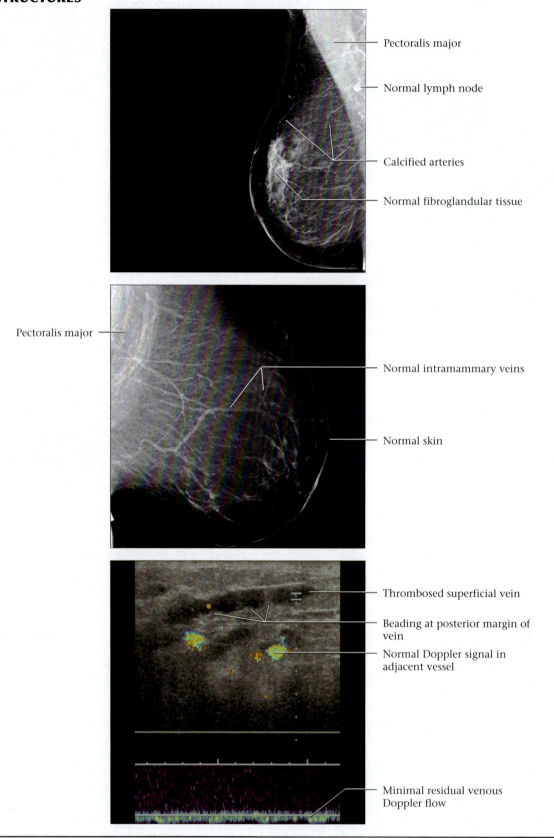

Pectoralis major

Normal lymph node

Calcified arteries

Normal fibroglandular tissue

Pectoralis major

Normal intramammary veins

Normal skin

Thrombosed superficial vein

Beading at posterior margin of vein

Normal Doppler signal in adjacent vessel

Minimal residual venous Doppler flow

(Top) Right MLO digital mammogram of an elderly post-menopausal women shows extensive but physiologic breast arterial calcification. When seen in younger patients, consideration should be given to systemic conditions such as diabetes, hypertension and premature vasculopathy. **(Middle)** Left MLO digital mammogram shows normal veins in a fatty-replaced breast. Veins do not calcify and are usually more curvilinear than arteries. When venous structures dilate or proliferate, coexisting conditions such as venous occlusive disease, heart failure or renal failure should be considered. **(Bottom)** Breast ultrasound shows a thrombosed superficial vein with beading, typical of superficial thrombosis (Mondor disease). Normal Doppler flow is seen in several normal and more posterior vessels. Minimal flow can be seen if there is only partial thrombosis or recanalization.

NEUROVASCULAR SUPPLY

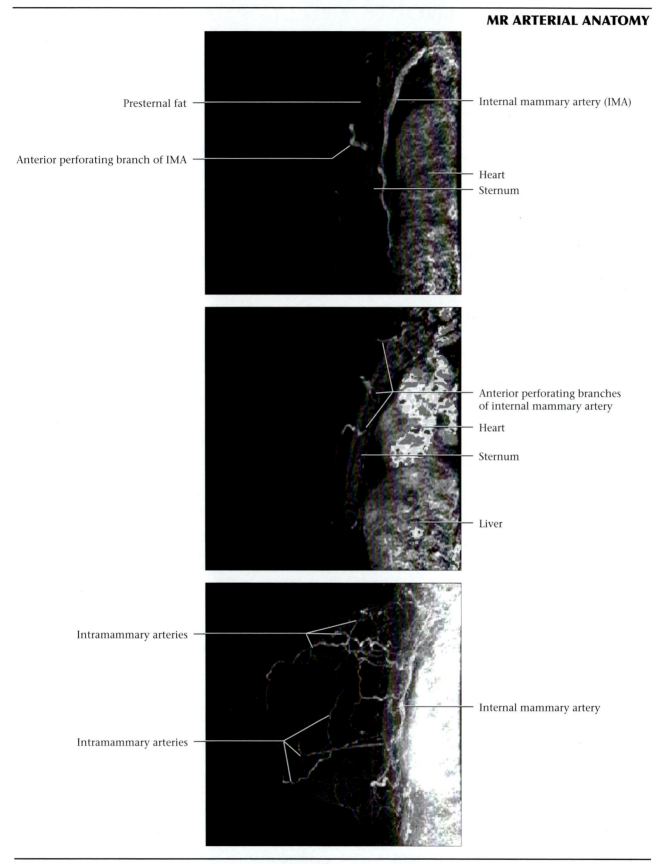

Presternal fat

Anterior perforating branch of IMA

Internal mammary artery (IMA)

Heart

Sternum

Anterior perforating branches of internal mammary artery

Heart

Sternum

Liver

Intramammary arteries

Internal mammary artery

Intramammary arteries

(Top) T1 SPGR FS MR shows internal mammary artery descending along the lateral surface of the sternum. These paired arteries provide 60% of the total arterial supply of the breast medially and centrally. **(Middle)** Sagittal T1 post-contrast SPGR FS MR with color enhancement shows anterior perforating branches of the internal mammary artery passing through the 2nd-4th intercostal spaces to supply the medial breast. **(Bottom)** Maximum intensity projection (MIP) generated from post-Gd T1 SPGR FS MR image shows rich vascular supply of the entire breast, normal in this case. MIP images can be used to define tumor vascularity and local extent of tumor within the breast. Asymmetric increased vascularity is often seen in breasts with cancer, with vessels directly feeding the tumor.

LYMPH NODES AND LYMPHATICS

General Concepts

Breast Lymphatic Drainage

- Deep breast tissues to superficial lymphatics to periareolar lymphatic (Sappey) plexus
- 75% of drainage via lateral and medial trunks extending from areola to axilla
  - Axilla drains to subclavian lymphatic trunk
- 25% of lymphatic drainage via internal mammary nodes
- Anastomotic lymphatic channels may communicate with contralateral skin and breast

Major Lymph Node Groups

Axillary Lymph Nodes

- **Axillary vein group**
  - Most lateral group
  - Lies medial and posterior to axillary vein
  - Consists of 4-6 nodes
- **Pectoral (anterior) group**
  - Projects at inferior margin of pectoralis minor muscle
  - Receives majority of breast lymphatic drainage
  - Drains primarily into central lymph node group but may drain directly into subclavicular group
  - Consists of 4-5 nodes
- **Scapular (subscapular) group**
  - Projects near posterior margin of axilla and lateral margin of scapula
  - Receives additional lymph flow from posterior neck, trunk and shoulder
  - Drains into central and subclavicular groups
  - Consists of 5-7 nodes
- **Central group**
  - Projects in axillary fat deep/posterior to pectoralis minor muscle
  - Drains to apical and infraclavicular groups
  - Most superficial and most easily palpable of axillary nodal groups
  - Consists of 3-4 nodes
- **Interpectoral (Rotter) group**
  - Between pectoralis major and pectoralis minor muscles
  - Drains into central and subclavicular groups
  - Consists of 1-4 nodes
- **Subclavicular (apical) group**
  - Medial and posterior to pectoralis minor muscle at apex of axilla
  - May be final common pathway of lymphatic drainage for all other axillary groups
  - Efferent lymphatics may join thoracic duct, internal jugular vein, subclavian vein or pass to deep cervical nodes
  - Consists of 6-12 nodes

Internal Mammary (Parasternal) Nodes

- In parasternal intercostal spaces; < 6 mm in diameter
- Predominantly drain far medial and deep medial breast
- Nodes in 1st-3rd intercostal spaces may be affected in metastatic breast cancer

Surgical Lymph Node Levels

- Level I
  - Lymph nodes lateral/inferior to pectoralis minor muscle
  - Includes scapular, axillary vein and pectoral groups
- Level II
  - Lymph nodes deep/posterior to pectoralis minor muscle
  - Includes central and interpectoral groups and possibly portions of subclavicular group
- Level III
  - Lymph nodes medial and superior to pectoralis minor muscle
  - Includes primarily subclavicular group
- Sentinel node evaluation: One to a few lower level I nodes
- Surgical axillary dissection: Level I and II nodes

Intramammary Lymph Nodes

- 25-28% of normal women have intramammary lymph nodes visible on mammography
- Can occur anywhere: Most common in far lateral, axillary, and posteromedial aspects of breast
- May be difficult to surgically distinguish intramammary lymph node in axillary tail from axillary lymph node

Imaging Issues

Mammography

- Normal lymph nodes
  - Circumscribed and variable size; short axis diameter may exceed 1 cm
  - Fatty hila usually visible
  - Oval, reniform shape
- Lowest level I lymph nodes may be seen on MLO views

Ultrasound

- Level I, level II and sometimes level III axillary nodes and sometimes internal mammary nodes can be seen
- Can help classify mammographically indeterminate lymph nodes
- Normal lymph nodes
  - Usually elliptical with definable long and short axes
  - Circumscribed, thin, hypoechoic cortex and hyperechoic fatty hila
  - Variable size: May be longer than 2 cm, esp. if fatty
  - Doppler often shows normal hilar vascularity
- Internal mammary nodes
  - Normal nodes may be visible in intercostal spaces
  - Smaller than axillary nodes: Average size 4-6 mm
  - Morphology difficult to assess: Size criteria more important

MR

- Characteristic reniform shape with fatty hilum
- Cortex usually hyperintense on T2WI FS
- Normal vessels may enter nodes via hila
- Often demonstrate physiologic rapid inflow and washout enhancement curves

LYMPH NODES AND LYMPHATICS

Normal axillary lymph node with fatty hilum

Pectoralis muscle

Normal fibroglandular elements

Skin

Normal fatty hilum

Sharp cortical margins

Normal vessels

Pectoralis major muscle

Metastatic lymph node

Pectoralis major

Retromammary fat

Primary breast cancer

Premammary fat

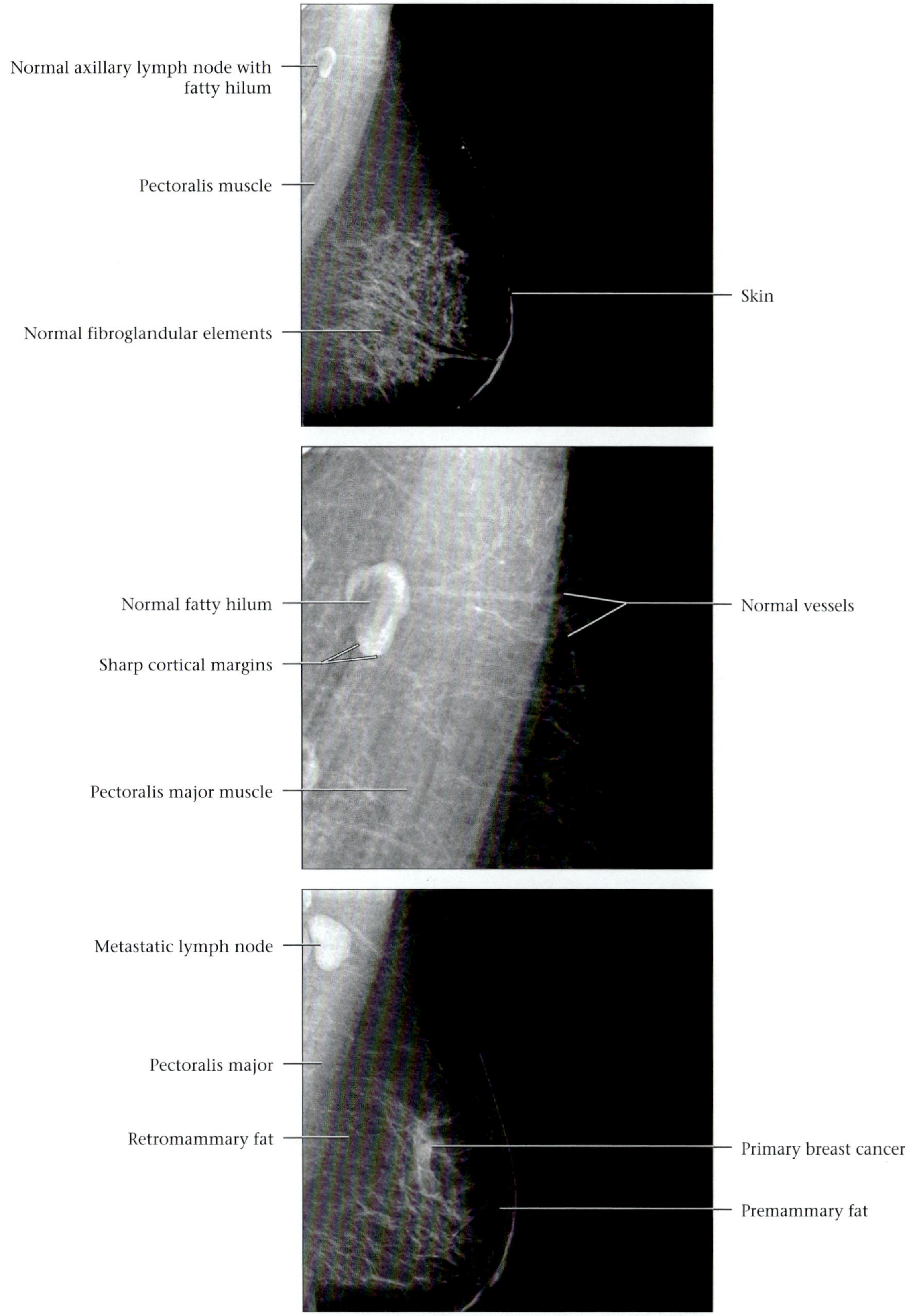

(Top) MLO digital mammogram shows a normal lymph node in the axillary region. Normal lymph nodes are circumscribed, most commonly have a reniform shape and usually have a visible fatty hilum. The most common locations for normal lymph nodes are the axilla, the upper-outer quadrant/axillary tail and extreme posteromedial breast. (Middle) Spot magnification view of the largest normal axillary lymph node shows a reniform shape, circumscribed cortex and a fatty hilum, hallmarks of a normal lymph node. (Bottom) The lymph node labeled was one of many involved with metastatic disease found at axillary dissection. It has lost its reniform shape, is exceedingly dense, and has no visible fatty hilum. Contrast this pathologically proven abnormal lymph node with the normal axillary lymph node in the top and middle images.

LYMPH NODES AND LYMPHATICS

ULTRASOUND, LYMPH NODE

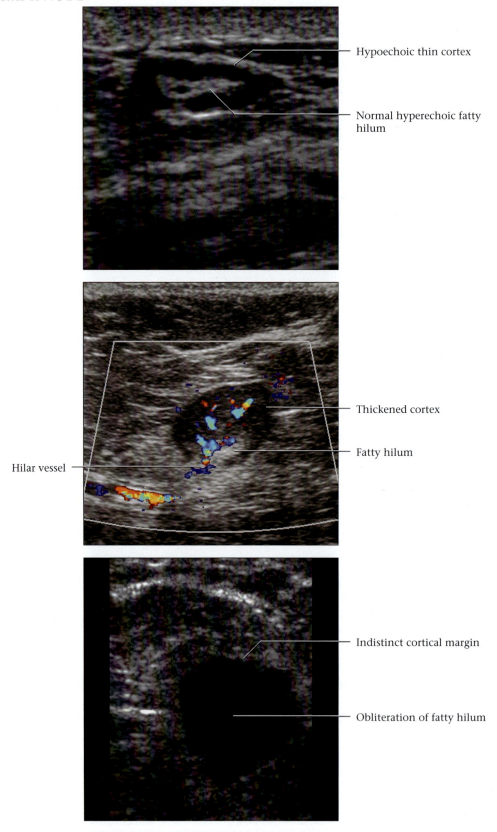

Hypoechoic thin cortex

Normal hyperechoic fatty hilum

Thickened cortex

Fatty hilum

Hilar vessel

Indistinct cortical margin

Obliteration of fatty hilum

(Top) Ultrasound shows a normal lymph node with a reniform configuration, hyperechoic fatty hilum and thin, well-circumscribed, hypoechoic cortex. Normal axillary nodes may exceed 2 cm in their long axis, especially if fatty replaced. Normal internal mammary lymph nodes are usually less than 6 mm in longest dimension. **(Middle)** Color Doppler ultrasound of a biopsy-proven, reactive axillary lymph node. The cortex is uniformly thickened but the fatty hilum and circumscribed contour remain. Note the vessel entering at the hilum. **(Bottom)** Note loss of the expected reniform configuration, obliteration of the fatty hilum, and extracapsular extension causing indistinctness of the cortical margin in this abnormal node. Fine needle aspiration biopsy yielded sheets of malignant cells consistent with breast cancer. The patient went directly to axillary dissection rather than a sentinel lymph node biopsy.

LYMPH NODES AND LYMPHATICS

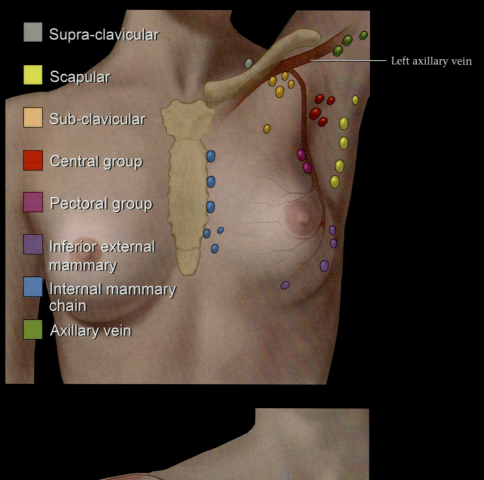

Supra-clavicular

Scapular

Sub-clavicular

Central group

Pectoral group

Inferior external mammary

Internal mammary chain

Axillary vein

Left axillary vein

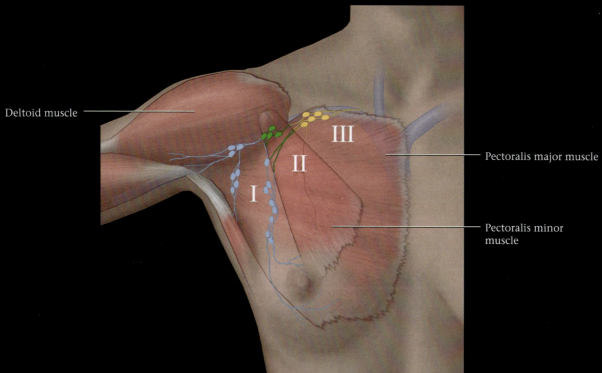

Deltoid muscle

Pectoralis major muscle

Pectoralis minor muscle

III

II

I

(Top) Each major lymph node group has well-defined anatomy. The axillary vein group is medial and posterior to the axillary vein, the pectoral group projects at the lower margin of the pectoral muscle, the scapular group projects at the intersection of posterior axilla & scapula, the central group projects posterior to pectoralis minor muscle into the axillary fat, the interpectoral group (not labeled) projects between pectoralis major and pectoralis minor, the subclavicular group projects at the apex of the axilla, the inferior external mammary group is lateral and inferior to the breast and the internal mammary chain in the parasternal intercostal spaces. **(Bottom)** Level I nodes (blue) are lateral/inferior to pectoralis minor. Level II nodes (green) are deep/posterior to pectoralis minor. Level III nodes (yellow) are medial and superior to pectoralis minor.

LYMPH NODES AND LYMPHATICS

MR, LYMPH NODE

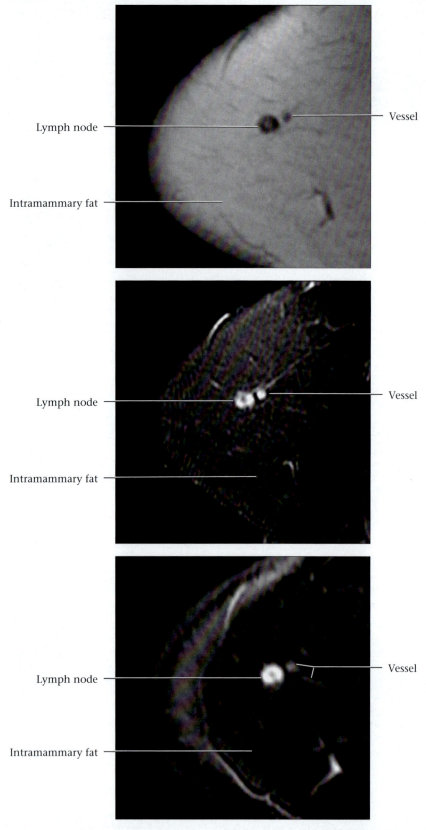

Lymph node — Vessel

Intramammary fat

Lymph node — Vessel

Intramammary fat

Lymph node — Vessel

Intramammary fat

(Top) First of three images of a normal intramammary lymph node. T1-weighted MR shows the characteristic reniform appearance. There is a high signal intensity fatty hilum surrounded by a low signal intensity cortex. An adjacent vessel is also seen. **(Middle)** On a T2WI FS, the cortex is hyperintense, while the signal from intramammary and nodal hilar fat are suppressed. **(Bottom)** A post-Gd fat-suppressed SPGR image shows enhancement of the cortex. Normal vessels enter the lymph node via the hilum. Normal lymph nodes will typically demonstrate rapid inflow and washout enhancement curves.

LYMPH NODES AND LYMPHATICS

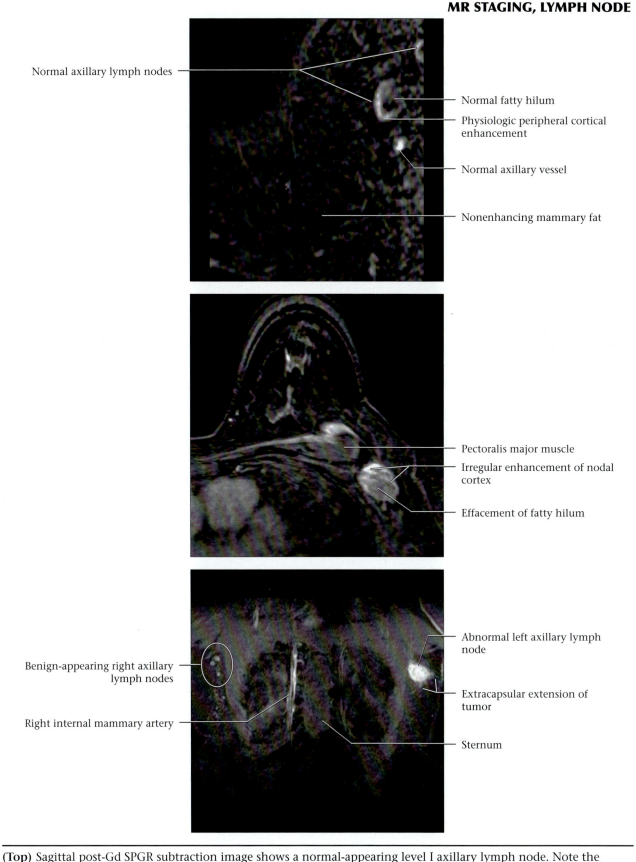

Normal axillary lymph nodes

Normal fatty hilum

Physiologic peripheral cortical enhancement

Normal axillary vessel

Nonenhancing mammary fat

Pectoralis major muscle

Irregular enhancement of nodal cortex

Effacement of fatty hilum

Benign-appearing right axillary lymph nodes

Right internal mammary artery

Abnormal left axillary lymph node

Extracapsular extension of tumor

Sternum

(Top) Sagittal post-Gd SPGR subtraction image shows a normal-appearing level I axillary lymph node. Note the reniform shape, circumscribed cortex and physiologic contrast enhancement at its periphery. This lymph node was proven histologically benign at the time of sentinel lymph node mapping. (Middle) Axial post-Gd SPGR subtracted image demonstrates an abnormal left axillary lymph node with surgically proven metastatic disease. There is loss of the normal reniform shape, obliteration of the fatty hilum and an irregular pattern of contrast enhancement throughout the lymph node. (Bottom) Coronal STIR image shows several small, benign-appearing right axillary lymph nodes and an enlarged, biopsy-proven metastatic left axillary lymph node. Its indistinct margins reflect extracapsular extension of tumor.

PART II
Imaging Modalities

Mammography: Positioning

Mammography: Screening

Mammography: Diagnostic

Mammography: Audit Benchmarks

High Risk Screening & Surveillance

Double Reading/CAD

Ultrasound

Magnetic Resonance Imaging

PET Imaging

Gamma Camera Imaging

MAMMOGRAPHY: POSITIONING

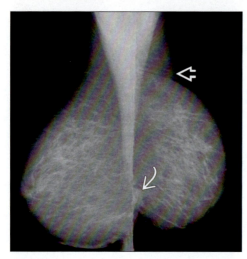

Screening MLO mammograms show poor positioning of left breast, with skin folds IMF region ➔ and axillary tail ⇥. The left pectoral muscle is not seen to level of the nipple. Read as negative in this 90 y/o.

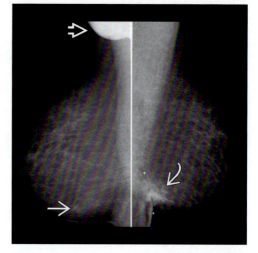

MLO views (same case) 2 yrs later show palpable spiculated mass left IMF ➔, missed before due to poor positioning. New focal asymmetry right ➔. Both = infiltrating ductal carcinoma. Note patient's chin ⇥.

TERMINOLOGY

Abbreviations
- Breast Imaging Reporting and Data System (BI-RADS®)
- Craniocaudal view (CC)
  - CC view with top of breast rolled laterally (CCRL)
  - CC view with top of breast rolled medially (CCRM)
  - Laterally exaggerated craniocaudal view (XCCL)
  - Medially exaggerated craniocaudal view (XCCM)
- Mediolateral oblique (MLO)
- Mediolateral view (ML)
- Lateromedial view (LM)
- Inframammary fold (IMF)
- Mammography Quality Standards Act (MQSA)

Definitions
- Interval cancer: Cancer becomes clinically evident in the interval between recommended screenings
  - Worse survival than screen-detected cancers
- Posterior nipple line (PNL): Line drawn from nipple perpendicular to pectoral muscle on MLO view, and from nipple to posterior edge of film on CC view

IMAGING ANATOMY

General Anatomic Considerations
- Nipple is the only fixed reference point
- Breasts composed of fat and fibroglandular tissue in variable proportions
  - More glandular tissue in upper outer quadrant than elsewhere
    - Axillary tail of Spence extends into axilla
    - More cancers in upper outer quadrant (~ half) than elsewhere
- Breast is a skin appendage: Can be pulled farthest from chest wall in a direction parallel to underlying muscle
  - Superior and medial breast are relatively fixed, inferior and lateral portions are more mobile
  - Move mobile surface toward a more fixed/immobile surface to optimize amount of tissue imaged on standard views

- MLO includes most of the axillary breast tissue, more of the breast included than on CC view
  - XCCL is complementary view of posterolateral breast
- On CC view, the opposite breast may prevent patient moving forward as much as possible
  - Depending on patient body habitus, opposite breast can be elevated onto cassette/digital detector to fully include posteromedial breast
  - Protuberant abdomen may have same effect: Better to image patient standing than seated when possible
  - CC view includes most posteromedial tissue

ANATOMY-BASED IMAGING ISSUES

Key Concepts or Questions
- Is the image quality acceptable?
  - Position
    - Assess depth of tissue seen: PNL depth on CC should be within 1 cm of depth on MLO
    - Fat should be seen posterior to parenchyma in both views: XCCL view(s) may be needed
    - Inferior extent of pectoral muscle at least to level of nipple on MLO view
    - Margin of pectoral muscle convex toward nipple
    - IMF elevated: No overlap between bottom of breast and upper abdomen
    - Pectoral muscle seen in about 30% of CC views
    - For CC view, nipple in midline
    - Nipple in profile both views (less important than including all tissue): Anterior compression MLO view ("tip shot") if necessary
  - Exposure
    - All glandular tissue penetrated adequately
    - Photocell set at densest portion of tissue
    - Lower kVp → better contrast; keep exposure < 200 mAs to minimize blur
  - Compression
    - Adequate compression prevents motion: Goal is at least "taut" and not painful
    - Less painful in first half of menstrual cycle

Keys to Quality Mammography

Maximize Compression
- Use small cassette whenever possible
- Maximum patient can tolerate
  - Reduces scatter, spreads out tissue better
  - Can use lower kVp (improving contrast), less radiation dose to patient
- Supplemental anterior MLO or 90° lateral view for better compression in large breasts

Optimize Exposure
- Lower kVp → better contrast; need to keep mAs < 200 to reduce motion blur
- If motion is limiting, e.g., known Ca++, then acceptable to ↑ kVp for shorter exposure

Optimize Positioning
- Elevate IMF prior to MLO exposure

- Bring in axillary tail tissue on CC view
- Include fat behind glandular tissue in both views
  - May need XCCL view to complete exam
- Include posterior tissue: Posterior nipple line should measure within 1 cm of same distance on CC vs. MLO view
- Eliminate skin folds
- Nipple in profile (less critical than including all tissue): Anterior tip view if needed

Experience and Continuing Education
- Technologist and radiologist must meet standards, e.g., MQSA in USA
- Regular feedback to technologist
- Radiologist ultimately responsible for image quality

Goal: < 2% repeat rate

- Less pain if compression gradually applied, patient assists
- Use small cassettes whenever possible
- Spreads out tissue
- Reduces amount of radiation needed
- Look at calcifications, margins should be sharp
- Cooper ligaments fine, linear structures should be sharp
- Inferior breast at inframammary fold is best place to check for motion, esp. on MLO view
- Viewing with magnification (either lens or electronic) improves conspicuity of motion blur

Imaging Approaches
- Screening mammography
  - CC and MLO views of each breast
  - Additional views performed as necessary to include all glandular tissue
    - XCCL if glandular tissue in lateral breast extends to edge of CC view
    - "Tip shot" if anterior tissue not well compressed due to thickness at chest wall
    - Overlapping CC, MLO views if breast too large to image on standard-size film/detector
- Diagnostic mammography
  - Examination is tailored to clinical question, performed under direct supervision of radiologist
  - Any number of views are used to answer the question
    - Is there a real abnormality?
    - If finding is real, what is the morphology and level of suspicion for cancer?
  - Final assessment may require additional modalities, e.g., ultrasound or (rarely) MR
  - Report should conclude with a BI-RADS final assessment and a management recommendation
    - Rare use of BI-RADS 0 if MR needed due to inconclusive mammogram and US, finding too vague to biopsy

Imaging Protocols
- MLO

- Cassette/digital receptor placed laterally, parallel to axis of pectoral muscle
  - Technologist manually pulls breast from lateral to medial then applies compression
  - IMF elevated and pulled forward as compression applied
- CC
  - Technologist should elevate cassette/digital receptor to maximum excursion of IMF
  - Minimizes distance compression paddle travels
  - Maximizes depth of tissue included in image
  - As compression applied lateral tissue "tugged" into field of view
  - Nipple central on CC view
- XCC
  - Patient rotates medially (XCCM) or laterally (XCCL) to include more tissue at posterior margins in CC projection
- "Tip shot": Anterior compression MLO view
  - Breast is thicker at chest wall than at nipple
  - Thickness of posterior tissue limits compression
  - Angled/tilting compression plates help compensate
  - Can also be performed in 90° lateral projection: Spreads tissue, additional information
- Axillary tail view
  - Variant on MLO projection with emphasis on lateral axillary tissue
  - Edge of cassette/digital detector along lateral chest wall
  - Central and medial tissue not included
- ML
  - 90° true lateral, orthogonal to CC, with cassette/digital detector at lateral breast
  - Does not include as much axillary tail but allows triangulation of lesions seen only on MLO
  - Important for milk of calcium calcifications (Ca++): Shows "teacup", layering configuration
- LM
  - 90° true lateral, with cassette/digital detector at medial breast
  - Goal is to better evaluate medial lesions
  - Medial lesions closer to detector → less risk of blur

MAMMOGRAPHY: POSITIONING

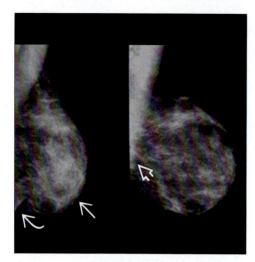

On initial MLO view (left), front of breast is drooping ("camel nose") ➡, with skin fold at IMF ➡. On repeat (right), tissue, including pectoral muscle ➡, is now fully included and well spread out (Courtesy LWB).

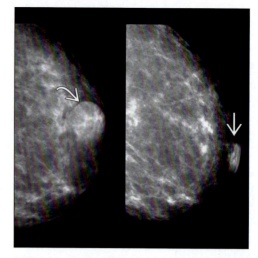

MLO mammograms show how nipple can mimic a mass (on left) ➡, and potentially obscure underlying pathology, when not in profile. Anterior tip view on right shows nipple in profile ➡.

- Rolled CC
  - Upper half of breast tissue rolled laterally (CCRL)
    - Lesion(s) in superior hemisphere move laterally, inferior lesion(s) move medially
    - Central lesion(s) does not move
  - Upper half of breast tissue rolled medially (CCRM)
    - Lesion in superior hemispheres moves medially
    - Lesion in inferior breast moves laterally
- Spot compression: Use of small compression paddle to increase local compression over a finding
  - ↑ Compression → ↓ thickness → improved resolution
  - Summation shadows can be proven normal
    - Alters the way parenchymal elements overlap
  - May use small cassette/detector in very large breasts
- Magnification: Geometric magnification of small objects within breast
  - 0.1 mm focal spot, breast farther from detector
  - Performed with patient standing
  - Image projects on larger area: Reduced noise, scatter → better resolution
  - Magnification of Ca++ → assess morphology, extent
  - Magnification of mass → assess margins, associated Ca++ if any
- Cleavage view
  - Both breasts placed on cassette/digital detector
  - Evaluates far posteromedial tissue
- "Lumpogram"
  - Performed for palpable mass, BB marker on mass
  - Skin over lesion in tangent, spot compression
  - Projects mass over subcutaneous fat rather than over dense tissue
    - Better ability to assess margins, overlying skin
  - US has replaced this technique in many centers

CLINICAL IMPLICATIONS

Clinical Importance

- In one series cancer detection 84% among patients with proper breast positioning; ↓ to 66% with poor positioning

  - Interval cancers more likely after images with poor positioning
    - Odds ratio 2.6
- Motion blurs Ca++ → missed diagnosis, esp. ductal carcinoma in situ (DCIS)
- Poor mobilization of breast → deep lesions may not be included in image
- Lesion(s) seen on one view only one cause of missed cancer
  - Measure distance from nipple to determine if included in other views
  - For very posterior lesions, may not have been included on both views due to variable positioning

RELATED REFERENCES

1. Majid AS et al: Missed breast carcinoma: pitfalls and pearls. Radiographics. 23(4):881-95, 2003
2. Taplin SH et al: Screening mammography: clinical image quality and the risk of interval breast cancer. AJR Am J Roentgenol. 178(4):797-803, 2002
3. Huynh PT et al: The false-negative mammogram. Radiographics. 18(5):1137-54; quiz 1243-4, 1998
4. Bradley FM et al: The sternalis muscle: an unusual normal finding seen on mammography. AJR Am J Roentgenol. 166(1):33-6, 1996
5. Eklund GW et al: Assessing adequacy of mammographic image quality. Radiology. 190(2):297-307, 1994
6. Bassett LW et al: Mammographic positioning: evaluation from the view box. Radiology. 188(3):803-6, 1993
7. Eklund GW et al: The art of mammographic positioning. Radiol Clin North Am. 30(1):21-53, 1992
8. Eklund GW et al: Art of positioning needs revival in mammography. Diagn Imaging (San Franc). 13(9):131-40, 1991
9. Brower TD: Positioning techniques for the augmented breast. Radiol Technol. 61(3):209-11, 1990
10. Berkowitz JE et al: Dermal breast calcifications: localization with template-guided placement of skin marker. Radiology. 163(1):282, 1987

IMAGE GALLERY

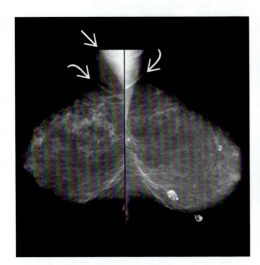
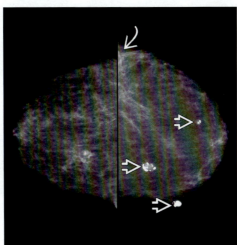

(Left) Screening MLO mammograms show poor positioning, with only a small portion of pectoral muscle (and thereby axillary tissue) included, not nearly to the level of the nipple, worse on the right ➡, in this 64 y/o. Bilateral skin folds are noted ➡. *(Right)* CC mammograms (same as on left) show calcifying fibroadenomas left breast ➡ and skin folds outer posterior left breast ➡. Ca++ were noted in the upper right breast prompting recall.

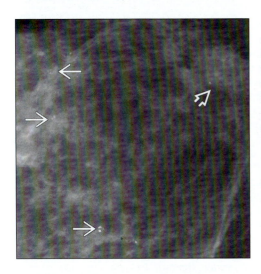
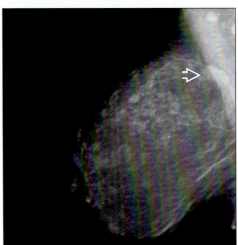

(Left) MLO mammography magnification upper posterior right breast (same as prior 2 images) shows multiple groups of rather coarse Ca++ ➡ (biopsy proven fibrocystic changes), as well as vague mass posteriorly ➡, noted at time of consult for Ca++ biopsy. *(Right)* Repeat right MLO view (same as prior 3 images) shows ill-defined mass right axillary tail ➡ which had initially been excluded from the screening views.

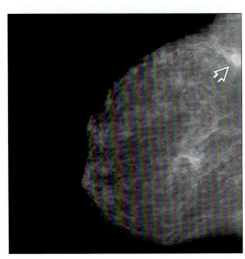
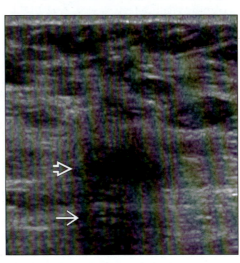

(Left) XCCL view of right breast (same case as prior 4 images) again shows irregular, dense mass axillary tail right breast ➡. *(Right)* Radial ultrasound (same as prior 5 images) shows irregular, hypoechoic mass ➡ with posterior shadowing ➡, corresponding to the mammographically-depicted mass. US-guided core biopsy showed infiltrating ductal carcinoma, grade II.

MAMMOGRAPHY: SCREENING

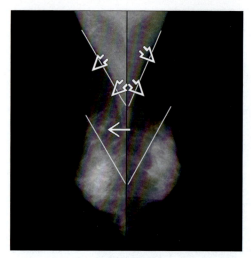

MLO mammography in an asymptomatic 51 y/o shows small suspicious asymmetry ➡ within the band (indicated by white lines) of fat between the pectoral fold ⬆➡ and posterior margin of the axillary tail.

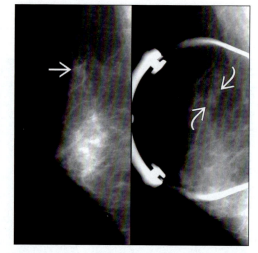

Lateral mammography (same case as left) confirms distortion in this region ➡, and a spot compression view (right image) confirms a small irregular mass ➡. Excision = 1 cm invasive ductal carcinoma.

TERMINOLOGY

Abbreviations

- SFM: Screen-film or analog mammography
  - X-ray photons converted to light by phosphor screens, exposed film processed chemically to create a visible image
- FFDM: Full field digital mammography
  - Flat panel detector to convert X-ray photons to digital signals and create an image
  - Computed radiography FFDM (CR-FFDM): Storage phosphor plate captures X-ray photons; laser plate scanner extracts digital image
- BI-RADS®: Breast Imaging Reporting and Data System

Definitions

- Mammographic screening: A proven **system** for early breast cancer detection and diagnosis
  - Sporadic or opportunistic screening goal: Detect early, preclinical breast cancer
  - Population or systematic screening goal: Reduce population mortality through early breast cancer detection and treatment
  - Accredited and audited quality assurance program, from screening to diagnosis
    - Images interpreted by MQSA-certified breast imager (USA) or equivalent
    - Must be backed up by accurate diagnostic assessment, expert image-guided needle biopsy, breast pathology, treatment
- Screening mammography: Periodic **examination** to detect preclinical asymptomatic breast cancer
  - Routine periodic mammography in asymptomatic women
  - ± Part of an integrated mammography screening program
  - Images interpreted by MQSA-certified breast imager (USA) or equivalent
- Mammography: Performed on dedicated x-ray units designed to image the whole breast

- Mammography x-ray tube with very fine focal spot, low kVp, special anode materials [Molybdenum (Mo) ± Rhodium (Rh), Tungsten (W)]
  - Rotating C-arm for different projections, compression device with compression paddles
  - Image capture stage with cassette holder and integrated grid (SFM), or digital flat plate detector and automatic exposure control (AEC) device (FFDM)
- SFM: Film serves as image display and storage device
  - Narrow dynamic range up to 100, limited by film grain, quantum noise and processing chemistry
  - Interpreted on high light output dedicated mammography film viewer or light box
  - Benefits: Very high spatial resolution [15-20 line pairs(lp)/mm], widely available, proven effective
  - Disadvantages: Only one physical copy; susceptible to QA errors, image degradation, damage, loss
- Digital mammography: Decouples image acquisition from display, storage and distribution
  - Direct capture reduces image acquisition time, increases patient throughput
  - Softcopy display: Images displayed, manipulated and interpreted on modality-based workstations using Food and Drug Administration (FDA; USA) approved 5 megapixel monitors
    - Workstation image interpretation slower than with hardcopy
  - Hardcopy display: Printing digitally acquired images on film; interpretation on light box/viewer
  - Benefits
    - Dynamic range (latitude) up to 10,000; 4096 gray-scale levels or more (12 bits/pixel)
    - Improves image contrast, tissue equalization and penetration, esp. dense breasts
    - More consistent than SFM; lower image noise; comparable or lower dose
    - Enables electronic image display, storage and transmission, telemammography
    - Novel technologies enabled by FFDM: Tomosynthesis, dual-energy subtraction contrast enhancement

MAMMOGRAPHY: SCREENING

Key Facts

Screening Mammography
- Periodic examination to detect preclinical asymptomatic breast cancer
- Optimal screening interval not well-defined; between 1 and 3 years depending on country, authority
- Sporadic screening: Detect clinically unsuspected breast cancer
- Systematic screening: Reduce population mortality from breast cancer
  - 30% mortality reduction for women over age 50; weaker evidence for age 40-49 group
  - Mortality reduction parallels reduction in node-positive cancers
- Sensitivity SFM ~ 98% in fatty breasts; < 50% in dense breasts
  - ~15% absolute ↑ sensitivity with FFDM in dense breasts
- Supplemental screening with US, MRI being evaluated in high-risk women

Quality Assurance (QA) Program Crucial
- MQSA in USA; equivalent programs in many countries and centers
- FFDM more consistent than SFM, but lower resolution

Systematic Expert Reading is Critical
- Readers should be appropriately trained and accredited (MQSA in USA)
- Batch (off-line) reading in a suitably quiet environment minimizes distraction
- Double reading (human-human, human-CAD) increases detection rate by 5-20%

  - Disadvantages
    - Very expensive: FFDM 3-5X and CR-FFDM 2-3X more costly than typical SFM
    - Lower spatial resolution than SFM: 100 μm pixel size = 5 lp/mm, 50 μm pixel size = 10 lp/mm
    - Limited PACS integration, high data storage requirements (1 view mammogram = 7-26 megabytes)
- On-line screening: Interpretation at time of examination with immediate provision of results
  - Main decision: Whether to perform additional imaging investigations immediately
  - Abnormal mammograms (BI-RADS 0,4,5) result in additional imaging or biopsy
- Off-line screening: Mammograms batch-read, either later or remotely, by one or more radiologists
  - Main decision: Recall for diagnostic assessment or return to routine screening
  - Abnormal mammograms (BI-RADS 0,4,5) result in woman being recalled for additional imaging or biopsy
  - Postal (or phone call) recommendation to return for additional investigation
- MQSA: Mammography Quality Standards Act (USA)
  - Federal law (1992) with stringent quality standards for all stages and personnel involved
  - Governed by FDA and/or state with required regular QA process and annual inspections

IMAGING ANATOMY

General Anatomic Considerations
- Dense (extremely and heterogeneously) breast tissue: Breast cancer risk factor, RR 1.8 - 5X, ↓ sensitivity as compared with fatty breasts
  - May be influenced by dietary phytoestrogen intake, genetics (lower RR in Asian women)
- FFDM vs. SFM: ↑ Breast cancer detection by 15% in dense breasts
  - Varying availability of FFDM depends on location, socioeconomic, political factors

    - Survey of 45 facilities in 3 USA states between 2001-2002: Only 5% used FFDM; 8% in 2005
    - Scandinavian and Dutch screening programs progressively converting to FFDM
    - Widespread in private centers in France (higher reimbursement than for SFM)

Critical Anatomic Structures
- Axillary fold/pectoral muscle: Should be visible on MLO view down to level of nipple
- Inframammary fold: Should be visible on MLO view
- Nipple: Should be in profile on all projections

ANATOMY-BASED IMAGING ISSUES

Key Concepts or Questions
- Breast compressed to ↓ motion, even out breast thickness, ↓ radiation dose

Imaging Approaches
- Standard 4-view screening study: MLO and CC views of each breast
- Additional views may be deemed necessary by technologist to adequately image the entire breast
- Large breasts require additional overlapping imaging to include all tissue
- Patients with silicone implants require additional implant-displaced (ID; Eklund) views

Imaging Protocols
- Screening mammography recommendations
  - USA: Begin at age 40 (general population)
  - Most population screening programs start screening at age 50
  - Screening intervals vary; no proven optimal interval
    - American College of Radiology (ACR), American Cancer Society (ACS): Every year
    - National Cancer Institute (NCI) and US Preventive Services Task Force (USPSTF): Every 1 to 2 years
    - Dutch, Scandinavian, Canadian, Australian, New Zealand Screening Programs: Every 2 years

MAMMOGRAPHY: SCREENING

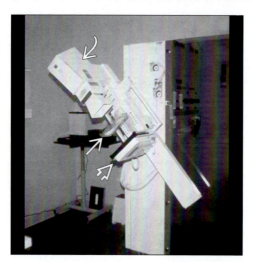

A typical SFM unit is depicted, with the tube gantry ➡ angulated. The film cassette holder ➡ is fixed, with a motor-controlled plastic compression plate above it ➡.

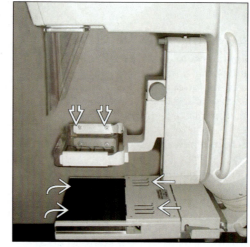

Close-up of another mammography unit shows the adjustable compression plate ➡ marked for AEC chamber positioning, and stage with cassette holder ➡ with integrated position markers ➡.

- ■ UK NHS National Breast Screening Program: Every 3 years
- Online screening mammographic interpretation
  - ○ High incidence of additional views and/or ultrasound (20-40%)
- Off-line dual reading: Standard of care for population-based programs (non-USA)
  - ○ Higher cancer detection rate (~90%) vs. single reader (mean 77%)
  - ○ Lower recall rate (typically 4-8%) compared to online or single reader screening
  - ○ Recent USA survey:15% screening mammograms double read; only 5% used computer-aided detection (CAD)
- Benefits of off-line reading: Decrease recall rate without ↓ in cancer detection; lower costs
- Main disadvantage of off-line reading: Inherent delays in reading and recall process
- USA trend toward off-line batch interpretation
  - ○ 1992: 20% of centers; more recent survey in 3 states: 84% of centers

PATHOLOGY-BASED IMAGING ISSUES

Key Concepts or Questions
- Benchmarks: Cancer detection rate of > 4/1000 screens, invasive cancer size < 1.4 cm, lymph node positivity < 20%, PPV > 25%, recall rate < 10%

CLINICAL IMPLICATIONS

Clinical Importance
- Six randomized controlled trials (RCTs) show benefit from screening mammography
  - ○ Endpoint: Death from breast cancer in women aged 40-70 receiving screening, compared with controls
    - ■ Breast cancer mortality reductions: 23%, 32%, 20% (Health Insurance Plan Project [HIP; USA], Swedish Two-County Trial, Edinburgh Trial)

- ■ 1997 meta-analysis of 40-49 age group: 5 Swedish trials, mortality reduction = 30%
- Mammographic screening contributed 28-65% to falling US breast cancer mortality, 1975-2000
  - ○ May not be effective if local incidence of breast cancer is very low

RELATED REFERENCES

1. Berry DA et al.: Effect of screening and adjuvant therapy on mortality from breast cancer. N Engl J Med 353:1784-92, 2005
2. Burnside ES et al: The use of batch reading to improve the performance of screening mammography. AJR 185:790-6, 2005
3. D'Orsi C et al: Current realities of delivering mammography services in the community: do challenges with staffing and scheduling exist? Radiology 235:391-5, 2005
4. Hendrick RE et al: Community-based mammography practice: services, charges, and interpretation methods. AJR 184:433-8, 2005
5. Pisano ED et al: Diagnostic performance of digital versus film mammography for breast-cancer screening. N Engl J Med 353:1773-83. 2005
6. Skaane P et al: Screen-film mammography versus full-field digital mammography with soft-copy reading: randomized trial in a population-based screening program - the Oslo II study. Radiology 232:197-204, 2004
7. Elmore JG et al: International variation in screening mammography interpretation in community-based programs. J Natl Cancer Inst. 95:1384-93, 2003
8. Tabar L et al: Beyond randomized trials: organized mammographic screening substantially reduces breast carcinoma mortality. Cancer 91:1724-31, 2001
9. Hendrick RE et al: Benefit of screening mammography in women aged 40-49: a new meta-analysis of randomized controlled trials. J Natl Cancer Inst Monogr 22:87-92, 1997

IMAGE GALLERY

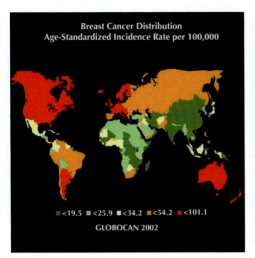

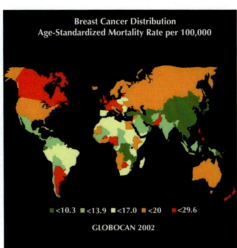

(Left) Graphic map of global age-standardized breast cancer incidence by country. Developed nations and cities usually have the highest incidence; this phenomenon is not understood. *(Right)* Graphic map of global breast cancer mortality shows highly variable mortality rates, not always linked to high incidence. This may reflect variable availability of high quality mammographic screening and adjuvant therapy.

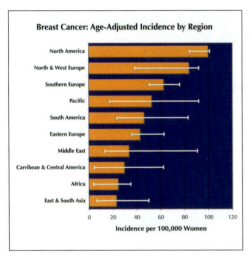

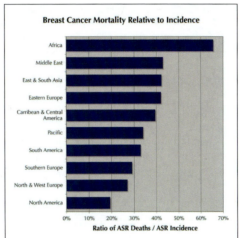

(Left) Chart indicates regional breast cancer incidences around the world. Error bars depict the range between countries with the highest and lowest incidence in each region; there is marked individual national variation. *(Right)* Chart shows the ratio of age-adjusted breast cancer mortality relative to incidence. Women in Western nations have better chance of survival than elsewhere, probably due to better screening and therapy.

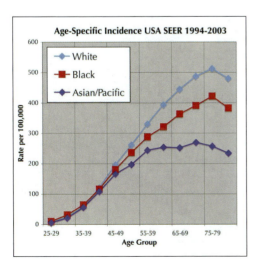

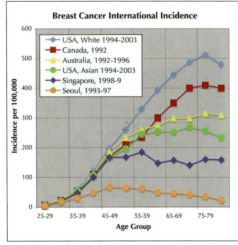

(Left) Chart shows age specific breast cancer incidence for USA, 1994-2003. White American women have highest incidence at every age of the 3 ethnic groups. Note curve divergence after 45-49 y/o. *(Right)* Chart shows age specific breast cancer incidence for various countries. USA, Canada, Australia show progressive rise after age 50; rise is not universal. Asians have ↑ incidence in USA than in Asia. Note curves diverge after age 50.

MAMMOGRAPHY: SCREENING

(Left) MLO mammography shows symmetrically positioned fatty breasts in a 58 y/o. The pectoral folds ⇥ extend to the level of the nipple ⇒, perpendicular to the plane of the fold. The inframammary fold ⇒ is not well seen however. *(Right)* CC mammography (same case as left) shows maximal inclusion of the breast on the image, confirmed by visualization of the pectoral muscles ⇥. The CC view should have the nipple ⇒ well centered, not rotated inwards.

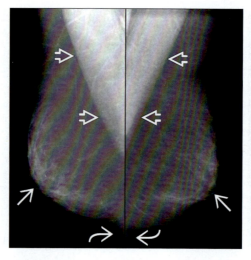

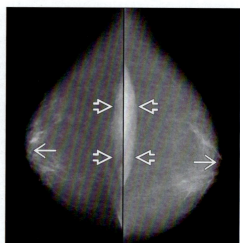

(Left) MLO mammography in a 44 y/o with small breasts show positioning difficulties. Despite exceptional inclusion of the pectoral folds ⇥, they do not reach the level of the nipple ⇥ on both sides. *(Right)* CC mammography (same case as left) shows no pectoral muscle posteriorly ⇥, not indicative of poor positioning. CC view measurement from nipple to chest wall should be within 1 cm of the MLO nipple-to-pectoralis distance (posterior nipple line) as is true in this case.

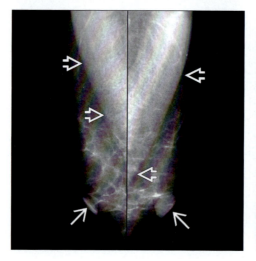

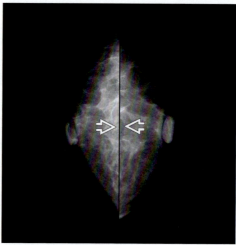

(Left) Tools of the trade for SFM reading. Large 2X magnifying glass ⇥ is essential. Plastic dome magnifier ⇒ permits up to 8X magnification. Viewer box ⇥ has corrective lenses and minimizes extraneous light. *(Right)* Typical setup for SFM batch reading with a mammographic multiviewer. Current study is hung below the previous study (or 2 year prior) for comparison. Bright light ⇥, magnifying lens ⇒ and mammographic box viewer ⇥ are on hand.

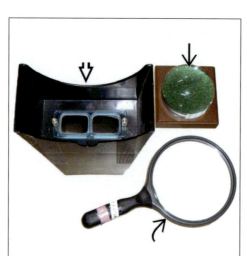

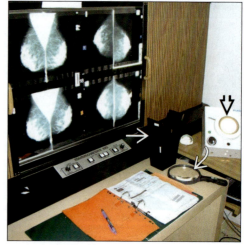

IMAGE GALLERY

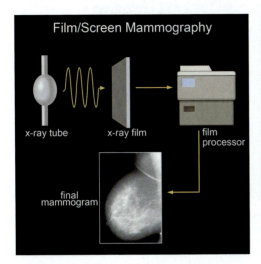

Film/Screen Mammography

x-ray tube · x-ray film · film processor · final mammogram

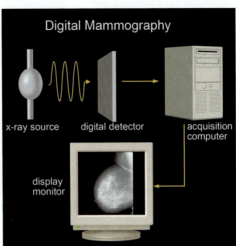

Digital Mammography

x-ray source · digital detector · acquisition computer · display monitor

(Left) The process for obtaining a SFM image is depicted in this graphic. While many basic steps are similar to SFM, FFDM (right image) decouples the image acquisition from the image display. *(Right)* Graphic shows basics of FFDM where the digital image may be adjusted as to brightness and contrast on a display monitor (workstation), permitting more flexible viewing, remote telemammography.

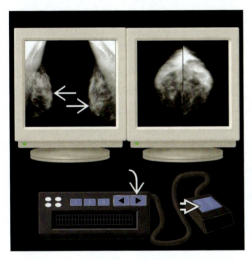

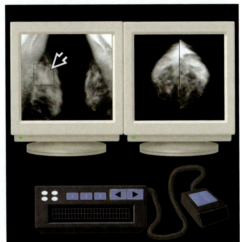

(Left) Graphic shows a typical layout for soft-copy workstation reporting of FFDM images. Programmable display allows personalized layouts as on these MLO views ➡. Image layouts are controlled by mouse ➡ or pre-programed buttons ➡ on the console. *(Right)* Graphic shows a virtual magnification glass ➡, which is mouse-controlled and easily manipulated manually. Detail is less than geometric magnification.

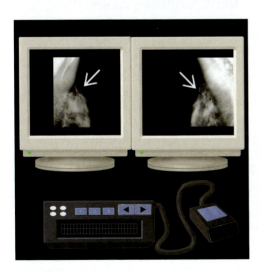

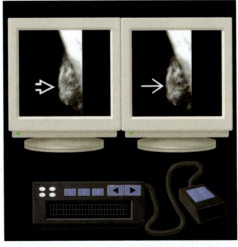

(Left) Graphic shows automatically zoomed views of upper MLO views ➡. This can be programmed into personalized 'hanging protocols' to ensure a predictable and consistent image presentation. *(Right)* Graphic shows side-by-side display of the right MLO view of a current ➡ and previous study ➡. Prior pre-loaded (pre-fetched) digital images can be reviewed either through customized hanging protocol or by individual image selection.

MAMMOGRAPHY: DIAGNOSTIC

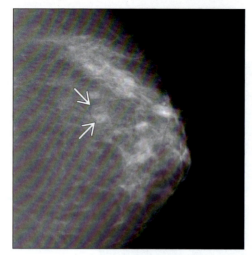

CC mammography on the left side in a 52 y/o woman shows a screen-detected rounded density with a partly well-circumscribed margin ➡. Additional workup views were requested.

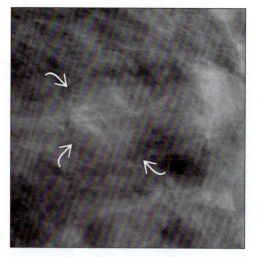

CC mammography magnification defines an almost complete mammographic halo ➡. Diagnostic mammography suggests this is benign. US showed a typical fibroadenoma.

TERMINOLOGY

Abbreviations
- BI-RADS®: Breast Imaging Reporting and Data System

Synonyms
- Mammography workup
- Additional mammographic views

Definitions
- Mammography used to evaluate a clinical or screen-detected breast abnormality
  - Additional problem-solving imaging views include: Magnification, spot compression, rolled, 'lumpograms' (with BB marker over palpable lesion), tangential, others
  - Exam includes on-site review by radiologist
  - Communication of results to patient

Indications
- Clinical abnormality
  - Lump, thickening, skin or nipple changes, nipple discharge, axillary mass, unknown primary malignancy
- Abnormal screening mammogram
  - "Recall": May be performed at time of on-line screening visit: Dictate separate paragraph for screening, indicating reason for additional views
- Short-interval follow-up of probably benign findings on prior mammogram
  - Typically initially performed at 6 months

Can be Performed as Diagnostic Mammogram
- Annual mammogram in women with personal history of breast cancer
- Annual mammogram in women with implants
- Breast pain
  - Focal, noncyclical may be appropriate
  - Cyclical pain essentially a normal variant, can be screening

Goals
- Problem solving: Patient leaves with final recommendation
  - Define extent and 3-D location of abnormalities
  - Perform US as needed at time of diagnostic mammography:
    - Separate paragraph detailing US findings
    - Integrated impression and recommendations
- BI-RADS 0, incomplete, essentially not used
  - Rare case will merit further evaluation with MRI if both mammography and US equivocal, lesion too vague to biopsy (e.g., asymmetry or possible distortion)

IMAGING ANATOMY

General Anatomic Considerations
- Mammography creates two-dimensional projections
- Breast is highly deformable, 3-dimensional structure
- Breast size, shape and glandular parenchymal distribution may be asymmetric
- Cooper ligaments, vessels, and parenchyma may overlap and simulate pathology (summation shadows)
- Lesions within the breast are mobile and deformable, may vary in shape and appearance with projection
- True lesion may be inadvertently displaced out of image during special views (e.g., spot compression)

Anatomic Relationships
- Identify distance from nipple in both projections

ANATOMY-BASED IMAGING ISSUES

Imaging Approaches
- Standard diagnostic mammogram includes routine CC and MLO views (which may have been performed initially as part of screening)
  - In women < 30 years of age, standard exam may be limited to MLO views only due to concern for radiation exposure

MAMMOGRAPHY: DIAGNOSTIC

Key Facts

Roles
- Confirmation of a mammographic finding
  - Is it real? 3-D localization if yes
  - Lesion characterization
    - CC and 90° lateral magnification views are best way to assess Ca++
- Use triangulation and specific views to localize screen-detected lesions
- Skillful use of additional views for better visualization of specific abnormalities
- Screen entirety of both breasts for other disease
  - Especially symptomatic women
- Short interval follow-up of mammographic abnormality, including initial follow-up after core biopsy

- 'Diagnostic' mammography should yield a final assessment and recommendation
  - Integrate mammographic and US findings
  - 11-16% of palpable masses occult on mammography: Liberal use of supplemental US
  - 25-40% of biopsies recommended → cancer

Pitfalls
- Dismissal of true lesion, esp. infiltrating cancer
  - Small invasive cancers can trap fat, thin on spot compression: US can help
- Area of interest not included on images
- Lesion hidden by overlying dense parenchyma
- Satisfaction of search
- Lack of comparison examinations
  - Prior studies ↑ cancer detection rate, PPV of biopsy

- If more than 4 months have elapsed since screening, consider obtaining routine views again
- True lateral view often obtained in patients with prior history of cancer
- Implant-displaced (ID; Eklund) views in women with implants
- Additional views as needed to address clinical symptoms and/or mammographic abnormalities

Imaging Pitfalls
- Abnormality visible on both views may not be the same lesion
- Area of interest not included on images
  - Problematic for spot compression views in large breasts: Use small cassette/detector instead of spot
  - Loss of landmarks on magnification views
    - Especially problematic for focal asymmetries: Use broad spot or 90° lateral view instead
- Satisfaction of search: May miss other pathology in same or contralateral breast

PATHOLOGY-BASED IMAGING ISSUES

Key Concepts or Questions
- Diagnostic mammography cannot exclude malignancy
  - Most palpable abnormalities (50-75%) are not clearly visible on mammography
  - Most visible lesions (esp. masses) cannot be definitively diagnosed by mammography alone, even with additional views
- Diagnostic mammography can underestimate disease extent significantly
  - "Tip-of-iceberg" problem, esp. in dense breasts
  - Extent of calcifications (Ca++) on magnification views predicts extent of DCIS to within 2 cm in 80-85% of cases

Imaging Approaches
- Palpable lesion
  - Standard 4-view mammography of both breasts

- BB marker over lesion, may need to be repositioned over mass prior to each exposure
  - Perform tangential view or "lumpogram"
    - Tape BB marker to skin over lesion, perform spot compression views in CC and LM projection with skin over lump in profile
- Alternate views performed to further evaluate lesion, solve specific imaging problem
  - Laterally exaggerated craniocaudal (XCCL) and axillary tail views for far lateral, axillary lesions
  - Inframammary fold view, cleavage views for far inferior or medial lesions respectively
  - Tangential skin views for skin masses
- Ca++: Magnification CC and 90° lateral views
  - Open or spot compression magnification
  - Skin localization can be performed if suspect dermal calcifications
- Mass: Spot compression or magnification views
  - US unless clearly a lymph node, oil cyst, calcifying fibroadenoma (FA)
- Focal asymmetry
  - Comparison to prior mammograms critical
  - Spot compression views to confirm true finding
  - US often helpful
- Use US liberally to complement mammography
- Lesion only visible on one view
  - Lesion should fall on a line or curved arc at the same distance from nipple on both CC and MLO views
  - Obtain true lateral view (and compare to CC and MLO views)
    - Triangulation: With MLO view in center, a line drawn through lesion in two views, extending across the third view, will intersect lesion location in third view
  - Slight changes in angulation or positioning in projection where lesion is most visible: Step oblique views
  - Rolled views, most commonly rolled CC views: Lesion moves with top or bottom of breast

Imaging Protocols
- Mediolateral (ML) or straight lateral (90°) view
  - Horizontal x-ray beam

MAMMOGRAPHY: DIAGNOSTIC

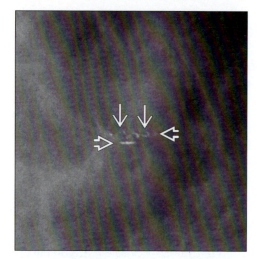

Lateral mammography magnification shows value of horizontal beam (90°) view. Clustered Ca++ ➡ in this 52 y/o show layering ⬆ due to milk-of-calcium. Ultrasound showed Ca++ in a cyst.

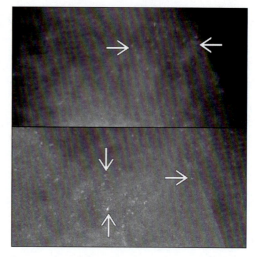

Images show close-up of standard mammogram (upper) and geometric magnification view (lower), which shows the Ca++ ➡ much more clearly in this 46 y/o. Core biopsy = sclerosing adenosis.

- ▪ Evaluation of dependent calcifications (milk of calcium)
- ○ Should be performed routinely for evaluation of most lesions and prior to needle localization for distance from skin
- ○ Allows perpendicular triangulation with CC view
- • Lateromedial (LM) view
  - ○ Medial lesions better seen (closer to cassette) than on MLO or ML
  - ○ Also horizontal beam, perpendicular to CC
- • Laterally exaggerated CC (XCCL) view
  - ○ As for CC but patient rotated inward so axillary tail tissue on CC view
- • Axillary tail (AT) or "Cleopatra" view
  - ○ Originally performed in semireclining position, now performed upright
  - ○ Aim: Isolate axillary tail, lateral breast
    - ▪ Compression along edge of breast and in axilla
    - ▪ Central and medial tissues should be excluded
    - ▪ Common error: Identical to MLO view if centering and compression too medial
- • Inframammary fold view
  - ○ Coned lateromedial view of inframammary fold with elevation of the breast
  - ○ For far inferior lesions not otherwise clearly seen
- • Cleavage view
  - ○ Vertical beam CC view of medial breast and cleavage
    - ▪ Breasts pushed together, then pulled forward
  - ○ For far medial posterior lesions
- • Angled recompression and rolled views
  - ○ Exploits deformable motion of breast and parallax to remove or demonstrate tissue overlap
  - ○ Use projection where abnormality is most visible initially
  - ○ Angled recompression: Slight (10-15 degree) tube/film angulation away from standard projection
  - ○ Rolled: Standard angulation, breast upper surface rolled medially (CCRM), laterally (CCRL) or forwards before compression

Imaging Pitfalls

- • Mammograms must be technically adequate: Responsibility of the radiologist

- • Lesion may not be able to be included on mammograms despite additional views: Low threshold for US
- • Inappropriate or inexpert use of additional views
- • "Diagnostic mammography" often not definitively diagnostic
  - ○ True lesion may appear to resolve or be artifactual
  - ○ Benign-looking mass or Ca++ can be malignant
  - ○ Malignant-looking mass or Ca++ can be benign

CLINICAL IMPLICATIONS

Clinical Importance

- • Most clinically palpable abnormalities should have mammographic evaluation
  - ○ Initial US in women < 30 yrs, pregnant, lactating: May be sufficient
    - ▪ Mammogram only if US suspicious and/or high clinical suspicion
  - ○ Unless technically impractical (e.g., huge fungating tumor)
- • Suspicious lesions should be confirmed histologically before definitive therapy initiated

RELATED REFERENCES

1. Sickles EA et al: Performance benchmarks for diagnostic mammography. Radiology. 235:775-90, 2005
2. Burnside ES et al: Differential value of comparison with previous examinations in diagnostic versus screening mammography. AJR. 179:1173-7, 2002
3. Kopans DB: Breast Imaging, 2nd Ed. Philadelphia: Lippincott-Raven. 171-210; 721-46, 1998
4. Faulk RM et al: Efficacy of spot compression-magnification and tangential views in mammographic evaluation of palpable masses. Radiology. 185:87-90, 1992
5. Sickles EA: Practical solutions to common mammographic problems: tailoring the examination. AJR. 151:31-9, 1988
6. Swann CA et al: Practical solutions to the problems of triangulation and preoperative localization of breast lesions. Radiology. 163:577-9, 1987

IMAGE GALLERY

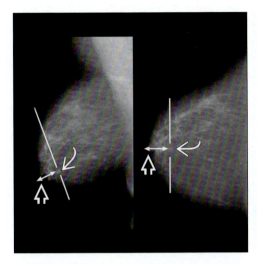
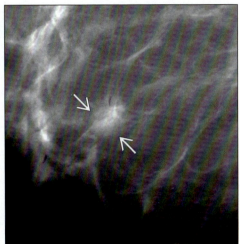

(Left) A line parallel to the pectoral fold on the MLO mammogram (left) and parallel to the film edge on the CC view (right) passes through a small mass ➔ at the same distance from the nipple ➔ in both views in this 56 y/o. *(Right)* MLO mammography magnification (same case as left) shows a mostly circumscribed oval mass ➔. This lesion was deemed mammographically benign.

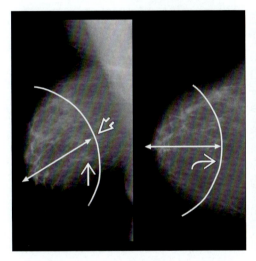
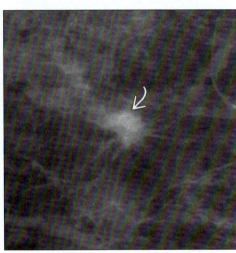

(Left) Mammography (same case as prior 2 images) shows a tiny spiculated asymmetry only on CC view (on right) ➔. The lesion should fall on an arc of same radius, centered on the nipple, in both views. Lesion did not correspond to focal asymmetry on MLO ➔, but rather a faint density posterosuperiorly ➔. *(Right)* CC mammography magnification (same as left) shows spiculated mass ➔. Excision = infiltrating ductal carcinoma (IDC).

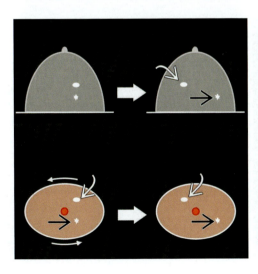
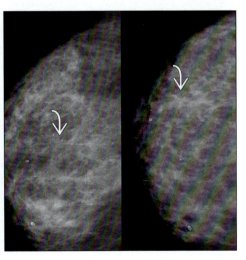

(Left) Graphic shows how CC rolled views (left breast illustrated) can determine if a lesion is in upper or lower breast. When top of breast is rolled medially (inferior images), a superior lesion ➔ moves medially, and an inferior lesion ➔ shifts laterally (upper images). *(Right)* CC mammography (left) in a 43 y/o shows subtle architectural distortion with two Ca++ ➔, which moved laterally on CCRL view (right) indicating location in the upper breast. Biopsy = IDC.

(Left) CC mammography spot compression shows an oval circumscribed mass ⮞, almost displaced out of the spot view in this 55 y/o woman. Care with positioning is crucial for mobile lesions. *(Right)* CC mammography in a 41 y/o woman with a palpable lump. Initial view (left) is normal. Penetrated lumpogram (right) with a BB ⮞ over the lump shows a focal asymmetry ⮞ corresponding to the lesion. Pure DCIS on excision.

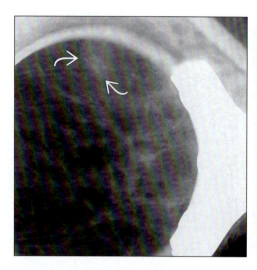 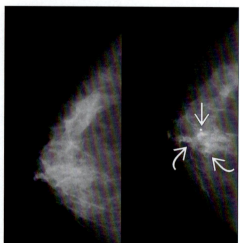

(Left) CC mammography magnification shows a group of indeterminate slightly irregular screen-detected Ca++ ⮞ in this 48 y/o. Some lucent centered Ca++ raised the possibility of dermal Ca++. *(Right)* CC mammography magnification (same case as on left), using a tangential skin view with very light exposure, shows these Ca++ to be clearly dermal ⮞ and benign. No further investigation was performed.

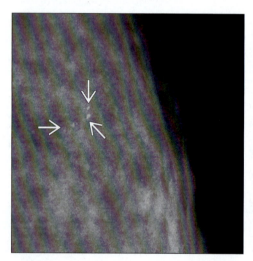 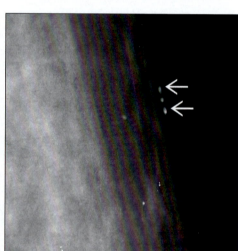

(Left) MLO mammography screening examination in this 47 y/o woman shows a very subtle area of architectural distortion ⮞ seen on the right MLO only, near the axillary tail. She was recalled for additional workup views. *(Right)* MLO mammography magnification with spot compression (same case as left) shows the abnormality to be persistent as an area of distortion with poorly defined central mass ⮞. US showed a focal mass; core biopsy showed IDC.

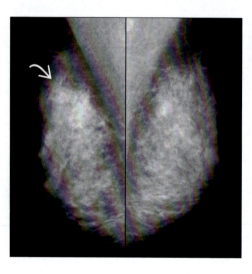 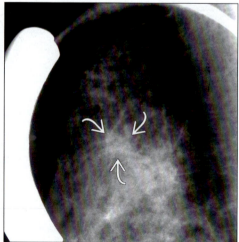

IMAGE GALLERY

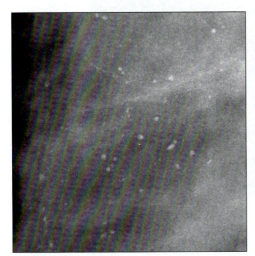
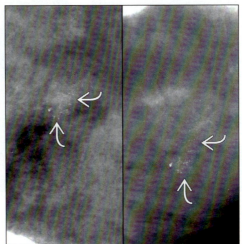

(Left) CC mammography magnification in a 47 y/o with screen-detected indistinct Ca++ shows scattered smooth dense well-defined Ca++ which are typically benign. *(Right)* In this 52 y/o woman with screen-detected indeterminate Ca++, magnification MLO (left) and CC (right) mammograms show these to be pleomorphic in morphology ➔, moderately suspicious, BI-RADS 4C. High-grade DCIS on biopsy.

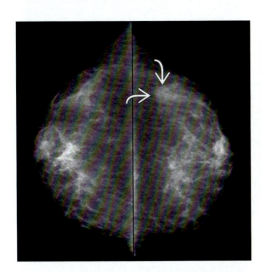
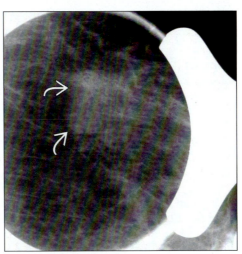

(Left) CC mammography screening shows a rounded asymmetry ➔ in the lateral left breast of a 59 y/o woman. This was also visible on the MLO view, and she was recalled for further diagnostic imaging. *(Right)* CC mammography spot compression (same case as left) shows an indistinct dense mass ➔ similar in density to surrounding tissue. Other views and ultrasound showed no lesion; interpretation = focal glandular asymmetry.

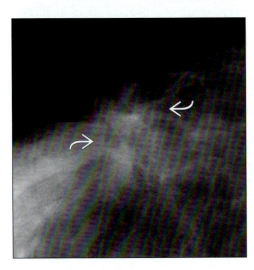
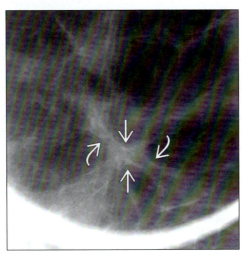

(Left) CC mammography magnification shows subtle architectural distortion in this 78 y/o woman with palpable thickening ➔. This persisted on a lateromedial view (not shown). *(Right)* Lateral mammography spot compression (same case as left) shows the benefit of spot compression, which reveals a spiculated mass ➔ with adjacent architectural distortion ➔. Core biopsy = infiltrating lobular carcinoma.

MAMMOGRAPHY: AUDIT BENCHMARKS

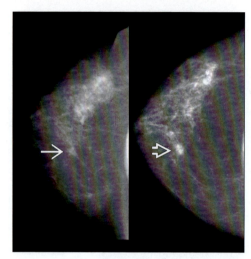

Mammography shows a FN mammogram in 2002 ➡️*, with the cancer being found on a mammogram in 2003* ⏩*. Utilization of an expanded audit enables review of such FN cases, thereby improving future outcomes.*

Chart of relationship among TP, FP, FN, BI-RADS categories, sensitivity and PPV in screening mammography.

TERMINOLOGY

Abbreviations
- Mammography Quality Standards Act (MQSA)
- Breast Imaging Reporting and Data System (BI-RADS®)
- True positive (TP)
- False positive (FP)
- True negative (TN)
- False negative (FN)
- Positive predictive value (PPV)
- Cancer detection rate (CDR)

Definitions
- Mammography audit: Assessment of all important performance parameters in both screening and diagnostic mammography
- Mammography audit benchmarks: Points of reference to which mammography performance measurements can be made
- Screening mammogram: One performed on an asymptomatic woman to detect early, clinically unsuspected breast cancer
- Diagnostic mammogram (first definition): Performed on a woman with clinical signs or symptoms that suggest breast cancer
- Diagnostic mammogram (second definition): Performed on a woman for whom further mammographic evaluation has been requested because of an abnormal screening mammogram
- BI-RADS final assessments used for audits
  - BI-RADS 0: Screening mammogram with finding for which additional evaluation is needed
    - Also known as recall or call-back
  - BI-RADS 1: Negative mammogram
  - BI-RADS 2: Mammogram with a benign finding
  - BI-RADS 3: Mammogram with a probably benign finding, for which short-interval follow-up suggested
    - Should not be applied directly from screening, but only after a screening-initiated diagnostic evaluation

- BI-RADS 4: Mammogram with a suspicious abnormality for which biopsy should be considered
- BI-RADS 5: Mammogram with a finding highly suggestive of malignancy, for which appropriate action should be taken
- BI-RADS 6: Mammogram with a known biopsy-proven malignancy, for which appropriate action should be taken
- Positive screening mammogram: One for which recall is initiated (i.e., BI-RADS 0) or that requires tissue diagnosis (BI-RADS 4 or 5)
  - Under MQSA, only BI-RADS 4 or 5 mammograms are included in this group
- Positive diagnostic mammogram: One requiring a tissue diagnosis (BI-RADS 4 or 5)
- Negative screening mammogram: One that is negative or has a benign finding (BI-RADS 1 or 2)
- Negative diagnostic mammogram: One that is negative or has a benign or probably benign finding (BI-RADS 1, 2 or 3)
- TP: Tissue diagnosis of cancer within 1 year after a positive mammogram (BI-RADS 0, 4 or 5)
  - Note: BI-RADS 0, 4, 5 are "positive" even if for an unrelated finding not at the site of cancer
  - Audit can be by breast or by patient; if by breast, must request permission to do so from FDA
- TN: No known tissue diagnosis of cancer within 1 year of a negative mammogram (BI-RADS 1 or 2 for screening; BI-RADS 1, 2 or 3 for diagnostic)
- FN: Tissue diagnosis of cancer within 1 year of a negative mammogram (BI-RADS 1 or 2 for screening; BI-RADS 1, 2 or 3 for diagnostic)
- FP: Three separate definitions
  - FP1: No known tissue diagnosis of cancer within 1 year of a positive screening mammogram (BI-RADS 0, 4 or 5)
  - FP2: No known tissue diagnosis of cancer within 1 year after recommendation for biopsy or surgical consultation (BI-RADS 4 or 5 on screening or diagnostic mammogram)

Key Facts

Current MQSA Audit is Not Sufficient
- Must perform an expanded audit for real value

Expanded Audit Assesses 3 Essential Goals
- Finding high % of cancers present (measure cancer detection rate, CDR, per 1,000 screening mammograms, and overall sensitivity)
- Finding high % of small, node-negative cancers (measure tumor size & LN negativity)
- Have low recall rate & requests for biopsy (measure recall rate & PPV)

Audit Data: Must Have Strict Separation of Screening and Diagnostic Mammograms
- Mixing of data renders analysis of both groups worthless

Improving Outcomes: Compare Audit Data to Screening Benchmarks
- Strive to achieve benchmarks: CDR of > 4, mean invasive cancer size of < 1.4 cm, LN positivity of < 20%, PPV_2 > 25%, and recall rate of < 10%
- If not doing so, identify areas requiring overall group improvement (review FNs, etc.)
- MOST IMPORTANT: Identify individual "outlier" who has significantly poorer performance
- Take action to improve outlier's skills, or remove outlier from mammography
- Be aware of the many variables in comparing to benchmark data before evaluating one's own audit data, especially the huge statistical variation when audit numbers are small

---

- FP_3: Benign tissue diagnosis within 1 year after recommendation for biopsy on the basis of a positive screening or diagnostic mammogram (BI-RADS 4 or 5)
- PPV: Three separate definitions
  - PPV_1: Percentage of all positive screening mammograms (BI-RADS 0, 4 or 5) that result in tissue diagnosis of cancer within 1 year
    - $PPV_1 = TP/(\text{\# of positive screening mammograms})$, or $PPV_1 = TP/(TP + FP_1)$
  - PPV_2: Percent of screening or diagnostic mammograms recommended for biopsy (BI-RADS 4 or 5) → tissue diagnosis of cancer within 1 year
    - $PPV_2 = TP/(\text{number of screening or diagnostic mammograms recommended for biopsy})$, or $PPV_2 = TP/(TP + FP_2)$
  - PPV_3: Percent of known biopsies done as a result of positive screening or diagnostic mammograms (BI-RADS 4 or 5) → tissue diagnosis of cancer within 1 year
    - $PPV_3 = TP/(\text{number of biopsies})$, or $PPV_3 = TP/(TP + FP_3)$
- Sensitivity: Probability of detecting a cancer when a cancer exists = number of cancers diagnosed after being identified at mammography in a population (within 1 year of the mammogram), divided by all cancers present in that population
  - Sensitivity = $TP/(TP + FN)$
- CDR: Number of cancers detected at mammography per 1,000 patients examined
  - Best when calculated for screening mammograms only, or separately for screening and diagnostic cases
- Raw data: Collected information on mammograms in the various BI-RADS categories and pathology results of all biopsies performed
- Derived data: Data calculated from raw data; used to assess overall performance

PATHOLOGY-BASED IMAGING ISSUES

Measuring Mammography Performance: The Audit
- Current audit requirements under MQSA are not sufficient
  - Track all positive mammograms for pathology outcomes
  - Seek information on all FN cases
  - Lead physician oversees entire Quality Assurance process
  - Perform audit at least yearly, collectively & by individual
- Expanded Audit: True measure of quality, efficacy & efficiency
  - Requires information to assess 3 essential goals
    - Find high % of cancers in screening population (measure sensitivity & CDR)
    - Find high % of small & node-negative cancers (measure tumor size & LN positivity)
    - Have low recall rate & requests for biopsy (measure recall rate & PPV)
  - Requires strict separation of screening and diagnostic cases
  - Raw data required
    - Audit dates, # of mammograms (screening & diagnostic separately), # of BI-RADS 0, 4, 5, biopsy results from BI-RADS 4 & 5 readings, pathology data on each cancer
  - Derived data calculated from raw data
    - First ascertain number of TN, TP, FP_1, FP_2, FP_3 cases
    - Then calculate PPV_1, PPV_2, PPV_3, & CDR
    - Can also calculate tumor size, LN positivity & recall rate
    - Need access to a tumor registry to more accurately calculate sensitivity
  - If cannot separate screening from diagnostic cases, can estimate expected clinical outcomes based on case mix

Sample of a raw data collection form used for performing an expanded audit. This is used for screening cases only.

Continuation (from previous image) of raw data collection form.

○ If can separate screening from diagnostic cases, should perform separate audit of diagnostic group as well (see Table)

Using Expanded Audit Data to Improve Outcomes: Benchmarking

- Cannot assess performance data in a vacuum
  ○ Compare to desirable goals & measured benchmarks
  ○ 1994 desirable goals based on experts' performance: Ideals toward which to strive
    ▪ Somewhat outdated by advances in technology
  ○ 2005-2006 Benchmark Data (see Table)
    ▪ Based on actual performance of over 1 million mammograms in U.S.
    ▪ Provide real snapshot of current mammography practice
    ▪ Excellent standard for comparison
- Using benchmark comparisons to improve future outcomes
  ○ Measure overall group performance and compare to benchmarks
    ▪ Goals: CDR of > 4 , mean invasive cancer size of < 1.4 cm, LN positivity of < 20%, PPV₂ > 25%, and recall rate of < 10%
    ▪ If not achieving these levels, look for ways to improve upon performance (review FNs, etc.)
  ○ Measure individual performance as well
    ▪ Compare to others in group
    ▪ All group members serving same population, so is valid to compare
  ○ Goal to assure no "outliers" in group
    ▪ Standout poor performer(s) require intervention
    ▪ Outliers → remedial training or stop interpreting mammograms: In best interests of individual, group, and patient
    ▪ Group must be prepared to take such action from outset of audit process; otherwise, no point in performing audit
  ○ Factors to consider in comparing benchmarks to one's own data
    ▪ Patient age, frequency of screening, risk factors can dramatically change audit data

- May be huge statistical variation in data obtained, especially when numbers are small
- Performance may vary from year to year, due to random chance
- No single metric should be evaluated in isolation (e.g., if recall rate high, but CDR equally high, overall performance may be deemed acceptable)

RELATED REFERENCES

1. Rosenberg RD et al: Performance benchmarks for screening mammography. Radiology. 241:55-66, 2006
2. Weaver DL et al: Pathologic findings from the Breast Cancer Surveillance Consortium: population-based outcomes in women undergoing biopsy after screening mammography. Cancer. 106(4):732-42, 2006
3. Sickles EA et al: Performance benchmarks for diagnostic mammography. Radiology. 235(3):775-90, 2005
4. D'Orsi CJ et al: Breast Imaging Reporting and Data System, BI-RADS: Mammography, 4th ed. Reston: American College of Radiology, 2003
5. Sohlich RE et al: Interpreting data from audits when screening and diagnostic mammography outcomes are combined. AJR Am J Roentgenol. 178(3):681-6, 2002
6. Dee KE et al: Medical audit of diagnostic mammography examinations: comparison with screening outcomes obtained concurrently. AJR Am J Roentgenol. 176(3):729-33, 2001
7. 21 CFA Part 16 and 900: Mammography quality standards; final rule. Federal register, Washington, DC: Government printing office. 62:55851-994, 1997
8. Linver MN et al: The mammography audit: a primer for the mammography quality standards act (MQSA). AJR Am J Roentgenol. 165(1):19-25, 1995
9. Bassett LW et al: Quality Determinants of Mammography. Clinical Practice Guideline No. 13. AHCPR Publication No. 95-0632. Rockville MD: Agency for Health Care Policy and Research, Public Health Service, U.S. Department of Health and Human Services, 1994
10. Sickles EA: Quality assurance. How to audit your own mammography practice. Radiol Clin North Am. 30(1):265-75, 1992
11. Tabar L et al: Update of the Swedish two-county program of mammographic screening for breast cancer. Radiol Clin North Am. 30(1):187-210, 1992

IMAGE GALLERY

PARAMETER TO BE CALCULATED	EQUATION*	RESULT
Number of True Positives (TP)	#5A + #6A	
Number of False Positives (FP) Three Definitions:		
FP₁	#2 - TP	
FP₂	#5B + #6B + #7	
FP₃	#5B + #6B	

PARAMETER TO BE CALCULATED	EQUATION*	RESULT
Positive Predictive Values (PPV) Three Definitions:		
PPV₁ (how often abnormal screens are cancer)	[TP]/[#2]	
PPV₂ (how often biopsies recommended are cancer)	[TP]/[TP + FP₂]	
PPV₃, or PBR (how often biopsies done are cancer)	[TP]/[TP + FP₃]	
Cancer Detection Rate	([TP]/[#1]) x 1000	
Percent Minimal Cancers (Invasive Cancers ≤ 1 cm, or DCIS) Found	([#8 + #10]/[TP]) x 100	
Percent Axillary Node-Positive Invasive Cancers Found	([#11]/[#9]) x 100	
Recall Rate	([#2]/[#1]) x 100	

(Left) Sample of a derived data calculation form for performing an expanded audit. This also applies to screening cases only. The numbers in the equations refer to the same numbers on the raw data form (prior 2 images). *(Right)* Continuation (from left) of derived data calculation form. This provides quantitative data of essential outcomes that determine mammography quality and efficiency in one's practice.

AUDIT DATA ANALYSIS – DESIRABLE GOALS (1994)

(SCREENING CASES ONLY)

PPV1	5-10%
PPV2	25-40%
Tumors found - stage 0 or 1	50%
Minimal cancers found	30%
LN Positivity	< 25%
CDR	2-10
Recall rate	≤ 10%
Sensitivity	85%
Mean Inv. Ca size (cm)	<1.5

2005-2006 BCSC SCREENING BENCHMARK DATA

	SCREEN RECALLS (Ref. 3)	SCREENING (Ref. 1)
PPV2	23%	25%
Tumors, 0 or 1	83%	76%
Min. Ca's	63%	52%
LN Positivity	16%	19%
CDR	3.1	4.4
Recall rate	12%	9.7%
Sensitivity	86%	80%
Mean Inv. Ca size (cm)	1.1	1.3

(Left) 1994 desirable goals for screening mammography (ref. 9). Actual current performance exceeds these goals (on right), likely due to advances in technology. *(Right)* Mean performance benchmarks for screening mammography, based on over 1 million mammogram interpretations in the U.S. performed 1996-2001. This provides an excellent standard of comparison for one's own practice.

Screen: Dx mix	Abn. findngs (%)	Pos. Bx findngs (%)	Ca Detect rate (per 1 K)
90:10	6	38	10
80:20	7	40	15
70:30	8	41	20
60:40	10	41	25
50:50	11	42	30
40:60	12	43	35
30:70	13	44	39
20:80	14	45	44
10:90	15	45	49

Screen: Dx mix	Nodal mets (%)	Stage 0 & 1 Ca (%)	Mean size invas. Ca (mm)
90:10	8	87	14.4
80:20	9	86	14.8
70:30	9	85	15.2
60:40	9	83	15.6
50:50	11	82	16.0
40:60	11	80	16.4
30:70	12	79	16.8
20:80	13	78	17.2
10:90	13	76	17.6

(Left) Table of outcomes data for relative mixes of screening and diagnostic mammography exams (ref. 5). *(Right)* Continuation (from previous image) of outcomes data for mixes of screening plus diagnostic mammography exams. These can be utilized as surrogate benchmarks for radiologists unable to completely separate screening from diagnostic studies for audit analysis.

MAMMOGRAPHY: AUDIT BENCHMARKS

IMAGE GALLERY

(Left) Table of outcomes data for screening plus diagnostic mammography for case mixes based on percent of cases evaluated for palpable masses (ref. 5). These can be utilized as surrogate benchmarks for radiologists unable to completely separate screening from symptomatic patients for audit analysis. *(Right)* Continuation of same outcomes data (from previous image).

Palp. Mass (%)	Abn. findngs (%)	Pos. Bx findngs (%)	Ca Detect rate (per 1 K)
2	7	40	15
5	8	41	18
10	9	43	24
15	9	44	29
20	10	44	35
30	12	46	35
50	15	51	68

Palp. Mass (%)	Nodal mets (%)	Stage 0 & 1 Ca (%)	Mean size invas. Ca (mm)
2	8	86	14.3
5	10	83	15.4
10	12	79	17.0
15	14	76	18.3
20	16	73	19.3
30	19	68	21.0
50	23	61	23.1

(Left) Table of audit summary results by radiologist shows the value of the expanded audit in detecting poor performance by an outlier individual. *(Right)* Continuation of the audit summary (see previous image) shows radiologist #6 had a CDR ⇒ barely half that of the next lowest person in the group. Remedial training was instituted, with subsequent improvement in performance.

RAD.	CASES READ	REC. FOR BX.	MALIG	B9
#1	11,904	245	93	151
#2	10,658	383	131	247
#3	5,665	131	35	94
#4	5,071	137	42	91
#5	4,667	127	33	92
#6	4,002	33	12	20
#7	3,284	74	25	47
#8	2,782	85	24	61
#9	2,067	44	16	25
#10	2,000	33	18	15
#11	1,944	52	18	33
#12	1,650	36	10	25
TOTALS	61,214	1,380	457	901

RAD.	FALSE NEGS.	SENS. %	PPV %	CANCERS PER 1000
#1	18	84	38	7.8
#2	7	95	35	12.3
#3	8	81	27	6.2
#4	2	95	32	8.3
#5	7	79	26	7.1
#6	4	75	38	⇒ 3.1
#7	8	76	35	7.6
#8	7	77	28	8.6
#9	1	94	39	7.7
#10	3	86	55	9.1
#11	2	90	35	9.3
#12	5	67	29	6.1
TOTALS	78	86	34	7.9

(Left) Chart of the CDR and positive biopsy rate (PPV3) by age from an audit of 110,000 patients. Note CDR of 4 and PPV3 of 25% are for 40-49 year age group ⇒, and each should be three times higher for ages 80 and over ⇒. Practice audit numbers, therefore, are dramatically affected by the age of the population being served. *(Right)* False negative mammogram (⇒ showing tumor) tracked through an audit. Reviewing FNs allows remedial training to be undertaken.

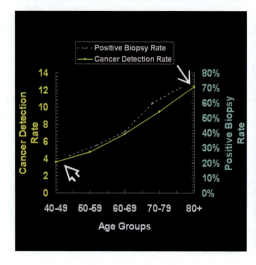

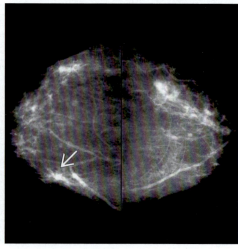

IMAGE GALLERY

5 YEAR INDIVIDUAL AUDIT: VARIABILITY WITH SMALL NUMBERS

YEAR	TOTAL CASES	TP	PPV3	SENSI-TIVITY	CDR
1998	1817	13	35%	81%	9.3
1999	998	4	13%	57%	4.0
2000	1852	16	28%	94%	8.6
2001	2412	11	22%	79%	4.6
2002	3012	33	52%	92%	11.0
5 YR TOTAL	**10,091**	**77**	**32%**	**86%**	**7.6**

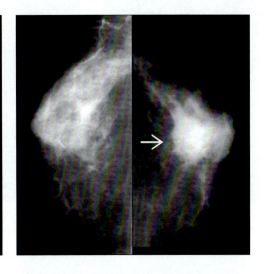

(Left) Audit of an individual's performance, 1998-2002. Note relatively small numbers for each year, and the dramatic swings in the audit results. This demonstrates the huge statistical variation one can expect in an individual audit when the numbers are small, even when overall performance is good. *(Right)* False negative mammogram (➡ shows tumor) tracked through an audit.

SCREENING & DIAGNOSTIC AUDIT DATA WITHIN ONE PRACTICE: COMPARISON (REF. 6)

	SCREENING DATA	DIAGNOSTIC DATA
Abnormal findings (Screen. BIRADS 0)	5.2%	14.4%
Biopsy performed	1.4%	11.9%
PPV3	36%	46%
CDR	5	55
Invasive tumor size	1.3 cm	2.6 cm
LN positivity	6%	33%

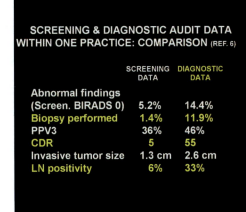
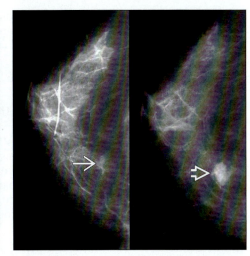

(Left) Chart of an audit summary within a radiology practice able to separate screening from diagnostic mammography cases (ref. 6). Note huge differences in many categories, especially CDR. Mixing of such data would severely corrupt audit results of both groups. *(Right)* Mammography shows a FN ➡, with the cancer diagnosed one year later ➡. Audits allow remedial training to be undertaken for individuals performing below expected standards.

2005-2006 BCSC SCREENING vs. DIAGNOSTIC BENCHMARKS

	2006 SCREENING DATA (Ref. 1)	2005 DIAGNOSTIC DATA (PALP. LUMP) (Ref. 3)
PPV2	25%	48%
Tumors, 0 or 1	76%	40%
Min. Ca's	52%	16%
LN positivity	19%	33%
CDR	4.4	47
Recall rate	9.7%	10%
Sensitivity	80%	84%
Inv. Ca size	1.3 cm	2.1 cm

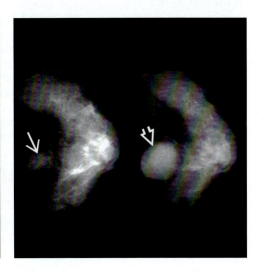

(Left) Chart of mean performance benchmarks for screening and diagnostic mammography, based on review of over 1 million mammogram interpretations in the U.S. performed between 1996 & 2001. Note huge differences in most categories, especially CDR. *(Right)* Mammography shows a FN ➡, with the cancer diagnosed one year later ➡. Audit allowed remedial training to be undertaken.

HIGH RISK SCREENING & SURVEILLANCE

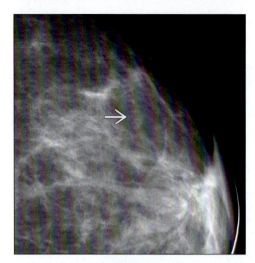

CC mammography close-up shows new cluster of punctate Ca++ ➡ in 36 y/o with prior lumpectomy & XRT for cancer 7 years earlier. Biopsy: DCIS. Mammography is the mainstay of surveillance.

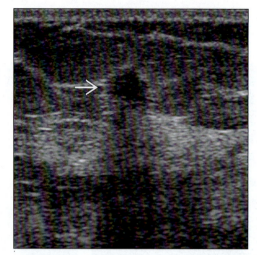

Ultrasound in this 51 y/o with dense breasts and negative mammogram shows irregular hypoechoic 5 mm mass ➡. Biopsy showed DCIS in a papilloma. Screening US in dense breasts remains controversial.

TERMINOLOGY

Definitions
- Relative risk (RR): Rate of developing breast cancer among women with risk factor compared to rate among women without risk factor
- Sojourn time: Time during which cancer could be detected on imaging, before clinically evident
- Interval cancer: Cancer clinically detected in interval between screenings
- Screening: Testing to detect cancer in women with no signs or symptoms of breast cancer
- Surveillance: Close observation of a person or group under suspicion
  - E.g., personal history of breast cancer, or other high risk; follow-up of probably benign findings
- Prevalence screen: First screen
- Incidence screen: Screens after the first, at the proscribed screening interval
- First-degree relative: e.g., Mother, father, sister, daughter
- Second-degree relative: e.g., Grandmother, aunt, niece
- Normal risk of breast cancer for women in USA: 1:8 if live to age 80
  - 1:200 by age 40; 1:50 by age 50
- High risk of breast cancer: Variably defined, usually at RR of at least 3x normal risk
  - Personal history of breast cancer: 8-10x risk
  - Prior atypical ductal hyperplasia (ADH): 4.5x risk
  - ADH and family history of breast cancer in first-degree relative: 7-13x risk
  - Prior lobular carcinoma in situ (LCIS): 8x risk in either breast
  - Prior atypical lobular hyperplasia (ALH): 3.1x risk, unilateral in 68%; contralateral in 24%
  - Strong family history
    - First degree relative diagnosed with breast cancer < age 50 (= surrogate measure of pre-menopausal)
  - > 20 or 25% lifetime risk of breast cancer
    - Gail, Claus models developed
    - Underestimate risk in African American women
  - > 1.7% 5-year risk of breast cancer by Gail model

- Prior radiation treatment (XRT) to chest or mediastinum < age 30
- BRCA-1 or BRCA-2 mutation carrier or suspected carrier
- ↑ Age, ≥ 60, defined as high risk in some trials

IMAGING ANATOMY

General Anatomic Considerations
- Dense breast tissue: Heterogeneously dense or extremely dense
  - > 50% parenchymal density
  - Increased breast density is risk factor: 1.8-5x risk
  - ↓ Mammographic sensitivity in dense breast tissue

PATHOLOGIC ISSUES

General Pathologic Considerations
- Proliferative breast disease
  - RR of breast cancer 1.5-2.0x, not high risk
  - Includes: Fibrocystic changes, excised radial scar, columnar cell changes without atypia, papilloma
- High-grade cancers: Short sojourn time (~ < 1 year)
- Low-grade cancers: Longer sojourn time (~ 2-5+ years)
- Higher rates of grade III histology in BRCA-mutation carriers: 46-62% of all cancers detected on MR

PATHOLOGY-BASED IMAGING ISSUES

Key Concepts or Questions
- No screening trials have proven mortality reduction specifically in high-risk women
- Mortality reduction closely parallels rate of reduction in node-positive cancers
  - Downstaging in tumor size
- Low-grade ductal carcinoma in situ (DCIS) ⇒ invasive cancer in 10-20 yrs in most cases
- High-grade DCIS ⇒ invasive cancer rapidly, ~ 1-4 yrs

Key Facts

Key Concepts in Screening
- Early detection of breast cancer will alter the natural history of the disease
  - Reduce mortality
  - More breast conservation, less harmful treatments
  - Benefits should be independent of method of detection
- To be effective, screening test must be widely available and cost-effective
- Healthy women will not be harmed
  - Induced biopsies, surgeries
- Mammography is only screening test proven to reduce breast cancer mortality

Goals of Screening
- Cancers detected are node negative

- Mean size of invasive cancers ≤ 1 cm

Issues Unique to High-Risk Women
- No screening trials to date have proven reduction in mortality specifically in high-risk women
- Higher prevalence of breast cancer: Higher yield of true positive examinations
- Many develop breast cancer at younger age, denser breast tissue

Rates of Breast Cancer Detection
- Mammography: 3-5 per 1000 women average risk
- US: 3-4 per 1000 in average risk women, dense breasts; 4.8-13 per 1000 women at increased risk
- MR: 10 per 1000 women with > 15% lifetime risk
  - 18-38 per 1000 women suspected BRCA mutation carriers

- Detection of DCIS may result in overtreatment
  - Estimate that 37% of DCIS detected on prevalence screen will not progress to invasive cancer
    - Possible overdiagnosis, harm from treatment
  - Estimate that < 4% of DCIS detected on incidence screens is nonprogressive
- Natural history of ALH and LCIS unclear: Possible precursors to invasive carcinoma

Imaging Approaches
- Mammography
  - 30-48% sensitivity in extremely dense breasts
  - Digital mammography: 15% ↑ cancer detection in dense breasts; not widely available
  - Stage and sensitivity worse in BRCA-mutation carriers and women < age 40 years
- Ultrasound after mammography
  - Women with fatty breasts excluded
  - 60-100% ↑ cancer detection in dense breasts
  - Labor intensive; physician performed in all but one study
  - Widely available technology; ~ 35% of centers offering
- MR after mammography
  - Requires injection of contrast; high cost
  - Less available; ~ 12% of centers offering

Imaging Protocols
- Annual mammography
  - Any other screening is supplemental to mammography
  - Begin 10 years before the age of diagnosis of first-degree relative
    - Begin by age 40 in all women
    - Not < age 25 years
  - Begin 8 years after XRT to chest or mediastinum if given < age 30 years
  - Begin at age 25 if known or suspected BRCA-mutation carrier
  - Usually a diagnostic examination in women with personal history of cancer
- Annual US: Data only on prevalence screens
  - Variable practice; ongoing studies

- ~ No detection benefit after MR screening
- Mean size of cancers detected 9-11 mm; 91% node negative when reported; < 2% DCIS
- Annual MR: Similar detection rates for prevalence and incidence screens
  - Becoming standard for known or suspected BRCA-mutation carriers
    - 5% of cancers detected in interval between screens: No data support more than annual frequency of MR screening
  - No data support MR screening of women of average risk with dense breasts
  - Sometimes staggered at 6 month intervals with mammography; ongoing studies
  - Across series: Mean size of cancers detected 1-2 cm; 82-91% node negative; 18-24% DCIS

Imaging Pitfalls
- Risk of false positives
  - Mammography: Data not specific to high risk; ~ 10% recall, 1-2% biopsy rate; 15-35% PPV of biopsy
  - US: Data not specific to high risk; 2.2-5.5% risk of biopsy (3.0% across series); 7-18% PPV of biopsy (11% across series)
  - MR: 9-17% suspicious or additional evaluation (14% across series); 8-50% PPV of biopsy (19% across series)

CLINICAL IMPLICATIONS

Clinical Importance
- BRCA-1 mutation carriers
  - Tumor suppressor gene on chromosome 17; autosomal dominant
  - Lifetime risk breast cancer: 50-85%
    - Often early age of onset
    - Second primary breast cancer 40-60%
  - Ovarian cancer risk 15-45%
  - Possible increased risk of other cancers (e.g. prostate)
- BRCA-2 mutation carriers
  - Tumor suppressor gene on chromosome 13; autosomal dominant

HIGH RISK SCREENING & SURVEILLANCE

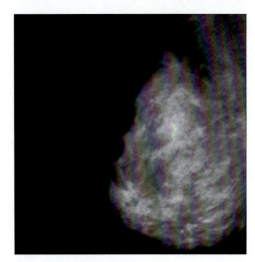

MLO mammography shows dense parenchyma in this 51 y/o woman.

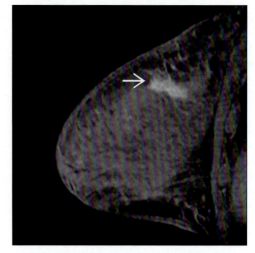

Sagittal T1 C+ subtraction MR (same patient as previous image) shows irregular regional enhancement in the upper left breast ➡. Targeted US-guided biopsy → intermediate grade DCIS.

- ○ Lifetime risk breast cancer: 50-85%
- ○ Male breast cancer 6%
- ○ Ovarian cancer: 10-20%
- ○ Increased risk of prostate cancer, melanoma, pancreatic cancer
- • Factors that increase likelihood of BRCA mutation
  - ○ Two or more cases of breast cancer on same side of family with onset < age 50 years
  - ○ Two or more cases of breast and ovarian cancer on same side of family, irrespective of age
  - ○ History of breast & ovarian cancer in same woman
  - ○ ≥ 3 cases of breast cancer on same side of family
  - ○ Family history of breast cancer diagnosed < age 35
  - ○ Bilateral breast cancer
  - ○ Male breast cancer
  - ○ Ashkenazi Jewish heritage

RELATED REFERENCES

1. Corsetti V et al: Role of ultrasonography in detecting mammographically occult breast carcinoma in women with dense breasts. Radiol Med (Torino). 111:440-8, 2006
2. Farria DM et al: Professional and economic factors affecting access to mammography: a crisis today, or tomorrow? Results from a national survey. Cancer. 104(3):491-8, 2005
3. Kuhl CK et al: Mammography, breast ultrasound, and magnetic resonance imaging for surveillance of women at high familial risk for breast cancer. J Clin Oncol. 23(33):8469-76, 2005
4. Leach MO et al: Screening with magnetic resonance imaging and mammography of a UK population at high familial risk of breast cancer: a prospective multicentre cohort study (MARIBS). Lancet. 365(9473):1769-78, 2005
5. Pisano ED et al: Diagnostic performance of digital versus film mammography for breast-cancer screening. N Engl J Med. 353(17):1773-83, 2005
6. Warner E et al: MRI surveillance for hereditary breast-cancer risk. Lancet. 365(9473):1747-9, 2005
7. Berg WA: Supplemental screening sonography in dense breasts. Radiol Clin North Am. 42(5):845-51, vi, 2004
8. Harvey JA et al: Quantitative assessment of mammographic breast density: relationship with breast cancer risk. Radiology. 230:29-41, 2004
9. Kriege M et al: Efficacy of MRI and mammography for breast-cancer screening in women with a familial or genetic predisposition. N Engl J Med. 351(5):427-37, 2004
10. Liberman L: Breast cancer screening with MRI--what are the data for patients at high risk? N Engl J Med. 351(5):497-500, 2004
11. Smith RA et al: The randomized trials of breast cancer screening: what have we learned? Radiol Clin North Am. 42(5):793-806, v, 2004
12. Duffy SW et al: The Swedish Two-County Trial of mammographic screening: cluster randomisation and end point evaluation. Ann Oncol. 14(8):1196-8, 2003
13. Morris EA et al: MRI of occult breast carcinoma in a high-risk population. AJR Am J Roentgenol. 181(3):619-26, 2003
14. Page DL et al: Atypical lobular hyperplasia as a unilateral predictor of breast cancer risk: a retrospective cohort study. Lancet. 361(9352):125-9, 2003
15. Tabar L et al: Mammography service screening and mortality in breast cancer patients: 20-year follow-up before and after introduction of screening. Lancet. 361(9367):1405-10, 2003
16. Yen MF et al: Quantifying the potential problem of overdiagnosis of ductal carcinoma in situ in breast cancer screening. Eur J Cancer. 39(12):1746-54, 2003
17. Michaelson JS et al: Predicting the survival of patients with breast carcinoma using tumor size. Cancer. 95(4):713-23, 2002
18. Podo F et al: The Italian multi-centre project on evaluation of MRI and other imaging modalities in early detection of breast cancer in subjects at high genetic risk. J Exp Clin Cancer Res. 21(3 Suppl):115-24, 2002
19. Brekelmans CT et al: Effectiveness of breast cancer surveillance in BRCA1/2 gene mutation carriers and women with high familial risk. J Clin Oncol. 19(4):924-30, 2001
20. Stoutjesdijk MJ et al: Prophylactic mastectomy in carriers of BRCA mutations. N Engl J Med. 345(20):1499; author reply 1499-500, 2001
21. Dershaw DD: Mammographic screening of the high-risk woman. Am J Surg. 180(4):288-9, 2000
22. Claus EB et al: The calculation of breast cancer risk for women with a first degree family history of ovarian cancer. Breast Cancer Res Treat. 28(2):115-20, 1993
23. Gail MH et al: Projecting individualized probabilities of developing breast cancer for white females who are being examined annually. J Natl Cancer Inst. 81:1879-86, 1989
24. Page DL et al: Atypical hyperplastic lesions of the female breast. A long-term follow-up study. Cancer. 55(11):2698-708, 1985

IMAGE GALLERY

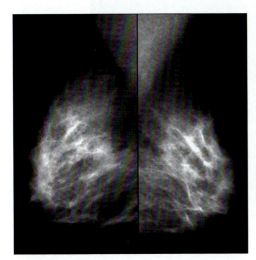
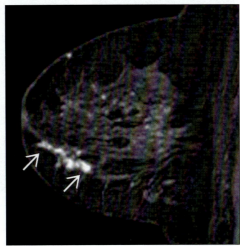

(Left) MLO mammography in this 47 y/o shows heterogeneously dense parenchyma. A recent left breast biopsy showed ADH in the upper outer quadrant and MR was requested for screening of the remainder of the breasts. (Right) Sagittal T1 C+ subtraction MR (same patient as previous image) shows clumped, linear enhancement in the 6:00 region left breast ➡, moderately suspicious for DCIS.

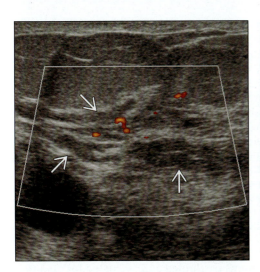
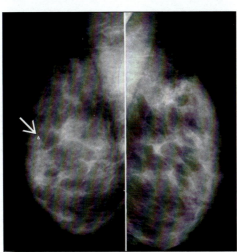

(Left) Power Doppler ultrasound near the left nipple (same patient as prior 2 images) shows multiple ducts distended with solid material ➡ and surrounding increased vascularity. US-guided biopsy showed intermediate-grade DCIS. (Right) MLO mammography in another 47 y/o with a strong family history of breast cancer shows dense parenchyma and is otherwise negative. Clip from MR-prompted biopsy (see next image) is noted ➡.

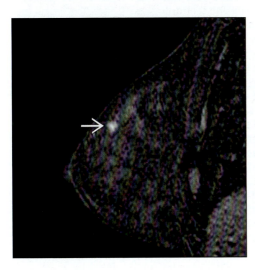
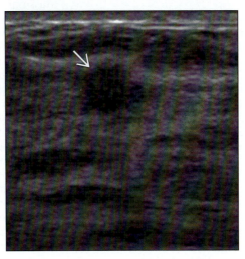

(Left) Sagittal T1 C+ subtraction MR (same patient as prior image) shows irregular 8 mm enhancing mass ➡. (Right) Ultrasound targeted to the MR abnormality (see previous image) shows an irregular 8 mm mass ➡, felt to correspond to the MR finding. US-guided biopsy (with clip placement) showed grade II invasive ductal carcinoma.

DOUBLE READING/CAD

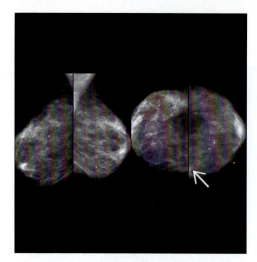

Bilateral screening mammogram in a 54 y/o initially interpreted by the breast imager as negative was marked by CAD ➡ alerting the imager to look again. The patient was recalled.

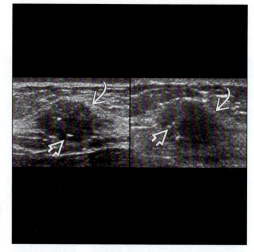

Ultrasound (same case as left) shows transverse (left) & sagittal (right) views of a hypoechoic irregular microlobulated mass ➡ with Ca++ ➡. Biopsy showed 1.5 cm infiltrating ductal carcinoma (IDC), grade II.

TERMINOLOGY

Abbreviations
- Computer-aided ("assisted") detection (CAD)
  - Distinguish from computer-aided diagnosis
- Breast Imaging Reporting and Data System (BI-RADS®)

Definitions
- **Double reading:** Two or more independent radiologists interpreting the same group of images
  - Discordant readings assigned assessment by consensus or arbitration
    - Consensus: Discussion among interpreting radiologists
    - Arbitration: Third radiologist makes independent decision
    - ↑ Perception (sensitivity) and ↑ specificity
  - May act on all cases indicated as abnormal from either reading
    - ↑ Perception (sensitivity) and ↓ specificity
- **Computer-aided detection**
  - Neural network-generated prompts (marks) highlight areas of concern, directing attention of interpreting radiologist
  - Analog films must be digitized; digitally acquired images directly interface with the CAD system
    - CAD marks are displayed on low-resolution images by pushing a button or on a paper printout
  - For digital mammography, CAD systems interface directly with the workstation on which mammograms are interpreted
    - CAD engaged by pushing a button on the workstation console; CAD marks displayed directly over the mammographic images
  - Recognized marks (e.g., circles or triangles) project over/near findings recognized by neural network
    - Densities with crossing lines that could be irregular or spiculated masses
    - Bright dots likely to be calcifications (Ca++)
  - Interpreting radiologist makes final determination as to assessment

- Negative or benign, return to screening interval (BI-RADS 1, 2)
- Abnormal, requires additional imaging evaluation (BI-RADS 0); recommend biopsy (BI-RADS 4, 5)
- Vast majority of CAD prompts are dismissed by interpreting radiologist
  - False positive prompts: CAD-generated prompts over areas where no visible suspicious lesion present
    - Variable rates of prompts per normal mammogram reported by different systems; lowest: Average of 0.5/image
- **Computer-aided diagnosis:** Computer-generated statistical assessment of imaging findings suggesting likelihood of malignancy based on comparison with large number of similar findings
- Recalled or "call-back" cases
  - Asymptomatic standard MLO and CC screening mammograms performed and evaluated for quality assurance by the technologists
  - Women arrive and leave the center without waiting for either verbal or written reports
  - Mammograms "batch-read" by a radiologist in a concentrated and focused setting
  - Mammograms are either deemed negative, benign (BI-RADS 1, 2) or abnormal (BI-RADS 0, 4, 5)
  - Women receive via mail or phone call either standard negative report or recommendation to return for additional imaging or biopsy
- **Recall rates:** Percentage of women with recommendation to return for further imaging following screening mammogram
  - Recall rate desired goal based on expert performance ("benchmarks") < 10%
    - Women with prior recent comparisons should have an overall recall rate 30% lower than those having an initial mammogram
  - Costs (financial and emotional) related to recall rates must be considered
  - Most recalled cases do not undergo biopsy: 10% recall, 1-2% biopsy rate; 15-35% PPV of biopsy

DOUBLE READING/CAD

Key Facts

Double "Reading" Screening Mammograms
- Human-human and human-computer algorithm (CAD) increase cancer detection rate
- Is not standard of care in the USA

Human-Human
- May increase perception or aid in interpretation
- Increase in expense; not and/currently billable
  - Additional radiologists
  - Person-power differs based on independent vs. consensus method

Human-CAD
- Aids in perception
- Prospective increase in cancer detection likely related to radiologist experience; little added yield for specialists

- Analog system ~ $55,000-200,000 based on mammography volume, display configuration
- Digital system ~ $55,000/digital acquisition system
- Marginal cost-effectiveness of adding CAD to a screening program
  - Medicare fee = $19 (2006)
    - Medicare reimbursement may be cut by 1/2 (information available summer 2006)
  - Mean cost per year of life saved: $19,508 based on a potential of 4% increase in early-stage cancers
- Time required
  - 25-76 seconds for screening mammogram interpretation
  - Adding CAD increases interpretation time 20-56%
  - 1 helpful (positive) CAD mark per 2,000-4,000 false positive marks
  - Too many false prompts reduces effectiveness

PATHOLOGIC ISSUES

General Pathologic Considerations
- With CAD, detection rate of invasive cancers ≤ 1 cm increased (one series)
  - Detection rate of in situ cancer declined 6.7%
  - Stage I invasive cancers strongly associated with detection by CAD
  - Mean age 5.3 years younger in women with CAD-detected cancer

PATHOLOGY-BASED IMAGING ISSUES

Key Concepts or Questions
- Factors affecting interpretive performance
  - Mammographic breast density, patient age, family history, personal history breast cancer influence likelihood of FP and FN results
  - Specialization in breast imaging improves performance
  - Volume: Minimum number required per year United Kingdom: 5,000; Netherlands: 3,000; British Columbia: 2,500; Australia: 2,000; USA: 480 (960 every 2 years)

Imaging Protocols
- Methods suggested to improve performance detecting breast cancer
  - Initial training and continuing medical education
  - Rigorous insistence on images of excellent quality
  - Comparison with prior mammograms
  - Standardized reporting; understanding and use of BI-RADS lexicon
  - Regular individual and group practice audits
  - Double reading: Human-human; human-CAD

Imaging Pitfalls
- Research needed to assess affect of new imaging technologies such as full-field digital on human performance of image interpretation

- Additional research may aid in clarifying root causes of errors
  - Fundamentally ambiguous image information (e.g., dense breast tissue) vs. problems related to perception, inattention, or decision making

CLINICAL IMPLICATIONS

Clinical Importance
- Double reading and CAD of particular applicability to screening mammography
  - Prevalence of cancer is low (0.3-0.7%)
  - Breast tissue architecture variable and complex
  - Findings are often subtle
  - Interpreting radiologists are vulnerable to fatigue and distraction

Expected Performance
- Retrospective evaluations of screen-detected cancers judged as missed on the prior mammogram
  - Non-blinded retrospective evaluation reports a range of missed cancers of 23-77%
  - Blinded retrospective studies report a range of 25-41%
- Effect of double reading on cancer detection
  - Increased breast cancer detection: Range 5-15%
  - Single series reports ↑ detection rate of 6.1% with an increase in recall rate of 1.5%
  - Additional 3% of cancers detected by a cursory "quick" batch-read by a second radiologist; recall rate ↑ 0.7%
  - Parenchymal distortion reported as most common mammographic finding of early cancers seen only on double reading
- Retrospective potential of cancer detection using CAD
  - 1,083 consecutive breast cancers detected on screening mammogram
    - CAD marked 98% of Ca++, 86% of masses
  - CAD showed potential to ↓ false negative rate (31% to 19%) following double reading by dedicated breast imagers

DOUBLE READING/CAD

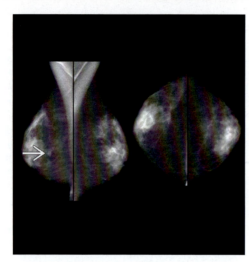

Bilateral screening mammogram in a 44 y/o shows a round mass ⇥ best seen on the MLO view. Interpreting breast imager detected the finding and patient was recalled. CAD did not mark the lesion.

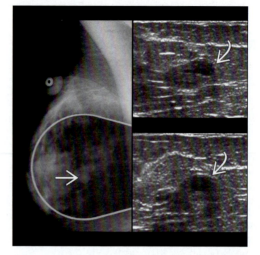

Spot compression (same as on left) shows mass ⇥, seen also in two views on US (right) ⇥. Biopsy showed intermediate-grade DCIS. Lesion likely not marked by CAD due to smooth margin, tissue density.

- Correctly marked 71% of findings considered in retrospect as ["actionable" (should have been either recalled or recommended for biopsy)] read as negative on previous screening mammograms
- Retrospective potential of cancer detection using CAD in cases deemed actionable or non-actionable by blinded panels of radiologists
  - 115 actionable cancers: CAD marked 86% of Ca++; 73% of masses
  - 172 non-actionable cancers: CAD marked 30%
- Prospective performance of CAD (4 studies with similar study designs)
  - Increase in detection rate of 7-20%
    - Percentage increase in recall rates (7.4-19.5%) either mirrored or < increase in cancer detection rates in most studies
- As of 2006, 3 CAD systems approved by Food and Drug Administration in USA
  - Varying sensitivity and specificity rates for marking cancers based on lesion type; variable reports of average marks per negative mammogram
    - Sensitivity for malignant Ca++ ~ 86-99%; only 57% malignant amorphous Ca++ detected (one series)
    - Sensitivity for masses ~ 43-85%
  - Algorithms most sensitive for spiculated masses
    - Vague or non-spiculated masses less commonly marked
    - Less than 1/2 of architectural distortion cases detected (one study)
  - No recognition of "developing" asymmetries per se
  - Reproducibility of CAD prompts for digitized analog films scanned and analyzed 3 times showed identical marking patterns in only 53%
  - Need to retain CAD-marked image information for medical legal purposes an unresolved question
  - 0.5-1 marks per image per negative mammogram
  - Assuming 5 cancers/1,000 screens, CAD adds ~ 20% ↑ detection benefit = 1/5 cancers = 1 cancer/1,000 screens

RELATED REFERENCES

1. Birdwell RL et al: Computer-aided detection with screening mammography in a university hospital setting. Radiology. 236:451-7, 2005
2. Burhenne LJW: Proficiency in mammography: interpretive skills, computer-aided detection, and double reading. Breast Imaging: RSNA Categorical Course in Diagnostic Radiology. 93-106, 2005
3. Cupples TE et al: Impact of CAD in a regional screening mammography program. AJR. 185:944-50, 2005
4. Soo MS et al: Computer-aided detection of amorphous calcifications. AJR. 184:887-92, 2005
5. Destounis SV et al: Can computer-aided detection with double reading of screening mammograms help decrease the false-negative rate? Initial experience. Radiology. 232:578-84, 2004
6. Feig SA et al: Changes in breast cancer detection and mammography recall rates after the introduction of a computer-aided detection system. (Comment). J Natl Cancer Inst. 96:1260-1, 2004
7. Lindfors KK et al: Computer aided detection of breast cancer: a study of cost-effectiveness (abstr). In: Radiological Society of North America Scientific Assembly and Annual Meeting Program. Oak Brook, Ill: Radiological Society of North America. 379, 2004
8. Baker JA et al: Computer-aided detection (CAD) in screening mammography: sensitivity of commercial CAD systems for detecting architectural distortion. AJR. 181:1083-8, 2003
9. Beam CA et al: Association of volume and volume-independent factors with accuracy in screening mammogram interpretation. J Natl Cancer Inst. 95:282-90, 2003
10. Beam CA. Interpretation error in mammography: taxonomy and measurement. Semin Breast Dis. 6:153-5, 2003
11. Harvey SC et al: Increase in cancer detection and recall rates with independent double interpretation of screening mammography. AJR. 180:1461-7, 2003
12. Sickles EA et al: Performance parameters for screening and diagnostic mammography: specialist and general radiologists. Radiology. 224:861-9, 2002
13. Freer TW et al: Screening mammography with computer-aided detection: prospective study of 12,860 patients in a community breast center. Radiology. 220:781-6, 2001

IMAGE GALLERY

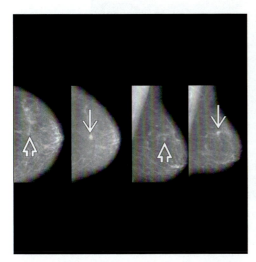 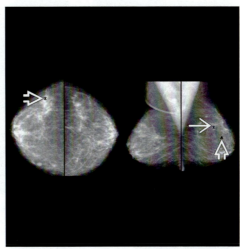

(Left) Two mammograms (CCs left, MLOs right) 13 mo apart in a 61 y/o show a grade I IDC ➡ detected on the more recent study. Unblinded expert review determined that the area ➡ did not warrant recall on the earlier study. (Right) CAD marks displayed on the mammogram prospectively interpreted as negative (same case as left) show a mark ➡ where the cancer later developed only on the MLO view. Two false positive marks ➡ are also present.

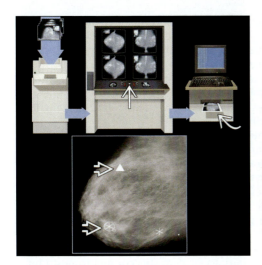 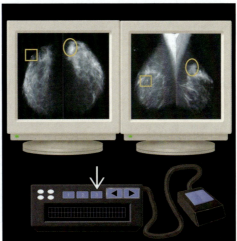

(Left) Upper images left to right show the process of digitizing analog films, hanging original films on an alternator and either engaging the CAD-marked images ➡ on a low-resolution monitor or printing the CAD-marked images on paper ➡. Lower image shows CAD marks ➡ projected over an MLO mammogram. (Right) Digitally acquired images may be assessed with CAD simply by depressing a pre-programed button ➡ on the key-pad.

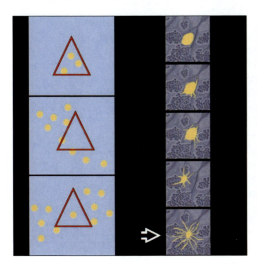 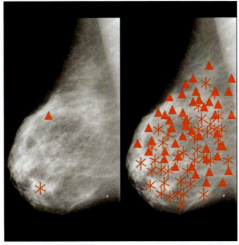

(Left) Left side images demonstrate a graphic of CAD marks projected over groups of Ca++. Right side, top to bottom, shows mass findings increasingly more likely to be marked by CAD. Density and crossing lines ➡ = most suspicious. (Right) Most CAD marks must be dismissed by the interpreter. Too many marks (exaggerated here for effect) limit interpretation of both marked and unmarked areas (Courtesy RAC).

ULTRASOUND

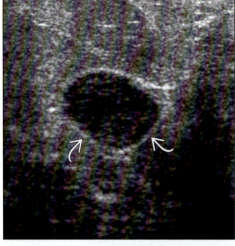

Radial ultrasound in a 24 y/o with a palpable mass shows a well circumscribed mass with a sharp echogenic border ➡. These are benign features. Excision at her request revealed fibroadenoma.

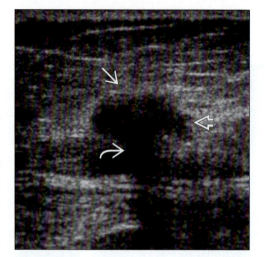

Radial ultrasound in a 60 y/o w/abnormal mammogram shows hypoechoic, indistinctly marginated mass ➡ with angular margins ➡ and distal acoustic shadowing ➡. Biopsy = invasive ductal cancer.

TERMINOLOGY

Abbreviations
- Core needle biopsy (CNB)
- Fine needle aspiration biopsy (FNAB)
- Time-gain-compensation curve (TGC)
- Positive predictive value (PPV): E.g., risk of cancer after positive test such as recommendation for biopsy
- Negative predictive value (NPV): E.g., number of women without cancer after a negative test result

Definitions
- Targeted US: Ultrasound directed to area of clinical, mammographic, or MRI abnormality
- Second-look US: US directed to abnormality, usually on MRI, where US had been performed earlier (e.g., before the MRI)
- Spatial compounding: Averaging of signal from multiple (usually off-angle) beams to reduce noise
  - Loss of posterior features
- Tissue harmonic imaging (THI): Insonate tissue at one frequency, receive at multiples of that frequency (usually 2X, e.g., 6 → 12MHz)
  - Preserves posterior features, reduces noise

General Performance Statistics US
- Not limited by breast density
- Phantom studies suggest reduced performance in very large breasts (> 5 cm thick while scanning) and deep lesions
- **Infiltrating ductal carcinoma (IDC)**
  - 96% sensitivity across three series (range 95-97%) vs. 84% for mammography (range 81-89%)
- **Infiltrating lobular carcinoma (ILC)**
  - 88% sensitivity across five series (range 82-94%) vs. 52% for mammography (range 34-72%)
- **Ductal carcinoma in situ (DCIS)**
  - Wide range of sensitivities, depending on gold standard: Up to 74%; < 50% sensitivity if MRI used to identify false negatives

Indications
- Palpable abnormality

- In combination with mammography, 97% sensitivity, 98.6% NPV across five series
- Opportunity for direct correlation of imaging and clinical findings
- Normal variant fatty lobulation, a common source of palpable concern
- Use US as initial test for women < 30 yrs or pregnant or lactating
  - Mammogram done first for women ≥ 30 yrs if not pregnant or lactating
- **Mammographic abnormality**
  - Mass, asymmetry, architectural distortion
  - Further evaluation, guide biopsy if needed
- **Pathologic nipple discharge**
  - 93% sensitivity vs. 68% for galactography (two series)
  - Central papilloma most common cause
  - 90% sensitivity to DCIS in this context (one study)
- **Guide biopsy**
  - ↑ Accuracy in sampling palpable masses
    - < 2% miss for US-CNB vs. 13% without US guidance
  - Nonpalpable masses, US-guided 14-g CNB sufficient in vast majority
    - Definitive result in 93% across multiple series
    - Poor performance for FNAB: 77% overall accuracy, 10% insufficient sample rate
  - Suspicious calcifications (Ca++) visible on US
    - US-visible Ca++ more likely malignant, more likely invasive carcinoma
    - Benefit to obtaining more material: Possible indication for vacuum-assisted US biopsy
  - Targeted US after MRI, highly variable performance
    - 23-89% success, average 55%
    - 6-14% rate malignancy among lesions not seen at targeted US: Need for MRI-guided biopsy
- **Guide aspiration**
  - Vast majority of cysts do not require intervention
  - Aspirate cysts if painful to patient if requested
    - Round, tense cysts most likely to be symptomatic
  - Aspirate/drain breast abscess: Catheter can be placed
- **US-guided localization for surgery**

ULTRASOUND

Breast Ultrasound

Key Questions
- Does a solid mass have malignant features?
  - Follow-up may be reasonable if benign-appearing: Further validation required
- Is there a correlate to a palpable mass?
- Is there a correlate to a mammographically occult abnormality detected on a breast MRI?
- Is there an occult cancer in a high-risk patient with dense breast tissue?
  - High-risk women 2-3x more likely to have cancer seen only on US
  - Sensitivity to breast cancer < 50 y/o with dense tissue < 50% for mammography, ~ 79% for US

Optimize Technique
- High frequency transducer, center frequency 10 MHz

- Gentle scan pressure, maximize detail in breast
- Poor technique may result in missed/delayed cancer diagnosis, unnecessary biopsies
- High reliability in lesion detection and characterization across experienced observers
- Real-time validation of findings by radiologist

Document Images Even if Study is Negative
- Palpable/mammographic finding: Annotated orthogonal views at finding site
- Screening: Representative 4-quadrant images + subareolar view

Interpretation
- Use of BI-RADS: US encouraged
- Integrate with mammographic and clinical findings: One combined assessment and recommendation

---

- Mark overlying skin, provide depth ± needle localization as well

US Can Be Helpful, Further Studies Ongoing
- **Supplemental screening for dense breasts**
  - 60-100% ↑ in cancer detection rates in dense breasts
  - Across 7 series, 3-4 cancers per 1000 average-risk women screened
  - 4.8-13 cancers per 1000 high-risk women screened
  - Average 3% risk of US-induced biopsy (range 2.2-5.5%)
  - 11% PPV of biopsy recommendation (range 7-18%)
- **Extent of disease in the breast**
  - Of those suspected to have unifocal cancer on mammography and clinically, ~ 48% of breasts have additional tumor foci at histopathology
  - Combined mammography + US depicts ~ 90% of all tumor foci
  - May underestimate tumor size, especially > 2 cm
- **Axillary nodal staging**
  - If node known to have metastasis pre-operatively, axillary node dissection performed directly without need for sentinel node biopsy
  - If node can be identified and sampled using FNAB or CNB to detect metastasis, sensitivity 90% (range 84-94%); specificity 99% (range 96-100%)
- **Intra-operative US**: May help achieve clear margins
- **Distinguishing recurrence from scar**
  - Lumpectomy scar should decrease over time, extend to skin incision
  - Recurrence tends to be convex, focal mass near scar

US Not Appropriate
- Not a substitute for mammographic screening
- Measuring response to treatment
  - Inaccurate for sizing large tumors
- Assessing chest wall invasion
  - Posterior shadowing obscures evaluation
- Saline breast implant integrity: Clinical diagnosis
- Silicone breast implant integrity better assessed by MRI
  - Sensitivity low for uncollapsed rupture
    - Folds can mimic rupture
  - Particularly poor for double lumen implants

- Note: Pathognomonic appearance of siliconoma ('snowstorm') can be helpful in documenting extracapsular silicone

ANATOMY-BASED IMAGING ISSUES

Anatomic Relationships
- Skin: ≤ 2 mm thick, hypoechoic
- Layer of subcutaneous fat/fat lobules
  - Serves as reference for echogenicity of other structures (hypo-, iso-, or hyperechoic to fat)
- Cooper ligaments: Hyperechoic, surround fat lobules, support parenchyma
  - Normally curvilinear: Straightening ± thickening imply architectural distortion
- Fibrotic (dense) parenchyma is typically hyperechoic
- Layer of prepectoral fat, musculature, ribs, chest wall

Imaging Protocols
- High frequency linear array transducer with center of frequency 10 MHz preferred
  - Color, power Doppler helpful
  - Spatial compounding, THI desirable
- Scan planes
  - Breast ducts are arranged radially from nipple
    - Lesions tend to grow along duct system
  - Scan in radial and antiradial (orthogonal to radial) planes for lesions
    - Maximal diameters in perpendicular planes
  - Survey scanning: Transverse and sagittal more efficient at covering entire breast
  - Images labeled with scan plane, clock face, distance from nipple in cm
    - Use transducer width (e.g. 38 or 50 mm) as measuring guide
- Positioning: Area of interest is as thin as possible
  - Supine for medial breast
  - Oblique with arm above head for lateral breast
  - Patient can elevate breast for inferior lesions
- Field of view to reach chest wall but not beyond
- Overall gain set so that fat is gray

ULTRASOUND

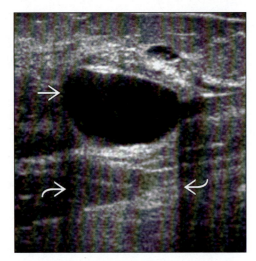

Anti-radial ultrasound in a 42 y/o with a palpable mass shows a circumscribed, anechoic mass ➡ with posterior enhancement ⬈, and imperceptible wall = simple cyst.

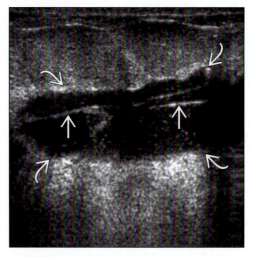

Radial ultrasound in a 63 y/o post lumpectomy with a fluctuant mass shows complex fluid ➡ with fibrin strands ➡ consistent with a seroma. The patient was reassured. Aspirate if there is concern for infection.

- ○ Too much gain creates artifactual echoes → cysts look complicated, complex, or solid
- ○ Too little gain→ masses look cystic, hypoechoic masses may "disappear"
- • Gradually increase TGC with increasing depth
  - ○ Compensates for absorption of sound by tissues
- • Set focal zone at lesion
  - ○ Most current transducers allow realtime scanning with multiple focal zones
  - ○ Once lesion identified, set single focal zone at that depth for maximum resolution
- • Gentle transducer pressure while scanning
  - ○ ↓ Tissue thickness → ↑ increased resolution
  - ○ Some shadowing is artifactual: Will ↓ or resolve with ↑ transducer pressure
  - ○ Light pressure better when evaluating flow
- • Change angle of scanning/insonation
  - ○ Important to see borders of masses, evaluate subareolar area
- • Correlate directly with clinical findings
  - ○ Annotate: 'Palpable', 'area indicated by patient', etc.
- • **Special techniques**
  - ○ Evaluation of lesion seen on one view
    - ▪ Look for sonographic correlate, if seen, place BB on skin
    - ▪ Repeat mammogram→confirm sonographic finding is mammographic finding
  - ○ Mark palpable lesions: "**Paper clip trick**"
    - ▪ Trap palpable mass between limbs of an unfolded paper clip
    - ▪ Shadowing from limbs of clip marks mass margins on images
    - ▪ Confirms that US finding = the palpable finding
    - ▪ Documents absence of US mass if scan negative
  - ○ "**Rolled nipple**" technique: Nipple discharge
    - ▪ Roll nipple over examiner's finger
    - ▪ Scan long axis of superficial aspect of nipple-areolar complex to look for distal intraductal mass
  - ○ Use standoff pad or glob of gel for superficial lesions
    - ▪ Transducers not optimally focused < 7 mm depth
- • **Color Doppler**

- ○ **Vocal fremitus**: Tissues vibrate when patient hums; movement → "color"
  - ▪ Mass vibrates < normal tissue → defect in color-filled background
- ○ Internal vascularity in solid masses
  - ▪ May help with identification of papilloma in distended duct
- • Must be familiar with US artifacts to avoid interpretation pitfalls

RELATED REFERENCES

1. Alvarez S et al: Role of sonography in the diagnosis of axillary lymph node metastases in breast cancer: a systematic review. AJR. 186:1342-8, 2006
2. Berg WA et al: Operator dependence of physician-performed whole breast sonography: Lesion detection and characterization. Radiology. in press, 2006
3. Dillon MF et al: The accuracy of ultrasound, stereotactic, and clinical core biopsies in the diagnosis of breast cancer, with an analysis of false-negative cases. Ann Surg. 242:701-7, 2005
4. Berg WA et al: Diagnostic accuracy of mammography, clinical examination, US, and MR Imaging in preoperative assessment of breast cancer. Radiology. 233:830-49, 2004
5. Berg WA: Supplemental screening sonography in dense breasts. Radiol Clin North Am. 42(5):845-51, vi, 2004
6. Berg WA: Rationale for a trial of screening breast ultrasound: American College of Radiology Imaging Network (ACRIN) 6666. AJR Am J Roentgenol. 180(5):1225-8, 2003
7. Mendelson EB et al: Breast Imaging Reporting and Data System, BI-RADS: Ultrasound, 1st ed. Reston: American College of Radiology. 2003
8. Soo MS et al: Sonographic detection and sonographically guided biopsy of breast microcalcifications. AJR. 180:941-8, 2003
9. Dennis MA et al: Breast biopsy avoidance: the value of normal mammograms and normal sonograms in the setting of a palpable lump. Radiology. 219(1):186-91, 2001
10. Stavros AT et al: Solid breast nodules: use of sonography to distinguish between benign and malignant lesions. Radiology. 196(1):123-34, 1995

IMAGE GALLERY

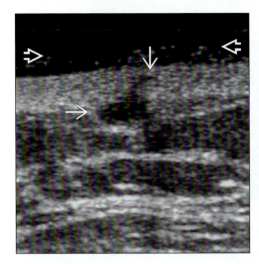

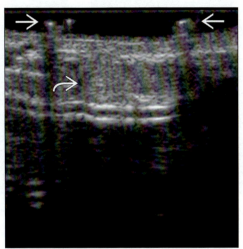

(Left) Radial ultrasound with gel "standoff" ➡ in a 57 y/o with a palpable skin lesion shows a sebaceous cyst ➡. Despite benign features on mammography and US, the patient insisted on excision which confirmed the diagnosis. (Right) Ultrasound in a 48 y/o post mastectomy and implant reconstruction for diffuse DCIS shows a paperclip ➡ on the skin anchoring a subtle palpable mass ➡. US-guided core biopsy = invasive cancer.

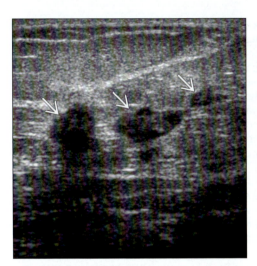

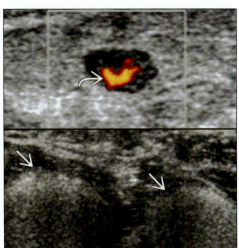

(Left) Radial ultrasound shows multiple masses ➡ extending along a ductal system in a 63 y/o with a palpable subareolar mass illustrating the importance of looking for multifocal tumor. Biopsy confirmed invasive cancer. (Right) Power Doppler ultrasound (upper image) shows a normal lymph node with hilar vessels ➡. Contrast this appearance with silicone-containing nodes ➡ in the axilla of a patient with ruptured implants (lower image).

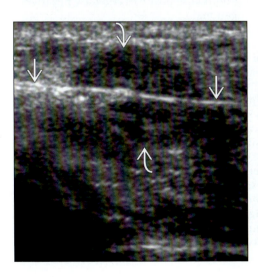

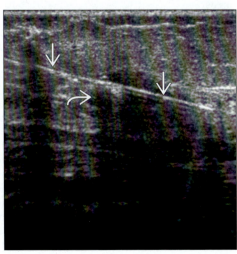

(Left) Transverse ultrasound shows a biopsy needle ➡ traversing a solid mass ➡ in the left breast during core biopsy. Needle position can be confirmed by an orthogonal view. (Right) Ultrasound shows a localization wire ➡ through a non-palpable cancer ➡. US guided localization allows more flexible lesion access than standard mammographic approaches and is faster and better tolerated by the patient.

MAGNETIC RESONANCE IMAGING

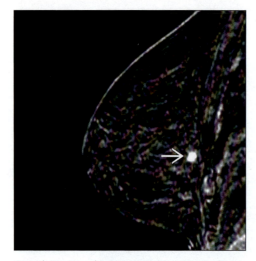

Sagittal T1 C+ subtraction MR in a 55 y/o known BRCA-1 carrier shows irregular 5 mm enhancing mass ➡ *at chest wall right breast. Mammogram was negative with heterogeneously dense tissue.*

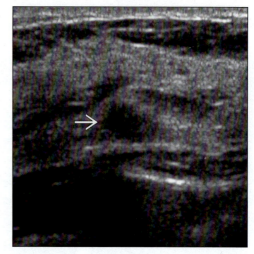

US targeted to MR finding (prior image) shows indistinctly-marginated, hypoechoic mass ➡ *at posterior depth, felt to correlate. US-guided biopsy showed grade II IDC. Bilateral mastectomy performed.*

TERMINOLOGY

Abbreviations
- Clinical breast examination (CBE)
- Field of view (FOV)
- Magnetic resonance (MR) imaging
- Magnetic resonance spectroscopy (MRS)
- Signal to noise ratio (SNR)

Definitions
- In-plane resolution: FOV divided by matrix
  - 32-36 cm FOV, 256 x 256 matrix → 1.25-1.4 mm resolution
  - Improved detail with 400 x 512 matrix
    - ↑ Imaging time to improve SNR (or go to higher field strength magnet)
- Maximum intensity pixel projection (MIP)
  - Performed on 3D-subtraction dataset post-contrast to see only the enhancing areas
- Region of interest (ROI), not < 3 pixels, of most suspicious areas of enhancing lesion(s)
- Neoadjuvant chemotherapy (NAT): Primary chemotherapy prior to surgical treatment

Indications
- **Evaluate local extent of disease** in patient with newly diagnosed cancer
  - Ipsilateral breast: 27-43% of breasts anticipating breast conservation surgery based on mammography & CBE have additional tumor foci on MR
    - Risk of false positives: Biopsy needed to confirm prior to altering surgical management
    - More accurate method for sizing breast malignancies than mammography: US, CBE
    - Most accurate imaging method to assess chest wall involvement: Enhancement of musculature
  - Contralateral breast: 3-6% rate of cancers occult on mammography & CBE
    - Similar additional yield with US
  - Particularly helpful in young women ≤ age 45, dense breasts, invasive lobular histology, > 2.5 cm known malignancy

- Particularly helpful with extensive intraductal component (EIC): 95% accuracy vs. 36% for mammography and US (one series)
- **Metastatic adenopathy, unknown primary**
  - 75-86% success in identifying primary after negative mammogram, US, and CBE
- **Positive margins at initial excision**
  - Absence of enhancement should not preclude reexcision
  - Irregular enhancing mass abutting seroma or elsewhere suspicious
  - ≤ 4 mm smooth enhancing rim around seroma expected acutely
    - Decreases over time
- **Suspected recurrence vs. scar**
- **Monitor response to NAT**
  - Correlates closely with pathologic extent of tumor
  - Potential for both false positives and false negatives
  - MRS investigational
    - Choline peak seen in malignancies, not benign lesions
    - Loss of choline peak may predict response within days of treatment, before change in size of tumor
    - Evaluation usually limited to one voxel, ≥ 1 cm³, 10-15 minute scan to acquire data, on-line selection of voxel
    - 3-4T scanners may facilitate
- **Evaluate silicone breast implant integrity**
  - Clinical significance of implant rupture controversial
- **High-risk screening**
  - Known or suspected BRCA-1 or BRCA-2 carrier
  - Other high-risk patients
  - In combination with mammography, 92% sensitivity overall
    - 9% of cancers seen only on mammography; 73% are DCIS
    - 49% of cancers seen only on MR; 24% DCIS
- Evaluation of **inconclusive mammogram ± US**
  - Possible suspicious finding, inadequately seen to target for biopsy
- **Pathologic nipple discharge**

MAGNETIC RESONANCE IMAGING

MR Image Interpretation

Parenchymal Evaluation for Cancer

- Sensitivity ~ 88%; half of false negatives = DCIS
- Appropriate scheduling: Days 7-14 of menstrual cycle
- Clear statement of indication
- Attention to technique: 1.5T or higher field strength
- Full standard breast imaging workup, including current mammography ± US
  ○ Review together with MR
- Use BI-RADS®: MR to describe findings
  ○ Track outcomes, especially BI-RADS 0, 4, 5
- Integrate all breast imaging findings
- Need MR-guided biopsy capability
  ○ Targeted US efficacious in many cases
  ○ Decide management within MR report if US recommended and lesion not seen
  ○ Suspicious enhancing lesions → MR-guided biopsy

Implants

- Location (subglandular, subpectoral)
- Type of implant
  ○ Silicone, double lumen, expander
  ○ Saline (MR done for other reasons)
- Integrity
  ○ Silicone external to implant shell = rupture
    ▪ Distinguish intracapsular (contained by hypointense scar capsule) or extracapsular rupture (STIR WS sequences help)
  ○ Varying degrees of shell collapse: Uncollapsed, partial, complete
  ○ Consultation with plastic surgeon
    ▪ Elective removal if ruptured
- Exam may also include contrast-enhanced parenchymal evaluation

---

○ Can be helpful if mammography, US ± galactography are all unrevealing

Contraindications

- Not a substitute for mammography ± US
  ○ Patient unwilling to have mammogram due to discomfort, fear of radiation, other
  ○ Gynecomastia: Mammography mainstay
  ○ Breast pain: Clinical evaluation, US if needed
- Probably benign findings on mammography ± US
  ○ Multiple bilateral circumscribed masses
- Suspicious findings on mammography ± US
  ○ MR should not be used to preclude biopsy, particularly for calcifications (Ca++)
  ○ Proceed directly to biopsy without MR
- Screening women at average risk of breast cancer
  ○ No data supports MR for this use; not cost-effective
- Saline implant integrity: Clinical diagnosis
- Facility lacks MR-guided biopsy capability (relative)
  ○ Arrangements in place for referral if needed
- Patient unable to have MR
  ○ Weight > 300 lbs; stout body habitus ≤ 300 lbs
  ○ Claustrophobia not able to be controlled by premedication (typically benzodiazepines)
  ○ Pacemaker, aneurysm clip, insulin pump, other metallic implant
    ▪ Isolated surgical clips cause artifact but patient can be scanned unless clips near vital structures (e.g., intracranial aneurysm)
    ▪ Metal worker with shard(s) possibly in orbit: X-ray to exclude metal fragments
    ▪ Metal will absorb energy, heat up, may move
  ○ Lack of IV access (parenchymal evaluation)
  ○ Patient uncooperative, unable to lie prone, unable to consent for contrast
  ○ Pregnancy (relative): Safety of Gd-contrast agents not widely established

---

ANATOMY-BASED IMAGING ISSUES

Key Concepts or Questions

- Patient questionnaire

○ No contraindications to MR
○ Consent for contrast injection (parenchyma)
○ Date of last menstrual period (parenchyma)
○ Symptoms, indication for examination
- Most recent prior breast imaging: Review together with MR
  ○ **Patient for parenchymal evaluation should have current mammogram first**
  ○ Initial US targeted to any mammographic ± clinical abnormality(ies) before MR
- Surgical history
- Pathology reports from recent biopsy(ies)

Imaging Approaches

- High spatial resolution to resolve mass margins: ≤ 1 mm in plane, ≤ 3 mm acquired slice thickness
- High temporal resolution (< 2.5 min to scan both breasts) to appreciate peak enhancement
  ○ Peak is typically ~ 90 seconds post-injection
- Need to see bright areas of Gd-enhancement; fatty breast tissue also bright on T1WI
  ○ Fat suppression
    ▪ Parenchyma may still be hyperintense
  ○ Subtract pre-contrast from post-contrast images
    ▪ Requires coregistration: No motion
- Schedule MR 7-14 days after onset of last menstrual period: ↓ Background parenchymal enhancement

Imaging Protocols

- Breast parenchymal evaluation
  ○ Dedicated phased array breast coil, ≥ 1.5T
  ○ Simultaneous bilateral acquisition, prone position
  ○ Axial or sagittal plane
  ○ T1WI without fat suppression
    ▪ Fat (e.g., fat necrosis, hila of lymph nodes) hyperintense
    ▪ Acute blood hyperintense
  ○ T2WI with fat suppression or STIR
    ▪ Fluid (e.g., cysts, seromas) hyperintense
    ▪ Myxoid fibroadenomas, mucinous carcinomas can appear hyperintense
  ○ 3D spoiled gradient echo volume acquisition (T1WI) with fat suppression

MAGNETIC RESONANCE IMAGING

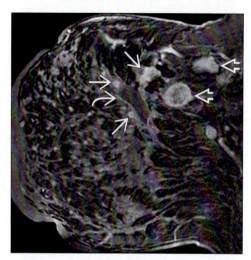

Sagittal T1 C+ FS MR after resection of a 2.8 cm IDC & 5% DCIS with margins positive for IDC shows seroma upper outer left breast ➡ and multiple irregular masses abutting seroma ➡. Metastatic nodes are noted ⇒.

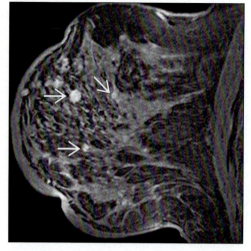

Sagittal T1 C+ FS MR of inner left breast (same as on left) shows additional irregular masses ➡. US-guided core biopsy confirmed multicentric IDC. MR can aid decision to proceed to re-excision or mastectomy.

- Resolution 1 mm x 1 mm x not more than 3 mm slice thickness
  - Pre-contrast: Establish appropriate field of view
  - If reposition patient, repeat pre-contrast imaging
  - Inject 0.1 mmol/kg Gd-contrast IV, ideally with power injector
  - Image both breasts within 2 minutes of injection
  - Image both breasts ≥ 5 minutes post-injection
  ○ Post-processing of 3D dataset
    - Subtract pre-contrast from post-contrast images at each time point
    - 3D MIP images from subtraction dataset
    - Optional: Computer-assisted parametric mapping (CAD) of kinetics
    - CAD includes thresholding: ≥ 50-60% enhancement in first 2 minutes
    - CAD color coding of 3-4 pixel areas of persistent, plateau, and washout kinetics
- Silicone implant evaluation: Noncontrast exam
  ○ Axial and sagittal FSE T2WI
    - 3-4 mm slice thickness
  ○ If extracapsular silicone suspected, silicone-only sequences
    - Water-suppressed STIR (STIR WS): Only silicone is bright

Imaging Pitfalls

- Avoid setting phase anteroposterior (AP) due to ↑ motion artifacts
- Remove any external metallic objects
  ○ Can "fly" into magnet: Risk to patient, staff, magnet
  ○ Cause magnetic field inhomogeneity, loss of signal
- Careful attention to positioning breast
  ○ Breast should be gently pulled into coil, spread out, nipple pointing forward
    - Facilitates correlation with other breast imaging
    - Inadequate to have patient position herself: Female technologist if possible
  ○ Gentle compression helpful to reduce motion
    - Avoid excess compression: Lack of contrast enhancement; lesion may not be seen at time of scheduled biopsy (recommend follow-up)
  ○ Breast should not contact edge(s) of coil

- Problematic with very large breasts
- Adequate fat suppression
  ○ Software automatically identifies the (usually) dominant water peak, saturates 220 Hz downfield (at 1.5T) where fat peak should be
  ○ In fatty breasts, trouble identifying water peak → saturates inappropriate frequency
  ○ Manual fine-tuning of fat suppression helpful
- Validate successful contrast injection: Heart, great vessels, liver enhance

RELATED REFERENCES

1. Schnall MD et al: Diagnostic architectural and dynamic features at breast MR imaging: multicenter study. Radiology. 238:42-53, 2006
2. Kuhl CK et al: Dynamic bilateral contrast-enhanced MR imaging of the breast: trade-off between spatial and temporal resolution. Radiology. 236:789-800, 2005
3. Kuhl CK et al: Mammography, breast ultrasound, and magnetic resonance imaging for surveillance of women at high familial risk for breast cancer. J Clin Oncol. 23:8469-76, 2005
4. Berg WA et al: Diagnostic accuracy of mammography, clinical examination, US, and MR imaging in preoperative assessment of breast cancer. Radiology. 233:830-49, 2004
5. Fischer U et al: The influence of preoperative MRI of the breasts on recurrence rate in patients with breast cancer. Eur Radiol. 14:1725-31, 2004
6. Lee JM et al: MRI before reexcision surgery in patients with breast cancer. AJR. 182:473-80, 2004
7. Ikeda DM et al: Breast Imaging Reporting and Data System, BI-RADS: Magnetic Resonance Imaging, 1st ed. Reston, American College of Radiology. 2003
8. Nunes LW et al: Update of breast MR imaging architectural interpretation model. Radiology. 219:484-94, 2001
9. Lee CH et al: Clinical usefulness of MR imaging of the breast in the evaluation of the problematic mammogram. AJR. 173:1323-9, 1999
10. Kuhl CK et al: Healthy premenopausal breast parenchyma in dynamic contrast-enhanced MR imaging of the breast: normal contrast medium enhancement and cyclical- phase dependency. Radiology. 203:137-44, 1997
11. Berg WA et al: Single- and double- lumen silicone breast implant integrity: prospective evaluation of MR and US criteria. Radiology. 197:45-52, 1995

PET IMAGING

Key Facts

Radiation Dose to Patient
- ~ 3-4 Rads for FDG PET
- Contraindicated in pregnancy
- Nursing mothers should pump breasts and discard milk for ~ 24 hours after FDG PET or PET CT

Primary Breast Cancer
- Results with whole body FDG PET poor
- Dedicated devices: Improved sensitivity with FDG PEM; studies ongoing
  - Potential roles being explored: Local extent of disease, response to treatment, early detection
- ↑ FDG uptake may predict worse prognosis

Axillary Lymph Node Status
- Whole body FDG PET unreliable
- Sentinel lymph node (SLN) biopsy standard

Metastases
- FDG PET more accurate than Tc-99m MDP bone scan for bone metastases
- Response on FDG PET CT predicts ↑ outcome

Biopsy
- Second look with US, MR used
- Radiotracer-guided biopsy methods being refined

Approved Indications for FDG PET (Medicare, 2002)
- Staging patients with distant metastasis(es)
- Restaging patients with locoregional recurrence or metastasis(es)
- Monitoring response to treatment: Locally advanced and metastatic breast cancer

---

- Patient should fast for ≥ 4 hours prior to study
  - False positives include fibroadenoma (FA), abscess, fat necrosis
  - False negatives: Small cancers (< 1 cm), low grade cancers, ILC
- FDG PEM
  - Same concerns as FDG PET for cardiac uptake and blood glucose level
  - False positives include FA, abscess, fat necrosis
  - False negatives: ILC, few low-grade cancers < 1 cm
  - Limited visualization of posterior breast
    - ~ 1 cm less tissue included than on mammography

IMAGING OF PRIMARY BREAST CANCER

Whole Body FDG PET
- Across 7 series, 214/289 (74%) of primary breast cancers depicted
- ↓ Sensitivity for cancers < 2 cm in size: 68% vs. 92% for 2-5 cm cancers (one series)
  - Only 3/12 (25%) of cancers < 1 cm depicted
  - ↓ Sensitivity to ILC: 35% vs. 76% for IDC (one series)
- SUV values for cancers typically 2-5 in cancers, vs. 1 for benign lesions
- Potential inadvertent detection of breast cancer on PET performed for other reasons
  - 6/533 (1%) of women had incidental suspicious breast lesions
    - 5/6: Invasive breast cancer
    - 1/6: Fibroadenoma

FDG PEM
- **Diagnostic performance with suspicious breast lesions**
  - One series: 77 women, 92 suspicious lesions, 48 cancers (median invasive size: 21 mm)
    - PEM depicted 43 (90%) cancers: 10/11 (91%) DCIS and 33/37 (89%) invasive cancers

- False negatives: 25 mm ILC, 3 mm grade II IDC plus DCIS, 6 mm IDC (tubular), 10 mm grade I IDC
  - ~ 40% ↑ background FDG uptake in dense breasts vs. fatty breasts
    - Not likely to obscure lesion detection, but further study warranted
    - Uptake does not appear to be hormonally sensitive, though further study is warranted

IMAGING OF LYMPH NODE METASTASES

Whole Body FDG PET for Axillary Nodal Metastases
- Multicenter study: Mean sensitivity 61% (range 54-67%), NPV 79%
- Average sensitivity ↓ when only one node involved: 46% vs. 64% when multiple nodes metastatic
- Reduced sensitivity to metastases from ILC: 25% vs. 64% for IDC
- Specificity 80%; PPV 62% for one suspicious axillary focus

STAGING FOR DISTANT METASTASES

Imaging Bone Metastases
- Bone scan with MDP: Lytic metastases may be missed
- Whole body FDG PET: Blastic bone metastases may be missed
  - Comparably high sensitivity: 95% FDG; 93% MDP
  - High specificity: 91% FDG vs. only 9% for MDP (one series)

FDG PET or PET CT
- Trend toward improved staging with PET CT
- Marginal improvement over restaging accuracy with PET alone

PET IMAGING

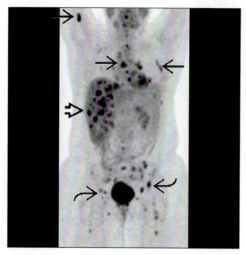

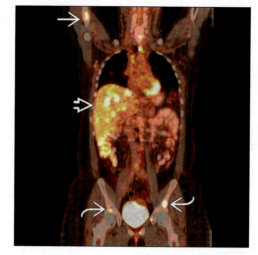

Coronal FDG PET shows diffuse metastases in liver ⬆, lymph nodes ➡ & bone ➡ in this 42 y/o treated for mixed IDC-ILC 8 years earlier, with known T11 metastasis. Rising CA27-29 levels prompting restaging.

Single coronal slice from fused PET CT (same as left) confirms liver ⬆, node ➡, & bilateral hip ➡ metastases.

- PET CT better initial staging accuracy than CT alone: 86% vs. 77% PET ↑ sensitivity and specificity over CT
  - ↑ Diagnostic confidence vs. PET alone in > 50% patients
- PET CT more accurate initial staging than PET alone: 90% vs. 79% (one series)

RESPONSE TO TREATMENT

Whole Body FDG PET
- Locally advanced breast cancer (LABC)
  - ↓ FDG uptake within 8 days of neoadjuvant chemotherapy treatment
  - 88% accuracy after first treatment
- Metastatic breast cancer
  - Visual and quantitative ↓ uptake after treatment predicts response
  - Negative post chemotherapy PET predicts ↑ survival: 24 months vs. 10 with positive PET (one study)
- Early prediction of responders: Potential to tailor individual therapies

Metabolic Flare
- Tamoxifen (TAM) and other selective estrogen receptor modifiers → transient estrogen-like stimulation of tumor growth in estrogen-receptor (ER) + breast cancer ("metabolic flare")
- Baseline ↑ FES tumor uptake in TAM responders, overlap with nonresponders
  - FES can be used to assess ER status of metastases
- ↑ FDG uptake 7-10 days after initiation of TAM predicts response: More reliable than FES uptake
- Granulocyte colony stimulating factor (GCSF)
  - Causes ↑ FDG uptake in marrow, ↓ uptake in normal tissues and potentially ↓ tumor uptake

RELATED REFERENCES

1. Berg WA et al: High-resolution fluorodeoxyglucose positron emission tomography with compression ("positron emission mammography") is highly accurate in depicting primary breast cancer. Breast J. 12:309-23, 2006
2. Cachin F et al: Powerful prognostic stratification by [18F] fluorodeoxyglucose positron emission tomography in patients with metastatic breast cancer treated with high-dose chemotherapy. J Clin Oncol. 24:3026-31, 2006
3. Korn RL et al: Unexpected focal hypermetabolic activity in the breast: significance in patients undergoing 18F-FDG PET/CT. AJR. 187:81-5, 2006
4. Kumar R et al: Clinicopathologic factors associated with false negative FDG-PET in primary breast cancer. Breast Cancer Res Treat. 98:267-74, 2006
5. Tatsumi M et al: Initial experience with FDG-PET/CT in the evaluation of breast cancer. Eur J Nucl Med Mol Imaging. 33:254-62, 2006
6. Dose Schwarz J et al: Early prediction of response to chemotherapy in metastatic breast cancer using sequential 18F-FDG PET. J Nucl Med. 46:1144-50, 2005
7. Fueger BJ et al: Performance of 2-deoxy-2-[F-18]fluoro-D-glucose positron emission tomography and integrated PET/CT in restaged breast cancer patients. Mol Imaging Biol. 7:369-76, 2005
8. Tafra L et al: Pilot clinical trial of 18F-fluorodeoxyglucose positron-emission mammography in the surgical management of breast cancer. Am J Surg. 190:628-32, 2005
9. Wahl RL et al: Prospective multicenter study of axillary nodal staging by positron emission tomography in breast cancer: a report of the staging breast cancer with PET Study Group. J Clin Oncol. 22:277-85, 2004
10. Vranjesevic D et al: Relationship between 18F-FDG uptake and breast density in women with normal breast tissue. J Nucl Med. 44:1238-42, 2003
11. Yang SN et al: Comparing whole body (18)F-2-deoxyglucose positron emission tomography and technetium-99m methylene diphosphonate bone scan to detect bone metastases in patients with breast cancer. J Cancer Res Clin Oncol. 128:325-8, 2002
12. Mortimer JE et al: Metabolic flare: indicator of hormone responsiveness in advanced breast cancer. J Clin Oncol. 19:2797-803, 2001
13. Wahl RL: Current status of PET in breast cancer imaging, staging, and therapy. Semin Roentgenol. 36:250-60, 2001
14. Avril N et al: Breast imaging with positron emission tomography and fluorine-18 fluorodeoxyglucose: use and limitations. J Clin Oncol. 18:3495-502, 2000
15. Schelling M et al: Positron emission tomography using [(18)F]Fluorodeoxyglucose for monitoring primary chemotherapy in breast cancer. J Clin Oncol. 18:1689-95, 2000

IMAGE GALLERY

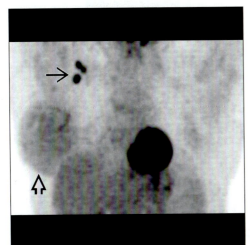

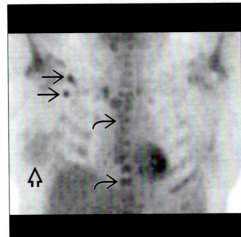

(Left) This 49 y/o is 2 months post right lumpectomy for 1.5 cm grade III IDC with 5/5 SLNs negative. Coronal MIP of FDG PET shows uptake in right subpectoral nodes ➡ (proven metastatic by US-guided FNA; SLN false negative). Diffuse right breast uptake ⬆➡ was post-surgical. (Right) Coronal MIP of FDG PET after 4 cycles chemotherapy (same as left) shows ↓ nodal ➡ and right breast ⬆➡ uptake. Marrow uptake ➡ is due to GCSF stimulation of marrow.

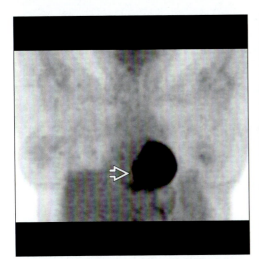

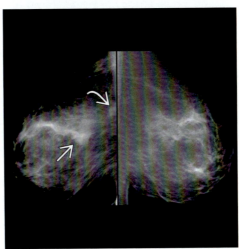

(Left) Coronal MIP of FDG PET 2 months later (same as prior) shows resolution of uptake in marrow, nodes, and right breast. Cardiac FDG uptake ⬆➡ is physiologic. Follow-up at one year showed no evidence of disease. (Right) MLO mammography shows focal asymmetry upper right breast ➡ in this 46 y/o who noted nodular thickening. US showed a mass, and biopsy showed grade II IDC with DCIS. Suspicious axillary node was also noted ➡ (metastatic).

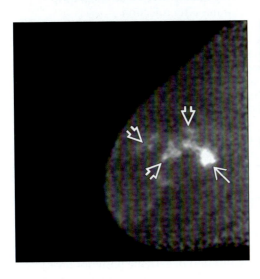

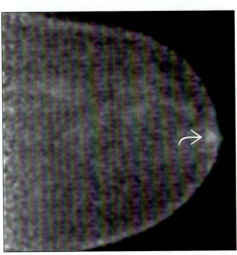

(Left) Single MLO slice from FDG PEM (same as prior) shows intense uptake in known cancer ➡ & clumped uptake anteriorly ➡ (also suspicious on MR). Mastectomy showed multifocal grade III IDC with extensive intraductal component. (Right) Single CC slice from left FDG PEM study (same case) shows physiologic uptake at nipple ➡; otherwise negative. US-prompted biopsy centrally showed tubular adenoma, true negative on PEM (Courtesy LT).

GAMMA CAMERA IMAGING

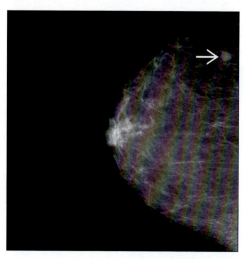

CC mammography shows new 1 cm irregular mass ➡ outer posterior right breast in this asymptomatic 58 y/o.

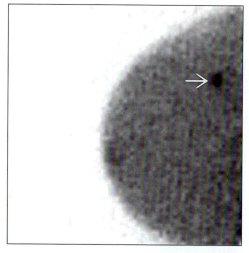

CC breast-specific gamma image following IV injection of 20 mCi MIBI (same as previous image) shows intense focal uptake ➡ in known mass. Histopathology showed 8 mm grade I IDC (Courtesy WLB).

TERMINOLOGY

Abbreviations
- Breast-specific gamma imaging (BSGI)
- Ductal carcinoma in situ (DCIS)
- Estrogen receptor (ER)
- Infiltrating ductal carcinoma (IDC)
- Infiltrating lobular carcinoma (ILC)
- Tc-99m methylene diphosphonate (MDP), used for bone scans
- Tc-99m sestamibi (MIBI) (Tc-99m methoxy-isobutyl isonitrile = Cardiolite = Miraluma, DuPont Pharmaceuticals, Wilmington, DE, USA)
- Sentinel lymph node (SLN) biopsy (SNB)
- Single photon emission computed tomography (SPECT), resolution ~ 12 mm
- Tetrofosmin: Tc-99m-1,2-bis[bis(2-ethoxyethyl)phosphino]ethane

Definitions
- Scintimammography: Gamma camera imaging of the breast using a standard whole body gamma camera ± modified positioning/tables
- BSGI: Gamma camera imaging of the breast using dedicated device ± gentle compression
  - MIBI and Tetrofosmin were developed for cardiac imaging and incidentally noted to be taken up in breast cancers
  - MIBI is taken up by mitochondria of cancer cells, as a substrate of P-glycoprotein 170 (product of multidrug resistance gene MDR1)
- Half-life: Time required for half the nuclei of a specific isotopic species to undergo radioactive decay
  - Tc-99m: 6 hours, gamma emitter
- Millicurie (mCi): 3.7×10^7 disintegrations per second (where 1 disintegration per second = 1 becquerel, Bq)
- Tc-99m sulfur colloid: Particulate radiotracer taken up by lymphatic system
- Lymphoscintigraphy = lymphatic mapping = sentinel node mapping: Gamma camera imaging following injection of Tc-99m sulfur colloid

- Identify location of first draining "sentinel" lymph node(s) (SLN)
- Lymphoscintigraphy allows identification of nonaxillary SLN
- Axillary SLN typically confirmed with intra-operative gamma probe

ANATOMY-BASED IMAGING ISSUES

Imaging Protocols
- MIBI
  - Inject 20-30 mCi MIBI iV into dorsalis pedis or antecubital vein
    - Preferential to inject distant from the site of known cancer/symptoms
  - BSGI: Dedicated device, gentle compression (~ 15 lbs), positioning analogous to mammography
  - Wait ~ 10 minutes after injection
  - Image for ~ 10 minutes per image, craniocaudal (CC) and mediolateral oblique (MLO) images: Total of ~ 40-45 minutes
- Sentinel node mapping (lymphoscintigraphy)
  - Tc-99m sulfur colloid, variable doses (0.1-10 mCi) and volumes (0.1-5 cc)
    - Massage for ~ 5-10 minutes after injection to facilitate uptake in lymphatics
  - Multiple routes of injection successful: Peritumoral, subdermal, subareolar
    - Only peritumoral injection will demonstrate nonaxillary SLN

Imaging Pitfalls
- MIBI
  - Uptake in heart, can cause "shine through" to posterior breast
  - Limited visualization of extreme posterior breast
  - Infiltration during iV injection → uptake in nodes
  - False positives include fibroadenomas, fat necrosis, fibrocystic changes
- Lymphoscintigraphy

Key Facts

Radiation Dose to Patient
- ~ 1-2 rads for MIBI scanning
- Contraindicated in pregnancy

Primary Breast Cancer
- MIBI, Tetrofosmin, other potential tracers
- Results with whole body cameras poor
- Dedicated devices: Improved sensitivity; studies ongoing

- Roles being explored: Pre-operative extent of disease, high-risk screening dense breasts

Axillary Lymph Node Status
- MIBI not useful in axillary staging: 79% sensitivity
- Tc-99m sulfur colloid ± blue dye → detection of SLN
- Successful identification of axillary SLN: 92-93% with combined radiocolloid and blue dye
- Lymposcintigraphy does not improve yield of SNB
  - Most centers do not excise internal mammary SLNs

- If inject peritumorally, upper outer quadrant breast cancer, potential for "shine through" from injection site → obscures axillary node imaging
- Can shield injection site
- Node full of metastatic disease may fail to take up sulfur colloid → false negative

IMAGING OF PRIMARY BREAST CANCER

MIBI or Tetrofosmin
- Not adversely affected by breast density
- **Breast-specific gamma-camera imaging** (BSGI)
  - **Performance with suspicious lesions**
    - 79-92% sensitivity with biopsy proven cancers
  - **Screening: MIBI**
    - Single study: 94 high-risk women with normal mammogram and clinical breast examination
    - 78 (83%) had normal scintimammograms
    - 16 (17%) abnormal scintimammograms: PPV 13%
    - Targeted US abnormal in 11; 2 showed cancer, 9 mm IDC plus DCIS each
    - Sources of false positives: Fibroadenomas (FA, n=7), fibrocystic changes (FCC, n=1), fat necrosis (n=1)
    - 6 month follow-up scintimammography normal in 5 with negative targeted US
- **Planar and SPECT scintimammography**
  - Insensitive to cancers < 1 cm

- Mean size of cancers depicted: 2.4 cm vs. 1.3 cm for false negatives
  - Sensitivity: 74% across several series
  - Specificity: 82%; PPV: 72%; NPV: 84%
  - SPECT performance not significantly better than planar imaging in small series
- Biopsy guidance
  - Targeted US or MR often helpful
  - Radiotracer-guided biopsy methods need refining

RELATED REFERENCES

1. Brem RF et al: Occult breast cancer: scintimammography with high-resolution breast-specific gamma camera in women at high risk for breast cancer. Radiology. 237:274-80, 2005
2. Rhodes DJ et al: Molecular breast imaging: a new technique using technetium Tc 99m scintimammography to detect small tumors of the breast. Mayo Clin Proc. 80(1):24-30, 2005
3. Taillefer R: Clinical applications of 99mTc-sestamibi scintimammography. Semin Nucl Med. 35(2):100-15, 2005
4. Brem RF et al: High-resolution scintimammography: a pilot study. J Nucl Med. 43:909-15, 2002
5. Khalkhali I et al: (99m)Tc sestamibi breast imaging for the examination of patients with dense and fatty breasts: multicenter study. Radiology. 222:149-55, 2002
6. Khalkhali I et al: Procedure guideline for breast scintigraphy. Society of Nuclear Medicine. J Nucl Med. 40:1233-5, 1999
7. Khalkhali I et al: Scintimammography: the complementary role of Tc-99m sestamibi prone breast imaging for the diagnosis of breast carcinoma. Radiology. 196:421-6, 1995

IMAGE GALLERY

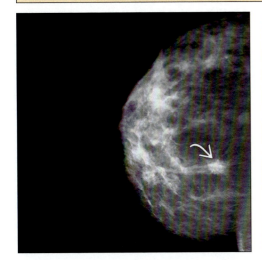
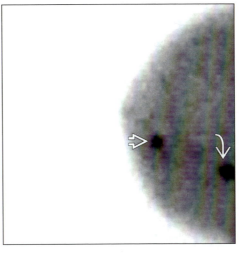

(Left) CC mammography shows spiculated mass ⟶ inner right breast in this 82 y/o asymptomatic woman. *(Right)* CC breast-specific gamma image following IV injection of 20 mCi MIBI (same as on left) shows intense uptake in known mass posteriorly ⟶. Unsuspected focal uptake was also seen in the retroareolar region ⟶. Both areas proved grade III IDC and DCIS on US-guided biopsy (Courtesy WLB).

PART III

Breast Cancer: Basic Treatment, Basic Tenets

Staging

Pathology

Surgery

Radiation Therapy

Oncology

STAGING

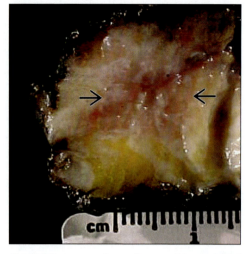

Picture of gross specimen shows a 1.2 cm (pT1c) cancer ➡. The tumor size (pT) is measurement of the invasive component only and it has to be verified microscopically.

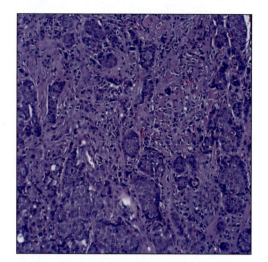

Medium power histopathology image (same case as previous) confirms the diagnosis of infiltrating carcinoma, and reveals that it was duct cell type, histologic grade II (H&E). Stage I (pT1c pN0 M0).

TERMINOLOGY

Abbreviations
- American Joint Committee on Cancer (AJCC)
- Union Internationale Contre le Cancer (UICC)
- Immunohistochemistry (IHC)
- Axillary lymph node(s) (ALN) dissection (ALND)
- Sentinel lymph node(s) (SLN) biopsy (SNB)
- Internal mammary lymph node(s) (IMN)
- Reverse transcriptase/polymerase chain reaction (RT-PCR)

Introduction to the Staging System
- Staging for breast cancer includes clinical and pathologic information based on the TNM system
  - T = Primary tumor
  - N = Regional nodes
    - N based on clinical findings, pN based on pathologic findings
  - M = Metastases
- Stage grouping may include any combination of clinical and pathologic classifications

Determining Tumor Size (T)
- T clinical size is taken from the most accurate determination either from physical exam or imaging studies within 4 months of diagnosis
- MR correlates best with tumor size
  - US correlates well with invasive tumor size, especially < 2 cm
- Definitions to classify the primary tumor (T) are the same for clinical and pathologic classification
- T pathological size (pT) measures the invasive component only
- After several core biopsies the true T size should be reconstructed from the original imaging studies and histological findings
- If multiple foci of microinvasion, only the size of the largest focus is used
  - Microinvasion: Extension of cancer cells beyond the basement membrane with no focus > 0.1 cm
- In multiple simultaneous ipsilateral cancers: T stage defined by the largest cancer

- Indicate (m) for multiple tumors, e.g., T1(m), or number of grossly recognizable multiple foci, e.g., T1(4): Largest invasive tumor is ≤ 2 cm, with 4 tumor foci identified
- Simultaneous bilateral tumors: Each staged separately
- Inflammatory carcinoma is a clinical diagnosis = T4d
- Dimpling of the skin, nipple retraction or other skin change, except as described under T4b and T4d may occur in T1, T2, or T3 without changing classification

Regional Lymph Nodes (N)
- If SNB is followed by ALND, the classification is based on the total number of dissected nodes
- Classification of pN0(i-) indicates no detectable tumor cells by either staining (H&E and IHC)
- Nodal metastases identified only by RT-PCR are classified as pN0(mol+) and believed to be clinically not significant
- Micrometastases: Tumor deposits greater that 0.2 mm but not greater than 2.0 mm; classified as pN1mi

Assessment of Distant Metastases
- Negative clinical history and physical exam are sufficient to designate as M0

CLINICAL IMPLICATIONS

Clinical Importance
- Breast cancer stage estimates prognosis
  - Lymph node status is most important prognostic factor
- Gauge for assessing success of screening programs
  - ↑ % Patients presenting as stage 0 or stage I from 42.5% in 1985 to 56.2% in 1995 (USA)
  - ↓ % Patients presenting as stage III or stage IV from 18.3% in 1985 to 11.6% in 1995 (USA)

TNM CLASSIFICATION

Primary Tumor (T)
- TX: Primary tumor cannot be assessed

STAGING

Stage Grouping/TNM Descriptors

Stage 0 (TisN0M0)

Stage I (T1*N0M0)

Stage IIA (T0N1M0, T1*N1M0, T2N0M0)

Stage IIB (T2N1M0, T3N0M0)

Stage IIIA (T0N2M0, T1*N2M0, T2N2M0, T3N1M0, T3N2M0)

Stage IIIB (T4N0M0, T4N1M0, T4N2M0)

Stage IIIC (Any T N3M0)

Stage IV (Any T Any N M1)
- T1* includes T1mic

TNM Descriptors
- Descriptors do not affect stage grouping; indicate cases needing separate analysis: "m" suffix and "y", "r" and "a" prefixes are used
- "m": Multiple primary tumors in a single breast, recorded in parentheses, e.g., pT(m)NM
- "y": Classification is performed during or following initial multimodality therapy (i.e., neoadjuvant chemotherapy, radiation therapy, or both)
  - "y" categorization is not an estimate of tumor prior to multimodality therapy (i.e., before initiation of neoadjuvant therapy)
- "r": Recurrent tumor when staged after a documented disease-free interval, identified by the "r" prefix, e.g., rTNM
- "a": Stage determined at autopsy, e.g., aTNM

- T0: No evidence of primary tumor
- Tis: Carcinoma in situ
  - Tis (DCIS): Ductal carcinoma in situ
  - Tis (LCIS): Lobular carcinoma in situ (not treated as cancer clinically)
  - Tis (Paget): Paget disease of the nipple with no tumor
    - Paget disease associated with a tumor is classified according to size of the tumor
- T1: Invasive tumor ≤ 2.0 cm in greatest dimension
  - T1mic: Microinvasion ≤ 0.1 cm in greatest dimension
  - T1a: Tumor > 0.1 cm but ≤ 0.5 cm in greatest dimension
  - T1b: Tumor > 0.5 cm but ≤1 cm in greatest dimension
  - T1c: Tumor > 1 cm but ≤ 2 cm in greatest dimension
- T2: Tumor > 2 cm but ≤ 5 cm in greatest dimension
- T3: Tumor > 5 cm in greatest dimension
- T4: Tumor of any size with direct extension to chest wall or skin, only as described below
  - T4a: Extension to chest wall, not including pectoralis muscle
  - T4b: Edema (including peau d'orange) or ulceration of the skin of the breast, or satellite skin nodules confined to the same breast
  - T4c: Both T4a and T4b
  - T4d: Inflammatory carcinoma

Regional Lymph Nodes (N)
- NX: Regional lymph nodes cannot be assessed (e.g., previously removed)
- N0: No regional lymph node metastasis
- N1: Metastasis in movable ipsilateral ALN
- N2: Metastases in ipsilateral ALN fixed or matted, or in clinically apparent* ipsilateral IMN in the absence of clinically evident ALN metastasis
  - N2a: Metastasis in ipsilateral ALN fixed to one another (matted) or to other structures
  - N2b: Metastasis only in clinically apparent* ipsilateral IMN and in the absence of clinically evident ALN metastasis

- N3: Metastasis in ipsilateral infraclavicular lymph node(s), or in clinically apparent* ipsilateral IMN(s) and in the presence of clinically evident ALN metastasis; or metastasis in ipsilateral supraclavicular lymph node(s) with or without ALN or IMN involvement
  - N3a: Metastasis in ipsilateral infraclavicular lymph node(s) and ALN
  - N3b: Metastasis in ipsilateral IMN and ALN
  - N3c: Metastasis in ipsilateral supraclavicular lymph node(s)

Regional Lymph Nodes (pN) †
- pNX: Regional lymph nodes cannot be assessed (e.g., previously removed or not removed for pathologic study)
- pN0: No regional lymph node metastasis histologically, no additional examination for isolated tumor cells (ITC)‡
  - pN0(i–): No regional lymph node metastasis histologically, negative IHC staining
  - pN0(i+): ITC identified histologically or by positive IHC staining, no cluster > 0.2 mm§
  - pN0(mol-): No regional lymph-node metastasis histologically, negative molecular findings (RT-PCR)
  - pN0(mol+): No regional lymph-node metastasis histologically, positive molecular findings (RT-PCR)
- pN1: Metastasis in 1-3 ALN, and/or in IMN with microscopic disease detected by SLN dissection but not clinically apparent*
  - pN1mi: Micrometastasis (> 0.2 mm, none > 2.0 mm)
  - pN1a: Metastasis in 1-3 ALN
  - pN1b: Metastasis in IMN with microscopic disease detected by SLN dissection but not clinically apparent*
  - pN1c: Metastasis in 1-3 ALN** and in IMN with microscopic disease detected by SLN dissection but not clinically apparent*
- pN2: Metastasis in 4-9 ALN, or in clinically apparent* IMN in the absence of ALN metastasis
  - pN2a: Metastasis in 4-9 ALN (at least one tumor deposit > 2.0 mm)

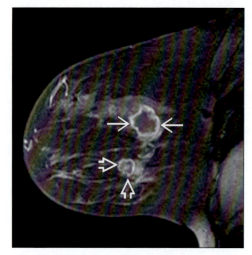

T1 C+ FS MR in a 48 y/o shows 2.6 cm known invasive carcinoma ➡ in lateral breast with a second 1.7 cm highly suspicious rim-enhancing mass ⇨ also noted. The largest invasive focus ➡ is used for T staging.

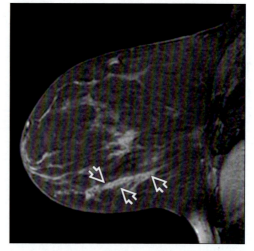

T1 C+ FS MR (same as prior) shows linear enhancement in medial breast suspicious for DCIS ⇨. MR-guided core biopsy showed intraductal papillomata & florid ductal hyperplasia: T2(m) N1 M0 (stage IIB).

○ pN2b: Metastasis in clinically apparent* IMN in the absence of ALN metastasis
- pN3: Metastasis in 10 or more ALN, or in infraclavicular lymph nodes, or in clinically apparent* ipsilateral IMN in the presence of 1 or more positive ALN; or in more than 3 ALN with clinically negative microscopic metastasis in IMN; or in ipsilateral supraclavicular lymph nodes
  ○ pN3a: Metastasis in 10 or more ALN (at least one tumor deposit > 2.0 mm), or metastasis to the infraclavicular lymph nodes
  ○ pN3b: Metastasis in clinically apparent* ipsilateral IMN in presence of 1 or more positive ALN; or in more than 3 ALN & in IMN with microscopic disease detected by SLN dissection but not clinically apparent*
  ○ pN3c: Metastasis in ipsilateral supraclavicular lymph nodes

Distant Metastasis (M)
- MX: Distant metastasis cannot be assessed
- M0: No distant metastasis
- M1: Distant metastasis

Notes
- *Clinically apparent is defined as detected by imaging studies (excluding lymphoscintigraphy) or by clinical examination
- †Classification is based on ALN dissection with or without SLN dissection
  ○ Classification based solely on SLN dissection without subsequent ALN dissection is designated (sn) for "sentinel node"
- ‡ITC: Single tumor cells or small cell clusters ≤ 0.2 mm, usually detected only by IHC or molecular methods but which may be verified on H&E stains
  ○ ITC do not usually show evidence of metastatic activity (e.g., proliferation or stromal reaction)
- §Definition of (i) was adapted in 2003 in order to be consistent with the updated UICC classification
- **If associated with more than 3 positive ALN, IMN metastases are classified as pN3b

Histologic Grade
- All invasive breast carcinomas, with exception of medullary carcinoma, should be graded
  ○ Grade is not part of the TNM system
- Nottingham combined histologic grade is recommended (Elston-Ellis modification of the Scarff-Bloom-Richardson grading system)

Residual Tumor (R)
- Tumor remaining in a patient after therapy with curative intent (e.g., surgical resection for cure) is categorized by a system known as R classification
  ○ RX: Presence of residual tumor cannot be assessed
  ○ R1: Microscopic residual tumor
  ○ R2: Macroscopic residual tumor

RELATED REFERENCES

1. Connolly JL: Changes and problematic areas in interpretation of the AJCC Cancer Staging Manual, 6th edition, for breast cancer. Arch Pathol Lab Med. 130:287-91, 2006
2. Singletary SE et al: Breast cancer staging: working with the sixth edition of the AJCC Cancer Staging Manual. CA Cancer J Clin. 56:37-47, 2006
3. Harris JR et al: Disease of the Breast. Philadelphia: Lippincott Williams & Wilkins, 2004
4. Greene FL et al: AJCC Cancer Staging Manual, 6th ed. New York, Springer, 2002
5. Fitzgibbons PL et al: Prognostic factors in breast cancer: College of American Pathologists Consensus Statement 1999. Arch Pathol Lab Med. 124:966-78, 2000
6. American Society of Clinical Oncology: 1997 update of recommendations for the use of tumor markers in breast and colorectal cancer. J Clin Oncol. 16:793-5, 1998
7. Elston CW et al: Pathological prognostic factors in breast cancer. I. The value of histological grade in breast cancer: experience from a large study with long-term follow-up. Histopathology. 19:403-10, 1991
8. Bloom HJ et al: Histological grading and prognosis in breast carcinoma: a study of 1049 cases of which 359 have been followed for 15 years. Br J Cancer. 11:359-77, 1957

IMAGE GALLERY

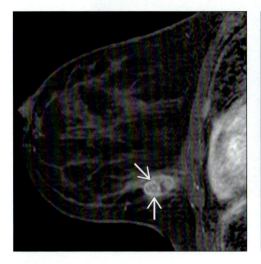
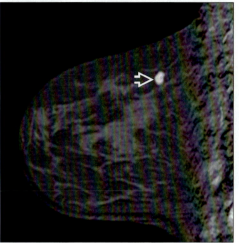

(Left) Sagittal T1 C+ FS MR shows primary malignancy ➡, grade III IDC, measuring 2.5 cm in greatest dimension (T2) in a 40 y/o woman. *(Right)* T1 C+ FS MR (same patient as previous image) shows a smaller enhancing mass in the upper outer quadrant ➡. Core biopsy with ultrasound guidance showed metastatic carcinoma within an intramammary lymph node (T2 N1 M0 = Stage IIB).

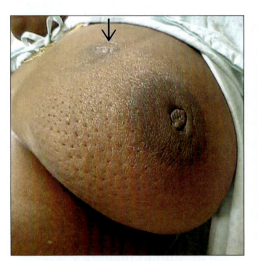
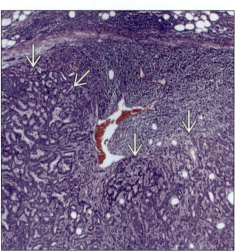

(Left) Clinical photograph of a 39-year-old woman shows inflammatory breast cancer (T4d) with skin ulceration, retraction ➡ and diffuse skin thickening with pitted appearance, described as resembling an orange peel (peau d'orange). *(Right)* Histopathology (same case as on left) shows metastatic carcinoma ➡ in a lymph node (H&E). Four of 9 ALN were positive for metastatic carcinoma (T4d pN2a M0 = Stage IIIB).

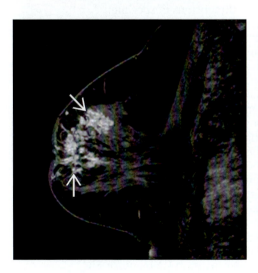
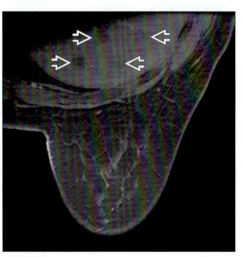

(Left) T1 C+ FS MR of the left breast in a 59 y/o shows a 5.0 cm enhancing breast cancer ➡, which was occult mammographically. *(Right)* T1 C+ FS MR (same patient as previous image) shows incidentally noted liver metastases ➡. Stage IV (T2 N1 M1).

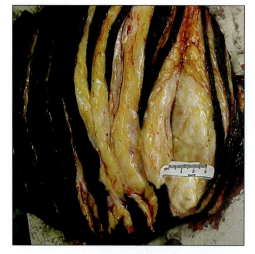

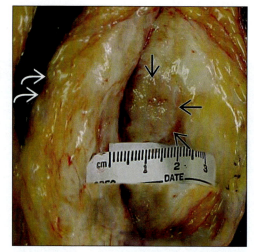

Gross pathology shows a modified radical mastectomy specimen from the black-inked posterior surface. The entire breast was sliced into 2 cm or less in thickness slices ("breadloafing"; sliced, like a loaf of bread).

Gross pathology, section shows (close-up of previous image) a circumscribed, 1.4 cm in diameter, pink-tan mass ➡, located 2.1 cm from the deep margin ➡. The mass was firm on palpation. Histology revealed IDC.

TERMINOLOGY

Abbreviations

- Lobular carcinoma in situ (LCIS)
- Ductal carcinoma in situ (DCIS)
- Not otherwise specified (NOS)
- Invasive ductal carcinoma (IDC)
- Invasive lobular carcinoma (ILC)
- Extensive intraductal component (EIC)
- Estrogen receptor (ER)
- Progesterone receptor (PR)
- Her-2/neu = c-erbB-2: Human epidermal growth factor receptor 2 gene
- Immunohistochemistry (IHC)
- Fluorescence in situ hybridization (FISH)
- American Joint Committee on Cancer (AJCC)

Definitions

- LCIS: Distention of lobule by monomorphic epithelial proliferation ± pagetoid spread in terminal ducts
- DCIS (intraductal carcinoma): Proliferation of malignant epithelial cells confined to ducts ± lobules, without light-microscopic evidence of invasion through the basement membrane
- Invasive carcinoma: Cancer cells infiltrate beyond the basement membrane
- Microinvasion: Extension of cancer cells beyond the basement membrane with no focus > 0.1 cm
- Extensive intraductal component (EIC): DCIS comprises a substantial portion of the main (infiltrating) tumor mass (~ ≥ 25%), with foci of DCIS also in surrounding tissue
  - ↑ Risk of local recurrence when surgical margins are not evaluated or focally involved

PATHOLOGIC ISSUES

Grading Criteria

- All invasive breast carcinomas, with the exception of medullary carcinoma, should be graded
  - This includes invasive lobular and mucinous carcinomas
- Grading system used must be specified in report: Nottingham combined histologic grade (Elston-Ellis modification of Scarff-Bloom-Richardson grading system) is recommended by AJCC
- Within each stage grouping there is a correlation between histologic grade and outcome

Staging Criteria

- TNM staging described by the AJCC
- Pathologic staging includes all data used for clinical staging plus data from surgical resection
- Imaging findings within 4 months of diagnosis are considered elements of staging

Surgical Pathology Report for Specimens with Breast Cancer Should Include

- Type and size dimensions of specimen
- Tumor location and extent
  - Size of invasive carcinoma
    - Pathologic tumor size (pT): Measurement of invasive component only; size is verified microscopically
    - After core biopsy, measuring residual lesion may result in underclassification of T component: Tumor size is reconstructed by combining imaging, core and excisional histopathologic findings
  - Size of DCIS; methods for estimating extent
    - Direct measurement on histologic slide
    - Submitting the entire specimen
    - Estimating % of tissue involved
  - Number of tumors; if multiple, measurement of distance apart
- Histologic type; grade and presence or absence of lymphovascular invasion (LVI) and/or EIC
- Status of microscopic margins
  - Distance and type of tumor to closest margin
- Status of lymph nodes (if dissection was performed)
- Presence and location of calcifications
  - In invasive cancer, DCIS, ± benign tissue
- Ancillary studies

PATHOLOGY

Histological Diagnoses on Surgical Pathology: Cancer Case Summary

Noninvasive Carcinoma
- LCIS (not treated as cancer clinically)
- DCIS, Paget disease without invasive carcinoma

Invasive Carcinoma
- IDC NOS (± EIC or ± Paget disease)
- ILC: Single file growth pattern, a monotonous population of small cells with very low grade nuclei, and low cell density
- Special types
  - Mucinous: Low grade nuclei and extracellular mucin in ≥ 90% of tumor; tumors with less extensive mucin = "IDC with mucinous features"
  - Tubular: Well differentiated tubules compose ≥ 90% of the tumor; low histologic grade
  - Papillary: Papillary architecture
- Medullary: Circumscribed border; high histologic grade with sheets of large, undifferentiated tumor cells; lymphoplasmacytic infiltrate between cellular nests, and scant fibrous stroma
- Adenoid cystic: Histologically similar to the salivary gland counterpart
- Secretory (juvenile): Produce milk-like material
- Apocrine: ≥ 90% of the carcinoma cells have features of apocrine cells
- Invasive cribriform: Minor (< 50%) component of tubular carcinoma may be admixed
- Carcinoma with metaplasia (squamous, spindle cell, cartilaginous/osseous or mixed type metaplasia)
- Other (neuroendocrine; lipid-rich; sebaceous; acinic cell; invasive micropapillary, etc.)
- Carcinoma type cannot be determined

- E.g., hormone receptor studies, special stains, prognostic assays, flow cytometry, FISH

Microscopic Evaluation and Special Studies
- Hematoxylin and eosin staining (H&E)
  - Widely used, two-stage stain: Hematoxylin is followed by a counterstain of red eosin; nuclei stain blue-black and cytoplasm, pink
- Hormone receptor studies
  - ER (and PR)
    - Nuclear hormone receptor; routinely determined by IHC on invasive carcinomas and DCIS
  - Her-2/neu (c-erbB-2) oncogene
    - Member of the epidermal growth factor receptor (EGFR) family; has been found to be altered in approximately 20% of breast cancers
    - Amplification of gene resulting in more than usual 2 copies of Her-2/neu gene (one on each copy of chromosome 17)
    - Usually IHC used as an initial screen, with FISH studies performed on cases with 2+ staining
    - Positive IHC study (i.e., 3+ IHC study): PPV for amplification by FISH is 94%
    - Negative IHC study (i.e., a score of 0 or 1): NPV for negative amplification by FISH is 96%
    - Indeterminate Her-2/neu status by IHC: 2+
- E-Cadherin
  - Tumor invasion suppressor gene involved in cell adhesion, located on chromosomal region 16q
  - Mutated (expression lost) in lobular breast cancers
- Other IHC studies
  - p53 antibody: Tumor suppressor gene; mutation leads to overexpression of p53 protein and to loss of cell proliferation control
  - Myoepithelial markers
    - Loss of myoepithelial layer supports the diagnosis of infiltrating carcinoma vs. in situ cancer, as well as the diagnosis of infiltrating carcinoma (especially tubular carcinoma) vs. sclerosing adenosis and other benign sclerosing lesions
    - Smooth muscle myosin heavy chain (SMM-HC) and p63 are the most sensitive and specific markers of myoepithelium
    - Other markers: Actin, cytokeratin 5, CD10, calponin
  - Markers of cell proliferation
    - MIB-1 (and Ki-67 antigen)
- Molecular diagnostic testing
  - Gene expression profiling: Identifies which specific genes are turned on or off in a tumor
  - Estimation of risk of recurrence and prediction whether stage I cancer will benefit from chemotherapy
    - OncotypeDX™: Currently under clinical trial
    - Possibility of "personalized treatment"

PATHOLOGY-BASED IMAGING ISSUES

Specimen Processing and Radiologic-Pathologic Correlation
- Radiologic-pathologic correlation is essential
  - Pathologic diagnosis must be concordant with impression from imaging studies
  - Discordant diagnoses must be reconciled, and this may require repeat biopsy
- Calcifications (Ca++)
  - Documented by specimen x-ray
  - Calcium phosphate crystals
    - Basophilic (purple) on H&E stain
    - Do not polarize
    - Seen with cysts, sclerosing adenosis, fibroadenomas, DCIS and invasive cancer
  - Calcium oxalate crystals
    - Pale and refractile clear or yellow crystals
    - Well visualized under polarized light
    - Seen in association with cysts but not cancer
  - Documentation of Ca++ at histopathology
    - If initial sections (levels) fail to reveal Ca++, deeper sections and x-ray of paraffin blocks may be helpful
    - Larger Ca++ may fall out of block during sectioning

PATHOLOGY

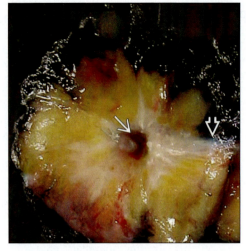

Gross pathology of infiltrating carcinoma. The small hemorrhagic cavity ⇒ is secondary to prior core needle biopsy. The specimen margins are inked. The tumor extends grossly into the margin ⇒.

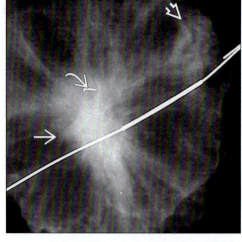

Specimen radiograph (same patient as previous image) shows the spiculated mass ⇒, core biopsy clip ⇒ and extension of the mass into the margin ⇒.

- ■ Smaller Ca++ may dissolve after > 24 hours in formalin
- • Core needle biopsy (CNB) and incisional biopsy
  - ○ Entire specimen submitted for histology (varies)
  - ○ CNB specimens suitable for IHC studies of hormone receptors and other biological markers
- • Excisional surgical biopsy (e.g., lumpectomy)
  - ○ Typically needle localization used to guide surgeon to the abnormality(ies)
  - ○ Specimen radiography: Documents presence of target and localizes suspicious area for histologic sections; also roughly estimates the closest margin
    - ■ Target must be identified by the pathologist
    - ■ Specimen is palpated for masses and correlated with radiograph
  - ○ Prior core biopsy site should be identified at histology by presence of hemorrhage and fibrosis
- • Mastectomy
  - ○ Breast divided into quadrants
  - ○ Entire breast sliced, and examined grossly for tumor or suspicious areas
- • Margin evaluation
  - ○ Surgeon orients the specimen by sutures, clips, diagram ± different ink colors
  - ○ Intact specimen is inked (usually by the pathologist)
  - ○ After inking, the specimen is sectioned
  - ○ Sections perpendicular to inked tissue edges: Distance from cancer to margin can be measured on the histopathology slide
  - ○ 'En face' sections: Specimen edge shaved; larger proportion of margin is examined but any tumor cells in shaved piece considered with margin: Potential for false positive margins
  - ○ Intraoperative evaluation of margins (frozen section or touch preparation) may detect focally positive margins that may be excised
- • Specimen sampling for microscopic examination
  - ○ All gross lesions and areas of mammographic abnormality are sampled
  - ○ Multiple lesions: Section between the lesions
  - ○ If no gross lesion, most fibrous areas are sampled

- ○ If excision is for atypical ductal hyperplasia (ADH), DCIS, or MR-guided, entire specimen should be submitted
- • Axillary lymph node dissection (ALND)
  - ○ Typical ALND: Level I and II nodes
  - ○ Average of 16 lymph nodes removed (range of averages across series = 11-23) up to 40 or more
  - ○ Nodes bivalved, submitted for histological analysis
  - ○ Report number of nodes removed, number involved by tumor, size of largest metastasis
- • Sentinel lymph node (SLN) biopsy
  - ○ Varying methods of processing
  - ○ SLN thinly sectioned and completely submitted
  - ○ Intraoperative frozen section or touch prep possible
    - ■ ALND is completed if SLN shows metastasis
  - ○ "Isolated tumor cells" (≤ 0.2 mm) of unknown significance
- • Micrometastasis: Metastasis > 0.2 mm and ≤ 2.0 mm
  - ○ Clinical significance is currently unknown

RELATED REFERENCES

1. Elledge RM et al: Clinical aspects of estrogen and progesterone receptors. In: Harris JR, Lippman ME, Morrow M, Osborne CK, editors. Diseases of the Breast. Philadelphia, Lippincott Williams & Wilkins. 603-17, 2004
2. Greene FL et al: AJCC Cancer Staging Manual. 6th ed. New York, Springer, 2002
3. Connolly JL et al: Predictors of breast recurrence after conservative surgery and radiation therapy for invasive breast cancer. Mod Pathol. 11:134-9, 1998
4. Schwartz GF et al: Consensus conference on the classification of ductal carcinoma in situ. The Consensus Conference Committee. Cancer. 80:1798-802, 1997
5. Berg WA: When is core breast biopsy or fine-needle aspiration not enough? Radiology.198:313-5, 1996
6. Rosen PP et al: Tumors of the Mammary Gland. Atlas of Tumor Pathology. 3rd Series, Fascicle 7. Washington DC, Armed Forces Institute of Pathology. 1993
7. Bennington JL et al: The Mammographically Directed Biopsy. Philadelphia, Hanley and Belfus, 1992
8. Schnitt SJ et al: Processing and evaluation of breast excision specimens. A clinically oriented approach. Am J Clin Pathol. 98:125-37, 1992

IMAGE GALLERY

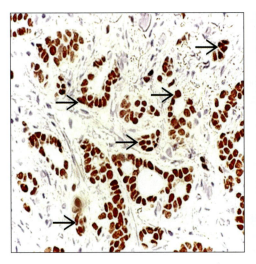

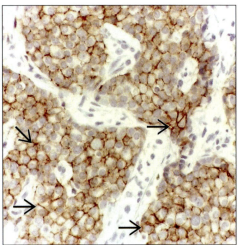

(Left) Low power histopathology shows IDC, with strong nuclear immunopositivity with antibodies for ER ➡. ER is a weak prognostic factor but a strong predictive factor for response to endocrine therapies. *(Right)* Her-2/neu overexpression is detected on the cell membranes, 3+ by IHC ➡ in this IDC. Equivocal (2+) results on IHC are further evaluated by FISH.

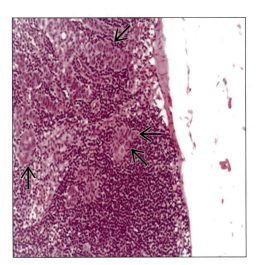

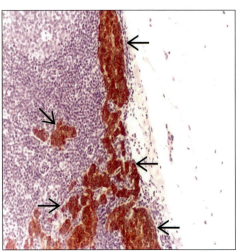

(Left) Routine H&E stained section of sentinel lymph node shows small clusters of tumor cells in subcapsular sinus area ➡. Lymph travels to the lymph node via afferent lymphatic vessels and drains into the node beneath the capsule into subcapsular sinus. *(Right)* Keratin-positive cancer cells highlighted by IHC ➡ in the same lymph node as previous image. The metastasis measured less than 2.0 mm in greatest dimension: Classified as micrometastasis.

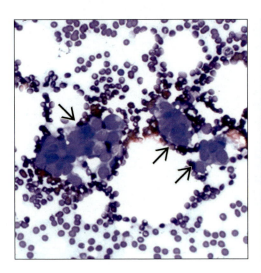

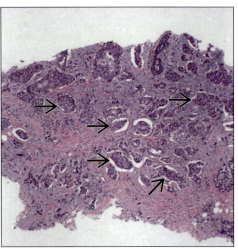

(Left) US -guided fine needle aspiration (FNAB) of a breast mass shows cellular smear with clusters of carcinoma cells ➡ (Giemsa x 200). With FNAB, usually the grade or presence of invasion cannot be determined. *(Right)* Core-needle biopsy (same mass as previous image) enables histologic diagnosis of high-grade IDC ➡, critical to planning subsequent treatment. In addition, hormone receptor status can be determined on CNB specimens.

(Left) Histopathology shows extension of DCIS into lobules, i.e., cancerization of lobules, resulting in solid expansion of the acini and ductules (low power H&E). Calcifications ➡. Differential diagnosis is often difficult between LCIS and solid DCIS, especially when DCIS involves lobules. *(Right)* IHC for E-cadherin is strongly positive (brown) in this example of DCIS with cancerization of the lobules. DCIS retains the ability to express E-cadherin whereas lobular tumors do not.

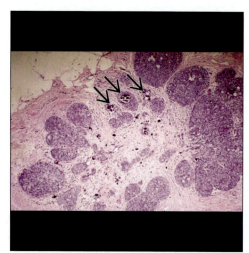
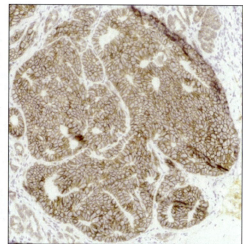

(Left) Histopathology shows LCIS, with distention of lobules by monomorphic cells ➡ and adjacent cysts ➘, one of which contains a calcium phosphate crystal ➴ (medium power, H&E). *(Right)* Histopathology, IHC for E-cadherin (same patient as previous image), shows staining of cyst walls ➘ and myoepithelial layer of lobules, but absence of staining in areas of LCIS itself ➡. E-cadherin is lost in lobular lesions.

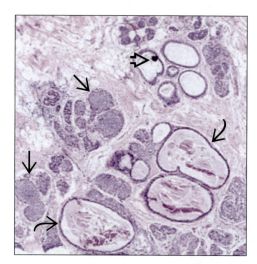
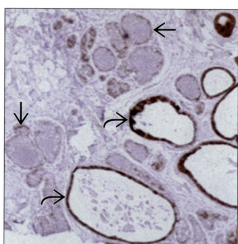

(Left) Histopathology of 11-g biopsy (H&E) shows duct hyperplasia, with focal streaming of cells within an area of bridging ➘. This just barely qualifies as ADH. Excision was benign. *(Right)* Histopathology of 11-g biopsy (different case than previous image) shows single duct profile typical of DCIS (H&E). As the diagnosis of DCIS requires at least 2 duct profiles, this was considered ADH. Excision was performed, confirming the diagnosis of DCIS.

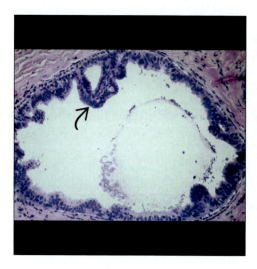
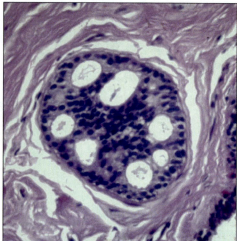

PATHOLOGY

IMAGE GALLERY

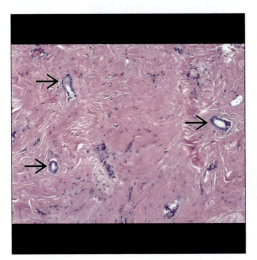

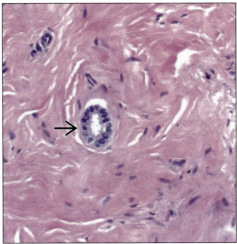

(Left) Histopathology shows tubular carcinoma. Nests of tumor (tubules) ➡ are separated by intense fibroblastic proliferation (medium power, H&E). *(Right)* Histopathology, high power, H&E (same patient as previous image) shows profile of a single tubule of tubular carcinoma ➡. Note there is only a single layer of epithelial cells, with no myoepithelial cell layer present.

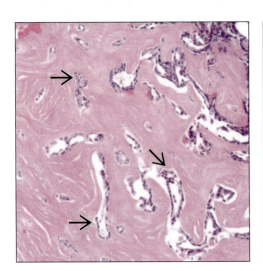

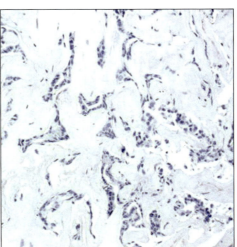

(Left) Histopathology shows tubular carcinoma (H&E). The neoplastic cells form a single cuboidal layer in small round to teardrop-shaped distorted ductules ➡ widely spaced in a fibrous stroma. *(Right)* Histopathology shows actin IHC stain (same case as previous image). There is absence of any brown staining, confirming absence of myoepithelial cell layer in the tubules of this case of tubular carcinoma.

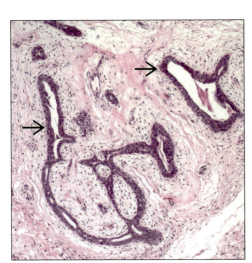

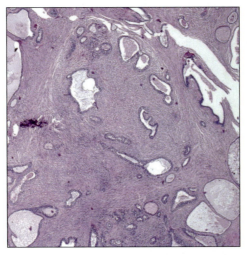

(Left) Cellular fibroadenoma. Cellular stroma surrounds glandular spaces ➡ lined by benign epithelial cells (H&E). The tumor was grossly well circumscribed. *(Right)* Phyllodes tumor (H&E). The distinction between cellular fibroadenoma and phyllodes tumor can be challenging on core biopsy. Excision is recommended when there is uncertainty. This tumor was grossly lobulated, resembling a leaf ("phyllodes": Leaf-like in Greek). (Last 12 images courtesy of OBI).

SURGERY

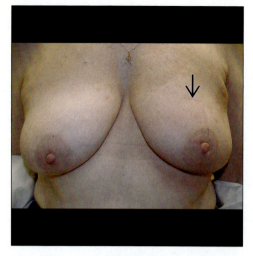

Clinical photograph shows an excellent cosmetic result 3 yrs after BCT for a T1 N0 breast cancer treated with lumpectomy (incision in upper left breast ➡) with ALND and whole breast XRT.

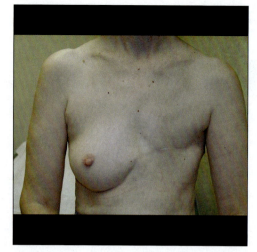

Clinical photograph shows patient 3 yrs status post MRM for a T2N1 left breast cancer. The patient chose not to have reconstruction, and wears an external prosthesis.

TERMINOLOGY

Abbreviations
- Axillary lymph node dissection (ALND)
- Sentinel lymph node (SLN) biopsy (SNB)
- Tamoxifen (TAM)
- National Surgical Adjuvant Breast and Bowel Project (NSABP)
- Disease free survival (DFS)
- Overall survival (OS)
- Estrogen receptor (ER)
- Radiation therapy (XRT)

Definitions
- Radical mastectomy (RM): Complete removal of the breast, pectoralis major & minor muscles, and complete ALND at all three levels
- Extended radical mastectomy: Radical mastectomy with dissection of internal mammary nodes (IMN)
- Modified radical mastectomy (MRM): Complete removal of breast and variable portion of axillary lymph nodes; pectoral muscles are left intact
- Total mastectomy (TM): Removal of all breast tissue only, without axillary lymph nodes
- Lumpectomy or partial mastectomy: Breast-conserving surgery with goal of removing breast cancer and surrounding margin of benign tissue
- Breast conserving treatment (BCT): Breast-conserving surgery followed by XRT
  - Typically lumpectomy in USA; more often quadrantectomy (sector resection) in Europe

HISTORY

Evolution of Mastectomy
- Radical mastectomy era (Early 1900s to late 1970s)
  - 1890s: Radical mastectomy pioneered by William Halsted at the Johns Hopkins Hospital
  - Wide en bloc resection: Belief that spread of disease was primarily via local lymphatics
  - 1950s: Wider resection with extended radical mastectomy (Urban): ↑ Morbidity, no benefit
- NSABP B-04 trial (1971-74)
  - Clinically node negative patients randomized to: 1) RM; 2) TM with axillary nodal XRT; 3) TM with axillary observation & delayed ALND if positive nodes develop
  - No difference in DFS at 25 yr follow-up
- Paradigm shift
  - Understanding that tumors spread systemically with resultant distant recurrence; can happen at any stage
  - Distant failure a result of pre-operative spread of cancer cells, not inadequate local surgery
  - Shift to less extensive local surgical procedures

Breast Conservation Treatment Trials
- Multiple trials have demonstrated equivalent survival with BCT and MRM (late 1970s & early 1980s)
  - NSABP B-06 trial: Patients randomized to BCT (with lumpectomy) or mastectomy, 20 yr follow-up
    - OS same: 46% with BCT & 47% with MRM
    - Local recurrence: 14% with BCT & 10% with MRM
  - Milan I trial: Patients randomized to BCT (with quadrantectomy) or mastectomy, 20 yr follow-up
    - OS same: 42% with BCT & 41% with MRM
    - Local recurrence: 9% with BCT & 2% with MRM
- Local recurrence with BCT
  - Rates in early trials 10-19%; more recent studies report 2-7% recurrence rates at 10 years
- Further ↓ in local recurrence rates with improving systemic chemo- and hormonal therapy (1980s)
  - NSABP B-13 trial: Node negative, ER- tumors
    - Surgery → by chemotherapy or no treatment
    - BCT subset 8 yr local recurrence 2.6% with chemotherapy vs. 13.4%
  - NSABP B-14 trial: Node negative, ER+ tumors
    - BCT followed by 5 yrs of TAM vs. placebo
    - 10 yr local recurrence 4.3% with TAM vs. 14.3% with placebo
- Pathologic studies of mastectomies thought to have unifocal tumor on mammography and clinically: 20% had additional tumor within 2 cm & 41% had > 2 cm beyond reference tumor (Holland)

Key Clinical Trials

NSABP B-04 trial
- Early 1970s: Showed that Halstedian concept of wide resection incorrect
- Clinically node negative patients randomized to 1) RM; 2) TM with nodal XRT; 3) TM with axillary observation with possible delayed ALND
- No difference in DFS at 25 yr follow-up

NSABP B-06 & Milan I Trials
- 1970s & 80s: Patients randomized to BCT or mastectomy
- Conducted in North America (NSABP B-06) & Europe (Milan I)
- Showed that BCT equivalent to MRM
- At 20 yr follow-up, OS same in both groups in both trials

- Local recurrence at 20 yrs slightly greater in BCT arm

NSABP B-14 Trial
- 1980s: Node negative ER+ tumors treated with BCT followed by TAM/placebo for 5 yrs
- TAM decreases ipsilateral breast recurrence with BCT

NSABP B-21 Trial
- 1 cm node negative patients post lumpectomy randomized to 1) XRT; 2) XRT + TAM; 3) TAM alone
- Showed that TAM not as good as XRT in BCT local recurrence, but TAM with XRT is of added benefit

NSABP B-32 & ALMANAC Trials
- Closed trials evaluating various aspects of SNB compared to ALND
- ALMANAC trial: ↓ Arm morbidity & ↑ quality of life after SNB compared to ALND

- ○ XRT effectively treats majority of occult foci
- Can XRT be omitted from BCT in select patients?
  - ○ XRT ↓ local recurrence risk in all patient subsets
  - ○ NSABP B-21 trial (1990s): Could TAM substitute for XRT?
    - ≤ 1 cm, node negative patients following lumpectomy randomized to: 1) XRT; 2) XRT with TAM; 3) TAM alone
    - Ipsilateral local recurrence rates at 8 yrs: 1) XRT, 9.3%; 2) XRT + TAM, 2.8%; 3) TAM alone, 16.5%
    - XRT better than TAM; XRT with TAM better than TAM alone
  - ○ Very small select group with small focus of low grade DCIS & wide margins of excision (using modified van Nuys index); controversial
  - ○ May consider in elderly (> 70 yrs old) and low risk: XRT would benefit, but mortality from other causes may make small decrease in local recurrence irrelevant

Axillary Lymph Node Evaluation
- Lymph node status is most important prognostic indicator for OS
- 75% of breast lymphatics drain to axilla, 25% to IMNs
  - ○ 10% incidence of IMN metastases with negative axilla; more common with medial & central tumors
- SNB: Removal of the first draining lymph node from a regional lymph node basin: If no tumor cells in SLN, remaining nodes presumed to be tumor free
  - ○ Early 2000s: NSABP B-32 trial, ALMANAC trial, ACOSOG-Z0011: Large studies evaluating its role
- ALND: Removal of level I and level II nodes
  - ○ Performed when patient known to have metastatic node(s) pre-operatively or SLN shows metastases other than isolated tumor cells

SOME IMPORTANT CONSIDERATIONS

Breast Conservation Treatment
- BCT still significantly underutilized

- Multifocality & multicentricity of tumors
  - ○ Mammographically occult tumor foci common: 48% across series; leaving such foci in breast may lead to recurrence, though majority of such foci are treated by XRT and adjuvant therapy
  - ○ Potential benefit of pre-operative imaging to assess extent of disease being evaluated, especially MR
    - Likely ↓ rate of positive margins, but further study warranted
    - Risk of false positives → additional biopsies, potentially mastectomies where patient could have had BCT
- Types of local recurrence
  - ○ True recurrence: Recurrence at site of primary tumor, within area that received XRT boost, usually in cases with close or positive margins, most frequently seen within first 5 yrs post treatment
  - ○ Marginal miss: Recurrence near site of primary tumor, adjacent to area of boost, usually in first 5 yrs
  - ○ Elsewhere recurrence: Tumor in ipsilateral breast away from original tumor, presumed to represent a new primary, risk same as for contralateral breast
- ↑ Risk local recurrence
  - ○ Younger patient age, BRCA-1 or -2 mutation carrier, margins of resection close or positive, ↓ extent of resection, no boost given with XRT, no adjuvant systemic therapy
- No influence on risk of local recurrence
  - ○ Tumor size, nodal metastases, invasive lobular carcinoma (ILC) histology
  - ○ These are adverse prognostic factors for systemic relapse, signify need for adjuvant systemic treatment

Sentinel Lymph Node Biopsy
- Safe and accurate method to determine axillary nodal status in experienced hands
  - ○ Use blue dye (peritumoral) and/or Tc-99m sulfur colloid (Tc-99m SC) injections (peritumoral, subdermal, or subareolar route)
- ↓ Morbidity compared to ALND
- Standard of care in clinically node negative patients
  - ○ Use even when palpable lymph nodes (these can be benign enlargements) unless positive pre-op FNAB

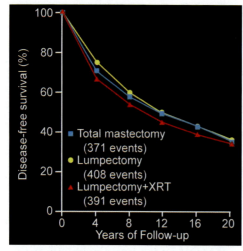
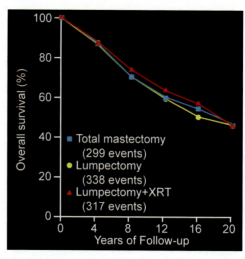
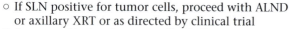

Results from the NSABP B-06 trial show no significant difference in DFS at 20 yrs of follow up. Local recurrence rates were 10.2% with MRM, 14.3% with lumpectomy + XRT & 39.2% with lumpectomy alone.

The overall survival in the three groups in the NSABP B-06 trial was also without significant difference at 20 yrs of follow-up.

- ○ If SLN positive for tumor cells, proceed with ALND or axillary XRT or as directed by clinical trial
- Relevance of isolated tumor cells (ITC) on immunohistochemistry (IHC) unclear
- Should micrometastases (focus of tumor cells > 0.2 mm and ≤ 2 mm) prompt adjuvant chemotherapy?
- Need for biopsy & staging of IMNs is controversial: Consider if it may change adjuvant XRT ± chemotherapy approach
  - ○ Peritumoral injection required to visualize IMNs

In Situ Carcinoma

- Ductal carcinoma in situ (DCIS): Local treatment as a cancer: BCT or mastectomy
  - ○ Considered precursor of invasive cancer
- Lobular carcinoma in situ (LCIS): Not treated as cancer
  - ○ Generally an incidental pathologic finding
  - ○ ↑ Cumulative long term & bilateral invasive breast cancer risk (8-10 fold increased risk, 1-2% per yr, lifetime risk of 30-40%)
    - Options: Close surveillance, chemoprevention, bilateral prophylactic mastectomy
  - ○ Loss of E-cadherin expression (protein involved with cell-to-cell adhesion)
  - ○ Excision typically recommended after core biopsy diagnosis
    - Upgrade more common if associated mass lesion or architectural distortion, possible DCIS on histology, pleomorphic LCIS
    - Do not need negative margins on excision
    - "Non-obligate" precursor to invasive lobular carcinoma

Immediate Reconstruction after Mastectomy

- No difference in local failure rates vs. delayed or no reconstruction
- Skin-sparing mastectomy: Mastectomy technique where most of the skin is preserved, used with immediate reconstruction; nipple areolar complex generally excised
  - ○ No increase in local recurrence rates
  - ○ Some preserve nipple areolar complex; controversial
    - 6-11% malignant involvement of nipple ± areola

- Problems with ischemia, lack of sensation, non-erectile nipple, difficulty with symmetry
- Post-mastectomy XRT influences immediate reconstruction choice
  - ○ Autologous flaps: Flap loss rare, but other problems are common, e.g., fibrosis, volume loss, fat necrosis
    - Delay reconstruction until after XRT
  - ○ Implants: Tolerate XRT very poorly
    - Can place tissue expanders, expand to desired size, XRT, then implant exchange

RELATED REFERENCES

1. Lyman GH et al: American Society of Clinical Oncology guideline recommendations for sentinel lymph node biopsy in early-stage breast cancer. J Clin Oncol. 23(30):7703-20, 2005
2. Fisher B et al: Tamoxifen, radiation therapy, or both for prevention of ipsilateral breast tumor recurrence after lumpectomy in women with invasive breast cancers of one centimeter or less. J Clin Oncol. 20(20):4141-9, 2002
3. Fisher B et al: Twenty-five-year follow-up of a randomized trial comparing radical mastectomy, total mastectomy, and total mastectomy followed by irradiation. N Engl J Med. 347(8):567-75, 2002
4. Fisher B et al: Twenty-year follow-up of a randomized trial comparing total mastectomy, lumpectomy, and lumpectomy plus irradiation for the treatment of invasive breast cancer. N Engl J Med. 347(16):1233-41, 2002
5. Veronesi U et al: Twenty-year follow-up of a randomized study comparing breast-conserving surgery with radical mastectomy for early breast cancer. N Engl J Med. 347(16):1227-32, 2002
6. Mariani L et al: Ten year results of a randomised trial comparing two conservative treatment strategies for small size breast cancer. Eur J Cancer. 34(8):1156-62, 1998
7. Dewar JA et al: Local relapse and contralateral tumor rates in patients with breast cancer treated with conservative surgery and radiotherapy (Institut Gustave Roussy 1970-1982). IGR Breast Cancer Group. Cancer. 76(11):2260-5, 1995
8. Holland R et al: Histologic multifocality of Tis, T1-2 breast carcinomas. Implications for clinical trials of breast-conserving surgery. Cancer. 56(5):979-90, 1985

IMAGE GALLERY

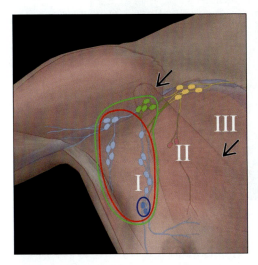

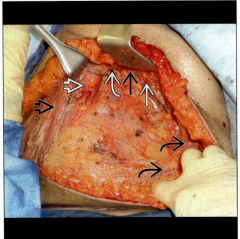

(Left) Depiction of axillary lymph node levels, defined in relation to the pectoralis minor muscle ➡. Blue oval: Typical SNB; red oval: Typical level I ALND; green oval: Typical level I & II ALND. (Right) Intra-operative photograph of ALND (with MRM). The pectoralis major ➡, latissimus dorsi ➡ muscles, and axillary vein ➡ are the limits of dissection. Level II of the axilla ➡ is behind pectoralis minor muscle ➡. The intercostobrachial nerve ➡ is preserved.

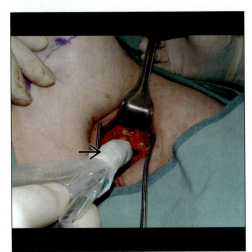

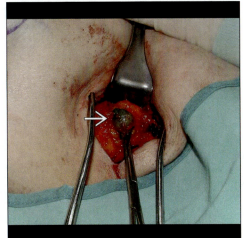

(Left) Intra-operative photograph shows an axillary SNB done in conjunction with a lumpectomy. A gamma probe ➡ is used to find the "hot" lymph node (Tc-99m SC used as SLN mapping agent). (Right) A blue dye was also used (same patient as on left), and a blue lymph node ➡ visually identified (node was also hot). This SLN was sent for intra-operative pathologic evaluation with a touch preparation.

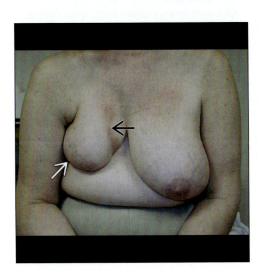

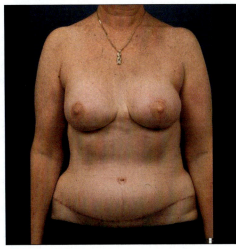

(Left) Clinical photograph of a patient who underwent BCT 22 years ago. Treatment was a very large right lumpectomy ➡ (scar at edge of breast contour) & XRT. The patient developed significant radiation necrosis ➡. The resulting cosmetic result is very poor. (Right) Clinical photograph of a patient who underwent bilateral prophylactic skin sparing total mastectomies with immediate deep inferior epigastric perforator (DIEP) flap reconstruction with excellent cosmetic outcome.

RADIATION THERAPY

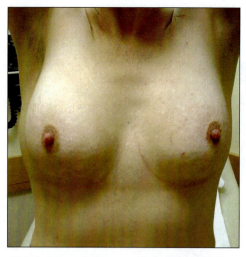

Clinical photograph shows excellent cosmesis 2 1/2 yrs after breast-conserving surgery and adjuvant XRT for a T2N1 lower outer quadrant right invasive tumor. Even with arms raised, there is no visible deformity.

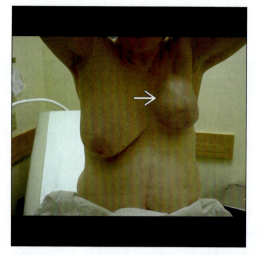

Clinical photograph shows marked asymmetry ➡ post left mastectomy, reconstruction, and chest and nodal XRT. The XRT was given with a tissue expander in place. A permanent implant is in place at this time.

TERMINOLOGY

Abbreviations

- APBI: Accelerated partial breast irradiation (shortened elapsed overall time)
  - Majority of recurrences occur at site of the initial cancer: Rationale for radiation directed more focally to lumpectomy site
  - Smaller treated volume permits an accelerated course typically over one week or less
  - More convenient for patient and decreases dose to normal tissue
- BCT: Breast-conserving treatment (lumpectomy + XRT)
- 1cGy: Centigray; 1/100 gray = 1 rad
- Rad: Radiation dose absorbed in tissue
- CALGB: Cancer and leukemia group B
- DVH: Dose volume histogram (quantitative expression of radiation dose to a given volume of structure)
- IDC: Infiltrating ductal carcinoma
- DCIS: Ductal carcinoma in situ
- IMRT: Intensity modulated radiotherapy
- MeV: Million electron volts (describes strength of electron beam energies)
- MLC: Multileaf collimator
- NSABP: National Surgical Adjuvant Breast and Bowel Project
- RTOG: Radiation Therapy Oncology Group
- WBI: Whole breast irradiation
- XRT: Radiation therapy

History

- 1902: First attempted use of ionizing XRT in treating breast cancer
- 1920: Understanding differential response of normal tissue vs. malignant tumors to XRT; understanding value of fractionation
- 1960s: Introduction of linear accelerators-versatile, rotational, photon and electron beams from same source; Iridium replaces radium as brachytherapy isotope of choice (more useful beam characteristics)

- 1980s: Exploration of dose modifying agents: Radiation sensitizers, radiation protectors, hyperthermia; investigation of altered fractionation schemes-hyperfractionation (2x/day) and hypofractionation (3x/week)
- 1990s: Three dimensional computer-generated isodose plans; immobilization devices
- 2000s: IMRT: Ability to create purposeful dose gradients within the target volume

External Beam Radiation

- Linear accelerator
  - Electron gun produces electron beam that accelerates down a waveguide to strike a tungsten target, producing photons of varying energies
- Photon therapy
  - 4-6 MeV X-rays are optimal for thickness of breast tissue to deliver desired dose at depth
  - Depth dose characteristics permit high dose deep in the breast while limiting dose to skin
  - Surgical clips placed at lumpectomy site improve target definition, particularly for boost dose; clips mark areas at high risk to facilitate XRT planning
- Electron beam therapy
  - Range of energies between 6 and 15 MeV available
  - Limited penetration in tissue; avoids potential problems of exit beam
  - Frequently used as boost following WBI at lumpectomy site; source is linear accelerator
- Isocenter
  - Center (directed toward tumor) of axis of rotation of linear accelerator
- Gantry
  - Machine component that houses wave guide; rotates about patient to permit customized treatment planning
- Collimator
  - Fits on end of gantry to modify beam shape
  - MLC are leaves that move independently to create further beam shaping

RADIATION THERAPY

Key Clinical Trials

NSABP Trial B-06
- Randomized trial of lumpectomy with or without XRT vs. mastectomy (1976); findings showed XRT necessary and breast conservation is safe
- At 20 yrs, risk of recurrent tumor ipsilateral breast = 14.3% with BCT compared with 39.2% lumpectomy without XRT (p < .001)

NSABP Trial B-17
- XRT as adjuvant treatment in management of DCIS (1985); addition of XRT decreased risk of both invasive and non-invasive recurrence
- At 8 yrs, non-invasive tumor recurrence reduced from 13.4 to 8.2% (p = .007)
- Reduction in invasive ipsilateral tumor from 13.4 to 3.9% (p < .0001)

CALGB 94-43
- Randomized trial of tamoxifen with XRT or tamoxifen alone following lumpectomy in women older than 70 yrs; adjuvant XRT may not be necessary in carefully selected elderly women

2000 Oxford Overview
- Meta-analysis of local therapy; improvement of local control with XRT resulted in improved overall survival
- 5 yr local recurrence with XRT 7% vs. 26% without; 15 yr overall mortality 49.5% without XRT, ↓ to 44.6% with XRT (p < .0001)

NSABP Protocol B-39 RTOG 0413
- Ongoing randomized trial of WBI vs. APBI

III

0

17

Brachytherapy
- Radiation delivered from a source rather than from a linear accelerator
  - Limited range of radiation permits greater normal tissue sparing than conventional external XRT
  - Can be intracavitary or interstitial; sources can be temporary or permanent
- High dose afterloading
  - Newer technique using temporary iridium sources permits XRT over a shorter time period while protecting radiation personnel
- Accelerated partial breast irradiation
  - Investigational; highly selective, early stage disease

Treatment Planning
- Simulator
  - Imaging device (fluoroscopic or CT-guided) that reproduces the actual treatment machine
  - Provides images for development of isodose plans on computer planning equipment
- 3D treatment planning
  - Standard of care today; able to fuse CT and PET images in generating targets
  - Dose can be calculated in multiple planes
- IMRT
  - Dose can be modulated across a treatment field in order to target areas at high risk while minimizing dose to surrounding normal tissue
- Boost treatment
  - Additional treatment to high risk areas (typically the lumpectomy site)
- Isodose plan
  - Graphic display of dose distribution; isodose line connects all points of the same dose; similar to isotherms on a weather map or altitude lines on a topographic map

Dose
- Unit is cGy which measures amount of radiation absorbed per unit of tissue
  - Expressed as fraction size and cumulative dose

- Fractionation: Total dose divided into smaller daily treatment typically over 5-7 weeks
  - Purpose: Allows normal tissue to repair sublethal damage whereas tumor cells do not share the same ability to repair cellular injury; result is differential killing of tumor cells while preserving normal cells in same irradiated volume
- Radiation target
  - Radiation results in DNA double strand breaks
  - Cell death occurs at time of attempted replication
  - Normal tissue has a greater ability to repair sublethal damage
- Total dose (WBI)
  - 4500-5000 cGy to the entire breast, additional 1000-1600 cGy (boost) to excisional site
  - Key is to give maximum dose to kill tumor cells with minimal damage to normal tissue
- Cumulative dose
  - Re-irradiation is not commonly performed due to concern for increased toxicity to normal tissues

Patient Setup
- Tattoo
  - Permanent pinpoint marks made with India ink to aid in repositioning patient on a regular basis; also used if question of retreatment or treatment of adjacent tissue(s) arises in the future
- Immobilization
  - Use of active or passive measures that facilitate accurate and prompt positioning of patient; "cradles" or molds can be custom made so patient can quickly find the same position on a daily basis

IMAGING ANATOMY

General Anatomic Considerations
- CT in the exact treatment position allows for computer planning to overlay isodose curves on the axial slices → idealize and customize the plan to a particular situation

RADIATION THERAPY

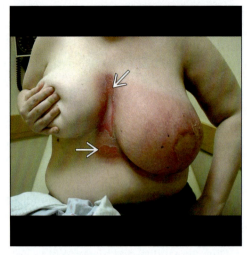

Clinical photograph shows desquamative radiation dermatitis ➡ predominantly in the inframammary fold region (an acute reversible complication) early in the course of a 5 week radiation treatment.

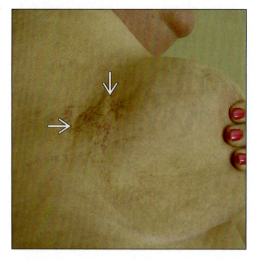

Clinical photograph 5 years after breast-conserving surgery and adjuvant radiation for DCIS in a 48 y/o. Telangiectasias ➡ (a permanent complication) are seen in the area of the radiation boost.

Critical Anatomic Structures
- Identification of the chest wall, lung, heart, and internal mammary nodes, in addition to breast tissue, is important in developing a treatment plan

CLINICAL IMPLICATIONS

Clinical Importance
- XRT standard following breast-conserving surgery
  - Additional fields are added to treat regional lymph nodes when multiple axillary nodes are involved with tumor
- Post-mastectomy XRT generally given when
  - ≥ 4 positive axillary lymph nodes
  - Primary tumors > 5 cm or when the skin or chest wall are involved
  - Locally advanced breast cancer (LABC)
  - Close or positive surgical margins
- Contraindications to breast-conserving surgery
  - Multicentric disease
  - Diffuse suspicious ipsilateral calcifications
  - Inability to obtain negative histologic margins after reasonable attempts at surgical excision/re-excision
- Contraindications to XRT
  - Collagen vascular diseases: Active systemic lupus or scleroderma
  - Prior irradiation to the breast(s) and/or chest
  - First or second trimester pregnancy

Function-Dysfunction
- Patient expectations
  - Whole breast XRT generally = 5-7 weeks 5 day/week treatments; generally well tolerated
  - Acute effects: During or in the immediate post-treatment period
    - Skin erythema, dry desquamation, moist desquamation, skin edema, breast edema
    - Fatigue
  - Late or delayed effects: Occur sometime following treatment completion

- Radiation pneumonitis: Increased risk with nodal XRT and systemic treatment
- Skin: Thickening or fibrosis; telangiectasias may occur late in high-dose areas
- Rib injury: Rarely rib fracture(s) may occur; breast and/or chest tenderness
- Cardiac: Premature coronary artery disease; unlikely with modern techniques; present day treatment shows survival advantage to XRT no longer overcome by ↑ in toxicity
- Lymphedema: Function of combined surgery and XRT to axilla; less common with sentinel node biopsy
- Brachial plexus: Injury rarely seen
- Radiation-induced malignancy: Incidence generally quoted at < 1% of long term survivors: Sarcomas most common

RELATED REFERENCES

1. Clarke M et al: Effects of radiotherapy and of differences in the extent of surgery for early breast cancer on local recurrence and 15-year survival: an overview of the randomized trials. Lancet. 366:2087-106, 2005
2. Hughes KS et al: Lumpectomy plus tamoxifen with or without irradiation in women 70 years of age or older with early breast cancer. N Engl J Med. 351:971-7, 2004
3. Fisher B et al: Twenty year followup of a randomized trial comparing total mastectomy, lumpectomy, and lumpectomy plus irradiation for the treatment of invasive breast cancer. N Engl J Med. 347:1233-41, 2002
4. Fisher B et al: Lumpectomy and radiation therapy for the treatment of intraductal breast cancer: findings from the NSABP B-17. J Clin Oncol. 16:441-52, 1998

RADIATION THERAPY

IMAGE GALLERY

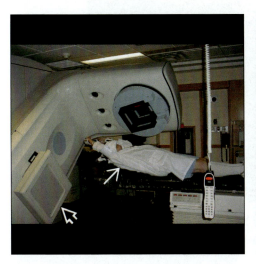

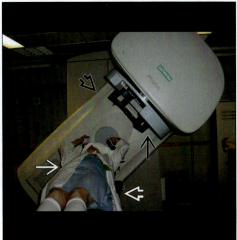

(Left) Patient reclines supine in customized body mold ➔ *for rapid, accurate, reproducible daily position. On-line portal imaging* ➔ *verifies pretreatment daily. (Right) Photograph of a supine patient* ➔ *positioned for right breast setup. Gantry* ➔ *of accelerator rotates around treatment couch* ➔ *, collimator head* ➔ *shapes the beam, and gantry angle is set for medial tangent beam.*

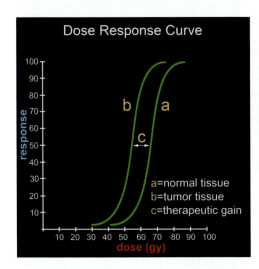

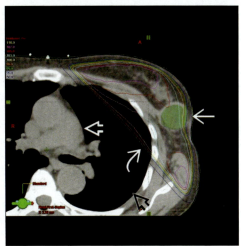

(Left) Dose response curve illustrates differential response of normal (curve "a") and tumor tissue (curve "b") to XRT. Dose-modifying agents attempt to increase the differential response, "c" = therapeutic gain. (Right) Schematic 3D treatment-planning CT shows isodose curves ➔ *reflecting medial and lateral beam arrangement. Target volume* ➔ *and breast tissue are within isodose lines. Mediastinum* ➔ *and lung* ➔ *are largely excluded (Courtesy Cytyc Corp.).*

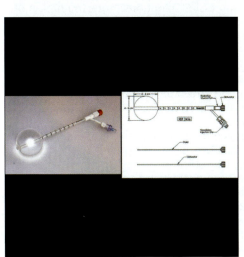

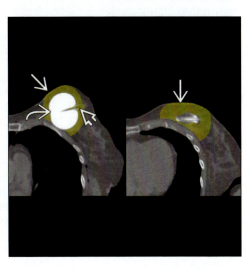

(Left) Photograph (left) and schematic (right) of a Mammosite™ intracavitary balloon catheter which is placed within a lumpectomy site where high dose XRT is introduced. (Right) Schematic 3D treatment-planning CT shows the target volume ➔ *, inflated balloon* ➔ *, and catheter* ➔ *(left) through which the radiation source is introduced. After completing treatment, the balloon is deflated (right) and catheter withdrawn (Courtesy Cytyc Corp.).*

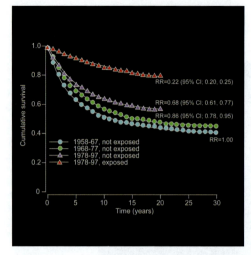

Time period	Screened or not	RR breast cancer death
1958-77	Unscreened	1.0
1978-97	Unscreened	0.84 (0.71-0.99)
1978-97	Screened	0.56 (0.49-0.64)

Figure shows survival among women exposed (red) or not exposed to screening mammography (other curves). Early detection reduces mortality from breast cancer (Tabar et al Lancet 361:1405-1410, 2003).

Table shows 44% ↓ in breast Ca mortality in 40-69 y/o women screened by mammography (same as left). 16% ↓ in mortality was attributable to improved breast cancer treatments compared to earlier time period.

TERMINOLOGY

Abbreviations
- Overall survival (OS)
- Disease-free survival (DFS): Time from randomization to treatment failure or death (any cause)
- Distant disease-free survival (DDFS)
- Tamoxifen (TAM)
- National Surgical Adjuvant Breast and Bowel Project (NSABP): Multicenter collaborative trials group

Definitions
- Neoadjuvant chemotherapy: "Primary" chemotherapy prior to surgery to shrink primary tumor and kill or inhibit growth of occult micrometastases
- Adjuvant chemotherapy: Chemotherapy after surgery to kill or inhibit growth of occult micrometastases
- Chemoprevention: Medication given to patients at high risk of cancer to reduce risk of developing cancer
- Dose-dense: Standard chemotherapy with shorter interval between cycles
- Prognostic factor: Predicts risk of relapse or death
  - If very favorable prognosis, treatment(s) may not be worth risks
  - If poor prognosis, benefits of treatment often outweigh risks
  - Clinical stage
  - Pathologic tumor size
  - Lymph node status
    - Isolated tumor cells in sentinel node: Unclear significance
  - Distant metastases
  - Gene expression array
    - 21 gene panel (Oncotype Dx™) validated on NSABP B-14 tumor blocks, recurrence risk score
    - For (ER+), stage I-II, node-negative breast cancers, predict patients most likely to benefit from systemic chemotherapy
    - Distant recurrence at 10 yrs: 7% (95% CI, 4-10) in low-risk [recurrence score (RS) < 18]; 14% (8-20) in intermediate risk (RS 18-30); and 31% (24-37) in high-risk group (RS > 30) in TAM-treated patients
    - RS correlates with OS, relapse-free interval, both in patients treated with TAM and those without
    - MammaPrint® array in Europe
  - Consider
    - Tumor grade, proliferation index, lymphovascular invasion (LVI)
- Predictive factor: Predicts sensitivity to specific treatment
  - Estrogen receptor (ER) ± progesterone receptor (PR) positive: Predicts response to hormonal therapy
  - Her-2/neu positive: Predicts response to trastuzamab (Herceptin)

PATHOLOGIC ISSUES

Classification
- Hormonal manipulation
  - Ovarian suppression: Oophorectomy, irradiation of ovaries, or by luteinizing hormone releasing hormone (LhRH) agonists/antagonists
    - For pre-menopausal women with ER+ tumors, 25% ↓ risk recurrence and mortality vs. no adjuvant therapy
    - Unclear if of added benefit when combined with TAM or ovarian toxic chemotherapy: Studies ongoing
  - Block estrogen receptor: Selective estrogen receptor modifiers (SERMs): TAM, raloxifene (Evista), toremifene (Fareston)
    - Both estrogen agonist and antagonist activities
    - Effective in pre- and post-menopausal women with ER+ tumors (~ 60-75% cancers are ER+, % increases with ↑ age of patient)
    - More effective when tumor both ER+ and PR+
  - Block estrogen production: Aromatase inhibitors (AIs): Anastrozole (Arimidex), letrozole (Femara), exemestane (Aromasin)
    - Effective only in post-menopausal women
    - AIs as initial adjuvant hormonal treatment or sequentially after TAM
    - Increased osteoporotic fractures

ONCOLOGY

Oncologic Management Strategies

Chemoprevention in High-Risk Women
- TAM or raloxifene: 49-72% reduction in risk of ER+ invasive cancer
- Fewer DCIS cases with TAM, but greater risk endometrial cancer, PE, DVT

Stage 0 Breast Cancer (DCIS)
- Consider 5 yrs TAM if ER+; AIs being studied

Stage I Breast Cancer
- ER+ cancers: TAM; AIs instead of or after TAM in post-menopausal women
- Select patients at high risk of recurrence may benefit from adjuvant chemotherapy

Stage II, III Breast Cancer
- Consider imaging to exclude distant metastases: PET CT or bone scan + CT chest, abdomen, pelvis
- Consider 3-6 months of adjuvant anthracycline-based therapy (may be more effective than CMF)
- ± Taxanes, dose dense regimen, Herceptin (if Her-2+)
- Consider neoadjuvant chemotherapy, esp. stage III
  - Reduced rates of positive margins
  - No effect on OS: Response predicts longer DFS
  - Consider adjuvant therapy post-operatively
- 5 yrs TAM for ER+ tumors; AIs instead of or after TAM in post-menopausal women

Stage IV Disease
- Palliative; systemic therapy protocols
- Herceptin for Her-2+ tumors
- TAM/AIs for ER+ tumors

- Targeted therapy: Her-2/neu receptor: Herceptin
  - Her-2/neu receptor overexpressed on cell membranes: 20-25% of invasive breast cancers
  - Epidermal growth factor (EGF) receptor type 2
  - Her-2/neu "positive": At least 2-3+ by immunohistochemistry or gene amplified by fluorescence in situ hybridization (FISH)
    - Adverse prognostic factor
  - Herceptin: Antibody to Her-2/neu receptor
    - Cardiac toxicity in up to ~ 4% of patients
    - High cost, availability may be problematic
    - Rare anaphylaxis
- Cytotoxic agents
  - Rapidly dividing cells of any type will be killed
    - Cancer cells, hematopoietic cells, hair follicles, gastrointestinal tract lining, ovarian function
  - Small risk of secondary leukemia
  - Antimetabolites: Fluorouracil ("F"), methotrexate ("M")
    - Inhibit synthesis of DNA precursors
  - Intercalaters: Anthracyclines, e.g., adriamycin ("A", doxorubicin), epirubicin ("E")
    - Intercalate into DNA, inhibit DNA synthesis
    - Cardiac toxicity
  - Alkylating agents: e.g., Cyclophosphamide ("C")
    - Damage DNA covalently; DNA repair deficient in cancer cells
  - Antimicrotubule agents: Taxanes, e.g., "T" = docetaxel (Taxotere), "PTX" = paclitaxel (Taxol)
    - Block microtubule depolymerization, inhibit cell division
    - Risk of neuropathy, allergic reaction

Staging Criteria
- Tumor, node, distant metastases (TNM)
  - X: Cannot be or not assessed, e.g., TX, NX, MX
  - Distinguish clinical (c) stage or pathologic (p) stage
  - T0: No evidence of primary tumor
  - Tis: Carcinoma in situ (ductal; lobular carcinoma in situ not treated as cancer)
  - T1: Invasive tumor ≤ 2 cm
    - T1mic: Microinvasion ≤ 0.1 cm
    - T1a: 0.1 cm < tumor size ≤ 0.5 cm
    - T1b: 0.5 cm < tumor size ≤ 1 cm
    - T1c: 1 cm < tumor size ≤ 2 cm
  - T2: 2 cm < invasive tumor size ≤ 5 cm
  - T3: Invasive tumor > 5 cm
  - T4: Tumor of any size with direct extension to
    - Chest wall (T4a), skin (T4b), both (T4c), or inflammatory carcinoma (T4d)
  - N0: No regional node metastases
  - N1: Metastasis in ipsilateral movable axillary node(s)
  - N2: Metastasis in ipsilateral fixed or matted axillary node(s) or clinically apparent internal mammary (IM) node(s)
  - N3: Metastasis in ipsilateral infraclavicular node(s) or clinically apparent IM node(s) with clinically evident axillary node(s); or metastasis ipsilateral supraclavicular node(s)
  - M0: No distant metastases
  - M1: Distant metastases
- Stage 0: Tis N0 M0 (DCIS)
- Stage I: T1 N0 M0
- Stage IIA: T0 N1 M0 or T1 N1 M0 or T2 N0 M0
- Stage IIB: T2 N1 M0 or T3 N0 M0
- Stage IIIA: T0 N2 M0 or T1 N2 M0 or T2 N2 M0 or T3 N1 M0 or T3 N2 M0
- Stage IIIB: T4 N0 M0 or T4 N1 M0 or T4 N2 M0
- Stage IIIC: Any T N3 M0
- Stage IV: Any T any N M1

Overview of Treatment Approaches
- Primary surgical treatment stage 0, I, II disease
  - Select stage I patients → systemic chemotherapy
  - Stage II: Adjuvant systemic chemotherapy if appropriate
- Consider neoadjuvant chemotherapy (NAT) if locally advanced (e.g., most stage III), followed by surgery
  - Consider NAT for larger T2 tumors, small breast
- Radiation therapy (XRT): Breast conservation, selected post-mastectomy patients
- Stage IV disease: Systemic chemotherapy protocols ± palliative local XRT ± surgery
- Hormonal therapy for ~ all ER+ tumors (begin during or after XRT)
- Herceptin for stage II-IV disease for Her-2+ tumors

ONCOLOGY

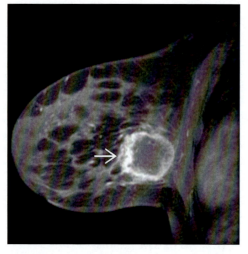

Sagittal T1 C+ FS MR shows rim-enhancing 5 cm mass ➡ in this 40 year old. US-guided biopsy = grade III IDC. MR is useful in pretreatment assessment of disease extent. (Courtesy DNS).

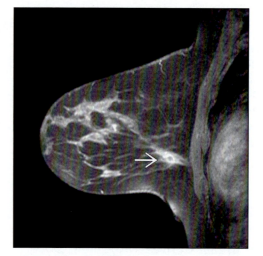

Sagittal T1 C+ FS MR (same as left) shows minimal residual enhancement ➡ after 4 cycles neoadjuvant chemotherapy. No residual tumor was found at lumpectomy (false positive MR) = complete response.

CHEMOTHERAPY RESULTS

Chemoprevention in High-Risk Women

- NSABP P-1: Tamoxifen for prevention of breast cancer
  - ↓ Risk of invasive breast cancer by 49% and DCIS by 50%
  - ↓ Risk spine and hip fractures
  - ↑ Risk endometrial cancer (risk ratio 2.53)
  - ↑ Risk of stroke, pulmonary embolism (PE), deep-vein thrombosis (DVT)
- NSABP P-2: Study of Tamoxifen and Raloxifene (STAR)
  - Raloxifene (Evista) as effective as tamoxifen at reducing risk of invasive breast cancer
  - Similar (↓) risk of osteoporotic fractures
  - Similar (↑) risk ischemic heart disease, stroke
  - Raloxifene: Trend to ↓ risk endometrial cancer (RR 0.62, 95% CI 0.35-1.08)
  - ↓ Thromboembolic events, cataracts with raloxifene

Adjuvant Chemotherapy: Early Breast Cancer

- 6 months CMF: ↓ Annual breast cancer death rate by 34% (SE 5) if diagnosed < age 50; 10% (SE 3) if 50-69 yrs old at diagnosis
- 3-6 months FAC or FEC: ↓ Annual breast cancer death rate 38% (SE 5) if diagnosed < age 50; 20% (SE 4) if 50-69 yrs old at diagnosis
  - May be more effective than CMF
- Addition of taxane with or after AC or EC improves OS
- Dose-dense regimens: Slight improvement in OS
- Herceptin: 50% ↓ recurrence & 33% ↓ mortality when combined with other adjuvant chemotherapy in Her-2+ breast cancer
- Addition of TAM for 5 years for ER+ disease: ↓ Annual breast cancer death rate by 31% (SE 3)
  - Regardless of chemotherapy, age or PR status
  - Five yrs treatment significantly more effective than 1-2 yrs
- Aromatase inhibitors (AIs) instead of TAM or sequentially
  - Arimidex, tamoxifen, alone or in combination (ATAC) trial: Benefits of Arimidex over TAM
    - Prolonged DFS, time to recurrence
    - Reduced distant metastases
    - 42% ↓ in contralateral breast cancers; 53% ↓ in ER+ second primaries
    - No benefit to combination with TAM
    - Other AIs vs. TAM: Similar results to ATAC
    - 3.6-4.6% absolute increase in DFS at 3-7 yrs
    - No evidence of survival benefit
  - Other studies: Slight benefit to initial TAM 2-5 yrs then switch to AIs; also more cost-effective

RELATED REFERENCES

1. Habel LA et al: A population-based study of tumor gene expression and risk of breast cancer death among lymph node-negative patients. Breast Cancer Res. 8:R25, 2006
2. Paik S et al: Gene expression and benefit of chemotherapy in women with node-negative, estrogen receptor-positive breast cancer. J Clin Oncol. 24:3726-34, 2006
3. Vogel VG et al: Effects of tamoxifen vs raloxifene on the risk of developing invasive breast cancer and other disease outcomes: the NSABP Study of Tamoxifen and Raloxifene (STAR) P-2 trial. JAMA. 295:2727-41, 2006
4. Early Breast Cancer Trialists' Collaborative Group: Effects of chemotherapy and hormonal therapy for early breast cancer on recurrence and 15-year survival: an overview of the randomised trials. Lancet. 365:1687-717, 2005
5. Howell A et al: Results of the ATAC (Arimidex, Tamoxifen, Alone or in Combination) trial after completion of 5 years' adjuvant treatment for breast cancer. Lancet. 365(9453):60-2, 2005
6. Romond EH et al: Trastuzumab plus adjuvant chemotherapy for operable HER2-positive breast cancer. N Engl J Med. 353:1673-84, 2005
7. Paik S et al: A multigene assay to predict recurrence of tamoxifen-treated, node-negative breast cancer. N Engl J Med. 351:2817-26, 2004
8. Singletary SE et al: Revision of the American Joint Committee on Cancer staging system for breast cancer. J Clin Oncol. 20:3628-36, 2002
9. Fisher B et al: Tamoxifen for prevention of breast cancer: report of the National Surgical Adjuvant Breast and Bowel Project P-1 Study. J Natl Cancer Inst. 90:1371-88, 1998
10. Early Breast Cancer Trialists' Collaborative Group. Ovarian ablation in early breast cancer: Overview of the randomised trials. Lancet. 348:1189-96, 1996

ONCOLOGY

IMAGE GALLERY

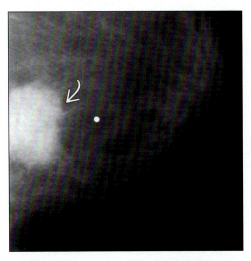

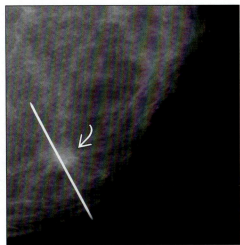

(Left) CC mammography shows 3.5 cm spiculated, palpable mass ⇗ posterior inner left breast in this 37 year old. Clinically this was fixed to the chest wall, though mammography is inadequate to assess this. Core biopsy showed grade II IDC & DCIS. *(Right)* CC mammography after 4 cycles AC shows marked shrinkage of the tumor ⇗, now nonpalpable. Needle-localized excision revealed an 1.7 cm residual (grade III) IDC & DCIS with clear margins.

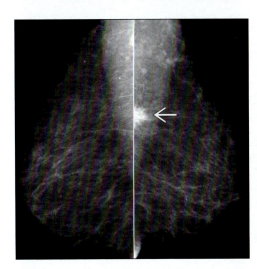

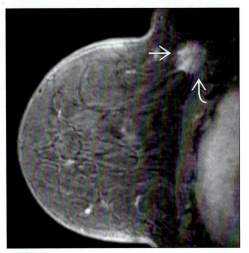

(Left) MLO mammography shows spiculated mass ➡, clinically fixed to the chest wall, in this 85 year old. US-guided 14-g core biopsy showed mixed IDC-ILC. *(Right)* Sagittal T1 C+ FS MR (same as left) shows enhancement of spiculated mass ➡ & pectoral muscle ⇗, compatible w/chest wall invasion. In view of age, direct excision performed, w/positive posterior margins despite resection of part of pectoral muscle. MR accurately depicts chest wall involvement.

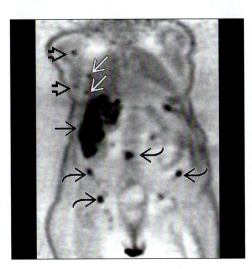

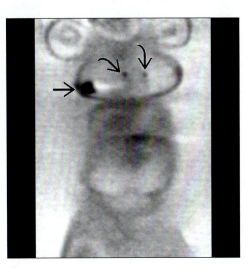

(Left) Coronal whole body FDG PET scan shows diffuse metastatic disease in the liver ➡, spine and pelvis ⇗, lung ➡, and right axilla ⇨ in this 78 year old woman who presented with back pain. (Courtesy MP). *(Right)* Anterior coronal FDG PET scan (same patient as previous) shows previously unknown primary right breast cancer ➡ and additional metastases ⇗. FDG PET and PET CT are effective for staging advanced breast cancer. (Courtesy MP).

PART IV
Diagnoses

Introduction and Overview 0

Lesion Imaging Characteristics 1

Histopathologic Diagnoses 2

Anatomic Considerations 3

Post-Operative Imaging Findings 4

Special Topics 5

Infections and Inflammation 6

Artifacts 7

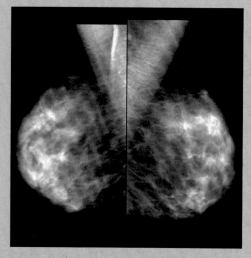

Mammography shows heterogeneously dense parenchyma in a 32 y/o with lump left breast. Mammogram itself is negative, but US is needed: BI-RADS 0. Preferably, US is performed at same visit.

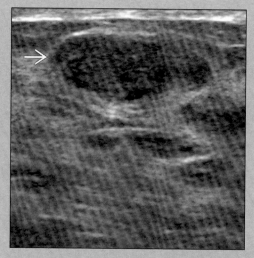

US (same patient as previous) shows a circumscribed, gently lobulated, slightly hypoechoic mass ➡. Biopsy was recommended: Integrated mammography + US report = BI-RADS 4A. Biopsy: Fibroadenoma.

TERMINOLOGY

Abbreviations
- BI-RADS®: Mammography = Breast Imaging Reporting and Data System for Mammography
  - Please note: Terms may undergo revision; please consult current edition of lexicon published by the American College of Radiology (ACR)
  - Minor modifications to phrasing have been made
- Mammography Quality Standards Act (MQSA)

Definitions
- A lexicon of terminology developed through the ACR
  - Standardized terms to describe breast density, mammographic findings, assessment, and management recommendations
- Includes guidance on report organization and audits
- Facilitates communication across facilities, disciplines
- Descriptors ≈ listed in order of ↑ risk malignancy
  - Consider combination of features → management
- Baseline = first mammogram

ANATOMY-BASED IMAGING ISSUES

Key Concepts or Questions
- Reason for examination must be clearly indicated
  - Screening or diagnostic
  - Describe prior breast procedures and results of biopsies, known risk factors
- Comparison to prior mammograms when possible

Imaging Protocols
- Standard CC and MLO views of both breasts
- Implant-displaced views also in women with implants
- Additional views may be obtained as needed
- Recommended: Describe views obtained in report

Breast Composition
- Almost entirely fat: Mostly fatty replaced
  - Mammographic sensitivity 97-98%
- Scattered fibroglandular densities
  - Can be further described as minimal or moderate

- Heterogeneously dense: ~ 51-75% glandular
  - "Which could obscure detection of small masses"
  - Mammographic sensitivity reduced: 64-70%
- Extremely dense: > 75% glandular
  - "Which lowers the sensitivity of mammography"
  - Mammographic sensitivity reduced: 30-48%
    - Masses obscured; most Ca++ still seen
- "Dense" = heterogeneously dense or extremely dense
  - > 1/2 of women < 50 years have dense breasts
  - ~ 1/3 of women ≥ 50 years have dense breasts
  - 15% improvement in sensitivity with digital mammography in dense breasts vs. film

Lesion Location
- Location: Give breast, clock face or quadrant or specific location, and depth
  - Clock Face: Superimpose clock on top of breast
    - 9:00 is outer right breast and inner left breast
  - Quadrant: Upper outer (UOQ); upper inner (UIQ); lower outer (LOQ); lower inner (LIQ)
  - Specific location
    - Subareolar = retroareolar (does not require depth)
    - Central = directly behind nipple
    - Axillary tail (does not require statement of depth)
- Depth: Divide breast into thirds nipple to chest wall
  - Anterior, middle, or posterior
  - Alternatively, give distance from nipple in cm

PATHOLOGIC ISSUES

Mass
- Use "focal asymmetry" on screening if finding seen on only one view, not clearly a three-dimensional mass
  - Diagnostic views, US, may reveal underlying mass
- Describe shape, margin, density
- Describe any associated findings

Calcifications
- Typically benign Ca++ need not all be described
  - Dermal, vascular, coarse, popcorn-like, secretory (large rod-like), round, lucent-centered, eggshell or rim, milk of calcium, suture, dystrophic

MAMMOGRAPHY BI-RADS® LEXICON AND USAGE

Key Facts

BI-RADS: Mammography Concepts
- Management based on worst feature(s) present
- Cancers usually have multiple suspicious findings
- To be "benign", lesion must lack any suspicious features and have specific benign appearance
- Screening generally BI-RADS 1, 2, or 0 assessment
  - Absent comparison films: Usually can be 1 or 2; code as BI-RADS "0" only if would need workup if finding(s) new or increasing
- Probably benign classification, BI-RADS 3, validated, often misused
  - Generally requires full diagnostic work-up first
  - Finding should have < 2% risk of malignancy based on literature ± internal audit
    - Circumscribed mass, baseline: If US shows cyst, BI-RADS 2

- Focal asymmetry, thins on spot compression: US can help exclude mass
    - Cluster of punctate Ca++ on baseline
  - Usually not for new or increasing findings
    - Except: Suspected hormonally-influenced asymmetries after full work-up
- Assessment guided by most suspicious finding(s) ± those needing acute work-up (e.g., known cancer but needs biopsy of another lesion → BI-RADS 4)

MQSA Requirements
- BI-RADS assessment included at end of report
  - Strongly recommended for other breast imaging
- System for tracking outcomes after abnormal reports (BI-RADS 0, 4, 5)
- Patient should receive lay letter summarizing results and recommendations

- Milk of calcium best demonstrated on CC and 90° lateral magnification views
    - Remainder of typically benign Ca++ rarely need further work-up
- Describe morphology, distribution if not typically benign
  - Magnification CC and 90° lateral views generally needed for adequate characterization

Architectural Distortion
- Lines or spiculations radiating from a point ± focal retraction at edge of parenchyma
- A standalone descriptor or associated finding

Special Cases
- Solitary dilated duct: Usually retroareolar, benign unless other suspicious findings
- Intramammary lymph node: Fat-containing, circumscribed, usually upper outer quadrant, ≤ 1 cm; can be anywhere in breast
  - When involved by tumor, cortex thickens, fatty hilum ↓ or gone, same adverse prognosis as axillary node metastasis
- Global asymmetry: Large (~ > 2 cm²) area of one breast is denser than contralateral breast
  - Requires clinical correlation, often normal variant
  - If palpable ± associated suspicious findings (e.g. Ca++ or distortion), merits workup
- Focal Asymmetry: Small (~ ≤ 2 cm²), relatively discrete area of tissue density
  - Asymmetry may be seen on one view or both views; "focal" typically on both views
  - Lacks border and conspicuity of a true mass
    - Spot compression, US may reveal underlying mass
  - More suspicious when new: Comparison to prior exams critical for such a finding
  - When due to normal variation, will usually demonstrate interspersed fat

Associated Findings
- Skin retraction, nipple retraction, skin thickening, trabecular thickening, skin lesion(s), axillary adenopathy

- Architectural distortion ± Ca++ may be seen alone or associated with a mass or asymmetry

PATHOLOGY-BASED IMAGING ISSUES

Mass Shape
- Round, oval, lobular, irregular

Mass Margin
- Circumscribed: At least 75% of margin is well-defined, with remainder no worse than obscured
  - < 2% risk of malignancy, BI-RADS 3, on baseline
  - Multiple, bilateral circumscribed masses BI-RADS 2
    - Any palpable, dominant, or suspicious mass → US
    - Cysts ± fibroadenoma(s) (FAs)
  - Biopsy if enlarges, suspicious feature(s), not a cyst
  - 12-13% of masses biopsied; 0-9% malignant
- Obscured: Margin hidden by overlying tissue
  - Used when margin believed to be circumscribed
  - Spot compression views ± US needed for further characterization
- Microlobulated: Short cycle undulations
  - 3-4% of masses biopsied; 17-50% malignant
- Indistinct: Ill-defined, suggests infiltration
  - 12-38% of masses biopsied; 44-60% malignant
- Spiculated: Radiating lines extend from mass
  - 15-40% of masses biopsied; 81-97% malignant
  - Invasive ductal carcinoma (IDC) NOS, invasive lobular carcinoma, tubular carcinoma; radial scar, post-surgical scar

Mass Density
- Compare to equal volume of fibroglandular tissue
- High, equal, low: Inconsistent across observers
  - High-density uncommon (6% of lesions biopsied), favors malignancy: 87% PPV one series
- Fat-containing: At least partially radiolucent
  - Overwhelmingly likely benign: Oil cyst, lipoma, fibroadenolipoma, galactocele, lymph node
  - Rarely, early malignancy can trap fat

MAMMOGRAPHY BI-RADS® LEXICON AND USAGE

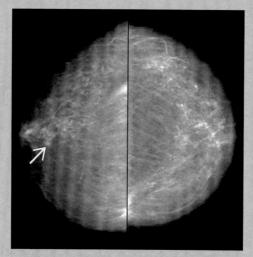

CC mammography shows subtle focal asymmetry ➡️ retroareolar right breast, BI-RADS 0 with need for comparison to prior mammograms, and spot compression if not shown stable.

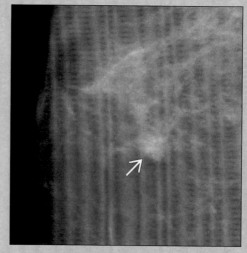

CC mammography spot compression (same patient as previous) shows subtle spiculated mass ➡️, new: BI-RADS 5. Biopsy: Grade II IDC. A focal asymmetry on screening can be a mass on additional views ± US.

Calcification Morphology

- If typically benign, use specific descriptors above
- Punctate: < 0.5 mm, round shape
  - Scattered, diffuse typically benign: Adenosis
  - Clustered on baseline, BI-RADS 3
  - New cluster BI-RADS 4; 11% malignant among Ca++ biopsied
- Coarse, heterogeneous: > 0.5 mm irregular Ca++
  - Calcifying FA, fibrosis, fat necrosis
  - 7% malignancy rate when biopsied
- Amorphous: Too small or hazy to define morphology
  - 20-26% rate of malignancy, usually low grade DCIS
- Fine pleomorphic: ≤ 0.5 mm irregular Ca++, vary in size and shape
  - 25-41% risk of malignancy among lesions biopsied
- Fine linear/branching: Thin linear, irregular or curvilinear Ca++, suggests filling of a duct lumen irregularly involved by tumor
  - > 80% risk of malignancy, often high grade DCIS

Calcification Distribution

- Diffuse, scattered: When bilateral, any morphology, usually benign
  - When unilateral, manage based on morphology
- Regional: Scattered in large volume, > 2 cm³
  - Consider morphology: Punctate favors benign
  - 4% of Ca++ biopsied; 46% malignant
- Grouped or clustered: ≥ 5 Ca++ in 1 cm³
  - 80% of Ca++ biopsied; 36% malignant
- Linear: Suggests Ca++ in a duct
  - Elevates suspicion of any morphology
  - 6% of Ca++ biopsied; 68% malignant
- Segmental: Ca++ in duct(s) ± branches
  - 7% of Ca++ biopsied; 74% malignant

Assessments, Recommendations

- 0: Incomplete, additional evaluation needed
  - Usually a screening assessment; rarely after diagnostic mammography ± US → MR needed
- 1: Negative, no lesion found, routine follow-up
  - Note: Common typically benign findings do not all require description (e.g., nodes, vascular Ca++)
- 2: Benign, routine follow-up
- 3: Probably benign, short interval (e.g. 6-month) follow-up
- 4: Suspicious, optional subdivision
  - Subdivision is not officially sanctioned by Food and Drug Administration
  - 4A = Low suspicion, consider biopsy
  - 4B = Intermediate suspicion, biopsy
  - 4C = Moderate suspicion, biopsy
- 5: Highly suggestive of malignancy, take appropriate action (typically biopsy)
- 6: Known biopsy-proven malignancy
  - Following neoadjuvant chemotherapy
  - Second opinion, outside imaging, prior to treatment
- Integrate US + mammography findings in one report
  - One combined assessment

RELATED REFERENCES

1. Burnside ES et al: The ability of microcalcification descriptors in the BI-RADS 4th edition to stratify the risk of malignancy. Radiologic Society of North America (abstr). 286, 2005

2. Hong AS et al: BI-RADS for sonography: positive and negative predictive values of sonographic features. AJR Am J Roentgenol. 184(4):1260-5, 2005

3. D'Orsi CJ et al: Breast Imaging Reporting and Data System (BI-RADS): Mammography, 4th ed. Reston: American College of Radiology, 2003

4. Rosen EL et al: Malignant lesions initially subjected to short-term mammographic follow-up. Radiology. 223(1):221-8, 2002

5. Varas X et al: Revisiting the mammographic follow-up of BI-RADS category 3 lesions. AJR Am J Roentgenol. 179(3):691-5, 2002

6. Vizcaino I et al: Short-term follow-up results in 795 nonpalpable probably benign lesions detected at screening mammography. Radiology. 219(2):475-83, 2001

7. Liberman L et al: The breast imaging reporting and data system: positive predictive value of mammographic features and final assessment categories. AJR Am J Roentgenol. 171(1):35-40, 1998

8. Sickles EA: Nonpalpable, circumscribed, noncalcified solid breast masses: likelihood of malignancy based on lesion size and age of patient. Radiology. 192(2):439-42, 1994

IMAGE GALLERY

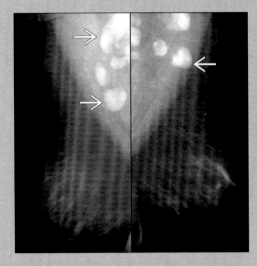
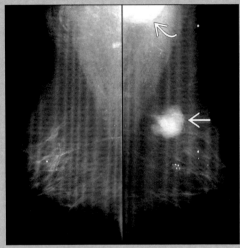

(Left) Screening MLO mammograms show bilateral large, dense axillary nodes ➡ in 57 y/o with known mycosis fungoides. The breasts are negative; BI-RADS 6, known malignancy, excluded from screening audits. *(Right)* 62 y/o with prior lymphoma had recent FNAB of left axillary mass ➡: Metastatic breast cancer. Mammography shows dense mass ➡ suspicious for the primary. BI-RADS 4C or 5, not 6, as biopsy of the breast mass is most acute problem.

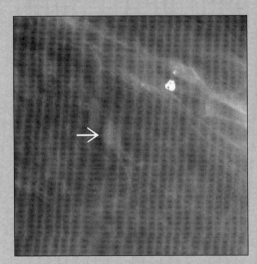
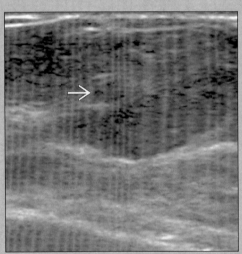

(Left) CC mammography magnification shows new, mostly circumscribed mass ➡ in this 61 y/o post lumpectomy and radiation 12 years earlier for invasive ductal cancer. *(Right)* US of the mammographic mass (same patient as previous) shows mostly circumscribed, oval, hypoechoic mass ➡. This was erroneously classified as BI-RADS 3. At 6 months, stable; at 12 months, larger. Biopsy: Papillary DCIS. BI-RADS 3 is not appropriate for new or enlarging solid masses.

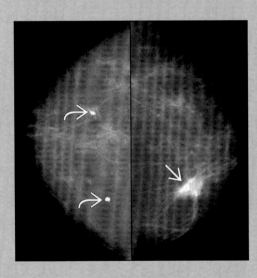
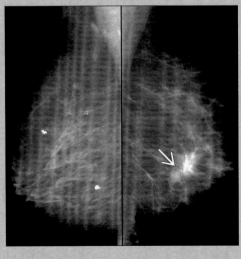

(Left) Screening CC mammograms show spiculated mass ➡ with distortion inner left breast & benign Ca++ on right ➡. *(Right)* MLO mammography (same as on left) confirms spiculated mass ➡. While most screening assessments are BI-RADS 1, 2, or 0, left breast mass is suspicious for cancer and can be coded BI-RADS 4 or 5 from screening. Direct communication with referring physician and patient is needed. Biopsy = grade III IDC.

ONE-VIEW-ONLY FINDINGS

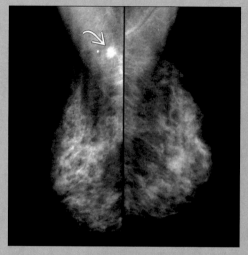

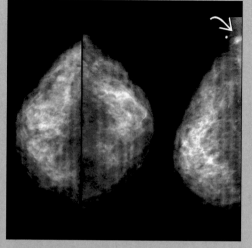

MLO mammography shows indistinctly marginated mass corresponding to palpable finding superimposed on axillary tail right breast ➔.

Routine CC views (left, same patient as previous image) do not include the palpable mass. XCCL view (right) is able to include the palpable mass axillary tail right breast ➔. Biopsy = 8 mm IDC.

TERMINOLOGY

Abbreviations
- Laterally exaggerated CC view (XCCL)
- Medially exaggerated CC view (XCCM)
- Craniocaudal view with the top of the breast rolled medially (CCRM)
- CC view with the top of the breast rolled laterally (CCRL)

Definitions
- Mammographic finding seen on either CC or MLO view
- Two types of findings most common
  - Focal asymmetry(ies) that could represent normal variant
  - Mass ± calcifications (Ca++) ± architectural distortion included on only one view due to its location
- Mass generally defined as space-occupying in two projections; potential mass seen in only one view usually described as "focal asymmetry"
- Summation shadow = summation artifact: Superimposition of normal breast structures in one view only, mimicking a true finding
- Step obliques: Images obtained in gradually increasing obliquity (e.g. 15°, 30°) for lesion seen in only CC view
- Posterior nipple line: Line drawn from nipple to perpendicular to pectoral muscle on MLO or back edge of film on CC view

IMAGING ANATOMY

General Anatomic Considerations
- Posteromedial breast only included on CC view
  - XCCM view can be used to maximize tissue included
  - Sternalis muscle is a normal variant in the posteromedial breast
    - Triangular or rounded structure at extreme medial chest wall

- Occurs in < 8% of population
- Unilateral twice as common as bilateral
- Axillary tail often included only on MLO view
  - XCCL view can include this area in CC projection
    - If tissue extends to posterior outer edge of CC mammogram, XCCL view should be routinely obtained by technologist to complete the exam
- Inframammary fold region often excluded from both views
  - Final step in positioning is elevation of the inframammary fold
- Lesions in or near the skin difficult to see on analog CC and MLO films due to relative overexposure at skin surface
  - Hotlight can help demonstrate superficial findings
  - Astute technologist can annotate skin lesions on patient history form ± place markers
  - Superficial findings may move a great deal between CC and MLO views

ANATOMY-BASED IMAGING ISSUES

Key Concepts or Questions
- First determine if finding is likely to have been included on the other projection or not
  - Posterior lesions are often excluded: Additional views ± US
  - Posterior nipple line should measure within 1 cm of the same between CC and MLO views
    - Repeat with better positioning when needed
- A focal asymmetry in one view may be able to be dismissed as summation artifact based on its appearance in the second routine view
  - If the area is clearly included
  - If there is corresponding tissue which clearly spreads out in the second view
  - If there is only minimal scattered density which is unlikely to obscure a true finding
  - Normal tissue should contain interspersed fat
- Comparison to prior mammograms particularly helpful for one-view-only asymmetries

ONE-VIEW-ONLY FINDINGS

Key Facts

Prevalence
- 3.3% of screening mammograms (Sickles)
- 85% one-view-only findings = focal asymmetries; another 11% are due to possible distortion
- 83% of all one-view-only findings are due to summation artifact
  - 56% dismissed as such from screening views
  - 69% of recalled asymmetries or possible distortions
- 1.8% of one-view-only findings malignant

Imaging Approach
- Optimize positioning to fully include breast tissue
  - Use small cassette/detector when possible
    - ↑ Compression, ↓ radiation dose, ↓ scatter
- Comparison to prior mammograms
  - Improve recognition of subtle new findings

- Reduce false positives
- Additional mammographic views
  - Spot compression → thins or persists
  - Establish three-dimensional location
- US of palpable findings
- Low threshold for US of focal asymmetries
  - Approximate location can be inferred even if seen on only one view
- Stereotactic biopsy usually feasible when indicated
- MR can be used for problem solving, rarely needed

Consider
- Early malignancies may partially thin on spot compression: US can be helpful
- Focal asymmetries overrepresented among missed cancers

- Helps reduce need for recall for stable focal asymmetries
  - Normal variant typically contains interspersed fat
- Stability should not preclude work-up of suspicious findings
- ~ 20% of neodensities malignant
  - Exclude hormone replacement therapy (HRT) as cause: Consider discontinuing HRT for 6 weeks and repeat
- Determine if the finding is real
  - Spot compression of focal asymmetries
    - Assure finding is included in the spot compression view
    - Repeat of the original projection can be helpful if the finding appears to dissipate
    - Use broad paddle or 8 x 10" cassette with good compression if spot compression ambiguous
    - If the finding persists, then additional projections may be warranted prior to US
    - Caution: Some small indistinctly margined masses may appear to thin with spot compression
    - Low threshold for US for further evaluation
  - Exclude skinfolds, artifacts mistaken for calcifications
- Triangulation
  - Used when a finding is seen in only two of the following three views: CC, MLO, and/or 90° lateral views (usually MLO and 90° lateral views)
  - With the MLO view displayed between CC and 90° lateral views, and the nipples aligned, a line drawn through the lesion in the two projections in which the lesion is visible will project onto the third view where the lesion should lie
  - Lateral lesions move lower from CC to MLO to 90° views
  - Medial lesions rise from CC to MLO to 90° views

Imaging Approaches
- Determine the three-dimensional location of the lesion by use of additional special projections ± US
- Rarely MR may be warranted in further evaluation

Imaging Protocols
- Appropriate next imaging derives from projection in which finding is well seen
- For a persistent concerning finding seen only on the CC view
  - CCRL or CCRM views or both
    - A lesion which moves with the top of the breast is superiorly located
    - Facilitates targeted US even if only seen in CC projection
  - Shallow oblique views
    - Step obliques can help establish location
  - US of pertinent region of breast
    - Can perform in mammographic template grid
    - Reproduce mammographic positioning by scanning in upright sitting position, holding breast as in CC view
  - Stereotactic biopsy is usually feasible
    - Vague asymmetries may be difficult to target
    - For extreme posterior lesions, arm can be pulled through opening in stereotactic table to help access posterior breast
- For a persistent lesion seen only on the MLO view
  - Posterior-superior lesions most often lateral: XCCL view can help depict in CC projection
    - Less commonly medial: XCCM view
    - High 12:00 location difficult to include on CC view: "Tuck" view emphasizing superior breast, excluding inferior breast
  - True lateral view
    - Can help with posterior-inferior lesions
    - Posterior-inferior lesions usually lower inner: US
    - Extreme posterior-superior breast tissue may be excluded
  - Rolled oblique views can be performed: e.g. Outer rolled superiorly, inner inferiorly
  - US of pertinent half of breast
  - Stereotactic biopsy often feasible
- MR for problem solving in unusual cases
  - Persistent subtle distortion in one view, US negative, no history of surgery or trauma, not easily biopsied

ONE-VIEW-ONLY FINDINGS

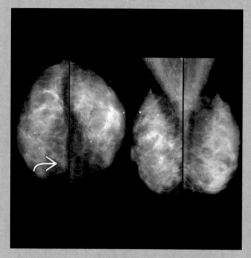

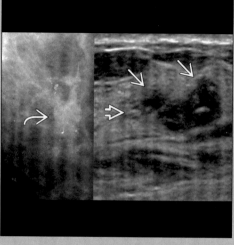

CC (left) and MLO (right) mammograms show new focal asymmetry with Ca++ posterior inner right breast, seen only on the CC view ⟳. This area could not be included on orthogonal projections.

Magnification CC view (left-hand image, same as previous) shows irregular mass ➔ with Ca++. US (on right) shows irregular hypoechoic mass ➔ with Ca++ ➔ at 2:00. US-biopsy = grade II IDC + DCIS.

- o New focal asymmetry equivocal after additional work-up, not easily biopsied
- o Not appropriate in lieu of biopsy for Ca++

Imaging Pitfalls

- Rolled views are only of value if finding will be displaced onto fatty tissue
  - o When projected onto dense tissue → obscured
- Review of prior mammograms in patients with cancer will show focal asymmetry at that site in > 50%
  - o Many quite subtle, mimic normal tissue
  - o Of those considered normal/benign even on retrospective review by majority of expert reviews, computer-assisted detection will mark ~ 30%

PATHOLOGIC ISSUES

General Pathologic Considerations

- Infiltrating lobular carcinoma (ILC)
  - o Majority of ILC mammographically subtle or occult
  - o Often seen in only one view: More commonly CC
  - o Subtle indistinct or spiculated mass ± distortion
  - o US helpful to depict and guide biopsy
    - ▪ Relatively inaccurate at determining size of ILC
  - o MR helps depict size and multifocal, multicentric, contralateral disease
    - ▪ Lobular carcinoma in situ (LCIS) a source of false positives
- Infiltrating ductal carcinoma (IDC) NOS
  - o Can rarely entrap fat
  - o Most one-view-only IDC due to extreme posterior location: Attention to positioning
    - ▪ Additional views, US as needed
- Ductal carcinoma in situ (DCIS)
  - o Most often manifest as Ca++
  - o May be seen in only one view due to extreme posterior location
  - o Motion artifact may cause blurring in one projection, obscure Ca++
    - ▪ Repeat with better compression
    - ▪ Small cassette/detector improves compression
    - ▪ True lateral view of area of interest

RELATED REFERENCES

1. Berg WA et al: Mammographic-sonographic correlation. Radiol. Clin North Am. In press, 2006
2. Ikeda DM et al: Computer-aided detection output on 172 subtle findings on normal mammograms previously obtained in women with breast cancer detected at follow-up screening mammography. Radiology. 230:811-9, 2004
3. Ikeda DM et al: Analysis of 172 Subtle Findings on Prior Normal Mammograms in Women with Breast Cancer Detected at Follow-up Screening. Radiology. 226(2):494-503, 2003
4. Shetty MK et al: Sonographic evaluation of focal asymmetric density of the breast. Ultrasound Q. 18(2):115-121, 2002
5. Brenner J: Asymmetric densities of the breast: strategies for imaging evaluation. Semin Roentgenol. 36(201-216, 2001
6. Butler RS et al: Sonographic evaluation of infiltrating lobular carcinoma. AJR. 172(2):325-330, 1999
7. Hussain HK et al: The significance of new densities and microcalcification in the second round of breast screening. Clin Radiol. 54(4):243-247, 1999
8. Lee CH et al: Clinical usefulness of MR imaging of the breast in the evaluation of the problematic mammogram. AJR. 173:1323-9, 1999
9. Sickles EA: Findings at mammographic screening on only one standard projection: outcomes analysis. Radiology. 208(2):471-475, 1998
10. Harvey JA et al: Previous mammograms in patients with impalpable breast carcinoma: retrospective vs blinded interpretation. 1993 ARRS President's Award. AJR. 161:1167-72, 1993
11. Brem RF et al: Template-guided breast US. Radiology. 184:872-4, 1992
12. Berkowitz JE et al: Equivocal mammographic findings: evaluation with spot compression. Radiology. 171(2):369-371, 1989
13. Sickles EA: Combining spot-compression and other special views to maximize mammographic information. Radiology. 173(2):571, 1989
14. Sickles EA: Practical solutions to common mammographic problems: tailoring the examination. AJR. 151:31-9, 1988
15. Swann CA et al: Localization of occult breast lesions: practical solutions to problems of triangulation. Radiology. 163(2):577-579, 1987

ONE-VIEW-ONLY FINDINGS

IMAGE GALLERY

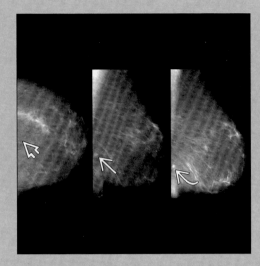

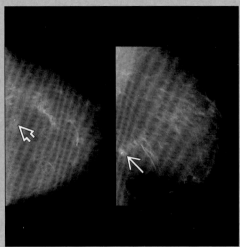

(Left) Triangulation of 6 mm IDC seen only on MLO view in a 71 year old. With the MLO view in the middle, and the nipples aligned, the expected location of the mass in the CC view can be inferred ➡ from its location in the MLO ➡ and 90° lateral views ➡ as a line can be drawn through any finding across the three views. *(Right)* Post-clip mammograms confirm the location of the mass and clip (same case as on left) on better-positioned CC ➡ and MLO ➡ views.

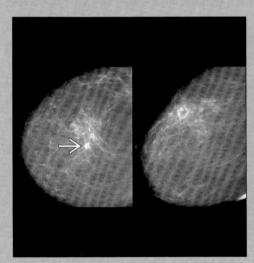

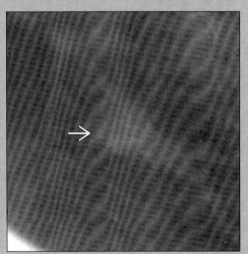

(Left) CC and MLO mammograms show new 8 mm focal asymmetry on CC view ➡, probably in the upper breast, but not well seen on the MLO view (right) in this 62 year old. *(Right)* CC mammography spot compression of the focal asymmetry (same as previous image) shows persistence of a spiculated 8 mm mass ➡, moderately suspicious for malignancy.

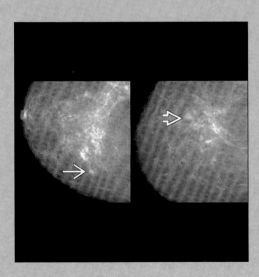

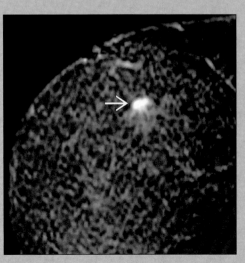

(Left) Rolled CC views were obtained (same as prior two images). On CCRM view, the mass moves medially ➡, with the upper breast. On CCRL view, the mass superimposes on an area of tissue density ➡. US was negative, and the mass could not be clearly seen on attempted stereotactic biopsy. *(Right)* Sagittal T1 C+ subtraction MR (same as previous) shows spiculated 8 mm mass in the upper breast ➡, biopsied successfully under MR guidance yielding DCIS with microinvasion.

ULTRASOUND BI-RADS® LEXICON AND USAGE

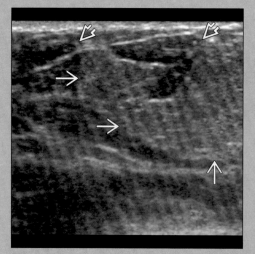

US shows homogeneously hyperechoic parenchyma ➡ in this 34 year old lactating woman. The subcutaneous fat ➡ remains normal in appearance.

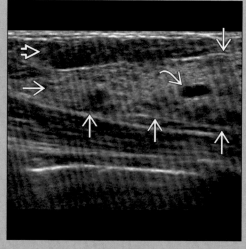

US shows subcutaneous fat ➡. The parenchyma ➡ shows heterogeneous echotexture with a small cyst ➡, typical of dense parenchyma with fibrocystic changes in this 41 year old.

TERMINOLOGY

Abbreviations
- Breast Imaging Reporting and Data System for breast ultrasound: BI-RADS®:US
  - Please note: Terms may undergo revision; please consult current edition of lexicon published by the American College of Radiology (ACR)
  - Minor modifications to phrasing have been made

Definitions
- Standardized terms to describe breast texture, abnormal findings, assessment and management recommendations
- Facilitates communication across facilities
- Facilitates tracking of patients and outcomes analysis
- Incidental finding: Seen only on US, no signs or symptoms of breast cancer
- Cyst: Anechoic, circumscribed mass with posterior enhancement, imperceptible wall, fluid-filled
  - Typical cysts are benign, BI-RADS 2
- Findings other than cysts or special cases require full description of features

Special Cases
- Unique diagnosis or finding
- Does not require description of margins, boundary, echo pattern, posterior features, or effect on surrounding tissue
- Mass in or on skin: Typically a benign finding such as sebaceous cyst, epidermal inclusion cyst, BI-RADS 2
- Complicated cyst: Special case only when nonpalpable, incidental, with imperceptible wall, mobile internal echoes, and/or fluid-debris level
  - In company of simple cysts, can be dismissed as benign finding(s): BI-RADS 2
  - Complicated cysts can be hypoechoic and indistinguishable from solid lesions: With this appearance, their features should be described, and may require surveillance, BI-RADS 3
  - If palpable or enlarging (e.g., on mammography), may require aspiration for symptomatic relief or to exclude abscess: BI-RADS 4A

- Distinguish from complex cystic (cystic and solid) lesion which merits biopsy
- Clustered microcysts: BI-RADS 2 or 3 depending on level of certainty in finding
- Intraductal mass: Usually a papilloma, requires biopsy, BI-RADS 4A
- Foreign body: Includes clip, coil, wire, catheter sleeve
  - Silicone granuloma = siliconoma = snowstorm appearance, rarely anechoic areas, BI-RADS 2
- Lymph node: Peripherally hypoechoic, centrally hyperechoic, circumscribed mass
  - Normal-appearing lymph nodes dismissed as benign, BI-RADS 2
  - Abnormal nodes: Focally thickened cortex ± diminutive fatty hilum ± indistinct margins suspicious
    - Enlarged node(s) with symmetrically thickened cortex favor benign, reactive adenopathy
    - Correlation with clinical history needed; reactive nodes due to known HIV benign, BI-RADS 2
  - New abnormal node BI-RADS 4, merits fine needle aspiration or core biopsy
  - Suspicious nodes in patient with known lymphoma BI-RADS 6, known malignancy

ANATOMY-BASED IMAGING ISSUES

Background Echotexture
- Homogeneous: Entirely hypoechoic fat lobules or entirely echogenic tissue (usually = extremely dense on mammography)
- Heterogeneous: Focally or diffusely variable in echotexture, may lower sensitivity of US

Labeling
- Orientation: Obtain orthogonal images of lesions
  - Radial: Along expected orientation of duct(s)
  - Antiradial: Perpendicular to radial
  - Transverse, sagittal
- Clock face
- Distance from nipple: Use width of transducer as guide (e.g., 38 or 50 mm)

ULTRASOUND BI-RADS® LEXICON AND USAGE

Key Facts

BI-RADS:US Concepts

- Descriptors for background echotexture, masses, calcifications, special cases, vascularity, and final assessments
- Terms parallel those in BI-RADS:Mammography when possible
  - Report should integrate mammographic and US findings, with one overall assessment and recommendation(s)
- Management based on worst feature(s) present
- Cancers generally have multiple suspicious findings
- To classify a lesion as benign, must lack any suspicious features and have specific benign features
- Probably benign classification requires further validation for US
  - Risk of malignancy not well established, likely < 2%

- For the few malignancies inadvertently followed, prognosis should not be adversely affected by delay in diagnosis
- Multiplicity and bilaterality of similar benign-appearing masses supports benignity
- Not appropriate if lesion new, enlarging, or generally if ipsilateral to cancer
- 6 month, 12 month, 24 month follow-up
  - Suspicious change or growth at any follow-up should prompt aspiration or biopsy
- Not usually appropriate for palpable findings
- Assessment and recommendations linked
  - If intervention recommended, code BI-RADS 4 or 5
- While BI-RADS assessments are not legally required for breast US, their use is strongly recommended
- Encourage tracking and outcomes analysis

- Annotate any clinical findings: Palpable, tender

PATHOLOGIC ISSUES

Masses

- Describe shape, orientation, margins, lesion boundary, echo pattern (echogenicity), posterior acoustic features
- Describe effect on surrounding parenchyma, skin
  - No effect
  - Duct changes
    - Describe dilated ducts (> 2 mm), focally narrowed ducts, intraductal extension of mass
  - Architectural distortion
    - Straightening or thickening of Cooper ligaments
    - Disruption of normal anatomic planes
  - Edema: Increased echogenicity of surrounding parenchyma ± dilated lymphatic channels
  - Skin thickening: Focal or diffuse; normal skin ≤ 2 mm, thicker in periareolar and inferior breast
  - Skin retraction: Skin surface is concave, pulled in
- May have associated calcifications

Calcifications

- Macrocalcifications: ≥ 0.5 mm in diameter
- Microcalcifications
  - Describe location as in a mass or in surrounding parenchyma or both

Vascularity

- If present, describe location (in or immediately adjacent to lesion; increased in surrounding tissue)

PATHOLOGY-BASED IMAGING ISSUES

Mass Shape

- Oval: Elliptical, egg-shaped, includes 2 or 3 gentle lobulations
  - 59% of masses going to biopsy; 16% malignant
  - 51% of benign masses ovoid; another 19% of benign masses 2-3 gentle lobulations

- Round: Spherical, ball-shaped, anteroposterior diameter = transverse diameter
  - Uncommon: < 1% of masses going to biopsy; 60-100% malignant
  - High grade invasive ductal carcinoma (IDC) can appear round, as can metastatic nodes, cysts
- Irregular: Neither round nor oval
  - 41% of masses going to biopsy; 62% malignant
  - 72% of malignancies have this appearance

Mass Orientation

- Parallel: Wider than tall; long axis parallel to skin
  - 73% of solid masses going to biopsy; 22% malignant
- Vertical: Not parallel; taller than wide; long axis perpendicular to skin; includes round lesions
  - Applies if any portion of lesion is vertical
  - 27% of solid masses going to biopsy; 69% malignant
  - 42-53% of malignancies have this feature

Mass Margin

- Circumscribed: Smooth, distinct margin
  - 44% of solid masses going to biopsy; 10% malignant
- Not circumscribed
  - Microlobulated: At least 3 short cycle undulations
    - 9% of solid masses going to biopsy; 51% malignant
    - Clustered microcysts can appear microlobulated
  - Indistinct: No abrupt transition to adjacent tissue
    - 26% of solid masses going to biopsy; 46% malignant
  - Angular: At least part of margin has sharp corners
    - 15% of solid masses going to biopsy; 60% malignant
  - Spiculated: Sharp projecting lines
    - 5% of solid masses going to biopsy; 86% malignant

Lesion Boundary

- Abrupt interface: No transition zone between mass and surrounding tissue
  - Indistinctly marginated masses lack an abrupt interface, may or may not have an echogenic rim
  - 85% of solid masses going to biopsy; 29% malignant

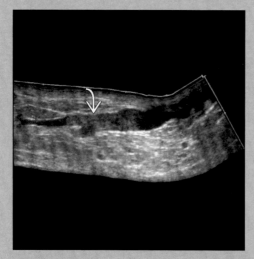

Intraductal masses ➘, as in this US of a 50 year old with clear nipple discharge, are a special case, and do not require further description of the mass features. BI-RADS 4A. Excision showed papillomas.

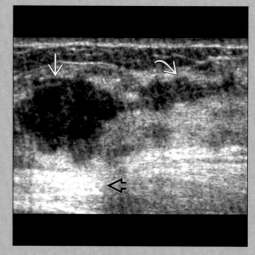

US of a 44 year old shows intraductal extension ➘ of an irregular, hypoechoic mass ➔ with posterior enhancement ➩. BI-RADS 5. IDC with extensive intraductal component.

- Echogenic halo (rim): Echogenic zone of transition between mass and surrounding tissue
  - May represent unresolved spiculations or edema
  - 15% of solid masses going to biopsy; 70% malignant

Echo Pattern = Internal Echogenicity

- Anechoic: Absence of internal echoes
  - Solid anechoic masses are suspicious: Metastatic nodes, high grade malignancies
  - 1% of solid masses going to biopsy; 50% malignant
- Hyperechoic: Homogeneously more echogenic than fat
  - Uncommon: 7% of benign lesions one series
  - 1% of solid masses going to biopsy; none malignant in two series
  - Most often normal variant fibrotic bands
  - Angiosarcomas, rarely lymphoma can be hyperechoic: Usually some hypoechoic component
- Complex cystic: Mixed cystic and solid components
  - Thick-walled (> 0.5 mm), thick internal septations, or intracystic mass
  - Usually merits biopsy; BI-RADS 4B, 23% malignant
  - Clinical history may suggest hematoma or fat necrosis: BI-RADS 3 appropriate in some cases
- Isoechoic: Equal to fat
  - 12% of solid masses going to biopsy; 16% malignant
- Hypoechoic: Less than fat
  - 80% of solid masses going to biopsy; 40% malignant
- Mixed hyper- and hypoechoic: Uncommon
  - Fibrosis, fat necrosis, fibroadenolipoma, cancer (rare)

Posterior Acoustic Features

- None: No posterior shadowing or enhancement
  - 42% of solid masses going to biopsy; 21% malignant
- Posterior enhancement: Increased echoes deep to lesion relative to adjacent tissue
  - 21% of solid masses going to biopsy; 33% malignant
- Posterior shadowing: Decreased echoes deep to lesion relative to adjacent tissue
  - Excludes refractive edge shadowing
  - 33% of solid masses going to biopsy; 52% malignant
  - 49% of malignancies have this feature
- Combined posterior enhancement and shadowing

  - 4% of solid masses going to biopsy; 50% malignant

Assessments and Recommendations

- Integrate with mammography, combined assessment
- Final assessment based on combination of features
- 0: Incomplete, additional evaluation needed
- 1: Negative, routine screening
- 2: Benign, routine screening
- 3: Probably benign, short-interval follow-up recommended
- 4: Suspicious, biopsy should be considered
  - 4A: Low suspicion
  - 4B: Intermediate suspicion
  - 4C: Moderately suspicious
- 5: Highly suggestive of malignancy, biopsy
- 6: Known malignancy, take appropriate action
  - Patient with a current known cancer
    - Following neoadjuvant chemotherapy
    - Second opinion review of outside imaging prior to treatment
    - Evaluating extent of disease on US ± MR

RELATED REFERENCES

1. Berg WA et al: Breast US: Cystic and probably benign breast lesions, in Categorical Course Syllabus: Breast Imaging, Ed. Feig SA. Oak Brook: RSNA. 115-24, 2005
2. Hong AS et al: BI-RADS for sonography: positive and negative predictive values of sonographic features. AJR Am J Roentgenol. 184(4):1260-5, 2005
3. Graf O et al: Follow-up of palpable circumscribed noncalcified solid breast masses at mammography and US: can biopsy be averted? Radiology. 233(3):850-6, 2004
4. Berg WA et al: Cystic lesions of the breast: sonographic-pathologic correlation. Radiology. 227(1):183-91, 2003
5. Mendelson EB et al: Breast Imaging Reporting and Data System: BI-RADS, Ultrasound, 1st ed. Reston, American College of Radiology, 2003
6. Baker JA et al: Sonography of solid breast lesions: observer variability of lesion description and assessment. AJR Am J Roentgenol. 172(6):1621-5, 1999
7. Stavros AT et al: Solid breast nodules: use of sonography to distinguish between benign and malignant lesions. Radiology. 196(1):123-34, 1995

ULTRASOUND BI-RADS® LEXICON AND USAGE

IMAGE GALLERY

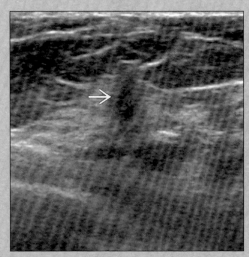
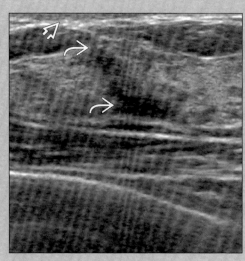

(Left) US shows vertically-oriented hypoechoic mass ➡ due to invasive ductal carcinoma, grade II, in this 57 year old woman. *(Right)* US shows vertically-oriented post-surgical scar ➡ at the site of prior abscess drainage in this 41 year old woman. The hypoechoic scar connected to a visible skin scar with focal skin thickening and skin retraction ➡.

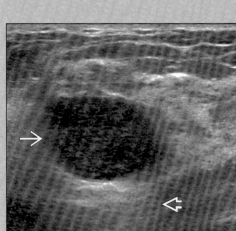
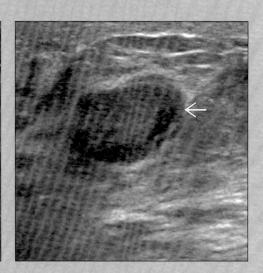

(Left) US shows circumscribed oval mass ➡ with posterior enhancement ➡ and low level echoes, compatible with a complicated cyst. In this 41 year old with multiple simple cysts, this is a benign finding, BI-RADS 2. *(Right)* US shows circumscribed oval, hypoechoic mass ➡. At baseline, when nonpalpable, this can be followed, BI-RADS 3. Further validation is needed to use BI-RADS 3 for palpable probable fibroadenomas (FA). Biopsy-proven FA.

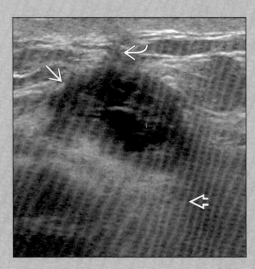
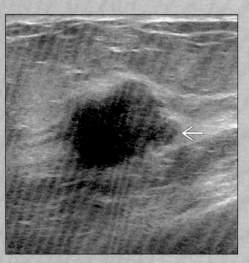

(Left) US shows complex cystic and solid mass ➡ with posterior enhancement ➡. A track ➡ to the overlying skin incision from reduction mammoplasty 3 months earlier suggests hematoma: BI-RADS 3. This decreased on 6 month follow-up. *(Right)* US shows indistinctly marginated complex cystic and solid mass ➡ in this 88 year old woman. This was new on mammography. BI-RADS 4B. Biopsy showed grade II IDC.

MR BI-RADS® LEXICON AND USAGE

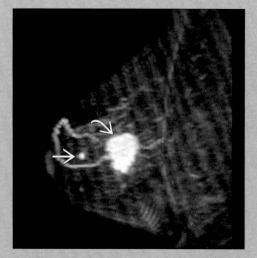

Sagittal MIP of T1 C+ subtraction MR shows satellite 5 mm enhancing focus ➔ 2 cm anterior to known lobulated cancer ➔ in this 61 year old. A satellite focus is suspicious. Biopsy: Multifocal ILC.

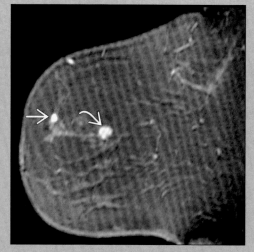

Sagittal T1 C+ FS MR shows smooth enhancing mass anteriorly ➔ (invasive ductal cancer), and lobulated mass with nonenhancing internal septations centrally ➔ (fibroadenoma). (Courtesy EAM)

TERMINOLOGY

Abbreviations

- BI-RADS®: MRI: Breast Imaging Reporting and Data System for Magnetic Resonance Imaging
  - Please note: Terms may undergo revision; please consult current edition of lexicon published by the American College of Radiology (ACR)
  - Minor modifications to phrasing have been made
- 3D SPGR FS: Three-dimensional spoiled gradient echo acquisition with fat suppression
- Maximum intensity pixel (MIP) projections: From 3D post-contrast subtraction dataset, 3D reconstruction of brightest pixels, essentially an MR angiogram
- Computer aided "detection" (CAD) = computer-assisted parametric mapping: Typically, thresholding based on % enhancement in first 2 minutes then color-coding by delayed kinetic behavior (persistent, plateau, washout)
- Region of interest (ROI); should be at least 3 pixels

Definitions

- Standardized terminology developed through the ACR
  - Lexicon to describe findings, associated findings, location, kinetics, assessment, and management recommendations
- Kinetics: Plot of signal intensity (SI) of lesion over time, following contrast injection
- Focus: Punctate, nonspecific enhancement, too small to characterize morphologically, usually < 5 mm
- Non-mass-like enhancement: Area, not a mass, whose internal enhancement results in a pattern discrete from surrounding parenchyma
  - Usually has interspersed fat or normal tissue

ANATOMY-BASED IMAGING ISSUES

Key Concepts or Questions

- Provide indication for examination
  - Detail prior biopsies, risk factors, symptoms (if any)

- Compare to recent prior mammography, US (when performed)
- Compare to prior breast MR (if applicable)

Imaging Protocols

- Describe technical factors
  - Magnet field strength (usually ≥ 1.5 T)
  - Coil: Dedicated breast coil, e.g., phased array
  - Describe which breast(s) scanned ± compression
  - Scan orientation (e.g., axial, sagittal) and types of sequences
    - Typically: T1WI; T2WI FS (or STIR); 3D SPGR FS pre- and post-contrast
  - Amount and type of contrast injected: Typically 0.1 mmol/kg Gd-contrast, preferably with power injector
  - Number of post-contrast acquisitions, time period imaged
  - Post-processing: Subtraction, MIPs, ± use of CAD

Imaging Pitfalls

- Describe limitations of examination
  - Hormonal influences: Include date of onset last menses in report for pre-menopausal women
    - Schedule in days 7-14 when possible: ↓ Parenchymal enhancement, false positives
    - Post-menopausal women on hormone replacement therapy: Include in history
  - Validate successful injection of contrast: Heart, great vessels, and liver enhance
  - Motion or other artifacts: Gentle compression helps
- Optional: Degree of parenchymal enhancement
  - None/minimal; mild; moderate; marked
  - Increased background enhancement may obscure detection of small masses
  - Parenchyma usually slower to enhance than cancer
    - Importance of rapid imaging (within 1-2 minutes) after contrast injection

Lesion Location

- Detail which breast (right, left, or bilateral)
- Location: Quadrant, subareolar, central, axillary tail

MR BI-RADS® LEXICON AND USAGE

Key Facts

General Principles
- Terms parallel BI-RADS: Mammography and BI-RADS: US when possible
- Not a substitute for full mammographic, US workup
  - Interpret together with mammogram, breast US
- Consider morphology > kinetics
- Management based on most suspicious feature(s)

Absence of Enhancement
- < 50-60% increase in signal within 1-2 minutes of injection dismissed
- 88% NPV in diagnostic setting
  - Nearly half of nonenhancing cancers = DCIS
- 99-99.6% NPV in screening setting
- Lesion seen on T1WI pre-contrast images
  - 4% malignant if no enhancement

Probably Benign
- Very low risk of malignancy, may be followed
- Concept requires further validation for MR
- Consider circumstances of exam
  - Higher risk malignant if satellite to known cancer
  - Follow-up problematic: Plan pregnancy, relocating
- 2.8% risk of malignancy across multiple series, varying criteria
- Proposed criteria (ACRIN 6666)
  - 1-2 smooth, oval mass(es), persistent or plateau kinetics, not suspicious on mammography or US
  - Solitary focus, persistent or plateau kinetics
    - 1/37 (3%) malignant one series
  - Patchy regional enhancement, persistent kinetics, no US correlate
  - Multiple, bilateral similar findings favor benign

- Depth: Distance from nipple, skin, or chest wall (in cm) as appropriate
- Include table position (e.g., R72) and/or series/slice # where finding best seen

PATHOLOGIC ISSUES

Mass
- Describe shape, margin, internal enhancement characteristics

Non-Mass-Like Enhancement
- Describe distribution, internal enhancement pattern, symmetry (if bilateral)

Associated Findings
- Nipple retraction or inversion, pre-contrast high duct signal, skin retraction, skin thickening (> 2 mm), edema, abnormal signal void (artifacts), cyst(s)
- Lymphadenopathy: Enlarged, rounded nodes, eccentrically thickened cortex, loss of fatty hila
  - Encourage positioning to include axilla
- Pectoralis muscle or chest wall invasion: Must see extension of suspicious enhancement into pectoralis or intercostal muscle(s) or rib(s); not sufficient to abut
- Hematoma/blood: Bright signal on pre-contrast T1WI
- Cyst: Circumscribed round or oval fluid-filled mass, imperceptible wall, bright on T2WI FS

Kinetics
- Sample and report ROI's of most rapidly enhancing ± most suspicious areas in lesion
- Initial phase: Change in SI within first 2 minutes of injection (before curve changes)
  - Suggested thresholds are listed; CAD programs vary
  - Slow: < 60% increase in SI within 2 minutes
  - Medium: 60-100% increase in SI within 2 minutes
  - Rapid: > 100% increase in SI within 2 minutes
- Delayed phase: Enhancement pattern
  - Persistent (Type I): Progressive, continued increase in signal over time; 6% malignant

  - Plateau (Type II): SI does not change over time after initial rise; flat (± 10%); 64% malignant
  - Washout (Type III): SI decreases after peaking; 87% malignant
    - Normal lymph nodes often show washout kinetics

PATHOLOGY-BASED IMAGING ISSUES

Mass Shape
- Round - spherical; oval - elliptical
- Lobulated: Undulating contour, scalloped
- Irregular: Uneven shape

Mass Margin
- Smooth: Circumscribed
  - Resolution of ~ 1 mm may be insufficient to identify subtle spiculation
  - 30% of masses → biopsy; 5-17% rate of malignancy; 20% of malignant masses
- Irregular: Neither smooth nor spiculated, may be ill-defined or indistinct; 23-32% malignant
- Spiculated: Radiating lines from margin, 80% malignant

Mass Internal Enhancement Characteristics
- Homogeneous: Confluent, uniform enhancement
- Heterogeneous: Nonuniform enhancement
- Rim enhancement: Greater at periphery
  - 8% of lesions → biopsy; 40-84% malignant
  - Invasive carcinoma; ruptured/inflamed cyst, abscess; fat necrosis
  - Thick, irregular rim, rapid enhancement, washout kinetics favor malignancy
- Dark internal septations = nonenhancing internal septations
  - 98% NPV; often fibroadenomas
- Enhancing internal septations
- Central enhancement: Greater in center of mass

Non-Mass-Like Distribution
- Focal Area: < 25% of quadrant in confined area

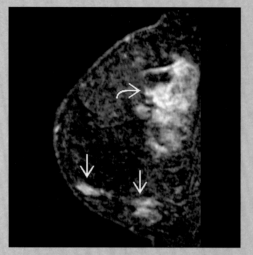

Sagittal T2WI FS MR shows patchy regional enhancement upper outer breast ➡ as well as linear enhancement inferiorly ➡.

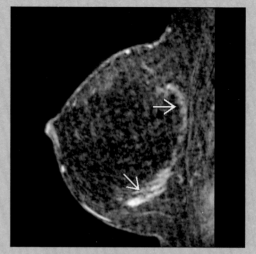

Sagittal T1 C+ FS MR (2 cm medial to previous image) shows linear enhancement ➡ is sheet-like and at periphery of breast tissue. Findings resolved on repeat scan 6 weeks later: Inflow phenomena.

○ Contains interspersed fat or normal glandular tissue
- Linear: In a line, not definitely a duct, may be sheet-like
- Ductal: In a line, pointing to nipple, can branch, conforming to a duct
  ○ 5% of all breast MR examinations
  ○ 20-59% malignant, usually clumped enhancement
  ○ > 75% of malignancies are ductal carcinoma in situ (DCIS)
- Segmental: Triangular region or cone with apex pointing to nipple
  ○ Suggests a duct and its branches, 67% malignant
- Regional: Geographic, ≥ 25% of quadrant
  ○ Symmetric regional favors benign etiology
  ○ At edges of parenchyma may be "inflow"
  ○ Cyclic dependency if normal variant
  ○ 47-50% malignant, often clumped morphology
- Multiple regions: ≥ 2 regions, patchy
- Diffuse: Uniform, even throughout breast

Non-Mass Internal Enhancement

- Homogeneous or heterogeneous
- Stippled/punctate: Round, tiny, dot-like
- Clumped: Cobblestone-like, confluent in areas, bunch of grapes, string of pearls
  ○ Favors DCIS, especially in linear or segmental distribution
- Reticular/dendritic: Strand-like
  ○ Can be seen with inflammatory carcinoma

Non-Mass Symmetry

- Symmetric: Mirror image, both breasts
- Asymmetric: More in one breast than the other

Assessments, Recommendations

- 0: Incomplete, additional evaluation needed
- 1: Negative, no lesion found, routine follow-up
- 2: Benign finding, routine follow-up
- 3: Probably benign, short interval follow-up
  ○ Optional 3A: Possibly hormonal, follow-up at different time in cycle, 2-6 weeks
  ○ Optional 3B: 6 month follow-up
- 4: Suspicious abnormality, optional subdivision

○ 4A: Low suspicion of malignancy, biopsy
○ 4B: Intermediate suspicion of malignancy, biopsy
○ 4C: Moderate suspicion of malignancy, biopsy
- 5: Highly suggestive of malignancy, take appropriate action (usually biopsy)
- 6: Known, biopsy-proven malignancy
  ○ Exam for local extent of disease and nothing suspicious beyond known cancer
  ○ Following neoadjuvant chemotherapy
  ○ Second opinion review of study from another facility prior to treatment
- Can give separate assessments by breast
- Track outcomes

RELATED REFERENCES

1. Liberman L et al: Does size matter? Positive predictive value of MRI-detected breast lesions as a function of lesion size. AJR Am J Roentgenol. 186(2):426-30, 2006
2. Schnall MD et al: Diagnostic architectural and dynamic features at breast MR imaging: multicenter study. Radiology. 238(1):42-53, 2006
3. Morakkabati-Spitz N et al: Diagnostic usefulness of segmental and linear enhancement in dynamic breast MRI. Eur Radiol. 15(9):2010-7, 2005
4. Kriege M et al: Efficacy of MRI and mammography for breast-cancer screening in women with a familial or genetic predisposition. N Engl J Med. 351(5):427-37, 2004
5. Warner E et al: Surveillance of BRCA1 and BRCA2 mutation carriers with magnetic resonance imaging, ultrasound, mammography, and clinical breast examination. JAMA. 292(11):1317-25, 2004
6. Ikeda DM et al: Breast Imaging Reporting and Data System, BI-RADS: Magnetic Resonance Imaging (BI-RADS®: MRI), 1st ed. Reston, American College of Radiology, 2003
7. Liberman L et al: Ductal enhancement on MR imaging of the breast. AJR Am J Roentgenol. 181(2):519-25, 2003
8. Liberman L et al: Probably benign lesions at breast magnetic resonance imaging: preliminary experience in high-risk women. Cancer. 98(2):377-88, 2003
9. Liberman L et al: Breast lesions detected on MR imaging: features and positive predictive value. AJR Am J Roentgenol. 179(1):171-8, 2002
10. Nunes LW et al: Update of breast MR imaging architectural interpretation model. Radiology. 219(2):484-94, 2001

IMAGE GALLERY

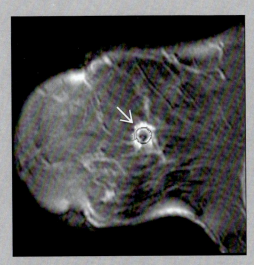

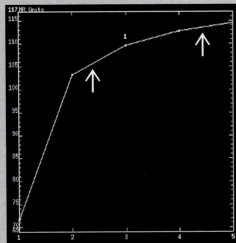

IV

0

17

(Left) Sagittal T1 C+ FS MR shows irregular, spiculated mass ➡ with central defect due to prior biopsy of this invasive ductal cancer. A large ROI had been drawn by the technologist. (Right) Kinetic curve of the ROI (see previous image) shows rapid initial enhancement and apparently persistent kinetics ➡.

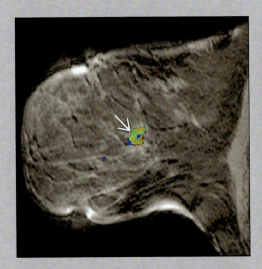

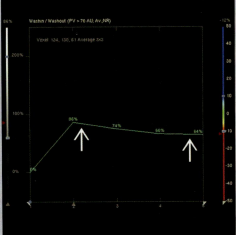

(Left) Sagittal T1 C+ FS MR with computer-assisted color-coded parametric mapping (CAD) over mass ➡ (same patient as previous 2 images) shows mixed kinetics (blue = persistent, green = plateau, red = washout). (Right) Representative kinetic curve (see previous image) shows washout kinetics ➡. ROI's 3-4 pixels in size are appropriate, with sampling and reporting of the most suspicious area of the lesion. Larger ROI's may result in erroneous interpretation.

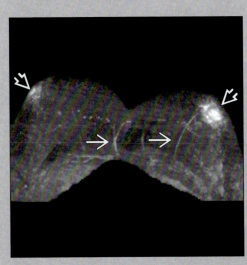

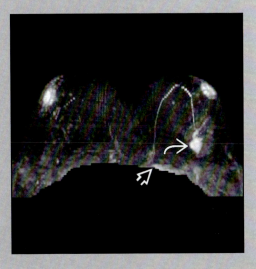

(Left) Axial MIP of T1 C+ subtraction MR shows normal variant nipple enhancement ⇗ as well as vascular enhancement ➡. (Right) Axial MIP of T1 C+ subtraction MR 5 days later (same patient as previous image) shows irregular enhancing mass left breast ➡ (known invasive ductal carcinoma). Poor contrast injection can be difficult to recognize clinically and on imaging. The cardiac bolus was better seen on the repeat scan ⇗.

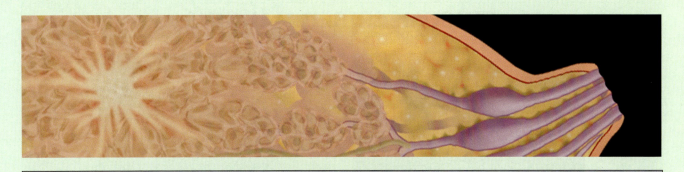

SECTION 1: Lesion Imaging Characteristics

CIRCUMSCRIBED MARGINS

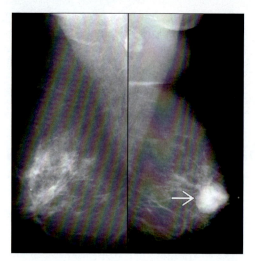

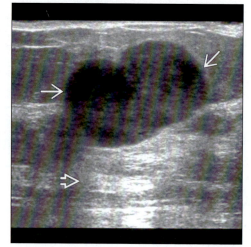

MLO mammography shows a 55 yo woman with an oval well-circumscribed 2.5 cm mass ➡ immediately behind left nipple. Her last mammogram was 3 years earlier & negative. US (right image) was performed.

Transverse ultrasound shows the lobulated circumscribed hypoechoic mass ➡ parallel to the skin with posterior enhancement ⬧. Excisional biopsy = 3 cm solid papillary and cribriform invasive carcinoma.

TERMINOLOGY

Abbreviations and Synonyms
- Well-defined margins (mammography, US)
- Smooth borders (MR)

Definitions
- Well-defined, sharply marginated with abrupt transition between lesion and surrounding tissue
- At least 75% of the margin must be well-defined, remainder no worse than obscured
- If any portion of margin is indistinct or spiculated, the mass should be so described and classified

IMAGING FINDINGS

General Features
- Best diagnostic clue
  - ≥ 75% of margin sharply defined on mammography
    - Up to 25% can be obscured by overlying tissue

Mammographic Findings
- CC and MLO views

- Identify multiplicity, bilaterality
- Examine mass(es) in both views
- < 25% of margin hidden by overlying tissue
- Isolated circumscribed mass
  - Compare to prior films if available
  - Additional views if new, enlarging, or on baseline
  - If suspect associated calcifications (Ca++), spot magnification CC and ML views
  - Spot compression and/or magnification views may also help characterize margins
  - Mediolateral view can demonstrate benign layering fat-fluid level (galactocele) or milk-of-calcium in cyst(s)
  - US unless clearly a benign lymph node (LN) or cyst with milk-of-calcium
  - US to guide biopsy if clearly suspicious
- Tangential view to demonstrate skin lesions
- Multiple bilateral, similar benign-appearing masses
  - Evaluate each mass completely
  - At least three masses, at least one in each breast
  - No suspicious findings
  - Can be assessed as BI-RADS 2 if all masses meet these criteria

---

DDx: Margins that may Appear Circumscribed

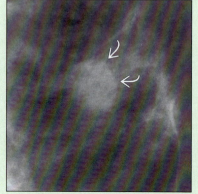

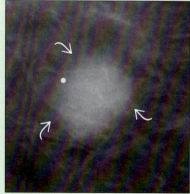

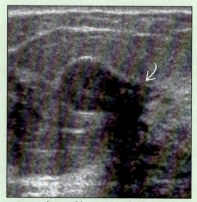

Obscured, Cyst

Indistinct, Cyst

Irregular, Infiltrating Lobular & FA

CIRCUMSCRIBED MARGINS

Key Facts

Terminology
- At least 75% of the margin must be well-defined, remainder no worse than obscured

Imaging Findings
- Spot compression and/or magnification views may also help characterize margins
- Mediolateral view can demonstrate benign layering fat-fluid level (galactocele) or milk-of-calcium in cyst(s)
- Evaluate each mass completely

Top Differential Diagnoses
- Simple Cyst(s)
- Oil Cyst
- Fibroadenoma (FA)
- Phyllodes Tumor

- Benign Lymph Node (LN)
- Epidermal inclusion cyst or sebaceous cyst
- Invasive ductal carcinoma (IDC) NOS
- Papillary ductal carcinoma in situ (DCIS)
- Metastases to breast
- Metastatic intramammary lymph node

Pathology
- 1.4% of circumscribed masses were malignant in study of screening mammograms

Clinical Issues
- Cysts, FA may fluctuate in size (hormonal changes)
- New, enlarging, and/or palpable circumscribed masses merit further evaluation
- Biopsy warranted for any concerning feature, despite other benign findings

- Bilateral waxing/waning masses generally benign: Cysts and/or fibroadenomas (FA)
  - Dominant or palpable mass merits US
- Worst margin characteristics should guide management

Ultrasonographic Findings
- Characterize palpable or mammographic finding
  - Suspicious findings: Indistinct or thick wall, posterior shadowing, taller than wide
- Optimize technique
  - Center frequency at least 10 MHz
  - Adjust gain for tissue-appropriate shades of gray
  - Conventional imaging for posterior features
  - Spatial compounding for margin evaluation
  - Tissue harmonic imaging may decrease artifactual echoes
- Posterior enhancement in solid masses
  - An indeterminate finding; seen in benign and malignant masses

MR Findings
- T1WI
  - Sequence depicts anatomy well: Smooth border
  - Fat hyperintense: Hilum of lymph node(s), oil cyst
  - Proteinaceous cysts and hematomas hyperintense
- T2WI FS
  - Most lesions isointense to glandular tissue
  - Hyperintensity generally benign
    - Cystic lesions hyperintense unless hemorrhagic
    - FA can be hyperintense
    - Mucinous carcinoma can be hyperintense
- T1 C+
  - Smooth margins 95% NPV for malignancy
  - Nonpalpable smooth enhancing masses represented 17% of malignancies in one series
  - Enhancement pattern
    - Rim-enhancement suspicious
    - Slow, progressive rim-enhancement: Inflamed cyst, abscess
    - Nonenhancing septations favor FA
  - Enhancing foci (< 5 mm) may have smooth margins but are too small to definitively characterize

- Spatial resolution lower than mammography
  - Margins may be artifactually "smoothed"

Imaging Recommendations
- Best imaging tool
  - Mammography
    - Spot compression views displace adjacent tissue
    - Magnification views if associated Ca++
  - US for further characterization

DIFFERENTIAL DIAGNOSIS

Simple Cyst(s)
- Anechoic, imperceptible wall, posterior enhancement
- Solitary or multiple; often bilateral
- Most common in perimenopausal women or those on hormonal therapy
- Aspirate for symptomatic relief or diagnostic uncertainty
- May show dependent milk-of-calcium or rim Ca++

Complicated Cyst(s)
- Imperceptible wall, posterior enhancement
- Homogeneous low-level echoes
- Fluid-debris level
- Mobile internal echoes
- Aspirate for symptomatic relief or diagnostic uncertainty

Oil Cyst
- Lucent mass (mammography) +/- peripheral Ca++

Fibroadenoma (FA)
- Oval, smooth or 2-3 gentle lobulations, hypoechoic, parallel to skin (US)
- Most common benign solid mass in young women (< 40 years old)
- May have associated popcorn Ca++

Complex Cystic Lesion
- Contains any of: Thick wall, thick septations, intracystic mass, mixed cystic and solid lesion
- 20% malignancy rate: Merit biopsy

CIRCUMSCRIBED MARGINS

Phyllodes Tumor
- Rapidly growing, can be multiple

Benign Lymph Node (LN)
- Reniform shape, notched fatty hilum

Other Benign Masses
- Hamartoma/fibroadenolipoma
  - Contains fat, soft tissue, rarely Ca++
- Lipoma
  - Low density; slightly hyperechoic on US
- Lactating adenoma
  - Patient pregnant or lactating
- Epidermal inclusion cyst or sebaceous cyst
  - Correlate with clinical exam, skin marker, tangential view

Malignancy
- Most malignant mass margins at least partially indistinct on close examination
- Invasive ductal carcinoma (IDC) NOS
  - 36% of grade III; 6% grade II; 18% grade I IDC NOS have circumscribed margins
- Medullary carcinoma
- Mucinous carcinoma
  - Dense (mammography); isoechoic (US)
- Papillary ductal carcinoma in situ (DCIS)
  - Most often intracystic mass (US)
- Metastases to breast
  - Carcinoid, melanoma most common
  - More often solitary than multiple, usually unilateral
- Metastatic intramammary lymph node
  - Breast primary most common
  - MR can be helpful if breast primary occult on mammography, US
  - Lymphoma: Other adenopathy, systemic disease

PATHOLOGY

General Features
- Etiology
  - 1.4% of circumscribed masses were malignant in study of screening mammograms
    - 9% malignancy rate among lesions going to biopsy

CLINICAL ISSUES

Presentation
- Most common signs/symptoms: Asymptomatic
- Other signs/symptoms: Palpable mass
- Cysts, FA may fluctuate in size (hormonal changes)
- History of trauma, surgery/biopsy
  - Hematoma, fat necrosis, oil cyst

Natural History & Prognosis
- Medullary and mucinous carcinoma better prognosis than grade III IDC NOS
- Circumscribed IDC NOS generally high grade

Treatment
- New, enlarging, and/or palpable circumscribed masses merit further evaluation
- Appropriate interval follow-up of BI-RADS 2 or 3
  - Bilateral multiple (at least 3, at least one in each breast) similar-appearing masses (mammography) = BI-RADS 2
  - Baseline solitary well-circumscribed mass (mammography) = individualized; BI-RADS 3
  - Solid mass(es) (US) parallel to skin, no more than 3 gentle lobulations, no malignant features may = BI-RADS 3
- Biopsy warranted for any concerning feature, despite other benign findings
  - Physical exam findings may dictate further management

DIAGNOSTIC CHECKLIST

Consider
- Multiplicity, bilaterality favor benign etiology

Image Interpretation Pearls
- Exclude any suspicious features

SELECTED REFERENCES

1. Morris EA et al: Breast MRI Diagnosis and Intervention. New York, Springer. 140-83, 2005
2. Sickles EA, et al. Performance benchmarks for diagnostic mammography. Radiology. 235:775-90, 2005
3. Graf O et al: Follow-up of palpable circumscribed noncalcified solid breast masses at mammography and US: can biopsy be averted? Radiology. 233:850-6, 2004
4. D'Orsi CJ et al: Breast Imaging Reporting and Data System: BI-RADS, Mammography, 4th ed. Reston, VA: American College of Radiology, 2003
5. Ikeda DM et al: Breast Imaging Reporting and Data System: BI-RADS, Magnetic Resonance Imaging, 1st ed. Reston, VA: American College of Radiology, 2003
6. Mendelson EB et al: Breast Imaging Reporting and Data System: BI-RADS, Ultrasound, 1st ed. Reston, VA: American College of Radiology, 2003
7. Liberman L et al: Breast lesions detected on MR imaging: features and positive predictive value. AJR Am J Roentgenol. 179(1):171-8, 2002
8. Lamb PM et al: Correlation between ultrasound characteristics, mammographic findings and histological grade in patients with invasive ductal carcinoma of the breast. Clin Radiol. 55(1):40-4, 2000
9. Leung JW et al: Multiple bilateral masses detected on screening mammography: assessment of need for recall imaging. AJR. 175:23-9, 2000
10. Liberman L et al: The breast imaging reporting and data system: positive predictive value of mammographic features and final assessment categories. AJR Am J Roentgenol. 171(1):35-40, 1998
11. Sickles EA: Management of probably benign lesions of the breast. Radiology. 193(2):582-3, 1994
12. Varas X et al: Nonpalpable, probably benign lesions: role of follow-up mammography. Radiology. 184(2):409-14, 1992

CIRCUMSCRIBED MARGINS

IMAGE GALLERY

Typical

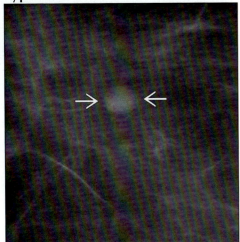 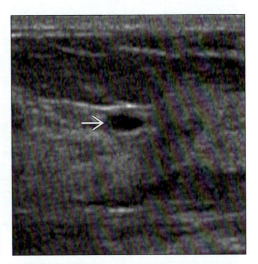

(Left) CC mammography spot compression shows an oval small mass with well-circumscribed margins ➔. An US was performed (right image). *(Right)* Anti-radial ultrasound of the mass shows the mammographic mass to be a simple cyst with imperceptible walls ➔. Despite the small size, this cyst was confidently interpreted as a BI-RADS 2, benign.

Typical

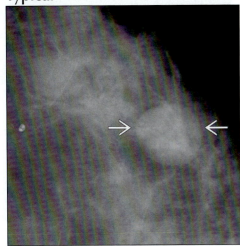 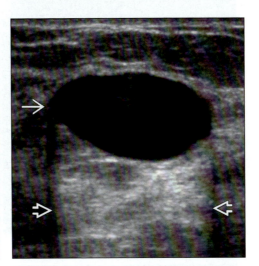

(Left) CC mammography spot compression shows a circumscribed mass ➔. *(Right)* Anti-radial ultrasound of the same mass as in left-hand image ➔ shows it to be anechoic and thin-walled, with circumscribed margins and posterior enhancement ⬌. This is a simple cyst, a benign finding, BI-RADS 2.

Typical

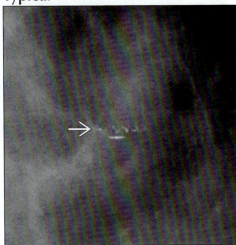 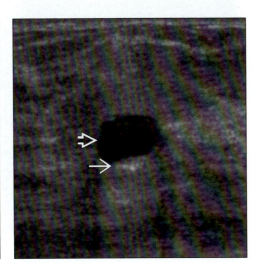

(Left) Lateral mammography magnification of a cluster of amorphous calcifications demonstrates layering of the calcifications ➔, compatible with milk-of-calcium. *(Right)* Transverse ultrasound of the mammographic finding (same patient as left-hand image) shows dependent calcifications ➔ within a circumscribed cyst ➔.

Typical

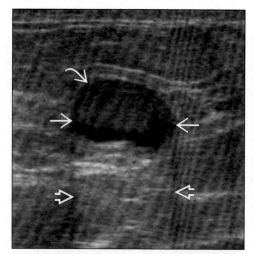

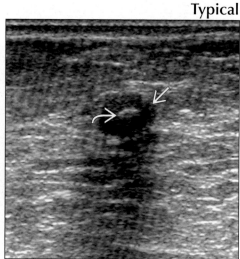

(Left) Radial ultrasound shows a galactocele with fat-fluid level ➡, edge refraction ➡, and thin wall ➡. *(Right)* Sagittal ultrasound shows a well-circumscribed mass ➡ with a coarse echogenic internal calcification ➡. Pathology showed a hyalinized fibroadenoma.

Typical

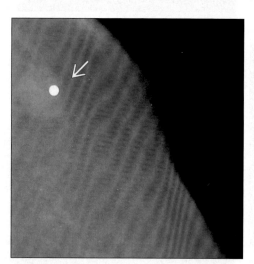

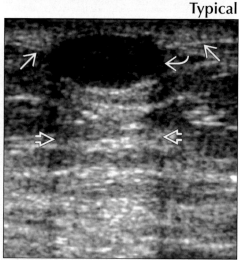

(Left) CC mammography shows a circumscribed mass ➡ corresponding to a palpable mass which is marked by a BB. *(Right)* Radial ultrasound confirms that the mass ➡ is intradermal ➡ and hypoechoic, with posterior enhancement ➡. This is either a sebaceous cyst or epidermal inclusion cyst.

Typical

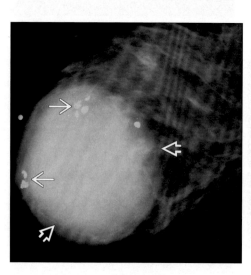

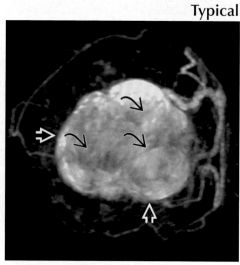

(Left) MLO mammography shows a large, circumscribed, dense mass ➡. Chunky, coarse, "popcorn" calcifications are noted within the mass ➡. MR was performed (right-hand image). *(Right)* Coronal MIP of T1 C+ subtraction MR shows the same smooth ➡ mass to be avidly enhancing, with hypointense septations ➡. Phyllodes tumor was confirmed at excision.

CIRCUMSCRIBED MARGINS

Typical

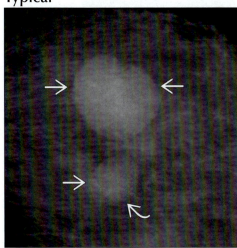

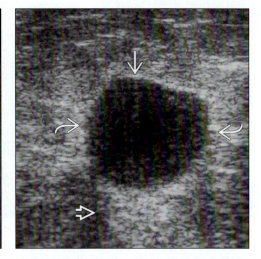

(Left) MLO mammography shows two dense, gently lobulated masses ➡, one which had a partially indistinct margin ➡. US was performed (right-hand image). *(Right)* Transverse ultrasound of the inferior mass (same patient as left-hand image) shows a hypoechoic mass ➡ with posterior enhancement ➡, and subtle spiculated margins ➡. US-guided biopsy confirmed medullary carcinoma in both masses.

Typical

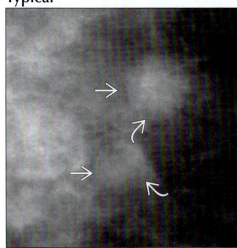

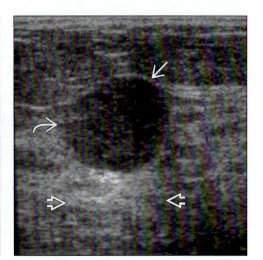

(Left) CC mammography shows two partially obscured ➡, partially circumscribed masses ➡. US was performed (right-hand image). *(Right)* Radial ultrasound of one of the two masses at left shows both sharp ➡ and microlobulated ➡ margins and posterior enhancement ➡. Both masses were metastatic carcinoid tumor.

Typical

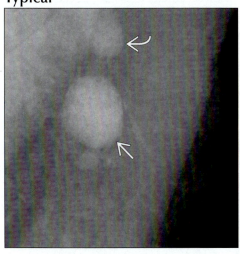

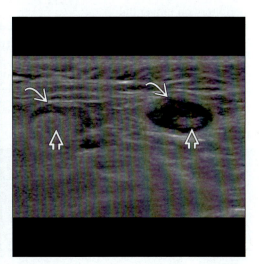

(Left) MLO mammography shows two circumscribed axillary masses. The inferior mass ➡ is dense and larger than the superior mass ➡. US was performed (right-hand image). *(Right)* Sagittal ultrasound shows the superior mass to have a thin hypoechoic cortex ➡ and a hyperechoic fatty hilum ➡ consistent with a LN. The inferior LN has a thicker cortex ➡ and the fatty hilum ➡ is compressed. The inferior LN was involved with B-cell lymphoma.

INTRAMAMMARY LYMPH NODE

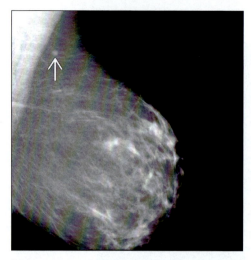

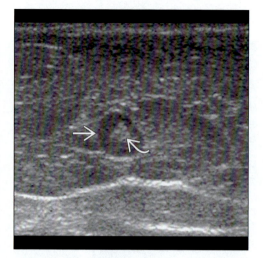

MLO mammography shows a small, well-circumscribed intramammary lymph node ➡ in the upper breast. The CC view (not shown) showed the location to be in the outer quadrant.

Transverse ultrasound shows the small, well-circumscribed intramammary lymph node with a hypoechoic cortex ➡ and an echogenic hilum ➡.

TERMINOLOGY

Abbreviations and Synonyms
- Intramammary lymph node (IMLN); intraparenchymal lymph node

Definitions
- Small, oval, smoothly-marginated, intraparenchymal breast mass with eccentric fatty hilum

IMAGING FINDINGS

General Features
- Best diagnostic clue
  - Mammographic reniform or lobulated mass with a fatty hilum or notch
    - Radiolucent fat seen in periphery on tangential view and centrally when en face
- Location
  - Upper outer quadrant most common
  - May be anywhere within the breast and may be multiple
- Size
  - Typically < 1 cm
    - Size less important than classic appearance

Mammographic Findings
- Mammography usually diagnostic

Ultrasonographic Findings
- Grayscale Ultrasound: Hypoechoic circumscribed small oval or reniform mass with echogenic hilum
- Color Doppler: Vascular hilum may be visible

MR Findings
- T1WI: Fatty hilum may be visible as high signal
- T2WI: Small oval mass cortex may have high signal
- T1 C+: Enhancement may be rapid and intense

DIFFERENTIAL DIAGNOSIS

Other Encapsulated Fat-Containing Well-Circumscribed Masses
- Lipoma
- Fibroadenolipoma
- Galactocele
- Group of cysts with intervening fat

DDx: Other Intramammary Lymph Node Examples

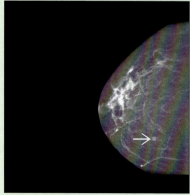

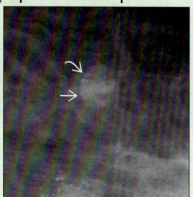

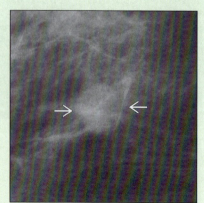

Medial Location

Breast Cancer Metastasis

Melanoma Metastasis

INTRAMAMMARY LYMPH NODE

Key Facts

Imaging Findings
- Mammographic reniform or lobulated mass with a fatty hilum or notch
- Upper outer quadrant most common
- T1 C+: Enhancement may be rapid and intense
- Grayscale Ultrasound: Hypoechoic circumscribed small oval or reniform mass with echogenic hilum

Top Differential Diagnoses
- Other Encapsulated Fat-Containing Well-Circumscribed Masses
- Well-Circumscribed, Non-Calcified Masses

Pathology
- Lymph node completely surrounded by breast tissue
- Epidemiology: Present in up to 47% of breasts
- Breast cancer IMLN involvement considered stage II

Well-Circumscribed, Non-Calcified Masses
- Cyst, fibroadenoma, lymphoma, metastases, primary carcinomas (uncommon)

PATHOLOGY

General Features
- General path comments
  - Lymph node completely surrounded by breast tissue
  - Enlargement
    - Neoplasm: Breast cancer, lymphoma, melanoma
    - Regional inflammation: Dermatitis
    - Infections: Fungal, tuberculosis
    - Foreign body reaction: Gold injections
    - Sinus histiocytosis
- Epidemiology: Present in up to 47% of breasts

Microscopic Features
- Fine needle aspiration: Lymphocytes
- Core biopsy: Lymphoid tissue, capsule, subcapsular sinuses

Staging, Grading or Classification Criteria
- Breast cancer IMLN involvement considered stage II
  - Even in absence of axillary lymph node involvement
- May be independent predictor of poor outcome
  - One study: 64% vs. 88% 5 year overall survival (P = 0.004)

CLINICAL ISSUES

Presentation
- Most common signs/symptoms: Asymptomatic finding on a mammogram

DIAGNOSTIC CHECKLIST

Image Interpretation Pearls
- Despite the fact that IMLNs can be in any breast quadrant, careful morphologic assessment should be given to any medially located breast mass

SELECTED REFERENCES
1. Shen J et al: Intramammary lymph node metastases are an independent predictor of poor outcome in patients with breast carcinoma. Cancer. 101:1330-7, 2004
2. Schmidt WA et al: Lymph nodes in the human female breast: a review of their detection and significance. Hum Pathol. 32:178-87, 2001
3. Rosen PP: Breast Pathology: Diagnosis by Needle Core Biopsy. Philadelphia, Lippincott Williams & Wilkins. Chapter 24, 247, 1999
4. Spillane AJ et al: Clinical significance of intramammary lymph nodes. Breast. 8:143-6, 1999

IMAGE GALLERY

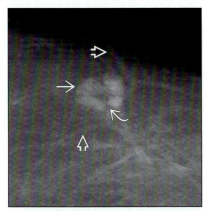
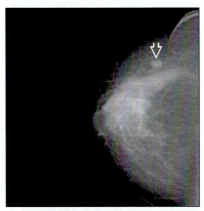
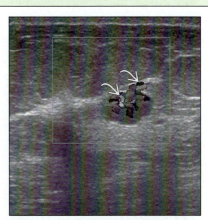

(Left) CC mammography shows a lobulated ➡ fat containing ➡ IMLN adjacent to vessels ➡ in lateral breast. IMLN had been mammographically stable for 5 years. *(Center)* CC mammography shows a circumscribed 1.1 cm smooth IMLN with an eccentric fatty hilum ➡. Slightly enlarged IMLN had reassuring benign features but an ultrasound was performed. *(Right)* Transverse color Doppler ultrasound (same case as left-hand image in black & white) shows vascular flow ➡ within the hilum. Atypical FNA led to a core biopsy which showed a normal IMLN.

OIL CYST

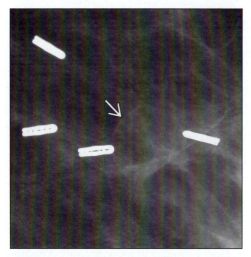

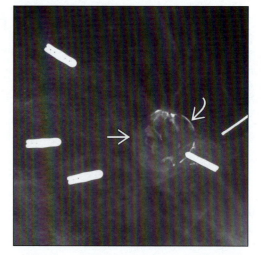

Lateral mammography magnification shows non-calcified oil cyst ➡ *at the site of scar and clips, 18 months post lumpectomy followed by radiation therapy in this 64 year old.*

Lateral mammography magnification 6 months later (same patient as left-hand image) shows development of peripheral rim calcifications ➡ *and slight decrease in size of the oil cyst* ➡.

TERMINOLOGY

Abbreviations and Synonyms
- Lipid cyst
- Liponecrosis microcystica calcificans, if < 3 mm
- Liponecrosis macrocystica calcificans, if ≥ 3 mm

Definitions
- Round to oval encapsulated lesion containing liquefied fat

IMAGING FINDINGS

General Features
- Best diagnostic clue
  - Round or oval lucent, smooth-bordered mass on mammography
  - Develops coarsening rim calcification over time
- Location
  - Can occur anywhere in breast or axilla
  - Subareolar region most common
  - Usually occurs in superficial tissues
    - Most vulnerable to trauma

- Size: Few mm to several cm in size

Mammographic Findings
- Round or oval well-circumscribed mass
  - Lucent
  - Thin capsule
  - Often calcifies: Rim, dystrophic, eggshell
  - Uniform, continuous eggshell calcification pathognomonic
  - Fat-fluid levels rarely detected
- Small lesion may be difficult to detect
  - Indistinguishable from normal surrounding fat and Cooper ligaments

Ultrasonographic Findings
- Grayscale Ultrasound
  - Well-circumscribed mass
    - Round to oval
  - Usually anechoic
    - Variable posterior acoustic features
  - May be hypoechoic or isoechoic
    - Variable posterior acoustic features
  - Occasionally complex
    - Septations
    - Internal echogenic bands

DDx: Fatty Masses

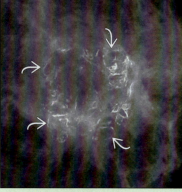

Fat Necrosis

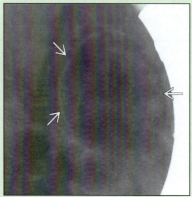

Lipoma

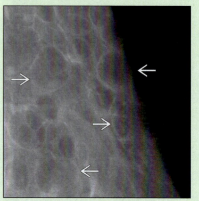

Steatocystoma Multiplex

OIL CYST

Key Facts

Terminology
- Lipid cyst
- Round to oval encapsulated lesion containing liquefied fat

Imaging Findings
- Round or oval lucent, smooth-bordered mass on mammography
- Develops coarsening rim calcification over time
- Can occur anywhere in breast or axilla
- Subareolar region most common
- Size: Few mm to several cm in size

Top Differential Diagnoses
- Fat Necrosis
- Lipoma
- Galactocele

Pathology
- General path comments: Non-suppurative, benign inflammatory process characterized by local adipose cell destruction
- Manifestation of post-traumatic fat necrosis
- Commonly occurs secondary to breast trauma

Clinical Issues
- Usually clinically occult
- Other signs/symptoms: May present as tender palpable mass or masses
- Age: All age groups
- No malignant potential

Diagnostic Checklist
- Appearance on US often more worrisome than mammography

- • Thickened walls
- • Mural nodules
- ○ May appear solid due to inspissated, echogenic fat
- ○ Fat in pure lipid cysts anechoic
- ○ Fat-fluid levels well depicted on ultrasound
  - • Due to partial resorption of water-soluble contents
  - • Change patient position to distinguish from mural nodule
- ○ Calcifications (Ca++) in rim
  - • Can cause shadowing
- • Color Doppler: Lack of Doppler-demonstrable blood flow

MR Findings
- T1WI: Well-defined, round to oval hyperintense mass
- T1 C+ FS: May demonstrate faint rim-enhancement along capsule

CT Findings
- CECT: No enhancement characteristics
- NECT
  - ○ Calcified, well-circumscribed, lucent mass
    - • May see calcified capsule

Imaging Recommendations
- Mammography

DIFFERENTIAL DIAGNOSIS

Fat Necrosis
- History of trauma or surgery
- Usually solid mass with central fat and surrounding and intervening inflammatory cell reaction
  - ○ Oil cyst is usually a subtype of fat necrosis with liquefied fat centrally
- Mammography may be diagnostic
  - ○ Often a central lucency associated with smooth, irregular, or sometimes spiculated margins
  - ○ Dystrophic Ca++ (coarse with lucent centers) may develop > 2 years following trauma/surgery
    - • Typically following lumpectomy and radiation therapy

- • May develop in fibrous capsule the body forms around silicone or saline implants
- ○ Coarse heterogeneous Ca++ near nipple common following breast reduction mammoplasty
- • Ultrasound internal echogenicity pattern variable
  - ○ Often heterogeneously hyperechoic
  - ○ May be anechoic
  - ○ Rim Ca++ may cause posterior acoustic shadowing

Lipoma
- Circumscribed fat-containing lesion
- Soft and freely movable
- Asymptomatic
- Usually unilateral
- Mammography is diagnostic in most cases
  - ○ Well-defined radiolucent mass
  - ○ May have areas of fat necrosis
  - ○ Apparent thin radiopaque capsule (no true capsule at pathology)
    - • Usually does not calcify
- Ultrasound
  - ○ Isoechoic to slightly hyperechoic mass
  - ○ Thin, echogenic capsule

Galactocele
- Fat-containing, well-circumscribed mass
- May demonstrate fat-fluid level
  - ○ Lateral projection mammography
  - ○ Ultrasound: Hyperechoic fat nondependent
- Ultrasound characteristics
  - ○ Low level internal echoes
  - ○ May see thin echogenic rim
  - ○ Variable acoustic enhancement

Steatocystoma Multiplex
- Rare cutaneous disorder
- Autosomal dominant
- Usually in adolescent or young men
- Multiple cutaneous intradermal cysts
  - ○ Mainly trunk, upper extremities
- Usually asymptomatic
  - ○ May become secondarily inflamed
- Soft to firm and smooth

OIL CYST

PATHOLOGY

General Features
- General path comments: Non-suppurative, benign inflammatory process characterized by local adipose cell destruction
- Etiology
  - Manifestation of post-traumatic fat necrosis
  - Commonly occurs secondary to breast trauma
    - Iatrogenic: Lumpectomy; post-mastectomy TRAM flap reconstruction; radiation therapy; reduction mammoplasty (minimized with free nipple graft technique); augmentation mammoplasty; implant removal; biopsy (open, core or FNA) and cyst aspiration
    - Injury: Blunt trauma; penetrating trauma; seatbelt injury
  - Not all cases thought to arise from fat necrosis
    - Steatocystoma multiplex: Round, well-circumscribed, intradermal masses; intradermal oil cysts; usually in adolescent or young men
  - Non-traumatic causes
    - Anticoagulant therapy
    - Infection
- Associated abnormalities
  - Post-surgical or post-traumatic scarring
  - Post-radiation edema

Gross Pathologic & Surgical Features
- Thick, oily material obtained at aspiration or surgery

Microscopic Features
- Early
  - Inflammatory changes: Foreign body giant cells, fat-filled macrophages, interstitial infiltration by plasma cells
  - Hemorrhage into fat
- Injury to adipose tissue → damage to fat cells releases lipid contents into interstitium → breakdown of lipids into liquefied fatty acids → fibrous capsule forms along capsule from fatty acid saponification
  - Calcium may precipitate along capsule from fatty acid saponification

CLINICAL ISSUES

Presentation
- Most common signs/symptoms
  - Usually clinically occult
    - Detected on screening mammography
- Other signs/symptoms: May present as tender palpable mass or masses
- Reduction mammoplasty
  - Often develops beneath scars
    - Around nipple
    - Vertical incision to inframammary fold

Demographics
- Age: All age groups
- Gender
  - Females more common than males
    - In males usually due to blunt trauma

- Ethnicity: No ethnic predilection

Natural History & Prognosis
- No malignant potential

Treatment
- No treatment necessary
- Biopsy not necessary if meets imaging criteria for oil cyst
- Aspiration and biopsy are best avoided due to irritating nature of oil cyst contents

DIAGNOSTIC CHECKLIST

Consider
- Appearance on US often more worrisome than mammography
  - Correlate with mammography
  - US alone may lead to unnecessary biopsy
  - If lesion fits clinical and strict mammographic criteria for benign oil cyst, routine follow-up

SELECTED REFERENCES

1. Berg WA et al: Cystic lesions of the breast: Sonographic-pathologic correlation. Radiology. 227:183-191, 2003
2. D'Orsi CJ et al: Breast Imaging Reporting and Data System: BI-RADS, Mammography, 4th ed. Reston, American College of Radiology, 2003
3. Park KY et al: Steatocystoma multiplex mammographic and sonographic manifestations. AJR. 180:271-4, 2003
4. Pui MH et al: Fatty tissue breast lesions. Clin Imaging. 27:170-5, 2003
5. Bilgen IG et al: Fat necrosis of the breast: Clinical, Mammographic and Sonographic Features. Eur Jour Rad. 39(2):92-9, 2001
6. Soo MS: Fat necrosis in the breast: Sonographic Features. Radiology. 206:261-96, 1998
7. Harvey JA et al: Sonographic features of mammary oil cysts. J Ultrasound Med. 16:719-24, 1997
8. Hogge JP et al: The mammographic spectrum of fat necrosis of the breast. Radiographics. 15:1347-56, 1995

OIL CYST

IMAGE GALLERY

Typical

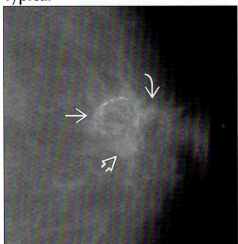

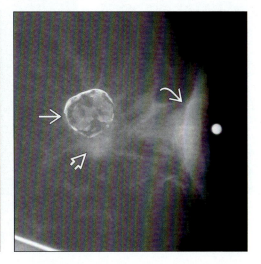

(Left) CC mammography 2 years following lumpectomy & radiation therapy for cancer shows calcifying oil cyst ➡ at the scar, with some adjacent density medially ➡ & anteriorly ➡. (Right) CC mammography spot compression 5 years post initial treatment surgery (same patient as left-hand image) shows coarsening of Ca++ around oil cyst ➡. Density medial to oil cyst ➡ has increased. Biopsy showed recurrent invasive ductal carcinoma. Nipple retraction is also noted ➡.

Typical

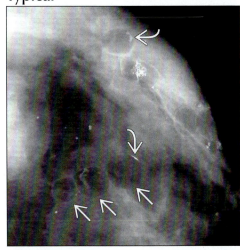

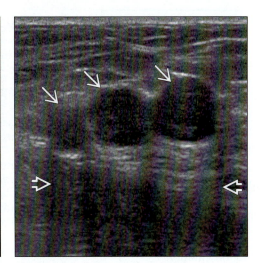

(Left) CC mammography shows multiple, round or oval circumscribed lucent masses ➡ compatible with oil cysts. Note peripheral calcification ➡ in some of the cysts. (Right) Radial ultrasound shows multiple, contiguous oil cysts, presenting as circumscribed masses ➡ with posterior enhancement ➡. Note homogeneous low level internal echoes.

Typical

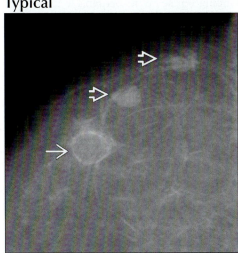

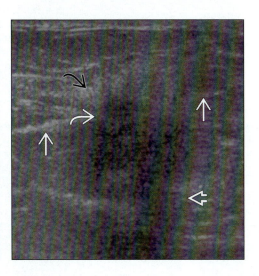

(Left) CC mammography shows benign, palpable oil cyst ➡. Note benign intramammary lymph nodes ➡. (Right) Anti-radial ultrasound. Without recognizing its benign characteristics on mammography, the oil cyst (left-hand image) had been aspirated by the woman's surgeon, causing an inflammatory, irregular hypoechoic mass ➡ with posterior shadowing ➡, tethering of Cooper ligaments ➡ and an echogenic rim ➡.

MICROLOBULATED MARGINS

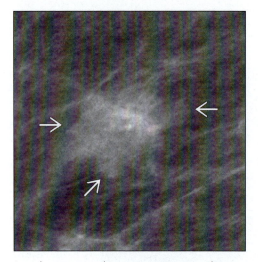

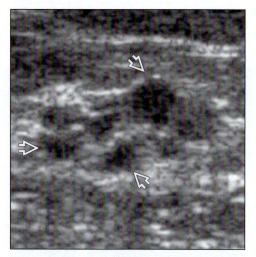

Lateral mammography spot compression shows a microlobulated ➡ mass. This image and US at right reprinted with permission. (Warner JK et al: AJR. 170:1375-79, 1998).

Radial ultrasound (same mass as left-hand image) shows clustered microcysts ➡. Biopsy revealed a terminal duct lobular unit with cystically dilated acini lined by apocrine metaplastic epithelium.

TERMINOLOGY

Definitions
• Short cycle undulations of mass margins

IMAGING FINDINGS

General Features
• Best diagnostic clue: 1-2 mm undulations/lobulations of mass surface

Mammographic Findings
• CC and MLO views
  ○ Check for multifocal/multicentric, bilateral disease
  ○ Search for axillary lymphadenopathy
  ○ Associated architectural distortion, skin retraction
• Spot compression views reduce obscuration
• Spot magnification views
  ○ May better depict microlobulation
  ○ Depict associated microcalcifications
• Tangential view to verify if skin lesion

Ultrasonographic Findings
• Spatial compounding for margins
• Clustered microcysts
  ○ Evaluate for associated solid component

MR Findings
• T1WI
  ○ Most masses isointense to parenchyma
  ○ Hyperintensity: Fat in mass, protein, or hemorrhage
• T2WI FS
  ○ Hyperintense masses usually benign
    ▪ Fibroadenoma (FA), lymph node, apocrine metaplasia
    ▪ Colloid (mucinous) carcinoma can be bright
  ○ Hypointense internal septations typically FA
• T1 C+ FS
  ○ Nonenhancing mass nearly always benign
  ○ Evaluate internal enhancement homogeneity
    ▪ Nonenhancing septae favors benign FA
  ○ Evaluate margin enhancement
    ▪ Rim-enhancement especially suspicious
  ○ Concerning morphology overrules benign kinetics
  ○ Assess for skin, pectoral muscle, chest wall invasion

DDx: Causes of Microlobulated Margins

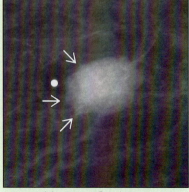

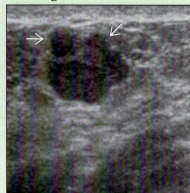

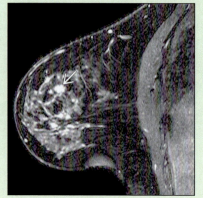

Mucinous Carcinoma

Lactating Adenoma

Papilloma

MICROLOBULATED MARGINS

Key Facts

Terminology
- Short cycle undulations of mass margins

Imaging Findings
- Best imaging tool: Spot magnification views and US

Top Differential Diagnoses
- Invasive ductal carcinoma
- Ductal carcinoma in situ (DCIS)
- Fibrocystic changes

- Apocrine metaplasia

Pathology
- 1% of all cancers are microlobulated

Diagnostic Checklist
- Clustered microcysts BI-RADS 2 or 3
- Solid, microlobulated mass BI-RADS 4, biopsy

Imaging Recommendations
- Best imaging tool: Spot magnification views and US

DIFFERENTIAL DIAGNOSIS

Malignancy
- Invasive ductal carcinoma
- Ductal carcinoma in situ (DCIS)

Clustered Microcysts
- Fibrocystic changes
- Apocrine metaplasia

Other Benign Lesions
- Fibroadenoma, fibroadenomatoid change
- Papilloma
- Lactating adenoma
  - Pregnant or lactating patient
- Tubular adenoma
- Nodular adenosis
- Phyllodes

PATHOLOGY

General Features
- Etiology
  - 17% of mammographically microlobulated masses going to biopsy are malignant

  - 67% of sonographically microlobulated masses going to biopsy are malignant
  - 1% of all cancers are microlobulated

Microscopic Features
- Expansion of terminal duct lobular unit
- Microinvasion of stroma

DIAGNOSTIC CHECKLIST

Consider
- Clustered microcysts BI-RADS 2 or 3
- Solid, microlobulated mass BI-RADS 4, biopsy

SELECTED REFERENCES

1. Hong AS et al: BI-RADS for sonography: positive and negative predictive values of sonographic features. AJR. 184:1260-5, 2005
2. D'Orsi CJ et al: Breast Imaging Reporting and Data System: BI-RADS, Mammography, 4th ed. Reston, American College of Radiology, 2003
3. Mendelson EB et al: Breast Imaging Reporting and Data System: BI-RADS, Ultrasound, 1st ed. Reston, American College of Radiology, 2003
4. Liberman L et al: The breast imaging reporting and data system: positive predictive value of mammographic features and final assessment categories. AJR. 171:35-40, 1998

IMAGE GALLERY

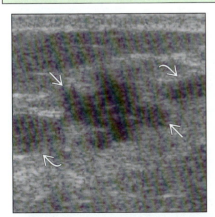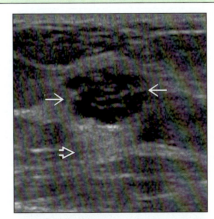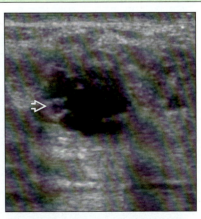

(Left) Radial ultrasound shows a microlobulated hypoechoic mass ➡, mammographically occult. US-guided biopsy showed invasive ductal carcinoma. Adjacent tubular masses ➡ were due to DCIS. *(Center)* Radial ultrasound shows clustered microcysts ➡, a benign finding. Posterior enhancement is noted ➡. *(Right)* Anti-radial ultrasound shows microlobulated anechoic mass ➡ with posterior enhancement, an unusual appearance for a simple cyst. Fusion of adjacent acini in the terminal duct lobular unit can result in a microlobulated appearance.

OBSCURED MARGINS

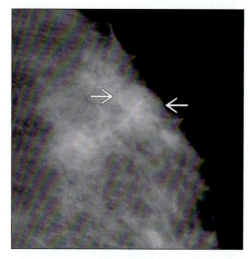

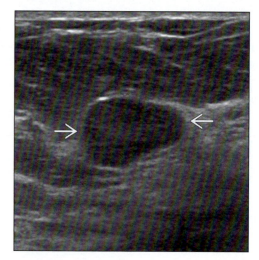

CC mammography spot compression shows a rounded mass ➡ whose margins remain mostly obscured by overlying tissue on spot compression. US was obtained for further characterization (right-hand image).

Radial spatial compounding ultrasound of the mass (left-hand image) shows a circumscribed, oval, slightly hypoechoic mass ➡. US-guided 14-g core biopsy confirmed fibroadenoma.

TERMINOLOGY

Definitions
- Margin hidden by superimposed or adjacent normal tissue on mammography
- Used when underlying mass is presumed to be circumscribed, but < 75% of the margin is visible
- Primarily a screening description: Spot compression usually reveals underlying margins
- Not used to refer to masses completely obscured (and thereby not detected) due to dense tissue

IMAGING FINDINGS

General Features
- Best diagnostic clue: Visualized margins are circumscribed, with tissue overlying > 25% of margin

Mammographic Findings
- CC and MLO views
  - Examine mass in both views
  - Visualized margins appear circumscribed, not indistinct
  - > 25% of margin hidden by overlying tissue
  - Identify multiplicity, bilaterality
  - Associated architectural distortion or calcifications require work-up
- Isolated partially obscured mass
  - Additional views if new, enlarging, or on baseline
  - Spot compression and/or ML views
  - If suspect associated calcifications, spot magnification CC and ML views
  - US for further characterization unless clearly lymph node
- Multiple bilateral partially circumscribed, partially obscured masses
  - At least 3 masses, at least one in each breast
  - No suspicious findings
  - Can be assessed as BI-RADS 2 if all masses meet these criteria
  - Dominant or palpable mass merits US
  - Fluctuating pattern suggests cysts
  - Coarse calcifications suggest fibroadenomas (FA)
- Worst margin characteristics should guide management

DDx: Masses with Partially Obscured Margins

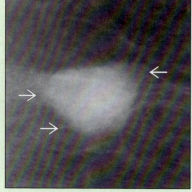

Mucinous Carcinoma

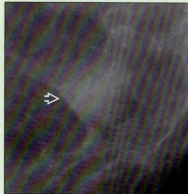

Atypical Papilloma

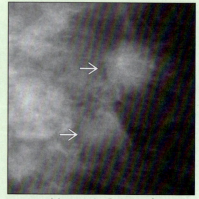

Metastatic Carcinoid

OBSCURED MARGINS

Key Facts

Terminology
- Margin hidden by superimposed or adjacent normal tissue on mammography
- Primarily a screening description: Spot compression usually reveals underlying margins

Imaging Findings
- Best diagnostic clue: Visualized margins are circumscribed, with tissue overlying > 25% of margin
- Additional views if new, enlarging, or on baseline
- Worst margin characteristics should guide management

Top Differential Diagnoses
- Cyst(s)
- Fibroadenoma
- Normal Variant Nodular Asymmetry

- Focal Fibrosis
- Phyllodes
- Papilloma(s)
- Invasive ductal carcinoma (IDC) NOS
- Papillary ductal carcinoma in situ (DCIS)
- Metastases

Pathology
- 5% of all masses going to biopsy

Diagnostic Checklist
- Spot compression mammographic views, US key
- Spot compression views less helpful if mass surrounded by dense tissue
- Multiple bilateral partially obscured, partially circumscribed masses generally benign
- Do not confuse obscured and indistinct margins

Ultrasonographic Findings
- Characterize palpable or mammographic finding
  - May demonstrate margins not seen on mammography
- Optimize technique for margins
  - Spatial compounding can be helpful
- Evaluate internal structure
  - Complicated cyst
  - Complex cystic lesion
- Multiple bilateral circumscribed solid masses benign or probably benign
- Guide biopsy if any suspicious findings

MR Findings
- T1WI: Most masses isointense to surrounding parenchyma
- T2WI FS
  - Cystic lesions hyperintense unless hemorrhagic
  - FA can be hyperintense
  - Mucinous carcinoma can be hyperintense
- T1 C+ FS
  - Nonenhancing mass > 98% predictive of benign etiology
  - Nonenhancing septations favor FA
  - Rim-enhancement suspicious

Imaging Recommendations
- Best imaging tool
  - Spot compression views useful
    - Displace adjacent tissue
    - Magnification views if suspect associated calcifications

DIFFERENTIAL DIAGNOSIS

Cyst(s)
- Solitary or multiple, often bilateral
- Most common in perimenopausal women or those on hormonal therapy
- Aspirate only for symptomatic relief or diagnostic uncertainty

- May show dependent milk-of-calcium

Complicated Cyst
- Homogeneous low level echoes
- Circumscribed, imperceptible wall
- Posterior enhancement
- May show fluid-debris level or other mobile debris
- Solitary or multiple, often in company of simple cysts

Oil Cyst
- Lucent mass
- Periphery may calcify
- History of surgery or trauma

Fibroadenoma
- 15% are multiple, often bilateral
- May develop coarse, "popcorn" calcifications as involute

Normal Variant Nodular Asymmetry
- Interspersed fat
- Thins on spot compression
- May appear hyperechoic on US, can be fibrotic

Focal Fibrosis
- Often hyperechoic or mixed hyper- and hypoechoic on US
- Can contain coarse, heterogeneous calcifications

Complex Cystic Lesion
- Any of: Thick wall, thick septations, intracystic mass, mixed cystic and solid lesion
- Merits biopsy
- Differential includes, fibrocystic changes, abscess, papillary lesions, malignancy

Phyllodes
- Rapidly growing
- Can be multiple
- "Cellular FA" on core biopsy may be a phyllodes tumor, consider excision

Lymph Node
- Notched fatty hilum

OBSCURED MARGINS

Papilloma(s)
- Intraductal or intracystic mass
- Merit biopsy
- May show associated amorphous or punctate calcifications
- Can be multiple

Other Benign
- Tubular adenoma
- Lactating adenoma
  - Patient pregnant or lactating
- Sclerosing adenosis
- Fibrocystic changes

Malignancy
- Suspicious features on any imaging should prompt biopsy
- Invasive ductal carcinoma (IDC) NOS
  - Look for partially indistinct margins, suspicious calcifications
- Medullary carcinoma
  - Partially indistinct margins
  - Can be complex cystic mass
- Colloid (mucinous) carcinoma
  - Dense on mammography
  - Often isointense to fat on US
  - Margins usually partially indistinctly marginated
- Papillary ductal carcinoma in situ (DCIS)
  - Most often intracystic mass
- Metastases
  - Usually unilateral
  - May be partially indistinctly marginated
- Lymphoma
  - Associated adenopathy
  - Usually partially indistinctly marginated
  - Often mixed hyper- and hypoechoic on US

PATHOLOGY

General Features
- Etiology
  - 5% of all masses going to biopsy
  - 33% rate of malignancy among obscured masses going to biopsy

CLINICAL ISSUES

Presentation
- Most common signs/symptoms
  - Asymptomatic, detected incidentally on mammogram
  - Palpable mass

Treatment
- Biopsy if concerning feature revealed by additional imaging

DIAGNOSTIC CHECKLIST

Consider
- Dense parenchyma obscures both detection and mass margins once mass is detected
  - > 50% of cancers may be completely obscured and go undetected in dense tissue on film screen mammography
  - Digital mammography shows improved sensitivity for women < 50 years old, pre- or perimenopausal, those with dense breasts
    - Windowing and leveling may help reveal underlying mass in areas of denser tissue

Image Interpretation Pearls
- Spot compression mammographic views, US key
  - Spot compression views less helpful if mass surrounded by dense tissue
  - US of greater benefit in characterizing mass margins in denser breasts
- US unless multiple bilateral similar findings
- Multiple bilateral partially obscured, partially circumscribed masses generally benign
  - Consider each mass on its own merits, carefully evaluating margins
  - All masses should be mostly circumscribed between CC and MLO views
  - Dominant or palpable mass(es) merit further evaluation with spot compression, US
  - If margins possibly indistinct, spiculated, or microlobulated, further evaluation warranted
- Do not confuse obscured and indistinct margins
  - Management based on most suspicious margin or other suspicious feature(s)

SELECTED REFERENCES

1. Hong AS et al: BI-RADS for sonography: positive and negative predictive values of sonographic features. AJR. 184:1260-5, 2005
2. Pisano ED et al: Diagnostic performance of digital versus film mammography for breast-cancer screening. NEJM. 353:1773-83, 2005
3. D'Orsi CJ et al: Breast Imaging Reporting and Data System: BI-RADS, Mammography, 4th ed. Reston, American College of Radiology, 2003
4. Bassett LW: Imaging of breast masses. Radiol Clin North Am. 38(4):669-91, vii-viii, 2000
5. Leung JW et al: Multiple bilateral masses detected on screening mammography: Assessment of need for recall imaging. AJR. 175:23-9, 2000
6. Liberman L et al: The breast imaging reporting and data system: positive predictive value of mammographic features and final assessment categories. AJR. 171:35-40, 1998
7. Sickles EA: Practical solutions to common mammographic problems: tailoring the examination. AJR Am J Roentgenol. 151(1):31-9, 1988

OBSCURED MARGINS

IMAGE GALLERY

Typical

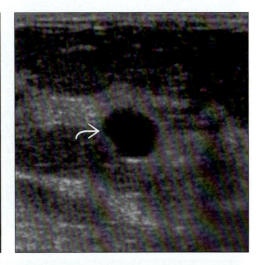

(Left) MLO mammography spot compression shows an oval mass with partially circumscribed margins ➡. At least 25% of the mass margins remain obscured ⮞ despite spot compression. *(Right)* Anti-radial ultrasound (same mass as left-hand image) shows a simple cyst ⮞, concordant in size and location with the mammographically-depicted mass, a benign finding (BI-RADS 2).

Variant

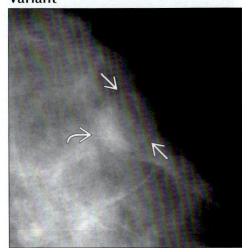
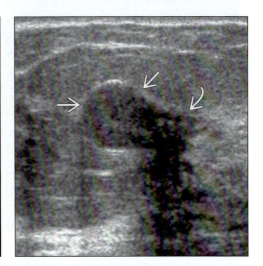

(Left) CC mammography shows a partially circumscribed ➡, partially obscured ⮞ mass. US was performed for further evaluation (right-hand image). *(Right)* Transverse ultrasound shows (same mass as left-hand image) to be partially circumscribed ➡, & partially irregular ⮞, and therefore suspicious. US-guided biopsy and excision showed a fibroadenoma involved by invasive lobular carcinoma.

Typical

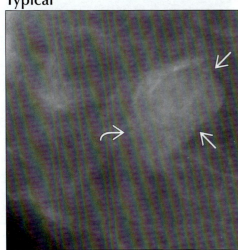
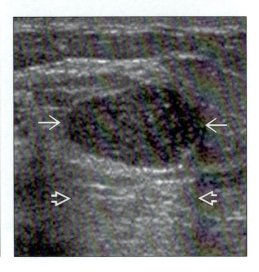

(Left) CC mammography in this 41 year old shows partially circumscribed ➡, partially obscured ⮞ mass on this baseline exam. US is recommended for further evaluation (right-hand image). *(Right)* Sagittal ultrasound shows the mass to be circumscribed ➡, oval, and hypoechoic with posterior enhancement ⮞, compatible with a fibroadenoma, and confirmed on US-guided core biopsy.

OBSCURED MARGINS

(Left) CC mammography spot compression shows a mass with partially circumscribed margins ➡. Posteriorly ➡, it is not clear whether the mass remains partially obscured by overlying tissue or is indistinctly marginated. *(Right)* Radial ultrasound (same mass at left) confirms partially circumscribed ➡ margins. Co-existing partially indistinct ➡, and partially microlobulated ➡ margins prompted biopsy, which showed grade III IDC NOS.

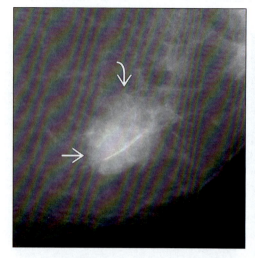
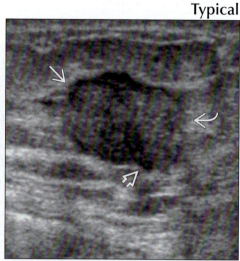

(Left) CC mammography of this 39 year old shows multiple bilateral partially circumscribed, partially obscured masses ➡. One of these in the upper outer left breast ➡ was noted to be enlarging compared to baseline mammogram 8 months earlier. *(Right)* MLO mammography (same patient as left-hand image) again shows multiple, bilateral similar masses ➡. These were initially considered BI-RADS 3. On follow-up, one had enlarged ➡ and was solid on US.

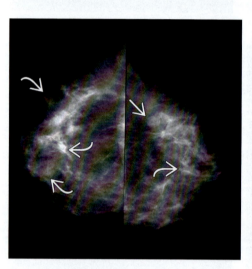
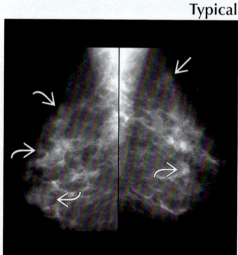

(Left) MLO mammography close-up (same patient as previous image) shows the enlarging mass to have mostly circumscribed margins ➡, though > 25% are obscured by an adjacent mass ➡. *(Right)* Sagittal MIP of T1 C+ subtraction MR (same patient as left-hand image) shows multiple smooth, oval, enhancing masses ➡. The most intensely enhancing mass ➡ corresponded to the enlarging mass, which was then biopsied under US showing fibroadenoma.

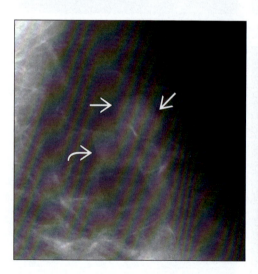
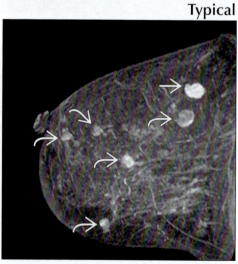

IV 1 20

OBSCURED MARGINS

Variant

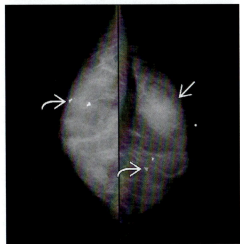

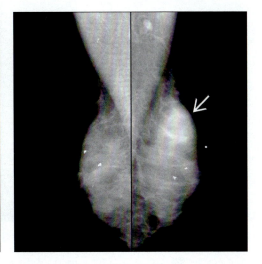

(Left) CC mammography shows a partially circumscribed, partially obscured mass ➡, corresponding to a palpable abnormality. A few coarse, typically benign calcifications are present ➡. *(Right)* MLO mammography (same patient as left-hand image) shows vague mass in upper breast ➡. Spot compression views were performed (see next 2 images).

Variant

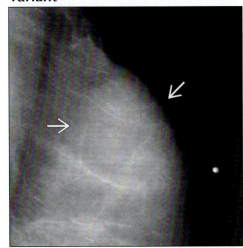

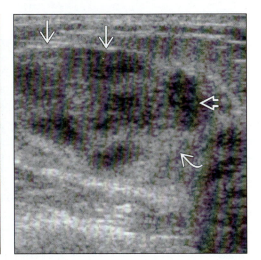

(Left) MLO mammography spot compression shows persistently obscured mass ➡. US is appropriate for further evaluation (right-hand image). *(Right)* Radial ultrasound (same patient as left-hand image) shows a mixed hyper- ➡ and hypoechoic ➡ mass which is partially circumscribed anteriorly ➡. US-guided biopsy showed lymphoma, primary to the breast.

Typical

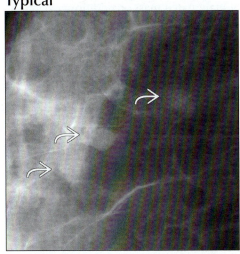

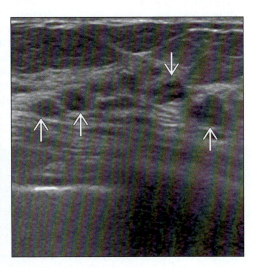

(Left) CC mammography close-up of this 39 year old shows multiple adjacent partially circumscribed, partially obscured masses ➡ in this woman with known papillomas. *(Right)* Radial ultrasound (same patient as left-hand image) shows multiple circumscribed, oval masses ➡. Core biopsies showed papillomas and atypical papillomas. Excision showed papillomas and papillary DCIS.

INDISTINCT MARGINS

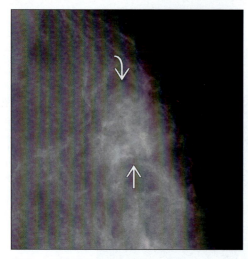 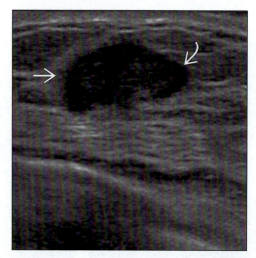

MLO mammography spot compression over a palpable mass in a 92 year old shows a partially circumscribed ➡, partially indistinctly marginated ➡ mass.

Transverse ultrasound (same mass as left) shows hypoechoic oval mass with partially circumscribed ➡ partially indistinct margins ➡. Management should be based on worst features: Biopsy showed IDC grade II.

TERMINOLOGY

Abbreviations and Synonyms
- Ill-defined, poorly-defined margins

Definitions
- Mammography: Demarcation between a mass and its surrounding tissue is not clearly defined
  ○ Any suggestion of poor margin definition raises the possibility of tumor infiltration
  ○ Distinguish from "obscured" margins
    ▪ Otherwise circumscribed margin camouflaged or obscured by overlapping tissue
  ○ Distinguish from focal asymmetry
    ▪ Spot compression views may reveal persistent, indistinctly marginated mass
- Ultrasound: Both mass and boundary zone lack discrete transition to surrounding tissue

IMAGING FINDINGS

General Features
- Best diagnostic clue: Poor definition of mass margin on mammography or ultrasound

Mammographic Findings
- CC and MLO views
  ○ Inspect fat-glandular interface carefully
  ○ Identify multiplicity, bilaterality
  ○ Check for skin thickening, nipple retraction
  ○ Check axillae for lymphadenopathy, axillary tail mass
  ○ Comparison to prior films aids detection of new asymmetries
- Spot compression views
  ○ Focal asymmetry on screening may prove to be an indistinctly marginated mass on additional views
  ○ Displace overlapping tissue which obscured margins on screening views
- Spot magnification compression views
  ○ A mass that appears circumscribed or obscured on screening views may prove to be indistinctly marginated on magnification views

DDx: Other Margin Characteristics

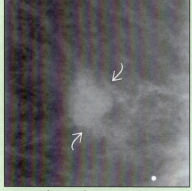 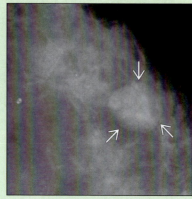 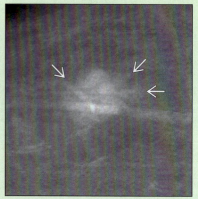

Obscured, IDC Grade III

Circumscribed, Cyst

Microlobulated, Apocrine Metaplasia

INDISTINCT MARGINS

Key Facts

Terminology
- Distinguish from "obscured" margins

Imaging Findings
- Best imaging tool: Spot compression mammographic views, US

Top Differential Diagnoses
- Invasive ductal carcinoma (IDC) NOS
- Mucinous or colloid IDC
- Invasive lobular carcinoma (ILC)
- DCIS
- Fibroadenoma (FA)
- Normal variant focal asymmetry
- Fibrocystic changes (FCC)
- Papilloma
- Ruptured cyst
- Abscess
- Pseudoangiomatous stromal hyperplasia (PASH)
- Fat necrosis

Pathology
- 44% mammographically indistinctly marginated masses malignant
- 60% of sonographically indistinctly-marginated masses malignant

Diagnostic Checklist
- Warrants BI-RADS 4 or 5 designation and biopsy unless a simple cyst on US
- Worst margin characteristics should guide management
- Should not be confused with focal asymmetry
- Indistinct mass is usually visible on two views

- ○ Characterize and determine extent of associated calcifications (Ca++) if any

Ultrasonographic Findings
- Grayscale Ultrasound
  - ○ Characterize palpable or mammographic finding
    - ▪ May demonstrate margins not seen on mammography
  - ○ Optimize technique for margins and posterior acoustic characteristics
    - ▪ Spatial compounding may "smooth" margins and limit visualization of posterior shadowing
    - ▪ Disengage spatial compounding to further evaluate margin characteristics and posterior features
    - ▪ Utilize appropriate high frequency transducer, adjust focal zone
  - ○ Invasive malignancy may cause loss of normal US interfaces
    - ▪ Thick, echogenic rim
    - ▪ May be due to invasion or peritumoral edema
  - ○ US can help evaluate extent
    - ▪ Multifocal, multicentric disease, adenopathy

MR Findings
- T1WI: Demonstrates overall architecture
- T1WI FS: Most lesions isointense to glandular tissue
- T1 C+ FS
  - ○ Enhancing lesions suggest possible malignancy
  - ○ Lower spatial resolution than mammography
    - ▪ Indistinct margins may appear "smoothed", leading to falsely benign assessment
    - ▪ Non-palpable smooth enhancing masses represented 17% of malignancies in one series
- Use MR for staging local extent, not in lieu of biopsy

Imaging Recommendations
- Best imaging tool: Spot compression mammographic views, US

DIFFERENTIAL DIAGNOSIS

Malignant Masses
- Most malignant mass margins are indistinct, microlobulated, or spiculated
- Invasive ductal carcinoma (IDC) NOS
  - ○ Most common indistinctly marginated carcinoma
  - ○ May have associated Ca++, often in ductal carcinoma in situ (DCIS) component
- Medullary IDC
  - ○ Oval or round mass with partially circumscribed margins
    - ▪ At least a portion of margin usually indistinct
  - ○ 5% of breast cancers
  - ○ Mean age 46-54
  - ○ Grow rapidly; locally aggressive
  - ○ Ca++ rare
  - ○ US: Hypoechoic well-defined mass; may have posterior acoustic enhancement
- Mucinous or colloid IDC
  - ○ Margins may appear fairly well-circumscribed
  - ○ Lobular or irregular shape; calcifications rare
  - ○ More common in postmenopausal woman
  - ○ Slow growing
  - ○ More favorable prognosis than IDC NOS
  - ○ US: Hypoechoic lobular mass; variable posterior acoustic characteristics
- Invasive lobular carcinoma (ILC)
  - ○ Most common presentation is spiculated mass
  - ○ May appear as a developing focal asymmetry with or without architectural distortion
  - ○ May be seen in only one mammographic view, CC more commonly
  - ○ US: Typically an irregular mass with intense posterior acoustic shadowing
  - ○ US: May be nearly anechoic with indistinct margins
- DCIS
  - ○ Usually Ca++: Fine linear, pleomorphic, amorphous
  - ○ Noncalcified mass an uncommon presentation
  - ○ Often solid type DCIS, usually low grade
- Metastases
  - ○ Usually unilateral, more often solitary than multiple

INDISTINCT MARGINS

- ○ Margins often partially circumscribed, but usually at least partially indistinct
- ○ Most common metastasis to breast = melanoma
- • Lymphoma
  - ○ May be fairly well-circumscribed
  - ○ Assess for associated lymphadenopathy

High Risk Lesions
- • Lobular carcinoma in situ (LCIS)
  - ○ Rarely visible on mammography
  - ○ LCIS can be an indistinctly marginated mass on US
- • Atypical papilloma

Benign Masses
- • Fibroadenoma (FA)
  - ○ Rarely: Malignancy involving FA
- • Normal variant focal asymmetry
  - ○ Can be difficult to distinguish from indistinctly marginated mass
  - ○ Concave margins
  - ○ Interspersed fat
  - ○ Thins on spot compression
  - ○ US: Hyperechoic oval or band-like
- • Fibrocystic changes (FCC)
  - ○ Mix of fibrosis, microcysts, adenosis, or sclerosing adenosis to varying degrees
  - ○ Can form discrete mass, often indistinctly marginated but not spiculated
  - ○ May show associated punctate, amorphous, heterogeneous Ca++
- • Papilloma
  - ○ May have associated punctate or amorphous Ca++
  - ○ Most common near nipple, often seen to be intraductal on US
  - ○ May present with clear or bloody nipple discharge
  - ○ Excision recommended when indistinctly marginated
    - ▪ Risk of atypical or malignant papillary lesion
- • Ruptured cyst
  - ○ Persistent rim-enhancing mass on MR, bright on T2WI
- • Abscess
  - ○ Tender, warm, palpable mass, overlying erythema
  - ○ Most common near nipple
  - ○ More common in lactating patient, diabetic, HIV, post-radiation or surgery
- • Pseudoangiomatous stromal hyperplasia (PASH)
  - ○ May have associated punctate or amorphous Ca++
- • Fat necrosis
  - ○ History of trauma or surgery
  - ○ Wide variety of appearances
  - ○ May develop Ca++ after 2-3 years
- • Hematoma/seroma
  - ○ History of trauma or surgery
  - ○ Collection on US with tract to overlying skin scar, may have septations, thick wall

PATHOLOGY

General Features
- • Etiology
  - ○ Tumor infiltration or peritumoral desmoplastic reaction

- ○ Edema surrounding traumatic or inflammatory process
- ○ 38% of mammographic masses going to biopsy were indistinctly marginated in one series
  - ▪ 44% mammographically indistinctly marginated masses malignant
- ○ 21% of US masses going to biopsy were indistinctly marginated in one series
  - ▪ 60% of sonographically indistinctly-marginated masses malignant

Microscopic Features
- • Invasive malignancy
  - ○ IDC: Extension from terminal ductal lobular unit into surrounding stroma
  - ○ ILC: Single-file growth or in sheets of cells

CLINICAL ISSUES

Presentation
- • Most common signs/symptoms: Asymptomatic, on screening
- • Other signs/symptoms: Palpable mass

DIAGNOSTIC CHECKLIST

Image Interpretation Pearls
- • Warrants BI-RADS 4 or 5 designation and biopsy unless a simple cyst on US
- • Worst margin characteristics should guide management
- • Stability of worrisome findings is not reassuring
- • Should not be confused with focal asymmetry
  - ○ Indistinct mass is usually visible on two views

SELECTED REFERENCES

1. Hong AF et al: BI-RADS for sonography: positive and negative predictive values of sonographic features. AJR. 184:1200-5, 2005
2. D'Orsi CJ et al: Breast Imaging Reporting and Data System: BI-RADS, Mammography, 4th ed. Reston, American College of Radiology, 2003
3. Mendelson EB et al: Breast Imaging Reporting and Data System: BI-RADS, Ultrasound, 1st ed. Reston, American College of Radiology, 2003
4. Berg WA et al: Breast Imaging Reporting and Data System: inter- and intraobserver variability in feature analysis and final assessment. AJR. 174:1769-77, 2000
5. Liberman L et al: The breast imaging reporting and data system: positive predictive value of mammographic features and final assessment categories. AJR. 171:35-40, 1998

INDISTINCT MARGINS

IMAGE GALLERY

Typical

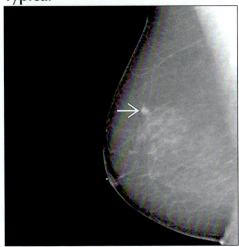

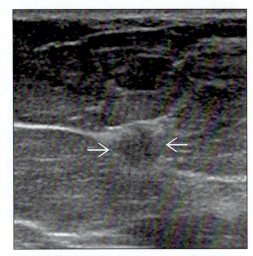

(Left) MLO mammography shows a new 8 mm mass with indistinct margins ➡. (Right) Transverse ultrasound (same mass as left-hand image) shows an indistinctly marginated hypoechoic mass ➡. US-guided biopsy demonstrated grade I infiltrating ductal carcinoma and low grade DCIS.

Typical

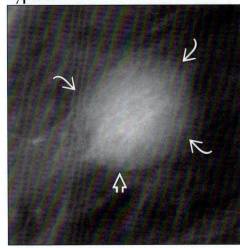

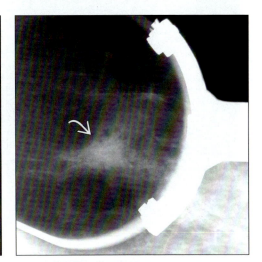

(Left) MLO mammography spot compression shows a mass with partially circumscribed ➡ and partially indistinct ➡ margins. On US this was a simple cyst. (Right) CC mammography spot compression shows an invasive lobular carcinoma, with typically indistinct margins ➡ and associated architectural distortion.

Typical

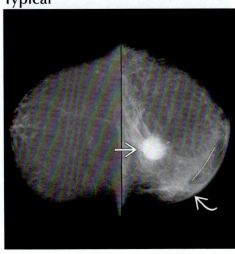

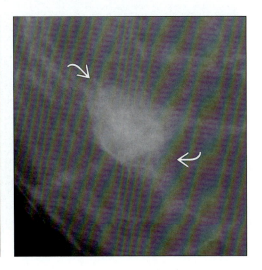

(Left) CC mammography shows a mass with indistinct margins ➡ and ipsilateral skin thickening ➡ from recent surgery. This post-surgical hematoma/seroma subsequently resolved. (Right) CC mammography spot compression in this 30 year old shows an indistinctly marginated mass ➡. US-guided biopsy showed FA.

Typical

(Left) CC mammography spot compression shows partially circumscribed ➡, partially indistinctly marginated ➡ mass which had been gradually enlarging in this 79 year old. US-guided biopsy showed low grade DCIS. *(Right)* Lateral mammography spot compression shows indistinctly marginated mass ➡. Biopsy showed an intramammary node involved with metastatic melanoma.

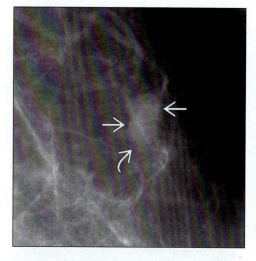

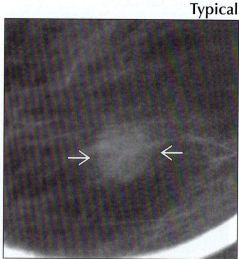

Typical

(Left) MLO mammography spot compression shows new indistinctly marginated mass ➡ in this 48 year old woman. Biopsy showed PASH. *(Right)* MLO mammography shows indistinctly marginated mass ➡ in this 68 year old. Biopsy showed stromal fibrosis.

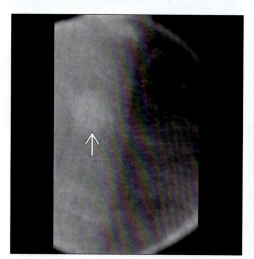

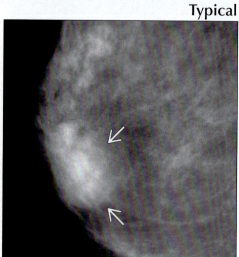

Typical

(Left) MLO mammography close-up in this 63 year old shows a dense, indistinctly marginated mass ➡. *(Right)* Transverse ultrasound (same mass as left-hand image) shows indistinctly marginated isoechoic mass ➡ with posterior enhancement ➡. US-guided core biopsy showed mucinous carcinoma.

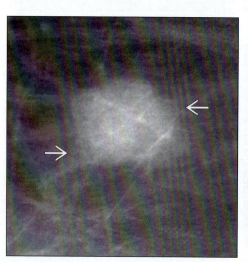

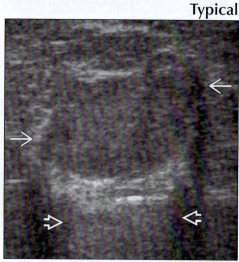

INDISTINCT MARGINS

Typical

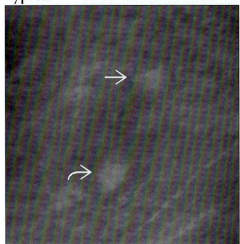

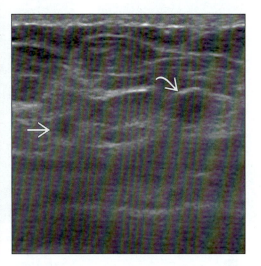

(Left) CC mammography spot compression in this 73 year old shows two adjacent indistinctly marginated masses, one of which was new ➡, and the other ➡ which was gradually enlarging over 8 years, with prior biopsy showing FCC. *(Right)* Anti-radial ultrasound again shows the two indistinctly marginated, nearly isoechoic masses ➡, ➡. US-guided biopsy and excision showed papillomas and sclerosing adenosis in each.

Typical

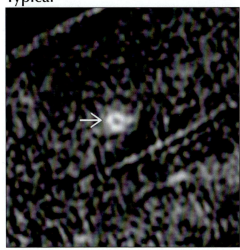

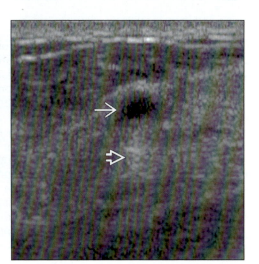

(Left) Sagittal T1 C+ subtraction MR in this 50 year old woman screening because of high risk shows a 4 mm rim-enhancing mass ➡. *(Right)* Radial ultrasound targeted to the MR abnormality (left-hand image) shows an indistinctly-marginated, thick-walled cystic lesion ➡ with posterior enhancement ➡. US-guided biopsy showed ruptured cyst.

Typical

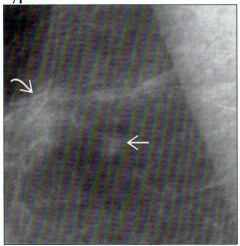

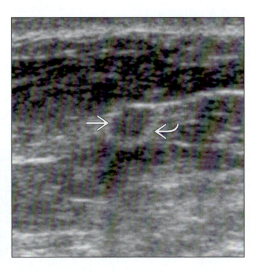

(Left) MLO mammography spot compression shows a 4 mm gradually enlarging indistinctly marginated mass ➡ adjacent to scar ➡ from lumpectomy surgery for cancer 7 years earlier in this 84 year old. *(Right)* Anti-radial ultrasound targeted to the mammographic abnormality (left-hand image) shows indistinctly marginated isoechoic mass ➡ with echogenic rim ➡, moderately suspicious for cancer. US-guided biopsy showed grade I IDC.

SPICULATED MARGINS

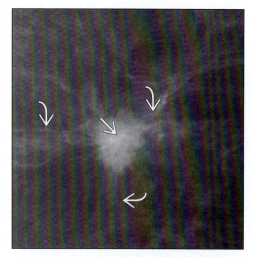

CC mammography magnification shows a spiculated mass ➡ as well as some subtle amorphous calcifications centrally ➡.

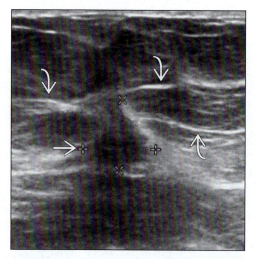

Radial ultrasound (same mass as left-hand image) shows a hypoechoic, irregular mass ➡ with tethering of Cooper ligaments ➡. Biopsy showed DCIS and IDC.

TERMINOLOGY

Abbreviations and Synonyms
- Stellate

Definitions
- Sharp lines radiating from the margin of a mass
- Distinguish from isolated architectural distortion without a central mass
  - Distortion, with retraction of parenchyma and tethering of Cooper ligaments, can be associated with a spiculated mass

IMAGING FINDINGS

General Features
- Best diagnostic clue: Centrally dense mass with radiating lines

Mammographic Findings
- CC and MLO views
  - Inspect fat-glandular interface carefully
  - Check for multifocal or multicentric disease, contralateral findings
  - Check for ancillary findings: Skin thickening, nipple retraction, lymphadenopathy
  - Prior comparison images aid in detection of subtle change
  - Stability of worrisome findings is not reassuring
  - Skin scar marker may be used to localize post-surgical findings
- Spot compression views
  - Confirm persistent mass
  - Reveal margins obscured by superimposed tissue
- Spot magnification compression views
  - May depict subtle spiculations or calcifications (Ca++)

Ultrasonographic Findings
- Grayscale Ultrasound
  - Mass known to be spiculated on mammography
    - US used to guide biopsy, not for characterization
  - Characterize palpable finding
    - May be initial exam in young women, especially if < 30 years old, pregnant/lactating patient

DDx: Causes of Spiculated Margins

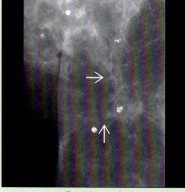

Fat Necrosis

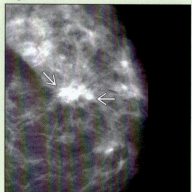

Biopsy Changes

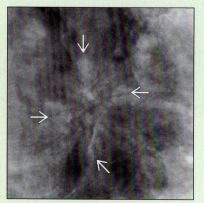

Radial Scar

SPICULATED MARGINS

Key Facts

Terminology
- Sharp lines radiating from the margin of a mass
- Distinguish from isolated architectural distortion without a central mass

Imaging Findings
- Spot compression magnification may demonstrate short spicules, calcifications
- US to guide biopsy, can use to evaluate disease extent
- MRI may depict extent of disease and contralateral malignancy

Top Differential Diagnoses
- Malignant Mass
- 2/3 of IDC NOS is spiculated
- Tubular carcinoma
- Post-Surgical Scar

- Radial Scar
- Fat Necrosis

Pathology
- IDC NOS: Most common spiculated malignancy

Clinical Issues
- Spiculation often signifies invasion of adjacent tissue
- Worse prognosis with increasing mass size
- Should prompt BI-RADS 4 or 5 designation and biopsy unless clearly due to scar or hematoma
- Radial scar usually warrants surgical excision

Diagnostic Checklist
- Avoid satisfaction of search
- Search for multifocal, multicentric, or contralateral disease

---

- If suspicious, bilateral mammogram needed for further work-up
  - Helpful to assess areas less accessible on mammogram
    - Far lateral axillary tail, far upper inner quadrant
  - Associated findings common
    - Irregular shape, posterior shadowing, duct extension, Ca++, architectural distortion, skin thickening or retraction
  - Evaluate abnormal or palpably enlarged lymph nodes
    - Loss of fatty hilum, convex/bulging contour, microcalcification
    - Consider fine needle aspiration biopsy (FNAB) to aid staging
  - Consider whole breast US to assess for multifocal or multicentric cancer
    - If using US to assess extent, evaluate contralateral breast
  - Spicule echogenicity variable
    - Hypoechoic spicules within echogenic fibrous tissue
    - Echogenic spicules within fat
  - Reduced visualization of mass margins perpendicular to US beam
    - Short unresolved spicules may appear as thick echogenic rim
    - Spatial compounding may increase conspicuity
  - Shadowing secondary to fibrous/desmoplastic reaction

MR Findings
- T1WI
  - Demonstrates overall architecture
    - Inspect for asymmetry or frank spiculation
  - Check for central hyperintensity within mass
    - Suggestive of fat necrosis (but not always present)
- T2WI FS
  - Centrally hyperintense spiculated mass
    - Post-surgical hematoma and/or seroma
- T1 C+
  - Enhancing spiculated margins 91% positive predictive value for malignancy

- Most common margin seen in malignancy
- Highly sensitive for malignancy

Imaging Recommendations
- Best imaging tool
  - Spot compression mammography in two projections
    - Spot compression magnification may demonstrate short spicules, calcifications
    - Verify presence of true mass, not focal asymmetry
  - US to guide biopsy, can use to evaluate disease extent
  - MRI may depict extent of disease and contralateral malignancy
    - Confirm finding seen on only one mammographic view
    - Helps depict extensive intraductal component (EIC) if present
    - Lack of enhancement should not deter biopsy: Tubular carcinoma, invasive lobular carcinoma (ILC) can be falsely negative
- Protocol advice
  - Optimize US technique
    - Disable spatial compounding feature to visualize shadowing
    - Increase frequency for superficial lesion conspicuity
    - Increase frequency to visualize tiny calcifications

DIFFERENTIAL DIAGNOSIS

Malignant Mass
- Invasive ductal carcinoma (IDC)
  - 2/3 of IDC NOS is spiculated
  - Associated ductal carcinoma in situ (DCIS) may be present, including EIC
  - Tubular carcinoma
    - Small mass, typically patient > 50 years old
- ILC
  - Findings often more subtle than IDC
  - May appear as focal asymmetry on routine views
- DCIS (rare)

SPICULATED MARGINS

Post-Surgical Scar
- History of benign biopsy
  - Often no residual finding
- History of lumpectomy and radiation
  - Overlying skin thickening/deformity
    - May be more prominent after radiation therapy
  - Appearances favoring scar over recurrence
    - Concave, extends to overlying skin scar
    - Most prominent on immediate post-op exam then decreases
    - MR: Should decrease in size, unusual to enhance > 18 months post-op
    - Dystrophic calcifications develop > 2 years post-op
  - Appearances favoring recurrence over scar
    - New pleomorphic or heterogeneous Ca++ in scar
    - MR: Increasing size and/or enhancement
    - Convex, nodular margins

Radial Scar
- Lacks central mass
- Imaging cannot differentiate from malignancy
  - Up to 25% associated with DCIS, tubular carcinoma

Fat Necrosis
- Variable appearance
- History of trauma, prior biopsy or surgery key to considering diagnosis
- Dystrophic Ca++ help suggest benignity
- Spiculation surrounding lucent center instead of mass
  - Most commonly fat necrosis
  - Overlapping appearance with radial scar, IDC engulfing fat

Hematoma
- History of trauma, biopsy, anticoagulation

Granular Cell Tumor
- Intermediate-risk mass

Other Benign Causes of Spiculation
- Fibromatosis
- Granulomatous mastitis
- Diabetic mastopathy
- Sarcoid

PATHOLOGY

General Features
- Etiology
  - IDC NOS: Most common spiculated malignancy
  - 81% PPV for malignancy on mammography
  - 86%-93% PPV for malignancy on US

Microscopic Features
- Malignant mass
  - IDC NOS
    - Invasion through basement membrane into interlobular stroma
    - Fibrosis, desmoplastic reaction causes spiculation
- Benign mass
  - Radial scar
    - Central fibrosis and elastosis, lucent center with entrapped fat

- Proliferation of ductal epithelium as well as fibroelastic tissue
  - Fat necrosis
    - Loss of blood supply, enzymatic fat breakdown
    - Peripheral distortion, lucent fatty center, late calcification

CLINICAL ISSUES

Presentation
- Most common signs/symptoms: Incidental mammographic finding
- Other signs/symptoms
  - Palpable mass
  - Skin dimpling, nipple retraction, axillary lymphadenopathy
  - Post-op changes

Natural History & Prognosis
- Spiculation often signifies invasion of adjacent tissue
  - Favors low grade histology, better prognosis than high grade
  - Worse prognosis with increasing mass size
- Tubular carcinoma: Better prognosis than IDC NOS

Treatment
- Should prompt BI-RADS 4 or 5 designation and biopsy unless clearly due to scar or hematoma
- Consider US-guided FNAB of axillary node
- Biopsy prior lumpectomy site if
  - Increase in size, density, or spiculation
  - New worrisome calcifications
- Radial scar usually warrants surgical excision

DIAGNOSTIC CHECKLIST

Image Interpretation Pearls
- Spot compression and/or magnification views
  - Persistence of mass and characterize margins
    - Search fat-glandular interface carefully
  - May demonstrate tiny spicules, Ca++
- Avoid satisfaction of search
  - Search for multifocal, multicentric, or contralateral disease

SELECTED REFERENCES

1. Hong AS et al: BI-RADS for sonography: positive and negative predictive values of sonographic features. AJR. 184:1260-5, 2005
2. Morris EA et al: Breast MRI Diagnosis and Intervention. New York, Springer. 140-183, 2005
3. D'Orsi CJ et al: Breast Imaging Reporting and Data System: BI-RADS, Mammography, 4th ed. Reston, American College of Radiology, 2003
4. Liberman L et al: The breast imaging reporting and data system: positive predictive value of mammographic features and final assessment categories. AJR. 171:35-40, 1998
5. Stavros AT et al: Solid breast nodules: use of sonography to distinguish between benign and malignant lesions. Radiology. 196:123-34, 1995

SPICULATED MARGINS

IMAGE GALLERY

Typical

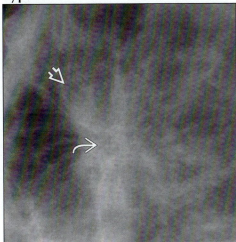

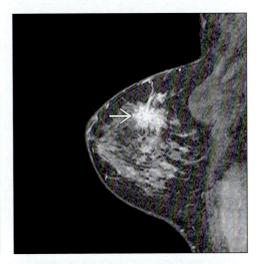

(Left) MLO mammography magnification shows architectural distortion ➡️ and central lucency ➡️. Histopathology showed radial scar with central fibroelastosis and adenosis along the spicules. (Right) Sagittal T1 C+ FS MR shows an enhancing irregular spiculated mass ➡️. Excisional histopathology included a radial scar, numerous papillomas and florid proliferative fibrocystic change.

Typical

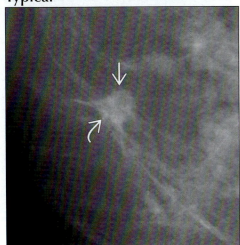

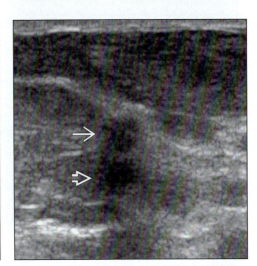

(Left) CC mammography spot compression shows a spiculated mass ➡️ with a few amorphous calcifications ➡️. (Right) Radial ultrasound (same mass as left-hand image) shows a spiculated, hypoechoic mass ➡️ with posterior shadowing ➡️. Biopsy confirmed grade II IDC NOS.

Typical

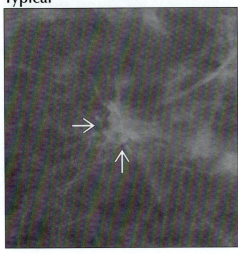

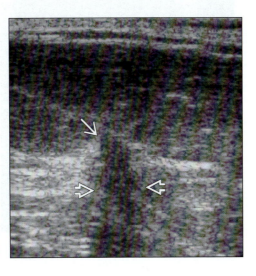

(Left) CC mammography magnification shows a 5 mm, spiculated mass ➡️. (Right) Transverse ultrasound (same mass as left-hand image) shows an irregular, hypoechoic mass ➡️ with posterior shadowing ➡️. US-guided biopsy and subsequent excision confirmed tubular carcinoma.

SPICULATED MARGINS

(Left) Mammography spot compression shows a subtle mass ➡ with peripheral spiculation ➡. *(Right)* Longitudinal ultrasound (same mass as left-hand image) shows spiculated margins ➡ and tethering of Cooper ligaments ➡. Biopsy confirmed IDC NOS.

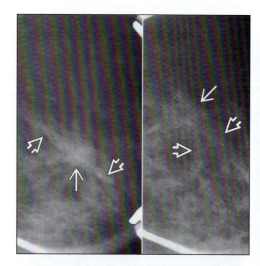
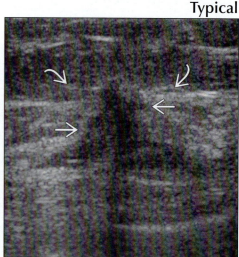

(Left) Serial 6 month follow-up mammograms (at times = 6 months, 12 months, 18 months, left to right) in this 50 year old status post lumpectomy and radiation therapy show increasing density at the lumpectomy site ➡. *(Right)* MLO mammography spot compression at the time of 18 month follow-up (same patient as left-hand image) shows persistent spiculated mass ➡. US-guided biopsy confirmed recurrent IDC.

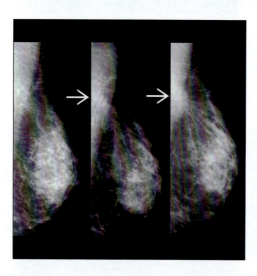
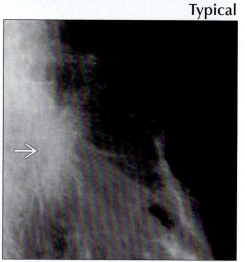

(Left) MLO mammography of a palpable area in the upper left breast of a 36 year old woman shows multiple spiculated masses ➡, the characteristics of which are better seen on the close-up MLO view (right-hand image). *(Right)* MLO mammography close-up shows at least 4 spiculated masses ➡. US-guided core biopsies confirmed multifocal invasive ductal carcinoma.

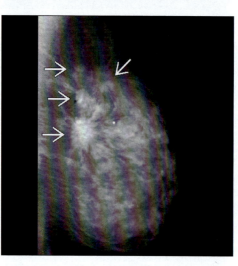
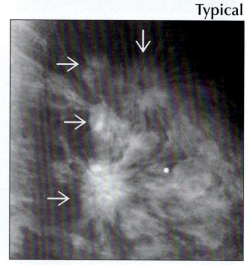

SPICULATED MARGINS

Typical

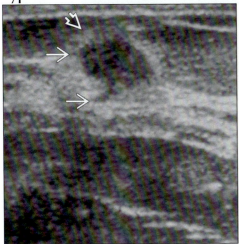 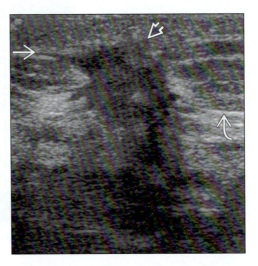

(Left) Sagittal ultrasound shows a subtle spiculated mass ➡ with echogenic rim ➡, which was palpable but mammographically-occult. Palpation-guided core biopsy showed papillomatosis, discordant, but not recognized as such. *(Right)* Sagittal ultrasound 4 years later (same mass as left-hand image) shows an irregular spiculated mass ➡ invading overlying skin ➡ with tethering of Cooper ligaments ➡. US-guided core biopsy = grade II IDC and DCIS.

Typical

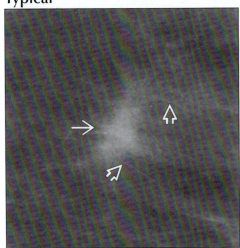 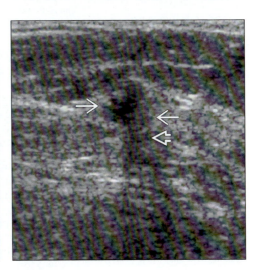

(Left) MLO mammography spot compression shows a new mass found on screening in a 78 year old woman. The mass is spiculated ➡ with associated architectural distortion ➡. An US (right-hand image) was performed. *(Right)* Radial ultrasound shows an irregular, hypoechoic, spiculated mass ➡ with minimal posterior shadowing ➡. Imaging findings highly suggestive of malignancy, BI-RADS 5. US-guided 14-g core biopsy = ILC.

Typical

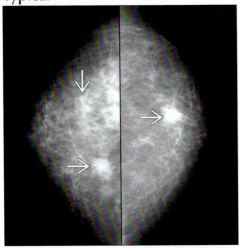 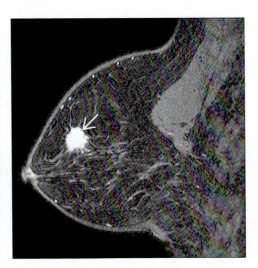

(Left) CC mammography shows bilateral spiculated masses ➡. Diffuse findings of mild edema (trabecular coarsening and overall increased breast density) are present in the right breast where multicentric IDC was present. *(Right)* Lateral T1 C+ FS MR of the same patient's left breast confirms the single spiculated mass ➡. Biopsy revealed a single grade II IDC.

COMPLICATED CYST

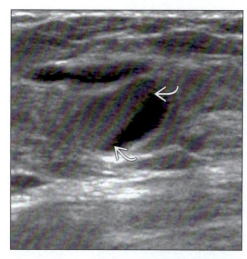

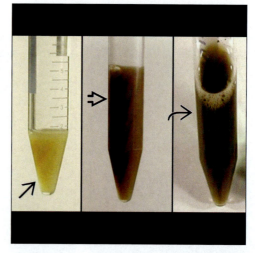

Ultrasound shows fluid-debris level ⟿ compatible with benign complicated cyst. Unless there are symptoms of infection, this can be dismissed as a benign finding, BI-RADS 2.

Cloudy brown fluid ⇨ is typical of a hemorrhagic cyst & should be sent for cytology. Cloudy yellow fluid ➔ can appear hypoechoic on US but can be discarded, as can green-black fluid ⤳.

TERMINOLOGY

Abbreviations and Synonyms
- Proteinaceous cyst

Definitions
- Cyst containing internal echoes on US
- No "complex" features (e.g., no thick wall, intracystic mass, thick septations, or solid component)
- If subsequently shown to be an oil cyst on mammography, it should be so described

IMAGING FINDINGS

General Features
- Best diagnostic clue
  - Fluid-debris level, imperceptible wall, on US or MR
  - Circumscribed mass, posterior enhancement, and
    - Mobile internal debris on US or
    - Homogeneous low level echoes on US
  - Usually in the company of simple cysts
- Location: Terminal duct lobular unit (TDLU)
- Morphology: Oval, round, or gently lobulated

Mammographic Findings
- Solitary or multiple circumscribed, partially obscured mass(es)
- Fluctuating pattern from one year to the next, with some regressing and others developing
  - Generally does not require further evaluation unless dominant or palpable finding(s) or tender

Ultrasonographic Findings
- Grayscale Ultrasound
  - Circumscribed oval, round, or gently lobulated mass(es)
  - Imperceptible wall
  - Posterior enhancement may not be seen when small (especially ≤ 5 mm)
    - More conspicuous without spatial compounding
  - Internal echoes can be any of the following or a combination of
    - Homogeneous low level echoes
    - Fluid-debris level
    - Mobile bright echoes
  - Individual microcysts within a cluster can be complicated
  - Usually in the company of simple cysts

DDx: Lesions that Mimic Complicated Cysts

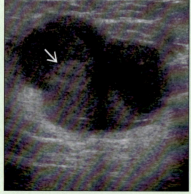

Papillary DCIS

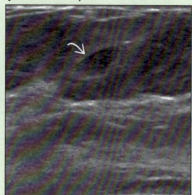

Papillary DCIS

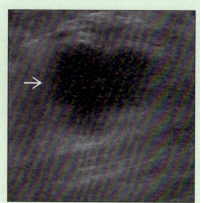

High Grade IDC

COMPLICATED CYST

Key Facts

Terminology
- Cyst containing internal echoes on US
- No "complex" features (e.g., no thick wall, intracystic mass, thick septations, or solid component)

Imaging Findings
- Fluid-debris level, imperceptible wall, on US or MR
- Circumscribed mass, posterior enhancement, and
- Mobile internal debris on US or
- Homogeneous low level echoes on US
- Usually in the company of simple cysts

Top Differential Diagnoses
- Simple Cyst with Artifactual Internal Echoes
- Abscess
- Galactocele
- Fibroadenoma

- Intracystic papillary DCIS
- Invasive ductal carcinoma (IDC)
- Fibrocystic Changes

Clinical Issues
- < 2% risk of malignancy if no complex features
- Fluctuating bilateral cysts and complicated cysts can be dismissed as benign, BI-RADS 2
- Asymptomatic complicated cyst with fluid-debris level or mobile internal echoes benign, BI-RADS 2
- Baseline or incidental finding on US, can follow at 6 months, probably benign, BI-RADS 3
- Aspirate and possible biopsy, BI-RADS 4 if
- Symptomatic relief (e.g., palpable, tender, possible abscess)
- Possibly solid and new or enlarging
- Complex cystic lesion

- Color Doppler: Power Doppler can impart energy to internal debris and facilitate recognition of its mobility

MR Findings
- T1WI
  - Oval, round, or gently lobulated smooth mass(es)
  - Signal characteristics depend on contents
    - Hyperintense suggests proteinaceous fluid or blood
  - May show fluid-debris level
- T2WI FS
  - Oval, round, or gently lobulated smooth mass
  - Signal characteristics depend on contents
    - Most are hyperintense on T2WI (fluid content)
    - Hypointense suggests proteinaceous fluid or blood
- T1 C+
  - Most show no enhancement
  - Progressive rim-enhancement can be seen with ruptured cysts
    - Ruptured cysts usually have thick or indistinct wall on US
    - Abscess can have identical appearance
    - Washout kinetics or irregular thick rim suggest carcinoma
- Inversion Recovery FSE: Similar to findings on T2WI

Imaging Recommendations
- Protocol advice
  - Fundamental US (without spatial compounding) facilitates recognition of posterior features
  - Power Doppler US or turn patient to cause internal debris to shift, better exclude solid mass
  - Tissue harmonic US can help exclude artifactual internal echoes

DIFFERENTIAL DIAGNOSIS

Simple Cyst with Artifactual Internal Echoes
- Usually anterior reverberation artifact
- Worse with cysts ≤ 8 mm

  - 14% of consensus cysts considered complicated cysts by another observer
  - 14% cysts considered solid by another observer
- Tissue harmonic imaging reduces artifact
- Appropriate gain and focal zone at mass

Proteinaceous Cyst
- Homogeneous low level echoes on US
- Bright on T1WI MR
- Fluid typically cloudy yellow on aspiration, can discard

Hemorrhagic Cyst
- Debris may appear tumefactive
- Bright on T1WI MR
- Bloody fluid should be sent for cytology
  - Can be due to papillary lesion
  - Surveillance suggested in 3-6 months to exclude underlying mass that bled; consider excision

Oil Cyst
- Lucent mass on mammography
- May show fluid-debris level

Abscess
- Associated edema
- Tender, may have erythema, usually near nipple

Galactocele
- Pregnant or lactating woman
- Fluid-debris level with nondependent fatty debris
- Can have echogenic fat plug

Fibroadenoma
- Hypoechoic or isoechoic to fat
- May show posterior enhancement, but less likely

Sebaceous Cyst or Epidermal Inclusion Cyst
- Within skin
- Benign finding, do not aspirate

Malignancy
- Ductal carcinoma in situ (DCIS)
  - Intracystic papillary DCIS

COMPLICATED CYST

- Can bleed and cause fluid-debris level obscuring mass
  - Circumscribed, solid mass (uncommon)
  - Usually manifest as intraductal calcifications on mammography
- Invasive ductal carcinoma (IDC)
  - High grade IDC NOS can present as nearly anechoic round or oval mass
    - Posterior enhancement often present
    - Margins can be partially circumscribed
    - Indistinct margins distinguish from complicated cyst
    - May show internal vascularity on color or power Doppler
    - Can be difficult to distinguish from complicated cyst when small, usually ≤ 5 mm
  - Any IDC can present as a complex cystic and solid mass
    - Thick wall, septations, or solid component distinguish from complicated cyst

Fibrocystic Changes
- Adenosis tumor
- Small cysts (≤ 5 mm) with apocrine metaplasia, usual hyperplasia, can appear hypoechoic

Intraductal Papilloma
- Intracystic mass
- Tumefactive debris can mimic

Ruptured/Inflamed Cyst
- Often thick-walled
- Indistinct margin
- Rim-enhancement on MR

PATHOLOGY

General Features
- Etiology
  - Proteins from cell turnover, hemorrhage, or pus
    - Rarely underlying malignancy can bleed
  - When multiple, more often apocrine cysts
- Epidemiology
  - ~ 1% prevalence on screening
  - ~ 2x risk of malignancy with history of multiple cysts, aspirations
- Associated abnormalities: Simple cysts

CLINICAL ISSUES

Presentation
- Most common signs/symptoms
  - Can be palpable and tender when arise rapidly
    - Usually round, tense and larger than 1 cm
- Other signs/symptoms
  - Erythema, tenderness can be due to abscess
  - Rarely communicate with duct, cause nipple discharge

Demographics
- Age: Peak in mid 40's to early 50's as with other cysts

Natural History & Prognosis
- Most complicated cysts regress spontaneously over weeks to years
- < 2% risk of malignancy if no complex features

Treatment
- Fluctuating bilateral cysts and complicated cysts can be dismissed as benign, BI-RADS 2
- Asymptomatic complicated cyst with fluid-debris level or mobile internal echoes benign, BI-RADS 2
- Asymptomatic, with homogeneous low level echoes
  - Baseline or incidental finding on US, can follow at 6 months, probably benign, BI-RADS 3
  - Circumscribed similar-appearing solid mass on baseline mammogram or incidental finding on US, probably benign, BI-RADS 3
- Aspirate and possible biopsy, BI-RADS 4 if
  - Symptomatic relief (e.g., palpable, tender, possible abscess)
  - Possibly solid and new or enlarging
  - Complex cystic lesion
    - Intracystic mass
    - Thick wall (≥ 0.5 mm)
    - Thick septations (≥ 0.5 mm)
    - Mixed cystic and solid
  - Cytology only for bloody fluid
  - Can inject air to decrease risk of recurrence of cyst

SELECTED REFERENCES

1. Berg WA et al: Operator dependence of physician-performed whole breast sonography: lesion detection and characterization. Radiology (in press), 2006
2. Berg WA et al: Cystic lesions of the breast: sonographic-pathologic correlation. Radiology. 227:183-191, 2003
3. Mendelson EB et al: Breast Imaging Reporting and Data System: BI-RADS, Ultrasound, 1st ed. Reston, American College of Radiology, 2003
4. Szopinski KT et al: Tissue harmonic imaging: utility in breast sonography. J Ultrasound Med. 22:479-487; quiz 488- 479, 2003
5. Gizienski TA et al: Breast cyst recurrence after postaspiration injection of air. Breast J. 8:34-37, 2002
6. Kolb TM et al: Comparison of the performance of screening mammography, physical examination, and breast US and evaluation of factors that influence them: an analysis of 27,825 patient evaluations. Radiology. 225:165-75, 2002
7. Buchberger W et al: Clinically and mammographically occult breast lesions: detection and classification with high-resolution sonography. Semin Ultrasound CT MR. 21:325-336, 2000
8. Hindle WH et al: Lack of utility in clinical practice of cytologic examination of nonbloody cyst fluid from palpable breast cysts. Am J Obstet Gynecol. 182:1300-05, 2000
9. Venta LA et al: Management of complex breast cysts. AJR. 173:1331-6, 1999
10. Bodian CA et al: The epidemiology of gross cystic disease of the breast confirmed by biopsy or by aspiration of cyst fluid. Cancer Detect Prev. 16:7-15, 1992
11. Ciatto S et al: The value of routine cytologic examination of breast cyst fluids. Acta Cytol. 31:301-4, 1987
12. Dixon JM et al: Natural history of cystic disease: the importance of cyst type. Br J Surg. 72:190-2, 1985

COMPLICATED CYST

IMAGE GALLERY

Typical

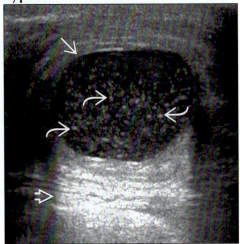
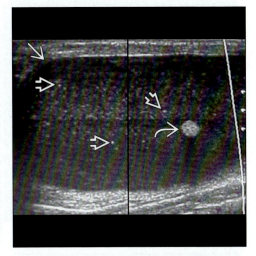

(Left) Radial ultrasound shows circumscribed mass ➡ with posterior enhancement ⇉ and mobile internal echoes with bright echogenic foci ➡ due to cholesterol crystals in this palpable complicated cyst. *(Right)* Sagittal ultrasound in this 19 year old who was post-partum shows circumscribed mass ➡ with tiny echogenic foci ⇉ as well as an echogenic fat plug ➡. At her request, this galactocele was aspirated.

Typical

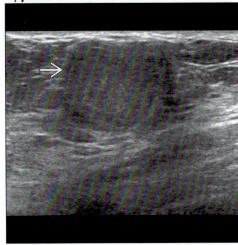
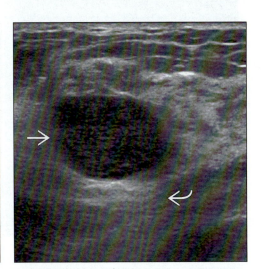

(Left) Ultrasound shows circumscribed mass ➡ with contents isoechoic to fat, mimicking a solid mass. 14-g core biopsy showed galactocele. *(Right)* Radial spatial compounding ultrasound shows homogeneous low level echoes in this circumscribed mass ➡ with posterior enhancement ⇗. Findings are typical of a complicated cyst, a BI-RADS 3 finding on baseline evaluation.

Variant

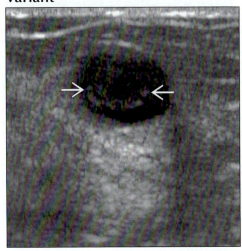
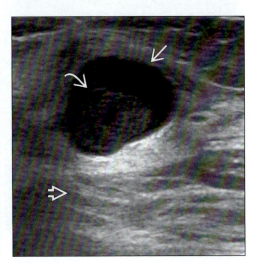

(Left) Anti-radial ultrasound shows an apparent intracystic mass ➡. US-guided aspiration showed greenish-black fluid typical of benign cyst contents, with resolution of the mass. *(Right)* Radial ultrasound shows tumefactive debris ➡ in this circumscribed mass ➡ with posterior enhancement ⇉. US-guided aspiration and cytology confirmed a hemorrhagic cyst.

Variant

(Left) Sagittal STIR MR shows smooth round mass ➡ with fluid-fluid level ➤. *(Right)* Sagittal T1WI MR again shows fluid-fluid level ➤. The more superior component is hyperintense on T1WI ➡ and hypointense on T2WI and inversion recovery (left-hand image, ➡), compatible with proteinaceous debris in a complicated cyst.

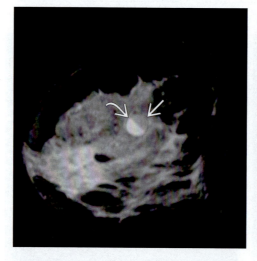
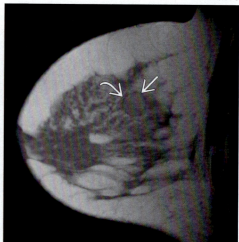

Typical

(Left) Anti-radial spatial compounding ultrasound shows mass whose margins are mostly circumscribed ➡ and partially indistinct ➤. Subtle posterior enhancement is noted ➡. *(Right)* Anti-radial ultrasound without spatial compounding (same mass as left-hand image) better depicts posterior enhancement ➡ though the margins now appear indistinct ➡. 20-g aspiration failed to yield fluid. 14-g biopsy showed cyst wall and proteinaceous debris.

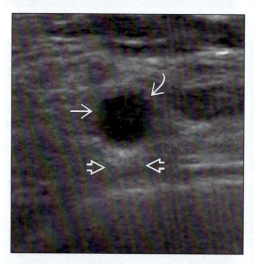
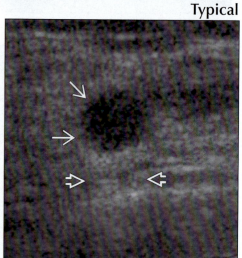

Variant

(Left) Radial ultrasound shows thick-walled ➡ cystic lesion with lobulated internal echoes ➤. Aspiration was performed (right-hand image). *(Right)* Gross pathology of aspirate shows cloudy yellow fluid with floating crystals ➡, usually cholesterol crystals, from this inflamed cyst. The contents are typical of benign cyst contents and were discarded.

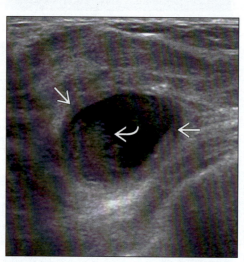
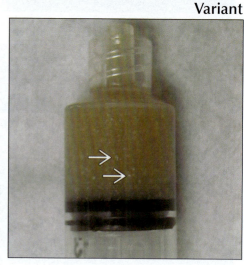

IV

1

38

COMPLICATED CYST

Variant

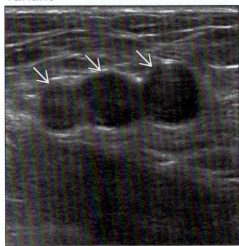 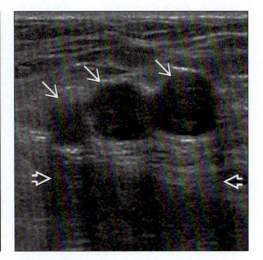

(Left) Radial spatial compounding ultrasound shows three adjacent circumscribed masses ➡ with homogeneous low level echoes. On US (right-hand image) these appear to be complicated cysts. *(Right)* Radial ultrasound without spatial compounding better depicts posterior enhancement ⇨ from these complicated cysts ➡. Mammography was performed (next image).

Variant

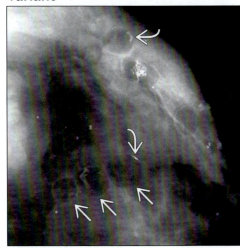 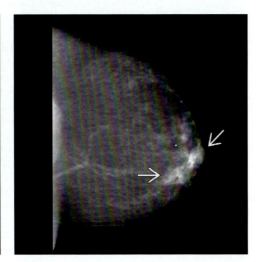

(Left) CC mammography shows the three adjacent complicated cysts (previous 2 images) ➡ are due to oil cysts in this patient s/p reduction mammoplasty. Some are calcifying peripherally ➡. These are benign findings, BI-RADS 2. *(Right)* CC mammography shows lobulated asymmetry ➡ corresponding to a palpable tender mass near the nipple. US was recommended (next image).

Variant

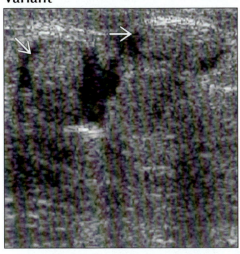 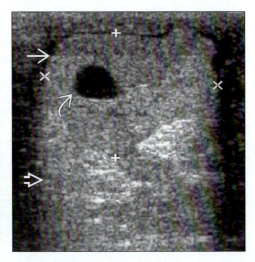

(Left) Transverse ultrasound shows cystic lesions or ducts with intracystic masses or debris ➡. Antibiotics were initiated and the patient returned 12 days later with enlarging painful mass (see next image). *(Right)* Transverse ultrasound performed at follow-up 12 days later shows enlarging, confluent mass with echogenic debris ➡, an anechoic component ➡, and posterior enhancement ➡. Aspiration yielded pus from this abscess.

CLUSTERED MICROCYSTS

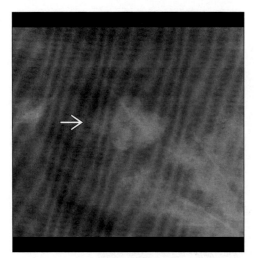

MLO mammography shows circumscribed microlobulated mass ➡ due to clustered microcysts.

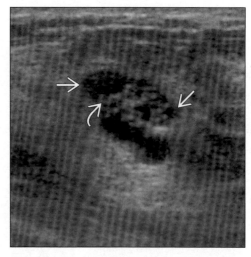

Radial ultrasound shows microlobulated cluster of tiny cysts ➡ due to dilated acini ranging from 1-4 mm in size. Thin intervening septations ➡ are due to walls of adjacent acini in the TDLU.

TERMINOLOGY

Definitions
- Cluster of tiny anechoic foci, individually 1-7 mm, with thin (< 0.5 mm) intervening septae
- No solid component

IMAGING FINDINGS

General Features
- Best diagnostic clue: Typical appearance on ultrasound of a cluster of tiny cysts with thin intervening septae
- Location: Lobular portion of terminal duct lobular unit (TDLU)
- Size: 5-30 mm, median 8 mm
- Morphology: Microlobulated mass

Mammographic Findings
- Circumscribed or partially obscured margins
- Microlobulated or oval shape
- Density equal to or lower than surrounding parenchyma
- May see milk-of-calcium in microcysts

Ultrasonographic Findings
- Grayscale Ultrasound
  - Circumscribed, microlobulated mass on US composed of multiple adjacent small cysts with thin intervening septae
  - May show posterior enhancement
  - Usually parallel orientation
  - "Fuzzy" internal border to individual microcysts can be seen with apocrine metaplasia
    - May be difficult to distinguish from complex cystic mass with thick septations (> 0.5 mm)
    - May require biopsy if uncertainty
  - May see dependent echogenic calcifications due to milk-of-calcium
  - Individual microcysts can be complicated microcysts
    - Fluid-debris level
    - Homogeneous low level echoes, difficult to distinguish from small solid component
  - Rarely can see communication to terminal duct
  - May see associated simple cysts
- Color Doppler: Usually no flow

MR Findings
- T1WI: Hypointense, equal to parenchyma

DDx: Complex Cystic and Solid Lesions

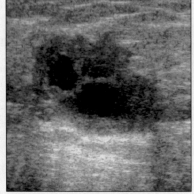

Medullary Carcinoma

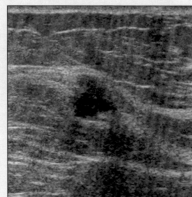

Grade III IDC

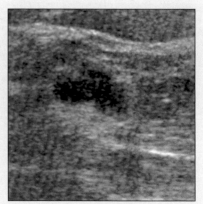

Invasive Lobular Cancer

CLUSTERED MICROCYSTS

Key Facts

Terminology
- Cluster of tiny anechoic foci, individually 1-7 mm, with thin (< 0.5 mm) intervening septae
- No solid component

Imaging Findings
- Circumscribed or partially obscured margins
- Microlobulated or oval shape
- Density equal to or lower than surrounding parenchyma
- May see milk-of-calcium in microcysts
- T2WI FS: Hyperintense, microlobulated mass on T2 or inversion recovery MR with hypointense internal septae
- T1 C+: With apocrine metaplastic epithelium, can see enhancement of septae
- May show posterior enhancement

- Individual microcysts can be complicated microcysts
- Best characterized on US

Pathology
- 38% apocrine metaplasia lining acini
- 38% fibrocystic changes

Clinical Issues
- Can be dismissed as benign (BI-RADS 2) when typical appearance
- Short interval follow-up (BI-RADS 3) if suboptimally seen or individual microcysts complicated
- Biopsy if discrete solid component, suspicious findings, rapid growth (BI-RADS 4)

- T2WI FS: Hyperintense, microlobulated mass on T2 or inversion recovery MR with hypointense internal septae
- T1 C+: With apocrine metaplastic epithelium, can see enhancement of septae
- Inversion Recovery FSE: Hyperintense, microlobulated mass with hypointense internal septae

Biopsy
- 14-g core biopsy under US guidance if associated solid component or thick walls
- 11-g or larger vacuum-assisted biopsy if associated suspicious calcifications
- May decrease in size while performing core biopsy
- Typically does not collapse with fine needle aspiration biopsy (FNAB)
  ○ Can show apocrine metaplastic epithelium
- Layering of microcalcifications dependently should preclude need for biopsy
  ○ True lateral magnification view will usually confirm layering of milk-of-calcium
  ○ May be necessary to wait up to five minutes for slowly sedimenting calcium to settle to bottom of microcysts
  ○ Sometimes layering only evident in prone position on stereotactic table

Imaging Recommendations
- Best imaging tool
  ○ Best characterized on US
    ▪ High-frequency (10-15 MHz) transducer necessary to resolve internal structure
- Protocol advice
  ○ Spatial compounding may help depict internal structure
    ▪ May lose posterior features
  ○ Posterior enhancement better seen on fundamental (native) imaging
  ○ Tissue harmonic imaging may help depict individual microcysts as anechoic
    ▪ Preserves posterior features
  ○ Use of gentle pressure encouraged to improve penetration with high-frequency transducers

DIFFERENTIAL DIAGNOSIS

Fibrocystic Changes
- May show milk-of-calcium in microcysts

Apocrine Metaplasia
- Most common appearance is clustered microcysts
- "Fuzzy" internal border to individual microcysts
- Can have associated punctate, amorphous, or heterogeneous calcifications

Papillary Apocrine Metaplasia
- Increased risk of malignancy
- More likely to have some solid component

Simple Cysts
- Group of several adjacent small cysts can have identical appearance

Complicated Cyst
- Debris can rarely mimic intervening septae

Ruptured/Inflamed Cyst(s)
- Usually thick, indistinct wall
- Rarely have intervening septae

Complex Cystic Lesion
- Presence of any of the following should prompt biopsy
  ○ Thick septations or thick wall (> 0.5 mm)
  ○ Indistinct or angular margins
  ○ Associated solid component
  ○ Intracystic mass
- Increased vascularity common
- Differential includes
  ○ Invasive ductal cancer (IDC, high grade most common)
  ○ Ductal carcinoma in situ (DCIS), usually papillary
  ○ Papilloma
    ▪ Most often intraductal mass near nipple
    ▪ May have associated nipple discharge (spontaneous clear or bloody)
  ○ Phyllodes tumor
    ▪ Predominantly solid with cystic foci
    ▪ Rapid growth

CLUSTERED MICROCYSTS

   ○ Abscess
      ▪ Tender, often palpable, overlying erythema

Microlobulated, Hypoechoic Solid Mass
- Differential includes: Fibroadenoma (FA), phyllodes, IDC, invasive lobular cancer (ILC), DCIS, lactating adenoma, tubular adenoma

Fat Necrosis
- History of trauma or surgery
- Central anechoic component(s) and peripherally hyperechoic on US
- Contains fat on mammography
- Develop peripheral rim-calcifications after several years

PATHOLOGY

General Features
- Etiology
   ○ Dilatation of multiple acini in TDLU
   ○ Part of the spectrum of benign cystic changes of the breast
- Epidemiology
   ○ 6% of breast US examinations
   ○ Most common in perimenopausal women
   ○ Nearly 50% of postmenopausal women with clustered microcysts are on hormonal therapy
- Associated abnormalities
   ○ 38% apocrine metaplasia lining acini
   ○ 38% fibrocystic changes
   ○ 4% of FA have cystic spaces, can be microcysts
      ▪ Phyllodes tumors more often have cystic spaces, rapid growth, otherwise resemble FA
   ○ Can have calcium oxalate crystals in microcysts (seen best on polarized light microscopy)
   ○ 21% simple cysts elsewhere in the breast(s)

Microscopic Features
- Bland epithelium or apocrine metaplasia (tall columnar epithelium) lining microcysts

CLINICAL ISSUES

Presentation
- Most common signs/symptoms: Usually an incidental finding on mammography or US or both
- Other signs/symptoms: Rarely palpable

Demographics
- Age: Median age 48, perimenopausal most common

Natural History & Prognosis
- 53% stable on 2 year follow-up
- 23% resolved on 2 year follow-up
- 18% decreased on 2 year follow-up
- 6% increased then were stable or resolved
   ○ Rapid growth (> 20% increase in diameter in 6 months) may indicate need for biopsy
- Individual microcysts can fuse and form larger cysts

Treatment
- Can be dismissed as benign (BI-RADS 2) when typical appearance
- Short interval follow-up (BI-RADS 3) if suboptimally seen or individual microcysts complicated
- Biopsy if discrete solid component, suspicious findings, rapid growth (BI-RADS 4)

DIAGNOSTIC CHECKLIST

Consider
- Careful attention to technique when performing US can help distinguish from solid mass
- Caution when new mass in post-menopausal patient not on hormone replacement therapy
   ○ Close surveillance required; may merit biopsy if uncertainty

Image Interpretation Pearls
- Any solid component or irregular, indistinct margins should prompt biopsy

SELECTED REFERENCES

1. Berg WA: Sonographically depicted breast clustered microcysts: is follow-up appropriate? AJR. 185:952-9, 2005
2. Berg WA: Breast ultrasonography: cystic lesions and probably benign findings. In Berg WA, Javit MC, eds. Women's Imaging: Strategies for Clinical Practice--Categorical course syllabus. (Leesburg, American Roentgen Ray Society). 95-102, 2004
3. Berg WA et al: Cystic lesions of the breast: sonographic-pathologic correlation. Radiology. 227:183-191, 2003
4. Kushwaha AC et al: Mammographic-pathologic correlation of apocrine metaplasia diagnosed using vacuum-assisted stereotactic core-needle biopsy: our 4-year experience. AJR. 180:795-8, 2003
5. Mendelson EB et al: Breast Imaging Reporting and Data System: BI-RADS, Ultrasound, 1st ed. Reston, American College of Radiology, 2003
6. Szopinski KT et al: Tissue harmonic imaging: utility in breast sonography. J Ultrasound Med. 22:479-487, 2003
7. Seo BK et al: Sonographic evaluation of breast nodules: comparison of conventional, real-time compound, and pulse-inversion harmonic images. Korean J Radiol. 3:38-44, 2002
8. Mendelson EB et al: Toward a standardized breast ultrasound lexicon, BI-RADS: Ultrasound. Semin Roentgenol. 36:217-225, 2001
9. Margolin FR et al: Microcystic calcifications at stereotactic breast biopsy. Breast J. 5:182-185, 1999
10. Venta LA et al: Management of complex breast cysts. AJR. 173:1331-1136, 1999
11. Warner JK et al: Apocrine metaplasia: mammographic and sonographic appearances. AJR. 170:1375-9, 1998
12. Linden SS et al: Sedimented calcium in benign breast cysts: the full spectrum of mammographic presentations. AJR. 152:967-71, 1989
13. Wellings SR et al: An atlas of subgross pathology of the human breast with special attention to possible precancerous lesions. J Natl Cancer Inst. 55:231-73, 1975

IMAGE GALLERY

Typical

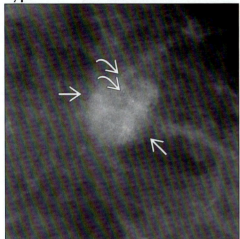
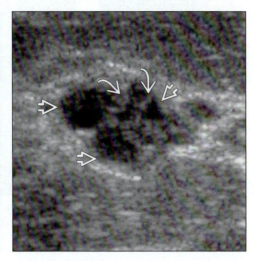

(Left) MLO mammography magnification view shows microlobulated mass ➡ with few punctate calcifications ➡. US was performed (next image). *(Right)* Radial ultrasound shows a microlobulated mass composed entirely of tiny anechoic spaces ➡ with intervening thin (< 0.5 mm) septations ➡, i.e., clustered microcysts. MR was also performed (next 2 images).

IV

1

43

Typical

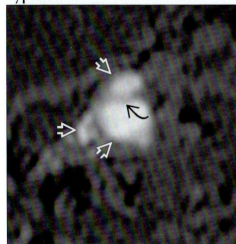
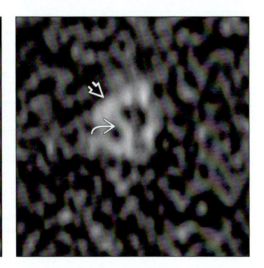

(Left) Sagittal inversion recovery FSE MR shows a microlobulated mass composed of hyperintense microcysts ➡ with thin intervening hypointense septations ➡. *(Right)* Sagittal T1 C+ subtraction MR shows rapid enhancement of internal septations ➡ and outer wall ➡. Biopsy (performed due to contralateral cancer) showed apocrine metaplasia.

Typical

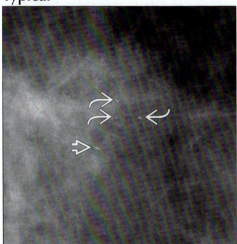
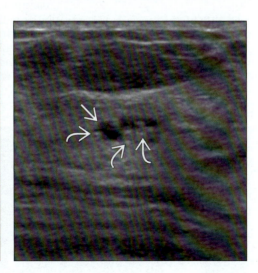

(Left) Lateral mammography magnification shows a loose cluster of punctate calcifications ➡ with one layering and clearly milk-of-calcium ➡. *(Right)* Anti-radial spatial compounding ultrasound shows clustered microcysts ➡ containing dependent milk-of-calcium ➡.

DUCT ECTASIA

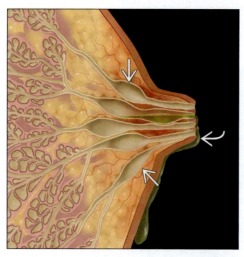

Graphic shows dilated major subareolar ducts ➡ and representation of nipple discharge ➡. Duct ectasia may be secondary to inflammation, obstruction or glandular atrophy and stasis.

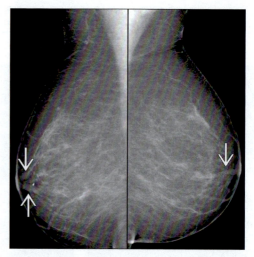

MLO mammography in a 67 year old asymptomatic woman shows bilateral tubular retroareolar densities ➡ c/w mildly dilated ducts, secondary to tissue atrophy in these fatty breasts (BI-RADS 1 or 2).

TERMINOLOGY

Abbreviations and Synonyms
- Mammary duct ectasia, mastitis obliterans

IMAGING FINDINGS

General Features
- Best diagnostic clue
  - Tubular or branching structure(s) most commonly in the subareolar regions of both breasts on mammography
  - One or more tubular structures may be seen away from the nipple
- Location: No clinical concern when bilateral and asymptomatic

Mammographic Findings
- Tubular radiopaque retroareolar structures
- Bilateral tubular or branching retroareolar ducts are benign unless there are physical findings
  - Spontaneous nipple discharge: Further work-up may include magnification views; US, ductography, MR
  - Orthogonal magnification mammography to look for microcalcifications
  - US: Assess for fluid-filled ducts without evidence for intraluminal mass
- Unilateral or single dilated duct may require further assessment
  - Comparison with old films to determine if a new finding
  - Orthogonal magnification mammography
  - US: Assess for intraluminal mass(es)
- Calcifications may be present within or around ducts
  - Benign secretory rod-like calcifications, some with lucent centers within or around ducts are benign
  - Suspicious forms (fine linear, pleomorphic, amorphous, punctate) suggesting a ductal distribution must be further evaluated
  - Possibly suspicious microcalcifications should be evaluated with orthogonal magnification mammography
- Tubular radiopaque structure away from the retroareolar region
  - May require magnification mammography, US
  - Papilloma, ductal carcinoma in situ (DCIS) may present with this finding

DDx: Tubular Structures

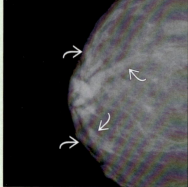

Dilated Ectatic Ducts

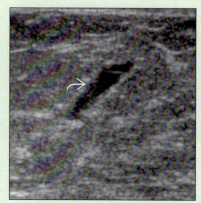

US, Fluid-Filled Duct

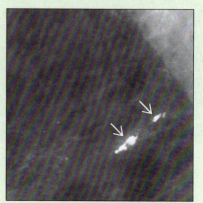

Single Dilated Duct, DCIS

DUCT ECTASIA

Key Facts

Imaging Findings
- Tubular or branching structure(s) most commonly in the subareolar regions of both breasts on mammography
- Calcifications may be present within or around ducts
- US: Anechoic fluid, or hypoechoic debris in dilated subareolar ducts

Top Differential Diagnoses
- Normal Variant
- Secretory Calcifications
- Papilloma
- Ductal Carcinoma in Situ (DCIS)

Pathology
- May be secondary to inflammation, obstruction, glandular atrophy and stasis

- Tissue atrophy
- Cigarette smoking, hyperprolactinemia, prolonged phenothiazine exposure

Clinical Issues
- Most common signs/symptoms: Asymptomatic screening mammogram finding
- Palpable retroareolar tubular structures
- Nipple discharge, spontaneous or with manipulation
- Yellow, green, brown, greenish-black
- Age: 42-85 reported range
- No known associated increased risk for breast cancer
- No further imaging when asymptomatic, multiple and without suspicious calcifications, masses or distortion
- Biopsy may be recommended if suspicious clinical or imaging characteristics

Ultrasonographic Findings
- Grayscale Ultrasound
  - US: Anechoic fluid, or hypoechoic debris in dilated subareolar ducts
    - Debris may be mobile
    - Repositioning the patient and waiting 2-5 minutes may be beneficial in demonstrating mobile nature
  - Intraluminal masses may be demonstrated
    - Debris may be difficult to differentiate from masses
    - Color or power Doppler may be beneficial
- Color Doppler: Vascular stalk may be seen with papillomas, papillary lesions

MR Findings
- T1WI: Retroareolar tubular structures may be bright when filled with proteinaceous or bloody fluid
- T2WI: Intraductal fluid may be bright
- T1 C+
  - May enhance
  - Intensity less than the normal nipple
  - Intraductal masses may enhance, some intensely
    - Papilloma
    - DCIS

DIFFERENTIAL DIAGNOSIS

Normal Variant
- Asymptomatic
- Symmetric bilateral dilatation typically of no clinical significance in postmenopausal women
- Dilatation may be somewhat asymmetric

Secretory Calcifications
- Benign, rod-like, coarse, linear mammographic calcifications
- Form either within ducts (may have lucent centers) or around ducts
- Unusual under the age of 60 years
- Typically bilateral
- Plasmacytic reaction to ductal retained secretion

- May present with a palpable mass

Papilloma
- May be central or peripheral
- Central lesions often present with spontaneous bloody nipple discharge
- Often multiple
- May appear as a mammographic mass with or without calcifications
  - Calcifications usually punctate or amorphous
- US: Intraluminal mass(es) within ectatic duct
  - Doppler may demonstrate vascular stalk
- MR patterns of enhancing papillomas variable
  - Small, smooth enhancing masses at ends of ectatic ducts
  - Irregular enhancing masses, some reported with rim-enhancement or spiculations
  - Occult on MR; not seen either with fat suppressed T2 or following contrast injection
- Can degenerate into atypical or malignant papillary lesions

Ductal Carcinoma in Situ (DCIS)
- Isolated single or multiple dilated duct(s) an uncommon presentation of DCIS
  - 4 of 300 nonpalpable breast cancers detected as single dilated ducts in one series
- Usually has associated calcifications (fine linear, pleomorphic, amorphous, punctate) in a linear distribution

Abscess
- Clinical constellation includes tenderness and palpable mass near the nipple
- Often begins in the subareolar ducts
- More common in pregnant and nursing women
- US demonstrates thick indistinct wall surrounding echogenic debris
- Clinical setting and aspiration usually diagnostic

Mondor Disease
- Thrombophlebitis of the superficial veins
- Self limited process

DUCT ECTASIA

- Typically associated with pain and a palpable cord

Granulomatous Lobular Mastitis
- No specific pathogenic organism
- Ducts filled with debris
- Associated irregular mass(es)

PATHOLOGY

General Features
- General path comments
  - Dilated major subareolar ducts
    - Occasional involvement of smaller ducts
  - Thick or granular secretions
- Etiology
  - May be secondary to inflammation, obstruction, glandular atrophy and stasis
  - Not related to parity or breast-feeding
- Epidemiology
  - Tissue atrophy
  - Cigarette smoking, hyperprolactinemia, prolonged phenothiazine exposure

Gross Pathologic & Surgical Features
- Grossly dilated, thick-walled ducts; thick or granular secretions

Microscopic Features
- Eosinophilic proteinaceous material, foam cells
- Inflammatory changes in ducts and surrounding tissue
- Epithelium may be thin; may be replaced by scar

CLINICAL ISSUES

Presentation
- Most common signs/symptoms: Asymptomatic screening mammogram finding
- Other signs/symptoms
  - Palpable retroareolar tubular structures
  - Pain
  - Nipple discharge, spontaneous or with manipulation
    - Yellow, green, brown, greenish-black

Demographics
- Age: 42-85 reported range

Natural History & Prognosis
- No known associated increased risk for breast cancer

Treatment
- No further imaging when asymptomatic, multiple and without suspicious calcifications, masses or distortion
- Spontaneous bloody nipple discharge requires further assessment
  - Clinical assessment
  - Spot and/or magnification mammographic views
  - US, grayscale and color Doppler
  - Ductography: Requires visibility of discharging duct on the day of the procedure to allow cannulation
  - MR
- Biopsy may be recommended if suspicious clinical or imaging characteristics

DIAGNOSTIC CHECKLIST

Image Interpretation Pearls
- Presence of a peripheral tubular mammographic structure should lead to further investigation
  - Finding may require biopsy
  - Papilloma, DCIS may manifest with this appearance

SELECTED REFERENCES

1. Daniel Bl et al: Magnetic resonance imaging of intraductal papilloma of the breast. Magn Reson Imaging. 21:887-92, 2003
2. Ammari FF et al: Periductal mastitis. Clinical characteristics and outcome. Saudi Med J. 23:819-22, 2002
3. Rosen PP: Rosen's Breast Pathology. Philadelphia, Lippincott Williams & Wilkins. Chapter 3, 33-9, 2001
4. Bassett LW et al: Diagnosis of Diseases of the Breast. Philadelphia, WB Saunders Co. Chapter 25, 413-4, 1997
5. Cardenosa G: Breast Imaging Companion. Philadelphia, Lippincott-Raven. 184-7, 1997
6. Huynh PT et al: Dilated duct pattern at mammography. Radiology. 204:137-41, 1997
7. Sickles EA: Mammographic features of "early" breast cancer. AJR. 143:461-4, 1984

DUCT ECTASIA

IMAGE GALLERY

Typical

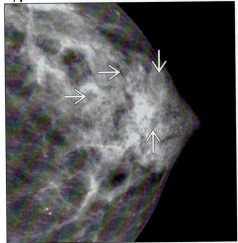

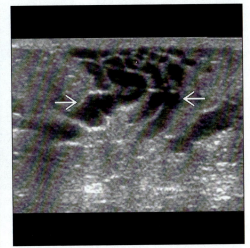

(Left) CC mammography photographic enlargement in an asymptomatic institutionalized woman shows markedly dilated ducts with internally lucent fat ➡ secondary to prolonged phenothiazine exposure. *(Right)* Transverse ultrasound in a lactating woman shows dilated ducts ➡ extending close to the skin surface where she palpated a "mass". Following nursing these previously milk-filled ducts were no longer visible.

Typical

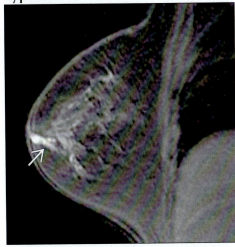

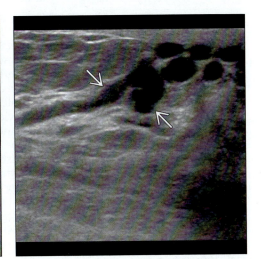

(Left) Sagittal pre-contrast T1WI FS shows hyperintense retroareolar duct ➡ in this 56 year old with ipsilateral invasive lobular cancer. No enhancement was evident on subtraction images. US was performed (right-hand image). *(Right)* Ultrasound shows no intraluminal filling defects in these mildly ectatic ducts ➡ in the retroareolar area. No further evaluation was performed.

Typical

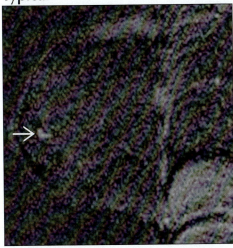

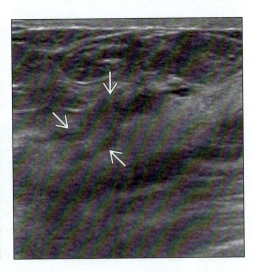

(Left) Sagittal T1 C+ subtraction MR performed to assess physical finding in opposite breast shows a V-shaped linear non-mass area of enhancement ➡. US was performed (right-hand image) targeted to the MR abnormality. *(Right)* Transverse ultrasound demonstrates the V-shaped region to be a focus of dilated ducts containing an intraluminal hypoechoic irregular mass ➡. US-guided core biopsy and excision showed sclerosed papilloma.

SIMPLE CYST

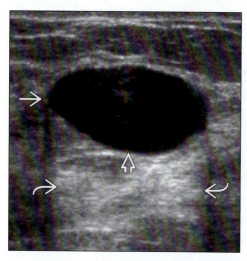 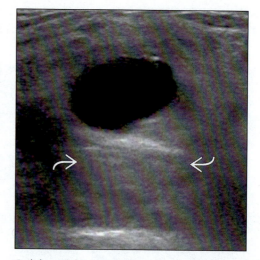

Anti-radial ultrasound demonstrates an anechoic, circumscribed mass ➡ with posterior acoustic enhancement ➡. The back wall of this simple cyst is very well-defined on US ➡. BI-RADS 2, benign.

Radial spatial compounding ultrasound shows a palpable, painful circumscribed, anechoic mass with posterior enhancement ➡, typical of a simple cyst that underwent aspiration at patient's request.

TERMINOLOGY

Definitions
- Fluid-filled round to oval structure lined by epithelium
- Distinguish from complicated cyst, complex cystic mass

IMAGING FINDINGS

General Features
- Best diagnostic clue: US: Circumscribed, round to oval anechoic mass with imperceptible wall and posterior enhancement
- Location: Anywhere in breast, not axilla
- Size
  - Microscopic to 5-6 cm
  - May fluctuate with menstrual cycle or hormone replacement therapy (HRT)

Mammographic Findings
- Well-circumscribed mass
  - Usually round or oval; occasionally lobulated
  - Low to equal density to parenchyma
  - Margins may be obscured by dense surrounding tissue
- Rim or eggshell calcification (Ca++) in cyst wall
- Single or multiple
  - May overlap on mammogram if multiple
- Intracystic calcium often detected on mammography = milk-of-calcium
  - Lateral view: Concave crescent densities, "teacup" calcifications, menisci
  - CC view: When seen en face, amorphous, smudgy
- Cannot distinguish from solid mass on mammography
- Often multiple, bilateral
  - Carefully evaluate individual mass margins
  - When at least 3 (with at least 1 in each breast), each circumscribed or at worst partially obscured, can be dismissed as benign finding
  - US for dominant or palpable mass

Ultrasonographic Findings
- Grayscale Ultrasound
  - Round or oval mass; occasionally lobulated
  - Circumscribed, imperceptible wall
  - Anechoic: Artifactual internal echoes can be seen

DDx: Circumscribed Masses

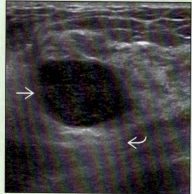 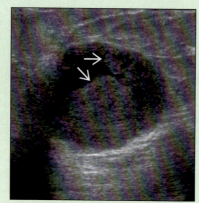 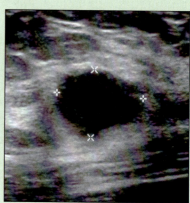

Complicated Cyst   *Intracystic Papillary DCIS*   *Grade III IDC*

SIMPLE CYST

Key Facts

Terminology
- Fluid-filled round to oval structure lined by epithelium

Imaging Findings
- Best diagnostic clue: US: Circumscribed, round to oval anechoic mass with imperceptible wall and posterior enhancement
- Location: Anywhere in breast, not axilla
- Cannot distinguish from solid mass on mammography
- US-guided aspiration when diagnostic uncertainty or for symptomatic relief
- Cytology only for bloody fluid

Top Differential Diagnoses
- Complicated Cyst

- Well-Circumscribed Carcinoma
- Metastatic or Reactive Lymph Node
- Fat Necrosis
- Post-Surgical Seroma

Pathology
- Thought to arise from obstructed ducts

Clinical Issues
- Most common mass in the female breast
- Rare in males
- Simple cysts have no malignant potential
- May proliferate under estrogenic stimulation
- Size may fluctuate with menstrual cycle; maximum size in premenstrual phase

- - Size < 5-8 mm may limit distinction of anechoic from markedly hypoechoic
    - If echoes present may be a complicated cyst
    - Adjacent or lobulated cysts: Can appear to have thin internal septations (< 0.5 mm)
  - Posterior enhancement
    - Acoustic enhancement helps ensure diagnosis
    - May be absent if cyst small or close to chest wall
  - Lateral edge refraction
    - Echo attenuation distal to lateral margins
  - Flattening occurs with transducer compression
    - Not observed with solid masses
  - US 96-100% accurate in diagnosing simple cyst
- Color Doppler: No observed flow

MR Findings
- T1WI: Smooth contour; low signal intensity
- T2WI: Extremely high, homogeneous signal intensity
- T1 C+: No enhancement

CT Findings
- CECT: No enhancement
- NECT: Fluid-density mass occasionally seen on chest CT; most, 10 HU; mean = 28 HU

Biopsy
- US-guided aspiration when diagnostic uncertainty or for symptomatic relief
  - Adjust needle to ensure complete aspiration
  - 20-22 gauge needle; if fluid thick, 16-18 gauge
- Cytology only for bloody fluid

Imaging Recommendations
- Best imaging tool: US with meticulous technique
- Protocol advice
  - Patients 30 years and older
    - Begin with mammography, supplement with US
  - Patients younger than 30: US first
  - US for new, enlarging, or palpable mass
    - Artificially increase gain to exclude internal echoes, then adjust down as appropriate
    - Document lesions with and without calipers to facilitate margin evaluation

  - High-resolution, high-frequency transducer
    - 10 MHz or higher suggested
    - Can detect cysts as small as 2-3 mm
    - Use lower frequency transducer (7.5 MHz) for deep cysts
  - Gentle compression, appropriate gain
  - Tissue harmonics
    - Helpful in reducing artifactual internal echoes
  - Spatial compounding
    - Improves margin definition
    - Decreases speckle and noise
    - Acoustic enhancement less apparent

DIFFERENTIAL DIAGNOSIS

Complicated Cyst
- Differentiation from simple cyst with reverberation echoes may be challenging

Well-Circumscribed Carcinoma
- Usually at least partially indistinctly marginated on mammography
- Hypoechoic, non-compressible on US
- Variable acoustic enhancement
- Invasive ductal carcinoma NOS, usually high grade
- Invasive lobular carcinoma (rarely)
- Ductal carcinoma in situ (DCIS)
  - Intracystic DCIS can mimic cyst when small (< 8 mm)

Metastatic or Reactive Lymph Node
- Diminutive fatty (echogenic) hilum
- Markedly hypoechoic, not anechoic; vascular
- Usually in axilla or axillary tail of breast

Fat Necrosis
- History of trauma or surgery
- Anechoic collections common
- Associated echogenic mass
- Surrounding edema
- Oil cysts usually hypoechoic or fluid-debris level
- Develop peripheral Ca++, lucent center

SIMPLE CYST

Post-Surgical Seroma
- Pertinent history; track to overlying skin scar
- Usually internal septations or fluid-debris level

PATHOLOGY

General Features
- General path comments
  - Cyst fluid rarely colorless
    - Often turbid yellow or green; may be dark gray/black
    - If brown, consider old hemorrhage
- Etiology
  - Thought to arise from obstructed ducts
  - Mechanism of obstruction controversial: Ductal vs. lobular origin
    - Ductal: Localized epithelial hyperplasia → duct obstruction; or inspissation/extrusion of duct contents into adjacent stroma → inflammation and/or fibrosis → periductal fibrosis → obstruction
    - Lobular: Atrophy of lobular epithelium → acinae coalesce → fluid-filled spaces → progressive dilatation → obliterated TDLU replaced by fluid-containing cyst

Microscopic Features
- Dilated lobular acini from fluid distention
- As with normal ducts, lined by two cell layers
  - Inner: Luminal, cuboidal epithelium
  - Outer: Myoepithelial
- Attenuated type: Flattened epithelium
  - Fluid transudate: High sodium, low potassium
- Apocrine type: Cyst lining shows apocrine metaplasia
  - Low sodium, high potassium; foamy cytoplasm
  - Bilateral and multiple, likely to recur

CLINICAL ISSUES

Presentation
- Most common signs/symptoms
  - Pain and tenderness
    - May be generalized or localized
    - Increased during premenstrual phase of cycle
  - Often asymptomatic
- Soft, fluctuant, freely movable on physical exam
  - Firm if under tension
- May develop or regress rapidly over many years
- Cannot distinguish from solid lesion on physical exam

Demographics
- Age
  - Can occur at any age; peak prevalence 35-50 years
  - 7% of postmenopausal women have cysts
    - More common in women on HRT, estrogen alone
- Gender
  - Most common mass in the female breast
  - Rare in males

Natural History & Prognosis
- Simple cysts have no malignant potential

- Increased risk of malignancy in women who have had multiple cyst aspirations
- May enlarge, persist several years then resolve spontaneously
- May proliferate under estrogenic stimulation
- Size may fluctuate with menstrual cycle; maximum size in premenstrual phase
- 20-50% of women found to have visible cysts at autopsy

Treatment
- Aspiration if painful or equivocal on imaging
  - Routine cytology not indicated for non-bloody fluid
- Post-aspiration air instillation reported to decrease recurrence
  - Equal volume of room air injected into cyst cavity
- Surgical excision rarely necessary
  - Only for painful reaccumulation, refractory to repeated aspiration, air injection

DIAGNOSTIC CHECKLIST

Consider
- Characterization of a mass as a simple cyst more difficult
  - Mass < 8 mm in mean diameter
  - Lesions deeper than 3 cm from skin: Gentle compression helps
- Margin assessment critical: Evaluate realtime and on US images without calipers

Image Interpretation Pearls
- Complicated cyst: Low level internal echoes, fluid-debris level, or mobile debris
  - Can be difficult to distinguish from solid mass: If new or enlarging, aspirate
- Complex cystic mass: Solid component, thick (> 0.5 mm) wall or septations, suspicious: Biopsy

SELECTED REFERENCES

1. Berg WA et al: Operator dependence of physician-performed whole breast sonography: lesion detection and characterization. Radiology in press, 2006
2. Berg WA et al: Cystic lesions of the breast: sonographic-pathologic correlation. Radiology. 227:183-91, 2003
3. Gizienski TA et al: Breast cyst recurrence after postaspiration injection of air. Breast J. 8:34-7, 2002
4. Leung JW et al: Multiple bilateral masses detected on screening mammography: assessment of need for recall imaging. AJR. 175:23-9, 2000
5. Stafford-Johnson DB et al: CT attenuation of fluid in breast cysts. Acad Radiol. 5:423-6, 1998
6. Brenner RJ et al: Spontaneous regression of interval benign cysts of the breast. Radiology. 193:365-8, 1994
7. Ciatto S: The value of routine cytologic examination of breast cyst fluids. Acta Cytol. 31:301-4, 1987
8. Hilton SV et al: Real-time sonography: application in 300 consecutive patients. AJR. 147:479-86, 1986

SIMPLE CYST

IMAGE GALLERY

Typical

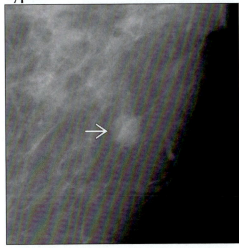

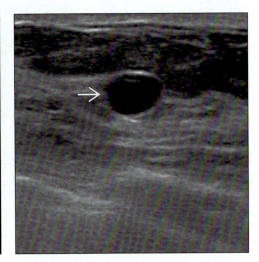

(Left) CC mammography magnification shows spot magnification of a new circumscribed, partially obscured mass ➡ in a post menopausal woman. Because the mass was new, US was performed (right-hand image). *(Right)* Radial ultrasound shows the mammographic abnormality to be a simple cyst ➡. Though unusual in the absence of hormone replacement, 7% of post-menopausal women not on HRT will have a cyst at some time.

Typical

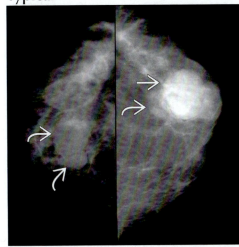

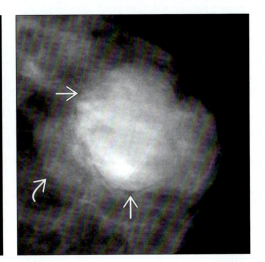

(Left) CC mammography shows multiple, fairly well-circumscribed bilateral masses ➡, with a dominant palpable lobulated left retroareolar mass ➡. *(Right)* CC mammography shows close-up view which confirms the circumscribed nature of the palpable mass ➡ and the smaller more posterior mass ➡ (left-hand image).

Typical

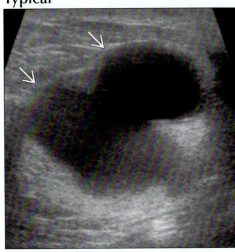

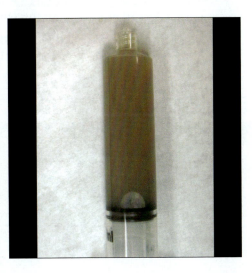

(Left) Transverse harmonic ultrasound shows palpable left retroareolar mass ➡ to be bilobed simple cyst. *(Right)* Specimen gross pathology shows contents of aspirated cyst: 17 cc cloudy, amber fluid, typical of a benign cyst. As with other non-bloody aspirates, it was discarded.

COMPLEX CYSTIC MASS

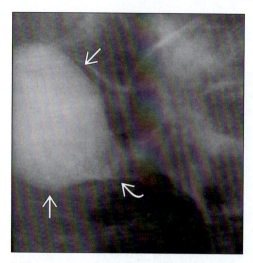

MLO mammography shows mostly circumscribed, dense mass ➡ in this 43 year old with a palpable mass. The anterior margin is focally indistinct ➡.

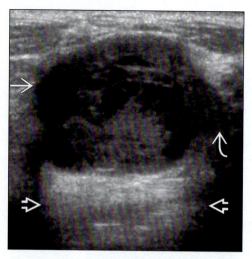

Ultrasound (same as left-hand image) shows complex cystic and solid mass ➡ with posterior enhancement ➡, partially indistinctly marginated ➡. Biopsy showed papillary DCIS, focally invasive at excision.

TERMINOLOGY

Definitions

- A mass with both cystic (anechoic) and solid (hypo-, iso-, or hyperechoic) components
- Any of the following in isolation or combination
  - Intracystic mass
  - Thick-walled (> 0.5 mm) cystic mass
  - Thick septations (> 0.5 mm) within an otherwise cystic mass
  - Predominantly solid mass with cystic (anechoic) areas within it
  - Mixed cystic and solid mass
- Distinguish from complicated cyst
  - Circumscribed, especially along back wall, imperceptible wall, posterior enhancement
  - Homogeneous low level echoes, mobile debris, or fluid-debris level without a mass
  - No solid component
- Distinguish from markedly hypoechoic mass with indistinct margins

IMAGING FINDINGS

General Features

- Best diagnostic clue: US appearance of partially cystic, partially solid mass
- Morphology: Can be circumscribed or not

Mammographic Findings

- Intracystic masses often circumscribed
- Thick-walled cystic masses or mixed cystic and solid masses often indistinctly marginated, may be irregular
- Evaluate for additional suspicious findings in both ipsilateral and contralateral breast
- Assess axillary nodes
- Associated calcifications (Ca++) uncommon: Best characterized by magnification CC and true lateral views
- Spot compression and/or magnification views can help characterize margins, but US is primary diagnostic tool for this entity

Ultrasonographic Findings

- Grayscale Ultrasound

DDx: Complex Cystic and Solid Masses

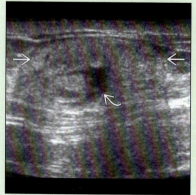

Fat Necrosis

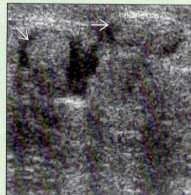

Abscess (Pus)

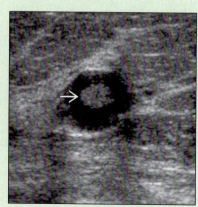

Intracystic Papilloma

COMPLEX CYSTIC MASS

Key Facts

Terminology
- Any of the following in isolation or combination
- Intracystic mass
- Thick-walled (> 0.5 mm) cystic mass
- Thick septations (> 0.5 mm) within an otherwise cystic mass
- Predominantly solid mass with cystic (anechoic) areas within it
- Mixed cystic and solid mass

Top Differential Diagnoses
- Invasive Ductal Carcinoma (IDC)
- Papillary Ductal Carcinoma in Situ (DCIS)
- Papilloma
- Fibrocystic Changes
- Ruptured Cyst
- Complex Fibroadenoma (FA)
- Phyllodes Tumor
- Apocrine Metaplasia
- Abscess
- Fat Necrosis
- Post-Surgical Seroma/Hematoma

Pathology
- Intracystic mass most often papillary: 22% rate of malignancy
- Thick-walled cystic mass most commonly high grade malignancy or abscess: 30% rate of malignancy
- Solid mass with cystic foci most commonly FCC or FA: 13% rate of malignancy

Clinical Issues
- Suspicious for malignancy and merits biopsy

- ○ Mass with both anechoic (cystic) and solid (hypo-, iso- or hyperechoic) components
  - ■ Thick (> 0.5 mm) indistinct wall or septations
  - ■ Intracystic mass or mixed solid and cystic mass
  - ○ Posterior enhancement common
  - ○ Exclude mobile debris mimicking intracystic mass if appropriate
    - ■ Reposition patient and wait 2-5 minutes
- Color Doppler
  - ○ Vascularity in solid component common
  - ○ Vascular stalk in papillary lesions

MR Findings
- T1WI
  - ○ Cystic component typically hypointense
    - ■ May be hyperintense if hemorrhagic or proteinaceous fluid
- T2WI FS: Cystic component hyperintense
- T1 C+
  - ○ Solid component will typically enhance
  - ○ Thick-walled cystic masses may show rim-enhancement
    - ■ Slow initial rise then persistent kinetics favors ruptured cyst
    - ■ Rapid initial rise then plateau or washout kinetics suspicious for malignancy
- Can be used to determine extent of disease for malignant lesions

Biopsy
- Aspiration of fluid can be performed: Send fluid for cytology only if bloody
- US-guided FNAB of solid component not reliable
  - ○ 10% insufficient rate for nonpalpable masses
  - ○ 4% false negative rate for nonpalpable masses
- US-guided core biopsy of solid component
  - ○ 97% sensitivity for malignancy
- Attempt to aspirate abscesses to resolution (under US guidance), may require 18-g needle for pus
  - ○ May require open drainage if > 3 cm

DIFFERENTIAL DIAGNOSIS

Invasive Ductal Carcinoma (IDC)
- Usually at least partially indistinctly marginated
- Most often high grade IDC NOS
  - ○ Can appear circumscribed
  - ○ Thick-walled cystic mass with central necrosis most common when complex
- Medullary carcinoma
  - ○ Most often thick-walled cystic mass when complex
  - ○ Can show eccentric cystic areas
- Mucinous (colloid) carcinoma
  - ○ Mixed cystic and solid components reported in 38% cases in one series

Papillary Ductal Carcinoma in Situ (DCIS)
- Synonymous with intracystic carcinoma
- Typically a circumscribed mass
- Can be hypervascular, often with vascular stalk
- Usually intracystic mass with at least focally thickened wall
- Can be solid type

Invasive Papillary Carcinoma
- Usually predominantly (intracystic) papillary DCIS with focal mural invasion
- Often irregular, dominant solid, hypervascular component
- May have thickened, nodular wall
- Usually at least partially indistinctly marginated

Papilloma
- Typically an intracystic or intraductal mass with imperceptible wall
- May have associated nipple discharge when close to the nipple

Fibrocystic Changes
- Mixed cystic and solid mass
- Solid component usually due to fibrosis
- Cystic component may show apocrine metaplasia
- Can have associated Ca++: Punctate, amorphous, heterogeneous, rarely linear, milk-of-calcium

COMPLEX CYSTIC MASS

Ruptured Cyst
- Thick-walled cystic mass
- Usually incidental on MR: Progressively rim-enhancing cyst

Complex Fibroadenoma (FA)
- Difficult to distinguish from phyllodes tumor
- Circumscribed margins
- Mixed cystic and solid mass

Phyllodes Tumor
- Usually circumscribed
- Rapid growth
- Mixed cystic and solid mass: Presence of cystic areas favors malignant phyllodes
- Cystic areas more common in phyllodes tumors than FA

Apocrine Metaplasia
- Clustered microcysts common
- Peak age mid 40's to early 50's
- Can have thick walls and thick septations due to tall columnar epithelium
  o May merit biopsy when appearance not typical
- Can have associated punctate or amorphous Ca++
  o May show layering (milk-of-calcium) on true lateral view
- Can enhance on MR

Abscess
- Usually tender, palpable mass, most often near nipple
- Thick, indistinct wall typical
- Echogenic debris = pus
- Aspiration usually diagnostic

Fat Necrosis
- History of trauma or surgery
- Anechoic fluid component
- Echogenic mass
- Surrounding edema (increased echogenicity)

Post-Surgical Seroma/Hematoma
- Appropriate history
- At surgical site, with track to overlying skin scar
- Can occur (1-3%) with percutaneous stereotactic or less commonly US-guided biopsy
  o More common with larger (> 14-g) bore devices or in patients on anticoagulation

Galactocele
- Pregnant or lactating woman
- Most common appearance = complicated cyst, e.g., fluid-debris level with echogenic debris (fat content)

PATHOLOGY

General Features
- Etiology
  o Intracystic mass most often papillary: 22% rate of malignancy
  o Thick-walled cystic mass most commonly high grade malignancy or abscess: 30% rate of malignancy

o Solid mass with cystic foci most commonly FCC or FA: 13% rate of malignancy

CLINICAL ISSUES

Presentation
- Most common signs/symptoms
  o Palpable or nonpalpable mass
    ▪ Abscess usually tender, may have overlying erythema
    ▪ Papillary lesions may have associated clear or less often bloody nipple discharge

Treatment
- Suspicious for malignancy and merits biopsy
  o US-guided core biopsy effective
    ▪ Papillary lesions generally merit excision
    ▪ Fluid can be aspirated: Cytology only if bloody
    ▪ Core biopsy of solid component
  o Excision an acceptable alternative to core biopsy

DIAGNOSTIC CHECKLIST

Image Interpretation Pearls
- Complicated cysts benign or probably benign: Circumscribed imperceptible wall, no solid component
- Complex cystic lesions suspicious: Indistinct or thick wall (> 0. 5 mm) and/or solid component

SELECTED REFERENCES

1. Cardenosa G: Ultrasound of cysts, cystic lesions, and papillary lesions. Radiologic Clinics N Amer in press, 2006
2. Fajardo LL et al: Stereotactic and sonographic large-core biopsy of nonpalpable breast lesions: results of the Radiologic Diagnostic Oncology Group V study. Acad Radiol. 11:293-308, 2004
3. Lam WW et al: Sonographic appearance of mucinous carcinoma of the breast. AJR. 182:1069-74, 2004
4. Berg WA et al: Cystic lesions of the breast: sonographic-pathologic correlation. Radiology. 227:183-91, 2003
5. Mendelson EB et al: Breast Imaging Reporting and Data System: BI-RADS, Ultrasound, 1st ed. Reston, American College of Radiology, 2003
6. Shetty MK et al: Sonographic findings in focal fibrocystic changes of the breast. Ultrasound Q. 18:35-40, 2002
7. Yilmaz E et al: Differentiation of phyllodes tumors versus fibroadenomas. Acta Radiol. 43:34-9, 2002
8. Pisano ED et al: Fine-needle aspiration biopsy of nonpalpable breast lesions in a multicenter clinical trial: results from the radiologic diagnostic oncology group V. Radiology. 219:785-92, 2001
9. Venta LA et al: Management of complex breast cysts. AJR. 173:1331-6, 1999
10. Soo MS et al: Fat necrosis in the breast: sonographic features. Radiology. 206:261-9, 1998
11. Warner JK et al: Apocrine metaplasia: mammographic and sonographic appearances. AJR. 170:1375-9, 1998
12. Liberman L et al: Benign and malignant phyllodes tumors: mammographic and sonographic findings. Radiology. 198:121-4, 1996

COMPLEX CYSTIC MASS

IMAGE GALLERY

Typical

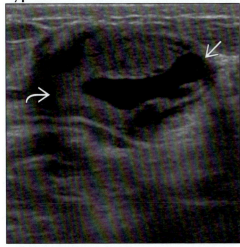
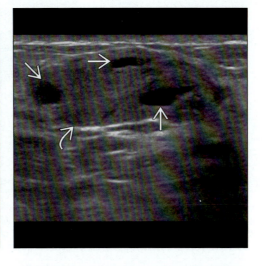

(Left) Radial ultrasound of a palpable mass in a 51 year old shows a circumscribed, oval mass with both solid ➡ and cystic ➡ components. *(Right)* Radial ultrasound at another level shows similar findings with both solid ➡ and cystic components ➡. Biopsy showed fibrocystic changes with apocrine metaplasia, duct ectasia, and stromal fibrosis.

Typical

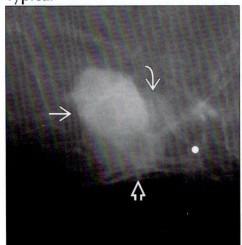
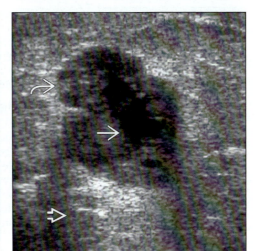

(Left) MLO mammography spot compression of a palpable mass in a 30 year old shows a partially circumscribed ➡, partially indistinctly marginated mass ➡ with overlying skin retraction ➡. *(Right)* Radial ultrasound (same mass as left-hand image) shows a thick-walled lobulated mass ➡ with central cystic component ➡ (due to necrosis), and posterior enhancement ➡. US-guided core biopsy and excision showed grade III invasive ductal carcinoma.

Typical

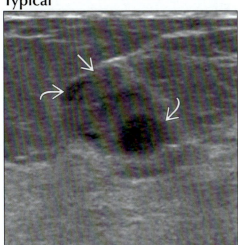
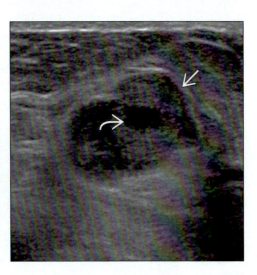

(Left) Anti-radial spatial compounding ultrasound in an asymptomatic 66 year old shows a mixed cystic ➡ and solid ➡ gently lobulated mass, with the solid component isoechoic to surrounding fat. US-guided biopsy showed complex FA with cysts, stable at 7 years of follow-up. *(Right)* Radial ultrasound in an asymptomatic 67 year old shows a mixed cystic ➡ and solid ➡ circumscribed, gently lobulated mass, which was new or enlarging. Biopsy showed phyllodes tumor.

INTRACYSTIC MASS

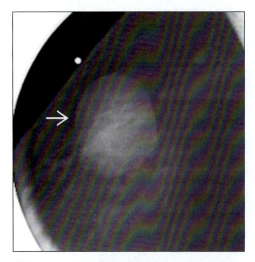

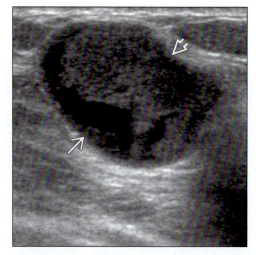

MLO mammography spot compression shows circumscribed, oval mass ➡ corresponding to a palpable mass in this 63 year old woman. US was performed (right-hand image). (Courtesy EAR).

Ultrasound shows complex cystic and solid mass with thick, indistinct wall ➡ and a large intracystic mass ➡ (hypervascular on color Doppler). Excision showed invasive papillary carcinoma. (Courtesy EAR).

TERMINOLOGY

Definitions
- Solid mass with a peripheral cystic (anechoic) component
- A subset of complex cystic masses
- Intracystic carcinoma synonymous with papillary ductal carcinoma in situ (DCIS)
  - For some pathologists, this is a gross diagnosis, and includes invasive papillary carcinoma

IMAGING FINDINGS

General Features
- Best diagnostic clue: US appearance
- Morphology: Usually peripherally circumscribed; intracystic mass can be oval, round, or irregular

Mammographic Findings
- Most often circumscribed mass
  - Indistinct margin suspicious for malignancy
- Can be obscured or occult due to overlying parenchyma

- Can be multiple, usually in one quadrant
- Associated calcifications (Ca++) uncommon
  - CC and true lateral magnification views to characterize Ca++ if present
  - Milk-of-calcium can be present, will layer on true lateral view

Ultrasonographic Findings
- Grayscale Ultrasound
  - Assess mobility of intracystic "mass"
    - Change patient position, wait 2-5 minutes
    - Mobile debris = benign
    - May reveal underlying mass
  - Posterior enhancement typical
  - Thick, nodular or indistinct margins increase suspicion for invasive component
  - Papillary lesions may be multiple, usually in same quadrant: Whole breast US recommended
- Color Doppler: Vascular stalk can be seen with papillary lesions

MR Findings
- T1WI
  - Hypointense
    - Bloody or proteinaceous fluid hyperintense

DDx: Lesions Mimicking Intracystic Masses

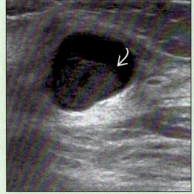

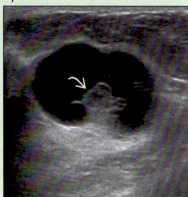

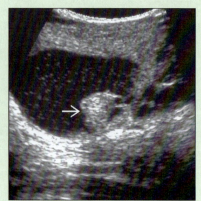

Hemorrhagic Cyst

Proteinaceous Debris

Galactocele, Normal Tissue

INTRACYSTIC MASS

Key Facts

Terminology
- Solid mass with a peripheral cystic (anechoic) component

Imaging Findings
- Morphology: Usually peripherally circumscribed; intracystic mass can be oval, round, or irregular

Top Differential Diagnoses
- Papilloma
- Atypical Papilloma
- Intracystic (Papillary) Ductal Carcinoma in Situ (DCIS)
- Invasive Papillary Carcinoma
- Tumefactive Debris in a Complicated Cyst
- Post-Surgical Seroma or Hematoma
- Abscess

- Adjacent normal parenchyma can (rarely) project into cyst and mimic intracystic mass

Pathology
- Etiology: 22% rate of malignancy in one series

Clinical Issues
- Intracystic mass is suspicious, merits tissue diagnosis, unless clearly due to tumefactive debris
- Initial aspiration to exclude tumefactive debris, then core biopsy of solid component
- Initial core biopsy if tiny mural nodule which may be obscured after aspiration
- Direct excision is reasonable
- Generally excise with result of papillary lesion on core

- T2WI FS
  - Fluid component hyperintense unless bloody or proteinaceous
  - Intracystic mass variable signal intensity
- T1 C+
  - Enhancement of intracystic mass, not fluid component
  - Rim-enhancement of thick-walled lesions
    - Malignancy usually shows rapid initial enhancement then plateau or washout kinetics

Biopsy
- Intracystic masses merit tissue diagnosis unless clearly due to mobile debris
- Variety of approaches are successful: US-guidance
  - Direct targeting of solid component initially
    - Favored by some if small mural nodule (< 5 mm)
    - Initial FNAB or core biopsy
  - Aspirate fluid, discard unless bloody, then core biopsy of solid component
  - Consider placing clip if difficult to visualize at conclusion of procedure
  - Direct excision with needle localization if nonpalpable
    - Initial core biopsy favored when malignancy suspected, i.e., especially for irregular or indistinctly-marginated masses
    - Allows single treatment surgery
    - Consider US-guided FNAB (or core biopsy) of node if suspect invasive carcinoma

Imaging Recommendations
- Best imaging tool: US to characterize and guide intervention
- Protocol advice: Whole breast US to evaluate for multiple similar masses

DIFFERENTIAL DIAGNOSIS

Papilloma
- Most often intraductal, can appear intracystic
- Usually round, oval, or frond-like intracystic mass

- Vascular stalk may be visualized on color or power Doppler
- Can degenerate into atypical or malignant lesion
- Can be multiple, peripheral
  - Increased risk of malignant degeneration
- May show associated Ca++: Usually punctate or amorphous
- May show associated nipple discharge, clear more often than bloody
  - More common when close to nipple

Atypical Papilloma
- Papilloma with cellular atypia or atypical ductal hyperplasia (ADH)
- Recommend excision, 36% rate of malignancy

Intracystic (Papillary) Ductal Carcinoma in Situ (DCIS)
- 0.6-0.8% of all breast cancer
- Intracystic mass itself irregular, can be hypervascular, vascular stalk
- Can bleed into mass causing fluid-debris level

Invasive Papillary Carcinoma
- Usually predominantly papillary DCIS with focal invasion
- Indistinct margin suggests invasive component
  - Evaluate axillary nodes on US, consider FNAB (or core biopsy) of axillary node
- Dominant, irregular solid component, often hypervascular
- May have thick-wall, mural nodularity

Invasive Ductal Carcinoma (NOS)
- Necrotic component can be anechoic, more often central than peripheral
  - Thick-walled (> 0.5 mm) complex cystic mass
- Usually solid mass with eccentric cystic foci rather than intracystic mass per se

Tumefactive Debris in a Complicated Cyst
- Usually adherent to wall

○ If freely mobile, or layers, can preclude aspiration or biopsy
• Hemorrhagic or proteinaceous debris
• Ruptured cyst with debris
  ○ Usually thick-walled, rim-enhancing mass on MR
  ○ Slow initial then persistent delayed enhancement, lack of internal enhancement

Post-Surgical Seroma or Hematoma
• History of surgery or biopsy
• Nodularity of adjacent tissue can mimic mass within collection
• Hemorrhagic debris can mimic mass

Abscess
• Tender, usually palpable mass, often near nipple
• Pus typically echogenic, can appear mass-like with anechoic surround
• Aspiration diagnostic and can be therapeutic
  ○ May require 18-g or even 16-g needle
• Often thick-wall, overlying skin thickening, edema

Galactocele
• Lactating or pregnant patient
• Fat-containing fluid relatively echogenic
• "Fatty plug" = echogenic intracystic mass
• Rare reports of milk fistula with biopsy
  ○ Aspiration can be safely performed for symptomatic relief

Lobulated Simple Cyst
• Adjacent normal parenchyma can (rarely) project into cyst and mimic intracystic mass
• Change angle of insonation, pressure

Fibrocystic Changes (FCC)
• Uncommon appearance
• Possibly discordant, consider excision
• Papillomatosis can appear mass-like

PATHOLOGY

General Features
• Etiology: 22% rate of malignancy in one series

Microscopic Features
• Variability distinguishing benign from atypical papillary lesions, no standardized criteria
  ○ Low threshold for recommending excision after core biopsy showing benign papilloma
• Invasive papillary carcinoma: Cells infiltrate breast tissue beyond duct wall

CLINICAL ISSUES

Presentation
• Most common signs/symptoms
  ○ Palpable or nonpalpable mass
  ○ Clear, or less often bloody nipple discharge
    ▪ 22-34% of patients with papillary carcinoma have nipple discharge

Demographics
• Age: Mean age at diagnosis of papillary carcinoma = 63-67 years

Natural History & Prognosis
• Papillary DCIS: Excellent prognosis

Treatment
• Intracystic mass is suspicious, merits tissue diagnosis, unless clearly due to tumefactive debris
  ○ Initial aspiration to exclude tumefactive debris, then core biopsy of solid component
  ○ Initial core biopsy if tiny mural nodule which may be obscured after aspiration
  ○ Direct excision is reasonable
• Generally excise with result of papillary lesion on core
  ○ 7% rate of malignancy after diagnosis of benign papilloma on core biopsy
  ○ 14% rate of malignancy after diagnosis of benign "equivocal" papillary lesion on core biopsy
  ○ 36% rate of malignancy with atypical papillary lesion on core biopsy

DIAGNOSTIC CHECKLIST

Consider
• Intracystic masses are most commonly papillomas, can be atypical or malignant papillary lesions
• Excision generally recommended for papillary lesions: Direct excision is reasonable

Image Interpretation Pearls
• Distinguish from complicated cyst, benign or probably benign: Imperceptible wall, homogeneous low level echoes, fluid-debris level, or mobile debris
• Intracystic masses are complex cystic masses, suspicious for malignancy, BI-RADS 4

SELECTED REFERENCES

1. Berg WA: Image-guided breast biopsy and management of high-risk lesions. Radiol Clin N Amer. 42:935-46, 2004
2. Berg WA et al: Cystic lesions of the breast: Sonographic-pathologic correlation. Radiology. 227:183-91, 2003
3. Jacobs TW et al: Nonmalignant lesions in breast core needle biopsies: to excise or not to excise? Am J Surg Pathol. 26:1095-110, 2002
4. Leung J et al: Benign papillary breast lesions diagnosed at large-core needle biopsy: correlation with surgical pathology and clinical outcome. AJR (abstr). 187:59-60, 2002
5. Liberman L et al: Case 35: Intracystic papillary carcinoma with invasion. Radiology. 219:781-4, 2001
6. Reynolds HE: Core needle biopsy of challenging benign breast lesions: A comprehensive literature review. AJR. 174:1245-50, 2000
7. Rosen PP: Papillary Carcinoma. In Rosen's Breast Pathology. Philadelphia, Lippincott-Raven. 335-54, 1997

INTRACYSTIC MASS

IMAGE GALLERY

Typical

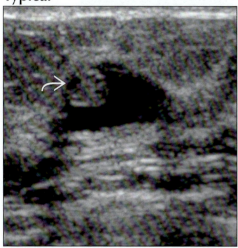

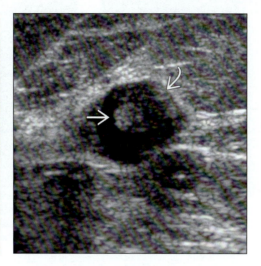

(Left) Radial ultrasound shows intracystic mass ➡ in this 44 year old with a mass on mammography. US-guided core biopsy and excision confirmed atypical papilloma. *(Right)* Ultrasound in a 47 year old shows an intracystic mass ➡ with focally thickened wall ➡. Initial core biopsy showed FCC and sclerosing adenosis, considered discordant. Excision showed sclerosed intraductal papilloma with incidental 3 mm DCIS 1 cm away from this mass.

Variant

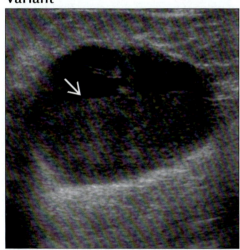

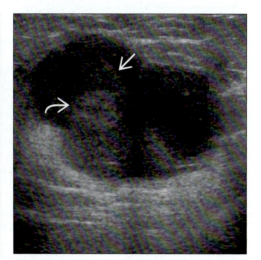

(Left) Ultrasound in this 53 year old with a palpable mass shows a circumscribed mass with fluid-debris level ➡, appearing to be a complicated cyst. *(Right)* Ultrasound with the patient positioned right side down shows mobility of the fluid-debris level ➡, and an echogenic round mass ➡ is now evident. Aspiration yielded blood. Core biopsy and excision of the solid component showed intracystic papillary DCIS.

Variant

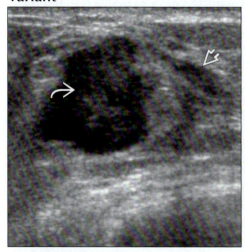

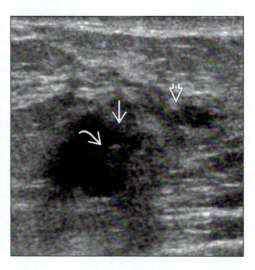

(Left) Ultrasound in a 71 year old shows an irregular intracystic mass ➡ with intraductal extension ➡. *(Right)* Ultrasound more anteriorly to mass on left shows a second intracystic mass ➡. The cyst wall is indistinct ➡, and an adjacent intraductal mass is seen ➡. The dominant mass (left image) proved IDC, grade III, with high grade DCIS and adjacent intracystic papillary DCIS (right image).

THICK-WALLED CYSTIC MASS

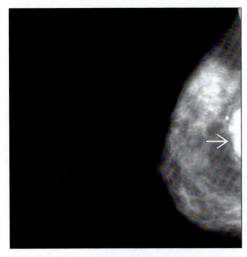

CC mammography in this 35 year old shows palpable, circumscribed mass ➡, partially included.

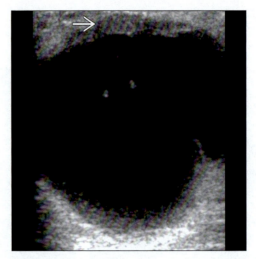

Sagittal ultrasound (same patient as left-hand image) shows thick-walled ➡, predominantly cystic mass. US-guided aspiration then core biopsy proved grade III IDC.

TERMINOLOGY

Abbreviations and Synonyms
- A subset of complex cystic masses

Definitions
- A sonographic definition, can also be seen on MR
- Internally cystic (fluid-containing, anechoic on US with posterior enhancement), outer wall > 0.5 mm, often indistinct
- May have associated thick septations or other internal solid components

IMAGING FINDINGS

General Features
- Best diagnostic clue: Cystic lesion with perceptible wall, > 0.5 mm thick, on US

Mammographic Findings
- Spot compression or magnification views helpful in characterizing margin

- Indistinctly marginated masses suspicious for malignancy
- Mass margins can be partially circumscribed, partially obscured
  - New, enlarging, or palpable circumscribed mass merits US
- Multiple, bilateral mostly circumscribed masses generally benign
  - Dominant or palpable mass still requires US evaluation
  - Evaluate each mass on its own merits: Indistinct margins require US evaluation
  - If one is found to be thick-walled cystic mass on US, it should still be deemed suspicious
- Magnification views to characterize associated suspicious calcifications
- Associated architectural distortion may be best perceived on spot compression or spot magnification views
- Overlying skin thickening or retraction seen best on tangential views over mass
- Evaluate for multifocal, multicentric, bilateral similar findings or other suspicious findings
- If suspicious findings present, evaluate for adenopathy

DDx: Complex Cystic Lesions with Thick Walls

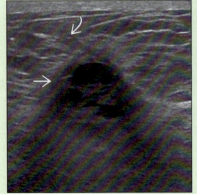

Post-Surgical Hematoma

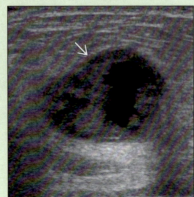

Adenomyoepithelioma

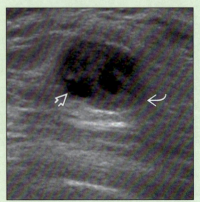

Ruptured Cyst

THICK-WALLED CYSTIC MASS

Key Facts

Terminology
- A subset of complex cystic masses
- Internally cystic (fluid-containing, anechoic on US with posterior enhancement), outer wall > 0.5 mm, often indistinct

Imaging Findings
- Best diagnostic clue: Cystic lesion with perceptible wall, > 0.5 mm thick, on US
- Indistinctly marginated masses suspicious for malignancy
- New, enlarging, or palpable circumscribed mass merits US
- Multiple, bilateral mostly circumscribed masses generally benign
- Rapid initial enhancement with subsequent plateau or washout favors malignancy

- Slow initial enhancement with persistent/progressive kinetics favors benign etiology
- Angular margins favor malignancy

Top Differential Diagnoses
- Ruptured or Inflamed Cyst
- Seroma or Hematoma
- Fat Necrosis
- Abscess
- When malignant, usually high grade IDC NOS
- Papillary Carcinoma
- Fibrocystic Changes
- Apocrine Metaplasia
- Phyllodes Tumor

Pathology
- 30% malignancy rate

- Trabecular thickening due to edema: Suggests abscess, fat necrosis, post-surgical collection

Ultrasonographic Findings
- Grayscale Ultrasound
  - Thick, hypoechoic wall (> 0.5 mm)
    - Angular margins favor malignancy
    - Indistinct or microlobulated margins of intermediate concern
    - Circumscribed margin can be benign or malignant
  - Internal structure
    - Anechoic
    - Internal septations may be present
    - Intracystic mass may be present
  - Can show fluid-debris level
    - Differential: Infection (e.g., pus), mass that has bled, proteinaceous debris in a ruptured cyst
  - Posterior enhancement usually present
  - Evaluate for surrounding edema: Diffuse increased echogenicity, dilated lymphatics
    - Differential: Abscess, fat necrosis
- Color Doppler: Internal flow or flow to wall on color or power Doppler is suspicious for malignancy

MR Findings
- T1WI
  - Fluid signal internally usually hypointense, can be hyperintense if bloody or proteinaceous
  - Fatty portion of fat necrosis will appear bright
- T2WI FS
  - Fluid signal internally usually hyperintense, can be hypointense if bloody or proteinaceous
  - Internal hypointense septations may be visible
  - Evaluate for other cystic lesions
  - May see associated edema with inflammatory or infectious conditions or due to lymphatic obstruction from nodal metastases
  - Mucinous (colloid) carcinoma can appear bright, but is solid
- T1 C+
  - Enhancement of wall usually seen
    - Rapid initial enhancement with subsequent plateau or washout favors malignancy

- Slow initial enhancement with persistent/progressive kinetics favors benign etiology
  - Lack of enhancement strongly predictive of benign etiology
  - Evaluate for suspicious nodes
  - Evaluate for multifocal, multicentric, bilateral disease
- Inversion Recovery FSE: Similar appearance to T2WI

Nuclear Medicine Findings
- PET: Rim uptake of FDG, black hole in cystic component

Biopsy
- US-guided core biopsy is favored approach
  - Can initially withdraw fluid under US guidance: Cytology only if frankly bloody
  - Need to deliberately sample solid components at core biopsy
  - Place clip if concerned about poor conspicuity post-biopsy, and to facilitate correlation with other imaging
  - Post clip-placement mammogram to confirm clip position

Imaging Recommendations
- Best imaging tool: Ultrasound with spatial compounding or tissue harmonic imaging
- Protocol advice: New, enlarging, or palpable mass merits US regardless of circumscribed margin on mammography

DIFFERENTIAL DIAGNOSIS

Ruptured or Inflamed Cyst
- Usually other cysts and/or complicated cysts present
- Round or oval shape
- Indistinct margins on US
- Gradually, progressively enhancing wall on MR
- Usually lack internal structure: Anechoic or hypoechoic due to proteinaceous debris

THICK-WALLED CYSTIC MASS

- Can develop rim calcifications

Seroma or Hematoma
- Usually post-operative or post-biopsy
- Internal track from scar should extend from collection to overlying skin scar
- Should decrease over time, but may be present for years
- May have mobile internal debris
- Smooth rim-enhancement ≤ 4 mm thickness on MR
  - Should decrease over time, rare beyond 18 months post surgery

Fat Necrosis
- Usually history of trauma or surgery
- Echogenic/hyperechoic rind and small fluid collection
- Associated edema
- Can develop rim or other calcifications over time
  - Calcifications usually develop after 2 years

Abscess
- Erythema, tender mass, surrounding edema
- Usually near nipple

Infiltrating Ductal Carcinoma (IDC)
- When malignant, usually high grade IDC NOS
- Can be mostly circumscribed
- Usually at least partially indistinctly marginated
- Evaluate for metastatic axillary adenopathy

Medullary Carcinoma
- Margins usually at least partially indistinct
- Usually associated internal septations or mass
- Evaluate for metastatic axillary adenopathy

Papillary Carcinoma
- Intracystic papillary carcinoma: Special type of ductal carcinoma in situ (DCIS)
- Usually intracystic mass with only focal wall thickening
- Can be focally invasive

Metastases
- Solitary or multiple masses, usually in one breast
- History of systemic primary
- Melanoma metastases can be cystic

Any Mass Post-Biopsy
- Appropriate history
- Defect in mass may fill with serum or blood
- May see associated edema, clip(s)

Fibrocystic Changes
- Mixed fibrosis, adenosis, and cystic changes with predominance of cystic change
- May have associated apocrine metaplasia in cystic component

Apocrine Metaplasia
- Can appear thick-walled with thick septations: Clustered microcysts with thick walls
- Biopsy indicated when thick-walled, can be papillary apocrine metaplasia
- May show associated punctate calcifications or milk-of-calcium

Phyllodes Tumor
- Usually mostly circumscribed, resembling fibroadenoma
- Solitary or multiple
- More often predominantly solid with cystic foci
- Cystic component may be more frequent with malignant phyllodes

PATHOLOGY

General Features
- Etiology
  - 30% malignancy rate
  - Necrotic center due to rapidly growing, usually high grade malignancy
  - Inflammation of wall due to infection or rupture

Gross Pathologic & Surgical Features
- Necrotic center may be evident with high grade malignancies

CLINICAL ISSUES

Presentation
- Most common signs/symptoms: Palpable or nonpalpable mass
- Other signs/symptoms: When due to abscess, erythema and thickening of skin, tender mass

Treatment
- Suspicious for malignancy, BI-RADS 4, and generally merits biopsy

SELECTED REFERENCES

1. Berg WA et al: Cystic lesions of the breast: sonographic-pathologic correlation. Radiology. 227:183-191, 2003
2. Mendelson EB et al: Breast Imaging Reporting and Data System: BI-RADS, Ultrasound, 1st ed. Reston, American College of Radiology, 2003
3. Liberman L et al: Case 35: intracystic papillary carcinoma with invasion. Radiology. 219:781-4, 2001
4. Nunes LW et al: Update of breast MR imaging architectural interpretation model. Radiology. 219:484-94, 2001
5. Lamb PM et al: Correlation between ultrasound characteristics, mammographic findings and histological grade in patients with invasive ductal carcinoma of the breast. Clin Radiol. 55:40-4, 2000
6. Leung JW et al: Multiple bilateral masses detected on screening mammography: assessment of need for recall imaging. AJR. 175:23-9, 2000
7. Soo MS et al: Fat necrosis in the breast: sonographic features. Radiology. 206:261-9, 1998
8. Warner JK et al: Apocrine metaplasia: mammographic and sonographic appearances. AJR. 170:1375-9, 1998
9. Liberman L et al: Benign and malignant phyllodes tumors: mammographic and sonographic findings. Radiology. 198:121-4, 1996
10. Wellings SR et al: An atlas of subgross pathology of the human breast with special reference to possible precancerous lesions. J Natl Cancer Inst. 55:231-73, 1975

THICK-WALLED CYSTIC MASS

IMAGE GALLERY

Typical

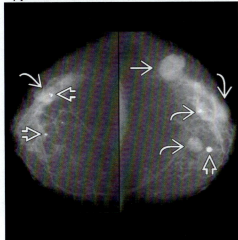

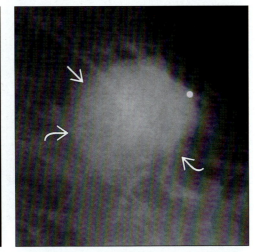

(Left) CC mammography in this 46 year old shows multiple bilateral mostly circumscribed masses ➡ and typically benign calcifications ➡. One mass ➡ is indistinctly marginated, seen better on spot compression view (right-hand image). *(Right)* MLO mammography spot compression confirms partially circumscribed ➡ and mostly indistinct margins ➡ to the palpable mass. US was performed (next image).

Typical

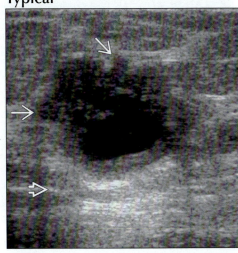

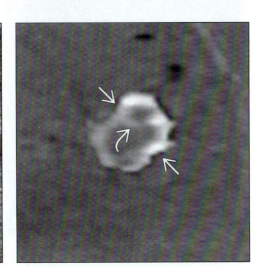

(Left) Anti-radial ultrasound shows the palpable mass (same patient as previous image) to be a thick-walled cystic mass with microlobulated margins ➡ and posterior enhancement ➡, moderately suspicious for malignancy. MR was performed (right-hand image). *(Right)* Coronal T1 C+ subtraction MR shows enhancing thick-walled mass ➡ with enhancing septations ➡. US-guided core biopsy and excision showed medullary carcinoma.

Variant

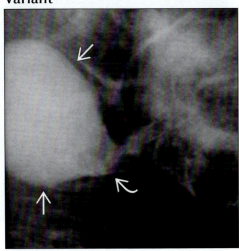

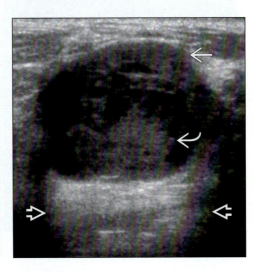

(Left) MLO mammography in this 43 year old shows mostly circumscribed ➡, partially indistinctly marginated ➡ mass. US was performed (right-hand image). *(Right)* Transverse ultrasound shows complex cystic mass which has thick wall anteriorly ➡ and a discrete intracystic mass ➡. Posterior enhancement is noted ➡. Biopsy showed papillary DCIS, microscopically invasive.

Variant

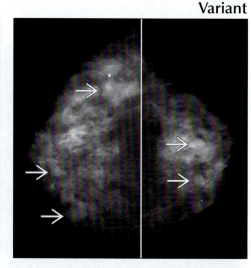

(Left) CC mammography in this 67 year old shows multiple, bilateral, mostly circumscribed masses ➡, fluctuating compared to mammogram obtained 3 years earlier (right-hand image). The largest mass is noted in the inner right breast ➡. *(Right)* CC mammography obtained three years earlier (same patient as left-hand image) shows some of the masses ➡ have resolved and some have developed.

Variant

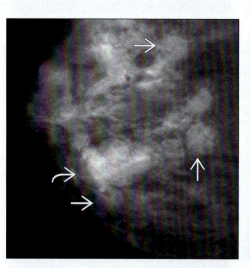 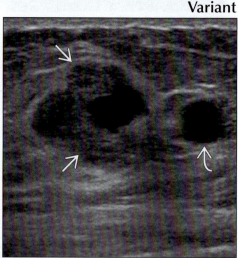

(Left) Close-up of CC current mammogram shows dominant circumscribed mass inner right breast ➡, new compared to prior mammogram (previous 2 images), as well as multiple smaller masses ➡. US was performed (right-hand image). *(Right)* US of dominant mass shows thick-walled cystic mass ➡ and adjacent cyst ➡. The other bilateral masses were cysts. Biopsy of thick-walled cystic mass showed borderline phyllodes tumor.

Typical

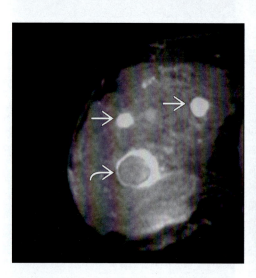 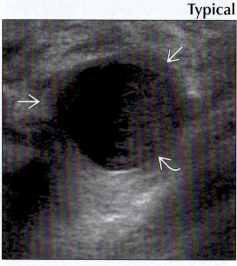

(Left) Sagittal T1 C+ FS MR of this 45 year old with prior breast cancer shows rim-enhancing mass ➡ as well as several other enhancing smooth masses ➡. *(Right)* Anti-radial ultrasound of the rim-enhancing mass (same patient as left-hand image) shows thick-walled ➡ cystic mass with mobile internal debris ➡. US-guided aspiration then core biopsy confirmed ruptured complicated cyst. Other two masses thought to be fibroadenomas.

IV

1

64

Typical

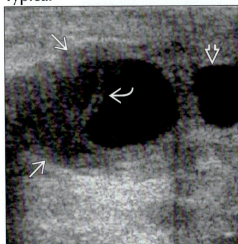 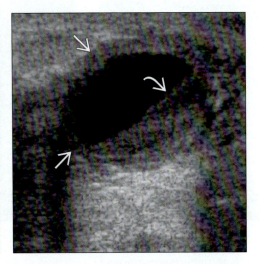

(Left) Right posterior oblique, transverse ultrasound of this palpable mass near the nipple in this 48 year old woman shows a thick-walled cystic mass ➡ with a thick internal septation ➡ and adjacent cyst ➡. *(Right)* Left posterior oblique, transverse ultrasound (same patient as left-hand image) shows internal debris ➡ within this mass ➡ which moves on repositioning the patient. Aspiration yielded pus, confirming abscess; cultures grew S. epidermidis.

Typical

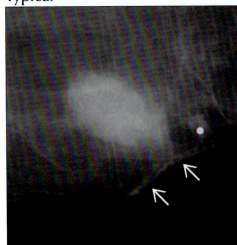 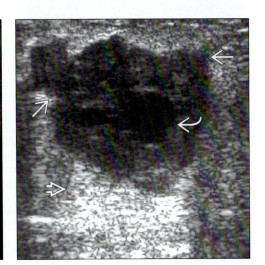

(Left) CC mammography spot compression over this palpable mass in a 30 year old shows a dense indistinctly marginated mass with overlying skin retraction ➡, BI-RADS 4C or 5. US was performed (right-hand image). *(Right)* Anti-radial ultrasound shows thick-walled, centrally cystic ➡ mass with angular ➡ margins and posterior enhancement ➡. US-guided core biopsy showed high grade IDC with central necrosis.

Typical

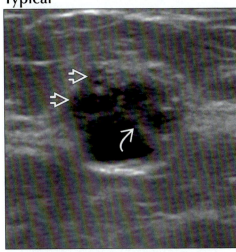 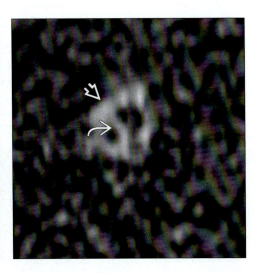

(Left) Anti-radial spatial compounding ultrasound in this 64 year old shows a complex cystic lesion with thickened walls ➡ and thick septations ➡, suspicious for malignancy. *(Right)* Sagittal T1 C+ subtraction MR (same patient as left-hand image) shows enhancement of the wall ➡ and septations ➡. Biopsy showed fibrocystic changes with apocrine metaplasia.

DYSTROPHIC CALCIFICATIONS

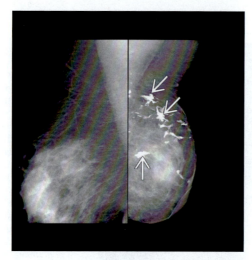

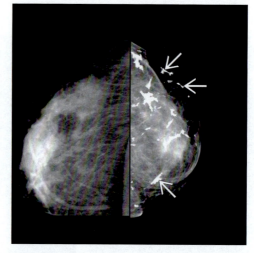

MLO mammography shows the left breast is smaller than the right and demonstrates extensive dystrophic calcifications ➡ *which are coarse, may have internal lucencies, and may be irregular in outline.*

CC mammography (same patient as left-hand image) demonstrates that some of the extensive dystrophic calcifications ➡ *are either within the subcutaneous tissue or skin.*

TERMINOLOGY

Abbreviations and Synonyms
- Heterotopic calcifications (Ca++)

Definitions
- Irregular, coarse, benign Ca++, typically following breast surgery or trauma

IMAGING FINDINGS

General Features
- Best diagnostic clue
  - Large irregular Ca++, may have lucent centers, at surgical site
  - Prior history of lumpectomy and radiotherapy
- Location
  - Typically adjacent to scar
  - May be subcutaneous, in the skin, very extensive
- Size: Typically coarse, > 0.5 mm, usually > 1 mm
- Morphology: Irregular, "lava-shaped"; commonly lucent-centered Ca++

Mammographic Findings
- Post-lumpectomy and radiation therapy
  - Focal skin tethering and distortion with irregular large Ca++
  - May be intermixed with suspicious Ca++ (recurrent malignancy)
- Post-implant
  - Dense irregular Ca++ in fibrous capsule adjacent to the implant
- Post benign surgical biopsy
  - Ca++ uncommon; < 50% mammograms show density or distortion at the biopsy site
- Can be scattered, no specific history of trauma

Ultrasonographic Findings
- Grayscale Ultrasound: Dense echogenic foci associated with hypoechoic scar, may shadow

MR Findings
- No specific MR findings; hypointense all sequences

Imaging Recommendations
- Best imaging tool: Mammography

DDx: Other Benign Coarse Calcifications

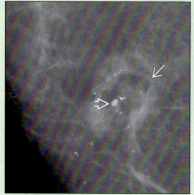

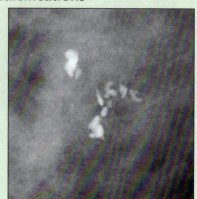

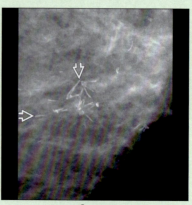

Fat Necrosis

Fibroadenoma

Suture

DYSTROPHIC CALCIFICATIONS

Key Facts

Terminology
- Irregular, coarse, benign Ca++, typically following breast surgery or trauma

Imaging Findings
- Large irregular Ca++, may have lucent centers, at surgical site
- Prior history of lumpectomy and radiotherapy
- Typically adjacent to scar
- Size: Typically coarse, > 0.5 mm, usually > 1 mm

- Protocol advice: If not characteristic, perform ML and CC magnification views

Top Differential Diagnoses
- Recurrent Malignancy
- Fat Necrosis
- Fibroadenomatous Calcifications

Clinical Issues
- No malignant potential or associations

- Protocol advice: If not characteristic, perform ML and CC magnification views

DIFFERENTIAL DIAGNOSIS

Recurrent Malignancy
- Post-lumpectomy cancer recurrence
- Typically suspicious (fine linear or pleomorphic), developing Ca++

Fat Necrosis
- Part of the spectrum of dystrophic Ca++
- Focal lucent-centered mass, oil cysts

Fibroadenomatous Calcifications
- Coarse, dense, irregular; no lucent center
- May have associated mass or density

PATHOLOGY

General Features
- Etiology
  - Nonspecific response to previous insult
  - Post-operative
    - Lumpectomy with radiation therapy
    - Post-reduction, post-liposuction
    - Post-silicone breast implant insertion or removal
    - Typically develop 3-5 years after treatment, in about 30% of women
  - Post-traumatic fat necrosis

Microscopic Features
- Usually some associated fibrosis

CLINICAL ISSUES

Presentation
- Most common signs/symptoms: Usually asymptomatic
- Other signs/symptoms: Fat necrosis can be palpable lump

Natural History & Prognosis
- No malignant potential or associations
- Coarsen over time

Treatment
- If characteristic, BI-RADS 2, benign; BI-RADS 3 for slightly atypical morphology
- Biopsy if morphology indeterminate or suspicious

SELECTED REFERENCES

1. Amin R et al: Subcutaneous calcification following chest wall and breast irradiation: a late complication. Br J Radiol, 75:279-82, 2002
2. Dershaw DD: Breast imaging and the conservative treatment of breast cancer. Radiol Clin North Amer. 40:501-16, 2002
3. Bilgen IG et al: Fat necrosis of the breast: clinical, mammographic and sonographic features. Eur J Radiol. 39:92-9, 2001

IMAGE GALLERY

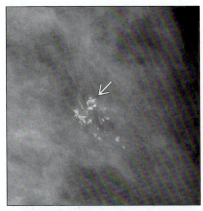 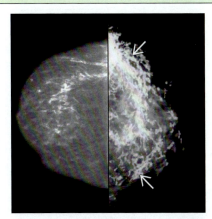 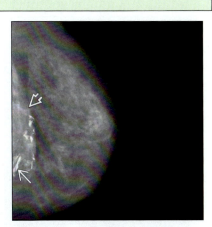

(Left) CC mammography magnification shows dense coarse irregular dystrophic calcifications, some with lucent centers ➡ at the site of prior lumpectomy. These had been stable for years. *(Center)* CC mammography shows a 52 yo woman's normal right breast and left breast post lumpectomy and radiotherapy. Most of the left glandular cone is involved by a reticular mesh of dense calcifications ➡. *(Right)* Lateral mammography shows dystrophic calcifications ➡ involving the retained fibrous capsule ➡ after breast implant removal (explantation).

MILK OF CALCIUM

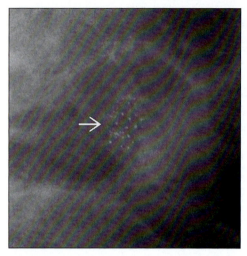

CC mammography magnification shows clustered Ca++ ➡ which are somewhat more discrete and clustered than typical microcyst Ca++.

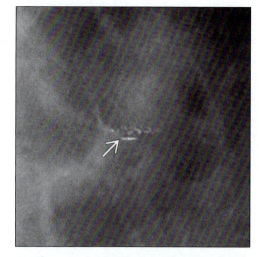

Lateral mammography magnification (same case as left-hand image) shows layering of most of the Ca++ with a linear interface ➡, suggesting a macrocyst with milk of calcium, a benign finding, BI-RADS 2.

TERMINOLOGY

Abbreviations and Synonyms
- Benign intracystic calcifications (Ca++)
- Sedimented Ca++
- Milk of calcium (MOC)

Definitions
- Very fine powdery, amorphous calcification particles precipitated into dilated lobules and microcysts
- Fine clustered Ca++ mobile within a macrocyst

IMAGING FINDINGS

General Features
- Best diagnostic clue: Differing shapes of Ca++ between CC and MLO views, more conspicuous in MLO view
- Location
  - Anatomy: Within dilated acini (microcysts) within terminal duct lobular unit (TDLU)
  - Usually in central to posterior glandular cone
  - Grouped, clustered or scattered through a segment
  - Rare behind nipple, in accessory tissue or glandular islands
- Size
  - Clusters of milk of calcium typically 10-20 mm diameter
  - In macrocysts, depends on cyst size
- Morphology
  - Shape
    - Rounded, fuzzy, amorphous on CC view
    - "Teacups": Crescentic or linear on horizontal beam views
  - Within macrocysts
    - Curvilinear distribution along dependent wall

Mammographic Findings
- Differing shapes and density of calcifications between MLO and CC projections
- Grouped or scattered
- Often coexist with punctate or amorphous Ca++, may all still be MOC but too small to perceive layering
- Can be admixed with malignant Ca++
  - Manage based on most suspicious forms present
- Magnification CC and ML views recommended

DDx: Calcifications Similar to Milk of Calcium

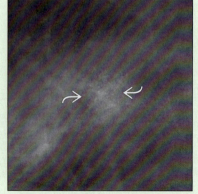

Amorphous, DCIS

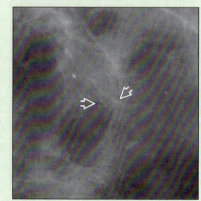

Punctate, FCC

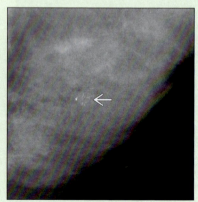

Pleomorphic, DCIS

MILK OF CALCIUM

Key Facts

Terminology
- Benign intracystic calcifications (Ca++)
- Sedimented Ca++

Imaging Findings
- Best diagnostic clue: Differing shapes of Ca++ between CC and MLO views, more conspicuous in MLO view
- Anatomy: Within dilated acini (microcysts) within terminal duct lobular unit (TDLU)
- Usually in central to posterior glandular cone
- Clusters of milk of calcium typically 10-20 mm diameter
- Rounded, fuzzy, amorphous on CC view
- "Teacups": Crescentic or linear on horizontal beam views

- Best imaging tool: Mammography with horizontal beam magnification views

Top Differential Diagnoses
- Ductal Carcinoma in Situ
- Atypical Ductal Hyperplasia (ADH)
- Lobular Neoplasia
- Fibrocystic Changes (FCC)

Pathology
- Calcium oxalate birefringent on polarized light microscopy

Diagnostic Checklist
- May coexist with malignant Ca++
- Manage based on most suspicious findings

- CC shows fuzzy, amorphous, rounded, calcific densities
  - Horizontal beam views show 1-3 mm crescentic (concave upwards) or linear densities
- Special views
  - Pendent or prone views sometimes required
  - Stereotactic prone positioning may reveal otherwise unrecognized particle layering; likely the affect of prone positioning over a longer period of time allowing Ca++ to settle within microcysts
- Unusual appearances
  - Layering within macrocysts
  - Unilateral clustered distribution
  - "Sand-like" appearance on CC

Ultrasonographic Findings
- Grayscale Ultrasound
  - Ca++ occasionally seen in clustered microcysts
  - Macrocysts may be present
    - Ca++ appear in curvilinear echogenic layer along dependent wall
    - Ca++ may float as punctate echoes in fluid

MR Findings
- MR not indicated for further evaluation of Ca++ per se

Biopsy
- Biopsy is not warranted unless there are associated suspicious forms
- If biopsy is inadvertently performed on Ca++ due to MOC, the Ca++ may not be visible on specimen radiography

Imaging Recommendations
- Best imaging tool: Mammography with horizontal beam magnification views
- Protocol advice: Perform appropriate horizontal beam films (LM, ML, prone)

DIFFERENTIAL DIAGNOSIS

Ductal Carcinoma in Situ
- Amorphous and punctate Ca++ due to MOC often coexist with typical MOC forms
- Amorphous Ca++ may be associated with low grade DCIS
  - Not gravitationally dependent
  - Grouped or clustered
  - More likely when Ca++ are new or increasing

Atypical Ductal Hyperplasia (ADH)
- Usually amorphous Ca++

Lobular Neoplasia
- Lobular carcinoma in situ (LCIS) usually adjacent to Ca++ which may appear amorphous
- Atypical lobular hyperplasia (ALH) also usually adjacent to Ca++

Fibrocystic Changes (FCC)
- Most common pathology found at biopsy for amorphous Ca++
- Ca++ typically in areas of usual duct hyperplasia, adenosis, or apocrine metaplasia
- Bland or apocrine metaplastic microcysts with MOC can be admixed with other FCC

Sclerosing Adenosis
- Ca++ often punctate
- May show associated mass

Fibroadenoma
- Early calcification forms may appear amorphous
- May show an associated mass

PATHOLOGY

General Features
- General path comments
  - Benign
  - Contained within dilated microcysts

MILK OF CALCIUM

Gross Pathologic & Surgical Features
- No specific features in microcystic milk of calcium
- Macrocyst(s) may be present

Microscopic Features
- Dilated acini (microcysts) with tiny calcium oxalate Ca++
- Ca++ may not be visible
  - May be lost in specimen preparation
  - Calcium oxalate birefringent on polarized light microscopy
- Rarely associated findings
  - Lipid cysts
  - Galactoceles
  - Adjacent malignancy (presumably incidental)

CLINICAL ISSUES

Presentation
- Most common signs/symptoms: Typically asymptomatic
- Other signs/symptoms
  - May present with lump or nipple discharge
    - Especially if macrocyst(s) present
    - Symptoms require further evaluation

Demographics
- Age: More common in peri- and postmenopausal women

Natural History & Prognosis
- Benign in isolation
- Rarely has adjacent malignancy; suspect if
  - Other more suspicious Ca++
  - Soft tissue masses

Treatment
- No specific treatment
- Reassurance and routine screening; BI-RADS 2, benign
- Short interval follow-up with BI-RADS 3, probably benign designation, may be appropriate if most of the Ca++ clearly layer and those few that do not appear punctate or amorphous
- Any suspicious calcification morphologies or worrisome associated mass(es) require biopsy for confirmation

DIAGNOSTIC CHECKLIST

Consider
- Carefully evaluate any Ca++ that do not layer
- May coexist with malignant Ca++
  - Manage based on most suspicious findings

Image Interpretation Pearls
- Rounded, fuzzy, hazy, amorphous on vertical beam (CC) films
- "Teacups" on horizontal beam (ML, LM) films
- Delaying the horizontal beam imaging for a few minutes may allow particles to settle for more confident assessment as MOC

SELECTED REFERENCES
1. D'Orsi CJ et al: Breast Imaging Reporting and Data System: BI-RADS, Mammography, 4th ed. Reston, American College of Radiology, 2003
2. Berg WA et al: Biopsy of amorphous breast calcifications; Pathologic outcome and yield at stereotactic biopsy. Radiology 221:495-501, 2001
3. Moy L et al: The pendent view: An additional projection to confirm the diagnosis of milk-of-calcium. AJR. 177:173-5, 2001
4. Ross BA et al: Milk of calcium in the breast: appearance on prone stereotactic imaging. Breast J. 7:53-5, 2001
5. Margolin FR et al: Microcystic calcifications at stereotactic breast biopsy. Breast J. 5:182-5, 1999
6. Liberman L et al: The breast imaging reporting and data system; positive predictive value of mammographic features and final assessment categories. AJR. 171:35-40, 1998
7. D'Orsi CJ et al: Mammographic feature analysis. Semin Roentgenol. 28(3):204-30, 1993
8. Truong LD et al: Calcium oxalate in breast lesions biopsied for calcification detected in screening mammography: incidence and clinical significance. Mod Pathol. 5:146-52, 1992
9. Tornos C et al: Calcium oxalate crystals in breast biopsies. The missing microcalcifications. Am J Surg Pathol. 14(10):961-8, 1990
10. Linden SS et al: Sedimented calcium in benign breast cysts: the full spectrum of mammographic presentations. AJR. 152:967-71, 1989

MILK OF CALCIUM

IMAGE GALLERY

Variant

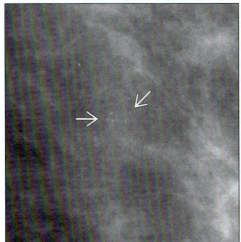

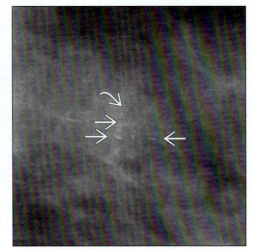

(Left) CC mammography magnification shows a cluster of subtle, amorphous, indistinct calcifications ➡. *(Right)* MLO mammography magnification (same case as left-hand image) shows layered calcifications ➡, compatible with milk of calcium. Few punctate Ca++ ➡ are likely benign.

Typical

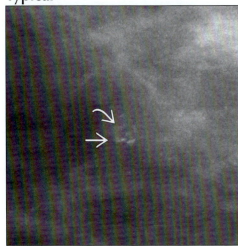

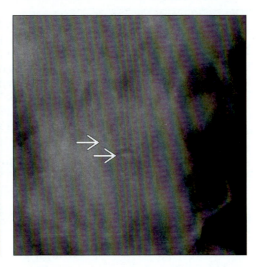

(Left) Lateral mammography magnification view of new Ca++ in 51 yo shows some layering ➡, though some Ca++ remain smudgy ➡ and indeterminate. Biopsy was recommended (right-hand image). *(Right)* Lateral spot mammogram obtained when positioning for planned stereotactic biopsy, after patient had lain prone for 5 minutes, shows definite layering of all Ca++ ➡, compatible with milk of calcium, a benign condition: Biopsy was canceled.

Variant

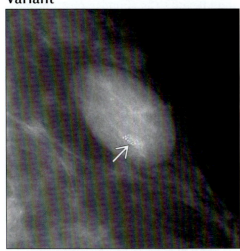

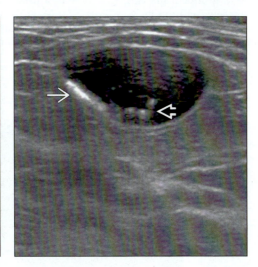

(Left) CC mammography shows smudgy amorphous and coarse calcifications ➡ within a circumscribed mass corresponding to a palpable abnormality. *(Right)* Radial ultrasound of the mass (same patient as on left-hand image) shows curvilinear Ca++ ➡ along the dependent wall of a large cyst as well as some floating mobile Ca++ ➡ due to milk of calcium.

ROUND CALCIFICATIONS

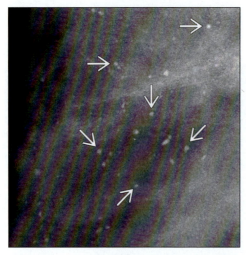

MLO mammography magnification shows scattered typical multiple sharply-defined rounded and ovoid Ca++ ➡, a benign finding, BI-RADS 2.

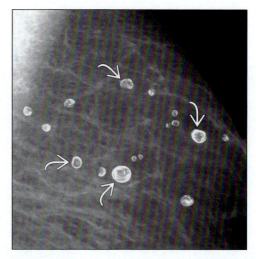

MLO mammography shows regional coarse round lucent-centered Ca++ ➡ in oil cysts.

TERMINOLOGY

Abbreviations and Synonyms
- Lobular or acinar calcifications (Ca++)

Definitions
- "Round": Smooth spherical or ovoid Ca++ ≥ 0.5 mm
  - When multiple, may vary in size
  - Can be considered benign when scattered
- "Punctate" refers to smaller, < 0.5 mm round smooth Ca++
  - Isolated cluster may warrant biopsy if new or with known ipsilateral cancer

IMAGING FINDINGS

General Features
- Best diagnostic clue: Scattered or grouped, smooth, ovoid, or spherical Ca++, easily seen without a magnifying lens
- Location: In glandular tissue, often acini; skin
- Size: 0.5-1 mm round Ca++ often formed in acini
- Morphology: Round or oval

Mammographic Findings
- Usually grouped, sometimes scattered
  - May be in multiple groups; may have slight shape heterogeneity
- When lucent-centered, may be in skin, oil cysts, or dystrophic
- May be intermixed with suspicious (pleomorphic, fine linear) Ca++
  - Biopsy associated suspicious forms

Ultrasonographic Findings
- Grayscale Ultrasound: Ca++ usually too small to detect unless within a mass

MR Findings
- Not indicated for characterization of Ca++

Imaging Recommendations
- Best imaging tool
  - Magnification ML and CC mammography if needed
  - Skin localization may be needed to prove dermal origin of clustered round Ca++

DDx: Other Round Microcalcifications

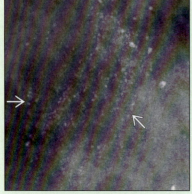

Columnar Cell Change

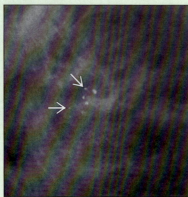

DCIS

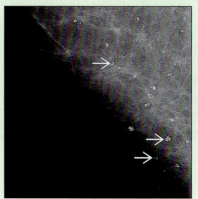

Dermal

ROUND CALCIFICATIONS

Key Facts

Terminology
- Lobular or acinar calcifications (Ca++)
- "Round": Smooth spherical or ovoid Ca++ ≥ 0.5 mm
- "Punctate" refers to smaller, < 0.5 mm round smooth Ca++

Imaging Findings
- Size: 0.5-1 mm round Ca++ often formed in acini
- Usually grouped, sometimes scattered

Top Differential Diagnoses
- Fibrocystic Change/Adenosis/Columnar Cell Change
- Skin Calcifications
- Ductal Carcinoma in Situ (DCIS)

Clinical Issues
- Typical appearance can be dismissed; BI-RADS 2, benign

DIFFERENTIAL DIAGNOSIS

Fibrocystic Change/Adenosis/Columnar Cell Change
- Round Ca++ often mixed with punctate and amorphous Ca++
- Usually scattered diffuse bilateral, clustered, or regional distribution
- May have associated mass or density

Skin Calcifications
- Classic polygonal shape with umbilicated centers
- Parasternal and axillary locations common
- Skin localization for less typical forms

Ductal Carcinoma in Situ (DCIS)
- Round Ca++ unusual; can be punctate Ca++ with some heterogeneity

Dystrophic, Oil Cysts
- Around lucent mass, > 1 mm

Skin Talc
- Usually typical distribution in skin pores
- Minimize through appropriate patient instruction

PATHOLOGY

General Features
- Epidemiology: Uncommon under 40

Microscopic Features
- Dilated lobular acini containing calcium oxalate

CLINICAL ISSUES

Presentation
- Most common signs/symptoms: Almost always screen-detected

Demographics
- Age: Usually perimenopausal and postmenopausal

Natural History & Prognosis
- No malignant potential if typical

Treatment
- Typical appearance can be dismissed; BI-RADS 2, benign

SELECTED REFERENCES

1. D'Orsi CJ et al: Breast Imaging Reporting and Data System: BI-RADS, Mammography, 4th ed. Reston, American College of Radiology, 2003
2. Frappart L et al: Different types of microcalcifications observed in breast pathology. Correlations with histopathological diagnosis and radiological examination of operative specimens. Virchows Arch A Pathol Anat Histopathol. 410:179-87, 1986
3. Sigfusson BF et al: Clustered breast calcifications. Acta Radiol Diagn (Stockh). 24:273-81, 1983

IMAGE GALLERY

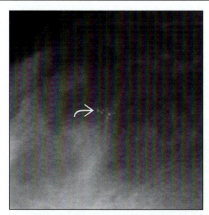 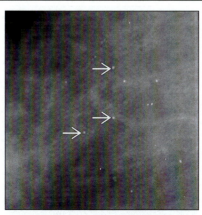 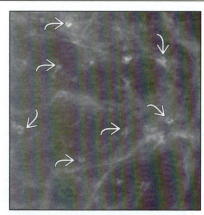

(Left) Lateral mammography magnification shows clustered round Ca++ which were proven to be within the skin ⇗. There is some heterogeneity of individual Ca++. *(Center)* MLO mammography shows scattered round calcifications ⇒. These had been stable for over four years, and are a benign finding, BI-RADS 2. *(Right)* CC mammography shows diffuse, scattered round, lobular Ca++ ⇒ that were present in both breasts, a benign finding.

SECRETORY CALCIFICATIONS

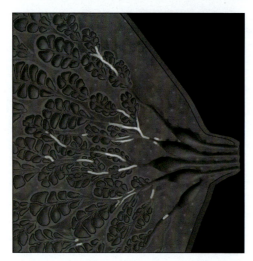

Graphic demonstrates typical secretory calcifications. Dense rod-like calcifications with some branching forms are seen in a ductal distribution directed toward the nipple.

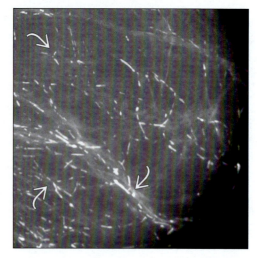

MLO mammography shows florid ductal secretory calcifications in the left breast. The branching pattern is particularly well seen ➔.

TERMINOLOGY

Abbreviations and Synonyms
- Plasma cell mastitis
- Mammary duct ectasia with secretory deposits

Definitions
- Benign calcifications (Ca++) in lumen or wall of dilated debris-filled ducts
- Large rod-like Ca++

IMAGING FINDINGS

General Features
- Best diagnostic clue: Dense, thick, continuous rod-like Ca++ in ductal pattern bilaterally
- Location: Radiating from nipple, ductal distribution
- Size: Typically ≥ 1 mm diameter, 3-10 mm long
- Morphology
  - Smooth, linear, rod-shaped or branching Ca++
  - May have lucent centers
  - Rounded or tubular forms, tapered ends, "cigar-shaped"

Mammographic Findings
- Radiate toward nipple, ductal pattern, branching
- Usually bilateral, may be extensive

Ultrasonographic Findings
- Grayscale Ultrasound: May see retroareolar hypo- to anechoic dilated ducts

MR Findings
- T1WI: Duct ectasia: Bright branching pattern pre-contrast if proteinaceous fluid

Imaging Recommendations
- Best imaging tool: Mammography; magnification CC and ML views to exclude more suspicious forms if atypical appearance

DIFFERENTIAL DIAGNOSIS

Ductal Carcinoma in Situ (DCIS)
- High grade DCIS with comedo necrosis
- Ca++ usually irregular, "casting" pattern
- Ductal pattern of small, fine linear, branching Ca++

DDx: Ductal Calcifications

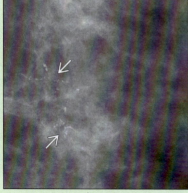

Branching DCIS

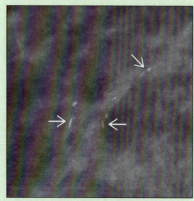

Fibroadenomatous

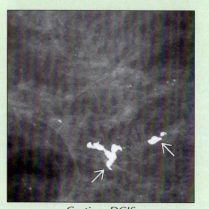

Casting, DCIS

SECRETORY CALCIFICATIONS

Key Facts

Terminology

- Benign calcifications (Ca++) in lumen or wall of dilated debris-filled ducts
- Large rod-like Ca++

Imaging Findings

- Best diagnostic clue: Dense, thick, continuous rod-like Ca++ in ductal pattern bilaterally
- Location: Radiating from nipple, ductal distribution
- Size: Typically ≥ 1 mm diameter, 3-10 mm long

Top Differential Diagnoses

- Ductal Carcinoma in Situ (DCIS)

Pathology

- Plasma cell mastitis: Usually premenopausal, prior pregnancy
- Mammary duct ectasia: Usually postmenopausal, unrelated to pregnancy

PATHOLOGY

General Features

- Etiology: Dystrophic or degenerative process
- Epidemiology
  - Plasma cell mastitis: Usually premenopausal, prior pregnancy
  - Mammary duct ectasia: Usually postmenopausal, unrelated to pregnancy
    - Atrophy, phenothiazines, hyperprolactinemia implicated

Gross Pathologic & Surgical Features

- Retroareolar dilated ducts
  - Contain thick, creamy, secretory material

Microscopic Features

- Type II Ca++ (calcium phosphate)
  - Nonbirefringent under polarized light
- Plasma cell mastitis
  - Ductal epithelial hyperplasia
  - Periductal intense plasma cell infiltrate
- Mammary duct ectasia
  - Moderate to marked retroareolar duct dilatation
  - Intraluminal debris
    - Amorphous or granular eosinophilic material
    - Lipid-containing foam cells ("colostrum cells") & desquamated epithelium
    - Cholesterol crystals and Ca++
  - Periductal lymphocytic inflammation

- Fibrosis and hyperelastosis cause duct wall thickening

CLINICAL ISSUES

Presentation

- Most common signs/symptoms
  - Most cases asymptomatic
  - Late nipple retraction not uncommon
  - May present with palpable thickening

Demographics

- Age: Uncommon < age 60

Treatment

- Benign finding, BI-RADS 2

SELECTED REFERENCES

1. D'Orsi CJ et al: Breast Imaging Reporting and Data System: BI-RADS, Mammography, 4th ed. Reston, American College of Radiology, 2003
2. Olson SL et al: Breast calcifications: analysis of imaging properties. Radiology. 169:329-32, 1988
3. Frappart L et al: Different types of microcalcifications observed in breast pathology. Correlations with histopathological diagnosis and radiological examination of operative specimens. Virchows Arch A Pathol Anat Histopathol. 410:179-87, 1986
4. Sickles EA: Breast calcifications: Mammographic evaluation. Radiology. 160:289-93, 1986

IMAGE GALLERY

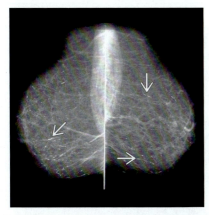 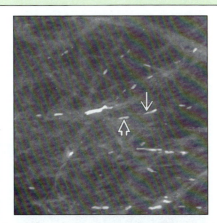 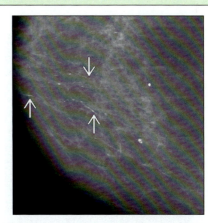

(Left) MLO mammography shows typical extensive bilateral secretory calcifications ➡. *(Center)* MLO mammography magnification shows the typical architecture of the rod-like calcifications. Some of the calcifications are tapered at the ends ➡; some are "cigar-shaped" ➡. *(Right)* CC mammography shows a single segment of smooth rod-like calcifications ➡. The distribution is of some concern, but the calcification morphology enables correct diagnosis.

VASCULAR CALCIFICATIONS

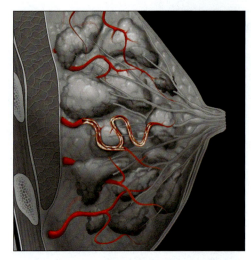

Graphic shows arteries depicted as serpiginous branching red structures, the central one of which has opposing walls partially calcified in a "tram track-like" fashion.

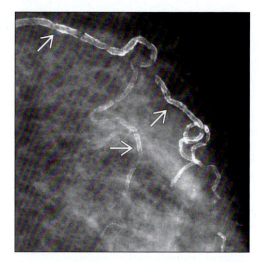

CC mammography shows typical serpiginous parallel-walled or "tram track" dense vascular wall calcifications ➡ in a left breast branching artery. Note peripheral location.

TERMINOLOGY

Abbreviations and Synonyms
- Breast arterial calcifications (BAC)

Definitions
- Calcification within the wall of breast arteries

IMAGING FINDINGS

General Features
- Best diagnostic clue
  - Serpiginous, linear and plaque-like calcifications (Ca++)
  - Parallel, "tram track" pattern along vessel wall
- Location
  - Anywhere in breast
  - Tend to be peripheral and superficial
- Size: Typically 1-3 mm diameter
- Morphology
  - Ca++ in parallel tracks
  - Tortuous or serpiginous configuration
  - Partly linear, partly plaque-like along vessel wall

- May have "dot dash", interrupted linear configuration
- May have "snake skin", patchy marbled mural plaque configuration

Mammographic Findings
- Typical calcifications easily recognized
- Atypical vascular Ca++ may mimic malignancy
  - May be limited to short segment
  - May be asymmetric along one wall, appearing linear, ductal
  - Rarely can appear clustered when early and in tortuous vessel

Ultrasonographic Findings
- Grayscale Ultrasound
  - Ca++ in wall of breast arteries not usually visible on US
  - Vessels seen as tubular anechoic structures, usually paired artery and vein
- Color Doppler: May show pulsatile flow on color or power Doppler

MR Findings
- Ca++ not visible

DDx: Linear Calcifications

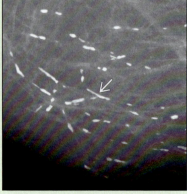

Secretory

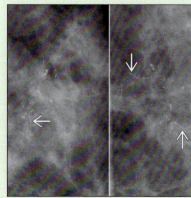

DCIS

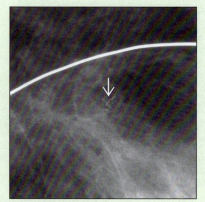

Fat Necrosis

VASCULAR CALCIFICATIONS

Key Facts

Terminology
- Breast arterial calcifications (BAC)
- Calcification within the wall of breast arteries

Imaging Findings
- Serpiginous, linear and plaque-like calcifications (Ca++)
- Parallel, "tram track" pattern along vessel wall
- Typical calcifications easily recognized
- Atypical vascular Ca++ may mimic malignancy
- Best imaging tool: Mammography

Top Differential Diagnoses
- Ductal Carcinoma in Situ (DCIS)
- Secretory Calcifications

Pathology
- General path comments: Calcifications in arterial media (medial sclerosis)
- Common in women with diabetes
- Common in women on dialysis
- 8-9% of all screening mammograms
- Increased frequency with increasing age

Clinical Issues
- Often considered clinically insignificant
- Large-scale study shows excess cardiovascular mortality if present
- No specific breast related treatment, a benign finding, BI-RADS 2
- Evaluation for other clinical factors may be useful, especially cardiovascular risk factors

- Enhancing vessels may be demonstrated on post-contrast scans
- Vessels bright on T2WI

Imaging Recommendations
- Best imaging tool: Mammography
- Protocol advice
  - Mammographic appearance usually typical
  - Magnification views sometimes helpful
  - Try to avoid during biopsy of adjacent suspicious lesions

DIFFERENTIAL DIAGNOSIS

Ductal Carcinoma in Situ (DCIS)
- Linear, often branching Ca++ in a ductal distribution
- Ducts typically arborize more than vessels
  - More branch points in ductal system
- May have irregular shape, casting configuration
- May show pleomorphic appearance
- Rarely serpiginous, never tortuous

Secretory Calcifications
- Smooth ≥ 1 mm rod-like branching Ca++
- Ca++ are either intraductal or within ductal walls
  - When within duct walls, may have lucent centers
- Typically bilateral and extensive
- Radiate toward the nipple

Fat Necrosis Calcifications
- Usually develop several years following trauma or surgery
- Most often curvilinear at edge of lucent mass/oil cyst
- Coarsen over time

Mondor Disease
- Self-limited superficial thrombophlebitis
  - Thoracoepigastric, lateral thoracic, or superior epigastric veins
- Located near the skin in the upper outer or inframammary breast and chest wall
- May calcify with a typical tram track appearance
- Often presents as a painful superficial mass or cord

- US may demonstrate noncompressible vein with clot
- Secondary to trauma, surgery, core biopsy procedures, injections; rarely due to underlying carcinoma (breast, lung)

Dermatomyositis
- A collagen-vascular disease
- Skin Ca++ may confound differentiation from vascular Ca++

Suture Calcifications
- At post-surgical site
- May see calcified knots
- Usually post radiation therapy

PATHOLOGY

General Features
- General path comments: Calcifications in arterial media (medial sclerosis)
- Etiology
  - Common in women with diabetes
    - 15% of diabetic women
  - Common in women on dialysis
    - Resolve or decrease after renal transplantation
  - Reduced in women who have taken hormone replacement therapy (HRT)
  - Significant (p < 0.05) relationship to various pathological clinical states
    - Relative risks (RR) defined compared to population without BAC
    - Albuminuria (RR 2.7)
    - Hypertension (RR 1.1)
    - Transient ischemic attack (TIA)/stroke (RR 1.4)
    - Thrombosis (RR 1.5)
    - Myocardial infarction (RR 1.8)
    - Diabetes for women 65 or older (RR 1.7)
  - Rarely with HIV (rare)
  - May rarely develop after neoadjuvant chemotherapy or pregnancy
- Epidemiology
  - 8-9% of all screening mammograms

VASCULAR CALCIFICATIONS

- ○ Increased frequency with increasing age
  - ▪ More common postmenopause
  - ▪ Uncommon under 50, even with diabetes

Gross Pathologic & Surgical Features
- No specific features

Microscopic Features
- Ca++ in media of small- to medium-sized arteries

CLINICAL ISSUES

Presentation
- Most common signs/symptoms: Asymptomatic, screen-detected

Demographics
- Age: Uncommon under age 50 years

Natural History & Prognosis
- Often considered clinically insignificant
- Reporting presence on mammogram is controversial
- Large-scale study shows excess cardiovascular mortality if present
  - ○ All women: 40% excess
    - ▪ Hazard ratio (HR) 1.4, $p < 0.05$
  - ○ Diabetic women: 90% excess
    - ▪ HR 1.9, $p < 0.05$
- Mammographically-detected vascular Ca++ correlated with coronary angiograms (recent study)
  - ○ Number of calcified vascular distributions within each breast rated as 0-3 and divided by number of breasts
  - ○ BAC score of ≥ 1.5 = odds ratio (OR) 1.9 for coronary artery disease (CAD) (> 50% stenosis)
  - ○ BAC > 2.5 did not confer any higher risk for CAD
  - ○ BAC reported as a risk factor for CAD independent of age
    - ▪ Recommendation: Radiologists should report presence of BAC
    - ▪ CAD risk factor screening and lifestyle modifications recommended for "any patient with BAC"

Treatment
- No specific breast related treatment, a benign finding, BI-RADS 2
- Evaluation for other clinical factors may be useful, especially cardiovascular risk factors
  - ○ Diabetes
  - ○ Renal function and albuminuria
  - ○ Hypertension
  - ○ Previous history of cardiovascular disease
  - ○ Family history of cardiovascular disease

DIAGNOSTIC CHECKLIST

Consider
- Recommend reporting of BAC when present
- Describe as "extensive" if at least 3 vascular distributions involved
- Suggest correlation with cardiac risk factor history if appropriate

Image Interpretation Pearls
- May cause large hematoma if unrecognized at time of biopsy
- Direct needle biopsy procedures away from obvious BAC if possible to avoid excessive bleeding

SELECTED REFERENCES

1. Bauerfeind I et al: Mondor's disease after bilateral axillary node biopsy. Arch Gynecol Obstet. 23:1-4, 2005
2. Doerger KM et al: Breast arterial calcification detected on mammography is a risk factor for coronary artery disease. Radiology. 225:553, 2005
3. Kim SM et al: Dystrophic breast calcifications in patients with collagen disease. Clin Imaging. 28:6-9, 2004
4. Pappo I et al: Mondor's disease of the axilla: a rare complication of sentinel node biopsy. Breast J. 10:253-5, 2004
5. Harris AT: Mondor's disease of the breast can also occur after a sonography-guided core biopsy. AJR. 180:284-5, 2003
6. Cox J et al: An interesting byproduct of screening: Assessing the effect of HRT on arterial calcification in the female breast. J Med Screen. 9:38-9, 2002
7. Jaberi M et al: Stereotactic vacuum-assisted breast biopsy: an unusual cause of Mondor's disease. AJR. 179:185-6, 2002
8. Shetty MK et al: Mondor's disease of the breast; sonographic and mammographic findings. AJR. 177:893-6, 2001
9. Feder JM et al: "Unusual breast lesions" radiologic-pathologic correlation. RadioGraphics. 19:511-26, 1999
10. Kemmeren JM et al: Breast arterial calcifications: Association with diabetes mellitus and cardiovascular mortality. Work in progress. Radiology. 201:75-8, 1996
11. van Noord PA et al: Mammograms may convey more than breast cancer risk: Breast arterial calcification and arteriosclerotic related diseases in women of the DOM cohort. Eur J Cancer Prev. 5:483-7, 1996
12. Evans AJ et al: Patterns of breast calcification in patients on renal dialysis. Clin Radiol. 45:343-4, 1992

VASCULAR CALCIFICATIONS

IMAGE GALLERY

Typical

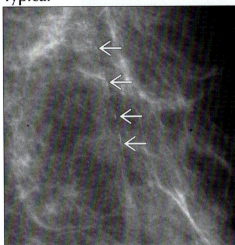 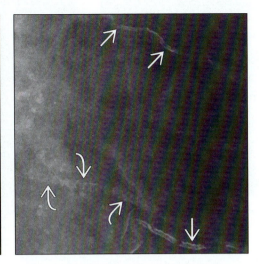

(Left) MLO mammography magnification shows linear "dot-dash" calcifications along one wall of an artery ➡. This is an early and more subtle manifestation of vascular calcification. *(Right)* MLO mammography magnification shows typical parallel "tram track" calcifications ➡. A larger vessel shows marbled, patchy calcifications, sometimes described as "snake skin" ➡.

Typical

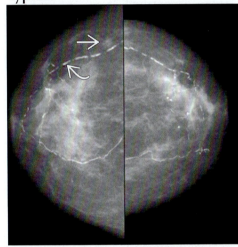 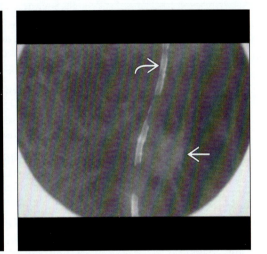

(Left) CC mammography shows a small spiculated mass ➡ adjacent to a calcified artery ➡. Core biopsy encountered marked bleeding; pathology showed both tumor and part of a calcified artery. *(Right)* Spot magnification view shows (same case as left-hand image) the spiculated mass ➡ immediately adjacent to the calcified artery ➡. Pathology showed grade I infiltrating ductal carcinoma and a piece of an arterial wall.

Variant

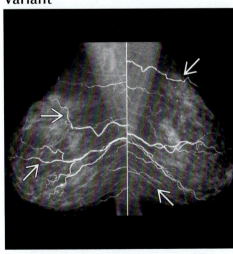 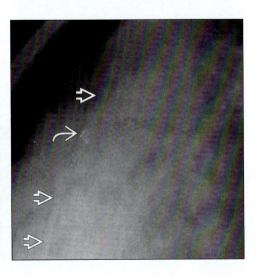

(Left) MLO mammography shows extensive vascular calcifications ➡ in a premenopausal woman, likely on the basis of HIV. *(Right)* Lateral mammography magnification view in a 53 year old shows short segment of vascular Ca++ ➡ superimposing on a mostly uncalcified vessel ➡. These could be mistaken for clustered Ca++.

COARSE HETEROGENEOUS CALCIFICATIONS

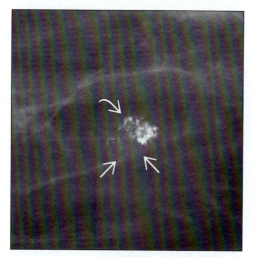

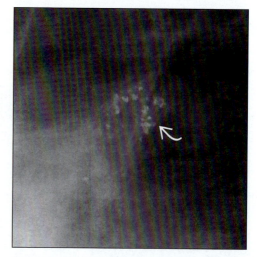

Lateral mammography magnification shows coarse heterogeneous calcifications ➡ in a low density mass ➡. Biopsy showed fibroadenoma.

Lateral mammography magnification shows coarse heterogeneous calcifications ➡ within a sclerosed fibroadenoma.

TERMINOLOGY

Abbreviations and Synonyms
- "Coral" type calcifications (Ca++)

Definitions
- Irregular, conspicuous Ca++, > 0.5 mm, tend to coalesce

IMAGING FINDINGS

General Features
- Best diagnostic clue: Clustered coarse irregular and coalescing Ca++ on mammography
- Location: Usually in stroma
- Size: > 0.5 mm
- Morphology: Variable in size and shape

Mammographic Findings
- Isolated cluster is of intermediate concern
- Multiple, bilateral similar groupings benign or probably benign
- May have associated mass or focal asymmetry
  - Can be early fibroadenomatoid Ca++
  - Multiple bilateral circumscribed masses favors fibroadenomas
  - Associated indistinctly marginated or spiculated mass should prompt biopsy

Ultrasonographic Findings
- Grayscale Ultrasound
  - Can be seen, especially when in mass
  - US not useful in characterization

MR Findings
- No role in further characterization
- When larger and coalescent, may see magnetization transfer artifact (signal void)

Imaging Recommendations
- Best imaging tool: Mammography
- Protocol advice: Magnification CC and ML views can help exclude more suspicious forms

DDx: Possible Etiologies

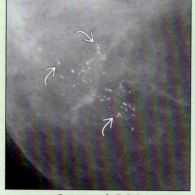

Segmental, DCIS

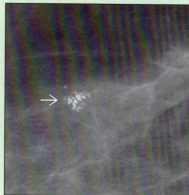

Stromal Fibrosis

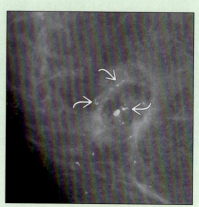

Fat Necrosis

COARSE HETEROGENEOUS CALCIFICATIONS

Key Facts

Terminology
- Irregular, conspicuous Ca++, > 0.5 mm, tend to coalesce

Imaging Findings
- Isolated cluster is of intermediate concern
- Multiple, bilateral similar groupings benign or probably benign
- Protocol advice: Magnification CC and ML views can help exclude more suspicious forms

Top Differential Diagnoses
- Fibroadenoma
- Stromal Fibrosis
- Fat Necrosis, Dystrophic
- Linear or segmental distribution suspicious for DCIS
- Invasive Ductal Carcinoma

Pathology
- Etiology: 7% rate of malignancy among Ca++ going to biopsy

DIFFERENTIAL DIAGNOSIS

Fibroadenoma
- May or may not show associated mass

Fibroadenomatoid Change
- May show associated asymmetry, less discrete than fibroadenoma

Stromal Fibrosis
- Often multiple, bilateral groupings

Fat Necrosis, Dystrophic
- Ca++ usually peripheral; central lucent mass
- History of trauma or surgery
- May have associated density, distortion

Ductal Carcinoma in Situ (DCIS)
- Linear or segmental distribution suspicious for DCIS

Invasive Ductal Carcinoma
- Associated spiculated or indistinct mass

PATHOLOGY

General Features
- Etiology: 7% rate of malignancy among Ca++ going to biopsy

Microscopic Features
- Can be in stroma or ducts

CLINICAL ISSUES

Presentation
- Most common signs/symptoms: Incidental finding on mammography

Treatment
- Biopsy usually warranted if solitary cluster on baseline mammogram
- Biopsy warranted if linear or segmental distribution, associated suspicious mass or Ca++
- Coarsening of individual Ca++ on follow-up, without increase in number, favors benign etiology

DIAGNOSTIC CHECKLIST

Image Interpretation Pearls
- Magnification views help exclude more suspicious forms

SELECTED REFERENCES

1. Burnside ES et al: The ability of microcalcification descriptors in the BI-RADS 4th edition to stratify the risk of malignancy. Radiologic Society of North America (abstr) p. 286, 2005
2. D'Orsi CJ et al: Breast Imaging Reporting and Data System: BI-RADS, Mammography, 4th ed. Reston, American College of Radiology, 2003

IMAGE GALLERY

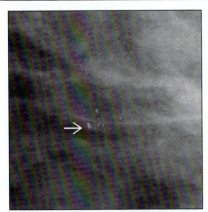 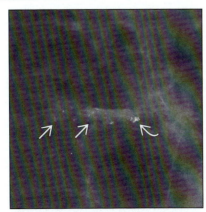 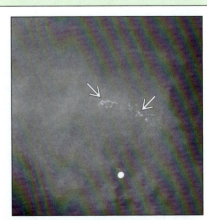

(Left) CC mammography magnification view shows cluster of coarse, heterogeneous calcifications ➡. Because they were new, they were biopsied, showing intermediate grade DCIS. *(Center)* CC mammography magnification shows coalescing amorphous ➡ and coarse heterogeneous calcifications ➡ with associated focal density. Biopsy showed hyalinized fibroadenoma. *(Right)* CC mammography magnification shows coarse heterogeneous calcifications ➡ in a linear distribution with associated mass/density. Biopsy showed invasive ductal cancer.

PUNCTATE CALCIFICATIONS

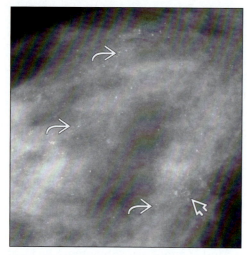

CC mammography magnification shows diffuse scattered punctate calcifications ➡. When present bilaterally, these are typically benign. Occasional clustering can be seen ➡.

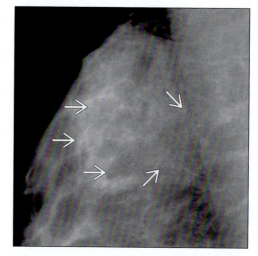

MLO mammography shows regional scattered punctate calcifications ➡ which had been stable for four years, compatible with benign etiology.

TERMINOLOGY

Definitions
- Round calcifications (Ca++) < 0.5 mm in size
- Term "round" Ca++ reserved for those 0.5 mm or larger in size

IMAGING FINDINGS

General Features
- Best diagnostic clue: Distribution is key factor in management
- Location: Acini of terminal duct lobular unit
- Size: < 0.5 mm
- Morphology: Uniformly round

Mammographic Findings
- Diffuse bilateral scattered are typically benign
  - Can see occasional clustering (5 or more in < 1 cc volume)
  - Can be admixed with round, amorphous or coarse heterogeneous Ca++
  - Magnification views not usually necessary
- Cluster (5 or more within < 1 cc volume)
  - Isolated cluster on baseline mammogram probably benign
  - New cluster often merits biopsy
  - Cluster may warrant biopsy if ipsilateral to cancer
  - Magnification CC and ML views recommended to exclude more worrisome morphology (e.g., pleomorphic)
  - Most often due to fibrocystic changes (FCC)
  - Can be milk-of-calcium; will layer on ML magnification view
- Multiple bilateral clusters
  - Usually due to FCC
  - Probably benign (BI-RADS 3) or benign (BI-RADS 2)
    - Further validation of outcomes is needed
- Regional (> 2 cc volume) usually benign
  - Magnification views recommended to exclude more worrisome forms
  - Can be atypical ductal hyperplasia (ADH)
  - Most often FCC, can be milk-of-calcium
- Linear distribution suspicious, merits biopsy
  - Magnification CC and ML views recommended
  - Often due to ductal carcinoma in situ (DCIS)

DDx: Other Calcifications

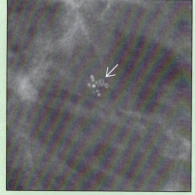

Round, Dermal

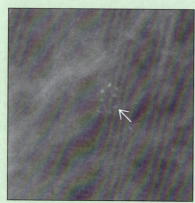

New, Pleomorphic, DCIS

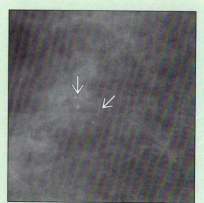

Linear, DCIS

PUNCTATE CALCIFICATIONS

Key Facts

Terminology
- Round calcifications (Ca++) < 0.5 mm in size

Imaging Findings
- Best diagnostic clue: Distribution is key factor in management
- Diffuse bilateral scattered are typically benign
- Isolated cluster on baseline mammogram probably benign
- Regional (> 2 cc volume) usually benign
- Linear distribution suspicious, merits biopsy
- Segmental distribution (duct and its branches) highly suggestive of malignancy, merits biopsy

Top Differential Diagnoses
- Fibrocystic Changes (FCC)
- Adenosis or sclerosing adenosis

- Columnar Cell Lesions
- Atypical Ductal Hyperplasia (ADH)
- Can rarely be within ALH or LCIS
- Ductal Carcinoma in Situ (DCIS)

Pathology
- Usually due to calcium phosphate
- Polarized light microscopy may be needed to identify when due to calcium oxalate

Diagnostic Checklist
- Management must be based on most worrisome morphology present
- Biopsy usually indicated if cluster is new or ipsilateral to cancer
- Magnification CC and ML views help exclude milk-of-calcium or more worrisome morphology

- Segmental distribution (duct and its branches) highly suggestive of malignancy, merits biopsy
  - Magnification CC and ML views recommended
  - Usually due to DCIS

Ultrasonographic Findings
- Grayscale Ultrasound
  - Punctate Ca++ not usually visible on US
    - May be visible on US when within a mass or cyst
    - Occasionally scattered echogenic foci in parenchyma

MR Findings
- T1WI: Not visible
- T2WI FS: When due to FCC, may see cysts
- T1 C+ FS
  - Findings will depend on etiology
    - DCIS may show slow, persistent, clumped, linear or segmental enhancement
    - FCC usually shows scattered foci of enhancement
- No role for MR in evaluation of Ca++ in lieu of biopsy

Nuclear Medicine Findings
- PET: No role for PET in evaluation of Ca++ in lieu of biopsy

Biopsy
- Stereotactic biopsy
  - Complete evaluation with CC and ML magnification views comparison to prior films may preclude need for biopsy (e.g., milk-of-calcium)
  - When biopsy, vacuum-assisted biopsy with at least 11-g system, retrieval of at least 10 specimens recommended
    - Ca++ can be adjacent to malignancy, ADH, or lobular neoplasia or within these entities, or both: Retrieval of greater amounts of material helps assure diagnostic sampling
    - Specimen radiograph required to assure retrieval of Ca++
    - Place specimens containing Ca++ in separate cassette or otherwise identify them for pathologist
    - Clip placement advocated to identify biopsy site

DIFFERENTIAL DIAGNOSIS

Fibrocystic Changes (FCC)
- Usually isolated cluster or diffuse bilateral
  - May be admixed with amorphous or coarse heterogeneous Ca++ or both
- Adenosis or sclerosing adenosis
  - Most common type of FCC to have punctate Ca++
  - May have associated oval or lobulated mass
- Apocrine metaplasia
  - May have associated microlobulated, low density mass on mammography
  - Often evident as clustered microcysts on US
- Milk-of-calcium (will layer on true lateral view)
  - May be admixed with other FCC or even malignancy
- Associated cysts on US
- Can be in areas of fibrosis (more often coarse heterogeneous Ca++)
- May see scattered echogenic foci in parenchyma on US

Columnar Cell Lesions
- Found in > 40% of biopsies for Ca++
- Of no known significance unless atypical

Dermal Calcifications
- Usually larger, round
- Often have lucent centers
- Tattoos can develop Ca++
- Skin localization with tangential magnification view can prove

Papilloma
- Usually within a small (< 5 mm) round or oval mass
- More often amorphous Ca++
- Often intraductal mass on US

Fibroadenoma (FA)
- Usually within a mass
- More often coarse, heterogeneous, or popcorn Ca++

PUNCTATE CALCIFICATIONS

Radial Scar

- Usually architectural distortion evident on mammography or US
- Ca++ usually in areas of associated epithelial proliferation such as adenosis
- When incidental adjacent to stereotactically-biopsied Ca++, may not require excision

Artifact

- Processor pick-off can mimic punctate Ca++
  - Repeat exposure if needed
- Talc or even deodorant on skin can mimic
  - Attentive technologist can preclude work-up

Atypical Ductal Hyperplasia (ADH)

- Isolated cluster or regional distribution, can be linear
- Often admixed with amorphous Ca++

Lobular Neoplasia

- More often associated with amorphous Ca++
- Ca++ usually adjacent to atypical lobular hyperplasia (ALH) or lobular carcinoma in situ (LCIS)
- Can rarely be within ALH or LCIS
- LCIS may be evident as a mass on US or MR

Ductal Carcinoma in Situ (DCIS)

- Suspect when calcifications in linear or segmental distribution
- Can be isolated cluster
- Most commonly cribriform or micropapillary subtypes
- Magnification views critical to assess extent
- Ca++ may be adjacent to DCIS

Following Intra-operative Radiotherapy (IORT)

- Single fraction ≈ 21 Gy delivered in operating room to lumpectomy site during cancer surgery
- Tend to develop punctate Ca++ within the treated area soon (< 6 months) after IORT
- Fat necrosis common: Lucent-centered mass
  - Over time usually develops curvilinear Ca++
  - Early on, some of the Ca++ may appear punctate

PATHOLOGY

General Features

- Etiology
  - Usually due to calcium phosphate
  - Can be due to calcium oxalate
  - Polarized light microscopy may be needed to identify when due to calcium oxalate
  - Uncommonly biopsied
    - In one series, of 320 Ca++ lesions biopsied, 11 (3.4%) showed punctate morphology
    - 1/11 (9%) proved malignant

CLINICAL ISSUES

Presentation

- Most common signs/symptoms: Incidental finding on mammography

DIAGNOSTIC CHECKLIST

Consider

- Uncommon to see only pure punctate Ca++, usually some other forms present
- Management must be based on most worrisome morphology present
- Comparison to prior mammograms can be helpful
- Biopsy usually indicated if cluster is new or ipsilateral to cancer

Image Interpretation Pearls

- Magnification CC and ML views help exclude milk-of-calcium or more worrisome morphology
- Distribution critical to management

SELECTED REFERENCES

1. D'Orsi CJ et al: Breast Imaging Reporting and Data System: BI-RADS, Mammography. 4th ed. Reston, American College of Radiology, 2003
2. Lawenda BD et al: Dose-volume analysis of radiotherapy for T1N0 invasive breast cancer treated by local excision and partial breast irradiation by low-dose-rate interstitial implant. Int J Radiat Oncol Biol Phys. 56:671-80, 2003
3. Schnitt SJ et al: Columnar cell lesions of the breast. Adv Anat Pathol. 10:113-24, 2003
4. Brenner RJ et al: Percutaneous core needle biopsy of radial scars of the breast: When is excision necessary? AJR. 179:1179-84, 2002
5. Jackman RJ et al: Stereotactic biopsy of nonpalpable lesions: determinants of ductal carcinoma in situ underestimation rates. Radiology. 218:497-502, 2001
6. Berg WA et al: Breast Imaging Reporting and Data System: inter- and intraobserver variability in feature analysis and final assessment. AJR. 174:1769-77, 2000
7. Liberman L et al: The breast imaging reporting and data system: positive predictive value of mammographic features and final assessment categories. AJR. 171:35-40, 1998
8. Selim A et al: Microscopic localization of calcifications in and around breast carcinoma: a cautionary note for needle core biopsies. Ann Surg. 228:95-8, 1998
9. Jackman RJ et al: Atypical ductal hyperplasia diagnosed at stereotactic breast biopsy: improved reliability with 14-gauge, directional, vacuum-assisted biopsy. Radiology. 204:485-8, 1997
10. Roubidoux MA et al: Women with breast cancer: Histologic findings in the contralateral breast. Radiology. 203:691-94, 1997
11. Baker JA et al: Breast imaging reporting and data system standardized mammography lexicon: observer variability in lesion description. AJR. 166:773-8, 1996
12. D'Orsi CJ et al: Mammographic feature analysis. Seminars Roentgenol. 28:204-30, 1993
13. Homer MJ et al: The relationship of mammographic microcalcification to malignancy: Radiologic-pathologic correlation. AJR. 153:1187-89, 1989
14. Berkowitz JE et al: Dermal breast calcifications: Localization with template-guided placement of skin marker. Radiology. 163:282, 1987
15. Sickles E: Breast calcifications: Mammographic evaluation. Radiology. 160:289-93, 1986
16. Colbassani Jr HJ et al: Mammographic and pathologic correlation of microcalcification in disease of the breast. Surg Gyn Obst. 155:689-96, 1982

PUNCTATE CALCIFICATIONS

IMAGE GALLERY

Typical

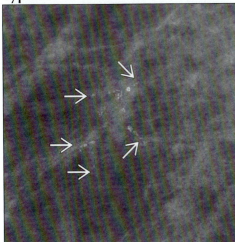

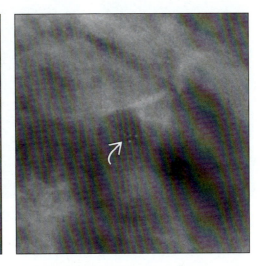

(Left) CC mammography magnification shows individually punctate calcifications ➡ in a linear, branching distribution suggesting filling of ducts, highly suggestive of malignancy, BI-RADS 5. Biopsy showed DCIS. *(Right)* CC mammography magnification shows punctate calcifications ➡ in a linear or "Y-shaped" distribution, moderately suspicious for malignancy, BI-RADS 4C. Stereotactic biopsy showed DCIS.

Variant

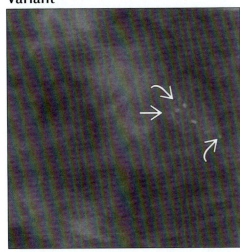

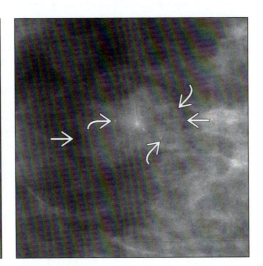

(Left) CC mammography magnification shows punctate calcifications ➡ inside of a low density mass ➡. Because this was a new finding, it was biopsied, showing calcifying fibroadenoma. *(Right)* CC mammography shows oval mass ➡ containing punctate ➡ and amorphous calcifications. Biopsy showed sclerosing adenosis.

Typical

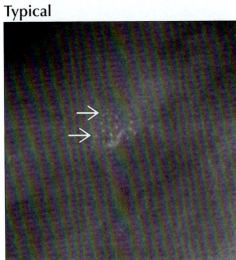

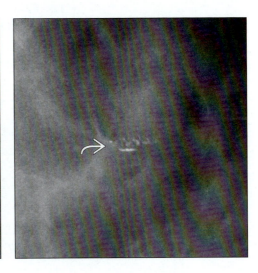

(Left) MLO mammography close-up shows cluster of microcalcifications individually punctate in morphology ➡. True lateral magnification view was performed (right-hand image). *(Right)* Lateral mammography magnification shows layering of calcifications ➡, compatible with milk-of-calcium, a benign condition.

AMORPHOUS CALCIFICATIONS

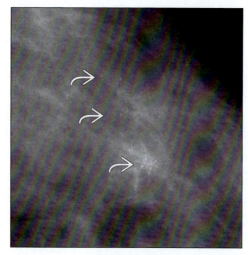

Lateral mammography magnification view shows clustered amorphous microcalcifications ➔ which proved to be due to ADH.

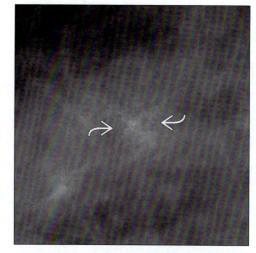

Lateral mammography magnification view shows clustered amorphous calcifications ➔ which showed low grade DCIS at excision.

TERMINOLOGY

Abbreviations and Synonyms
- Indistinct calcifications (Ca++)

Definitions
- Indistinct calcifications sufficiently small that a more specific morphologic classification cannot be assigned

IMAGING FINDINGS

General Features
- Best diagnostic clue: Tiny, fuzzy, hazy, indistinct Ca++ on mammography
- Location: Terminal duct lobular unit, can be within microcysts
- Size: < 0.1 mm

Mammographic Findings
- Magnification CC and 90° lateral views required for characterization
  - Layering in 90° lateral view diagnostic of milk-of-calcium, a benign condition
  - May see associated cyst(s) or clustered microcysts
  - Can have mixture of fibrocystic changes, milk-of-calcium, and malignancy
- Distribution guides management
  - Diffuse, bilateral, scattered punctate and amorphous Ca++ benign
  - Clustered, regional suspicious, BI-RADS 4B
  - Linear or segmental distribution moderately suspicious, BI-RADS 4C
- May be stable over multiple years and still be malignant or high risk lesion
- May be associated with other more suspicious forms or suspicious mass

Ultrasonographic Findings
- Grayscale Ultrasound: Not identified on US except when coalescent, usually in an associated mass

MR Findings
- MR not indicated in further evaluation unless known to be malignant

Biopsy
- Stereotactic biopsy

DDx: Associated Calcifications

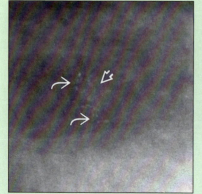

Pleomorphic, DCIS

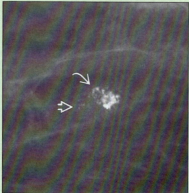

Coarse Heterogeneous, FA

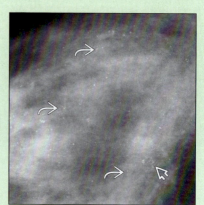

Diffuse Punctate, Benign

AMORPHOUS CALCIFICATIONS

Key Facts

Terminology
- Indistinct calcifications sufficiently small that a more specific morphologic classification cannot be assigned

Imaging Findings
- Best diagnostic clue: Tiny, fuzzy, hazy, indistinct Ca++ on mammography
- Diffuse, bilateral, scattered punctate and amorphous Ca++ benign
- Clustered, regional suspicious, BI-RADS 4B
- Linear or segmental distribution moderately suspicious, BI-RADS 4C
- May be stable over multiple years and still be malignant or high risk lesion
- MR not indicated in further evaluation unless known to be malignant
- Grayscale Ultrasound: Not identified on US except when coalescent, usually in an associated mass
- CC and 90° lateral magnification views required
- Milk-of-calcium will layer on 90° lateral view, benign

Top Differential Diagnoses
- Fibrocystic Change (FCC): 60%
- Milk-of-calcium definitively benign
- 20% of amorphous Ca++ yield ADH, atypical lobular hyperplasia (ALH), or lobular carcinoma in situ (LCIS)

Pathology
- 20% malignant
- 90% of malignancies DCIS, usually low grade
- 10% of malignancies are IDC, usually associated mass
- Polarized light microscopy improves visualization of calcium oxalate

- In prone position, Ca++ due to milk-of-calcium can be shown to layer, biopsy not needed
- Targeting successful in over 90% of cases
- Specimen radiography required to assure Ca++ retrieval
- Needle localization and excision
  - Required for result of high risk lesion or malignancy at stereotactic biopsy even if no residual Ca++
  - Specimen radiography required to assure Ca++ retrieval
  - Post-operative mammogram to assure complete removal if malignant
- Fine needle aspiration not appropriate
  - High rate of insufficient samples

Imaging Recommendations
- Best imaging tool: Mammographic magnification views
- Protocol advice
  - CC and 90° lateral magnification views required
  - Milk-of-calcium will layer on 90° lateral view, benign
    - Delayed 90° lateral (2-5 minutes) can help with subtle particulate
    - Some will only be shown to layer in prone position (e.g., on stereotactic table)
    - Manage based on most suspicious Ca++: I.e. those that do not layer

DIFFERENTIAL DIAGNOSIS

Fibrocystic Change (FCC): 60%
- Most common result at biopsy of amorphous Ca++
- Milk-of-calcium definitively benign
- Typically in areas of usual duct hyperplasia, adenosis, or apocrine metaplasia

Atypical Ductal Hyperplasia (ADH)
- Most common appearance for ADH
- Requires excision: 18% malignant at excision after ≥ 10 samples, 11-g

- 20% of amorphous Ca++ yield ADH, atypical lobular hyperplasia (ALH), or lobular carcinoma in situ (LCIS)

Lobular Neoplasia
- LCIS usually adjacent to Ca++
- ALH usually adjacent to Ca++, may also contain them

Ductal Carcinoma in Situ (DCIS)
- Usually low grade
- More likely when Ca++ are new or increasing or in linear or segmental distribution

Invasive Ductal Carcinoma
- Usually has associated mass
- Usually low grade NOS or tubular
- Usually associated DCIS

Sclerosing Adenosis
- More often punctate morphology
- May show associated mass

Papilloma
- Will usually show an associated mass

Fibroadenoma (FA)
- Early Ca++ in FA can appear amorphous
- Often associated with coarse, heterogeneous Ca++
- May show an associated mass, usually oval or gently lobulated

Amorphous Ca++ in a Lymph Node
- Gold injections with trapped gold mimicking Ca++
- Metastatic ovarian carcinoma
- Metastatic breast carcinoma

PATHOLOGY

General Features
- Etiology
  - 60% benign, usually FCC
    - Associated mass suggests papilloma, FA, or sclerosing adenosis
  - 20% malignant

AMORPHOUS CALCIFICATIONS

- 90% of malignancies DCIS, usually low grade
- 10% of malignancies are IDC, usually associated mass
  - 20% high risk lesions (ADH, ALH, LCIS)
    - Ca++ usually within ADH
    - Ca++ usually adjacent to ALH or LCIS

Microscopic Features

- Ca++ may be in ducts or microcysts
- Often calcium oxalate crystals in benign disease
  - Usually found in microcysts, milk-of-calcium
  - Colorless, birefringent, difficult to see on routine H&E microscopy
  - Polarized light microscopy improves visualization of calcium oxalate
- Often calcium phosphate crystals in malignancies
  - High density, dark blue on routine H&E staining
- Can be in both benign and malignant areas interspersed: 35% of malignancies
- Can be only adjacent to malignancy: 16% of malignancies

CLINICAL ISSUES

Presentation

- Most common signs/symptoms
  - Seen only on mammography
  - Rarely associated with a palpable mass

Treatment

- Almost certainly benign when diffuse and bilateral
- Multiple, bilateral clustered amorphous Ca++ probably benign
  - Consider biopsy of dominant, most numerous grouping
- Management of multiple, unilateral clustered amorphous Ca++ can be problematic
  - Biopsy of most dominant or suspicious cluster recommended
  - Manage other similar groupings based on those results
- Biopsy if clustered and not milk-of-calcium
- Biopsy if regional, linear, or segmental distribution

DIAGNOSTIC CHECKLIST

Consider

- Stability, even for 4 years, does not assure benign etiology
- Reduced sensitivity for computer-aided detection (CAD) of amorphous Ca++
  - CAD detects 86-99% of all malignant Ca++
  - CAD case sensitivity of 57% for malignant amorphous Ca++ and 29% for high-risk lesions manifest as amorphous Ca++

Image Interpretation Pearls

- Biopsy nearly always indicated unless diffuse bilateral or multiple bilateral clusters or clearly milk-of-calcium

SELECTED REFERENCES

1. Soo MS et al: Computer-aided detection of amorphous calcifications. AJR. 184:887-92, 2005
2. D'Orsi CJ et al: Breast Imaging Reporting and Data System: BI-RADS, Mammography, 4th ed. Reston, American College of Radiology, 2003
3. Jackman RJ et al: Atypical ductal hyperplasia: can some lesions be defined as probably benign after stereotactic 11-gauge vacuum-assisted biopsy, eliminating the recommendation for surgical excision? Radiology. 224:548-54, 2002
4. Berg WA et al: Atypical lobular hyperplasia or lobular carcinoma in situ at core-needle breast biopsy. Radiology. 218:503-09, 2001
5. Berg WA et al: Biopsy of amorphous breast calcifications: pathologic outcome and yield at stereotactic biopsy. Radiology. 221:495-503, 2001
6. Jackman RJ et al: Stereotactic breast biopsy of nonpalpable lesions: determinants of ductal carcinoma in situ underestimation Rates. Radiology. 218:497-502, 2001
7. Darling ML et al: Atypical ductal hyperplasia and ductal carcinoma in situ as revealed by large-core needle breast biopsy: results of surgical excision. AJR. 175:1341-6, 2000
8. Brem RF et al: Atypical ductal hyperplasia: histologic underestimation of carcinoma in tissue harvested from impalpable breast lesions using 11-gauge stereotactically guided directional vacuum-assisted biopsy. AJR. 172:1405-7, 1999
9. Liberman L et al: The breast imaging reporting and data system; positive predictive value of mammographic features and final assessment categories. AJR. 171:35-40, 1998
10. Pisano ED et al: Rate of insufficient samples for fine-needle aspiration for nonpalpable breast lesions in a multicenter clinical trial: The Radiologic Diagnostic Oncology Group 5 Study. The RDOG5 investigators. Cancer. 82:679-88, 1998
11. Selim A et al: Microscopic localization of calcifications in and around breast carcinoma: a cautionary note for needle core biopsies. Ann Surg. 228:95-8, 1998
12. Burbank F: Stereotactic breast biopsy of atypical ductal hyperplasia and ductal carcinoma in situ lesions: improved accuracy with directional, vacuum-assisted biopsy. Radiology. 202:843-47, 1997
13. Jackman RJ et al: Atypical ductal hyperplasia diagnosed at stereotactic breast biopsy: improved reliability with 14g directional vacuum-assisted biopsy. Radiology. 204:485-88, 1997
14. Berg WA: When is core breast biopsy or fine-needle aspiration not enough? Radiology. 198:313-15, 1996
15. Lev-Toaff AS et al: Stability of malignant breast microcalcifications. Radiology. 192:153-6, 1994
16. D'Orsi CJ et al: Mammographic feature analysis. Semin Roentgenol. 28:204-230, 1993
17. Stomper P et al: Atypical hyperplasia: frequency and mammographic and pathologic relationships in excisional biopsies guided with mammography and clinical examination. Radiology. 189:667-71, 1993
18. Truong LD et al: Calcium oxalate in breast lesions biopsied for calcification detected in screening mammography: incidence and clinical significance. Mod Pathol. 5:146-52, 1992
19. Tornos C et al: Calcium oxalate crystals in breast biopsies. the missing microcalcifications. Am J Surg Pathol. 14:961-8, 1990
20. Homer MJ et al: The relationship of mammographic microcalcification to malignancy: Radiologic-pathologic correlation. AJR. 153:1187-89, 1989
21. Colbassani JH et al: Mammographic and pathologic correlation of microcalcification in disease of the breast. Surg Gyn Obst. 155:689-96, 1982

AMORPHOUS CALCIFICATIONS

IMAGE GALLERY

Typical

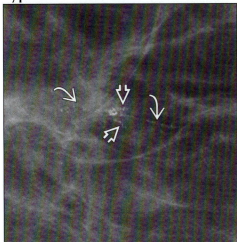

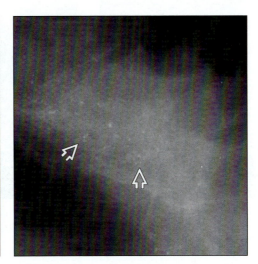

(Left) CC mammography magnification view shows amorphous calcifications in a linear distribution ➡, in a duct and its branches ⇨. Biopsy showed low grade DCIS. *(Right)* CC mammography magnification view shows regional amorphous microcalcifications ⇨. These were increasing. Biopsy showed infiltrating and intraductal carcinoma.

Variant

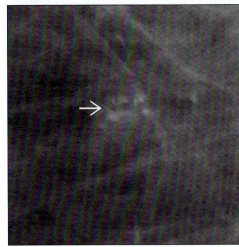

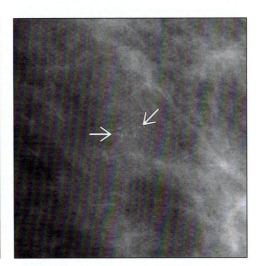

(Left) CC mammography magnification view shows smudgy, indistinct calcifications ➡, a variant of amorphous calcifications. Biopsy showed low grade DCIS. *(Right)* CC mammography magnification view shows clustered amorphous microcalcifications ➡. These layered on 90° lateral view, compatible with milk-of-calcium.

Variant

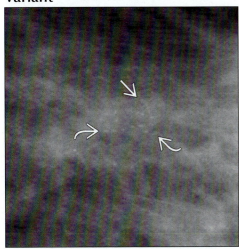

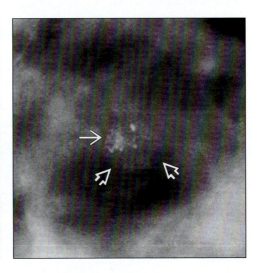

(Left) Lateral mammography magnification view shows clustered amorphous calcifications ➡ and milk-of-calcium ➡. Biopsy showed calcium oxalate crystals in microcysts (on polarized microscopy), and columnar cell changes. *(Right)* CC mammography magnification view shows clustered amorphous and punctate calcifications ➡ within a 4 mm circumscribed nodule ⇨. Biopsy showed intraductal papilloma.

FINE LINEAR CALCIFICATIONS

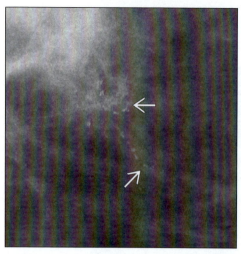

CC magnification view shows linear and branching distribution of individually fine linear calcifications ➡, highly suggestive of malignancy, BI-RADS 5. Biopsy showed DCIS.

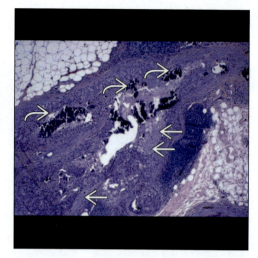

Histopathology of high grade DCIS with central comedo necrosis ➡ and calcifications ➡ (H&E x 100).

TERMINOLOGY

Abbreviations and Synonyms
- Branching, casting, dot-dash calcifications (Ca++)

Definitions
- Thin, irregular calcifications that appear linear but are discontinuous, measuring < 0.5 mm in diameter
- Used to define individual calcification morphology, not distribution per se

IMAGING FINDINGS

General Features
- Best diagnostic clue: Linear and irregular branching calcifications, conforming to ductal pattern at mammography
- Location: Distribution of calcifications follows ductal anatomy
- Size: Individual calcifications measure < 0.5 mm in diameter

- Morphology: The morphology of "Y" or "V"-shaped irregular individual calcifications suggests filling of a duct (casting)

Mammographic Findings
- True lateral and CC magnification views for characterization and extent
- Extent of carcinoma correlates closely with calcification extent on mammography
  - Can underestimate DCIS extent in 15-20% of patients

Ultrasonographic Findings
- Grayscale Ultrasound
  - Calcifications alone occasionally seen on US
  - Calcifications within a mass
    - Often invasive component
    - Pure DCIS may manifest as sonographic mass with or without calcifications
  - Can direct US-guided biopsy when visible on US

MR Findings
- T1 C+
  - Not helpful in characterizing calcifications

DDx: Fine Linear Calcifications

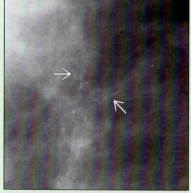

DCIS

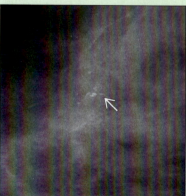

Milk-of-Calcium (ML View)

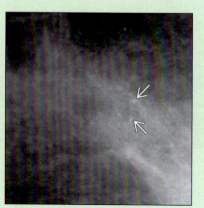

Fat Necrosis

FINE LINEAR CALCIFICATIONS

Key Facts

Terminology
- Branching, casting, dot-dash calcifications (Ca++)
- Thin, irregular calcifications that appear linear but are discontinuous, measuring < 0.5 mm in diameter

Imaging Findings
- Best diagnostic clue: Linear and irregular branching calcifications, conforming to ductal pattern at mammography
- Extent of carcinoma correlates closely with calcification extent on mammography
- Management must always be based on the most suspicious features, i.e., the most suspicious individual calcifications, distribution or interval change

- Post-excision (pre-radiation) magnification mammography to exclude residual malignant calcifications

Top Differential Diagnoses
- Ductal Carcinoma in Situ (DCIS)
- Fibroadenoma (FA)
- Fat Necrosis
- Fibrocystic Change (Milk-of-Calcium)
- Secretory Disease/Plasma Cell Mastitis

Clinical Issues
- High grade DCIS is likely diagnosis

Diagnostic Checklist
- Biopsy of the most suspicious area of calcifications is warranted

- ○ MR may demonstrate linear clumped enhancement in the area of the calcifications
- ○ May be useful in evaluating extent of disease in patients with known cancer

Biopsy
- Vacuum-assisted large (11g or larger) core needle biopsy with 10-12 samples is recommended
  - ○ Clip placement to facilitate localization for surgery
- Direct biopsy to associated mass or asymmetry to help sample associated invasive component if present
- Bracket needle localization of areas > 2 x 2 cm if conservation planned

Imaging Recommendations
- Best imaging tool: True lateral and CC magnification mammography with a 0.1-mm focal spot
- Management must always be based on the most suspicious features, i.e., the most suspicious individual calcifications, distribution or interval change
- Post-excision (pre-radiation) magnification mammography to exclude residual malignant calcifications

DIFFERENTIAL DIAGNOSIS

Ductal Carcinoma in Situ (DCIS)
- Fine linear calcifications in clustered or segmental distribution are almost always due to high grade DCIS

Invasive Cancer
- Infiltrating ductal carcinoma (IDC)
  - ○ Associated extensive intraductal component (EIC) suspected when mass and segmental fine linear calcifications
- Mucinous carcinoma

Fibroadenoma (FA)
- Early calcifications in involuting FA may mimic carcinoma
- Ca++ more often coarse, heterogeneous
- Associated circumscribed oval or lobulated mass common

Fat Necrosis
- Prior history of trauma or surgery
- Early calcifications can appear suspicious for malignancy
- Mammographic evolution of fat necrosis
  - ○ Dystrophic calcifications coarsen
  - ○ Oil cysts with peripheral curvilinear calcification
- Membranous fat necrosis
  - ○ Cystic spaces lined by hyaline membranous structures showing distinctive histochemical staining characteristics
  - ○ May be associated with irregular or linear clustered calcifications

Fibrocystic Change (Milk-of-Calcium)
- Fuzzy, amorphous on CC
- Layering, menisci on true lateral magnification view, BI-RADS 2

Secretory Disease/Plasma Cell Mastitis
- Calcifications typically are smooth, parallel-walled, > 1 mm, denser, than in DCIS
  - ○ Early forms may appear fine linear
- Usually bilateral

Arterial Calcification (Monckeberg Medial Calcific Sclerosis)
- Ring-like calcification of vascular media of small- to medium-sized vessels without intimal thickening
- "Railroad track" Ca++: Linear parallel calcifications in vessel wall, BI-RADS 2, benign
- Atypical patterns: Clustered calcifications in a curved and branching pattern

Atypical Ductal Hyperplasia (ADH)
- Usually means lesion inadequately sampled, excision required

Lactational/Postlactational
- Occasional linear and linear-branching patterns suggestive of ductal distribution pattern, bilateral
- MR may show patchy, regional, heterogeneous enhancement

FINE LINEAR CALCIFICATIONS

- Because of the possibility of DCIS usually biopsy is performed
- Histopathology shows lactational changes with coarse calcifications associated with benign ducts

Stromal Fibrosis
- Commonly appears as an enlarging solid mass or developing density
- In 9% a cluster of calcifications is detected
- Usually coarse heterogeneous Ca++, can be linear

Chondroid or Osseous Metaplasia
- Primary: No associated neoplasm or underlying medical condition; non-neoplastic, rare
- Within breast neoplasms (fibroadenoma, carcinoma or osteogenic sarcoma); associated mass

Skin Artifacts
- Soap or talc in skin lesion: Superficial, correlate with clinical findings
- Tattoo: Ca++ maintain fixed relationship to each other

Epidermal Inclusion Cyst
- Circumscribed mass in skin
- Rarely associated with heterogeneous calcifications

Basal Cell Carcinoma (BCC)
- BCC shows histopathological evidence of calcifications in over one fifth of the cases
- Usually the upper inner quadrants of the breasts are exposed to sun
- Skin lesion usually identifiable, sometimes vague

Amyloidosis
- Few reported cases, mostly as palpable masses, spiculated at imaging: "Amyloid tumor"
- Rare manifestation is clustered fine, linear and branching calcifications

Papilloma
- Usually amorphous or punctate Ca++, rarely linear

PATHOLOGY

General Features
- General path comments: Almost always due to high grade intraductal (comedo) carcinoma
- Etiology: Usually calcification of necrotic debris in ducts involved by high grade DCIS (comedocarcinoma)

Gross Pathologic & Surgical Features
- If comedocarcinoma, caseating yellow debris "comedones"

Microscopic Features
- DCIS: Malignant epithelial cells with pleomorphic nuclei within ducts
- Central necrosis with calcification

CLINICAL ISSUES

Natural History & Prognosis
- High grade DCIS is likely diagnosis

- Increased risk of associated invasive component when area of calcifications > 2. 5 cm

Treatment
- Vast majority of fine linear Ca++ are moderately suspicious (BI-RADS 4C) or highly suggestive of malignancy (BI-RADS 5), warrant biopsy
- If likely to be early secretory, FA, or fat necrosis, short-interval follow-up reasonable (BI-RADS 3)
- If malignant, surgical excision

DIAGNOSTIC CHECKLIST

Consider
- Fine linear morphology is suspicious regardless of distribution
- Associated findings
- Change from previous films, if available
- Direct initial biopsy to areas with associated density or mass to sample invasive component if present

Image Interpretation Pearls
- Biopsy of the most suspicious area of calcifications is warranted

SELECTED REFERENCES

1. Gombos EC et al: Basal cell carcinoma of the skin presenting as microcalcifications on screening mammography. The Breast J. 11:149, 2005
2. Saxena A et al: Monckeberg medial calcific sclerosis mimicking malignant calcification pattern at mammography. J Clin Pathol. 58:447-8, 2005
3. Haj et al: Membranous fat necrosis of the breast: diagnosis by minimally invasive technique. The Breast J. 10:504, 2004
4. D'Orsi CJ et al: Breast Imaging Reporting and Data System: BI-RADS, Mammography, 4th ed. Reston, American College of Radiology, 2003
5. Gulsun M et al: Evaluation of breast microcalcifications according to Breast Imaging Reporting and Data System criteria and Le Gal's classification. Eur J Radiol. 47:227-31, 2003
6. Stomper PC et al: Mammographic predictors of the presence and size of invasive carcinomas associated with malignant microcalcification lesions without a mass. AJR. 181:1679-84, 2003
7. Thurfjell MG et al: Nonpalpable breast cancer: Mammographic appearance as predictor of histologic type. Radiology. 222:165-70, 2002
8. Diaz-Bustamante T et al: Primary amyloidosis of the breast presenting solely as microcalcifications. AJR. 177:903-4, 2001
9. Stucker DT: New bilateral microcalcifications at mammography in a postlactational woman: Case report. Radiology. 217:247-250, 2000
10. Dershaw DD et al: Patterns of mammographically detected calcifications after breast-conserving therapy associated with tumor recurrence. Cancer. 79:1355-61, 1997
11. Holland R et al: Microcalcifications associated with ductal carcinoma in situ: Mammographic-pathologic correlation. Semin Diagn Pathol. 11:181-92, 1994
12. Bassett LW: Mammographic analysis of calcifications. Radiol Clin North Am. 30:93-105, 1992
13. Lanyi M: [Pattern analysis of 5641 microcalcifications in 100 mammary duct carcinomas: polymorphism] [Article in German] Rofo. 139:240-8, 1983

FINE LINEAR CALCIFICATIONS

IMAGE GALLERY

Variant

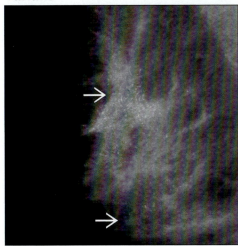

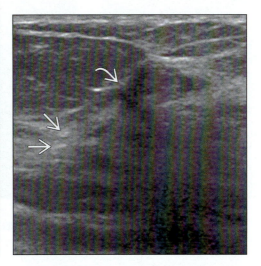

(Left) MLO mammography magnification shows diffuse fine linear calcifications throughout most of the right breast ➡, highly suggestive of malignancy, BI-RADS 5. (Right) Ultrasound (same patient as left-hand image) revealed an irregular, hypoechoic mass with posterior shadowing ➡ and a few calcifications in a duct ➡. US-guided core biopsy showed IDC and DCIS. Mastectomy confirmed extensive DCIS and a grade II IDC.

Typical

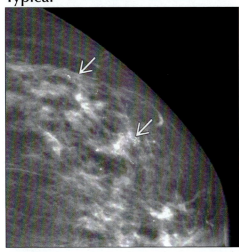

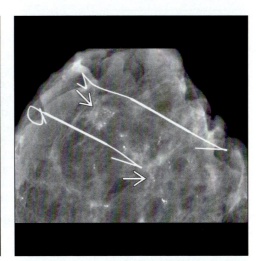

(Left) CC mammography magnification shows segmental fine, linear calcifications ➡, new when compared to the prior mammograms. Core biopsy showed ADH approaching DCIS, and excision was recommended (right-hand image). (Right) Specimen radiograph of the surgical specimen shows that most of the calcifications ➡ were removed, showing DCIS (comedo, solid, cribriform), intermediate nuclear grade.

Typical

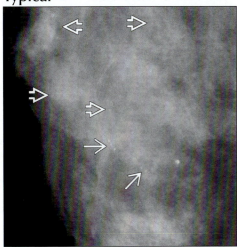

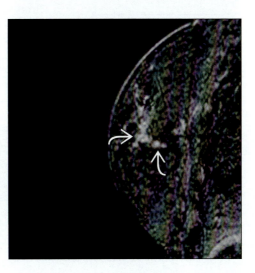

(Left) CC mammography magnification CC view of the upper inner right breast shows a few fine linear ➡ and punctate calcifications ➡. Because the calcifications were new, core biopsy was performed showing high grade DCIS. (Right) Sagittal T1 C+ subtraction MR (same patient as left-hand image) shows segmental clumped enhancement ➡, compatible with extensive DCIS. The patient underwent mastectomy, confirming the MR findings.

PLEOMORPHIC CALCIFICATIONS

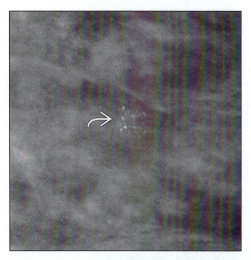

CC mammography magnification shows tightly clustered shard-like pleomorphic calcifications ➔. Stereotactic core biopsy diagnosed high grade DCIS. Because of the dense tissue, MR was performed.

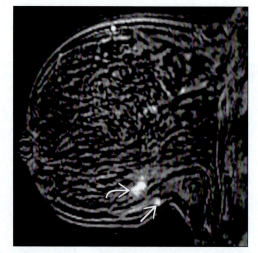

Sagittal T1 C+ subtraction MR shows clumped enhancement ➔ only at the site of the biopsy proven DCIS. Skin enhancement ➔ is at the site of the recent stereotactic biopsy.

TERMINOLOGY

Abbreviations and Synonyms

- Heterogeneous, granular calcifications (Ca++); "shard-like" Ca++

Definitions

- Irregular calcifications of varying sizes & shapes; usually < 0.5mm in size
- Smaller and less defined than heterogeneous coarse Ca++
- Typically denser and more conspicuous than amorphous Ca++
- Neither benign nor typically malignant
  - Linear and linear branching Ca++ are more suspicious for malignancy

IMAGING FINDINGS

General Features

- Best diagnostic clue: Small irregular Ca++ of different shapes & sizes
- Size: Usually < 0.5 mm in size

- Morphology: Variable shapes and sizes

Mammographic Findings

- Ca++ of different size & morphology
- Mammography findings are considered suspicious and warrant recommendation for biopsy
- Magnification orthogonal views (typically CC and ML) recommended to evaluate both morphology and distribution
  - Clustered (5 or more within < 1 cc volume)
  - Linear distribution (suggests ductal distribution)
  - Segmental distribution (suggests ductal distribution)
  - Regional or diffuse multiple bilateral groups (unlikely to represent a ductal process)

Ultrasonographic Findings

- Grayscale Ultrasound
  - Ca++ alone usually not seen on US
  - Ca++ within masses are more conspicuous
  - Ultrasound may identify a hypoechoic mass within a region of Ca++ and direct biopsy toward possible invasive tumor component

MR Findings

- T1 C+

DDx: Other Suspicious Calcification Morphologies

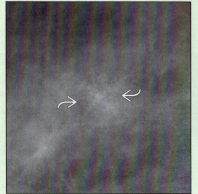

Amorphous, DCIS

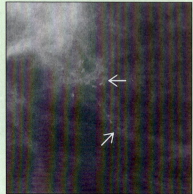

Fine Linear, DCIS

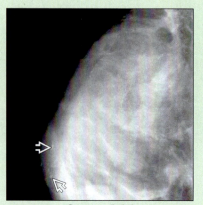

Casting, DCIS

PLEOMORPHIC CALCIFICATIONS

Key Facts

Terminology
- Heterogeneous, granular calcifications (Ca++); "shard-like" Ca++
- Typically denser and more conspicuous than amorphous Ca++

Imaging Findings
- Mammography findings are considered suspicious and warrant recommendation for biopsy
- MR may demonstrate mass or non-mass enhancement patterns in the areas of the calcifications
- Vacuum-assisted large core needle with 10-12 samples recommended

Top Differential Diagnoses
- Ductal Carcinoma in Situ (DCIS)

- Atypical Duct Hyperplasia
- Fat Necrosis

Pathology
- Overall have an intermediate, 25-40% risk of malignancy; BI-RADS 4B or 4C

Clinical Issues
- Most common signs/symptoms: Incidental mammographic finding
- If DCIS, progression to invasion in 33-50% cases

Diagnostic Checklist
- Careful assessment of Ca++ morphology revealing pleomorphic findings should not result in a BI-RADS 3 short interval follow-up

- ○ Not helpful in characterizing calcifications
- ○ MR may demonstrate mass or non-mass enhancement patterns in the areas of the calcifications
  - ■ Ill-defined enhancing masses; linear clumped enhancement; regional foci of enhancement
  - ■ Biopsy findings may be benign or malignant
- ○ May be beneficial when breast cancer is diagnosed to evaluate extent of disease; surveillance for recurrence

Nuclear Medicine Findings
- PET
  - ○ No role for PET in the characterization of mammographically detected suspicious calcifications
  - ○ May be used for breast cancer staging and assessment of recurrent breast cancer

Biopsy
- Stereotactic biopsy
  - ○ Diagnostic evaluation with magnification mammography essential prior to intervention
  - ○ Vacuum-assisted large core needle with 10-12 samples recommended
    - ■ Suspicious calcifications may be related to ductal carcinoma in situ (DCIS) and adjacent to invasive tumor, atypical duct hyperplasia (ADH), or lobular neoplasia
    - ■ Specimen radiography is required to determine successful target retrieval
    - ■ Core samples without Ca++ are more likely to miss the diagnosis of breast cancer than those with Ca++
  - ○ When Ca++ covers a large area, biopsy two areas far removed one from the other
    - ■ Clip placement advocated to identify biopsy site
    - ■ Localization with more than one wire prior to surgical biopsy may be beneficial in removing visible calcifications
    - ■ Bracketing does not ensure clear histologic resection margins

Imaging Recommendations
- Best imaging tool: Magnification mammographic CC and ML orthogonal images
- Protocol advice
  - ○ Magnification mammography for morphology characterization and pattern of distribution
    - ■ Obtain views in orthogonal planes
    - ■ Biopsy recommended
    - ■ If malignant, post-excision orthogonal magnification mammography to assess for residual Ca++ if a large area was involved

DIFFERENTIAL DIAGNOSIS

Ductal Carcinoma in Situ (DCIS)
- Literature reports that 53% of pleomorphic Ca++ in DCIS are associated with noncomedo subtypes

Atypical Duct Hyperplasia
- Imaging findings are nonspecific
- Ca++ are the most common imaging finding prompting biopsy
- Ca++ more often amorphous than pleomorphic

Fat Necrosis
- Pleomorphic irregular small Ca++ may be early manifestation of what will develop into coarse Ca++
- May be associated with a lucent mass

Fibroadenoma
- Early eccentric Ca++ associated with involuting fibroadenoma may appear pleomorphic and suspicious

Papilloma
- Mammographic findings include grouped small irregular Ca++

Fibrocystic Change
- Pleomorphic Ca++ usually in areas of fibrosis

PLEOMORPHIC CALCIFICATIONS

PATHOLOGY

General Features
- General path comments
  - Malignancy probability rate of pleomorphic Ca++ based on distribution
    - Linear 80%
    - Segmental 60%
    - Clustered 40%
    - Regional 40%
  - Overall have an intermediate, 25-40% risk of malignancy; BI-RADS 4B or 4C
  - Pleomorphic Ca++ associated more with noncomedo than comedo DCIS
  - Comedo DCIS more likely to be associated with
    - Microinvasion
    - Absence of estrogen receptors
    - Over-expression of Her-2/neu oncogene
    - Angiogenesis of surrounding stroma
  - Extent of Ca++ in comedo DCIS correlates well with pathologic size
- Etiology
  - Ca++ in DCIS are formed by
    - Necrotic cells that have not yet coalesced to form linear casts (comedo)
    - Calcified secretions in the cribriform spaces (noncomedo)
  - Ca++ in benign entities
    - Luminal secretions
    - Fibrocollagenous stroma
- Epidemiology
  - Atypia found on percutaneous biopsy requires open excisional biopsy
    - 50% upgraded to DCIS/invasion at surgery (14 gauge)
    - 20% upgraded to DCIS/invasion at surgery (11 gauge)
  - 60-75% of pleomorphic Ca++ referred for biopsy are benign
  - Pleomorphic Ca++ have an intermediate risk for malignancy

Microscopic Features
- Ca++ mostly found in ducts

CLINICAL ISSUES

Presentation
- Most common signs/symptoms: Incidental mammographic finding

Natural History & Prognosis
- If DCIS, progression to invasion in 33-50% cases
- Unable to prospectively identify lesions that will progress to invasive cancer

Treatment
- None for benign biopsy findings
- Mastectomy for > 2.5 cm DCIS if negative margins cannot be achieved
- Breast conservation alone for < 2.5 cm DCIS
  - Recurrence 2-7% per year
    - ~ 50% invasive carcinoma

- Breast conservation & whole breast radiation therapy for < 2.5 cm DCIS
  - Recurrence lower 1-2% per year
    - ~ 50% invasive carcinoma
  - Recommended treatment due to lower recurrence rate

DIAGNOSTIC CHECKLIST

Consider
- Comparison to prior mammograms should be done with care
  - Suspicious findings should be biopsied despite stability of imaging findings

Image Interpretation Pearls
- Careful assessment of Ca++ morphology revealing pleomorphic findings should not result in a BI-RADS 3 short interval follow-up
  - 45% of 51 malignancies found in lesions incorrectly classified as category 3 were clustered calcifications

SELECTED REFERENCES

1. Bassett LW et al: Diagnosis of Diseases of the Breast. 2nd ed. Philadelphia, WB Saunders Co. 120, 2005
2. Lomoschitz FM et al: Stereotactic 11-gauge vacuum-assisted breast biopsy: influence of number of specimens on diagnostic accuracy. Radiology. 232:897-903, 2004
3. Margolin FR et al: Stereotactic core breast biopsy of malignant calcifications: diagnostic yield of cores with and cores without calcifications on specimen radiographs. Radiology. 233:251-54, 2004
4. D'Orsi CJ et al: Breast Imaging Reporting and Data System: BI-RADS, Mammography, 4th ed. Reston, American College of Radiology, 2003
5. Liberman L et al: Breast Imaging Reporting and Data System: BI-RADS, Radiol Clin N Am. 40:409-30, 2002
6. Rosen EL et al: Malignant lesions initially subjected to short-term mammographic follow-up. Radiology. 223:221-28, 2002
7. Liberman L et al: Bracketing wires for preoperative breast needle localization. AJR. 177:565-72, 2001
8. Liberman L et al: Stereotaxic 14-gauge breast biopsy: how many core biopsy specimens are needed? Radiology. 192:793-5, 1994
9. Stomper PC et al: Ductal carcinoma in situ: the mammographer's perspective. AJR. 162:585-91, 1994
10. Stomper PC et al: Ductal carcinoma in situ of the breast: correlation between mammographic calcification and tumor subtype. AJR. 159:483-5, 1992

PLEOMORPHIC CALCIFICATIONS

IMAGE GALLERY

Typical

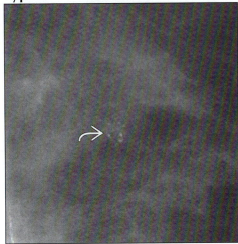
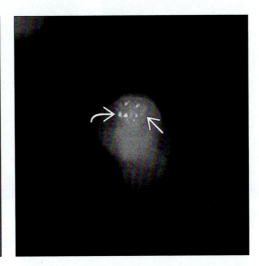

(Left) Lateral mammography magnification shows a small cluster of calcifications ➥ varying in shapes (triangular and shard-like forms) characterized as pleomorphic. Stereo core biopsy was performed. *(Right)* Specimen mammography magnification shows pleomorphic ➥ mixed with amorphous forms ➥ in this core biopsy specimen. Pathology showed fibrocystic change and apocrine metaplasia.

Typical

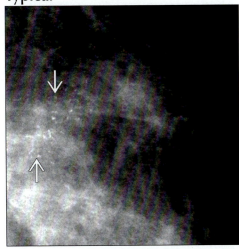
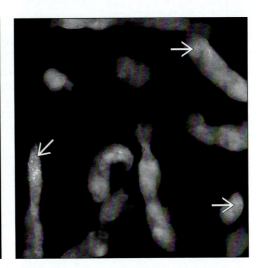

(Left) CC mammography shows a large group of mammographically detected pleomorphic calcifications ➥ without associated mass. The patient underwent stereotactic core biopsy. *(Right)* Specimen radiograph shows pleomorphic calcifications in numerous 11-gauge core biopsy specimens ➥. Pathology showed high grade DCIS with comedo necrosis.

Typical

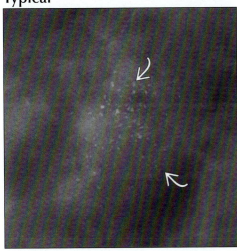
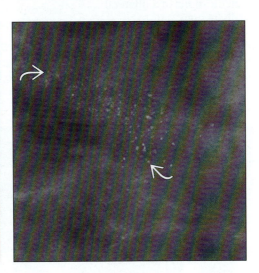

(Left) CC mammography magnification shows a regional distribution (> 2 cc volume not conforming to a duct distribution) of pleomorphic calcifications ➥. Shard-like forms are prominent. *(Right)* Lateral mammography magnification shows suspicious morphology ➥ which, despite the less suspicious distribution pattern, correctly prompted biopsy. Pathology was high grade DCIS with necrosis.

DIFFUSE DISTRIBUTION OF CALCIFICATIONS

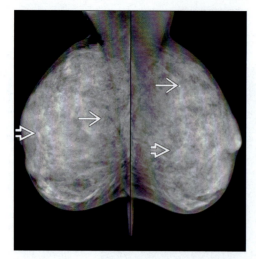

MLO mammography shows dense tissue throughout both breasts. Innumerable bilateral round ➡ and punctate ⬌ calcifications are present in a diffuse distribution.

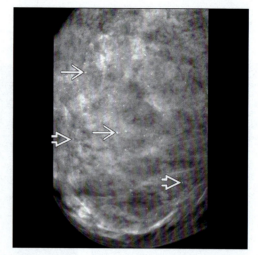

Mammography MLO close-up (same patient as left-hand image) better demonstrates some of the innumerable bilateral diffuse round ➡ and punctate ⬌ calcifications.

TERMINOLOGY

Abbreviations and Synonyms
- Scattered calcifications (Ca++)

Definitions
- Ca++ distributed randomly throughout one or both breasts; areas of random clustering are likely; bilateral distribution pattern favors benign entities

IMAGING FINDINGS

General Features
- Best diagnostic clue
  - Bilateral mammography demonstrates similar benign appearing calcifications throughout one or both breasts
  - Punctate and amorphous calcifications in a bilateral diffuse distribution are usually benign
  - Suspicious Ca++ morphology warrants biopsy regardless of the diffuse distribution pattern
- Size: Usually punctate (< 0.5 mm), round (< 1 mm), amorphous (hazy, variable in size)
- Morphology: Usually smooth, round, amorphous

Imaging Recommendations
- Best imaging tool: Bilateral mammogram
- Protocol advice
  - On baseline mammogram, may perform magnification views directed toward Ca++ clusters
  - Final management based on most suspicious finding, either Ca++ morphology or distribution

DIFFERENTIAL DIAGNOSIS

Adenosis
- Premenopausal
- Terminal ductal lobular unit (TDLU) proliferation

Sclerosing Adenosis
- Typically postmenopausal
- Sclerosis and loss of glandular formation; less conspicuous epithelial cells than in florid adenosis

Fibrocystic Change
- A spectrum of proliferative abnormalities largely derived from the TDLUs

---

DDx: Other Diffuse Ca++ Cases

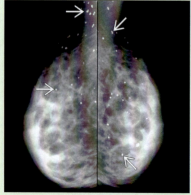

Dermal Ca++

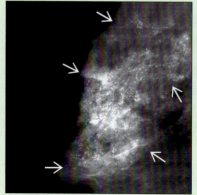

High Grade DCIS

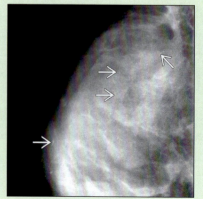

Extensive DCIS

DIFFUSE DISTRIBUTION OF CALCIFICATIONS

Key Facts

Terminology
- Ca++ distributed randomly throughout one or both breasts; areas of random clustering are likely; bilateral distribution pattern favors benign entities

Imaging Findings
- Suspicious Ca++ morphology warrants biopsy regardless of the diffuse distribution pattern
- Size: Usually punctate (< 0.5 mm), round (< 1 mm), amorphous (hazy, variable in size)

- Best imaging tool: Bilateral mammogram

Top Differential Diagnoses
- Adenosis
- Fibrocystic Change

Clinical Issues
- No biopsy necessary for diffuse bilateral morphologically benign appearing Ca++

- Ca++ typically within areas of fibrosis

Skin Calcifications
- Usually lucent-centered polygonal shapes; often in groups
- Most commonly seen in the parasternal skin, the inframammary fold, the axilla, and the areola

Extensive Ductal Carcinoma in Situ (DCIS)
- Ca++ associated with DCIS are typically linear, pleomorphic or amorphous in morphology
- Will often have associated mass due to invasive component; US may be helpful to identify a mass

PATHOLOGY

General Features
- Etiology
  - Calcifications may form in luminal secretions, in areas of fibrosis, and in areas of DCIS with or without comedonecrosis
  - Extensive diffuse bilateral Ca++ described in a post-lactational woman
    - Intraductal milk stasis +/- post-lactation apoptosis

CLINICAL ISSUES

Presentation
- Most common signs/symptoms: Asymptomatic screening mammogram

- Other signs/symptoms
  - Palpable masses associated with the spectrum of fibrocystic change
  - Palpable masses associated with invasive cancer and/or extensive DCIS

Natural History & Prognosis
- Fibrocystic proliferative lesions have a slight increase in the lifetime risk of invasive carcinoma
  - Risk increases as proliferation increases

Treatment
- No biopsy necessary for diffuse bilateral morphologically benign appearing Ca++
- Biopsy, typically percutaneous, for any suspicious Ca++ morphology regardless of diffuse distribution pattern

SELECTED REFERENCES
1. D'Orsi CJ et al: Breast Imaging Reporting and Data System: BI-RADS, Mammography, 4th ed. Reston, American College of Radiology, 2003
2. Stucker DT et al: New bilateral microcalcifications at mammography in a postlactational woman: case report. Radiology. 217:247-50, 2000
3. Sickles EA: Breast calcifications: mammographic evaluation. Radiology. 160:289-92, 1986

IMAGE GALLERY

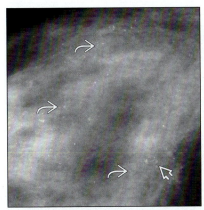
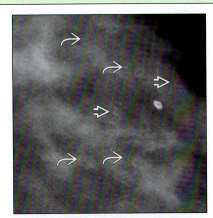
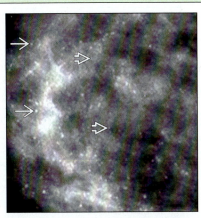

(Left) CC mammography magnification shows diffuse punctate ➜ and amorphous ⮞ calcifications present throughout both extremely dense breasts, and assessed as BI-RADS 2. Benign. *(Center)* CC mammography magnification shows diffuse scattered punctate ➜ and amorphous ⮞ calcifications. Both breasts showed the same benign pattern, a BI-RADS 2. *(Right)* CC mammography magnification shows diffuse round ➜ and punctate ⮞ calcifications throughout dense tissue. Bilateral similar findings were present, consistent with benign etiology.

CLUSTERED DISTRIBUTION

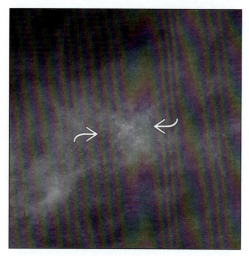

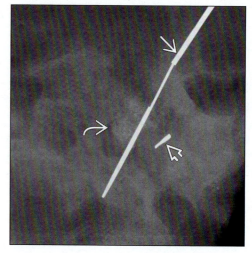

Lateral mammography magnification shows a cluster of amorphous microcalcifications ➡ only a few of which were sampled at core biopsy. Pathology found fibrocystic change, felt to be possibly discordant.

Specimen mammography magnification (same as left image) following needle localization ➡ & surgical excision proved low grade DCIS with microcalcifications ➡ adjacent to post biopsy marker ➡.

TERMINOLOGY

Abbreviations and Synonyms
- Grouped calcifications (Ca++)

Definitions
- A group of ≥ 5 calcifications within < 1 cc volume of breast tissue
- Clustered distribution is most common pattern, and is of intermediate concern

IMAGING FINDINGS

General Features
- Location: Within terminal ductal lobular unit (TDLU), ducts, stroma, masses, skin
- Morphology
  - Clustered Ca++ can be of any morphology
    - Individual calcification morphology critical for management; manage based on worst forms
  - Assessment of cluster shape
    - "V" or "swallowtail" shape suggest filling of duct, spectrum with linear, segmental, suggests DCIS

Mammographic Findings
- Close inspection of both breasts to detect Ca++
- Spot magnification orthogonal mammographic views (ML or LM and CC) to characterize Ca++ morphology and extent
- Evaluate for associated masses, architectural distortion, other findings

Ultrasonographic Findings
- Small clusters Ca++ difficult to identify unless in mass
- May find associated mass within larger groups of Ca++
  - US may then guide biopsy procedure

MR Findings
- Not indicated for evaluation of Ca++ per se
  - Can be used to determine extent of DCIS

Biopsy
- Percutaneous biopsy
  - Stereotactic 11-gauge vacuum-assisted biopsy with ≥ 10 samples most common method
  - Specimen radiography to confirm Ca++ retrieval
  - US may be used to guide biopsies if Ca++ visible

DDx: Other Distribution Descriptor Examples

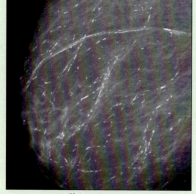

Diffuse, Secretory

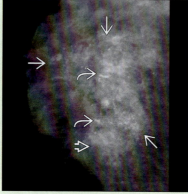

Regional, ADH

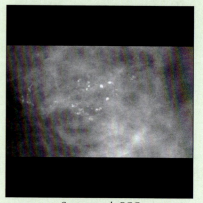

Segmental, FCC

CLUSTERED DISTRIBUTION

Key Facts

Terminology
- A group of ≥ 5 calcifications within < 1 cc volume of breast tissue
- Clustered distribution is most common pattern, and is of intermediate concern

Imaging Findings
- Location: Within terminal ductal lobular unit (TDLU), ducts, stroma, masses, skin
- Clustered Ca++ can be of any morphology
- Assessment of cluster shape

Top Differential Diagnoses
- Fibrocystic changes (FCC)
- Sclerosing adenosis
- Fibroadenoma (FA)
- Fat necrosis

- Atypical ductal hyperplasia (ADH)
- Lobular neoplasia
- Ductal carcinoma in situ (DCIS)

Clinical Issues
- Most common signs/symptoms: Asymptomatic mammogram finding
- Management driven primarily by Ca++ morphology
- Suspicious linear, pleomorphic, or amorphous morphologies require biopsy (BI-RADS, 4)

Diagnostic Checklist
- When multiple bilateral clusters are similar in their benign or probably benign calcification morphologies, imaging surveillance, BI-RADS 2 or 3, is appropriate

Imaging Recommendations
- Best imaging tool: Spot magnification orthogonal mammographic views (ML or LM and CC)
- Protocol advice
  - Two projection magnification views help confirm that a true cluster is present rather than overlapping Ca++ projecting as a cluster on one view
  - True lateral magnification view more beneficial than MLO magnification to identify layering of milk-of-calcium

DIFFERENTIAL DIAGNOSIS

Benign Lesions
- Fibrocystic changes (FCC)
  - Calcification morphology often amorphous, punctate; may be pleomorphic
  - Ca++ in areas of usual duct hyperplasia, adenosis, apocrine metaplasia, or stroma
  - Milk-of-calcium particles within microcysts
- Sclerosing adenosis
  - Ca++ often punctate or amorphous
  - Associated mass may be present
- Fibroadenoma (FA)
  - Early-forming Ca++ may be amorphous
  - Later Ca++ often coarse and heterogeneous, "popcorn"
  - May or may not see an associated mass
- Fibroadenomatoid changes
  - Benign breast lesion with features of FA and FCC
  - Ca++ usually stromal: Coarse heterogeneous, pleomorphic, granular, or rod-shaped
- Fat necrosis
  - Ca++ common
    - May be dystrophic: Coarse, irregular, often with lucent center
    - May be curvilinear: Within oil cyst wall
    - May be pleomorphic
- Papilloma
  - Ca++ may be amorphous, punctate or coarse
  - Typically associated with a mass

- Benign breast tissue
  - Ca++ of varying morphologies may be associated with benign ducts
- Dermal calcifications
  - Polygonal shapes with umbilicated centers
  - Most common in parasternal, areolar, or axillary location
  - When typical, dismiss as benign finding, BI-RADS 2
  - Confounding morphologies may require further evaluation with a skin localization procedure

High Risk Lesions
- Atypical ductal hyperplasia (ADH)
  - Ca++ often amorphous; may be punctate, pleomorphic, linear
  - Excision required after this result on core: 18% malignant after 11-g biopsy
- Lobular neoplasia
  - Lobular carcinoma in situ (LCIS) and atypical lobular hyperplasia (ALH) usually adjacent to Ca++
    - Ca++ may be amorphous, punctate, pleomorphic

Malignant Lesions
- Ductal carcinoma in situ (DCIS)
  - Ca++ may be linear, pleomorphic, amorphous, punctate
  - Careful attention to distribution may suggest a subtle more suspicious linear or segmental pattern
  - Amorphous and punctate Ca++ more likely related to low grade rather than high grade DCIS
- Invasive ductal carcinoma (IDC)
  - Ca++ may be linear, pleomorphic, amorphous, punctate
  - Usually has associated mass
  - Ca++ usually associated with DCIS

PATHOLOGY

General Features
- Etiology
  - Calcium phosphate most common form of calcium in breast tissue

- Typically medium to high density
- Frequently associated with malignancy
  - Calcium oxalate can be present in breast tissue
    - Amorphous morphology with low to medium density
    - Reported to be exclusively associated with benign lesions
  - Clustered Ca++ may contain both calcium phosphate and oxalate
    - Presence of calcium phosphate makes malignancy more likely
- Epidemiology
  - Relative risk (RR) of breast cancer in women with Ca++ on mammogram compared to those without
    - With calcifications RR = 1.68

CLINICAL ISSUES

Presentation
- Most common signs/symptoms: Asymptomatic mammogram finding

Natural History & Prognosis
- Distribution patterns may be stratified from those favoring benign etiology to those highly suggestive of malignancy
  - Diffuse/scattered favors benign, especially if bilateral
  - Multiple bilateral similar clusters usually benign
  - Clustered, regional of intermediate concern
    - Management driven primarily by Ca++ morphology
  - Linear, segmental moderate to highly suspicious
- Individual Ca++ morphology can be stratified on risk of malignancy
  - Round nearly always benign, can be dermal
  - Punctate probably benign (< 2% risk) on baseline; consider biopsy if new, 11% malignant
  - Coarse heterogeneous of low suspicion, 7% malignant
  - Amorphous of intermediate concern, 20-24% malignant
  - Pleomorphic of intermediate concern, 28-37% malignant
  - Fine linear and branching moderately suggestive of malignancy, 55-81% malignant
- 80% of Ca++ going to biopsy are clustered
- In cases of suspicious Ca++ at lumpectomy site found to represent recurrent breast cancer
  - Distribution reported as clustered in 73%
  - > 10 linear Ca++ in 68%; 77% had pleomorphic forms

Treatment
- Dependent on morphological appearance of the Ca++ and patient history
  - Round or punctate smooth Ca++ likely to be benign
    - May be followed at 6 months (BI-RADS 3) if baseline finding
    - May be returned to screening (BI-RADS 2) if stable from prior mammograms
  - New clustered punctate Ca++ merit consideration of biopsy

  - Suspicious linear, pleomorphic, or amorphous morphologies require biopsy (BI-RADS, 4)
- Indeterminate or suspicious findings undergoing biopsy are treated based on the pathology findings

DIAGNOSTIC CHECKLIST

Consider
- Management based on most suspicious Ca++ morphology present
- Multiple clusters must be evaluated individually for worrisome calcification morphology
- When multiple bilateral clusters are similar in their benign or probably benign calcification morphologies, imaging surveillance, BI-RADS 2 or 3, is appropriate

Image Interpretation Pearls
- When evaluating a cluster for possible milk-of-calcium, 90° lateral view is best to evaluate for layering of calcium within microcysts

SELECTED REFERENCES

1. Burnside ES et al: The ability of microcalcification descriptors in the BI-RADS 4th edition to stratify the risk of malignancy. Radiologic Society of North America (abstr) p. 286, 2005
2. D'Orsi CJ et al: Breast Imaging Reporting and Data System: BI-RADS, Mammography, 4th ed. Reston, American College of Radiology, 2003
3. Berg WA et al: Atypical lobular hyperplasia or lobular carcinoma in situ at core-needle breast biopsy. Radiology. 218:503-09, 2001
4. Berg WA et al: Biopsy of amorphous breast calcifications: pathologic outcome and yield at stereotactic biopsy. Radiology. 221:495-503, 2001
5. Bilgen IG et al: Fat necrosis of the breast: clinical, mammographic an sonographic features. Eur J Radiol. 39:92-9, 2001
6. Kamal M et al: Fibroadenomatoid hyperplasia: a cause of suspicious microcalcifications on mammographic screening. AJR. 171:1331-4, 1998
7. Liberman L et al: The Breast Imaging Reporting and Data System: positive predictive value of mammographic features and final assessment categories. AJR 171:35-40, 1998
8. Dershaw DD et al: Patterns of mammographically detected calcifications after breast-conserving therapy associated with tumor recurrence. Cancer. 79:1355-61, 1997
9. Hamby LS et al: Management of mammographic indeterminate lesions. First place winner of the Conrad Jobst Award in the Gold Medal paper competition. Am Surg. 9:4-8, 1993
10. Thomas DB et al: Mammographic calcifications and risk of subsequent breast cancer. J Natl Cancer Instit. 85:230-5, 1993
11. Winston JS et al: Calcium oxalate is associated with benign breast tissue. Can we avoid biopsy? Am J Clin Pathol. 100:488-92, 1993
12. Lanyi M: Diagnosis and Differential Diagnosis of Breast Calcifications. Berlin, Springer-Verlag, 1988
13. Sickles E: Breast calcifications: mammographic evaluation. Radiology. 160:289-93, 1986

CLUSTERED DISTRIBUTION

IMAGE GALLERY

Typical

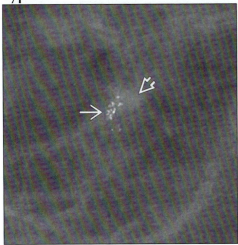 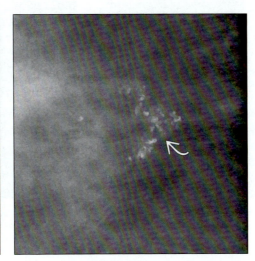

(Left) CC mammography magnification magnification shows a cluster of pleomorphic calcifications ➡ with minimal associated density ➡. Stereotactic bx = fibroadenoma with calcifications. *(Right)* CC mammography magnification shows clustered coarse, heterogeneous calcifications likely benign ➡, but with some increase in number in this 58 yo woman; BI-RADS 4A. Biopsy = sclerosed fibroadenoma.

Typical

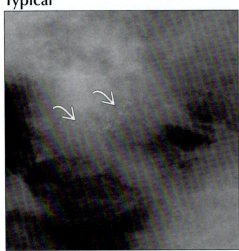 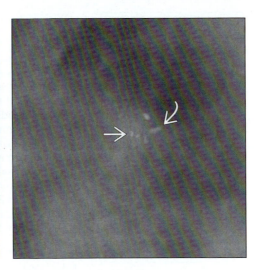

(Left) Lateral mammography magnification shows subtle, clustered amorphous calcifications ➡ of intermediate concern, BI-RADS 4B. Both stereotactic biopsy and excision showed ADH and fibrocystic change. *(Right)* CC mammography magnification shows a cluster of microcalcifications that are pleomorphic ➡ and linear ➡, moderately suspicious for malignancy, BI-RADS 4. Core biopsy = intermediate grade DCIS.

Typical

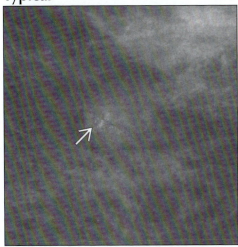 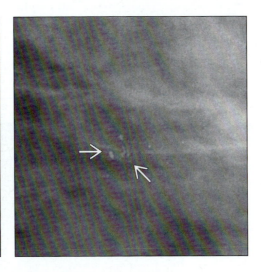

(Left) Lateral mammography magnification shows clustered amorphous microcalcifications ➡ with minimal associated density. Although relatively stable on comparison 5 years earlier, suspicious appearance led to biopsy = low grade DCIS. *(Right)* CC mammography magnification shows a cluster of rather coarse calcifications ➡ in a 48 yo woman. Despite the morphology, the fact that these were new prompted biopsy, showing intermediate grade DCIS.

REGIONAL DISTRIBUTION

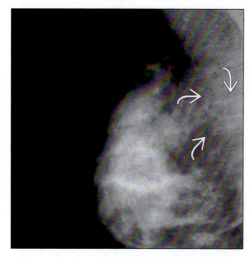

MLO mammography shows regional round calcifications ➡, seen better on photographic close-up view (right-hand image).

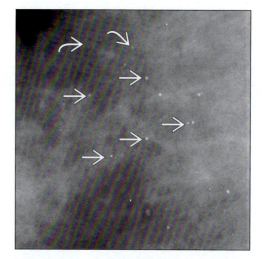

MLO mammography shows individual calcifications are punctate ➡ and round ➡. These had been stable for four years and are presumed benign.

TERMINOLOGY

Abbreviations and Synonyms
- Geographic, patchy

Definitions
- Used to describe calcifications (Ca++) distributed over a large (> 2 cc) volume of breast tissue, not in expected distribution of a duct
- May involve most of a quadrant or more than one quadrant
- Geographic enhancement on MR (≥ 25% of quadrant) not conforming to a ductal distribution
- Can be solitary or multiple regions
- "Global asymmetry" describes regional or diffuse asymmetric density on mammography

IMAGING FINDINGS

General Features
- Best diagnostic clue: Geographic distribution of calcifications or MR enhancement over large volume of tissue

- Size: > 2 x 1 cm area

Mammographic Findings
- Distribution itself is nonspecific
- When Ca++ follow ductal distribution, describe as linear or segmental not regional
- Magnification CC and ML views to characterize extent and individual Ca++ morphology
  - Management is based primarily on worst individual Ca++ morphology
- Associated asymmetry increases level of suspicion
  - US to evaluate for underlying mass, guide biopsy if appropriate
- Associated architectural distortion, skin thickening, skin retraction are suspicious for malignancy
- Bilaterality favors benign etiology

Ultrasonographic Findings
- Grayscale Ultrasound
  - Can help identify underlying mass in setting of regional highly suspicious calcifications
    - Calcifications visible on US more likely malignant
    - Calcifications visible on US more likely associated with invasive component
    - Direct biopsy to underlying mass

DDx: Distributions Similar to Regional

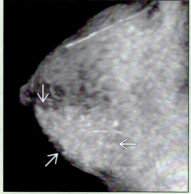

Segmental, DCIS on MR

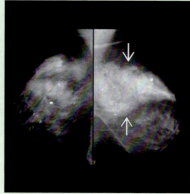

Global Asymmetry, Benign

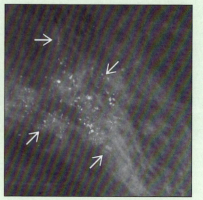

Segmental, DCIS

REGIONAL DISTRIBUTION

Key Facts

Terminology
- Used to describe calcifications (Ca++) distributed over a large (> 2 cc) volume of breast tissue, not in expected distribution of a duct
- Geographic enhancement on MR (≥ 25% of quadrant) not conforming to a ductal distribution

Imaging Findings
- Distribution itself is nonspecific
- Management is based primarily on worst individual Ca++ morphology
- Bilaterality favors benign etiology
- Magnification CC and ML views to depict individual calcification morphology and extent
- Perform MR at days 7-14 of menstrual cycle when possible and applicable

Top Differential Diagnoses
- Ductal Carcinoma in Situ (DCIS)
- Associated mass or asymmetry suggests invasive component
- Atypical Ductal Hyperplasia (ADH)
- Fibrocystic Changes (FCC)
- Invasive Ductal Carcinoma (IDC)
- Mixed IDC and DCIS with large area > 2 cm of malignant Ca++
- Fibrosis
- Dystrophic, Fat Necrosis
- Normal Variant

Pathology
- 46% malignancy rate among regional Ca++ biopsied
- 21-47% malignancy rate among MR regional enhancement biopsied

- US appropriate to evaluate palpable abnormalities
- Consider bilateral whole breast US if index lesion suspicious and parenchyma dense

MR Findings
- T1WI
  - Evaluate for areas of tissue with interspersed fat in areas which subsequently enhance
    - Suggests normal variant
- T2WI FS
  - Normal variant tissue may be edematous (slight increased signal)
  - May see small cysts in regional fibrocystic changes (FCC)
- T1 C+
  - Distinguish from segmental enhancement: Triangular/cone radiating toward nipple
  - Solitary or multiple geographic regions of enhancement
    - Slow initial enhancement, with persistent or progressive delayed enhancement, favors benign etiology (92% NPV)
    - Rapid initial enhancement, with delayed plateau or washout kinetics favors malignancy
  - Regional enhancement at periphery of parenchyma suggests normal variant inflow phenomenon
  - Clumped enhancement suspicious for ductal carcinoma in situ (DCIS) regardless of distribution
    - Usually requires biopsy even if second look US negative
  - Internal enhancement which is confluent or heterogeneous (separated by areas of fat) is less worrisome than clumped
    - Second look US helpful to guide management
    - Absence of correlate on US favors benign etiology
- Inversion Recovery FSE: Similar appearance to T2WI

Biopsy
- Stereotactic biopsy
  - Target most suspicious calcifications, ≥ 10 specimens with ≥ 11-g vacuum-assisted device
- US-guided biopsy
  - Target associated mass when present

- MR-guided biopsy
  - If suspicious and cannot be seen mammographically or on second-look US
- Needle localization
  - Bracketed needle localization of extremes of region if malignant on core biopsy
    - Helps achieve clear margins

Imaging Recommendations
- Best imaging tool: Mammography
- Protocol advice
  - Magnification CC and ML views to depict individual calcification morphology and extent
  - Perform MR at days 7-14 of menstrual cycle when possible and applicable

DIFFERENTIAL DIAGNOSIS

Ductal Carcinoma in Situ (DCIS)
- Individual Ca++ usually pleomorphic or fine linear
- Associated mass or asymmetry suggests invasive component
- Clumped regional enhancement on MR favors DCIS

Atypical Ductal Hyperplasia (ADH)
- Individual Ca++ usually amorphous to punctate
- Excision needed due to risk of sampling error on core biopsy

Atypical Lobular Hyperplasia (ALH) or Lobular Carcinoma in Situ (LCIS)
- Usually an incidental finding on sampling of amorphous Ca++
- Excision often recommended due to potential risk of adjacent unsampled malignancy

Fibrocystic Changes (FCC)
- Individual Ca++ most often punctate and amorphous
- Often background scattered groupings of similar Ca++ in one or both breasts

REGIONAL DISTRIBUTION

Invasive Ductal Carcinoma (IDC)

- Usually associated asymmetry or mass
- IDC NOS or tubular carcinoma
- Mixed IDC and DCIS with large area > 2 cm of malignant Ca++

Fibrosis

- Often multiple regions of enhancement on MR
- Clustered or scattered coarse heterogeneous Ca++ more common than regional Ca++
- Spectrum from oval mixed echogenicity mass to irregular hypoechoic mass on US

Dystrophic, Fat Necrosis

- History of trauma or surgery
- Calcifying oil cysts, coarse, round lucent centered Ca++
- May have associated architectural distortion at site of post-surgical scar
- Associated mass, if any, contains central fat

Normal Variant

- Premenopausal patient or woman on hormone replacement therapy
- MR enhancement in normal tissue
  - Most often at periphery of parenchyma (inflow)
  - Can correlate with areas of asymmetries seen mammographically

PATHOLOGY

General Features

- Etiology
  - 7% of mammographic Ca++ going to biopsy
  - 46% malignancy rate among regional Ca++ biopsied
  - 12-14% of biopsies prompted by MR are due to regional enhancement
  - 21-47% malignancy rate among MR regional enhancement biopsied

CLINICAL ISSUES

Presentation

- Most common signs/symptoms: Asymptomatic, on screening
- Other signs/symptoms
  - Palpable thickening
  - Bloody nipple discharge uncommon, suggests malignancy in this setting

Treatment

- If malignant, initial core biopsy then excision with clear margins
  - Bracket needle localization may be needed if > 2 cm of malignant Ca++ or MR enhancement
- Post-excision mammogram to assure complete removal of malignant Ca++ prior to radiation therapy

DIAGNOSTIC CHECKLIST

Consider

- US to help identify invasive component if individual Ca++ suspicious for malignancy

Image Interpretation Pearls

- Management primarily based on individual Ca++ morphology
  - Regional punctate Ca++ on baseline mammogram, BI-RADS 3, probably benign
  - Regional amorphous Ca++ of intermediate concern, BI-RADS 4B, biopsy recommended
  - Regional pleomorphic Ca++ moderately suspicious, BI-RADS 4C, biopsy recommended
  - Regional fine linear Ca++ highly suggestive of malignancy, BI-RADS 5, biopsy recommended
- Internal enhancement pattern, location, and pre-test risk of disease factor into MR management
  - Clumped regional enhancement suspicious for malignancy, BI-RADS 4C, biopsy recommended
  - Progressive enhancement at periphery of parenchyma suggests possible normal variant, BI-RADS 3A
    - Consider repeat study in 6 weeks at optimal timing in menstrual cycle (days 7-10)
  - Regional enhancement in patient at high risk or with known cancer is of greater concern, often merits biopsy

SELECTED REFERENCES

1. Schnall MD et al: Diagnostic architectural and dynamic features at breast imaging: multicenter study. Radiology. 238:42-53, 2006
2. D'Orsi CJ et al: Breast Imaging Reporting and Data System: BI-RADS, Mammography, 4th ed. Reston, American College of Radiology, 2003
3. Ikeda DM et al: Breast Imaging Reporting and Data System: BI-RADS, Magnetic Resonance Imaging, 1st ed. Reston, American College of Radiology, 2003
4. Soo MS et al: Sonographic detection and sonographically guided biopsy of breast microcalcifications. AJR. 180:941-8, 2003
5. Liberman L et al: Breast lesions detected on MR imaging: features and positive predictive value. AJR. 179:171-8, 2002
6. Liberman L et al: Bracketing wires for preoperative breast needle localization. AJR. 177:565-72, 2001
7. Nunes LW et al: Update of breast MR imaging architectural interpretation model. Radiology. 219:484-94, 2001
8. Liberman L et al: The breast imaging reporting and data system: positive predictive value of mammographic features and final assessment categories. AJR. 171:35-40, 1998
9. Kuhl CK et al: Healthy premenopausal breast parenchyma in dynamic contrast-enhanced MR imaging of the breast: normal contrast medium enhancement and cyclical-phase dependency. Radiology. 203:137-44, 1997
10. Gluck BS et al: Microcalcifications on postoperative mammograms as an indicator of adequacy of tumor excision. Radiology. 188:469-72, 1993
11. Holland R et al: Extent, distribution, and mammographic/histological correlations of breast ductal carcinoma in situ. Lancet. 335:519-22, 1990

IMAGE GALLERY

Typical

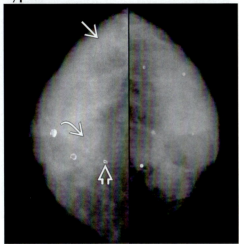

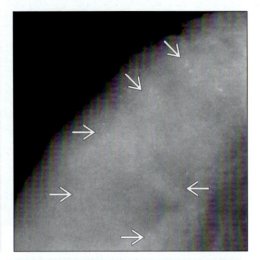

(Left) CC mammography in this 53 year old shows regional amorphous Ca++ in the outer right breast ➡. Loosely clustered amorphous calcifications in the central right breast ➡ had previously been biopsied (with clip, ➡) showing FCC. (Same patient as next 3 images). *(Right)* CC mammography magnification shows regional amorphous calcifications ➡, of intermediate suspicion, BI-RADS 4B. US was performed due to dense tissue (next image).

Typical

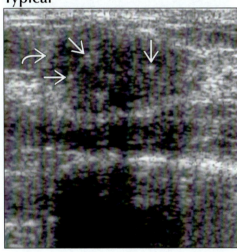

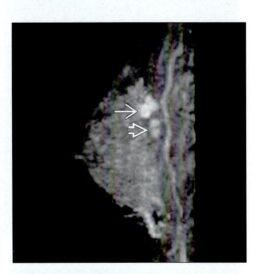

(Left) Anti-radial ultrasound shows lobulated hypoechoic mass ➡ containing microcalcifications ➡, corresponding to area of regional Ca++ seen on mammography. US-guided biopsy showed tubular carcinoma. *(Right)* Sagittal MIP of T1 C+ subtraction MR shows lobulated enhancing mass ➡ due to tubular carcinoma, as well as adjacent enhancement in area of known FCC ➡.

Typical

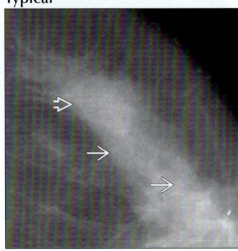

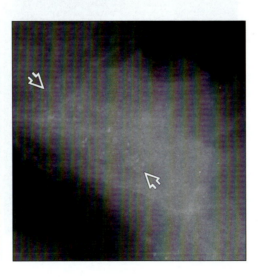

(Left) CC mammography magnification in this 70 year old shows regional amorphous calcifications ➡ (which were increasing) as well as a few loosely scattered punctate calcifications ➡. *(Right)* CC mammography magnification close-up (same patient as left-hand image) better shows regional amorphous calcifications ➡ with associated asymmetry. Needle-localized excision showed a 2.5 cm IDC and DCIS.

Typical

(Left) Sagittal T1 C+ subtraction MR in this 53 year old shows regional enhancement in the upper breast ➡. *(Right)* Sagittal T1 C+ subtraction MR of an adjacent level (same patient as left-hand image) shows the enhancement to be patchy ➡ with interspersed fat ➡. This was appropriately biopsied, showing stromal fibrosis, concordant with imaging findings.

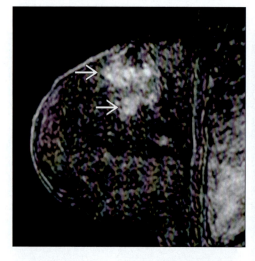
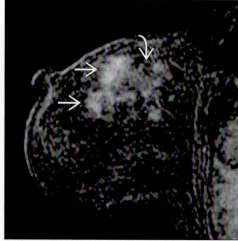

Typical

(Left) MLO mammography in this 77 year old shows regional coarse, benign calcifications in the upper left breast ➡. Focal asymmetry in the upper right breast ➡ proved to be infiltrating ductal carcinoma diagnosed two years later. *(Right)* CC mammography close-up (same patient as left-hand image) better depicts the regional round benign calcifications right breast ➡. A degenerating fibroadenoma with popcorn calcification is also noted ➡.

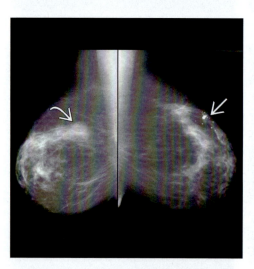
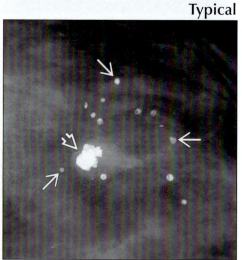

Typical

(Left) CC mammography in this 44 year old shows regional calcifications ➡. *(Right)* CC mammography magnification (same patient as left-hand image) shows individual calcifications to be punctate ➡. The patient had prior excision of similar calcifications showing FCC, and these had been stable for over 5 years, compatible with benign etiology.

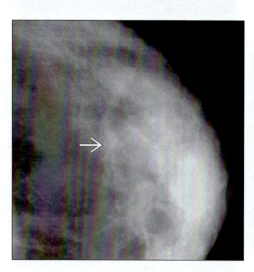
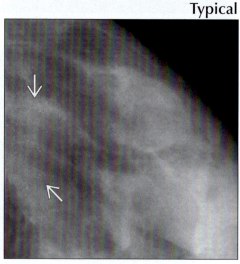

Typical

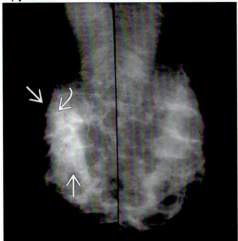
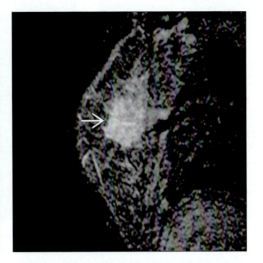

(Left) MLO mammography In this 39 year old shows global asymmetry ➡ with pleomorphic calcifications ⇗ in the area of palpable concern marked with BB's. Stereotactic biopsy showed IDC + DCIS. *(Right)* Sagittal T1 C+ subtraction MR (same patient as left-hand image) shows regional enhancement ➡ in the area of known cancer. Mastectomy showed a 6.5 cm grade III IDC with scattered DCIS.

Typical

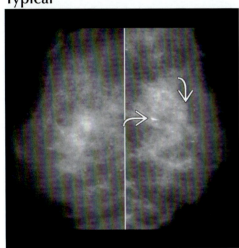
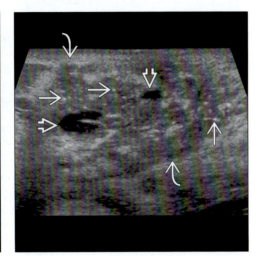

(Left) Lateral mammography close-ups in this 48 year old woman show diffuse bilateral, scattered punctate and amorphous calcifications, many of which layer on the left, compatible with milk-of-calcium ⇗. *(Right)* Radial ultrasound (same patient as left-hand image) shows regional heterogeneous echotexture ⇗ in the 12:00 axis right breast, with associated calcifications ➡ and small cysts ⇨, distinct from other areas. US-guided biopsy showed FCC.

Typical

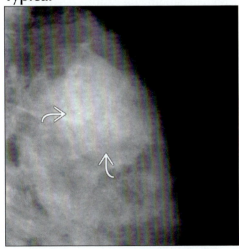
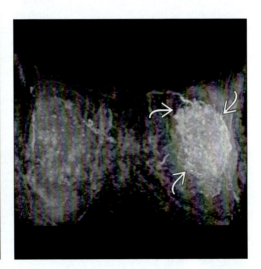

(Left) MLO mammography in this 53 year old shows regional amorphous Ca++ ⇗ and asymmetry. Stereotactic biopsy showed ADH with Ca++. MR was performed (right-hand image). *(Right)* Coronal MIP of T1 C+ subtraction MR (same patient as left-hand image) shows regional enhancement ➡ in most of the upper outer left breast and portions of the lower outer and upper inner left breast. Excision confirmed ADH, extending to the margins.

LINEAR DISTRIBUTION

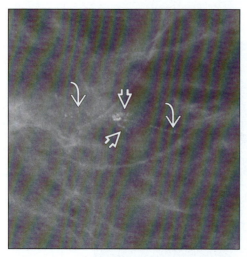

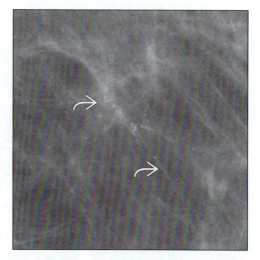

CC mammography magnification shows amorphous calcifications in a linear distribution ⬈, suggesting filling of a duct. Partial filling of a few small branches is also seen ⬈.

Lateral mammography magnification view (same patient as left-hand image) confirms the findings of amorphous calcifications in a linear distribution ⬈. Biopsy showed low grade DCIS.

TERMINOLOGY

Abbreviations and Synonyms
- "Ductal" distribution largely overlaps with "linear" distribution

Definitions
- Calcifications (Ca++) arrayed in a line, suggests deposits in a duct
- Includes "Y" distribution with duct and its branch
- On MR, non-mass enhancement in a line, not definitely a duct, may be sheet-like in three dimensions
- "Segmental" preferred when involves expected course of a duct and multiple branches
- Not used to describe known vascular distribution, i.e., vascular Ca++
- Distinguish from "curvilinear": Suggests at the periphery of a round or oval mass, favors benign etiology
- "Fine linear or branching" used to describe individual Ca++ morphology, not distribution

IMAGING FINDINGS

General Features
- Best diagnostic clue: Discontinuous or continuous structures arrayed in a line
- Location
  - Usually intraluminal in duct(s)
  - Usually radiating toward the nipple, in expected ductal distribution

Mammographic Findings
- Magnification CC and true lateral views to characterize individual morphology and extent
  - Ca++ typical of secretory disease (smooth, rod-like, ≥ 1 mm in diameter) are benign, BI-RADS 2
  - When curvilinear at edge of lucent mass, e.g. oil cyst, compatible with fat necrosis, benign or probably benign depending on history, degree of confidence in findings
  - Punctate, amorphous Ca++ in linear distribution suspicious for ductal carcinoma in situ (DCIS), usually low grade
  - Pleomorphic Ca++ in linear distribution suspicious for intermediate to high grade DCIS

DDx: Calcifications Mimicking Linear Distribution

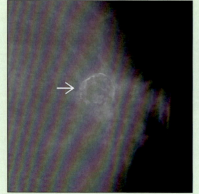

Curvilinear: Oil Cyst

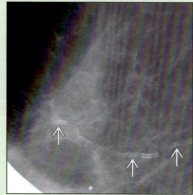

Parallel Linear: Vascular

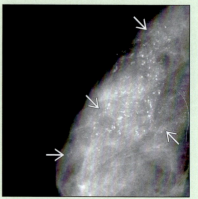

Segmental: EIC

LINEAR DISTRIBUTION

Key Facts

Terminology
- Calcifications (Ca++) arrayed in a line, suggests deposits in a duct
- On MR, non-mass enhancement in a line, not definitely a duct, may be sheet-like in three dimensions

Imaging Findings
- US-guided biopsy of associated mass can help sample invasive component

Top Differential Diagnoses
- Ductal Carcinoma in Situ (DCIS)
- Fine linear or branching Ca++ favor high grade DCIS
- Less often amorphous or punctate Ca++ in a linear distribution, favors low grade DCIS
- Atypical Ductal Hyperplasia (ADH)

- Associated mass or asymmetry suggests invasive tumor, usually invasive ductal carcinoma (IDC)
- Extensive Intraductal Component (EIC)
- Papilloma(s)

Pathology
- 68% of linear Ca++ biopsied proved malignant in one series
- 31-85% malignancy rates among linear, ductal MR enhancement biopsied

Clinical Issues
- Bracketed needle localization if > 2-2.5 cm in length
- Post-operative mammogram to assure removal of all malignant Ca++ prior to radiation therapy

---

- ○ Fine linear Ca++ in linear distributions suspicious for high grade DCIS
- Extent of Ca++ correlates with extent of DCIS in 85% of cases
- Associated mass or asymmetry suggests invasive component: US can help guide biopsy
- Assess for associated architectural distortion, adenopathy, skin thickening or retraction, multifocal, multicentric, bilateral disease
- Management based on worst feature present: Linear distribution moderately suspicious for malignancy unless individual Ca++ clearly smooth, secretory

Ultrasonographic Findings
- Grayscale Ultrasound
  - ○ Less than 50% of DCIS is visible on US in most series
  - ○ Ca++ rarely seen in absence of associated mass
    - ■ Ca++ within a duct suggests DCIS
  - ○ Malignant Ca++ more often visible
  - ○ When seen on US, more likely invasive
    - ■ US-guided biopsy of associated mass can help sample invasive component
- Color Doppler: Increased vascularity favors malignancy

MR Findings
- T2WI FS: Hyperintensity in ductal distribution is nonspecific, can be seen with DCIS
- T1 C+
  - ○ Tubular enhancement suggesting a duct
    - ■ Can be due to intraluminal mass(es), e.g., papillary lesions
  - ○ Clumped enhancement in linear distribution
    - ■ Strongly suggests DCIS
    - ■ May show slow initial enhancement, progressive or plateau kinetics in delayed phase
  - ○ Sheet-like enhancement
    - ■ Can appear linear on a single slice
    - ■ Continues as a plane across multiple images
    - ■ Usually due to normal variant, inflow phenomenon
  - ○ Not used to describe vascular enhancement per se
- Can help determine extent of DCIS

- Not used to characterize Ca++ per se

Biopsy
- Sampling with vacuum-assisted device, ≥ 11-g, at least 10 samples
- Specimen radiography to assure Ca++ retrieval when Ca++ targeted
- Clip placement to facilitate localization for excision if needed
- Target associated mass when possible to facilitate pre-operative identification of invasive component if any
  - ○ US guidance can be particularly helpful with broad areas (> 2.5 cm) of suspicious Ca++ and density

DIFFERENTIAL DIAGNOSIS

Ductal Carcinoma in Situ (DCIS)
- Fine linear or branching Ca++ favor high grade DCIS
- Pleomorphic Ca++
- Less often amorphous or punctate Ca++ in a linear distribution, favors low grade DCIS
- Associated density or mass suggests possible invasive component

Atypical Ductal Hyperplasia (ADH)
- Excision required after this result on core biopsy
  - ○ Frequent upgrade to DCIS or invasive carcinoma at excision
    - ■ 18% after 11-g vacuum-assisted biopsy
    - ■ 45% after 14-g core biopsy
- Amorphous and punctate Ca++ in linear distribution can be ADH, but much more likely to be DCIS

Lobular Carcinoma in Situ (LCIS)
- Duct extension of LCIS can cause linear enhancement on MR
- Typically occult on mammography
  - ○ Linearly distributed Ca++ are usually DCIS, not LCIS
  - ○ Diagnosis of LCIS should be questioned: E-cadherin staining lost in lobular lesions
- Excision often required after this result on core biopsy

LINEAR DISTRIBUTION

Infiltrating Carcinoma
- Ca++ usually in DCIS component
- Associated mass or asymmetry suggests invasive tumor, usually invasive ductal carcinoma (IDC)

Extensive Intraductal Component (EIC)
- Duct extension directly from invasive tumor mass
- DCIS represents at least 25% of main tumor mass
- MRI particularly helpful to assess extent
- Increased risk of recurrence only if incompletely resected

Fibrocystic Changes
- Usual duct hyperplasia
- Fibrosis
- Sclerosing adenosis

Ruptured/Inflamed Duct
- Usually near the nipple
- Asymptomatic

Papilloma(s)
- Intraductal mass(es), can have punctate or amorphous Ca++
- May present with bloody or clear nipple discharge

Fat Necrosis
- Typically curvilinear Ca++ at periphery of fatty mass(es)
- Coarsen over time
- Usually begin to see Ca++ 18-24 months after trauma or surgery

PATHOLOGY

General Features
- Etiology
  - 6% of all Ca++ going to biopsy in one series
  - 68% of linear Ca++ biopsied proved malignant in one series
  - 21-23% of biopsies prompted by MR
  - 31-85% malignancy rates among linear, ductal MR enhancement biopsied
  - 62% of pure DCIS showed linear/ductal enhancement on MR in one series
    - 34% of pure DCIS irregular enhancing mass on MR

CLINICAL ISSUES

Presentation
- Most common signs/symptoms
  - Usually asymptomatic
  - Thickening in area(s) of DCIS
  - Palpable lump more common with associated invasive tumor
- Other signs/symptoms: Bloody or clear nipple discharge with papillomas, less often DCIS

Natural History & Prognosis
- Depends on underlying etiology

Treatment
- Complete excision of malignant Ca++
- Bracketed needle localization if > 2-2.5 cm in length
  - Even if all Ca++ excised, clear margins in only 44% in one series
  - Post-operative mammogram to assure removal of all malignant Ca++ prior to radiation therapy
- "Clear margins" for DCIS may include 2-10 mm of normal tissue
- With broad area of DCIS (> 2.5 cm)
  - Consider MR for more complete assessment of extent if still felt to be candidate for conservation surgery
  - Consider sentinel lymph node biopsy due moderate likelihood of associated invasive component
- Treatment appropriate to tumor type, stage

DIAGNOSTIC CHECKLIST

Consider
- Management based on most suspicious findings present
- Linear distribution moderately suspicious for DCIS

Image Interpretation Pearls
- Findings conforming to expected course of a duct
- Unless secretory, view as suspicious with recommendation for biopsy

SELECTED REFERENCES

1. Menell JH et al: Determination of the presence and extent of pure ductal carcinoma in situ by mammography and magnetic resonance imaging. The Breast J. 11:382-90, 2005
2. Morakkabati-Spitz N et al: Diagnostic usefulness of segmental and linear enhancement in dynamic breast MRI. Eur J Radiol. 15:2010-7, 2005
3. Berg WA: Image-guided breast biopsy and management of high-risk lesions. Radiol Clin N Am. 42:935-46, 2004
4. Liberman L et al: Ductal enhancement on MR imaging of the breast. AJR. 181:519-25, 2003
5. Liberman L et al: Breast lesions detected on MR imaging: features and positive predictive value. AJR. 179: 171-8, 2002
6. Bilgen IG et al: Fat necrosis of the breast: clinical, mammographic and sonographic features. Eur J Radiol. 39:92-9, 2001
7. Liberman L et al: Bracketing wires for preoperative breast needle localization. AJR. 177:565-72, 2001
8. Nunes LW et al: Update of breast MR imaging architectural interpretation model. Radiology. 219:484-94, 2001
9. Liberman L et al: The Breast Imaging Reporting and Data System: positive predictive value of mammographic features and final assessment categories. AJR. 171:35-40, 1998
10. Gluck BS et al: Microcalcifications on postoperative mammograms as an indicator of adequacy of tumor excision. Radiology. 188:469-472, 1993
11. Holland R et al: Extent, distribution, and mammographic/histological correlations in ductal carcinoma in situ. Lancet. 335:519-22, 1990

LINEAR DISTRIBUTION

IMAGE GALLERY

Typical

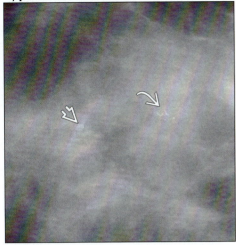 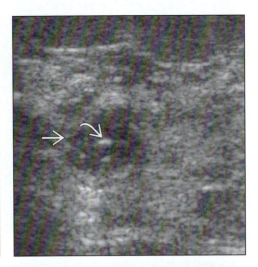

(Left) CC mammography magnification in this 73 year old shows fine linear calcifications in linear distribution ➔, highly suggestive of malignancy, BI-RADS 5. Smudgy calcifications posteriorly ➔ were due to DCIS. *(Right)* Radial ultrasound (targeted to linear Ca++ left-hand image) show microlobulated mass ➔ surrounding echogenic Ca++ ➔. US-guided biopsy showed grade II IDC + DCIS.

Typical

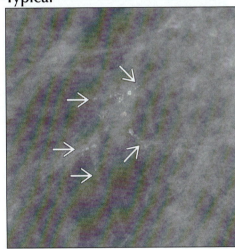 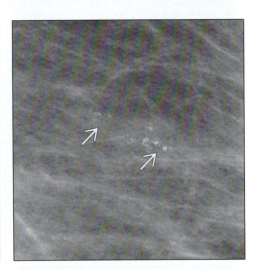

(Left) CC mammography magnification in this 54 year old shows individually punctate calcifications in a linear and branching distribution ➔ suggesting filling of a duct and branches. *(Right)* Lateral mammography magnification (same patient as left-hand image) confirms linear distribution of the calcifications ➔, moderately suspicious for malignancy. Biopsy showed intermediate grade DCIS.

Typical

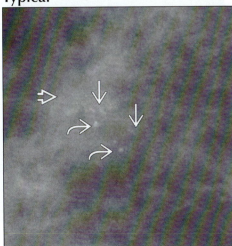 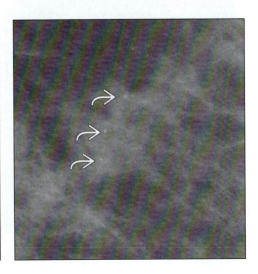

(Left) CC mammography magnification in this 68 year old woman shows amorphous ➔, round ➔, and fine linear calcifications ➔ in a linear and even branching distribution. *(Right)* Lateral mammography magnification (same patient as left-hand image) shows a few punctate and round calcifications ➔ in a linear distribution. Management should be based on the worst features, i.e., the linear distribution: Biopsy showed intermediate grade DCIS.

Variant

(Left) Lateral mammography magnification in this 80 year old shows irregular, coarse, casting calcifications in a linear/ductal distribution ➡. Several areas of pleomorphic calcifications are also noted in a linear or even segmental distribution ⏩. *(Right)* Sagittal ultrasound (same as left-hand image) shows linear calcifications ➡ in a duct, with posterior shadowing ⏩. Biopsy showed low grade DCIS.

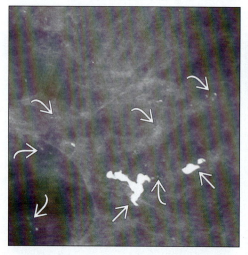
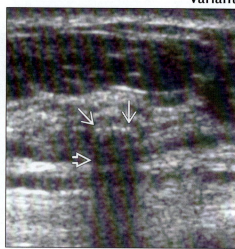

Typical

(Left) Sagittal MIP of T1 C+ subtraction MR in this 53 year old evaluated for contralateral breast pain shows incidental linear enhancement in the anterior breast ➡. Vascular enhancement is also noted ⏩. *(Right)* Targeted US (same patient as left-hand image) shows linear-branching hypoechoic mass ➡ near the nipple, felt to correspond to the MR finding. Biopsy showed intraductal papilloma.

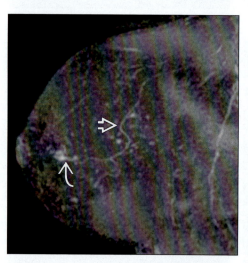
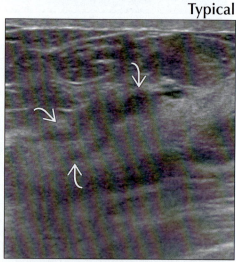

Typical

(Left) T1 C+ subtraction MR in this 61 year old with known high grade DCIS shows clumped linear enhancement ➡, more extensive than the distribution of Ca++ on mammography. *(Right)* Sagittal STIR MR (same patient as left-hand image) shows hyperintensity ➡ in the ducts involved by high grade DCIS. Hyperintensity on T2WI should not dissuade biopsy of suspicious findings.

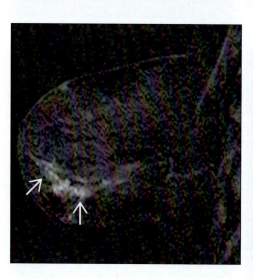
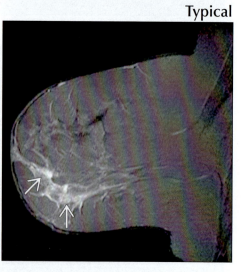

LINEAR DISTRIBUTION

Typical

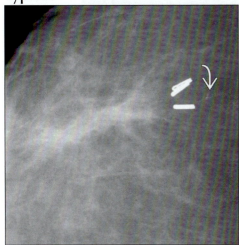

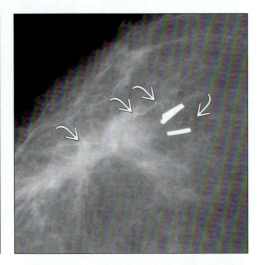

(Left) MLO mammography in this 51 year old 18 months post lumpectomy and radiation therapy for DCIS shows a single fine linear, branching Ca++ ➡ at the scar, which was overlooked. *(Right)* Lateral mammography magnification view (same patient as left-hand image) 6 months later shows marked increase in linear and branching Ca++ ➡ in a linear distribution. Stereotactic biopsy confirmed recurrent DCIS.

Typical

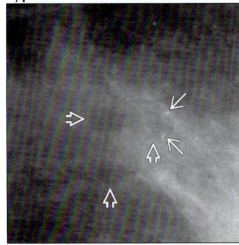

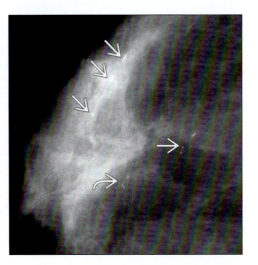

(Left) CC mammography magnification shows fine linear Ca++ ➡ in a linear or curvilinear distribution, possibly at the periphery of a lucent mass ➡ at this site of lumpectomy for cancer two years earlier. Biopsy showed fat necrosis with Ca++. *(Right)* CC mammography in another patient shows a few smooth, rod-like, linear Ca++ ➡ in a linear distribution, as well as a solitary branching Ca++ ➡ in this 79 year old with early secretory Ca++, a benign finding, BI-RADS 2.

Variant

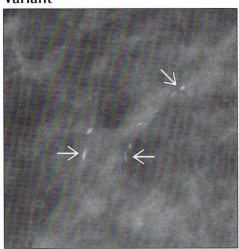

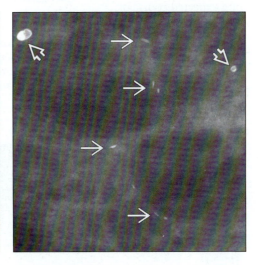

(Left) CC mammography magnification in this 68 year old shows smooth, coarse, linear calcifications in a linear distribution ➡. There is minimal associated density. *(Right)* Lateral mammography magnification (same patient as left-hand image) shows smooth, coarse linear Ca++ in a linear distribution ➡. Biopsy showed fibroadenomatous changes. A few dystrophic Ca++ are also noted ➡.

SEGMENTAL DISTRIBUTION

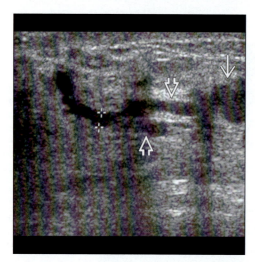

Transverse ultrasound shows an irregular mass ➡, known IDC, with intraductal extension over a duct segment and its branches ➡. The intraductal component was DCIS.

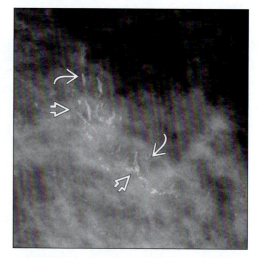

Lateral mammography magnification shows linear, casting ➡ and coalescent amorphous Ca++ ➡ in a segmental distribution suggesting filling of a duct and its branches. Histopathology showed high grade DCIS.

TERMINOLOGY

Abbreviations and Synonyms
- Linear and branching distribution

Definitions
- Calcification (Ca++) deposits in a duct or multiple ducts and their branches
- Involves one or multiple segments or lobes of the breast
- Enhancement on MR in a single ductal system

IMAGING FINDINGS

General Features
- Best diagnostic clue: Ca++ or MR enhancement radiates toward the nipple along expected course of ductal system(s)
- Morphology
  - Following a linear and branching distribution
  - Triangular region or cone with apex directed to nipple
  - Describe individual calcification morphology as well

Mammographic Findings
- Calcifications follow expected course of a duct or ducts and their branches
- Unless secretory Ca++, distribution suggests malignancy
- Magnification CC and ML views recommended for further characterization of morphology and extent unless secretory
- Punctate and/or amorphous calcifications suspicious
- Pleomorphic or fine linear calcifications highly suggestive of malignancy
- Presence of associated mass or asymmetry suggests invasive component
- Describe any associated architectural distortion, skin thickening, or skin retraction

Ultrasonographic Findings
- Grayscale Ultrasound
  - Slightly less than 50% of ductal carcinoma in situ (DCIS) visualized
    - Can see intraductal calcifications; difficult to determine extent on US
  - Calcifications seen on US more likely malignant

DDx: Causes of Segmental Calcifications

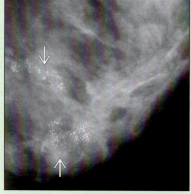

DCIS

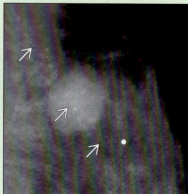

DCIS with IDC

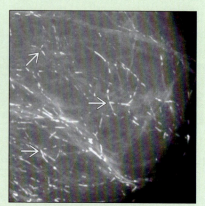

Benign Secretory

SEGMENTAL DISTRIBUTION

Key Facts

Terminology
- Calcification (Ca++) deposits in a duct or multiple ducts and their branches
- Involves one or multiple segments or lobes of the breast
- Enhancement on MR in a single ductal system

Imaging Findings
- Best diagnostic clue: Ca++ or MR enhancement radiates toward the nipple along expected course of ductal system(s)
- Unless secretory Ca++, distribution suggests malignancy
- Punctate and/or amorphous calcifications suspicious
- Pleomorphic or fine linear calcifications highly suggestive of malignancy

- US can help target biopsy if associated mass, likely invasive component
- Protocol advice: Magnification CC and ML views help define extent and morphology of Ca++

Top Differential Diagnoses
- Ductal Carcinoma in Situ (DCIS)
- Extensive Intraductal Component (EIC)
- Invasive Ductal Carcinoma (IDC), NOS
- Secretory calcifications: Usually bilateral, coarse, smooth, rod-like, ≥ 1 mm in diameter

Clinical Issues
- 74% segmental calcifications malignant
- 34-67% segmental MR enhancement malignant; specificity 96%

- ○ Calcifications seen on US more likely associated with a mass due to an invasive component
  - US can help target biopsy if associated mass, likely invasive component
- Color Doppler: May see increased vascularity when malignant

MR Findings
- T1 C+
  - ○ Triangular region or cone of enhancement with apex pointing toward nipple
  - ○ Clumped segmental enhancement is typical of DCIS
  - ○ May see associated mass or masses when invasive component present
  - ○ Distribution itself is suspicious, regardless of kinetic behavior

Nuclear Medicine Findings
- PET
  - ○ Whole body PET insensitive to DCIS
  - ○ Dedicated breast PET depicts 80-90% of DCIS
    - Triangular uptake of FDG with apex toward nipple
    - Linear and branching uptake of FDG

Biopsy
- Stereotactic biopsy
  - ○ Diagnosis by initial 11-g stereotactic biopsy, ≥ 10 specimens, reduces number of operations for malignant calcifications
  - ○ Result of atypical ductal hyperplasia requires excision
- US-guided biopsy
  - ○ Can target associated mass: Likely invasive component
  - ○ Rarely, calcifications can be biopsied under US-guidance
- MR-guided biopsy
  - ○ If lesion cannot be seen mammographically or on second-look US
- Needle localization
  - ○ Bracketed needle localization of extremes of segment can help achieve clear margins

- ○ Complete removal of calcifications can be achieved in 81% of bracketed localizations with median lesion size 3.5 cm
  - Despite excision of calcifications, clear margins only achieved in 44%
- ○ Post-operative mammogram to assure complete removal of calcifications prior to radiation therapy

Other Modality Findings
- Galactography can show extent of process in duct system
  - ○ Nipple discharge, inject discharging duct
  - ○ Papillomas most common
    - Intraductal mass or masses
  - ○ DCIS
    - Irregular filling defects, narrowing of duct(s)

Imaging Recommendations
- Best imaging tool: Mammography
- Protocol advice: Magnification CC and ML views help define extent and morphology of Ca++

DIFFERENTIAL DIAGNOSIS

Ductal Carcinoma in Situ (DCIS)
- Fine linear, pleomorphic, amorphous, punctate, and/or coarse heterogeneous calcifications
- Extent of calcifications on mammography 85% accurate in predicting extent of DCIS
  - ○ Micropapillary subtype most often multifocal, underestimated on mammography, higher risk positive margins

Extensive Intraductal Component (EIC)
- Associated invasive cancer, can be microinvasive
  - ○ Often associated mass on mammography, US, MR
- DCIS represents at least 25% of tumor present
- Additional separate foci of DCIS beyond the main tumor mass
- High risk of positive margins at excision
- MR helpful in defining extent of disease

SEGMENTAL DISTRIBUTION

Invasive Ductal Carcinoma (IDC), NOS
- Usually associated mass or density (asymmetry) on mammography
- Typically well seen on US

Invasive Lobular Carcinoma (ILC)
- Multifocal masses due to ILC, with or without lobular carcinoma in situ (LCIS), rare to have Ca++
- May show intraductal extension

Secretory Calcifications
- Secretory calcifications: Usually bilateral, coarse, smooth, rod-like, ≥ 1 mm in diameter
- Benign finding due to calcifications in wall or lumen of duct
- Previously known as plasma cell mastitis, chronic inflammation of ducts
- Unusual before age of 60 years

Fibrocystic Changes (FCC)
- Bilateral retroareolar fibrosis (rarely)

Multiple Papillomas
- Intraductal masses
- Can be extensive throughout one ductal system
- Increased risk of malignancy when peripheral, multiple
  - Excision recommended

PATHOLOGY

General Features
- Etiology
  - Excess production of calcium phosphate from rapidly dividing tumor cells in DCIS
  - Cell death with calcification of necrotic material in duct lumina in DCIS or invasive carcinoma
  - Secretory calcifications (plasma cell mastitis)
    - Secretions in duct lumen petrify, dense smooth rod-like concretions
    - Calcification in wall of duct, centrally lucent
  - Micropapillary and cribriform low grade DCIS usually amorphous or punctate calcifications
  - Fine linear or branching calcifications usually high grade DCIS
  - Pleomorphic calcifications usually intermediate or high grade DCIS
- Associated abnormalities: Associated mass or asymmetry suggests invasive component

CLINICAL ISSUES

Presentation
- Most common signs/symptoms
  - Most often asymptomatic
  - Palpable mass, skin thickening and/or retraction may be present with carcinoma
- Other signs/symptoms
  - Bloody nipple discharge usually papilloma(s), up to 13% have DCIS or invasive tumor
  - Spontaneous clear nipple discharge usually papilloma(s)

Demographics
- Age: DCIS peak incidence early 50's

Natural History & Prognosis
- 5% of mammographic lesions going to biopsy
  - 74% segmental calcifications malignant
- 5% of MR exams: Segmental enhancement; 7% of MR lesions biopsied
  - 34-67% segmental MR enhancement malignant; specificity 96%

Treatment
- If malignant, initial core biopsy then excision with clear margins
  - Bracket needle localization may be needed if > 2 cm of malignant calcifications or MR enhancement
- No treatment needed for secretory calcifications

DIAGNOSTIC CHECKLIST

Consider
- Large area, > 2.5 cm, of suspicious calcifications likely to have an invasive component: Consider US

Image Interpretation Pearls
- Segmental distribution is suspicious for malignancy unless smooth, secretory calcifications

SELECTED REFERENCES

1. Liberman L et al: MRI-guided 9-gauge vacuum-assisted breast biopsy: initial clinical experience. AJR. 185:183-193, 2005
2. Morakkabati-Spitz N et al: Diagnostic usefulness of segmental and linear enhancement in dynamic breast MRI. Eur Radiol. 15:2010-2017, 2005
3. D'Orsi CJ et al: Breast Imaging Reporting and Data System: BI-RADS, Mammography, 4th ed. Reston, American College of Radiology, 2003
4. Ikeda DM et al: Illustrated Breast Imaging Reporting and Data System: BI-RADS, Magnetic Resonance Imaging, 1st ed. Reston, American College of Radiology, 2003
5. Soo MS et al: Sonographic detection and sonographically guided biopsy of breast microcalcifications. AJR. 180:941-8, 2003
6. Liberman L et al: Breast lesions detected on MR imaging: features and positive predictive value. AJR. 179:171-178, 2002
7. Liberman L: Percutaneous image-guided core breast biopsy. Radiol Clin North Am. 40:483-500, 2002
8. Liberman L et al: Bracketing wires for preoperative breast needle localization. AJR. 177:565-572, 2001
9. Liberman L et al: Calcifications highly suggestive of malignancy: comparison of breast biopsy methods. AJR. 177:165-172, 2001
10. Liberman L et al: The breast imaging reporting and data system: positive predictive value of mammographic features and final assessment categories. AJR. 171:35-40, 1998
11. Gluck BS et al: Microcalcifications on postoperative mammograms as an indicator of adequacy of tumor excision. Radiology. 188:469-472, 1993
12. Holland R et al: Extent, distribution, and mammographic/histological correlations of breast ductal carcinoma in situ. Lancet. 335:519-522, 1990

IMAGE GALLERY

Typical

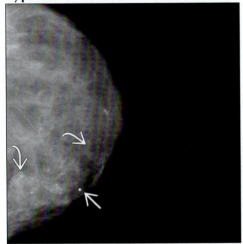 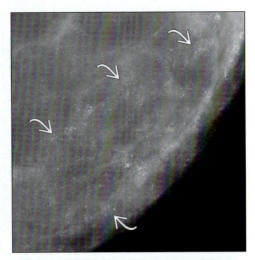

(Left) CC mammography in this woman with a palpable mass ➡, shows segmental pleomorphic calcifications and associated asymmetry ➡, seen better on magnification view (right-hand image). *(Right)* CC mammography magnification shows pleomorphic calcifications in a segmental distribution ➡, highly suggestive of malignancy. US was performed over the palpable mass (next image).

Typical

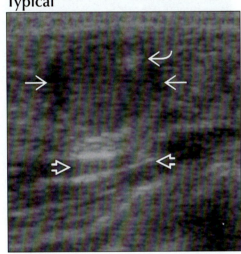 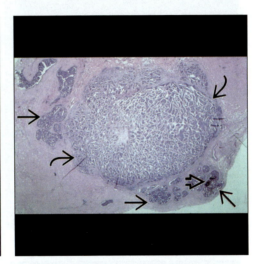

(Left) Radial ultrasound of palpable mass (previous image) shows hypoechoic mass ➡ with echogenic calcification ➡ & posterior enhancement ➡. US-guided core biopsy showed IDC & DCIS. *(Right)* Histopathology (same as previous 2 images) shows a 1 cm IDC ➡ corresponding to US-depicted mass, with extensive associated DCIS ➡ in the area of segmental calcifications ➡, i.e., an EIC. US helped direct sampling of invasive component.

Typical

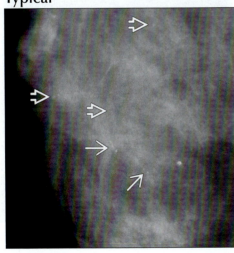 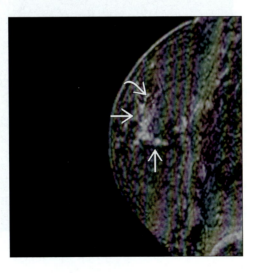

(Left) CC mammography magnification shows subtle fine linear calcifications ➡ in a linear distribution. Stereotactic biopsy yielded high grade DCIS. Clustered punctate and pleomorphic calcifications ➡ were also in DCIS. *(Right)* Sagittal T1 C+ subtraction MR (same patient as left-hand image) shows segmental, clumped enhancement ➡ as well as clip artifact ➡ from core biopsy. Mastectomy confirmed extensive high grade DCIS.

Typical

(Left) CC mammography magnification shows coarse, heterogeneous calcifications ➡ in a segmental distribution, highly suggestive of malignancy, BI-RADS 5. US (right-hand image) was performed as the patient was not a candidate for stereotactic biopsy. *(Right)* Anti-radial ultrasound (same patient as left-hand image) shows intraductal calcifications ➡ in several ducts. US-guided 14-g core biopsy showed high grade DCIS.

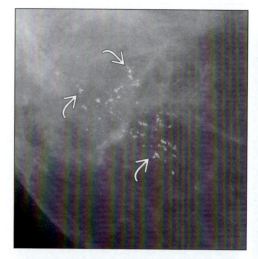
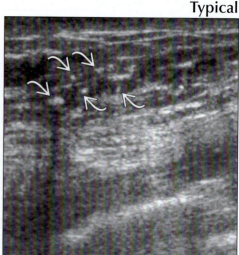

Typical

(Left) CC mammography of a woman with bloody nipple discharge shows global, nodular, triangular asymmetry central left breast ➡. Galactography was performed (right-hand image). (Same patient as next 3 images). *(Right)* CC galactography fills a duct and its branches in the distribution of the asymmetry. There is distention of the major duct and pruning of the terminal ducts ➡.

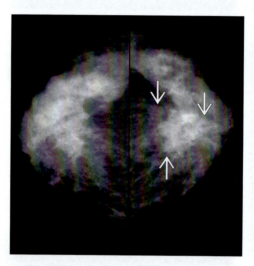
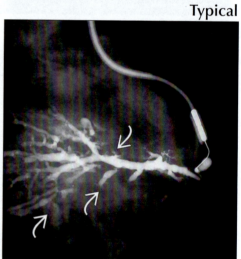

Typical

(Left) Sagittal T1 C+ subtraction MR (same patient as previous 2 images) shows clumped, segmental enhancement ➡, suspicious for DCIS. *(Right)* Anti-radial ultrasound shows a subtle tubular and nodular, slightly hypoechoic, irregular mass ➡ in the area of mammographic asymmetry and MR enhancement (left-hand image). US-guided biopsy showed high grade DCIS.

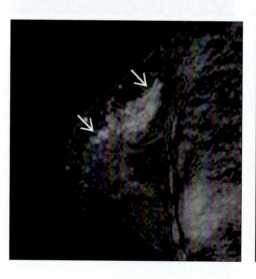
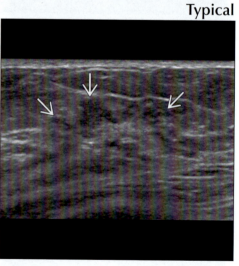

SEGMENTAL DISTRIBUTION

Variant

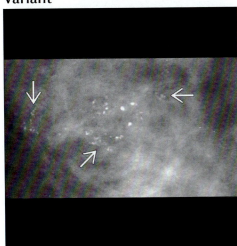

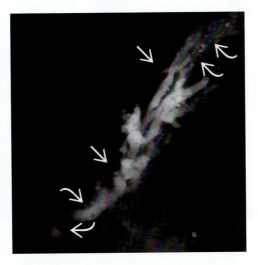

(Left) CC mammography magnification shows coarse heterogeneous calcifications ➡ in a segmental distribution. Histopathology showed fibrocystic changes with calcifications in benign ducts. *(Right)* Lateral galactography in this woman with bloody nipple discharge shows multiple intraductal masses ➡ over an entire segment (duct and its branches) ➡. Excision showed multiple papillomas.

Variant

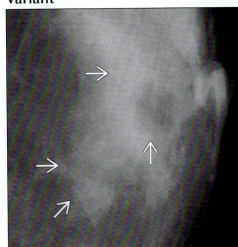

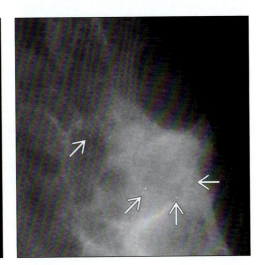

(Left) CC mammography magnification shows subtle punctate calcifications in a segmental distribution ➡, seen also on true lateral magnification view (right-hand image). *(Right)* Lateral mammography magnification again shows subtle punctate calcifications in a segmental distribution ➡. While individual morphology is not suspicious, the distribution prompted biopsy. Excision and mastectomy confirmed DCIS.

Typical

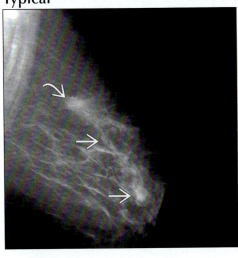

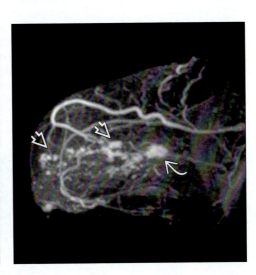

(Left) MLO mammography shows indistinctly marginated mass ➡. US-guided biopsy showed ILC. In retrospect, there is a subtle band of asymmetry extending toward the nipple ➡. *(Right)* Sagittal T1 C+ SPGR MIP MR (same as left-hand image) shows multiple enhancing masses ➡ in a segmental distribution, as well as the known ILC ➡. Second look US after MR depicted additional masses, and extensive ILC was confirmed by biopsy.

ARCHITECTURAL DISTORTION

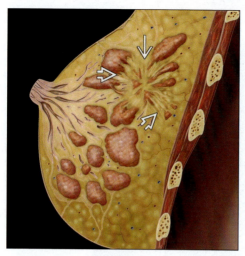

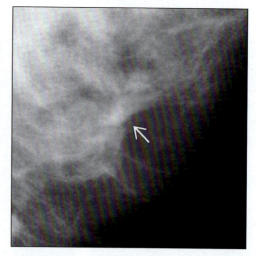

Graphic shows distortion ➡ of breast tissue with spiculations ⏩ emanating from a point. No central mass is present.

CC mammography magnification shows a single view finding of architectural distortion ➡ with parenchymal contour angulation and a pulling in of the tissue in an asymptomatic 49 year old. Biopsy = grade II IDC.

TERMINOLOGY

Abbreviations and Synonyms
- Puckering; "tent sign"

Definitions
- Alteration of the normal breast architecture with thin spiculations radiating from a point without a definite mass; focal retraction or distortion may be seen at the parenchymal margin
- Can be a primary finding or associated with a mass, asymmetry, or calcifications (Ca++)

IMAGING FINDINGS

General Features
- Best diagnostic clue
  - Linear opacities radiating from a focal area or point without obvious central mass
    - Disruption of normal tissue planes; tethering and possibly thickening of Cooper ligaments on US
- Location
  - Can be anywhere in breast, uncommon behind nipple
  - Best perceived at edge of parenchyma on mammography
    - Axillary tail and upper outer quadrant, especially on MLO view
    - Posterior boundary of glandular tissue, especially on CC view

Mammographic Findings
- Tissue straightening, angulation with "pulling in" ("edge" or "tent" sign)
- May be seen in only one view
- Additional evaluation required if scar becoming more prominent
  - Spot compression views to confirm persistent finding, may reveal frank spiculated mass
  - True lateral view, rolled CC views as needed to identify 3D location
  - Tangential view can help identify overlying skin thickening and/or retraction, may allow visualization of underlying mass at edge of parenchyma

DDx: Additional Examples of Architectural Distortion

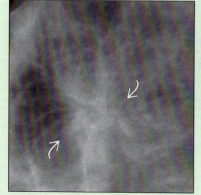

Radial Scar

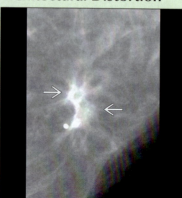

Infiltrating Ductal Cancer

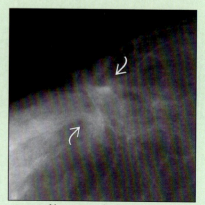

Infiltrating Lobular Cancer

ARCHITECTURAL DISTORTION

Key Facts

Terminology
- Alteration of the normal breast architecture with thin spiculations radiating from a point without a definite mass; focal retraction or distortion may be seen at the parenchymal margin
- Can be a primary finding or associated with a mass, asymmetry, or calcifications (Ca++)

Imaging Findings
- Tissue straightening, angulation with "pulling in" ("edge" or "tent" sign)
- Additional evaluation required if scar becoming more prominent
- Spiculated enhancement or distortion around enhancing lesion
- Associated suspicious mass central to architectural distortion

- Distortion alone (without a central mass) may be better diagnosed with excisional rather than percutaneous biopsy

Top Differential Diagnoses
- Post-Surgical Scar
- Fat Necrosis
- Infiltrating Ductal Carcinoma (IDC)
- Radial Scar (Radial Sclerosing Lesion, RSL)
- Infiltrating Lobular Carcinoma (ILC)
- Normal Overlapping Breast Tissues

Diagnostic Checklist
- Judicious use of prior mammograms for comparison may aid in the identification of subtle features and slowly growing lesions
- Stability of suspicious findings is not reassuring

- Magnification views (CC, ML or LM) to characterize associated Ca++
- US can help depict associated mass, guide biopsy
- Evaluate for additional associated findings: Skin thickening, nipple retraction, lymphadenopathy
- MRI may be helpful for further evaluation of vague architectural distortion, one view only, occult on US
- Length of radiating spicules may suggest possibility of radial scar [radial sclerosing lesion, (RSL)]
  - Long, > 1 cm radiating lines without an obvious central dense mass may suggest, but is not diagnostic
  - Short radiating lines emanating from a central density more suggestive of infiltrating carcinoma

Ultrasonographic Findings
- Grayscale Ultrasound
  - Thickening and tethering of Cooper ligaments
  - Associated suspicious mass central to architectural distortion
  - Post-surgical scar
    - Track to overlying skin incision
    - Fluid collection can be present for years
    - Concave borders
  - Optimize technique
    - Turn off spatial compounding to better depict posterior features
  - Helpful in assessment of areas less accessible to mammography positioning
    - Far lateral (axillary tail); far medial (upper inner quadrant)
  - Evaluate suspicious lymph nodes
    - Increase in cortex/fatty hilum ratio; bulging convex cortical contour
    - Frank loss of fatty hilum
    - Consider fine needle aspiration or core biopsy to aid staging

MR Findings
- T1WI
  - May demonstrate tissue distortion
  - Check for central bright signal suggestive of fat necrosis (or hemorrhage)

- Overlying skin thickening, skin retraction easily seen
- T2WI
  - Bright signal may be visible in post-operative seroma sites for months to years
  - Post-surgical and/or post-radiation edema: Dilated lymphatics hyperintense
- T1 C+
  - Spiculated enhancement or distortion around enhancing lesion
  - Distorted post-biopsy scar
    - Normal scar can enhance for up to 18 months, sometimes longer
    - Thin rim (≤ 4 mm) of enhancement around seroma is usually granulation tissue
    - Lack of enhancement is reassuring, nearly 100% NPV
    - Recurrent or residual tumor: Irregular, enhancing mass most common

Biopsy
- Percutaneous core biopsy
  - Distortion alone (without a central mass) may be better diagnosed with excisional rather than percutaneous biopsy
  - US-guided core biopsy effective if associated mass

Imaging Recommendations
- Best imaging tool: Mammography with spot compression and/or magnification
- Additional mammographic views if not explained by prior surgery
- US correlation to identify associated mass and direct biopsy
- MRI may aid in problem solving for both malignant and benign disease findings
  - Aid in confirming findings seen on only one mammographic view
  - Establish extent of disease, contralateral occult disease in cases of malignant findings
  - Differentiate scar from tumor

ARCHITECTURAL DISTORTION

DIFFERENTIAL DIAGNOSIS

Post-Surgical Scar
- Correlation with historical location of prior surgery crucial
- Distortion extends to overlying skin
- Typically irregular, hypoechoic mass on US (appearance nonspecific; may be indistinguishable from carcinoma)
- Stabilizes or becomes less conspicuous with time; may develop dystrophic Ca++, usually after several years
- Most will not enhance on MR > 18 months post-operatively
  - Some scars enhance over a much longer time period

Fat Necrosis
- History of trauma, prior biopsy or surgery: Including reduction mammoplasty
- Spiculation surrounding lucent center rather than a frank mass
- Overlapping appearance with radial scar, infiltrating carcinoma

Infiltrating Ductal Carcinoma (IDC)
- Often presents as spiculated or indistinctly marginated mass with or without associated architectural distortion
- Spiculations without central mass may be infiltrating cancer
- Associated suspicious Ca++ increase possibility of the presence of IDC, can be in associated DCIS component

Radial Scar (Radial Sclerosing Lesion, RSL)
- Often presents as spiculations without central mass
  - Cannot reliably differentiate from carcinoma on imaging findings alone
- Often excised for accurate diagnosis; up to 25% associated with DCIS, tubular carcinoma

Infiltrating Lobular Carcinoma (ILC)
- Growth pattern (single file cells) often results in more subtle findings than IDC
- Spiculated mass most common mammographic appearance
- May present as isolated architectural distortion
- Can be seen on only one mammographic view, more often CC
- Ca++ rare
- US can help depict subtle ILC

Normal Overlapping Breast Tissues
- Resolves with spot compression/additional imaging

Other Benign Causes
- Sclerosing adenosis: Benign proliferative process with fibrosis
  - Associated distortion usually due to associated RSL
- Focal fibrosis; fibromatosis
- Diabetic mastopathy: Long history; usually type I, insulin dependent
- Hematoma: History of trauma, anticoagulation

PATHOLOGY

General Features
- Etiology: When malignant, radiating spicules suggest stromal invasion

Gross Pathologic & Surgical Features
- Area of focal fibrotic distortion
- Frank spiculated mass

Microscopic Features
- Low power shows radiation of linear collagenous fibrosis from central area or lesion

CLINICAL ISSUES

Presentation
- Most common signs/symptoms
  - Post-operative surveillance mammogram
  - Asymptomatic screening mammogram
  - Palpable thickening or mass

Natural History & Prognosis
- Distortion from scarring worst on first post treatment mammograms

Treatment
- Based on lesion histology
- Radial scar presenting as architectural distortion merits excision after core biopsy
  - 4-12% rate of malignancy at excision

DIAGNOSTIC CHECKLIST

Image Interpretation Pearls
- Judicious use of prior mammograms for comparison may aid in the identification of subtle features and slowly growing lesions
- Stability of suspicious findings is not reassuring
- Avoid satisfaction of search
  - Additional findings may be present either within or adjacent to areas of distortion

SELECTED REFERENCES

1. D'Orsi CJ et al: Breast Imaging Reporting and Data System: BI-RADS, Mammography, 4th ed. Reston, American College of Radiology, 2003
2. Mendelson EB et al: Breast Imaging Reporting and Data System: BI-RADS, Ultrasound, 1st ed. Reston, American College of Radiology, 2003
3. Brenner RJ et al: Percutaneous core needle biopsy of radial scars of the breast: when is excision necessary? AJR. 179:1179-84, 2002
4. Krishnamurthy R et al: Mammographic findings after breast conservation therapy. Radiographics. 19 Spec No:S53-62; quiz S262-3, 1999
5. Venta LA et al: Imaging features of focal breast fibrosis: mammographic-pathologic correlation of noncalcified breast lesions. AJR. 73:309-16, 1999

ARCHITECTURAL DISTORTION

IMAGE GALLERY

Typical

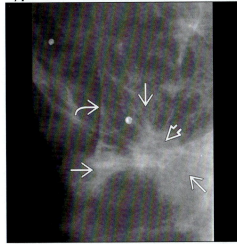 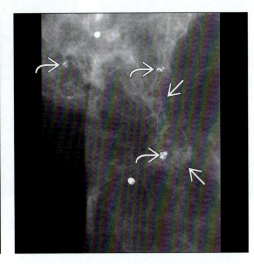

(Left) CC mammography magnification 4 years after lumpectomy and radiation shows the lumpectomy site to be distorted ➡ with central lucency ➡. Skin thickening ➡ at the incision site is present. *(Right)* CC mammography magnification (same case as left-hand image) 5 years post treatment demonstrates distortion ➡ now with an increase in coarse and dystrophic calcifications ➡. Findings are typical of benign post-surgical scar.

Typical

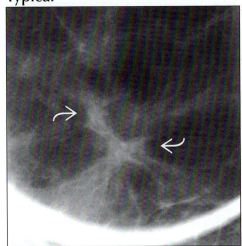 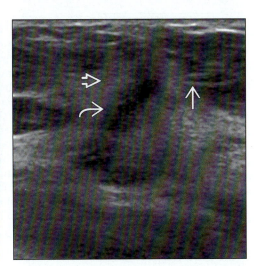

(Left) Lateral mammography magnification of a palpable thickening shows an area of architectural distortion ➡ in a 49 yo woman without history of prior surgery or trauma. US (right-hand image) was performed. *(Right)* Radial spatial compounding ultrasound shows an irregular vertically oriented hypoechoic mass ➡ with an irregular echogenic rim ➡ and associated tethering of Cooper ligaments ➡. US-guided biopsy = ILC.

Typical

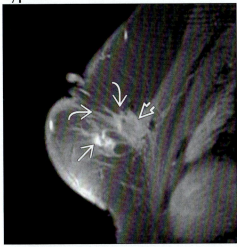 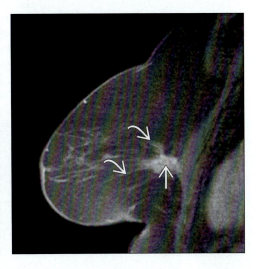

(Left) Sagittal T1 C+ FS MR shows distortion ➡ and an enhancing mass ➡ anterior to post-surgical site ➡ 18 months after lumpectomy and radiation. Biopsy of the enhancing mass = IDC. *(Right)* Sagittal T1 C+ FS MR shows distortion ➡ and abnormal enhancement of a lumpectomy scar ➡ 10 years after treatment. US-guided core = fibrosis which was discordant. Excisional biopsy = recurrent IDC.

ASYMMETRIES

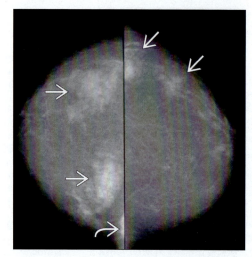

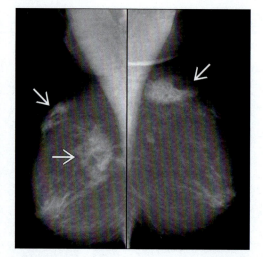

CC mammograms shows scattered focal & global asymmetries ➡ containing interspersed fat, compatible with normal variant, seen also on MLO views (next image). Note normal variant sternalis muscle ➡.

MLO views again show scattered focal and global asymmetries ➡, compatible with normal variant. On baseline study, short-interval follow-up can be considered. When stable, these are benign findings.

TERMINOLOGY

Abbreviations and Synonyms
- Focal density = focal asymmetry
- Developing density, neodensity = new focal asymmetry

Definitions
- Focal asymmetry = focal density on mammography, lacking the borders, conspicuity, and three-dimensionality of a mass
- Global asymmetry = regional or diffuse increase in density in one breast compared to similar area in opposite breast
- Not related to congenital asymmetry in breast size

IMAGING FINDINGS

General Features
- Location: Normal variant asymmetries most common in axillary tail of breast

Mammographic Findings
- Focal asymmetry
  - Present in one or both views
  - Spot compression views if new or increasing
  - Step oblique, rolled views, true lateral view can help in further evaluation
  - US may show suspicious mass or normal variant
- Global asymmetry
  - If palpable, merits further evaluation with spot compression, US
- Clinical findings, history, prior films needed
- Evaluate for associated suspicious calcifications or architectural distortion
- Additional imaging may reveal an underlying mass

Ultrasonographic Findings
- Grayscale Ultrasound
  - Normal variant can appear echogenic or mixed hyper- and isoechoic to fat
  - Hypoechoic mass suspicious for malignancy
  - Other findings depend on etiology, e.g., abscess, fat necrosis

DDx: Associated Findings

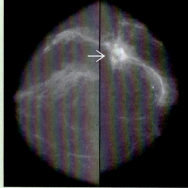

Architectural Distortion (IDC)

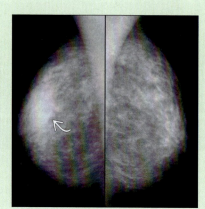

Palpable, IDC

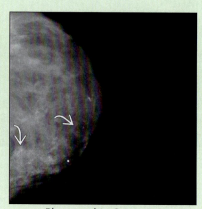

Pleomorphic Ca++, EIC

ASYMMETRIES

Key Facts

Terminology
- Focal asymmetry = focal density on mammography, lacking the borders, conspicuity, and three-dimensionality of a mass
- Global asymmetry = regional or diffuse increase in density in one breast compared to similar area in opposite breast

Imaging Findings
- Comparison to prior mammograms critical
- Developing asymmetries require explanation and often additional imaging
- Associated architectural distortion or suspicious calcifications generally prompt biopsy

Top Differential Diagnoses
- Normal Variant

- Summation Artifact
- Hormonal Influences
- Infiltrating Ductal Carcinoma (IDC)
- Infiltrating Lobular Carcinoma (ILC)
- Inflammatory Carcinoma
- Post-Surgical, Post-Radiation Changes
- Infection

Pathology
- Usually summation artifact or normal variant
- 20% of neodensities due to malignancy
- Present on 3-5% of screening mammograms
- 10% of women have normal variant tissue in axillary tail of Spence, often asymmetric

Diagnostic Checklist
- Common cause of missed cancer on screening

MR Findings
- T1WI
  - Soft tissue with interspersed fat (high signal)
  - Mimics mammographic findings
- T2WI FS: May show mild increased signal due to edema in premenopausal patients and women on hormones
- T1 C+ FS
  - Normal variant may show enhancement, usually gradual and persistent, similar to other parenchyma
  - Best to image on days 7 to 10 of menstrual cycle to avoid false positive enhancement
  - Enhancement depends on underlying etiology: Malignancy, infection, fat necrosis can all enhance

Imaging Recommendations
- Best imaging tool: Comparison mammograms, additional mammographic views
- Protocol advice
  - Comparison to prior mammograms critical
  - Developing asymmetries require explanation and often additional imaging
    - Spot compression views helpful
    - If seen only on CC view, rolled CC views to displace onto fatty area of breast
    - If seen only on MLO view, true lateral view to triangulate
    - Tangential view of palpable findings to identify overlying skin thickening or retraction
    - Targeted US if finding persists or is suspicious on initial views
  - Clinical breast examination (CBE) directed to global asymmetries helps guide management
  - Associated architectural distortion or suspicious calcifications generally prompt biopsy

DIFFERENTIAL DIAGNOSIS

Normal Variant
- Contains interspersed fat
- Usually nonpalpable

- Stable compared to prior mammograms
- Tail of Spence (axillary tail) most common
- Sternalis muscle
  - Focal, usually triangular asymmetry medial posterior breast on CC view only
  - 8% of patients, bilateral in 30%

Summation Artifact
- One view only, due to superimposed normal structures
- Thins on spot compression

Hormonal Influences
- Combined estrogen and progesterone (HRT) therapy
  - 21-43% of patients develop increased density
  - Can be focal or generalized and bilateral
  - Reduces mammographic sensitivity
  - Can discontinue HRT, repeat mammogram 6-8 weeks later
- Endogenous in perimenopausal patients
- Lactation, pregnancy usually generalized increase in density

Stromal Fibrosis
- Usually echogenic or mixed hyper-, hypoechoic on US

Infiltrating Ductal Carcinoma (IDC)
- Developing focal asymmetry
- May have associated architectural distortion or suspicious calcifications
- Persists on spot compression, hypoechoic mass on US

Infiltrating Lobular Carcinoma (ILC)
- Developing focal asymmetry
- Associated architectural distortion common
- Persists on spot compression, hypoechoic mass on US

Ductal Carcinoma in Situ (DCIS)
- Uncommon cause of focal asymmetries
- Usually has associated calcifications
  - Areas of asymmetry may reflect invasive component with extensive DCIS [extensive intraductal component, (EIC)]

Inflammatory Carcinoma
- Associated skin thickening, peau d'orange
- Associated trabecular thickening, adenopathy
- Punch biopsy of skin should confirm diagnosis

Post-Surgical, Post-Radiation Changes
- Most prominent on first post-surgical exam, focal at site of surgery, should decrease on follow-up
- Global asymmetry due to edema, with trabecular and skin thickening
- May develop calcifications due to fat necrosis, usually at least two years after surgery

Infection
- Associated erythema, tenderness, skin thickening
- Mastitis: Focal or global asymmetry due to edema
  - Should improve with 2 week course of antibiotics directed to skin organisms
- Abscess: Usually discrete hypo- or hyperechoic collection on US
- May show ipsilateral adenopathy

Other Edema
- Trabecular thickening
- Increased echogenicity and dilated lymphatics on US
- Congestive heart failure, anasarca, fluid overload
  - Usually bilateral, can be asymmetric when lie one side down preferentially
- Lymphatic or vascular obstruction, e.g., mass in axilla

Trauma
- Appropriate history should be present
- Associated edema, fluid collections, fat necrosis

Fibroadenolipoma (Hamartoma)
- Contains interspersed fat, encapsulated

Gynecomastia
- Male patient, flame-shaped density behind nipple
- 70% unilateral, and if bilateral, usually asymmetric

PATHOLOGY

General Features
- Etiology
  - Usually summation artifact or normal variant
  - Differential includes neoplastic, infectious, traumatic causes, HRT
  - 20% of neodensities due to malignancy
- Epidemiology
  - Present on 3-5% of screening mammograms
  - 10% of women have normal variant tissue in axillary tail of Spence, often asymmetric

CLINICAL ISSUES

Presentation
- Most common signs/symptoms: Incidental finding on mammography
- Other signs/symptoms: Associated suspicious clinical or imaging findings should prompt biopsy

Natural History & Prognosis
- Depends on underlying etiology

DIAGNOSTIC CHECKLIST

Consider
- Common cause of missed cancer on screening

Image Interpretation Pearls
- Interspersed fat favors normal variant
- Comparison to prior mammograms recommended

SELECTED REFERENCES

1. Gozzi G et al: Screening mammography interpretation test: more frequent mistakes. Radiol Med (Torino). 109:268-79, 2005
2. Shah NR et al: Postmenopausal hormone therapy and breast cancer: a systematic review and meta-analysis. Menopause. 12:668-78, 2005
3. D'Orsi CJ et al: Breast Imaging Reporting and Data System: BI-RADS, Mammography, 4th ed. Reston, American College of Radiology, 2003
4. Shetty MK et al: Sonographic evaluation of focal asymmetric density of the breast. Ultrasound Q. 18:115-21, 2002
5. Brenner J: Asymmetric densities of the breast: strategies for imaging evaluation. Semin Roentgenol. 36:201-16, 2001
6. Cheung KL et al: Palpable asymmetrical thickening of the breast: a clinical, radiological and pathological study. Br J Radiol. 74:402-6, 2001
7. Colacurci N et al: Effects of different types of hormone replacement therapy on mammographic density. Maturitas. 40:159-64, 2001
8. Rutter CM et al: Changes in breast density associated with initiation, discontinuation, and continuing use of hormone replacement therapy. JAMA. 285:171-6, 2001
9. Kushwaha AC et al: Primary inflammatory carcinoma of the breast: Retrospective review of mammographic findings. AJR. 174:535-8, 2000
10. Pearson KL et al: Efficacy of step-oblique mammography for confirmation and localization of densities seen on only one standard mammographic view. AJR. 174:745-52, 2000
11. Hussain HK et al: The significance of new densities and microcalcification in the second round of breast screening. Clin Radiol. 54:243-7, 1999
12. Lee CH et al: Clinical usefulness of MR imaging of the breast in the evaluation of the problematic mammogram. AJR. 173:1323-9, 1999
13. Sickles EA: Findings at mammographic screening on only one standard projection: outcomes analysis. Radiology. 208:471-5, 1998
14. DiPiro PJ et al: Seat belt injuries of the breast: findings on mammography and sonography. AJR. 164:317-320, 1995
15. Cyrlak D et al: Mammographic changes in postmenopausal women undergoing hormonal replacement therapy. AJR. 161:1177-83, 1993
16. Harvey JA et al: Previous mammograms in patients with impalpable breast carcinoma: retrospective vs blinded interpretation. AJR. 161:1167-72, 1993
17. Mendelson EB: Evaluation of the postoperative breast. Radiol Clin North Am. 30:107-38, 1992
18. Mendelson EB et al: Infiltrating lobular carcinoma: mammographic patterns with pathologic correlation. AJR. 153:265-71, 1989
19. Adler DD et al: Accessory breast tissue in the axilla: mammographic appearance. Radiology. 163:709-11, 1987

ASYMMETRIES

IMAGE GALLERY

Typical

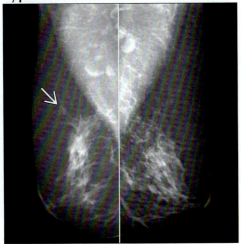 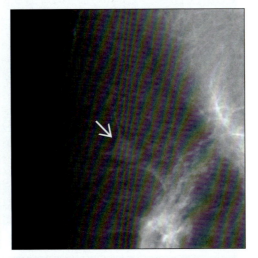

(Left) MLO mammography shows focal asymmetry ➡ upper right breast, seen only on the MLO view, new compared to prior study obtained 2 years earlier. (Same patient as next 3 images). *(Right)* MLO mammography spot compression shows persistence of the focal asymmetry ➡ noted on MLO view (left-hand image). Developing asymmetries are suspicious and merit further evaluation.

Typical

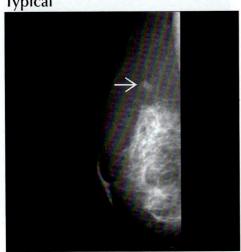 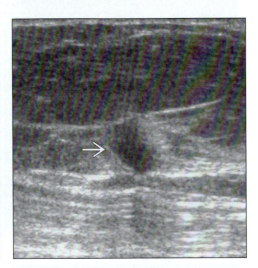

(Left) Lateral mammography shows the finding to be an ill-defined mass ➡ in the upper right breast, not visible on the CC or XCCL projection. By triangulation this would be in the 12:00 position. US was performed (right-hand image). *(Right)* Radial ultrasound shows vertically-oriented, indistinctly-marginated hypoechoic mass ➡ at 12:00 position, corresponding to the mammographic asymmetry. Biopsy showed grade I IDC.

Typical

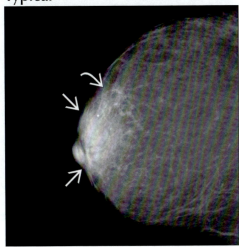 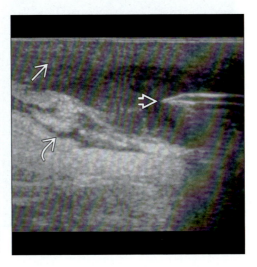

(Left) CC mammography shows global asymmetry ➡, skin thickening, and trabecular thickening ➡ in the anterior breast in this diabetic patient with a tender palpable mass at the nipple. US was performed (right-hand image). *(Right)* Radial ultrasound shows skin thickening ➡, diffuse increased echogenicity due to edema, dilated lymphatics ➡, and a hypoechoic abscess collection which is being drained under US guidance (➡ shows needle tip).

Typical

(Left) MLO mammography shows focal asymmetry upper left breast ➽ developing in this woman who began HRT one month earlier. *(Right)* MLO mammography prior to initiation of HRT (same patient as left-hand image) shows minimal scattered fibroglandular density with minimal underlying focal asymmetry ➽ which became more prominent with HRT.

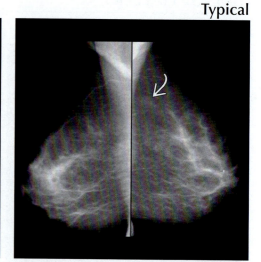

Typical

(Left) MLO mammography obtained three years later (same patient as previous image) shows diffuse bilateral progression of HRT-induced increase in parenchymal density. *(Right)* CC mammography in a woman who had sustained a motor vehicle accident shows band-like asymmetry in the inner left breast ➽, seen also on MLO views (next image).

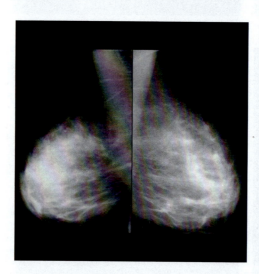

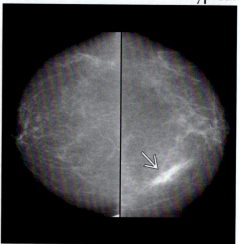

Typical

(Left) MLO mammography shows the band-like asymmetry to spread out in the upper left breast ➽. US was performed for further evaluation (right-hand image). *(Right)* Radial ultrasound shows increased echogenicity superficially ➽ with a central echogenic mass ➽ containing a tiny anechoic collection ➽, compatible with fat necrosis.

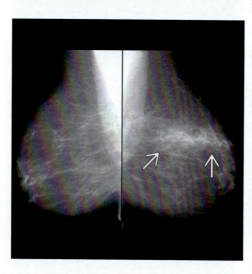

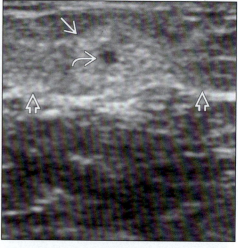

ASYMMETRIES

Typical

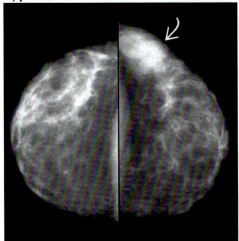 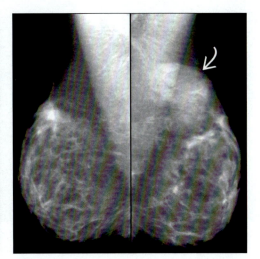

(Left) CC mammography shows global asymmetry ⇥ outer left breast, seen also on MLO view (right-hand image). *(Right)* MLO mammography shows the global asymmetry ⇥ to be in the upper posterior left breast. Because this was palpable, spot compression and US were performed (see next 2 images).

Typical

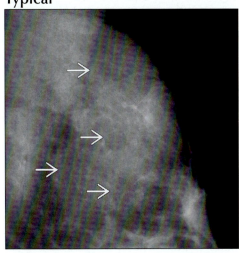 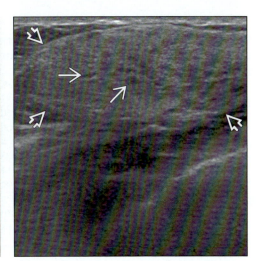

(Left) MLO mammography spot compression of the asymmetry (previous image) shows persistent asymmetry with interspersed fat ⇥ evident both mammographically and sonographically (right-hand image). *(Right)* Anti-radial ultrasound shows ovoid hyperechoic mass ⇥ with interspersed fat ⇥. The appearance is consistent with normal variant fibrotic tissue, confirmed on biopsy performed due to clinical concern.

Typical

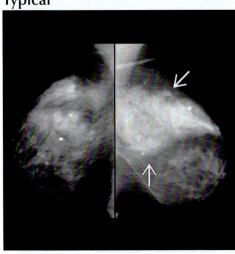 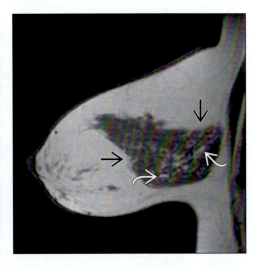

(Left) MLO mammography shows global asymmetry upper left breast ⇥ which had been stable for over 2 years. MR was performed (right-hand image). *(Right)* Sagittal T1WI MR shows concave tissue ⇥ with interspersed fat ⇥. No abnormal enhancement was seen on post-contrast images, compatible with normal variant.

TRABECULAR THICKENING

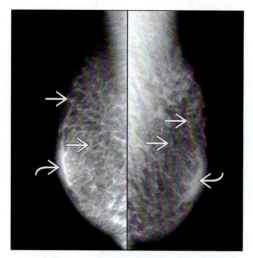

MLO mammography shows diffuse bilateral trabecular thickening ➡ in this 68 year old male with congestive heart failure and fluid overload. Gynecomastia is present ➡.

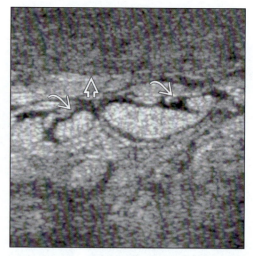

Transverse ultrasound in a 70 year old woman with CHF shows diffuse increased echogenicity, dilated lymphatics ➡, and skin thickening ➡.

TERMINOLOGY

Abbreviations and Synonyms
- Trabecular coarsening
- Synonymous with the generic imaging findings of edema

Definitions
- Linear/reticular coarsening of fibrous septae including Cooper ligaments
- Typically associated with generalized increase in breast density and skin thickening

IMAGING FINDINGS

General Features
- Location: Diffuse or focal
- The diagnostic dilemma is between benign inflammatory process and inflammatory cancer

Mammographic Findings
- Coarsening of trabecular markings

- ○ Trabecular thickness can be compared to the contralateral breast or to same area on prior mammograms
- ○ Detection may be difficult due to subtle changes
- Edema-related diffuse increased density typically pronounced around areola and dependent portions of the breast(s)
- Associated skin thickening (> 2 mm) is common
- Assess for associated mass, suspicious calcifications, architectural distortion
- Evaluate for adenopathy
- Density in the treated breast should be worst on first post-treatment mammogram and decrease thereafter
  - ○ Increasing density may suggest recurrence

Ultrasonographic Findings
- Grayscale Ultrasound
  - ○ Findings are not specific for inflammatory or tumoral infiltration
    - Generalized increased echogenicity due to edema
    - Dilated anechoic branching lymphatic channels
  - ○ May identify mammographically occult mass or underlying abscess
    - US-guided biopsy or aspiration/drainage

DDx: Causes of Trabecular Thickening

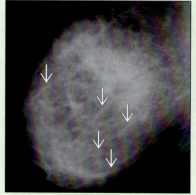

Inflammatory Cancer

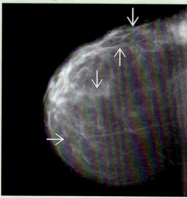

Mastitis

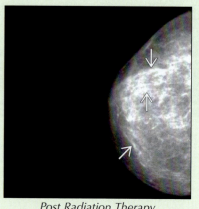

Post Radiation Therapy

TRABECULAR THICKENING

Key Facts

Terminology
- Linear/reticular coarsening of fibrous septae including Cooper ligaments

Imaging Findings
- Location: Diffuse or focal
- The diagnostic dilemma is between benign inflammatory process and inflammatory cancer
- Coarsening of trabecular markings
- Trabecular thickness can be compared to the contralateral breast or to same area on prior mammograms

Top Differential Diagnoses
- Generalized body edema
- Venous thrombosis
- Obstruction of lymphatic drainage

- Acute infection/mastitis
- Post surgical
- Post radiation therapy
- Inflammatory breast cancer (T4d)
- Invasive lobular cancer
- Locally recurrent breast cancer
- Hematoma, fat necrosis

Pathology
- Etiology: Trabecular thickening is most often due to dilated lymphatics from edema

Diagnostic Checklist
- Density in the treated breast should decrease on follow-up
- Increasing density at lumpectomy site may be due to recurrence

- ○ Evaluate axillary nodes
  - US-guided FNAB of suspicious node
  - If lymphoma is being considered, core biopsy specimen should be placed in saline for processing
- Color Doppler: Increased flow is not specific: Occurs in inflammation and in diffusely infiltrating tumor

MR Findings
- T2WI FS: Trabeculae show increased signal intensity due to edema
- T1 C+
  - ○ Trabecular and skin enhancement together with trabecular thickening: Principal etiologies
    - Tumoral infiltration, e.g., inflammatory carcinoma
    - True inflammation
  - ○ DCIS may show clumped, ductal enhancement
  - ○ Invasive cancer: Mass with rapid enhancement and washout or plateau kinetics
  - ○ Recurrent tumor usually enhances
  - ○ Normally no enhancement of scar on MR after 18 months post treatment
    - Rarely fat necrosis can enhance for years
- Inversion Recovery FSE: Similar to findings on T2WI

Nuclear Medicine Findings
- PET
  - ○ Malignancy and inflammatory conditions show FDG uptake
  - ○ Can help distinguish scar from recurrent tumor
  - ○ Dedicated breast PET: Improved resolution and sensitivity

DIFFERENTIAL DIAGNOSIS

Bilateral
- Edema
  - ○ Generalized body edema
    - Congestive heart failure (CHF), volume overload, peripheral edema (Anasarca)
    - Hypoalbuminemia (renal failure and hepatic failure)

  - ○ Venous thrombosis
    - Superior vena cava, subclavian vein or axillary vein thrombosis
  - ○ Obstruction of lymphatic drainage
    - Lymphoma: Enlarged axillary lymph nodes, can be unilateral
    - Metastatic disease in axillary lymph node(s): Often unilateral
    - Benign enlargement of axillary nodes (reactive to infection or inflammation)
    - Mechanical obstruction (e.g., pacemaker)
- Unilaterality or asymmetry of the finding of trabecular thickening and edema still may support the diagnosis of a systemic problem
- Bilateral (inflammatory) breast cancer: Very rare

Unilateral
- All the etiologies that cause bilateral disease may occur unilaterally or asymmetrically
- Acute infection/mastitis
  - ○ Tender, erythematous breast, skin thickening
  - ○ Most common near nipple, lactating breast
  - ○ Staphylococcus aureus (most common), or Staphylococcus epidermidis
  - ○ US can help depict underlying abscess
- Post treatment changes
  - ○ Post surgical
    - Excisional biopsy for benign conditions: Often resolves completely
    - Lumpectomy for cancer
    - Axillary dissection (causes diminished lymphatic drainage)
  - ○ Post radiation therapy
    - Diffuse radiation-induced trabecular thickening is seen secondary to edema within weeks after beginning of radiation therapy
    - Focal scarring and fibrosis months after radiation therapy, may increase up to 3 years and then attains stability
    - Accelerated partial breast irradiation: Focal scarring and fibrosis are more prominent and diffuse thickening is less frequent
  - ○ Radiation recall

TRABECULAR THICKENING

- Appears as acute radiation reaction in a previously irradiated field triggered by drugs (cytotoxics and other drugs, such as tamoxifen)
- Skin biopsy might be necessary for definitive diagnosis
- Breast cancer
  - Inflammatory breast cancer (T4d)
    - Peau d'orange, erythema
    - Up to two thirds of affected patients show trabecular thickening on mammography
    - Axillary adenopathy frequent
    - Diagnosis by punch biopsy of skin: Tumor emboli detected in dermis
    - US to depict associated mass, guide biopsy if dermal biopsy nondiagnostic
    - Despite the name, not associated with any significant inflammatory cell infiltration
    - Dermal lymphatic invasion without characteristic clinical picture is insufficient to qualify as inflammatory breast cancer
  - Pregnancy-associated breast cancer
  - Invasive lobular cancer
  - Locally recurrent breast cancer
    - Trabecular thickening should decrease on post treatment follow-up
    - Increasing density at lumpectomy site or diffusely may suggest recurrence
- Lymphoma (diffuse breast infiltration is a rare manifestation of lymphoma)
- Hematoma, fat necrosis
  - Clinical history, ecchymosis
    - Trauma
    - Anticoagulation
    - Bleeding diathesis
- Chronic infection/mastitis
  - Granulomatous mastitis, including specific causes such as tuberculosis
  - Chronic bacterial
  - Hydatid disease
  - Syphilis
- Other benign entities
  - Amyloidosis

PATHOLOGY

General Features
- Etiology: Trabecular thickening is most often due to dilated lymphatics from edema

CLINICAL ISSUES

Presentation
- Most common signs/symptoms
  - Increasing breast size and firmness
  - Skin thickening (wheals or ridging of the skin; if extreme, peau d'orange)
- Other signs/symptoms
  - Erythema, pain: Mastitis vs. inflammatory carcinoma
  - Axillary adenopathy

- Mass, skin retraction, nipple retraction favor malignancy

Natural History & Prognosis
- Depends on underlying etiology

Treatment
- In patients with possible mastitis vs. inflammatory carcinoma
  - Two week course of antibiotics directed to skin organisms
  - Lack of response should prompt punch biopsy

DIAGNOSTIC CHECKLIST

Consider
- Look for associated imaging findings
  - Axillary lymphadenopathy
  - Associated mass, architectural distortion, suspicious calcifications favor malignancy
  - Skin or nipple retraction favor malignancy
- Clinical symptoms, prior history, treatment
  - Erythema, other signs of inflammation
  - Volume overload
  - Arteriosclerosis
  - Pacemaker

Image Interpretation Pearls
- Density in the treated breast should decrease on follow-up
  - Increasing density at lumpectomy site may be due to recurrence

SELECTED REFERENCES

1. Kwak JY et al: Unilateral breast edema: spectrum of etiologies and imaging appearances. Yonsei Med J. 46:1-7,2005
2. Singer EA et al: Tamoxifen-induced radiation recall dermatitis. Breast J. 10:170-1, 2004
3. Ahn BY et al: Pregnancy- and lactation-associated breast cancer: mammographic and sonographic findings. J Ultrasound Med. 22:491-7; quiz 498-9, 2003
4. D'Orsi CJ et al: Breast Imaging Reporting and Data System: BI-RADS, Mammography, 4th ed. Reston, American College of Radiology, 2003
5. Gunhan-Bilgen I et al: Inflammatory breast carcinoma: mammographic, ultrasonographic, clinical, and pathologic findings in 142 cases. Radiology. 223:829-38, 2002
6. Chung SY et al: Imaging findings of metastatic disease to the breast. Yonsei Med J. 42:497-502, 2001
7. Fu K et al: Mammographic findings of diffuse amyloidosis and carcinoma of the breast. AJR. 177:901-2, 2001
8. Philpotts LE et al: Mammographic findings of recurrent breast cancer after lumpectomy and radiation therapy: comparison with the primary tumor. Radiology. 201:767-71, 1996
9. Dershaw DD: Evaluation of the breast undergoing lumpectomy and radiation therapy. Radiol Clin North Am. 33:1147-60, 1995
10. Dershaw DD et al: Inflammatory breast carcinoma: mammographic findings. Radiology. 190:831-4, 1994
11. Mendelson EB: Evaluation of the postoperative breast. Radiol Clin North Am. 30:107-38, 1992

TRABECULAR THICKENING

IMAGE GALLERY

Typical

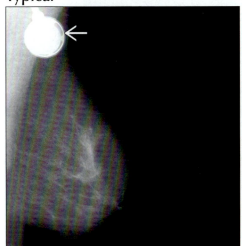

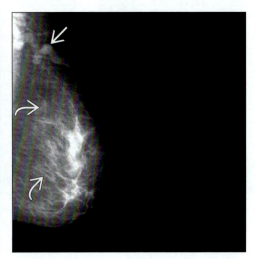

(Left) Left MLO view demonstrates the port ➡ of an indwelling subclavian catheter used for chemotherapy. *(Right)* MLO three years later (same patient as left-hand image), a left lateral mammogram demonstrates vascular dilatation ➡ and diffuse findings of breast edema including trabecular thickening ➡. There was subclavian vein occlusion, a complication related to the central venous catheter.

Typical

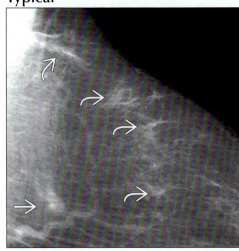

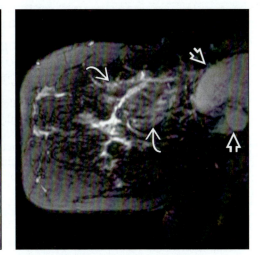

(Left) MLO mammography shows focal trabecular thickening in the upper outer left breast ➡. An ill-defined parenchymal mass was also seen ➡. *(Right)* On inversion recovery MR image (same patient as left-hand image), bulky adenopathy due to lymphoma was noted in the left axilla ➡. Edema was also seen in the upper outer left breast ➡, explaining the trabecular thickening seen mammographically.

Typical

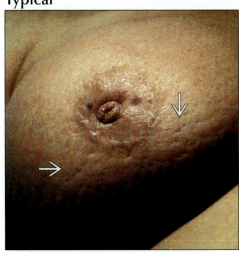

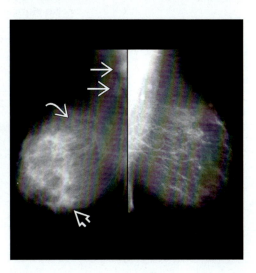

(Left) Clinical photograph of this 44 year old shows erythematous breast with peau d'orange ➡. *(Right)* MLO mammography (same patient as left-hand image) shows trabecular thickening ➡, ill-defined mass ➡, and axillary adenopathy on the right side ➡. Punch biopsy showed inflammatory carcinoma.

TUBULAR DENSITY

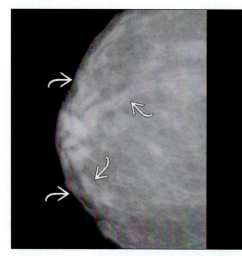

Bilateral CC mammograms show tubular densities representing dilated ducts ⇗ in the subareolar regions of both breasts.

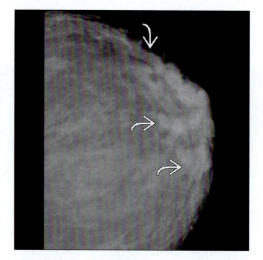

Subareolar ductal ectasia ⇗ is common, often bilateral, and can be dismissed as a benign finding in the absence of symptoms.

TERMINOLOGY

Abbreviations and Synonyms
• Tubular opacity, solitary dilated duct

Definitions
• Solitary dilated or branching soft tissue structure on mammogram

IMAGING FINDINGS

General Features
• Best diagnostic clue: Tubular or branching soft tissue density on mammography

Mammographic Findings
• Single or branching tubular structure(s)
• Evaluate for suspicious calcifications

Ultrasonographic Findings
• Grayscale Ultrasound
  ○ US indicated if new or associated nipple discharge
  ○ Dilated fluid-filled duct(s)
  ○ Evaluate for intraductal mass(es)

• Color Doppler: Distinguish vascular origin, intraluminal clot

MR Findings
• T1WI: Ducts may demonstrate high signal due to proteinaceous fluid
• T2WI FS
  ○ Fluid-filled ducts are bright
  ○ Ducts may show variable signal (fluid with variable protein content)
• T1 C+: Ductal carcinoma in situ (DCIS) may show nodular (clumped) or linear enhancement in ductal distribution

DIFFERENTIAL DIAGNOSIS

Duct Ectasia
• Dilated fluid-filled retroareolar duct(s)
• No clinical concern, BI-RADS 2, when asymptomatic, bilateral
• Possibly post-inflammatory, can develop secretory calcifications

DDx: Causes of Tubular Density

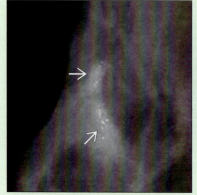

Ductal Carcinoma in Situ

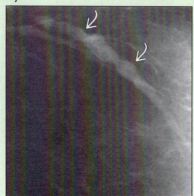

Mondor Disease

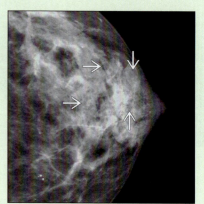

Fat Within Dilated Ducts

TUBULAR DENSITY

Key Facts

Terminology
- Solitary dilated or branching soft tissue structure on mammogram

Top Differential Diagnoses
- Duct Ectasia
- Ductal Carcinoma in Situ (DCIS)
- Papilloma(s)
- Abscess
- Fat Necrosis, Scar

- Mondor Disease
- Tortuous Vessel

Diagnostic Checklist
- Look for associated ductal calcifications
- Bilateral subareolar duct ectasia benign
- Asymptomatic solitary dilated duct benign or probably benign
- Intraductal mass or suspicious calcifications merit biopsy

Ductal Carcinoma in Situ (DCIS)
- Occasionally causes duct distention
- Often associated pleomorphic or fine linear Ca++

Papilloma(s)
- Intraductal mass(es)
- Nipple discharge
- May contain amorphous or punctate calcifications
- US useful when periareolar
- MR or galactography helpful when peripheral

Abscess
- Tender, possibly erythematous, edematous
- Mixed echogenicity collection on US

Fat Necrosis, Scar
- Post reduction mammoplasty scar, especially 6:00 axis
- Associated dermal calcifications

Mondor Disease
- Superficial thrombophlebitis
- Usually associated with pain and a palpable cord
- May see distended vein and sometimes intraluminal clot on US

Tortuous Vessel
- Collateral flow due to more central obstruction
- Arteriovenous fistula for dialysis, increased flow

Granulomatous Mastitis
- Tubular, nodular densities composed of collection of histiocytes, due to chronic inflammation

PATHOLOGY

General Features
- Etiology: Varies with cause of duct distention

DIAGNOSTIC CHECKLIST

Consider
- Look for associated ductal calcifications

Image Interpretation Pearls
- Bilateral subareolar duct ectasia benign
- Asymptomatic solitary dilated duct benign or probably benign
- Intraductal mass or suspicious calcifications merit biopsy

SELECTED REFERENCES

1. D'Orsi CJ et al: Breast Imaging Reporting and Data System: BI-RADS, Mammography, 4th ed. Reston, American College of Radiology, 2003
2. Yanik B et al: Imaging findings in Mondor's disease. J Clin Ultrasound. 31:103-7, 2003
3. Harris AT: Case 41: Ductal carcinoma in situ. Radiology. 221:770-3, 2001
4. Huynh PT et al: Dilated duct pattern at mammography. Radiology. 204:137-141, 1997
5. Sickles EA: Mammographic features of 300 consecutive nonpalpable breast cancers. AJR. 146:661-3, 1986

IMAGE GALLERY

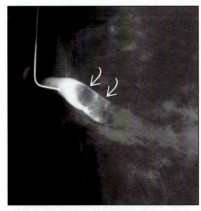
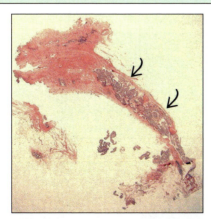
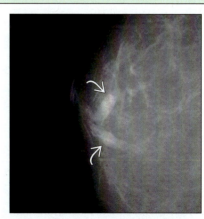

(Left) Galactography shows multiple papillomas, highlighted by contrast material ➤. Papillomas may cause tubular densities but more commonly appear as mass-like and nodular opacities. *(Center)* The patient underwent duct excision. Low power histopathology (H&E) shows multiple benign intraductal papillomas ➤. *(Right)* CC mammography from another woman shows two adjacent tubular structures in the retroareolar right breast ➤. US confirmed that the tubular structures are dilated ducts, a benign finding.

ANECHOIC (US)

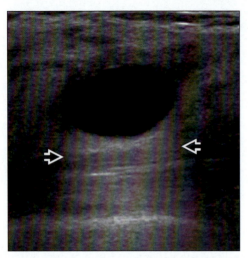

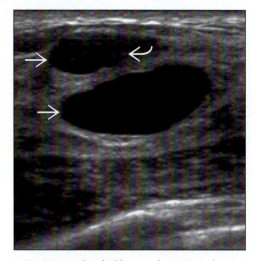

Ultrasound shows typical benign cyst: Circumscribed, anechoic mass with posterior enhancement ➡.

US in 30 yo with palpable mass shows 2 simple cysts ➡. Anterior cyst shows reverberation artifacts ➡ paralleling flat, anterior wall of cyst, recognized as artifactual by changing pressure & angle of insonation.

TERMINOLOGY

Abbreviations and Synonyms
- "Cystic" implies at least partially anechoic

Definitions
- Devoid of internal echoes (US)
  - Artifactual internal echoes can be present
  - Anterior reverberation artifact most common
- Distinguish from markedly hypoechoic (suspicious)

IMAGING FINDINGS

General Features
- Best diagnostic clue
  - Absence of any internal structure on US
  - With excess gain, may see homogeneous low level echoes due to protein content of cyst fluid
    - Any evidence of intracystic mass, irregular shape, or thick wall should prompt aspiration or biopsy

Mammographic Findings
- In woman 30 years old and over, CC and MLO mammograms should be obtained
- Mammogram in woman < 30 years of age with suspicious findings on US
- Evaluate mass margins
- Assess for multiplicity, bilaterality (favors benign)
- Identify any suspicious calcifications
  - CC and ML magnification views for further characterization
  - A mass containing calcifications is not anechoic

Ultrasonographic Findings
- Grayscale Ultrasound
  - Distinguish artifactual internal echoes from internal structure
    - Anterior reverberation artifact parallels anterior wall of structure
    - Deep (> 3 cm) cysts, especially < 8 mm in size, may appear hypoechoic
  - Distinguish markedly hypoechoic (suspicious) from anechoic (cystic)
  - Distinguish uniformly anechoic findings from complex cystic/solid or intraductal masses

DDx: Markedly Hypoechoic Masses

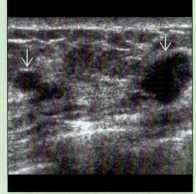

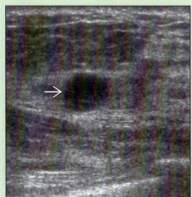

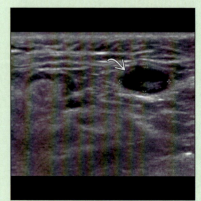

Multifocal ILC

Grade III IDC

Node, B-Cell Lymphoma

ANECHOIC (US)

Key Facts

Terminology
- "Cystic" implies at least partially anechoic
- Devoid of internal echoes (US)
- Artifactual internal echoes can be present
- Distinguish from markedly hypoechoic (suspicious)

Imaging Findings
- Anterior reverberation artifact parallels anterior wall of structure
- Deep (> 3 cm) cysts, especially < 8 mm in size, may appear hypoechoic
- Manage findings/mass based on worst features
- Absent internal flow in anechoic mass
- Appropriate gain: Fat appears medium gray throughout field of view
- Gentle compression to minimize breast thickness
- Document mass without calipers to evaluate margins

Top Differential Diagnoses
- Duct(s)
- Simple cyst
- Post-surgical seroma
- Cortex of reactive lymph node(s)
- High grade IDC can appear circumscribed, anechoic, with posterior enhancement
- Invasive lobular carcinoma (ILC)

Diagnostic Checklist
- Smaller lesions, < 8 mm, difficult to distinguish anechoic from hypoechoic
- Lower threshold for aspiration of smaller lesions, especially if new, palpable, or in high risk patient

○ Evaluate mass margins
- Circumscribed margin, imperceptible wall favors cyst
- Indistinct margin suspicious, as is thick wall to otherwise cystic lesion
○ Posterior features
- Enhancement nonspecific: Cysts, malignancies, other
○ Associated findings: Architectural distortion with post-surgical collection, malignancy
○ Manage findings/mass based on worst features
- Color Doppler
○ Absent internal flow in anechoic mass
○ Presence of flow suspicious for malignancy unless structure is a vessel

MR Findings
- T1WI
○ Fluid containing structures usually hypointense
○ Hyperintense: Proteinaceous fluid or blood
- T2WI FS: Hyperintense mass: Cyst, post-surgical collection, rarely malignancy
- T1 C+ FS
○ Cysts will not enhance
○ Thin rim (≤ 4 mm) of enhancement is within normal at edges of post-surgical collection
- Nodular or thicker enhancement may portend residual tumor if margins were positive
- Evaluate remainder of breast for additional suspicious findings if exam performed for positive margins

Imaging Recommendations
- Best imaging tool: US with proper technique
- Protocol advice
○ Optimize US technique
- Appropriate gain: Fat appears medium gray throughout field of view
- Time-gain compensation increases gradually with increasing depth
- Focal zone at lesion
- Gentle compression to minimize breast thickness

- Can artificially turn up gain to exclude internal mass, then adjust back down as appropriate
- Changing angle of insonation can reduce artifactual internal echoes
- Use of high frequency linear array transducers: Center frequency at least 10 MHz for detail of mass margins
- Document mass without calipers to evaluate margins
- Tissue harmonic imaging can help decrease artifactual internal echoes
- Transiently reducing center frequency to 5-7 MHz can help penetrate deeper cysts
- Posterior features better appreciated on fundamental imaging, without spatial compounding

DIFFERENTIAL DIAGNOSIS

Normal Anatomy
- Duct(s)
○ Tubular structure(s) near nipple
○ May be dilated as normal variant
- Blood vessels
○ Tubular structure
○ Color or power Doppler will show flow
- Lymphatics
○ Not normally visible on US
○ Edema
- Tubular, branching, fluid-filled lymphatics
- Skin thickening > 2 mm
- Trabecular thickening on mammography

Benign Findings
- Simple cyst
○ Circumscribed, imperceptible wall, posterior enhancement, and anechoic
○ Artifactual internal echoes can be seen
○ May be difficult to reliably characterize as anechoic when smaller than 8 mm
○ More difficult to characterize as anechoic with increasing depth, especially > 3 cm

ANECHOIC (US)

- Post-surgical seroma
  - Proper history
  - Granulation tissue at edges
  - Usually some internal septations or fluid-debris level
  - Track to overlying skin scar
- Fat necrosis
  - Fat necrosis typically mixed hyper- and anechoic mass
  - Surrounding edema
  - History of trauma or surgery
- Ruptured/inflamed cyst
  - Thick-walled, indistinct margins on US
  - Often a rim-enhancing mass on MR
    - Hyperintense on T2WI
    - Slow initial enhancement then persistent kinetics
    - Often in company of simple cysts
  - Can have fluid-debris level
- Sebaceous cyst
  - Skin lesion, usually mixed echogenicity
- Abscess
  - Tender, palpable mass, typically near nipple
  - Usually some internal echoes and/or debris
  - Thick and/or indistinct wall may be present
  - Aspirate for diagnosis and treatment; antibiotics directed to skin organisms
- Silicone "cyst"
  - Proper history: Silicone implants or injection silicone oil
  - Within areas of snowstorm appearance due to extracapsular silicone, small collections can appear anechoic
- Cortex of reactive lymph node(s)
  - Cortex can appear markedly hypoechoic
    - HIV
    - Sarcoid, psoriasis, rheumatoid arthritis, other inflammatory
    - Mastitis
  - Retain fatty hilum though it may be compressed
- Breast implants
  - Saline implant anechoic
    - Small amount of anechoic fluid adjacent to implant is normal
  - Silicone often appears anechoic in intact implant
    - Appears deeper than it really is due to slower speed of sound in silicone than tissue
    - Thick band of anterior reverberation artifact usually seen
    - Presence of internal echoes is nonspecific, can be seen in intact and ruptured implants
    - Radial folds of shell cause band-like internal echoes, a normal finding

Malignant Findings

- Invasive ductal carcinoma (IDC), NOS
  - Magnification views, US will usually reveal indistinct margins
  - High grade IDC can appear circumscribed, anechoic, with posterior enhancement
- Invasive lobular carcinoma (ILC)
  - Magnification views, US will usually reveal indistinct margins, irregular shape
- Metastatic adenopathy
  - Markedly hypoechoic, not anechoic

- Can have loss of fatty hilum, hypervascular
- Lymphoma
  - Lymphomatous nodes markedly hypoechoic
    - May or may not retain fatty hila
    - Usually bilateral, systemic disease

PATHOLOGY

General Features

- Etiology
  - Anechoic features result from lack of interfaces from which sound beam reflects
  - Lack of internal scattered and reflected waves; absence of internal texture or structure
  - Fluid in cysts can contain protein, desquamated cells, hemosiderin; particles often too small for reflection of sound wave

CLINICAL ISSUES

Presentation

- Most common signs/symptoms: Asymptomatic
- Other signs/symptoms: Palpable, often tender, mass

DIAGNOSTIC CHECKLIST

Consider

- Smaller lesions, < 8 mm, difficult to distinguish anechoic from hypoechoic
  - Lower threshold for aspiration of smaller lesions, especially if new, palpable, or in high risk patient
- The deeper the lesion, the less reliably it can be characterized as cystic

Image Interpretation Pearls

- Appropriate gain required to distinguish markedly hypoechoic masses (suspicious) from anechoic (cystic)
- Multiple, bilateral similar-appearing rounded masses favors benign etiology
- Careful attention to mass margins, with management based on most suspicious features

SELECTED REFERENCES

1. Berg WA et al: Lesion detection and characterization in a breast US phantom: results of the ACRIN 6666 investigators. Radiology. 239:693-702, 2006
2. Berg WA et al: Operator dependence of physician-performed whole breast sonography: lesion detection and characterization. Radiology in press, 2006
3. Berg WA et al: Cystic lesions of the breast: sonographic-pathologic correlation. Radiology. 227:183-91, 2003
4. Mendelson EB et al: Breast Imaging Reporting and Data System: BI-RADS, Ultrasound, 1st ed. Reston, American College of Radiology, 2003
5. Soo MS et al: Fat necrosis in the breast: sonographic features. Radiology. 206:261-9, 1998
6. Hilton SV et al: Real-time breast sonography: application in 300 consecutive patients. AJR. 147:479-86, 1986

ANECHOIC (US)

IMAGE GALLERY

Variant

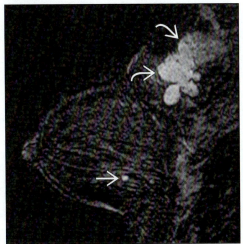
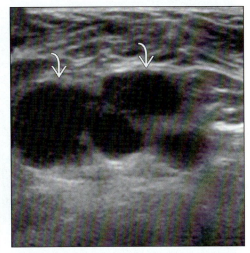

(Left) Sagittal T1 C+ subtraction MR in this 41 year old shows bulky, palpable, enhancing adenopathy ➡, proven metastatic consistent with breast primary. Small enhancing focus in the breast ➡ showed benign (fibrocystic changes). (Right) Ultrasound (same patient as on left) shows the lobulated masses ➡ in the axilla. These were misinterpreted as anechoic cysts, despite the presence of internal vascularity (which was described, below left).

Variant

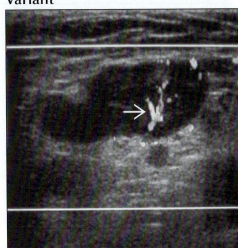
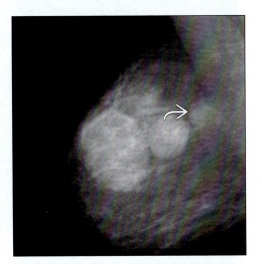

(Left) Color Doppler ultrasound shows internal vascularity ➡ within these markedly hypoechoic metastatic axillary nodes (same patient as above). (Right) MLO mammography in this 45 year old with known cysts shows multiple partially circumscribed, partially obscured masses (which were bilateral). One was tender ➡.

Variant

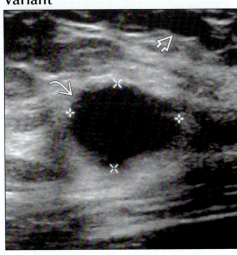
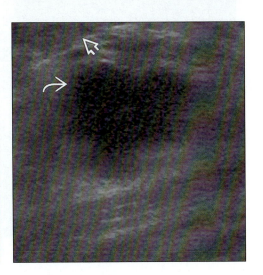

(Left) Initial US of tender mass (same as above right) shows apparently anechoic mass ➡ with posterior enhancement, interpreted as a cyst. FNA by a surgeon was suspicious. US was repeated (lower left). Note the fat appears black ➡. (Right) Follow-up US (same as on left) with proper contrast and gain shows the mass ➡ is hypoechoic with indistinct margins. US-guided core biopsy showed grade III IDC. Note that fat now appears appropriately medium gray ➡.

ANECHOIC (US)

(Left) Sagittal ultrasound in this 56 year old shows an irregular mass ➡ which was thought to be a cyst. In retrospect, there are a few internal echoes ➡, and the irregular shape is suspicious. Calipers on the images hamper evaluation of margins. *(Right)* Sagittal US, same image as on left with calipers edited out, more clearly demonstrates the irregular mass margins ➡. FNA showed suspicious cells. Biopsy confirmed IDC.

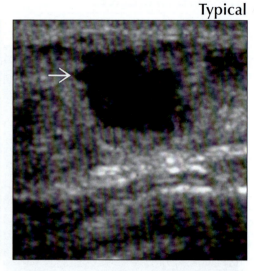

(Left) Radial ultrasound shows an anechoic, circumscribed simple cyst ➡ in another patient. *(Right)* Radial US (same mass as left-hand image) with excess gain shows minimal homogeneous low level echoes ➡. With current equipment, proteinaceous fluid in cysts can show such echoes, but there is no evidence of an intracystic mass or thick wall.

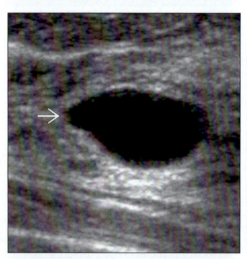
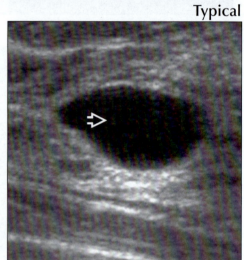

(Left) Ultrasound shows nearly anechoic dilated lymphatics ➡, skin thickening ➡, and diffuse increased background echogenicity, due to edema in this patient with congestive heart failure. *(Right)* Transverse ultrasound in this 55 year old shows anechoic dilated ducts ➡ near the nipple, a benign finding.

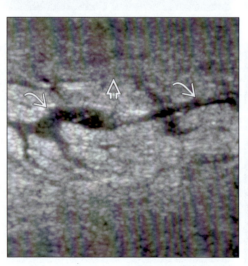
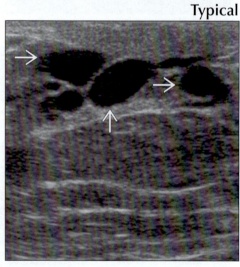

IV

1

142

Typical

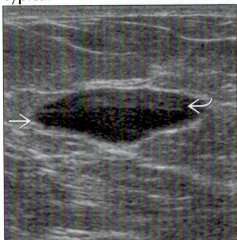 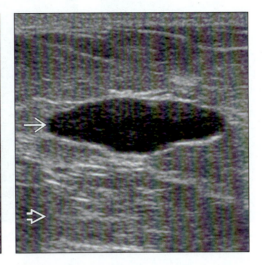

(Left) Transverse ultrasound shows a simple cyst ➡ with anterior reverberation artifact ➡. *(Right)* Transverse US (same lesion as left-hand image) with harmonic imaging applied shows reduction in artifactual internal echoes in the cyst ➡. Posterior enhancement is faintly seen ➡.

Variant

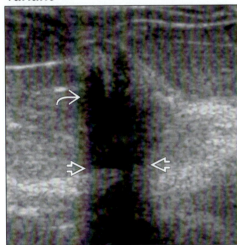 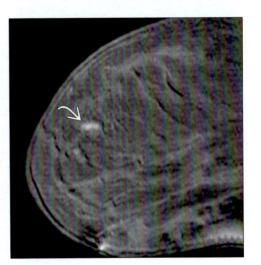

(Left) Radial ultrasound shows irregular, markedly hypoechoic mass ➡ with posterior shadowing ➡. Biopsy showed granular cell tumor, confirmed at excision. *(Right)* Sagittal T1 C+ FS MR in this 38 year old with clear nipple discharge and prior negative duct excision shows tubular enhancing mass ➡.

Typical

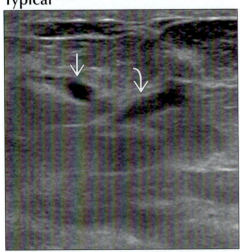 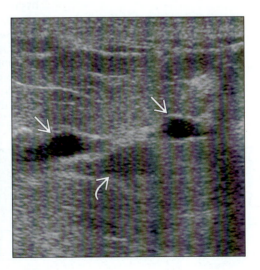

(Left) Transverse US directed to the MR abnormality (previous image) shows several adjacent ducts ➡. Minimal low level echoes in the deeper duct ➡ were felt to be artifactual. *(Right)* Transverse US (same as on left-hand image) with tissue harmonic imaging shows anechoic normal ducts ➡. The adjacent duct is now clearly hypoechoic ➡ and was felt to correspond to the MRI abnormality. US-guided biopsy showed papilloma.

HYPERECHOGENICITY (US)

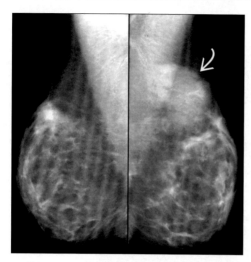

MLO mammography shows palpable global asymmetry axillary tail left breast ➡. US was performed (right-hand image).

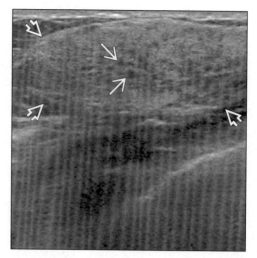

Anti-radial ultrasound shows oval, hyperechoic mass ➡ (containing minimal interspersed fat ➡), in area of mammographic asymmetry. US-guided core biopsy showed stromal fibrosis.

TERMINOLOGY

Abbreviations and Synonyms
- Hyperechoic, echogenic

Definitions
- Defined by US appearance: Increased echogenicity relative to fat
- Distinguish homogeneously hyperechoic from mixed hyper- and hypoechoic lesions
- Echogenic halo: Indistinct echogenic rim or transition zone between lesion and surrounding tissue
  - Distinguish from thin echogenic pseudocapsule (benign)
- Echogenic foci due to calcifications (Ca++) or other etiologies

IMAGING FINDINGS

General Features
- Best diagnostic clue: Brighter (whiter) than surrounding fat on US

Mammographic Findings
- Can show fatty nature of some hyperechoic masses
  - Fatty hilum in lymph nodes
  - Lipoma
  - Some fat necrosis
- Characterize Ca++ morphology
- Characterize mass with hyperechoic rim
  - Rim itself may have no mammographic correlate
- Trabecular thickening on mammography: Edema

Ultrasonographic Findings
- Grayscale Ultrasound
  - Assess homogeneity of echo pattern of hyperechoic masses
    - Homogeneously hyperechoic favors benign
    - Normal ducts and TDLUs within mass can appear hypoechoic (≤ 4 mm) yet mass still classified as homogeneously hyperechoic
    - Heterogeneous: Mixed hyper- and hypoechoic mass, indeterminate
  - Background hyperechogenicity due to edema
    - Dilated lymphatics
    - Skin thickening (> 2 mm)
  - Echogenic rim/halo

DDx: Mixed Hyper- and Hypoechoic Masses

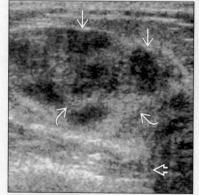

Non-Hodgkin Lymphoma

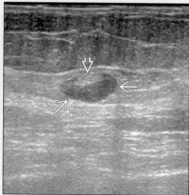

Benign Lymph Node

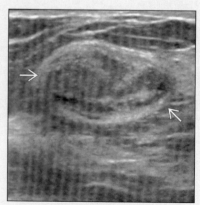

Stromal Fibrosis

HYPERECHOGENICITY (US)

Key Facts

Terminology
- Hyperechoic, echogenic
- Defined by US appearance: Increased echogenicity relative to fat
- Distinguish homogeneously hyperechoic from mixed hyper- and hypoechoic lesions
- Echogenic halo: Indistinct echogenic rim or transition zone between lesion and surrounding tissue
- Echogenic foci due to calcifications (Ca++) or other etiologies

Top Differential Diagnoses
- Focal atrophic breast tissue
- Lipoma
- Hemangioma
- Silicone granuloma

- Fat necrosis
- Focal fibrosis
- Benign lymph node
- Abscess
- Hamartoma/fibroadenolipoma
- Lymphoma or leukemia in breast
- Sarcomas
- Edema
- Ca++ within a suspicious mass favors IDC
- Ca++ within a duct favors ductal carcinoma in situ (DCIS)

Pathology
- 7% of benign masses are hyperechoic
- Nearly 100% NPV when homogeneously hyperechoic, circumscribed

- - Evaluate margins of underlying mass
  - Echogenic foci
    - Ca++: Determine location in duct or suspicious mass vs. parenchyma
    - US cannot characterize Ca++ morphology: Correlate with mammography
    - Cholesterol crystals mobile in complicated cysts
    - Clips from surgery or core biopsy
    - Air, will cause "dirty" shadowing, usually mobile when pressure applied
  - Evaluate for associated adenopathy
    - Lymphoma or leukemia
    - Metastatic adenopathy: Consider US-guided FNAB of suspicious node(s)
    - Mastitis or abscess
  - Normal Cooper ligaments are hyperechoic
- Color Doppler
  - Diffuse increased vascularity suggests inflammatory process
    - Mastitis, abscess, or inflammatory carcinoma

MR Findings
- T1WI
  - Fatty masses hyperintense on T1WI
    - Fatty hilum in lymph nodes
    - Lipoma
    - Some fat necrosis
- T2WI FS
  - Fatty masses hypointense
  - Edematous trabeculae hyperintense
- T1 C+
  - Fat necrosis can enhance at least up to 18 months following trauma or surgery and occasionally longer
  - Cortex of lymph nodes will enhance
  - Malignancies will enhance

Imaging Recommendations
- Best imaging tool: Ultrasound

DIFFERENTIAL DIAGNOSIS

Homogeneously Hyperechoic Mass
- Focal atrophic breast tissue
  - Concave, band-like
  - May correspond to mammographic asymmetry
  - Intensely hyperechoic
- Lipoma
  - Circumscribed, oval mass
  - Only slightly hyperechoic to adjacent fat
  - Fatty on mammography
- Hemangioma
  - Associated syndromes: Klippel-Trenaunay-Weber
  - Bluish pigmentation of skin, varicosities
- Silicone granuloma
  - Patient with history of silicone breast implant and extracapsular rupture
  - "Snowstorm" appearance with echodense noise deep to mass
- Angiolipoma

Heterogeneously Hyperechoic Mass
- Fat necrosis
  - History of trauma or surgery
  - Surrounding edema, skin thickening
  - Focal anechoic collections
  - Can develop Ca++, usually > 2 years after trauma
    - Rim Ca++ around oil cysts
  - Fat-containing on mammography
  - Track to overlying skin scar if post-surgical
- Focal fibrosis
  - Usually has interspersed fat (decreased echogenicity)
  - May have associated coarse heterogeneous calcifications
- Benign lymph node
  - Thin hypoechoic cortex
  - Echogenic hilum
- Abscess
  - Tender, palpable mass, may have erythema
  - Usually near nipple
  - Pus itself can be hyperechoic
  - Interspersed hypo- or anechoic areas

HYPERECHOGENICITY (US)

- ○ Surrounding edema
- Hamartoma/fibroadenolipoma
  - ○ Mixed hyper- and hypoechoic mass
  - ○ Not very discrete on US
  - ○ Characteristic fat-containing mass on mammography
- Lymphoma or leukemia in breast
  - ○ Primary lymphoma of breast or involving breast most often mixed hyper- and hypoechoic mass
  - ○ Usually have known systemic lymphoma or leukemia
  - ○ Often marked adenopathy, may be bilateral
  - ○ Broad echogenic halo can be seen
- Infiltrating ductal carcinoma (IDC)
  - ○ Coalescent Ca++ in IDC can appear echogenic
    - ▪ IDC NOS
    - ▪ Tubular carcinoma
  - ○ Echogenic rim around hypoechoic, usually irregular, mass
    - ▪ Associated architectural distortion, tethering of Cooper ligaments
    - ▪ Radial scars lack echogenic rim
    - ▪ Halo in 58% of breast cancers in one series
    - ▪ Infiltrating lobular carcinoma (ILC) can show echogenic halo as well
- Sarcomas
  - ○ Angiosarcoma most common
  - ○ Can be mixed hyper- and hypoechoic
  - ○ Often multiple masses

Diffuse Hyperechogenicity
- Edema
  - ○ Dilated lymphatics
  - ○ Skin thickening (> 2 mm)
  - ○ Trabecular thickening on mammography
- Normal variant dense parenchyma
  - ○ Heterogeneous with admixed fat
  - ○ Correlate with mammogram
- Inflammatory Carcinoma
  - ○ Clinically: Peau d'orange, erythema
  - ○ Focal irregular hypoechoic mass(es)
  - ○ Adenopathy
  - ○ Increased vascularity

Echogenic Foci
- Fibroadenoma (FA) with popcorn Ca++
  - ○ Hypo- or isoechoic mass with discrete echogenic foci
  - ○ May see shadowing from Ca++
  - ○ Characteristic appearance on mammography
- Malignancy
  - ○ Ca++ within a suspicious mass favors IDC
  - ○ Ca++ within a duct favors ductal carcinoma in situ (DCIS)
- Complicated cyst
  - ○ Mobile echogenic debris usually cholesterol crystals or milk-of-calcium
  - ○ Rim Ca++ can occur
- Galactocele
  - ○ Fatty plug
  - ○ Fluid-debris level with nondependent echogenic fat
  - ○ Diffusely slightly hyperechoic due to fat content
- Clips following surgery or core biopsy
- Air
  - ○ History of procedure, penetrating trauma

- ○ Mobile, usually cause "dirty" shadowing broader than echogenic area
- ○ Infection in proper clinical setting

PATHOLOGY

General Features
- Etiology
  - ○ 7% of benign masses are hyperechoic
  - ○ Nearly 100% NPV when homogeneously hyperechoic, circumscribed
  - ○ Source of increased echogenicity varies
    - ▪ Edema: Background increased echogenicity, dilated lymphatics
    - ▪ Halo may be due to edema or desmoplastic reaction around malignancy

CLINICAL ISSUES

Presentation
- Most common signs/symptoms: Incidental finding, asymptomatic
- Other signs/symptoms
  - ○ Erythema, tenderness, skin thickening suggest mastitis or abscess
  - ○ Skin or nipple retraction suggest malignancy
  - ○ History of silicone implants, trauma, or surgery may help distinguish etiology

DIAGNOSTIC CHECKLIST

Consider
- Solid mass with irregular echogenic rim 2.6x more likely to be malignant than one without

Image Interpretation Pearls
- Distinguish location of hyperechogenicity
  - ○ Hyperechoic mass (favors benign)
  - ○ Echogenic rim around mass (suspicious)
  - ○ Echogenic foci within mass (management depends on mass itself)
  - ○ Increased background echogenicity (suggests edema)

SELECTED REFERENCES

1. Cawson JN: Can sonography be used to help differentiate between radial scars and breast cancers? Breast. 14:352-9, 2005
2. Paulinelli RR et al: Risk of malignancy in solid breast nodules according to their sonographic features. J Ultrasound Med. 24:635-41, 2005
3. Mendelson EB et al: Breast Imaging Reporting and Data System: BI-RADS, Ultrasound, 1st ed. Reston, American College of Radiology, 2003
4. Soo MS et al: Fat necrosis in the breast: Sonographic features. Radiology. 206:261-9, 1998
5. Stavros AT et al: Solid breast nodules: use of sonography to distinguish between benign and malignant lesions. Radiology. 196:123-34, 1995

HYPERECHOGENICITY (US)

IMAGE GALLERY

Variant

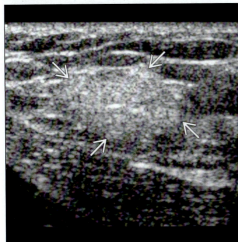

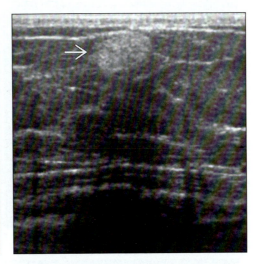

(Left) Transverse ultrasound targeted to a palpable mass in a 24 year old shows hyperechoic, irregular mass ➡. In view of the irregular margins and clinical findings, biopsy was performed, showing low grade angiosarcoma. *(Right)* Transverse ultrasound of superficial mass in a 41 year old shows homogeneously hyperechoic mass ➡. US-guided biopsy showed hemangioma.

Typical

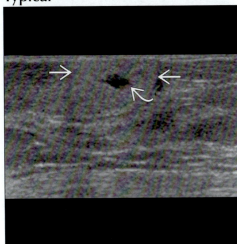

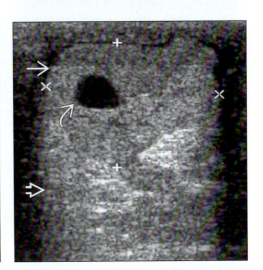

(Left) Ultrasound of palpable mass in an immunocompromised woman shows mostly hyperechoic mass ➡ with central anechoic collection ➡. US-guided biopsy, prompted by clinical findings, showed fat necrosis. *(Right)* Ultrasound of palpable, tender mass in a 42 year old shows predominantly echogenic mass ➡ with anechoic area within it ➡ and posterior enhancement ➡. Aspiration yielded pus, compatible with abscess.

Typical

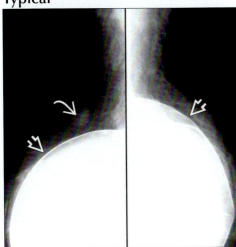

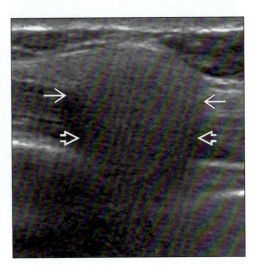

(Left) MLO mammography shows subglandular saline implants ➡ with a dense mass adjacent to the right breast implant ➡. This 56 year old woman had a ruptured silicone implant removed on the right side. *(Right)* Sagittal ultrasound of the mass adjacent to the implant (same patient as left-hand image) shows echogenic mass ➡ with "snowstorm" appearance ➡ typical of silicone granuloma.

Typical

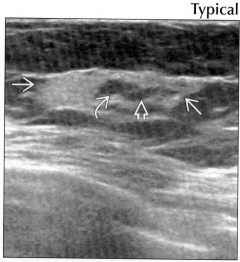

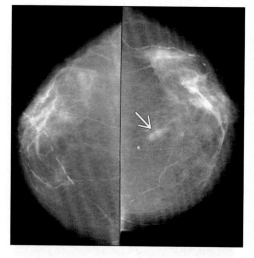

(Left) CC mammography in this 83 year old shows focal asymmetry central left breast ➡. *(Right)* Anti-radial ultrasound targeted to the mammographic abnormality (same patient as left-hand image) shows ovoid echogenic area ➡ with normal TDLU ➡ and duct ➡. Findings are compatible with normal variant atrophic breast tissue and have been stable on follow-up.

Typical

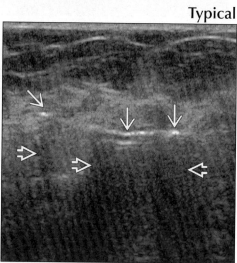

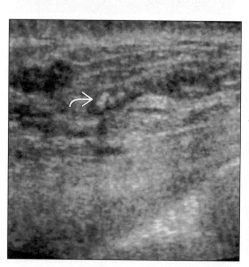

(Left) Anti-radial ultrasound in this 84 year old shows echogenic foci ➡ within a duct, highly suggestive of DCIS with comedonecrosis and Ca++. US-guided core biopsy confirmed high grade DCIS with Ca++. *(Right)* Ultrasound image obtained during core biopsy in a different patient shows linear echogenic tracks ➡ with minimal posterior shadowing ➡, due to air along the track of the 14-g core biopsy. These echoes were mobile on real-time imaging.

Variant

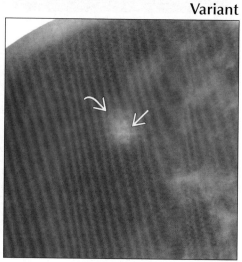

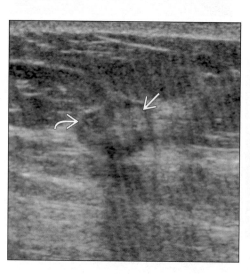

(Left) Ultrasound in this 57 year old with prior breast cancer shows irregular mass ➡ which is peripherally isoechoic to fat and centrally hyperechoic ➡. *(Right)* Lateral mammography magnification (same patient as left-hand image) shows spiculated mass ➡ corresponding to the mass seen on US. Central hyperechogenicity was due to coalescent amorphous Ca++ ➡. US-guided biopsy showed tubular carcinoma.

Typical

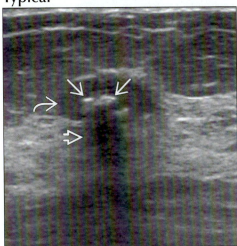
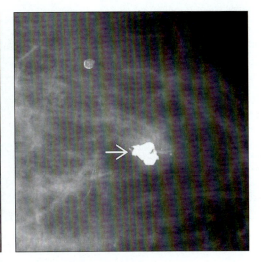

(Left) Ultrasound in this 62 year old shows coarse echogenic Ca++ ➡ within an ovoid, hypoechoic mass ➘, compatible with FA as seen mammographically. Posterior shadowing is seen from the Ca++ ➡. *(Right)* CC mammography (same patient as left-hand image) shows a partially obscured, partially circumscribed mass containing popcorn Ca++ ➡ compatible with degenerating fibroadenoma.

Typical

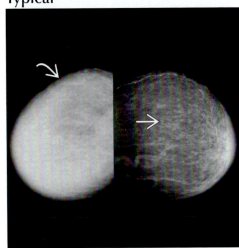
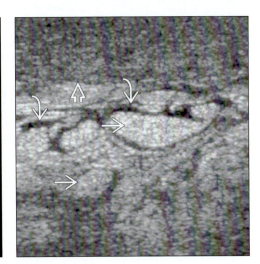

(Left) CC mammography in this 70 year old with congestive heart failure shows global asymmetry with a dense, swollen right breast ➘ and diffuse trabecular thickening on the left ➡. *(Right)* Transverse ultrasound (same patient as left-hand image) shows diffuse increased echogenicity ➡, dilated lymphatics ➘, and skin thickening ➡, due to edema, greater on the right than the left.

Variant

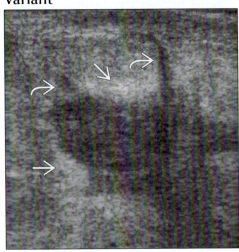
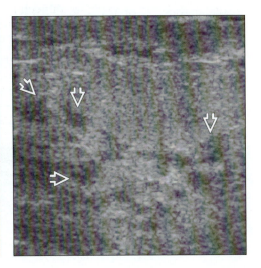

(Left) Transverse ultrasound In this 38 year old with known acute myelogenous leukemia shows spiculated, hypoechoic mass ➘ with echogenic halo ➡. *(Right)* Transverse ultrasound (same patient as left-hand image) shows diffuse increased parenchymal echogenicity and multiple tiny, hypoechoic masses ➡. US-guided core biopsy of the dominant palpable mass showed leukemic infiltrate compatible with chloroma.

HYPO & ISOECHOIC MASSES (US)

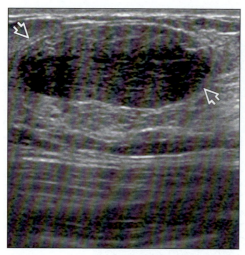

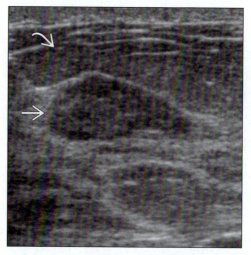

Ultrasound shows circumscribed hypoechoic mass ⮞. US-guided core biopsy diagnosed a fibroadenoma.

Ultrasound in a 30 year old with palpable mass shows an oval mass ⮞ isoechoic (equal in grayness) to surrounding fat ⮞. US-guided biopsy showed a fibroadenoma.

TERMINOLOGY

Abbreviations and Synonyms
- Echogenicity: Echo pattern

Definitions
- Internal echogenicity of mass assessed in relationship to fat in the breast, not to fibroglandular tissue or generic surrounding tissue
  - Hypoechoic: Less than the fat within the subcutaneous and pre-pectoral tissues of the breast
    - Distinguish from markedly hypoechoic: One of the "malignant" US features with ≥ 50% chance of malignancy
  - Isoechoic: Equal to fat
  - Hypo- and isoechoic patterns are common among benign and malignant lesions
    - Mildly hypo- to isoechoic solid masses: 527 of 625 (84%) of benign and 38 of 125 (30%) of malignant masses (single series)
    - Useful only in combination with other features
  - Echogenicity can have homogeneous or heterogeneous (mixed) echotexture

- "Mixed" echogenicity typically implies both hypo- and hyperechoic areas within mass

IMAGING FINDINGS

General Features
- Best diagnostic clue
  - These descriptors relevant only to US
  - Evaluate grayness of mass after coarse gain settings set for fatty breast tissue
    - Echogenicity of fat in pre-pectoral tissues must equal fat in subcutaneous tissues
    - Adjust time-gain compensation (TGC) curve to equalize fatty tissues throughout all depths of the breast tissue
- Size: Echogenicity of very small lesions, < 2 mm, difficult to assess due to scattering of echoes
- Morphology: Hypoechoic and isoechoic features can be seen in masses of all shapes and sizes

Mammographic Findings
- Isoechoic and hypoechoic masses: Soft tissue density masses on MLO and CC views

DDx: Heterogeneous, Mixed Echogenicity Masses

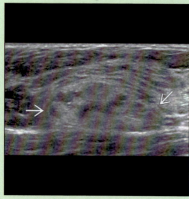

Fibroadenolipoma

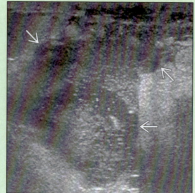

Abscess

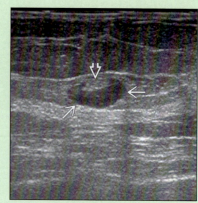

Lymph Node

HYPO & ISOECHOIC MASSES (US)

Key Facts

Terminology
- Internal echogenicity of mass assessed in relationship to fat in the breast, not to fibroglandular tissue or generic surrounding tissue
- Hypoechoic: Less than the fat within the subcutaneous and pre-pectoral tissues of the breast
- Isoechoic: Equal to fat
- Hypo- and isoechoic patterns are common among benign and malignant lesions

Imaging Findings
- Isoechoic lesions may be difficult to perceive when surrounded by fatty tissue
- Tissue harmonics and/or compound imaging may improve lesion detectability and characterization

Top Differential Diagnoses
- Normal anatomy/variants
- Complicated cyst
- Fibroadenoma (FA): 96% reported as mildly hypo- to isoechoic to fat
- Intramammary lymph node
- Ductal carcinoma in situ (DCIS): 35 of 65 (54%) reported as isoechoic (single series)
- Invasive ductal carcinoma (IDC)
- Invasive lobular carcinoma (ILC)

Clinical Issues
- Symptomatic: Palpable mass
- Asymptomatic: Screening mammogram

- Margins may be circumscribed, obscured, indistinct, microlobulated, spiculated
  - May be of any size, shape; single or multiple
- Spot compression and/or magnification views may better delineate margin characteristics, evaluate for associated calcifications

Ultrasonographic Findings
- Grayscale Ultrasound
  - Assess internal mass texture in relationship to surrounding fatty tissue
  - Determine if mass of homogeneous internal echotexture or mixed echogenicity
  - Isoechoic lesions may be difficult to perceive when surrounded by fatty tissue
    - Determine margins of lesion on real-time evaluation with 360° rotation to rule in isoechoic mass
    - Assess for edge refraction
    - Tissue harmonics and/or compound imaging may improve lesion detectability and characterization
- Color Doppler: Internal vascularity may be helpful to exclude complicated cyst and establish concern for solid mass

MR Findings
- T1WI
  - Cysts hypointense to parenchyma
    - May be hyperintense if hemorrhagic or contain proteinaceous fluid
- T2WI
  - Cysts hyperintense
  - Solid masses may be hyperintense: Some fibroadenomas, intramammary lymph nodes; mucinous carcinoma (rare)
- T1 C+ FS
  - Simple cysts do not enhance
  - Ruptured or inflamed cysts may show rim-enhancement
  - Fibroadenomas often enhance
    - May enhance somewhat early; typically persistent rather than wash-out enhancement pattern
    - May demonstrate nonenhancing septations

- Most invasive carcinomas enhance
  - Avid early enhancement followed by either wash-out or plateau of enhancement

Imaging Recommendations
- Best imaging tool: An US characteristic by definition
- Protocol advice
  - Dynamic range affects lesion contrast
    - Too narrow a dynamic range and markedly hypoechoic masses will appear anechoic
    - Too wide a dynamic range and hypoechoic masses will appear isoechoic to fat and may go undetected
    - Optimal range usually 55-70 dB, may require real-time adjustment
  - Gain affects lesion contrast
    - Accentuates effects of improper dynamic range
    - Too little gain and hypoechoic solid masses may be mistaken for cysts

DIFFERENTIAL DIAGNOSIS

Hypoechoic and Isoechoic Masses
- Normal anatomy/variants
  - Isoechoic glandular ridges: Palpable and nonpalpable
    - Often firmer than surrounding subcutaneous fat
  - Fat lobules
    - Elongate; can be palpable when there is a paucity of overlying subcutaneous fat
    - Typically demonstrate internal echogenic striations
  - Secretory changes: In pregnant or lactating women
    - Hypo- or hyperechoic depending on the nature of the secretions
    - Typically soft and compressible
  - Gynecomastia: Variable appearances
    - Subareolar hypoechogenicity: Nodular early phase; no associated posterior acoustic shadowing
    - As fibrosis develops, breast parenchyma echogenicity increases
- Benign masses

- ○ Complicated cyst
  - May be homogeneously hypoechoic
  - Can be indistinguishable from solid masses; US-guided aspiration (with biopsy if solid) may be necessary if new, enlarging, palpable, or for symptomatic relief
- ○ Fibroadenoma (FA): 96% reported as mildly hypo- to isoechoic to fat
  - 3% markedly hypoechoic; 1% completely or partially hyperechoic
  - Homogeneous or heterogeneous echotexture
  - 2-4% have cystic areas; cystic change and rapid growth more common in phyllodes tumor
- ○ Intramammary lymph node
  - Oval hypo- to isoechoic thin cortex surrounding an echogenic (fatty) hilum
- ○ Lipoma
  - Isoechoic or mildly hyperechoic oval mass
- ○ Papilloma
  - Typically hypoechoic with posterior acoustic enhancement
  - Most often intraductal or intracystic mass
  - Calcifications may develop: Usually punctate or amorphous
- ○ Fibroadenolipoma (hamartoma)
  - Lucent fat-containing portions of mass on mammography, mostly circumscribed
  - Oval mass, can blend in with surrounding tissue on US
  - Areas of mixed hypoechoic, isoechoic, and hyperechogenicity (due to fat); may be homogeneously hypoechoic
- ○ Abscess: Usually of mixed echogenicity, symptomatic
  - Surrounding increased echogenicity due to edema
  - Posterior enhancement
- ○ Seroma/post surgical change: Variable appearances; extends to overlying skin scar
- • Malignant masses
  - ○ Ductal carcinoma in situ (DCIS): 35 of 65 (54%) reported as isoechoic (single series)
    - 10-20% present as mass, usually hypoechoic
    - Intermediate grade DCIS reported as most likely to be isoechoic
  - ○ Invasive ductal carcinoma (IDC)
    - Markedly hypoechoic favors malignancy
    - Irregular, not circumscribed, may show echogenic halo; posterior features variable
    - May be homogeneous or heterogeneous; may have associated calcifications
    - 133 of 488 (27%) reported as isoechoic (single series)
  - ○ Invasive lobular carcinoma (ILC)
    - Architectural distortion common
  - ○ Lymphoma
    - Usually mixed hypo- and hyperechoic; can be homogeneously hyperechoic or hypoechoic

- ○ Symptomatic: Palpable mass
  - Mass may or may not be discernible on mammogram
  - Ultrasound indicated in work-up
  - Assessment for biopsy should be based on clinical and imaging assessment of palpable mass
  - If intervention indicated, US-guided procedure more likely diagnostic than clinically-guided sampling
- ○ Asymptomatic: Screening mammogram
  - Ultrasound indicated if mass new, larger, features suspicious of malignancy; guide in biopsy planning and performance

Treatment

- • Circumscribed oval or gently lobulated hypo- or isoechoic mass with minimal enhancement or no posterior features < 2% risk of malignancy in one series
  - ○ One series showed no malignancies among palpable, noncalcified masses which were also circumscribed on mammography

DIAGNOSTIC CHECKLIST

Consider

- • Isoechoic masses may be quite subtle: Attention to posterior features, architectural distortion, appropriate dynamic range can be helpful

Image Interpretation Pearls

- • Technical developments which decrease artifacts (e.g., tissue harmonic imaging) may render solid masses more conspicuous

SELECTED REFERENCES

1. Bassett LW et al: Diagnosis of Diseases of the Breast. Philadelphia, Elsevier Saunders. Chapter 29, 543-49, 2005
2. Graf O et al: Follow-up of palpable circumscribed noncalcified solid breast masses at mammography and US: can biopsy be averted? Radiology. 233:850-6, 2004
3. Stavros AT: Breast Ultrasound. Philadelphia, Lippincott Williams & Wilkins. Chapter 13, 539-41; 571-75, 2004
4. Stavros AT: Breast Ultrasound. Philadelphia, Lippincott Williams & Wilkins. Chapter 4, 71-5, 2004
5. Stavros AT: Breast Ultrasound. Philadelphia, Lippincott Williams & Wilkins. Chapter 5, 115-7, 2004
6. Mendelson EB et al: Breast Imaging Reporting and Data System: BI-RADS, Ultrasound, 1st ed. Reston, American College of Radiology, 2003
7. Szopinski KT et al: Tissue harmonic imaging: utility in breast sonography. J Ultrasound Med. 22:479-87, 2003
8. Stavros AT et al: Solid breast nodules: use of sonography to distinguish between benign and malignant lesions. Radiology. 196:123-134, 1995

CLINICAL ISSUES

Presentation

- • Most common signs/symptoms

IMAGE GALLERY

Typical

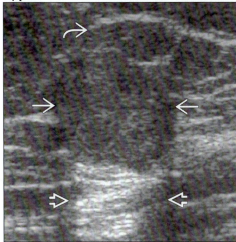

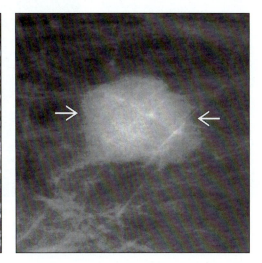

(Left) Sagittal ultrasound in this 63 year old shows a mass ➡ which is isoechoic to adjacent fat ➡, and quite inconspicuous except for its posterior enhancement ➡. (Right) MLO mammography (same mass as left-hand image) shows a dense, indistinctly marginated mass ➡. US-guided biopsy showed mucinous carcinoma.

Typical

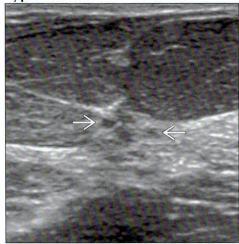

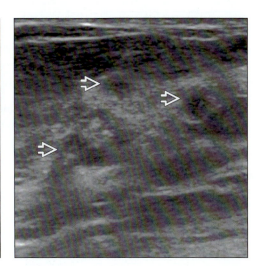

(Left) Transverse ultrasound shows an isoechoic, lobulated mass ➡ confirmed on real-time with 360° rotation of transducer. US-guided biopsy showed invasive ductal carcinoma. (Right) Radial ultrasound shows suspicious isoechoic masses ➡ in a woman with biopsy proven infiltrating lobular carcinoma. US-guided biopsy = multicentric invasive lobular carcinoma.

Typical

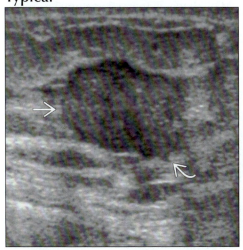

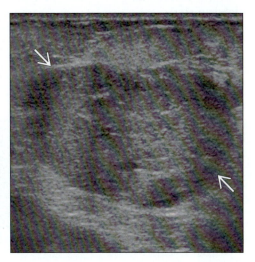

(Left) Radial ultrasound shows hypoechoic, oval mass ➡ with angular margins ➡ in this 46 year old. Biopsy showed high grade infiltrating ductal carcinoma. (Right) Radial ultrasound of a palpable finding in a lactating woman shows hypoechoic oval mass ➡. Biopsy showed benign lactational changes. There is global increased echogenicity of the surrounding tissue.

LESION ORIENTATION (US)

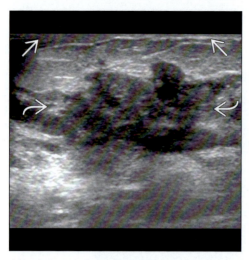

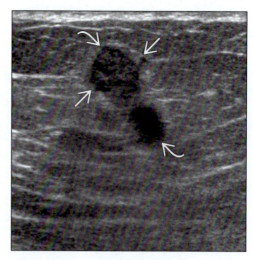

Sagittal ultrasound of a large palpable mass shows an irregular hypoechoic mass ➡ oriented parallel with the skin ➡. At mastectomy, 4.2 cm of high grade DCIS was found.

Ultrasound shows a taller-than-wide hypoechoic mass with AP diameter ➡ greater than the width ➡. US-guided biopsy showed IDC.

TERMINOLOGY

Abbreviations and Synonyms
- Orientation = longest lesion axis
- Parallel = "wider-than-tall" = horizontal orientation
- Vertical = not parallel = "taller-than-wide" = perpendicular orientation

Definitions
- Orientation = long axis of mass relative to skin
  - Parallel = long axis of mass is parallel to skin
    - Ratio of anteroposterior (AP) to longest horizontal lesion diameter is < 1 in all planes
    - Seen in both benign and malignant lesions
  - Vertical, "taller-than-wide" = long axis of mass is vertical or perpendicular to skin
    - Ratio of AP to horizontal lesion diameter is ≥ 1 in at least one plane
    - Includes round lesions, i.e. those with no long axis (AP same as horizontal diameter)
    - If any portion of the mass is vertical in orientation in any scanning plane, then consider it vertically oriented
    - Suggestive of malignancy; rarely benign

IMAGING FINDINGS

General Features
- Best diagnostic clue: US appearance of long axis orientation of mass vs. skin
- Location
  - Determine lesion axis in the central part of the mass
    - Longest axis is usually within the central part

Imaging Recommendations
- Best imaging tool: Description of lesion axis or orientation is specific to US
- Protocol advice
  - Under US, determine three dimensional shape
  - If mass is irregular in shape, rotate transducer through 180° over mass to determine longest axis
  - This descriptor is not specific enough to differentiate benign from malignant
    - Other US imaging findings must be taken into account: Mass shape, margin characteristics, posterior acoustic characteristics

---

DDx: Other Benign Examples of Lesion Orientation

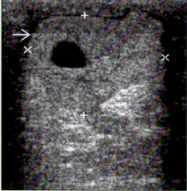

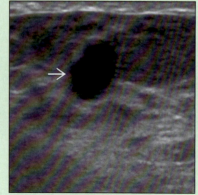

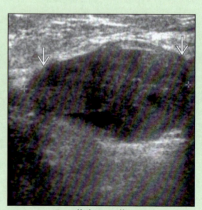

Parallel, Abscess

Vertical, Cyst

Parallel, Papilloma

LESION ORIENTATION (US)

Key Facts

Terminology
- Parallel = "wider-than-tall" = horizontal orientation
- Vertical = not parallel = "taller-than-wide" = perpendicular orientation
- Orientation = long axis of mass relative to skin

Imaging Findings
- Best imaging tool: Description of lesion axis or orientation is specific to US

Top Differential Diagnoses
- Parallel: Most Common Among Benign and Malignant Lesions
- Cysts
- Fibroadenoma (FA)
- Papilloma
- Malignancy

- Vertical, "Taller-than-Wide": Suspicious for Malignancy
- Invasive ductal carcinoma, not otherwise specified (IDC, NOS)
- Invasive lobular carcinoma (ILC)
- Radial scar: Radial sclerosing lesion (RSL)
- Surgical scar
- Fat necrosis

Clinical Issues
- Vertical orientation is suspicious and generally merits aspiration if possibly a cyst, with biopsy if solid
- Any malignant features (without antecedent history such as surgery or trauma) should result in recommendation for biopsy

DIFFERENTIAL DIAGNOSIS

Parallel: Most Common Among Benign and Malignant Lesions
- Significant overlap between benign and malignant masses
- Cysts
  - Mammography: Oval, circumscribed mass
  - Ultrasound: Typically oval, anechoic; complicated cysts may be hypoechoic
    - May be round, particularly when small, hemorrhagic or inflammatory
  - MR
    - T1: Low signal unless hemorrhagic
    - T2: Bright signal unless hemorrhagic as these are fluid-containing structures
    - T1 contrast-enhanced: Typically do not enhance; wall can enhance if ruptured or inflamed
- Fibroadenoma (FA)
  - Mammography may demonstrate a calcified or noncalcified mass
  - Margins usually circumscribed or obscured, can be indistinct
  - Shape may be oval or gently lobulated
  - Echogenic septations may be present
    - May correlate with nonenhancing septations on contrast-enhanced MR
  - MR findings include both T2 fat-saturated and contrast-enhanced sequences
    - T2 sequence may demonstrate a mass with bright signal: More common in cellular or myxoid types
    - Contrast-enhanced sequences demonstrate smooth enhancing mass
    - Persistent or plateau rather than wash-out kinetics are more typical
    - May show nonenhancing septations: Strongly favors FA
- Papilloma
  - Most commonly in subareolar ducts: Intraductal or intracystic mass
- Malignancy
  - Parallel orientation possible for both irregular and oval-shaped masses
  - Invasive ductal carcinoma
  - Ductal carcinoma in situ (DCIS)
  - Invasive lobular carcinoma

Vertical, "Taller-than-Wide": Suspicious for Malignancy
- Overlap between benign and malignant masses, though favors malignancy
- Suggests growth in an anterior, usually superficial, terminal duct lobular unit (TDLU)
- Vertical orientation rarely seen in lesions larger than 1 cm
- Malignancy
  - Invasive ductal carcinoma, not otherwise specified (IDC, NOS)
    - Mammography: Most commonly spiculated mass/architectural distortion
    - Ultrasound: Most commonly hypoechoic mass with irregular margins
    - MR: Most commonly brightly enhancing spiculated mass
  - Invasive lobular carcinoma (ILC)
    - Mammography: Architectural distortion/irregular mass; asymmetry; may not be perceptible
    - Ultrasound: Irregular hypoechoic mass, often with architectural distortion
    - MR: Usually irregular enhancing mass; less often dendritic-like area of enhancement without focal dominant mass
    - May have associated or adjacent lobular carcinoma in situ (LCIS)
  - DCIS
    - 10-20% present as mass with or without calcifications
    - Tubular, oval, microlobulated, or irregular mass
    - About half of DCIS visible on US, more often high grade
- Radial scar: Radial sclerosing lesion (RSL)
  - Indistinguishable by all imaging from malignancy
  - Diagnosis must be made by biopsy, histopathology

LESION ORIENTATION (US)

- ○ Mammography: Architectural distortion, spiculated, lucent center
- ○ Ultrasound: Ill-defined hypoechoic mass
  - Can be associated with thick echogenic halo
  - Architectural distortion
- ○ MR: Irregular, often spiculated, enhancing mass
- Surgical scar
  - ○ Clinical history and location of skin scar key to this diagnosis
  - ○ At US, track extension of finding to disrupted dermal fascial plane
  - ○ May be associated with seroma
    - Prominent and may persist for years following lumpectomy and radiation therapy
    - Persistent seroma > 1 year less common following benign biopsy
- Fat necrosis
  - ○ Anechoic areas with surrounding echogenic (edematous) tissue
  - ○ History of trauma or surgery
  - ○ Often fat-containing lucencies on mammography
- Cyst
  - ○ Can have vertical orientation when develop in anterior TDLU's
  - ○ Vertically-oriented cysts generally merit aspiration as difficult to distinguish from markedly hypoechoic solid mass
- Abscess
  - ○ Associated with skin thickening and tissue edema
  - ○ Tender, usually palpable mass, often near nipple
  - ○ Often mixed hyper- and anechoic collection

PATHOLOGY

General Features
- Etiology
  - ○ Parallel: Growth along the fascial planes
    - Most benign lesions show this growth pattern
    - Malignancies usually also grow in this pattern
    - 73% of all lesions going to US biopsy; 22% malignant
  - ○ Taller than wide: Growth that disrupts fascial planes or in anterior TDLU's
    - Growth pattern suggests malignant process
    - < 2% of benign lesions have this orientation
    - 27% of all lesions going to US biopsy; 69% malignant
    - 41% of malignancies had some vertical orientation
  - ○ Mass with vertical orientation 4.9x more likely malignant than a parallel mass

CLINICAL ISSUES

Presentation
- Most common signs/symptoms: Palpable or nonpalpable mass

Natural History & Prognosis
- US findings consistent with high NPV (99%) have been described

- ○ Markedly and uniformly hyperechoic: Typically represents fibrous tissue
- ○ Well-circumscribed mass parallel to skin ("wider-than-tall") with three or fewer gentle lobulations and a thin echogenic pseudocapsule: Typically FA
- ○ The finding of even one malignant feature, e.g. vertical orientation, usually merits aspiration or biopsy

Treatment
- Parallel orientation is common among benign and malignant lesions
- Vertical orientation is suspicious and generally merits aspiration if possibly a cyst, with biopsy if solid
- Any malignant features (without antecedent history such as surgery or trauma) should result in recommendation for biopsy
  - ○ Margins not circumscribed, thickened irregular rim or halo, marked hypoechogenicity, posterior shadowing

DIAGNOSTIC CHECKLIST

Consider
- Circumscribed margin (previously thin pseudocapsule) reported as most important sonographic finding predictive of solid mass benignity
- Statistically significant association with breast cancer reported for margins not circumscribed, irregular shape, round or vertical orientation, marked hypoechogenicity and no or decreased posterior sound transmission

Image Interpretation Pearls
- For parallel masses, management mostly dependent on margins and shape
- A mass which is vertical in orientation in any plane is usually suspicious, regardless of other benign features

SELECTED REFERENCES

1. Cawson JN: Can sonography be used to help differentiate between radial scars and breast cancer? Breast. 14:352-9, 2005
2. Hong AS et al: BI-RADS for sonography: positive and negative predictive values of sonographic features. AJR. 184:1260-5, 2005
3. Stavros AT: Breast Ultrasound. Philadelphia, Lippincott Williams & Wilkins. Ch 12:45-527, 2004
4. Mendelson EB et al: Breast Imaging Reporting and Data System: BI-RADS, Ultrasound, 1st ed. Reston, American College of Radiology, 2003
5. Zonderland HM et al: Ultrasound variables and their prognostic value in a population of 1103 patients with 272 breast cancers. Eur Radiol. 10:1562-8, 2000
6. Skaane P et al: Analysis of sonographic features in the differentiation of fibroadenoma and invasive ductal carcinoma. AJR. 171:1159-60, 1998
7. Stavros AT et al: Solid breast nodules: use of sonography to distinguish between benign and malignant lesions. Radiology. 196:123-34, 1995
8. Fornage BD et al: Fibroadenoma of the breast: sonographic appearance. Radiology. 172:671-5, 1989

LESION ORIENTATION (US)

IMAGE GALLERY

Typical

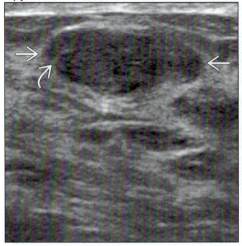
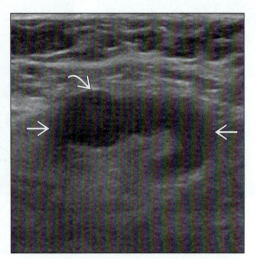

(Left) Radial ultrasound of a palpable mass in a 32 year old shows an oval, circumscribed, isoechoic mass ➡, parallel to the skin, containing an echogenic septation ➡. Biopsy showed FA. *(Right)* Sagittal ultrasound shows axillary node ➡ with markedly thickened cortex ➡, proven metastatic in this 37 year old with grade III IDC + DCIS. Orientation is parallel to skin.

Variant

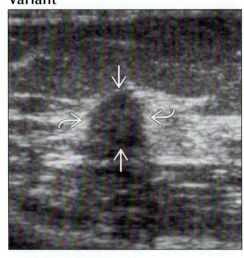
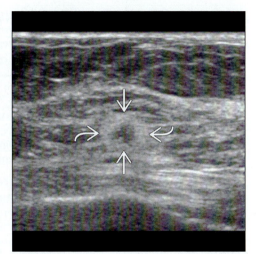

(Left) Transverse ultrasound in this 54 year old shows an indistinctly-marginated hypoechoic mass whose horizontal diameter ➡ is equal to its vertical (AP) diameter ➡. This is considered vertical orientation. Biopsy showed IDC + DCIS. *(Right)* Transverse ultrasound shows irregular mass with echogenic rim and parallel orientation. The longest horizontal diameter ➡ is greater than AP diameter ➡. US-guided biopsy showed IDC.

Typical

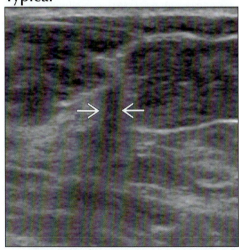
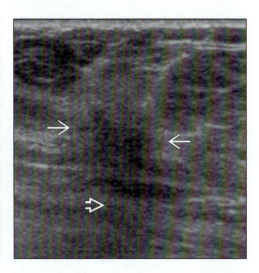

(Left) Anti-radial ultrasound shows vertically-oriented, irregular, hypoechoic mass ➡ in this 56 year old woman. *(Right)* Radial ultrasound (same mass as left-hand image) shows apparent horizontal orientation to mass ➡, with posterior shadowing ➡. Because the mass is vertically oriented in one plane, it is judged "taller-than-wide". US core biopsy showed 4 mm ILC + LCIS.

POSTERIOR ENHANCEMENT (US)

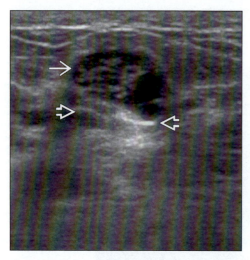

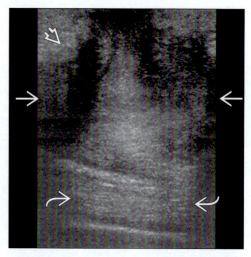

Anti-radial ultrasound of a non-palpable breast mass shows an oval, circumscribed, cluster of microcysts ➡ with posterior enhancement ⮞. This is a benign finding, BI-RADS 2.

Transverse ultrasound shows a symptomatic irregular 3.6 x 2.8 x 3.2 cm mixed hyper- and hypoechoic abscess ➡ with thick margins ⮞ and posterior enhancement ⮞ that responded to antibiotics.

TERMINOLOGY

Abbreviations and Synonyms
- Increased through transmission of sound, decreased attenuation

Definitions
- Posterior enhancement: Increase in echoes (brighter echotexture) in tissues posterior to lesion relative to adjacent tissues at comparable depth
- Distinguish from other posterior features
  - "No posterior acoustic features": No shadowing or enhancement
    - Echogenicity of the area immediately behind the mass is not different from that of adjacent tissue at the same depth
  - "Posterior shadowing": Decreased posterior echoes, attenuation of sound transmission through the lesion
  - "Combined pattern": Both posterior enhancement and posterior shadowing

IMAGING FINDINGS

General Features
- Best diagnostic clue: An indeterminate US finding
- Size
  - Width of enhancement is relative to size (width) of lesion
  - If lesion very small, particularly in AP direction, less apt to see this feature
- Morphology: Lesion shape has no specific influence over presence or absence of posterior enhancement

Mammographic Findings
- Masses with posterior enhancement usually seen as soft tissue density masses on MLO and CC views
- Margins may be circumscribed, obscured, indistinct, microlobulated, spiculated
  - May be of any size, shape; single or multiple
- Spot compression and/or magnification views may better delineate margin characteristics, evaluate for associated calcifications

DDx: Other Posterior Acoustic Characteristics

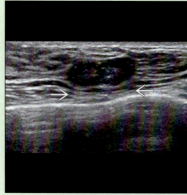

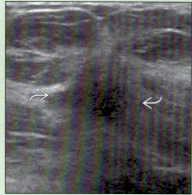

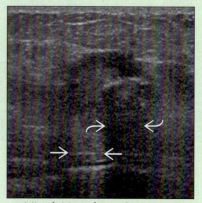

No Affect, DCIS

Shadowing, Invasive Lobular

Mixed, Metaplastic Carcinoma

POSTERIOR ENHANCEMENT (US)

Key Facts

Terminology
- Posterior enhancement: Increase in echoes (brighter echotexture) in tissues posterior to lesion relative to adjacent tissues at comparable depth

Imaging Findings
- Best diagnostic clue: An indeterminate US finding
- Inappropriate TGC curve may falsely simulate feature

Top Differential Diagnoses
- Normal Anatomy/Anatomic Variants
- Benign Lesions: Cystic
- Benign Lesions: Solid
- Fibroadenoma (FA)
- Papilloma
- Complex Cystic Masses: May be Benign or Malignant
- Malignant Lesions: Solid

- Invasive ductal carcinoma, not otherwise specified (IDC, NOS)
- Medullary carcinoma
- Mucinous carcinoma

Pathology
- Present in 23% of lesions going to US biopsy
- 36% malignant

Clinical Issues
- Most common signs/symptoms: Both asymptomatic and symptomatic

Diagnostic Checklist
- Posterior enhancement alone does not distinguish cystic from solid or differentiate benign from malignant solid masses

Ultrasonographic Findings
- Grayscale Ultrasound: Evaluate mass margins, shape, internal structure, associated calcifications, together with posterior features
- Color Doppler: Internal vascularity excludes a cyst

MR Findings
- T1WI
  - Proteinaceous or hemorrhagic cysts may be hyperintense
  - Masses typically isointense to glandular tissue
- T2WI FS: Fluid containing cysts, some cellular fibroadenomas and rare mucinous carcinomas are hyperintense
- T1 C+
  - Enhancement characteristics based on etiology of lesion
  - Simple cysts do not enhance
  - Inflamed or ruptured cysts may show rim-enhancement
  - Fibroadenomas may show gradual enhancement without washout characteristics
  - Malignant masses typically show rapid enhancement followed by either washout or plateau kinetics

Imaging Recommendations
- Best imaging tool: Ultrasound feature only
- Protocol advice
  - Use fundamental imaging or harmonic imaging to see posterior features
  - Spatial compounding reduces posterior features due to off-angle beams not directly traversing lesion
  - Set focal zone at lesion
  - Inappropriate TGC curve may falsely simulate feature

DIFFERENTIAL DIAGNOSIS

Normal Anatomy/Anatomic Variants
- Ectatic ducts

  - Fluid-filled tubular retroareolar structures may demonstrate posterior enhancement
- Secretory changes: Typically in pregnant or lactating women
  - Degree of fluid determines in part the presence of posterior enhancement

Benign Lesions: Cystic
- Simple cysts
  - Anechoic, circumscribed, oval or gently lobulated
  - 25% of cysts may not show enhancement
- Complicated cysts
  - Characteristics of simple cysts but with internal low level echoes, fluid-debris level
    - Galactocele is a complicated cyst typically with a fluid-debris level or echogenic debris
  - If internal echoes are mobile, reassured as to cystic nature of the mass
  - May require aspiration to differentiate from solid mass
- Clustered microcysts

Benign Lesions: Solid
- Fibroadenoma (FA)
  - Typically demonstrate benign US findings
    - No evidence of any malignant features
    - Parallel to skin, smooth, oval or no more than 3 gentle lobulations, circumscribed
- Papilloma
  - Typically a hypoechoic soft compressible mass
  - Enhancement decreases as these neoplasms age
- Fibroadenolipoma (hamartoma)
  - Encapsulated fat-containing mammographic mass
  - Oval often hypoechoic mass, can blend in with surrounding tissue on US
- Phyllodes
  - Usually circumscribed, hypoechoic
  - Rapid growth vs. FA
  - May contain cystic areas

Complex Cystic Masses: May be Benign or Malignant
- Both cystic and solid components present

POSTERIOR ENHANCEMENT (US)

- ○ Post-operative seroma or hematoma - (benign); correlate with clinical history
- ○ Thick-walled cystic mass = high grade malignancy (30%)
- ○ Intracystic mass 22% rate of malignancy; most often papillary
- ○ Solid mass with cystic foci most commonly fibrocystic change or fibroadenoma; 13% rate of malignancy
- ○ Abscess: Tender, palpable, often near nipple
- Enhancement from cystic portion: May show mixed posterior features

Malignant Lesions: Solid
- Invasive ductal carcinoma, not otherwise specified (IDC, NOS)
  - ○ Typically markedly hypoechoic with irregular shape and at least partially indistinct margins
  - ○ Of 120 women with IDC (single series), 22% showed acoustic enhancement
    - ■ 36% of high grade, 9% of low and intermediate grade IDC
  - ○ Of 19% or lactating women 26-49 yrs old, 12 (63%) demonstrated posterior enhancement (single series)
- Medullary carcinoma
  - ○ Most are markedly hypoechoic with posterior enhancement a reliable finding
    - ■ Likely on the basis of internal cellularity and limited desmoplastic fibrous reaction
- Mucinous carcinoma
  - ○ Often isoechoic to fat and difficult to recognize
  - ○ Lesions > 1.5 cm typically show posterior enhancement
- Ductal carcinoma in situ (DCIS)
  - ○ Limited detectability of DCIS by US
  - ○ Five of 70 (7%) with posterior enhancement (single series)
    - ■ Intracystic papillary DCIS more likely posterior enhancement
- Lymphoma
  - ○ Hypoechoic well-defined to irregular oval masses with mixed internal echogenicity
  - ○ Variable posterior enhancement or shadowing
- Metastatic adenopathy

PATHOLOGY

General Features
- Etiology
  - ○ Relative lack of attenuation of US beam by lesion compared to surrounding tissues at comparable depth
    - ■ Result is increase in penetration and resulting echoes from tissues deep to the lesion, which appear brighter (whiter) than adjacent tissue
  - ○ Present in 23% of lesions going to US biopsy
    - ■ 36% malignant

Staging, Grading or Classification Criteria
- Not a finding specific to staging, grading or classification

CLINICAL ISSUES

Presentation
- Most common signs/symptoms: Both asymptomatic and symptomatic

DIAGNOSTIC CHECKLIST

Consider
- Posterior enhancement alone does not distinguish cystic from solid or differentiate benign from malignant solid masses
- Difficult to demonstrate posterior enhancement from small cysts < 5 mm or with spatial compounding on

Image Interpretation Pearls
- Final assessment must be based on all features present
- Simple cyst must be anechoic, circumscribed (especially back wall), with posterior enhancement
  - ○ Characterization of mass as a simple cyst less reliable for lesions < 8 mm in size or deeper than 3 cm from skin
- Must take into account clinical correlation and other lesion imaging characteristics
  - ○ Any possibly malignant feature, i.e., marked hypoechogenicity, margin irregularities, vertical orientation, microcalcifications, should prompt intervention
  - ○ Other indeterminate US findings: Isoechogenicity, mild hypoechogenicity, normal sound transmission, heterogeneous and homogeneous internal echotexture

SELECTED REFERENCES

1. Hong AS et al: BI-RADS for sonography: positive and negative predictive values of sonographic features. AJR. 184:1260-5, 2005
2. Stavros AT: Breast Ultrasound. Philadelphia, Lippincott Williams & Wilkins. Chapter 14, 641-8, 2004
3. Ahn BY et al: Pregnancy-and lactation-associated breast cancer: mammographic and sonographic findings. J Ultrasound Med. 22:491-7, 2003
4. Berg WA et al: Cystic lesions of the breast: Sonographic-pathologic correlation. Radiology. 227:183-91, 2003
5. Mendelson EB et al: Breast Imaging Reporting and Data System: BI-RADS, Ultrasound, 1st ed. Reston, American College of Radiology, 2003
6. Woo KM et al: US of ductal carcinoma in situ. Radiographics. 22:269-81, 2002
7. Lamb PM et al: Correlation between ultrasound characteristics, mammographic findings and histological grade in patients with invasive ductal carcinoma of the breast. Clin Radiol. 55:40-4, 2000
8. Stavros AT et al: Solid breast nodules: use of sonography to distinguish between benign and malignant lesions. Radiology. 196:123-34, 1995
9. Hilton SV et al: Real-time breast sonography: application in 300 consecutive patients. AJR. 147:479-86, 1986

POSTERIOR ENHANCEMENT (US)

IMAGE GALLERY

Typical

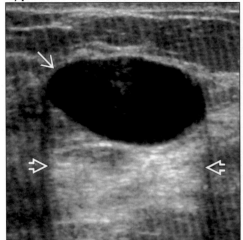 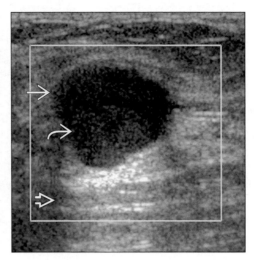

(Left) Anti-radial ultrasound of a palpable mass shows findings of a simple cyst ➡. Anechoic, circumscribed, with posterior enhancement ⏩, BI-RADS 2, benign. *(Right)* Radial color Doppler ultrasound shows a circumscribed mass ➡ with internal echoes ➡ and posterior enhancement ⏩ and no flow. US-guided aspiration revealed a hemorrhagic cyst.

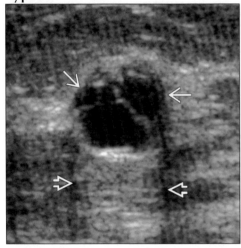 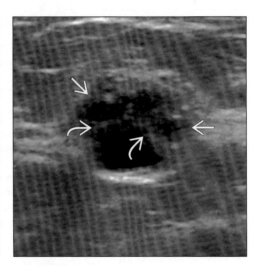

(Left) Anti-radial ultrasound shows a microlobulated mass c/w a microcyst ➡ with posterior enhancement ⏩ visible on the gray scale image, but not seen with spatial compounding (right-hand image). *(Right)* Anti-radial spatial compounding ultrasound shows no posterior acoustic features, but the internal structure ➡ of the clustered microcysts ➡ is slightly better visualized. BI-RADS 2, benign.

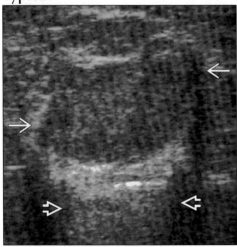 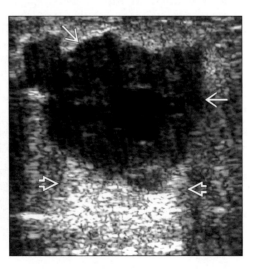

(Left) Transverse ultrasound shows an isoechoic irregular mass ➡ with posterior enhancement ⏩. US-guided core biopsy = mucinous carcinoma. *(Right)* Anti-radial ultrasound of a palpable mass shows an irregular thick-walled, centrally cystic mass ➡ with posterior enhancement ⏩ suspicious for malignancy, BI-RADS 4C. US-guided bx = grade III IDC with central necrosis.

POSTERIOR SHADOWING (US)

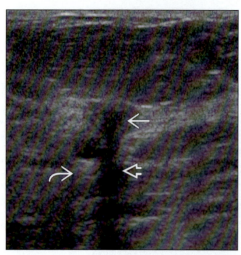
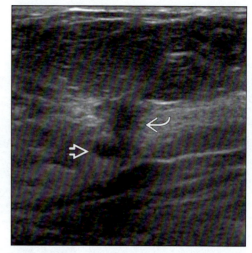

Radial ultrasound shows indistinctly-marginated hypoechoic mass ➡ with marked posterior shadowing ➡. An adjacent cyst with posterior enhancement ➡ is noted.

Spatial compounded US (same mass as left image) better depicts subtly spiculated margins ➡. Posterior shadowing is no longer evident, nor is enhancement from cyst ➡. Biopsy showed grade I IDC & DCIS.

TERMINOLOGY

Abbreviations and Synonyms
• Posterior attenuation; acoustic shadowing

Definitions
• Posterior shadowing: Decreased echoes deep to a structure
  ○ Attenuation of ultrasound beam with resulting decrease in echoes in tissue posterior to mass/anatomy relative to adjacent tissues at comparable depth
  ○ Calcifications larger than 1-2 mm can cause shadowing
• Does not include refractive edge shadowing
  ○ At edges of curved mass or ligaments perpendicular to the US beam, refraction of sound waves around the curved surface results in decrease in echoes in tissue directly deep to the curved surface relative to surrounding tissue
  ○ Thin (1-2 mm) stripe of shadowing tangential to surface of mass which is perpendicular to beam

IMAGING FINDINGS

General Features
• Best diagnostic clue
  ○ Tissues behind the structure, perpendicular to insonating beam, appear darker than surrounding tissue
  ○ May not visualize posterior margin of mass if central shadowing is very strong
    ■ Occurs with marked attenuation of US beam
    ■ Suggests marked fibrosis in mass
  ○ Posterior shadowing less apparent with compound, spatial imaging
    ■ Off-angle beam(s) are no longer perpendicular, no longer absorbed or blocked
    ■ Posterior margin of mass better seen with compound imaging
    ■ Can help evaluate tissues deep to mass: Possible chest wall invasion

Mammographic Findings
• Suspicious findings on US, such as shadowing, merit correlation and further evaluation with mammography

DDx: Dismissably Benign Shadowing

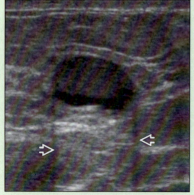
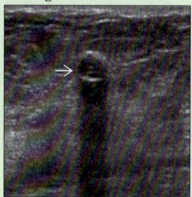
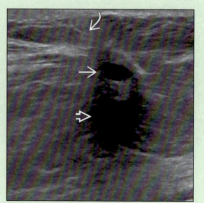

Refractive Edge, Galactocele

Calcifying Oil Cyst

Post-Surgical Scar, Seroma

POSTERIOR SHADOWING (US)

Key Facts

Terminology
- Posterior attenuation; acoustic shadowing
- Posterior shadowing: Decreased echoes deep to a structure
- Does not include refractive edge shadowing

Imaging Findings
- Posterior shadowing less apparent with compound, spatial imaging
- Multifocal, multicentric, or bilateral findings
- Distinguish source of shadowing: Echogenic Ca++ vs. mass itself

Top Differential Diagnoses
- Interface of fat lobules
- Fibroadenoma (FA): Popcorn calcifications will shadow

- Fat necrosis
- Fibrosis
- Invasive Ductal Carcinoma (IDC) NOS
- Invasive Lobular Carcinoma (ILC)
- Post-Surgical Scar
- Radial Sclerosing Lesion (RSL)

Pathology
- 53% malignant
- < 5% of benign masses show shadowing

Clinical Issues
- Unless caused by coarse, benign Ca++ or scar, shadowing is suspicious and should generally prompt biopsy

- When malignancy suspected, bilateral mammogram needed
  - Assess for calcifications (Ca++), typically benign
    - Coarse, popcorn Ca++ in a degenerating fibroadenoma (FA), typically benign
    - Curvilinear peripheral Ca++ around lucent mass, suggesting fat necrosis
    - Dystrophic Ca++ at scars
  - Assess for suspicious Ca++
    - Merit magnification CC and true lateral views to assess morphology, distribution, extent
  - Mass margins
    - Most commonly indistinct or spiculated masses
    - Mass may be obscured by dense tissue
    - Calcifying FA or cyst may be circumscribed and show shadowing on US
  - Associated or isolated architectural distortion
    - Correlate with any surgical scar sites
  - Multifocal, multicentric, or bilateral findings
  - Absence of a mammographic correlate should not deter biopsy of a sonographically suspicious finding

Ultrasonographic Findings
- Grayscale Ultrasound
  - Posterior shadowing unique to ultrasound
  - Distinguish source of shadowing: Echogenic Ca++ vs. mass itself
    - Macrocalcifications may suggest FA if mass circumscribed, oval
    - Rim calcification of an oval mass suggests calcified cyst (can be oil cyst)
    - Shadowing from mass itself is suspicious: Characterize visualized margins, shape
- Color Doppler
  - Can depict increased vascularity to underlying mass
  - Presence of vascularity may correlate with increased likelihood of malignancy

MR Findings
- T1 C+
  - Can use to assess extent of malignancy

  - Can be used for further characterization of areas of shadowing, possible distortion, too vague to discretely biopsy

Imaging Recommendations
- Best imaging tool: Feature unique to US due to interaction of sound waves in tissues
- Protocol advice
  - Rocking (heel-toe) movement of probe will allow visualization of tissues deep to shadowing
  - Spatial compounding reduces posterior shadowing
    - Has same effect as "rocking motion" of probe by changing angle(s) of the US beam(s)
  - Artifactual shadowing can occur with inadequate transducer pressure
    - Angle probe so that pectoralis fascial plane is parallel to transducer face
  - Nipple-areolar complex can shadow
    - Off-angle scan behind nipple
  - Harmonic imaging preserves posterior features and may accentuate shadowing

DIFFERENTIAL DIAGNOSIS

Normal Structures
- Nipple-areolar complex
  - Eliminate any air
  - Slight changes in angle or pressure will usually resolve this
- Ribs
  - Location, elongate when turn appropriately
- Interface of fat lobules
  - Refractive edge shadowing and/or focal areas of shadowing
  - Increase pressure, change angle of insonation, should resolve

Coarsely Calcifying Masses
- Correlate with mammographic findings
- Fibroadenoma (FA): Popcorn calcifications will shadow
- Fat necrosis
  - May show peripheral curvilinear calcifications

○ Usually centrally lucent mass on mammography
   ▪ Can appear dense and irregular: Merits biopsy
○ Includes calcifying oil cyst
○ Appropriate history of trauma or surgery
• Dystrophic calcifications in scar
   ○ Implant capsule commonly calcified
   ○ Silicone injections or granulomata
• Unusual Malignancies: E.g., metaplastic carcinoma with osteoid matrix

Fibrosis

• Normal variant dense parenchyma can have identical appearance
• Can be mixed echogenicity or markedly hypoechoic
• Oval or irregular
• Difficult to establish concordance in dense breast with highly suspicious appearance
• May show associated fibrocystic changes (FCC)

Invasive Ductal Carcinoma (IDC) NOS

• Acoustic shadowing in 71% of low grade tumors compared to 28% of high grade tumors
• Overall 49-58% show shadowing

Invasive Lobular Carcinoma (ILC)

• Irregular, hypoechoic, shadowing mass in 58-61% of ILC
• Another 15% focal shadowing alone, without discrete mass

Post-Surgical Scar

• Track to overlying skin incision site
• May have associated fluid collection
• Should decrease over time
• Shadowing more common in lumpectomy, post-radiation scars than benign surgical scars

Radial Sclerosing Lesion (RSL)

• Shadowing more common when RSL associated with malignancy

Diabetic Mastopathy

• Long-standing (> 20 year) type I diabetes
• Hard clinically, dense on mammography
• Irregular, ill-defined, hypoechoic, with shadowing

Galactocele

• Fatty plug can appear echogenic with shadowing

Air

• Usually introduced during biopsy, along track, mobile
• "Dirty shadowing", not band-like, no "edges"

Fibromatosis (Rare)

• Locally aggressive, can invade chest wall
• Treat with wide local excision

Granulomatous Mastitis (Rare)

• Irregular, hypoechoic mass, mimics malignancy

PATHOLOGY

General Features

• Etiology

○ Increased tissue interfaces within mass, e.g., mixture of desmoplastic response and tumor, or blocked sound transmission, e.g. calcifications
○ 34% of all masses going to US-guided biopsy showed shadowing in one series
   ▪ 53% malignant
○ < 5% of benign masses show shadowing
○ Mass showing shadowing is 3.9x more likely malignant than one without

CLINICAL ISSUES

Treatment

• Unless caused by coarse, benign Ca++ or scar, shadowing is suspicious and should generally prompt biopsy

DIAGNOSTIC CHECKLIST

Consider

• Exclude artifactual shadowing

SELECTED REFERENCES

1. Cawson JN et al: Can sonography be used to help differentiate between radial scars and breast cancers? Breast. 14:352-9, 2005
2. Hong AS et al: BI-RADS for sonography: positive and negative predictive values of sonographic features. AJR. 184:1260-5, 2005
3. Watermann DO et al: Ultrasound morphology of invasive lobular breast cancer is different compared with other types of breast cancer. Ultrasound Med Biol. 31:167-74, 2005
4. Selinko VL et al: Role of sonography in diagnosing and staging invasive lobular carcinoma. J Clin Ultrasound. 32:323-32, 2004
5. Mendelson EB et al: Breast Imaging Reporting and Data System: BI-RADS, Ultrasound, 1st ed. Reston, American College of Radiology, 2003
6. Memis A et al: Granulomatous mastitis: imaging findings with histopathologic correlation. Clin Radiol. 57:1001-6, 2002
7. Samardar P et al: Focal asymmetric densities seen at mammography: US and pathologic correlation. Radiographics. 22:19-33, 2002
8. Seo BK et al: Sonographic evaluation of breast nodules: Comparison of conventional, real-time compound, and pulse-inversion harmonic images. Korean J Radiol. 3:38-44, 2002
9. Wong KT et al: Ultrasound and MR imaging of diabetic mastopathy. Clin Radiol. 57:730-5, 2002
10. Lamb PM et al: Correlation between ultrasound characteristics, mammographic findings, and histological grade in patients with invasive ductal carcinoma of the breast. Clin Radiol. 55:40-44, 2000
11. Butler RS et al: Sonographic evaluation of infiltrating lobular carcinoma. AJR. 172:325-30, 1999
12. Georgian-Smith D et al: From the RSNA refresher courses. Freehand interventional sonography in the breast: Basic principles and clinical applications. Radiographics. 16:149-61, 1996
13. Stavros AT et al: Solid breast nodules: Use of sonography to distinguish between benign and malignant lesions. Radiology 196:123-34, 1995

POSTERIOR SHADOWING (US)

IMAGE GALLERY

Typical

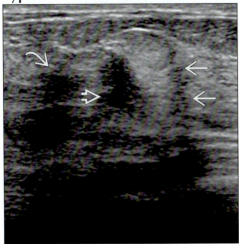 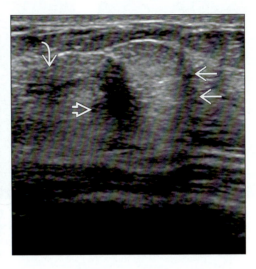

(Left) Ultrasound shows 3 forms of shadowing: Attenuation by tumor (IDC) ⮕; refractory from curved Cooper ligaments ➡, and artifactual shadowing ⮕. (Right) Ultrasound with greater pressure applied (same as on left) shows persistent tumoral shadowing (IDC) ➡ and refractory shadowing ➡, but previously noted artifactual shadowing ⮕ is gone.

Typical

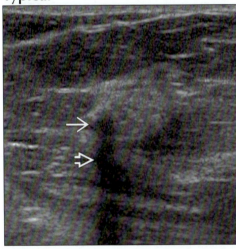 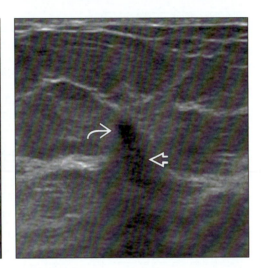

(Left) Screening US shows a hypoechoic 4 mm mass ➡ with marked posterior shadowing ⮕ in this 56 year old with personal history of cancer 5 years earlier. US biopsy showed stromal fibrosis. This lesion was gone at 6 month follow-up. (Right) Ultrasound shows a hypoechoic 4 mm mass ➡ with posterior shadowing ⮕ in this 49 year old with a spiculated mass on screening mammogram. Biopsy showed grade I IDC + DCIS.

Typical

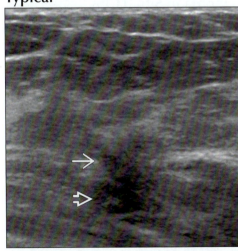 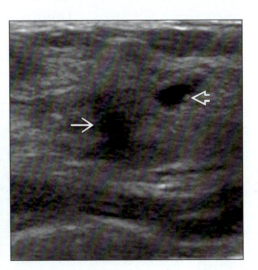

(Left) Ultrasound shows vague 6 mm hypoechoic mass ➡ and posterior shadowing ⮕ in this 56 year old with architectural distortion on mammography. US-guided biopsy showed ILC. (Right) Screening ultrasound in a 47 year old shows vague area of focal shadowing ➡ without a discrete mass. This is not at the interface of lobules. US-guided biopsy showed ILC. Incidental adjacent cyst ⮕ is seen.

CLUMPED (MR)

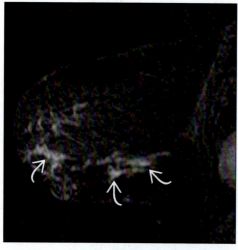

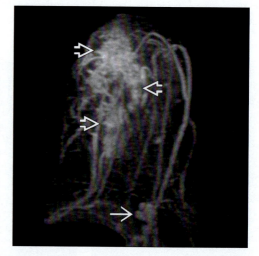

Sagittal T1 C+ subtraction MR of a 61 yo woman shows clumped enhancement in a segmental distribution ➡. Appearance is suspicious; shown to be more extensive on MIP images (right-hand image).

Axial MIP of T1 C+ subtraction MR shows the suspicious findings ➡. Mastectomy confirmed extensive high grade DCIS. Enhancing nodes ➡ not necessarily indicative of tumor; sentinel node negative.

TERMINOLOGY

Abbreviations and Synonyms
- Beaded, cobblestone-like, string of pearls, bunch of grapes

Definitions
- Rapid, non-mass enhancement on MR, typically with plateau kinetics
  - Linear/ductal: In a line pointing toward nipple, may show branching
  - Segmental: Cone of enhancement with apex pointing toward nipple
  - Regional: Large geographic area, not conforming to ductal distribution
  - Focal area: < 25% of quadrant, confined area

IMAGING FINDINGS

General Features
- Best diagnostic clue: Small, round or irregular clumps of enhancement in distribution suggestive of branching ductal system(s)

Imaging Recommendations
- Best imaging tool
  - Dynamic high-resolution contrast-enhanced MR
    - 75-88% sensitivity for mammographically occult DCIS
- Protocol advice: Spatial and temporal resolution equally important; need high speed MR

DIFFERENTIAL DIAGNOSIS

Ductal Carcinoma in Situ (DCIS)
- Majority (65-70%) of MRI detected DCIS visible as non-mass enhancement, 60% as clumped

Infiltrating Ductal or Lobular Carcinoma
- Especially when associated with extensive intraductal component (EIC)

Lobular Carcinoma in Situ (LCIS)
- May have associated invasive lobular carcinoma (ILC)

Fibrocystic Changes (FCC)
- Fibrosis, usual duct hyperplasia

DDx: Other Etiologies Presenting with Clumped Enhancement

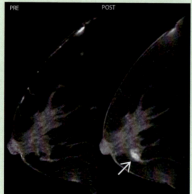

Fibrosis, Duct Ectasia

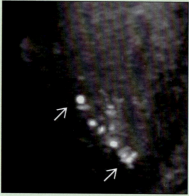

ILC, LCIS

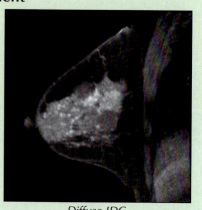

Diffuse IDC

CLUMPED (MR)

Key Facts

Terminology
- Beaded, cobblestone-like, string of pearls, bunch of grapes
- Rapid, non-mass enhancement on MR, typically with plateau kinetics

Top Differential Diagnoses
- Ductal Carcinoma in Situ (DCIS)
- Majority (65-70%) of MRI detected DCIS visible as non-mass enhancement, 60% as clumped

- Infiltrating Ductal or Lobular Carcinoma
- Lobular Carcinoma in Situ (LCIS)
- Fibrocystic Changes (FCC)
- Atypical Ductal Hyperplasia (ADH)
- Other Benign

Diagnostic Checklist
- Clumped ductal enhancement is most frequently associated with DCIS

Atypical Ductal Hyperplasia (ADH)
- Severe atypia, bordering on DCIS

Other Benign
- Papilloma(s), chronic inflammation, ruptured duct, hemangiomas

PATHOLOGY

General Features
- Etiology: Neovascularity and vascular permeability
- Epidemiology: Positive predictive value of lesions with clumped enhancement: 30-41%, majority are DCIS
- Associated abnormalities: May correlate with calcifications on mammogram

Microscopic Features
- Imaging characteristics may be related to heaped up tumor cells in ducts involved with in situ cancer

CLINICAL ISSUES

Natural History & Prognosis
- Dependent on histologic diagnosis

Treatment
- Suspicious finding, usually merits biopsy
  - MRI-guided biopsy with clip placement
  - Consider bracket localization if > 2 cm area for excision

DIAGNOSTIC CHECKLIST

Image Interpretation Pearls
- Clumped ductal enhancement is most frequently associated with DCIS

SELECTED REFERENCES

1. Morakkabati-Spitz N et al: Diagnostic usefulness of segmental and linear enhancement in dynamic breast MRI. Eur Radiol. 15(9):2010-7, 2005
2. Ikeda DM et al: Breast Imaging Reporting and Data System: BI-RADS, Magnetic Resonance Imaging, 1st ed. Reston, American College of Radiology, 2003
3. LaTrenta LR et al: Breast lesions detected with MR imaging: utility and histopathologic importance of identification with US. Radiology. 227(3):856-61, 2003
4. Liberman L et al: Ductal enhancement on MR imaging of the breast. AJR. 181:519-25, 2003
5. Nakahara H et al: A comparison of MR imaging, galactography and ultrasonography in patients with nipple discharge. Breast Cancer. 10(4):320-9, 2003
6. Neubauer H et al: High grade and non-high grade ductal carcinoma in situ on dynamic MR mammography: characteristic findings for signal increase and morphological pattern of enhancement. Br J Radiol. 76(901):3-12, 2003
7. Tuncbilek N et al: Evaluation of tumor angiogenesis with contrast-enhanced dynamic magnetic resonance mammography. Breast J. 9(5):403-8, 2003
8. Liberman L et al: Breast lesions detected on MR imaging: features and positive predictive value. AJR. 179:171-8, 2002

IMAGE GALLERY

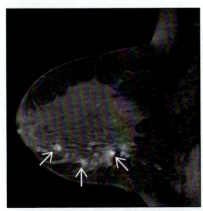 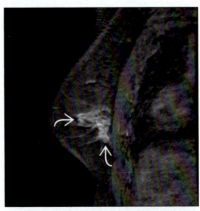 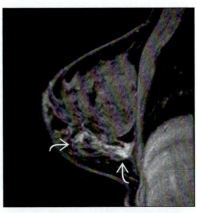

(Left) Sagittal T1 C+ FS MR shows clumped enhancement in ductal distribution ➡ in 48 year old with recently diagnosed IDC. Biopsy of anterior and posterior areas showed DCIS. *(Center)* Sagittal T1 C+ FS MR shows irregular clumped enhancement in a regional distribution ➡ in this 45 year old with invasive cancer and associated DCIS. *(Right)* Sagittal T1 C+ FS MR shows segmental enhancement ➡, in 33 year old with positive family history, palpable nodularity in upper breast & negative mammogram. MR-directed biopsy showed DCIS.

FOCI (MR)

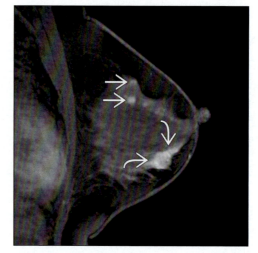

Sagittal T1 C+ FS MR in a woman with a contralateral invasive ductal carcinoma shows an incidental solitary 2 mm enhancing focus ➔. No further action was taken; stable mammogram 1 year later.

Sagittal T1 C+ FS MR of the left breast in a patient with malignant axillary nodes and IDC ➔ shows two remote enhancing foci ➔. No second look US findings; they were treated as benign.

TERMINOLOGY

Abbreviations and Synonyms
- Punctate focal enhancement
- Early literature, no longer used: Incidental enhancing lesions (IEL's), unidentified bright objects (UBO's)

Definitions
- Tiny spots of contrast-enhancement
- Too small to characterize morphologically, ≤ 5 mm

IMAGING FINDINGS

General Features
- Best diagnostic clue: Isolated rounded spots of contrast-enhancement
- Location: Anywhere in breast
- Size
  - Up to 5 mm diameter
  - Larger lesions are masses or non-mass enhancement
- Morphology
  - Typically round or oval, smooth, sharply-defined
  - No adjacent parenchymal distortion

Mammographic Findings
- Infrequent mammographic correlate, not generally helpful

Ultrasonographic Findings
- Grayscale Ultrasound
  - May see evidence of fibrocystic changes: Small cysts, echogenic calcifications
  - Malignant foci may be visible: US can be used to guide biopsy
  - Lack of US correlate not reliable for benign etiology

MR Findings
- T1WI
  - Typically occult, isointense to parenchyma
  - Rarely may visualize eccentric fatty hilum indicative of small lymph node
- T2WI FS
  - Hyperintensity on T2WI (or STIR) favors benign etiology
    - Usually fibrocystic changes (FCC)
    - Papillary ductal carcinoma in situ (DCIS), mucinous carcinoma can be hyperintense
- T1 C+ FS

DDx: Irregular Enhancing Nodules

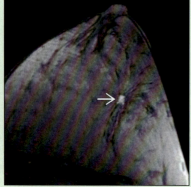

Radial Scar

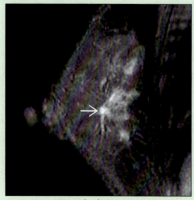

Invasive Lobular Carcinoma

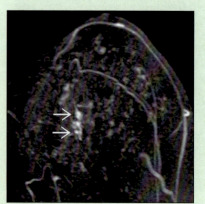

Lobular Carcinoma in Situ

FOCI (MR)

Key Facts

Terminology
- Tiny spots of contrast-enhancement
- Too small to characterize morphologically, ≤ 5 mm

Imaging Findings
- Typically round or oval, smooth, sharply-defined

Top Differential Diagnoses
- Hormonal or Cyclical Focal Enhancement
- Fibrocystic Changes (FCC)
- Benign Neoplasm
- Atypical Ductal Hyperplasia
- Lobular Carcinoma in Situ (LCIS)
- Ductal Carcinoma in Situ (DCIS)

Pathology
- Malignancy in 1/37 (2.7%) lesions < 5 mm (one series)
- 6% or more of women undergoing high risk screening have foci
- Synchronous with carcinoma elsewhere (20%)

Clinical Issues
- Incidental finding
- Asymptomatic
- Frequency declines with age
- Level of suspicion increases with age
- Majority resolve spontaneously on follow-up MR
- Risk of malignancy depends on clinical scenario
- < 50% benign in same quadrant as synchronous primary cancer

- ○ Describe kinetics of enhancement
  - Initial phase (first 2 minutes post injection): Slow (< 60%), medium (60-100%), rapid (> 100%)
  - Delayed phase (after 2 minutes, when curve starts to change): Persistent, plateau = flat (+/- 10%), washout
  - Most malignancies show rapid initial enhancement
  - Washout can be seen with normal lymph nodes; otherwise suspicious
  - Persistent kinetics favors benign etiology
- ○ Assess multiplicity, bilaterality
  - Scattered bilateral foci favors benign etiology
- ○ Are there suspicious findings in the same breast? Same quadrant?
- ○ Distribution of multiple foci itself can be suspicious
  - Multiple foci in a linear or segmental distribution suspicious for DCIS or other malignancy

Imaging Recommendations
- Best imaging tool: Gadolinium-enhanced dynamic temporally resolved MR
- Protocol advice
  - ○ Analysis improves with higher spatial resolution
    - Better definition with high resolution scans: ≤ 2 mm slice thickness, < 1 mm in-plane resolution
  - ○ Attention to optimal timing in menstrual cycle
    - Fewest false positives days 7-10 after onset of menses

DIFFERENTIAL DIAGNOSIS

Hormonal or Cyclical Focal Enhancement
- Normal breast tissue
- Varies from cycle to cycle and within cycle
- Minimized in weeks 2-3 of menstrual cycle
  - ○ Consider repeating scan at days 7-10 if possible
- May have suspicious contrast-enhancement kinetics
- Exogenous hormone replacement therapy can cause similar findings
- Tamoxifen can suppress hormonal enhancement

Fibrocystic Changes (FCC)
- May have associated apocrine metaplasia, usual hyperplasia, sclerosing adenosis
- Cysts on T2WI
- Frequent cause of foci: Often multiple, scattered, bilateral
- Can be evident as a mass or region of enhancement

Benign Neoplasm
- Fibroadenoma
- Papilloma

Radial Scar/Complex Sclerosing Lesion
- Adjacent parenchymal distortion

Atypical Ductal Hyperplasia
- May be more irregular in shape

Lobular Carcinoma in Situ (LCIS)
- Usually more irregular in shape

Ductal Carcinoma in Situ (DCIS)
- Often clumped linear or segmental enhancement
- Can be regional, even stippled
- Multiple foci in linear, segmental, or regional distribution can be DCIS

Invasive Carcinoma
- Tiny lobular or ductal carcinoma
- Often adjacent distortion
- May accompany dominant invasive carcinoma [satellite nodule(s)]

PATHOLOGY

General Features
- Etiology
  - ○ Localized hypervascularity and increased vascular permeability
  - ○ Malignancy in 1/37 (2.7%) lesions < 5 mm (one series)

FOCI (MR)

- Mammographically occult, lesions going to biopsy, independent of kinetics
- Epidemiology
  - 6% or more of women undergoing high risk screening have foci
  - 6% of MR-detected, mammographically occult lesions going to biopsy
  - Synchronous with carcinoma elsewhere (20%)
    - In same quadrant, tend to be malignant (~ 75%)
    - In other quadrants, usually benign (~ 85%)

Gross Pathologic & Surgical Features
- Usually not palpable at excision

Microscopic Features
- Those of underlying pathology
- Correlation with MR requires serial 5 mm slices and slice-by-slice comparison
- Immunohistochemical stains may show increased capillary vessel density

CLINICAL ISSUES

Presentation
- Most common signs/symptoms
  - Incidental finding
    - Especially in high risk screening
  - Asymptomatic

Demographics
- Age
  - Frequency declines with age
  - Level of suspicion increases with age
    - Almost always benign in premenopausal women unless satellite to malignancy
    - Occasionally malignant in postmenopausal women

Natural History & Prognosis
- Majority resolve spontaneously on follow-up MR
- Risk of malignancy depends on clinical scenario
  - > 95% benign in high risk screening
  - > 85% benign in quadrants away from synchronous primary cancer
  - ~ 70% benign when for evaluation of prior equivocal breast imaging (one series)
  - < 50% benign in same quadrant as synchronous primary cancer

Treatment
- Many foci can be dismissed as benign
  - Particularly when scattered, bilateral
  - Corresponding cystic changes on T2WI
- Possibly hormonal, consider repeat
  - At optimal time in menstrual cycle (days 7-10)
  - 6 weeks after stopping exogenous hormone replacement
- Solitary focus in high risk patient likely merits 6 month follow-up; further study needed
- When satellite to a known or presumed malignancy, merits further evaluation (e.g., targeted US), often biopsy

DIAGNOSTIC CHECKLIST

Consider
- Appropriate management predicated on indication for exam (pre-test risk of malignancy)
- May disappear with neoadjuvant or adjuvant chemotherapy or radiation treatment; disappearance could be secondary to malignant lesion(s) responding to treatment or variations in the appearance of foci based on timing of MR examination

Image Interpretation Pearls
- Parametric enhancement analysis not very reliable
  - Benign lesions may enhance with suspicious kinetics
  - ~ 2/3 all findings with rapid enhancement, early peak, and washout are malignant
  - < 6-10% with persistent enhancement are malignant
  - Reflects degree of hypervascularity, vascular permeability

SELECTED REFERENCES

1. Liberman L et al: Does size matter? Positive predictive value of MRI-detected breast lesions as a function of lesion size. AJR Am J Roentgenol. 186(2):426-30, 2006
2. Yabuuchi H et al: Incidentally detected lesions on contrast-enhanced MR imaging in candidates for breast-conserving therapy: Correlation between MR findings and histological diagnosis. J Magn Reson Imaging. 23(4):486-92, 2006
3. Delille JP et al: Physiologic changes in breast magnetic resonance imaging during the menstrual cycle: perfusion imaging, signal enhancement, and influence of the T1 relaxation time of breast tissue. Breast J. 11(4):236-41, 2005
4. Sadowski EA et al: Frequency of malignancy in lesions classified as probably benign after dynamic contrast-enhanced breast MRI examination. J Magn Reson Imaging. 21(5):556-64, 2005
5. Tozaki M et al: High-spatial-resolution MR imaging of focal breast masses: interpretation model based on kinetic and morphological parameters. Radiat Med. 23(1):43-50, 2005
6. Liberman L et al: Probably benign lesions at breast magnetic resonance imaging: preliminary experience in high-risk women. Cancer. 98:377-88, 2003
7. Heinig A et al: Suppression of unspecific enhancement on breast magnetic resonance imaging (MRI) by antiestrogen medication. Tumori. 88(3):215-23, 2002
8. Yuh EL et al: Clinical outcomes of incidental enhancing lesions detected on contrast-enhanced breast MRI. Radiology. 225:325-6 (abstr), 2002
9. Brown J et al: Incidental enhancing lesions found on MR imaging of the breast. AJR Am J Roentgenol. 176(5):1249-54, 2001
10. Nunes LW et al: Breast MR imaging: interpretation model. Radiology. 202(3):833-41, 1997

FOCI (MR)

IMAGE GALLERY

Typical

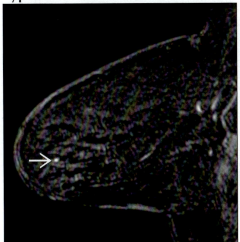
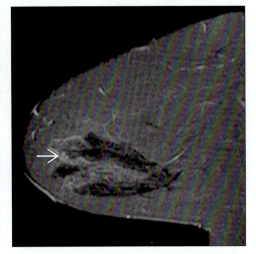

(Left) Sagittal T1 C+ subtraction MR of the right breast shows a solitary 3 mm enhancing focus ➡ with rapid enhancement kinetics. STIR image shown on the right. **(Right)** Sagittal STIR MR shows vague hyperintensity at site of enhancing focus ➡. This was considered probably benign, BI-RADS 3, and, at 6 month follow-up MR, had resolved.

Variant

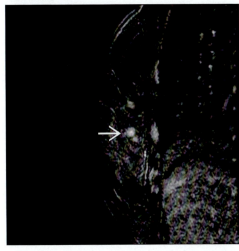
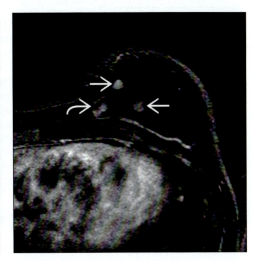

(Left) Sagittal T1 C+ FS MR shows a persistent enhancing focus ➡ in this woman undergoing high risk MRI screening. No US lesion was visible and mammography was normal. MR guided biopsy = sclerosing adenosis. **(Right)** Axial T1 C+ subtraction MR in another patient shows two satellite enhancing foci with benign enhancement kinetics ➡ adjacent to a proven carcinoma ➡. After neoadjuvant chemotherapy, these lesions disappeared.

Variant

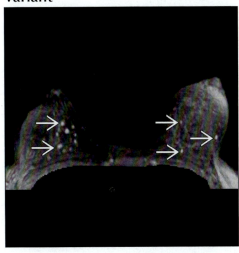
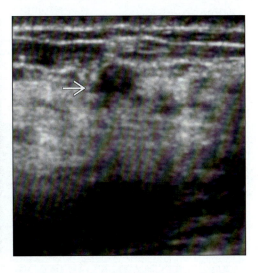

(Left) Axial MIP of T1 C+ subtraction MR in a patient with proven current right breast invasive lobular carcinoma at 3 minutes after contrast shows numerous 2-4 mm enhancing foci in both breasts ➡. **(Right)** Ultrasound of the right breast (same case as left-hand image) shows one of multiple 2-5 mm irregular hypoechoic masses ➡. At mastectomy, a 3 mm focus invasive lobular carcinoma and multiple foci of LCIS were found.

NONENHANCING INTERNAL SEPTATIONS (MR)

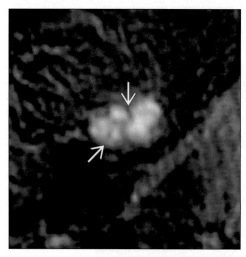

Sagittal T1 C+ subtraction MR shows a known fibroadenoma appearing as a lobulated enhancing mass on MR, with prominent nonenhancing internal septations ➡.

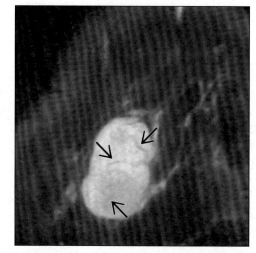

Axial T1 C+ FS MR shows a large ovoid sharply defined enhancing fibroadenoma with multiple prominent internal dark curvilinear lines ➔ representing incomplete fibrous septations.

TERMINOLOGY

Abbreviations and Synonyms
- Dark internal septa

Definitions
- Internal fibrous bands which do not enhance following contrast injection

IMAGING FINDINGS

General Features
- Best diagnostic clue: Linear and curvilinear nonenhancing dark lines within an enhancing focal mass lesion
- Size: < 1 mm thickness
- Morphology
  ○ Curvilinear or straight lines
  ○ May form apparent lobules within an enhancing mass

Imaging Recommendations
- Best imaging tool: High-resolution fat suppressed contrast-enhanced MR
- Protocol advice
  ○ Detection sensitivity increases with increasing spatial resolution
  ○ High spatial resolution acquisitions preferable
    - Unilateral imaging may provide higher spatial resolution
    - No diagnostic difference between 2D or 3D acquisitions
  ○ High temporal resolution not critical

DIFFERENTIAL DIAGNOSIS

Fibroadenoma
- Seen in 25% of fibroadenomas with in-plane resolution of 1.25 x 1.25 mm
- Seen in 50% of fibroadenomas with in-plane resolution of 0.80 x 0.60 mm
- Smooth, oval or gently lobulated mass(es)

DDx: Invasive Carcinoma

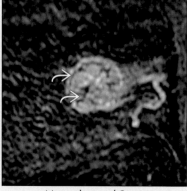

Nonenhanced Septa

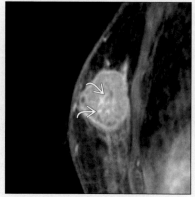

Enhancing Septa

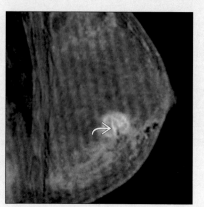

Enhancing Septa

NONENHANCING INTERNAL SEPTATIONS (MR)

Key Facts

Imaging Findings

- Best diagnostic clue: Linear and curvilinear nonenhancing dark lines within an enhancing focal mass lesion
- Size: < 1 mm thickness
- Best imaging tool: High-resolution fat suppressed contrast-enhanced MR
- Detection sensitivity increases with increasing spatial resolution

Top Differential Diagnoses

- Fibroadenoma
- Invasive Ductal Carcinoma
- Phyllodes Tumour

Pathology

- Etiology: Hypovascular fibrous bands within a mass

Invasive Ductal Carcinoma

- More often have enhancing internal septa
- Rarely may have nonenhancing internal septa

Phyllodes Tumour

- Usually homogeneous enhancement; may have nonenhancing septations

Intracystic Papillary Carcinoma

- Spaces between fronds of tumor may mimic septa

PATHOLOGY

General Features

- Etiology: Hypovascular fibrous bands within a mass
- Epidemiology: Sporadic, idiopathic

Gross Pathologic & Surgical Features

- Whitish firm bands within solid mass lesion

Microscopic Features

- Fibrous internal septa
- Paucity of blood vessels within septa

CLINICAL ISSUES

Presentation

- Most common signs/symptoms: Palpable or nonpalpable mass

Demographics

- Age: Usually premenopausal

Natural History & Prognosis

- Septa have no intrinsic clinical significance
- Prognosis is that of underlying lesion

DIAGNOSTIC CHECKLIST

Image Interpretation Pearls

- Manage based on worst feature: Irregular margins should prompt biopsy

SELECTED REFERENCES

1. Kuhl CK et al: Dynamic bilateral contrast-enhanced MR imaging of the breast: trade-off between spatial and temporal resolution. Radiology. 236(3):789-800, 2005
2. Tozaki M et al: High-spatial-resolution MR imaging of focal breast masses: interpretation model based on kinetic and morphological parameters. Radiat Med. 23(1):43-50, 2005
3. Daniel B et al: Magnetic Resonance Imaging of Breast Cancer and MRI-guided Breast Biopsy. Chapter 7 in Breast Imaging: The Requisites, Ikeda DM (ed.). Philadelphia, Elsevier Mosby, 2004
4. Nunes LW et al: Update of breast MR imaging architectural interpretation model. Radiology. 219(2):484-94, 2001
5. Hochman MG et al: Fibroadenomas: MR imaging appearances with radiologic-histopathologic correlation. Radiology. 204(1):123-9, 1997

IMAGE GALLERY

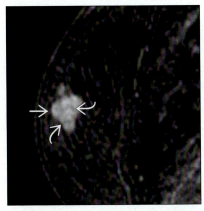 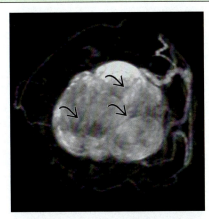 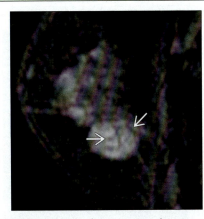

(Left) Sagittal T1 C+ subtraction MR shows a known lobulated fibroadenoma ➡ in the lower inner breast with nonenhancing internal septa on MR ➡. *(Center)* Coronal MIP of T1 C+ subtraction MR shows an intensely enhancing large mass with nonenhancing internal septations ➡. Core biopsy and wide excision showed phyllodes tumor. *(Right)* Sagittal T1 C+ subtraction MR shows a fibroadenoma with nonenhancing internal septations ➡ in a woman with multiple masses in the same breast, including a carcinoma.

RIM-ENHANCEMENT (MR)

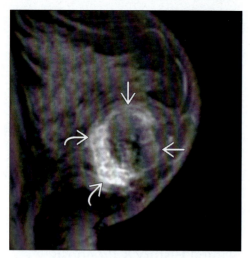

Sagittal T1 C+ FS MR shows a large IDC as a hypoenhancing ovoid mass ➡ with an eccentric thick enhancing rim ➡ posteriorly.

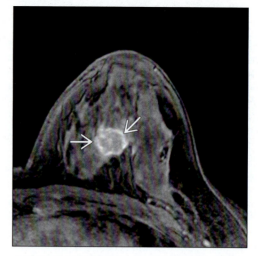

Axial T1 C+ FS MR shows a round irregular invasive ductal carcinoma with thick irregular rim-enhancement ➡. This is accentuated by central tumor washout on this delayed scan.

TERMINOLOGY

Abbreviations and Synonyms
- Edge enhancement

Definitions
- Enhancement on MR more pronounced at the periphery of a mass
- Appears earlier or more intensely than elsewhere in the mass

IMAGING FINDINGS

General Features
- Size: Variable thickness, 1-3 mm typically
- Morphology
  - Smooth and uniform rim in benign lesions
  - Irregular or variable thickness in infection, malignancy

Mammographic Findings
- Mass may be visible: Assess margins, associated findings

Ultrasonographic Findings
- Grayscale Ultrasound
  - "Second look" US moderately effective in targeting lesion for biopsy after MRI
    - Absence of a correlate on US should not preclude biopsy
    - Up to 14% rate of malignancy among lesions not seen on second look US
  - Thick-walled cystic masses will usually show rim-enhancement on MR
  - Surrounding increased echogenicity suggests edema: Post-operative or infection
- Color Doppler: Hypervascularity of periphery of mass may be demonstrated

MR Findings
- T2WI FS
  - Cysts will appear hyperintense
  - Proteinaceous cysts of intermediate signal
  - Hemorrhagic cysts of low or intermediate signal depending on how acute
  - Central necrosis in high grade malignancies may be hyperintense
  - Mucinous carcinoma can be hyperintense

DDx: Additional Examples of Rim-Enhancement

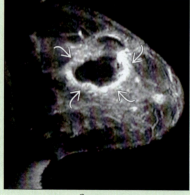

Seroma

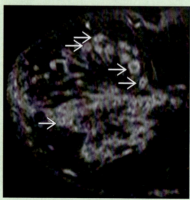

Diffuse, Recurrent IDC

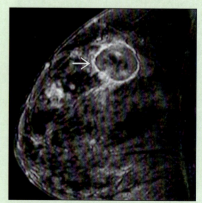

Multifocal Metaplastic Osteosarcoma

RIM-ENHANCEMENT (MR)

Key Facts

Terminology
- Enhancement on MR more pronounced at the periphery of a mass

Imaging Findings
- Size: Variable thickness, 1-3 mm typically
- Smooth and uniform rim in benign lesions
- Irregular or variable thickness in infection, malignancy
- PET: Rim-enhancement = uptake of 18-FDG in rim of mass, can be seen on PET imaging of malignancies
- Best imaging tool: Dynamic high-resolution contrast-enhanced MR
- Spatial and temporal resolution are equally important

Top Differential Diagnoses
- Invasive Ductal Carcinoma (IDC) NOS

- Medullary Carcinoma
- Seroma: Usually smooth, thin margin ≤ 4 mm
- Ruptured or Inflamed Cyst
- Abscess
- Granulomatous Mastitis (Rare)

Pathology
- 8-16% of MR-depicted masses going to biopsy showed rim-enhancement
- 84% PPV for malignancy in multicenter experience

Clinical Issues
- For invasive cancer, indicates worse prognosis
- Rim-enhancement of a solid mass is suspicious, merits biopsy

---

  - Hyperintense edema in inflammatory carcinoma, abscess, mastitis
- T1 C+ FS
  - Smooth, thin (≤ 4 mm) rim with slow, persistent kinetics favors benign etiology in proper setting
  - Irregular, thick rim favors malignancy
  - Assess for multifocal, multicentric, bilateral disease

Nuclear Medicine Findings
- PET: Rim-enhancement = uptake of 18-FDG in rim of mass, can be seen on PET imaging of malignancies

Imaging Recommendations
- Best imaging tool: Dynamic high-resolution contrast-enhanced MR
- Protocol advice
  - Spatial and temporal resolution are equally important
    - As central portion of mass fills in, may no longer appreciate rim-enhancement: Need for complete imaging through breast(s) within 1.5-2 minutes post injection
  - Combine dynamic lower resolution and delayed high-resolution MR
  - Use high speed MR methods to obtain both high temporal and spatial resolution
    - Parallel imaging
    - Spiral, radial or elliptical k-space acquisition
  - Difficult to appreciate rim-enhancement on 3D reconstructions [maximum intensity pixel projection (MIP)]
  - Fewer false positives for residual cancer 28-35 days post surgery, though emphasis is on remainder of breast(s)

DIFFERENTIAL DIAGNOSIS

Invasive Ductal Carcinoma (IDC) NOS
- Irregular thick margin
- Rapid intense rim-enhancement and delayed centripetal enhancement highly specific

- Delayed rim-enhancement with centrifugal progression in carcinomas with expansive growth pattern and high marginal vessel density
- High grade IDC may show rim-enhancement due to central necrosis

Medullary Carcinoma
- Can be complex cystic mass with thick wall, rim-enhancement on MR
- May be partially circumscribed, usually at least partially indistinctly marginated

Mucinous Carcinoma
- Hyperintense on T2WI

Seroma
- Seroma: Usually smooth, thin margin ≤ 4 mm
- Should decrease on follow-up
- Slow prolonged enhancement, variable intensity
- Nonenhancing central fluid collection
- Hyperintense on T2WI & STIR
- Nodular, discrete enhancement suggests residual tumor
  - Granulation tissue can have identical appearance
- Reduced false positive enhancement 28-35 days after surgery
- Emphasis is on remainder of breast (multifocal, multicentric disease) in patient evaluated for positive margins
- Enhancement > 18 months post surgery uncommon but does happen

Ruptured or Inflamed Cyst
- Nonenhancing central fluid collection
- Hyperintense on T2WI & STIR
- Thin (< 3 mm), smooth rim
- Usually in the company of simple cysts
- Slow initial enhancement, persistent delayed enhancement
- Indistinct, thick wall on US

Abscess
- Nonenhancing central fluid collection
- Prolonged slow intense enhancement, slow washout

RIM-ENHANCEMENT (MR)

- Hyperintense on T2WI, STIR
- Most often near nipple, tender, palpable, may have erythema
- Associated edema on T2WI
- May see associated skin thickening (> 2 mm)
- US-guided aspiration/drainage for diagnosis and treatment

Granulomatous Mastitis (Rare)

- Irregular thick margin
- Central nonenhancing collection(s)
- Slow prolonged intense enhancement
- Hyperintense on T2WI, STIR and diffusion weighted MR

Other Thick-Walled Cystic Masses

- Fibrocystic changes (rare)
- Invasive or intracystic papillary carcinoma
  - Usually predominantly intracystic mass
  - Can have focal wall thickening
- Phyllodes tumor (Rare)

Metaplastic Carcinoma (Rare)

- Mammary carcinomas with metaplasia

Sarcoma (Rare)

- Angiosarcomas most common; arise de novo in breast more than in any other organ

Hemangiomas (Rare)

- Typically in pectoral muscle, chest wall, may see in liver
- Phleboliths

PATHOLOGY

General Features

- Etiology
  - Peripheral vascularization of lesion
    - Neo-vascularity of invasive tumors may lead to vessel leakiness
  - Central necrosis, fibrosis or ischemia
  - 8-16% of MR-depicted masses going to biopsy showed rim-enhancement
    - 84% PPV for malignancy in multicenter experience

Microscopic Features

- Factor VIII or CD34 immunohistochemical staining shows increased microvascular density at lesion margin
- Combination of hypervascularity, distribution and degree of fibrosis, expression pattern of vascular endothelial growth factor (VEGF)

CLINICAL ISSUES

Presentation

- Most common signs/symptoms: Thickening or mass, either clinically or image-detected
- Other signs/symptoms: May be tender or painful, especially abscess

Natural History & Prognosis

- Depends on underlying condition
- For invasive cancer, indicates worse prognosis

Treatment

- Rim-enhancement of a solid mass is suspicious, merits biopsy

DIAGNOSTIC CHECKLIST

Consider

- Importance of both spatial and temporal resolution on contrast-enhanced breast MR
- Tender mass may represent infection, abscess

Image Interpretation Pearls

- Thin smooth rim (≤ 4 mm) with slow, persistent kinetics, at edges of fluid-collection (seroma) or cyst favors benign etiology
- Irregular, thick rim or internal solid components favor malignancy

SELECTED REFERENCES

1. Schnall MD et al: Diagnostic architectural and dynamic features at breast MR imaging: multicenter study. Radiology. 238:42-53, 2006
2. Tozaki M et al: High-spatial-resolution MR imaging of focal breast masses: interpretation model based on kinetic and morphological parameters. Radiat Med. 23:43-50, 2005
3. Lee JM et al: MRI before reexcision surgery in patients with breast cancer. AJR. 182:473-80, 2004
4. Ikeda DM et al: Breast Imaging Reporting and Data System: BI-RADS, Magnetic Resonance Imaging, 1st ed. Reston, American College of Radiology, 2003
5. LaTrenta et al: Breast lesions detected with MR imaging: utility and histopathologic importance of identification with US. Radiology. 227:856-61, 2003
6. Semple SI et al: Correlation of MRI/PET rim enhancement in breast cancer: a delivery related phenomenon with therapy implications? Lancet Oncol. 4:759, 2003
7. Szabo BK et al: Invasive breast cancer: correlation of dynamic MR features with prognostic factors. Eur Radiol. 13:2425-35, 2003
8. Liberman L et al: Breast lesions detected on MR imaging: Features and positive predictive value. AJR. 179:171-8, 2002
9. Nunes LW et al: Update of breast MR imaging architectural interpretation model. Radiology. 219:484-94, 2001
10. Frei KA et al: MR imaging of the breast in patients with positive margins after lumpectomy: influence of time interval between lumpectomy and MR imaging. AJR. 175:1577-84, 2000
11. Matsubayashi R et al: Breast masses with peripheral rim enhancement on dynamic contrast-enhanced MR images: correlation of MR findings with histologic features and expression of growth factors. Radiology. 217:841-8, 2000
12. Heywang-Köbrunner SH et al: Contrast-enhanced MRI of the breast after limited surgery and radiation therapy. J Comput Assist Tomogr. 17:891-900, 1993

IMAGE GALLERY

Typical

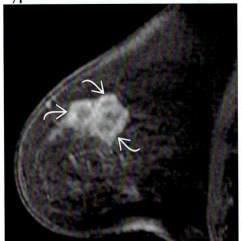
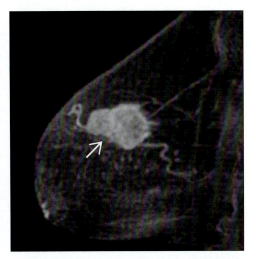

(Left) Sagittal T1 C+ FS MR shows rim-enhancement of this trilobed mass →, known to be grade III IDC in this 71 year old who noted a lump in her breast. (Right) Sagittal MIP of T1 C+ subtraction MR shows the enhancing mass →, but it is difficult to appreciate rim-enhancement on this 3D reconstruction, which better shows the surface of the mass than its internal structure.

Variant

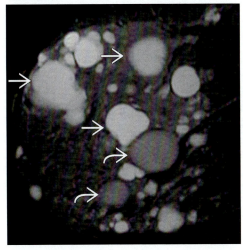
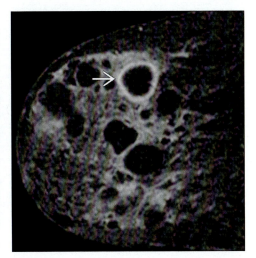

(Left) Sagittal STIR MR in this 52 year old shows multiple cysts →, some of which are of intermediate signal → compatible with proteinaceous content. (Right) Sagittal T1 C+ subtraction MR (same as left-hand image) shows smooth, progressive rim-enhancement at the edge of one of the cysts →, compatible with ruptured/inflamed cyst, a benign finding in this setting.

Typical

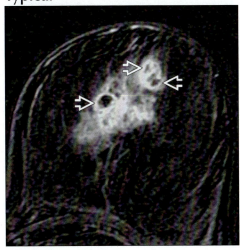
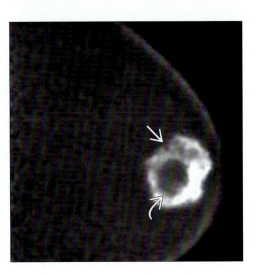

(Left) Axial T1 C+ subtraction MR in a patient with granulomatous mastitis shows strong irregular central enhancement with microabscesses showing prominent rim-enhancement →. (Right) Sagittal positron emission mammogram shows heterogeneous, irregular uptake of 18-FDG in the rim → of this 6 cm grade III IDC. Lack of central tracer uptake → was due to central necrosis. (Courtesy LPA via Naviscan PET Systems, Inc.).

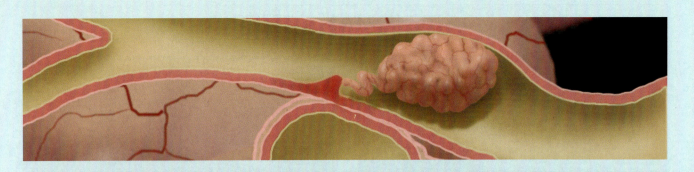

SECTION 2: Histopathologic Diagnoses

ADENOMAS, OTHER

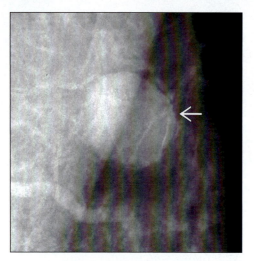

MLO mammography shows a circumscribed mass ➡ in the left breast axillary tail region in a 51 year old.

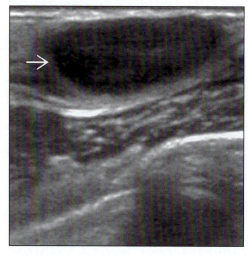

Ultrasound shows circumscribed, hypoechoic oval mass ➡ (same as on left) resembling a fibroadenoma. US-guided 14-g core biopsy showed tubular adenoma.

TERMINOLOGY

Abbreviations and Synonyms
- Pure adenoma, tubular adenoma

Definitions
- Benign, well-defined proliferation of ductules with sparse intervening stroma

IMAGING FINDINGS

General Features
- Best diagnostic clue: Mammography ± US: Circumscribed mass

Mammographic Findings
- Characteristics similar to those of fibroadenoma (FA)
  - Circumscribed mass: Oval; lobulated; round
  - May be partially indistinctly marginated
- Microcalcifications may be present
  - Tightly packed punctate and amorphous microcalcifications
  - Unlike FA, no "popcorn" calcifications reported

Ultrasonographic Findings
- Grayscale Ultrasound
  - Characteristics similar to FA
    - Circumscribed mass: Oval; lobulated; round
    - May be partially indistinctly marginated
    - Homogeneously hypoechoic
    - May have echogenic rim

MR Findings
- No reported specific characteristics
- Likely similar to fibroadenoma

DIFFERENTIAL DIAGNOSIS

Fibroadenoma (FA)
- Statistically more common
- Unlike adenoma, occasional "popcorn" calcifications
- Abundant stroma typical of FA

Lactating Adenoma
- Pregnant and lactating women
- May represent tubular adenoma with lactational change

DDx: Masses that Resemble Pure Adenomas

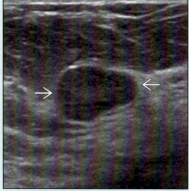

Fibroadenoma

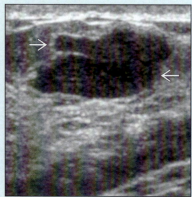

Lactating Adenoma

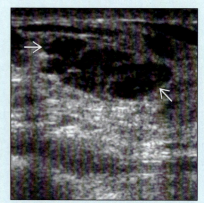

Fibroadenomatoid Changes

ADENOMAS, OTHER

Key Facts

Terminology

- Pure adenoma, tubular adenoma
- Benign, well-defined proliferation of ductules with sparse intervening stroma

Imaging Findings

- Best diagnostic clue: Mammography ± US: Circumscribed mass

Top Differential Diagnoses

- Fibroadenoma (FA)
- Lactating Adenoma
- Circumscribed Carcinoma

Diagnostic Checklist

- Young women: Similar to noncalcified FA on mammogram and US
- Older women: May mimic suspicious mass ± calcifications

- Prominent tubular and lobular elements with secretory activity

Phyllodes Tumor

- US findings similar; cystic spaces favor phyllodes tumor
- Mean age mid 40s

Circumscribed Carcinoma

- Typically high grade invasive ductal carcinoma
- May appear nearly anechoic with thick wall

PATHOLOGY

General Features

- General path comments
  - Other "adenomas" not "pure", unrelated to FA
    - Apocrine, pleomorphic, ductal, and nipple adenoma

Gross Pathologic & Surgical Features

- Nonencapsulated circumscribed mass

Microscopic Features

- Closely packed round or oval glandular structures
  - Single layer of epithelium
  - Intact basal layer of myoepithelial cells
  - Scant stroma
  - Resembles tubular adenosis
- Microcalcifications may be present
  - Formed from secretions in dilated acinar glands

CLINICAL ISSUES

Presentation

- Most common signs/symptoms: Painless, mobile mass
- Typically women of reproductive age; 90% < age 40
- No association with exogenous hormones or pregnancy

Natural History & Prognosis

- Excellent; no reported increased breast cancer risk

Treatment

- Percutaneous core biopsy may provide definitive diagnosis

DIAGNOSTIC CHECKLIST

Image Interpretation Pearls

- Young women: Similar to noncalcified FA on mammogram and US
- Older women: May mimic suspicious mass ± calcifications

SELECTED REFERENCES

1. Rosen PP: Rosen's Breast Pathology. 2nd ed. Philadelphia, Lippincott Williams & Wilkins. 167, 2001
2. Soo MS et al: Tubular adenomas of the breast: imaging findings with histologic correlation. AJR. 174:757-61, 2000
3. Cardenosa G: Breast Imaging Companion. Philadelphia, Lippincott-Raven. 252, 1997

IV

2

3

IMAGE GALLERY

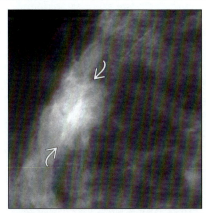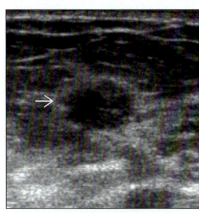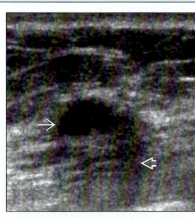

(Left) CC mammography spot compression in a 57 year old shows a microlobulated mass ➡. (Center) Radial ultrasound (same patient as on left) confirms a microlobulated, hypoechoic mass ➡. US-guided 14-g core biopsy showed tubular adenoma. (Right) Ultrasound directed to a mammographic asymmetry in another patient demonstrates an indistinctly-marginated, hypoechoic mass ➡ with minimal posterior shadowing ➡. US-guided core biopsy showed ductal adenoma, concordant.

ADENOSIS, SCLEROSING ADENOSIS

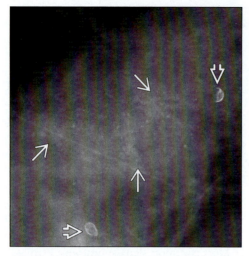

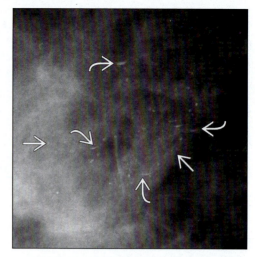

CC mammography magnification shows regional amorphous calcifications ➡ as well as a few incidental coarse, benign, dystrophic calcifications ➡.

Lateral mammography magnification (same patient as left) confirms layering of milk-of-calcium ➡, but not of others ➡. Biopsy showed fibrocystic changes and sclerosing adenosis with microcalcifications.

TERMINOLOGY

Abbreviations and Synonyms
- Blunt duct adenosis = adenosis
- Radical sclerosing lesion (RSL)

Definitions
- Adenosis: Expanded lobules with increased number of acini/ductules
  - Within pathologic spectrum of fibrocystic breast disease
- Sclerosing adenosis (SA): Combination of stromal sclerosis and adenosis
- Nodular subtypes form solid masses
  - Nodular adenosis, adenosis tumor
  - Nodular sclerosing adenosis
- Microglandular adenosis (MGA): Extremely rare variant of adenosis
  - Proliferation of ductules lacking myoepithelial cell layer but retaining basement membrane
  - Background collagenous stroma
- Distinguish from adenomas: Back-to-back glands without intervening stroma

IMAGING FINDINGS

General Features
- Best diagnostic clue
  - Microcalcifications (Ca++): Clustered or scattered, amorphous ± punctate
    - Less common: Oval circumscribed mass ± Ca++
  - May be incidental finding on biopsy
  - Imaging findings vary among pathologic subtypes
    - SA: Ca++ found in 47%, most common morphology = amorphous
- Size: Masses usually small, average 12-25 mm
- Often admixed with other elements of fibrocystic ± proliferative changes: Usual duct hyperplasia, fibrosis, cystic changes, apocrine metaplasia, RSL
- SA especially can be admixed with atypical lesions and malignancies

Mammographic Findings
- Ca++ most common finding
  - More common in sclerosing adenosis than simple adenosis
  - Amorphous ± round, punctate Ca++ > pleomorphic

DDx: Calcifications Resembling Those in Adenosis

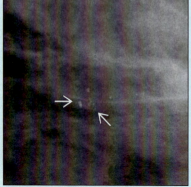

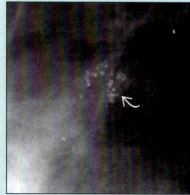

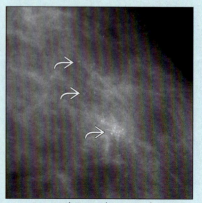

Ductal Carcinoma in Situ

Fibroadenoma

Atypical Ductal Hyperplasia

ADENOSIS, SCLEROSING ADENOSIS

Key Facts

Terminology
- Adenosis: Expanded lobules with increased number of acini/ductules
- Sclerosing adenosis (SA): Combination of stromal sclerosis and adenosis

Imaging Findings
- Amorphous ± round, punctate Ca++ > pleomorphic
- Nodular sclerosing adenosis subtype
- 59% circumscribed, 29% indistinct, 12% partially obscured oval or round solid mass ± Ca++

Top Differential Diagnoses
- Invasive Ductal Carcinoma NOS
- Ductal Carcinoma in Situ (DCIS)
- Atypical Ductal or Lobular Hyperplasia (ADH, ALH)
- Tubular carcinoma mimic at histopathology

- Presence of actin, p63 in myoepithelial cell layer in adenosis and SA (lost in tubular carcinoma)
- Radical Sclerosing Lesion (RSL)
- Adenoma

Clinical Issues
- Glandular proliferation most common in pre- and perimenopausal women

Diagnostic Checklist
- Discordant suspicious findings are not attributable to adenosis/SA alone, merit re-biopsy
- Pleomorphic or linear branching Ca++ ± linear, segmental distribution of Ca++
- Frankly spiculated or indistinct margins, distortion

  - 60% amorphous/indistinct; 27% pleomorphic; 13% punctate among biopsied SA (one series)
  - Clustered or diffuse distribution > regional
- Nodular sclerosing adenosis subtype
  - 59% circumscribed, 29% indistinct, 12% partially obscured oval or round solid mass ± Ca++
  - Less commonly irregular mass with indistinct margins
  - May be spiculated in combination with RSL: Excision warranted
  - Appearance may be indistinguishable from malignancy
- Other findings
  - Asymmetry, architectural distortion, spiculation may be seen in microglandular adenosis (MGA, uncommon)
- May be mammographically occult

Ultrasonographic Findings
- Grayscale Ultrasound: Nodular form: Oval, circumscribed, hypoechoic solid mass ± Ca++

MR Findings
- T1 C+ FS
  - Typically indistinguishable from parenchyma
  - Approximately 30% enhance

Biopsy
- At core biopsy, may be difficult to recognize associated RSL
  - Only 3 of 6 associated RSL were prospectively recognized (one series)
  - When manifest as a mass or distortion with RSL, excision warranted
- Fine linear or branching Ca++ morphology discordant with result of SA on core biopsy: Excise
- Linear or segmental distribution of any Ca++ morphology discordant: Excise

Imaging Recommendations
- Best imaging tool: Mammography ± spot magnification views for Ca++

- Protocol advice: 90° magnification view can help distinguish from milk-of-calcium

DIFFERENTIAL DIAGNOSIS

Invasive Ductal Carcinoma NOS
- Spiculation, distortion favor malignancy

Ductal Carcinoma in Situ (DCIS)
- Pleomorphic Ca++, linear or segmental Ca++ favor DCIS

Atypical Ductal or Lobular Hyperplasia (ADH, ALH)
- Can have amorphous Ca++

Fibroadenoma
- Overlap in appearances of masses ± Ca++

Pathologic Mimics
- Tubular carcinoma mimic at histopathology
  - Presence of actin, p63 in myoepithelial cell layer in adenosis and SA (lost in tubular carcinoma)
- Radical Sclerosing Lesion (RSL)
  - Adenosis, SA frequently associated with RSL
  - Central fibroelastosis distinguishes RSL
  - When manifest as spiculated mass or distortion, excision recommended
- Adenoma
  - Back to back glands without intervening stroma

PATHOLOGY

General Features
- Etiology
  - Possibly stimulated by estrogen
    - Exogenous (i.e. hormone replacement therapy)
    - Endogenous (i.e. obesity)
- Epidemiology
  - Adenosis: 6-17% at autopsy

ADENOSIS, SCLEROSING ADENOSIS

○ SA: 3% of breasts at autopsy; 12% of benign surgical biopsies

Gross Pathologic & Surgical Features
• Nonspecific findings

Microscopic Features
• Proliferation of glandular elements (lobules and ductules)
  ○ +/- Stromal fibrosis (sclerosing component)
  ○ Process similar to breast changes in pregnancy/lactation
  ○ Adenosis may represent failure of involution of lactational changes
  ○ Focal or diffuse
• Adenosis: Hyperplastic lobules contain numerous acini
  ○ Overall lobular architecture is preserved
  ○ Acini elongated, distorted
  ○ Benign-appearing double layer of apocrine epithelium
  ○ Preserved myoepithelial layer, unlike invasive carcinoma
  ○ GCDFP-15 (gross cystic disease fluid protein) stain strongly positive (marker of apocrine differentiation)
• Sclerosing adenosis: Fibrosis of surrounding supportive stromal tissue may trap glands
  ○ Distorted, narrowed glandular elements
  ○ Ca++ may form in compressed acini
  ○ Myoepithelial layer retained: Actin (1A4), p63, CD10 stains positive
• MGA (rare)
  ○ Haphazard proliferation of small round glands: Mimics well-differentiated carcinoma
  ○ Lacks myoepithelial cell layer
  ○ Glands are surrounded by an intact basement membrane (BM)
    ■ Because of abundant collagenous stroma around tubules, BM is often difficult to detect
    ■ BM positive with laminin and collagen type IV immunostains
    ■ Proliferation markers negative: Ki-67 and p53

CLINICAL ISSUES

Presentation
• Most common signs/symptoms
  ○ Incidental finding on mammography
    ■ Amorphous ± punctate Ca++ or oval mass or both
  ○ Palpable mass, mastalgia uncommon

Demographics
• Age
  ○ Glandular proliferation most common in pre- and perimenopausal women
    ■ Mean age 37-44 years
    ■ MGA mean age 45-55 years

Natural History & Prognosis
• Excellent prognosis
• No definite malignant transformation
  ○ 1.7-2.5x increased risk of invasive carcinoma
  ○ 6x increased risk for invasive carcinoma if ADH as well

• Lobular carcinoma in situ (LCIS) can develop in adenosis, or may secondarily involve areas of adenosis
  ○ LCIS: High-risk marker for future malignancy
• DCIS less commonly develops

Treatment
• Radiologic-pathologic discordance may necessitate excision
  ○ Presence of atypia generally warrants excision

DIAGNOSTIC CHECKLIST

Consider
• Biopsy recommendation based on imaging characteristic level of suspicion

Image Interpretation Pearls
• Important to assess radiologic-pathologic correlation
  ○ Discordant suspicious findings are not attributable to adenosis/SA alone, merit re-biopsy
    ■ Pleomorphic or linear branching Ca++ ± linear, segmental distribution of Ca++
    ■ Frankly spiculated or indistinct margins, distortion

SELECTED REFERENCES
1. Bassett LW et al: Diagnosis of Diseases of the Breast. 2nd ed. Philadelphia, Elsevier Saunders. 439-42, 2005
2. Guinebretiere JM et al: Normal and pathological breast, the histological basis. Eur J Radiol. 54(1):6-14, 2005
3. Gill HK et al: When is a diagnosis of sclerosing adenosis acceptable at core biopsy? Radiology. 228:50-7, 2003
4. Markopoulos C et al: Adenosis tumor of the breast. Breast J. 9(3):255-6, 2003
5. Resetkova E et al: Ten-year follow-up of mammary carcinoma arising in microglandular adenosis treated with breast conservation. Arch Pathol Lab Med. 127:77-80, 2003
6. Gunhan-Bilgen I et al: Sclerosing adenosis: mammographic and ultrasonographic findings with clinical and histopathological correlation. Eur J Radiol. 44:232-8, 2002
7. Sabate JM et al: Microglandular adenosis of the breast in a BRCA1 mutation carrier: radiological features. Eur Radiol. 12:1479-82, 2002
8. Rosen PP: Rosen's Breast Pathology. 2nd ed. Philadelphia, Lippincott Williams & Wilkins. 139-51, 2001
9. DiPiro PJ et al: Mammographic and sonographic appearances of nodular adenosis. AJR. 175:31-4, 2000
10. Cyrlak D et al: Breast imaging case of the day. Florid sclerosing adenosis. Radiographics. 19:245-7, 1999
11. Rosen PP: Microglandular adenosis. A benign lesion simulating invasive mammary carcinoma. Am J Surg Pathol. 7:137-44, 1983

ADENOSIS, SCLEROSING ADENOSIS

IMAGE GALLERY

Typical

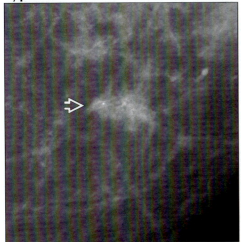
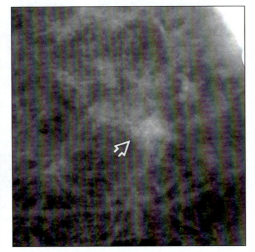

(Left) CC mammography shows an ill-defined mass ⇨ or focal asymmetry. (Right) CC mammography spot compression of the abnormality at left shows partial thinning on spot compression view ⇨. This was biopsied stereotactically, yielding adenosis.

Typical

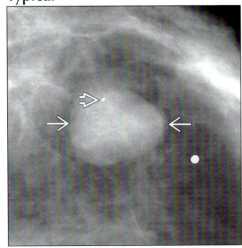
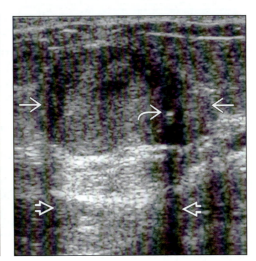

(Left) CC mammography shows a palpable lump (marked with a BB) corresponding to a circumscribed, oval mass ⇨ containing a single coarse calcification ⇨. (Right) US (same mass as on left), shows hypoechoic circumscribed mass ⇨ with posterior enhancement ⇨. The calcification is again evident ⇨. US-guided 14-g core biopsy showed sclerosing adenosis in this 38 year old.

Typical

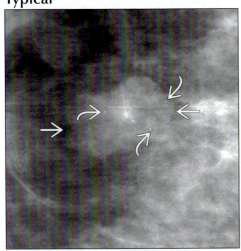
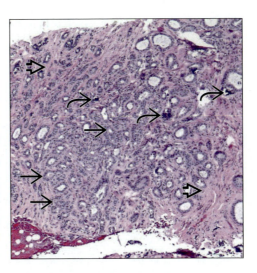

(Left) CC mammography (same patient as previous two images) shows partially circumscribed low density mass ⇨ containing a few punctate Ca++ ⇨. (Right) Micropathology, low power, H&E of core biopsy specimen (same as on left) shows nodular adenosis ⇨ with surrounding sclerosis ⇨, i.e. nodular sclerosing adenosis. A few calcifications are noted ⇨ (case from reference 3).

APOCRINE METAPLASIA

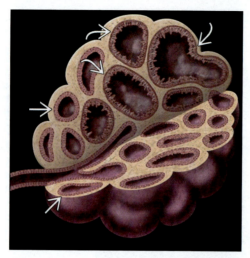

Graphic shows TDLU with some of the acini ⇗ dilated and lined by tall columnar, apocrine metaplastic secretory epithelium, as well as many normal acini ➡.

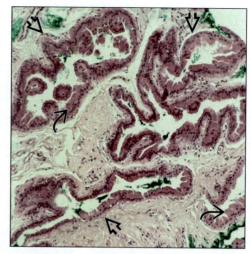

Micropathology, low power, H&E shows dilated acini ⇗ lined by columnar epithelium ➡ with abundant granular, eosinophilic cytoplasm, i.e. apocrine metaplasia.

TERMINOLOGY

Abbreviations and Synonyms
- Apocrine metaplasia (AM)

Definitions
- Dilated acini lined by columnar type secretory epithelium with granular, eosinophilic cytoplasm

IMAGING FINDINGS

General Features
- Best diagnostic clue: Clustered microcysts on US, especially if "fuzzy" border internally
- Location: Lobular portion of terminal duct lobular unit (TDLU) in dilated acini
- Size: Ranges from microscopic to several cm
- Morphology
  - Micro- or macrolobulated mass
  - Clustered pleomorphic, punctate, or amorphous calcifications
    - Can see milk-of-calcium in microcysts
  - Clustered microcysts on US
  - Microlobulated mass with cysts, enhancing internal septations on MR

Mammographic Findings
- Circumscribed microlobulated or macrolobulated low density mass on mammography
  - Same appearance as bland clustered microcysts
  - Indistinct margins should prompt biopsy
- Clustered pleomorphic, punctate, or amorphous calcifications without a mass
  - Nonspecific appearance
  - Milk-of-calcium may occur in microcysts

Ultrasonographic Findings
- Grayscale Ultrasound
  - Clustered microcysts on US
  - Complete overlap in appearances with bland fibrocystic change (FCC) without AM
  - Rarely, individual microcysts may be filled with proteinaceous debris (complicated microcysts)
  - Rarely, individual microcysts may show milk-of-calcium

DDx: Associated Findings

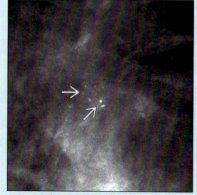

Fibrocystic Change, AM

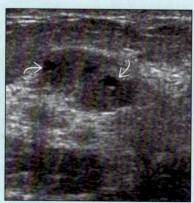

Fibroadenoma, AM

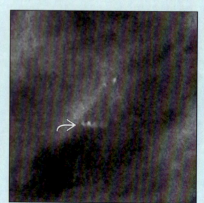

Milk-of-Calcium

APOCRINE METAPLASIA

Key Facts

Terminology
- Dilated acini lined by columnar type secretory epithelium with granular, eosinophilic cytoplasm

Imaging Findings
- Best diagnostic clue: Clustered microcysts on US, especially if "fuzzy" border internally
- Circumscribed microlobulated or macrolobulated low density mass on mammography
- Clustered pleomorphic, punctate, or amorphous calcifications without a mass
- Milk-of-calcium may occur in microcysts
- Microlobulated mass with rim-enhancement and enhancing internal septations on MR
- High frequency US transducer, at least 10 MHz, needed to resolve microcysts

Top Differential Diagnoses
- Fibrocystic Change (FCC)
- Complete overlap in appearances of FCC and AM at mammography and US
- Papillary DCIS can rarely present as microlobulated mass with microcysts

Pathology
- Not premalignant itself

Clinical Issues
- Age: Most common in women 40-50's
- Biopsy if associated solid component on US, rapidly enlarging
- More suspicious if new mass in postmenopausal woman

MR Findings
- T1WI FS: Microlobulated mass of clustered microcysts (hyperintense) with dark septations when large enough mass to resolve (usually > 5 mm)
- T1 C+ FS
  - Microlobulated mass with rim-enhancement and enhancing internal septations on MR
    - Dilated acini correspond to nonenhancing microcysts
    - Internal septations correspond to adjacent walls of acini with thickened AM epithelium

Biopsy
- Stereotactic core biopsy often necessary when manifest as calcifications
- Following US-guided core biopsy (when performed), majority of lesions will decrease in size
- US-guided FNA cytology usually diagnostic
  - Rarely can fluid be aspirated from microcysts

Imaging Recommendations
- Best imaging tool: Most often incidental finding on US
- Protocol advice
  - High frequency US transducer, at least 10 MHz, needed to resolve microcysts
  - Magnification CC and true lateral views required when manifest as calcifications

DIFFERENTIAL DIAGNOSIS

Fibrocystic Change (FCC)
- Complete overlap in appearances of FCC and AM at mammography and US
- Areas of AM may show associated bland cystic change, fibrosis, and adenosis (FCC)
- Milk-of-calcium can be present in areas of AM or bland FCC

Usual Ductal Hyperplasia
- Microscopically bland, cuboidal epithelium

Ductal Carcinoma in Situ (DCIS)
- Rapidly enlarging mass
- New or increasing pleomorphic or amorphous calcifications
- Papillary DCIS can rarely present as microlobulated mass with microcysts

AM within other Benign Lesions
- Fibroadenomas (FA)
  - Cystic areas within FA can show AM or bland epithelium
  - Presence of cystic spaces in FA should prompt biopsy as cystic areas more common in phyllodes tumors
- Sclerosing adenosis
- Papillomas
- Complex sclerosing lesions

AM Admixed with Neoplasms
- Phyllodes tumors
- Apocrine carcinoma, both in situ and infiltrating
- Other breast cancer

PATHOLOGY

General Features
- General path comments
  - Apocrine cells are result of metaplastic alteration of epithelial cells and are a usual component of FCC
  - AM is a possible progenitor of cyst formation
    - Gross cystic disease fluid protein (GCDFP-15) is produced by metaplastic apocrine cells
  - Secretory type epithelium produces fluid, dilating acini
  - Microcysts may fuse to form larger cysts
  - The apocrine phenotype is observed in a spectrum of lesions
    - Benign apocrine change: Frequent; recognized to show nuclear atypia (large nuclei)
    - Apocrine adenoma: Nodular adenosis with AM

APOCRINE METAPLASIA

- Atypical apocrine hyperplasia: Threefold or more variation in nuclear size
- Atypical apocrine adenosis may mimic apocrine DCIS or invasive apocrine carcinoma
- Apocrine DCIS: Some pathologists suggest a working classification of DCIS with five subtypes: High, intermediate and low grade, with apocrine and micropapillary DCIS as separate categories; apocrine DCIS can be admixed with all structural types of DCIS
- Invasive apocrine carcinoma: 0.3-4 % reported incidence; composed of sheets of large tumor cells with eosinophilic cytoplasm and distinct cell margins; Immunohistochemically, apocrine carcinomas express GCDFP-15 and androgen receptor, and are negative for ER, PR
- Epidemiology
  - Found in 50% of breasts at autopsy
  - Not premalignant itself
    - More common in breasts with cancer
  - Proliferative lesion with 1.3-2 x increased risk of developing breast cancer
  - Complex papillary apocrine metaplasia associated with 3.1 x relative risk of cancer
  - Atypical apocrine metaplasia associated with 5.5 x relative risk of cancer
    - May be a precursor of apocrine carcinoma
- Associated abnormalities
  - Often associated with bland FCC
  - May show associated milk-of-calcium within microcysts
  - Complex papillary apocrine metaplasia is associated with atypical ductal hyperplasia

Microscopic Features

- Apical snouting (cytoplasmic protrusions) usually seen
- Dilated acini lined by columnar epithelium
- Granular, eosinophilic cytoplasm with round, basally located nuclei
- Involves the lobular portion of the terminal duct lobular unit

CLINICAL ISSUES

Presentation
- Most common signs/symptoms
  - Incidental new or enlarging low density oval or microlobulated mass on mammography
  - Incidental clustered microcysts on US

Demographics
- Age: Most common in women 40-50's

Natural History & Prognosis
- 53% of clustered microcysts stable at 2 years
- 41% decreasing or gone at 2 years
- Rarely cystic spaces fuse to form larger cysts

Treatment
- Annual follow-up if well seen as clustered microcysts in perimenopausal woman
- Short interval (6 month) follow-up for masses thought to be clustered microcysts but less certain

- Biopsy if associated solid component on US, rapidly enlarging
  - More suspicious if new mass in postmenopausal woman
- Biopsy when manifest as indeterminate or suspicious calcifications
- Excise after core biopsy result of atypical apocrine hyperplasia
  - May be upgraded to apocrine DCIS or even invasive apocrine carcinoma at excision

DIAGNOSTIC CHECKLIST

Consider
- Presence of solid component should prompt biopsy
- Presence of suspicious calcifications should prompt biopsy
- Rapid clinical enlargement should prompt biopsy

Image Interpretation Pearls
- Clustered microcysts without a solid component do not require biopsy

SELECTED REFERENCES

1. Berg WA: Sonographically-depicted breast clustered microcysts: is follow-up appropriate? AJR. 185:952-9, 2005
2. Berg WA et al: Cystic lesions of the breast: sonographic-pathologic correlation. Radiology. 227:183-191, 2003
3. Kushwaha AC et al: Mammographic-pathologic correlation of apocrine metaplasia diagnosed using vacuum-assisted stereotactic core needle biopsy: our 4-year experience. AJR. 180:795-8, 2003
4. Warner JK et al: Apocrine metaplasia: mammographic and sonographic appearances. AJR. 170:1375-9, 1998
5. Page DL et al: Papillary apocrine change of the breast: associations with atypical hyperplasia and risk of breast cancer. Cancer Epidemiol Biomarkers Prev. 5:29-32, 1996
6. Seidman JD et al: Atypical apocrine adenosis of the breast: a clinicopathologic study of 37 patients with 8.7 year follow-up. Cancer. 77:2529-37, 1996
7. Tavassoli FA et al: Intraductal apocrine carcinoma: A clinicopathologic study of 37 cases. Mod Pathol. 7:813-8, 1994
8. Haagensen D Jr: Is cystic disease related to cancer? Am J Surg Pathol. 15:687-694, 1991
9. Yates AJ et al: Apocrine carcinoma and apocrine metaplasia. Histopathology. 13:228-231, 1988
10. Wellings SR et al: Apocrine cystic metaplasia: subgross pathology and prevalence in cancer-associated versus random autopsy breasts. Hum Pathol. 18:381-6, 1987
11. Wellings SR et al: An atlas of subgross pathology of the human breast with special reference to possible precancerous lesions. JNCI. 55:231-273, 1975

APOCRINE METAPLASIA

IMAGE GALLERY

Typical

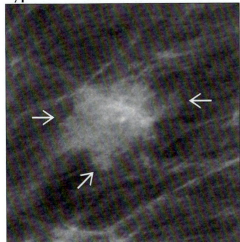

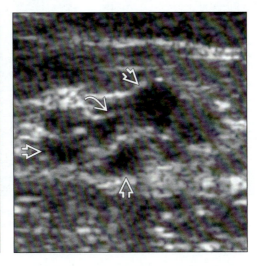

(Left) Lateral mammography spot compression view shows microlobulated mass ➡ on baseline mammogram. *(Right)* Radial ultrasound shows the mass (same as on left-hand image) ➡ to correspond to clustered microcysts ➡ with intervening thin (< 0.5 mm) septations. Biopsy showed apocrine metaplasia.

Typical

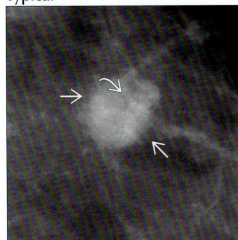

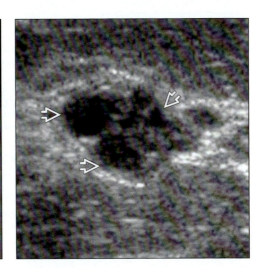

(Left) MLO mammography magnification view shows indistinctly marginated mass ➡ containing a few punctate calcifications ➡. *(Right)* Radial ultrasound shows the mammographically-depicted mass (left-hand image) to correspond to subtle clustered microcysts ➡. MR was performed (next image).

Typical

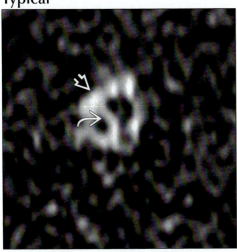

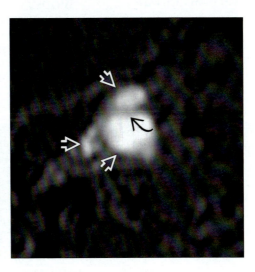

(Left) Sagittal T1 C+ subtraction MR (previous image) shows a microlobulated mass ➡ with enhancing septations ➡, hyperintense on IR (right-hand image). *(Right)* Sagittal T2WI FS MR shows microlobulated mass composed of small cysts 1-7 mm in size ➡ with intervening thin (< 0.5 mm) septations ➡. Biopsy showed AM.

COLUMNAR CELL LESIONS

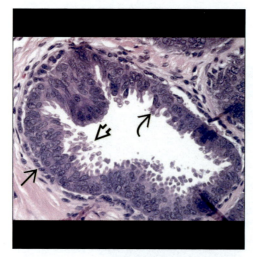

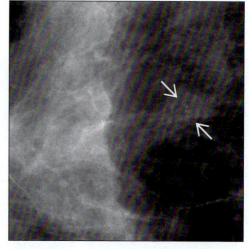

Micropathology, low power, H&E shows columnar cell change with hyperplasia ➡. The luminal tips of cells (i.e., apical) ➡ are pinching off vacuoles (secretions) ➡, into the dilated acinar lumen.

CC mammography with photographic magnification shows new clustered punctate calcifications ➡ in a 53 year old on screening exam. Core biopsy: Columnar cell change with atypia and numerous calcifications.

TERMINOLOGY

Abbreviations and Synonyms
- Columnar cell lesions (CCL)
- Columnar alteration with apical snouts and secretions (CAPSS)
- Columnar cell change (CCC) or CAPSS: Blunt duct adenosis; metaplasie cylindrique
- Columnar cell hyperplasia (CCH): Hyperplastic unfolded lobules; hypersecretory hyperplasia

Definitions
- Metaplastic change in epithelium of terminal duct lobular unit (TDLU) from low cuboidal epithelium to tall columnar epithelium
  - Luminal aspect of cells pinching off vacuoles: "Apical snouts and secretions"
- Spectrum of lesions
  - Distinguish benign CCC/CCH from CCL with associated cellular atypia
  - CCH: More than one cell layer focally
- Flat epithelial atypia (FEA): A CCL with a single layer of cells with apical secretions, cytologic atypia, nuclei turned (i.e., "flat"), disorganized

  - Considered neoplastic proliferation, type of atypical ductal hyperplasia, possibly a precursor of low grade ductal carcinoma in situ (DCIS) and tubular carcinoma

IMAGING FINDINGS

General Features
- Best diagnostic clue: Punctate or round microcalcifications (Ca++) on mammography
- Location: TDLU

Mammographic Findings
- Clustered or regional punctate and round Ca++
- Seldom seen with masses
- Frequently coexists with other proliferative lesions, other types of Ca++

Biopsy
- Percutaneous vacuum-assisted biopsy of indeterminate/suspicious Ca++
  - Usually stereotactic guidance
  - At least 10 specimens
  - Specimen radiography to confirm Ca++ retrieval

DDx: Other Calcifying Lesions

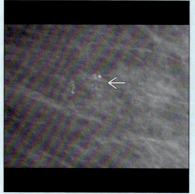

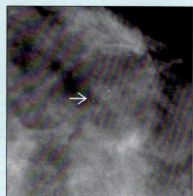

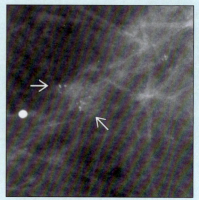

Low Grade DCIS

Apocrine Metaplasia

Stromal Calcifications

COLUMNAR CELL LESIONS

Key Facts

Terminology
- Columnar alteration with apical snouts and secretions (CAPSS)
- Columnar cell change (CCC) or CAPSS: Blunt duct adenosis; metaplasie cylindrique
- Metaplastic change in epithelium of terminal duct lobular unit (TDLU) from low cuboidal epithelium to tall columnar epithelium
- Spectrum of lesions
- Distinguish benign CCC/CCH from CCL with associated cellular atypia
- Flat epithelial atypia (FEA): A CCL with a single layer of cells with apical secretions, cytologic atypia, nuclei turned (i.e., "flat"), disorganized

Top Differential Diagnoses
- Fibrocystic changes (FCC)

- Atypical ductal hyperplasia (ADH)
- Ductal carcinoma in situ (DCIS)
- Usual intraductal hyperplasia
- Lactational changes

Pathology
- Found in 40% of biopsies for mammographic Ca++
- Frequent adjacent proliferative lesions with Ca++
- FEA may be precursor to DCIS and tubular carcinoma

Clinical Issues
- CCL with atypia and/or FEA found on CNB should be excised, similar to ADH on CNB

Diagnostic Checklist
- Benign columnar cell change common on biopsy of punctate Ca++, of no known significance

---

○ Post-biopsy CC and 90° lateral mammograms

Imaging Recommendations
- Best imaging tool: Mammography
- Protocol advice: Spot compression magnification views in CC and 90° lateral projections

DIFFERENTIAL DIAGNOSIS

Mammographic Differential
- Fibrocystic changes (FCC)
  ○ Sclerosing adenosis, apocrine metaplasia
  ○ Milk of calcium: Layering on ML view
- Atypical ductal hyperplasia (ADH)
- Atypical lobular hyperplasia (ALH) or lobular carcinoma in situ (LCIS)
  ○ Usually incidental, adjacent to biopsied Ca++
  ○ Can be associated with punctate and amorphous Ca++
- Ductal carcinoma in situ (DCIS)
  ○ Cribriform DCIS can have punctate Ca++
  ○ More often pleomorphic, linear, or fine-branching Ca++

Pathologic Differential
- Usual intraductal hyperplasia
- Lactational changes
- Tubular carcinoma
- DCIS
- ADH
- Flat epithelial atypia
- Columnar cell change/hyperplasia with atypia

PATHOLOGY

General Features
- Genetics
  ○ No mutations found in simple columnar cell change or CCH

○ Combined genomic hybridization (CGH) studies: Progressive mutational allelic imbalance with atypical hyperplastic columnar cell changes
  ■ Damage of loci at 9q, 10q, 17p, and 17q: Like DCIS and invasive cancer, CCC with atypia is likely part of molecular neoplastic progression
  ○ CCL with atypia often shows staining for keratin 19, estrogen receptor, progesterone receptor, and variably cyclin D1 (features seen in some DCIS, but not normal controls)
- Epidemiology
  ○ Increasing frequency of CCL due to more frequent biopsy of Ca++
  ○ Found in 40% of biopsies for mammographic Ca++
- Associated abnormalities
  ○ Frequent adjacent proliferative lesions with Ca++
  ○ FEA may be precursor to DCIS and tubular carcinoma
    ■ Cribriform and micropapillary DCIS subtypes most common
    ■ Up to 44% of tubular carcinomas can show associated FEA
    ■ Lobular neoplasia frequently shows associated FEA

Gross Pathologic & Surgical Features
- Often multifocal
- Rarely associated with mass

Microscopic Features
- Distended, unfolded TDLU lined by columnar cells, prominent apical snouts and intraluminal secretions
  ○ Columnar cell change (CCC): Acini lined by single layer of columnar cells oriented perpendicular to basement membrane (picket fence appearance); ovoid nuclei; ± apical snouts and luminal secretions (not prominent); ± Ca++
  ○ Columnar cell hyperplasia: Stratified columnar cells (at least focally more than 1 layer) with formation of small tufts; perpendicular orientation of cells and nuclei relative to basement membrane; exaggerated apical snouts; luminal secretions may be abundant; Ca++ usually present, may be psammomatous

COLUMNAR CELL LESIONS

- ○ Columnar cell hyperplasia with atypia: Architectural atypia with bridging and/or cytologic atypia
- ○ Flat epithelial atypia: Acini lined by single layer columnar cells with cytologic atypia and little architectural complexity; perpendicular orientation lost; rounded nuclei turned ("flat"), paralleling basement membrane; snouts/secretions may be prominent; Ca++ (psammomatous) often present
- On low power, distinct blue hue represents tightly packed columnar cells, usually in lesions with atypia
- CCL lack architectural complexity with micropapillary tufts, rigid arcades, and secondary (Roman) bridges: Such findings raise possibility of ADH or DCIS
- Multiple subtypes of CCL often coexist in same biopsy sample, creating diagnostic dilemmas
- ○ Deeper levels may show associated carcinoma
- Ca++ present in 56-74% cases

CLINICAL ISSUES

Presentation

- Most common signs/symptoms
  - ○ Asymptomatic, screen-detected punctate Ca++
  - ○ Incidental finding at histopathology on biopsy of more suspicious Ca++
  - ○ Rarely found in association with palpable lump, considered incidental

Demographics

- Age: 35-50 year old women

Natural History & Prognosis

- CCL with atypia on core biopsy (CNB): Approximately 1/3 show LCIS, ADH, or even DCIS at excision
- Slowly evolving lesions; inadequate data to evaluate long term history and outcome

Treatment

- CCL without atypia requires no further work up or treatment
- CCL with atypia and/or FEA found on CNB should be excised, similar to ADH on CNB
  - ○ Treatment depends on final pathology

DIAGNOSTIC CHECKLIST

Consider

- Benign columnar cell change common on biopsy of punctate Ca++, of no known significance
- Often admixed with proliferative, atypical, and malignant lesions

Image Interpretation Pearls

- CCL with atypia is analogous to ADH
  - ○ Excise after such a core biopsy diagnosis
    - ▪ Risk of adjacent unsampled malignancy
  - ○ Marker of high risk of subsequent cancer, usually DCIS
- FEA on core biopsy requires excision
  - ○ Risk of adjacent unsampled malignancy
  - ○ Marker of high risk

SELECTED REFERENCES

1. Dabbs DJ et al: Molecular alterations in columnar cell lesions of the breast. Mod Pathol. 19(3):344-9, 2006
2. O'Malley FP et al: Interobserver reproducibility in the diagnosis of flat epithelial atypia of the breast. Mod Pathol. 19(2):172-9, 2006
3. Ho BC et al: Flat epithelial atypia: concepts and controversies of an intraductal lesion of the breast. Pathology. 37(2):105-11, 2005
4. Sahoo S et al: Triad of columnar cell alteration, lobular carcinoma in situ, and tubular carcinoma of the breast. Breast J. 11(2):140-2, 2005
5. Simpson PT et al: Columnar cell lesions of the breast: the missing link in breast cancer progression? A morphological and molecular analysis. Am J Surg Pathol. 29(6):734-46, 2005
6. Simpson PT et al: Molecular evolution of breast cancer. J Pathol. 205(2):248-54, 2005
7. Tan PH et al: Pathological diagnosis of columnar cell lesions of the breast: are there issues of reproducibility? J Clin Pathol. 58(7):705-9, 2005
8. Tremblay G et al: Overexpression of estrogen receptors in columnar cell change and in unfolding breast lobules. Breast J. 11(5):326-32, 2005
9. Viale G: Histopathology of primary breast cancer 2005. Breast. 14(6):487-92, 2005
10. Nasser SM: Columnar cell lesions: current classification and controversies. Semin Diagn Pathol. 21(1):18-24, 2004
11. Saqi A et al: Columnar cell lesions: fine-needle aspiration biopsy features. Diagn Cytopathol. 31(6):370-5, 2004
12. Sewell CW: Pathology of high-risk breast lesions and ductal carcinoma in situ. Radiol Clin North Am. 42(5):821-30, v, 2004
13. Siziopikou KP et al: The emerging biological and clinical significance of the columnar cell lesions of the breast. Diagn Cytopathol. 31(6):369, 2004
14. Hoda SA et al: Evolving entities and changing concepts in breast pathology. Breast Cancer. 10(4):294-300, 2003
15. Schnitt SJ et al: Columnar cell lesions of the breast. Adv Anat Pathol. 10(3):113-24, 2003
16. Schnitt SJ: The diagnosis and management of pre-invasive breast disease: flat epithelial atypia--classification, pathologic features and clinical significance. Breast Cancer Res. 5(5):263-8, 2003
17. Tavassoli FA et al: Intraductal proliferative lesions.World Health Organization Classification of tumors. Pathology and genetics of the breast and female genital organs. Lyon: IARC Press, 2003
18. Vincent-Salomon A: [Columnar lesions: a frequent diagnosis in breast pathology!] Ann Pathol. 23(6):593-6, 2003
19. Gomez-Aracil V et al: Papillary neoplasms of the breast: clues in fine needle aspiration cytology. Cytopathology. 13(1):22-30, 2002
20. Jacobs TW et al: Nonmalignant lesions in breast core needle biopsies: to excise or not to excise? Am J Surg Pathol. 26(9):1095-110, 2002
21. Moinfar F et al: Genetic abnormalities in mammary ductal intraepithelial neoplasia-flat type ("clinging ductal carcinoma in situ"): a simulator of normal mammary epithelium. Cancer. 88(9):2072-81, 2000
22. Rosen PP: Columnar cell hyperplasia is associated with lobular carcinoma in situ and tubular carcinoma. Am J Surg Pathol. 23(12):1561, 1999
23. Fraser JL et al: Columnar alteration with prominent apical snouts and secretions: a spectrum of changes frequently present in breast biopsies performed for microcalcifications. Am J Surg Pathol. 22(12):1521-7, 1998
24. Azzopardi JG et al: Problems in breast pathology. Major Probl Pathol. 11:i-xvi, 1-466, 1979

COLUMNAR CELL LESIONS

IMAGE GALLERY

Typical

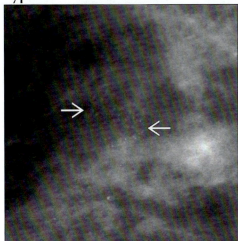
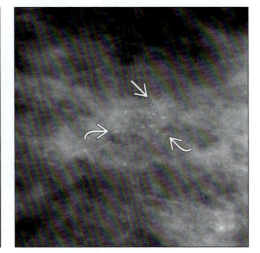

(Left) CC mammography magnification shows faint, clustered amorphous calcifications ➡, new when compared with prior mammogram. *(Right)* Lateral mammography magnification (same patient as previous image) shows layering of some of the Ca++ ➡; others remain amorphous ➡. Biopsy showed calcium oxalate crystals in microcysts and columnar cell change.

Typical

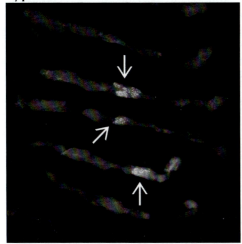
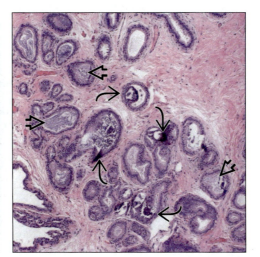

(Left) Specimen mammography of core biopsy for screen detected Ca++ in a 50 year old shows tightly clustered amorphous Ca++ in several cores ➡. Pathology: Columnar cell change. *(Right)* Micropathology, low power, H&E shows typical appearance of columnar cell change with luminal secretions ➡ and associated Ca++ ➡ in another patient with mammographic Ca++.

Typical

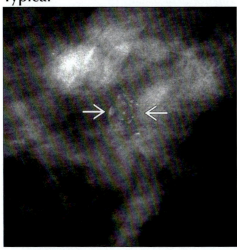
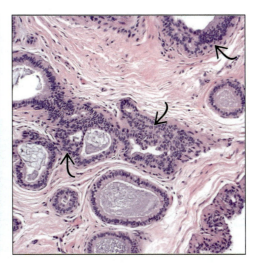

(Left) Lateral mammography magnification shows a 4 mm cluster of heterogeneous microcalcifications ➡. Subsequent core needle biopsy revealed columnar cell hyperplasia with mild atypia, benign at excision. *(Right)* Micropathology, low power, H&E of biopsy specimen of another patient whose screening mammogram showed similar Ca++ shows columnar cell change with some areas of hyperplasia ➡.

CYSTS, RUPTURED/INFLAMED

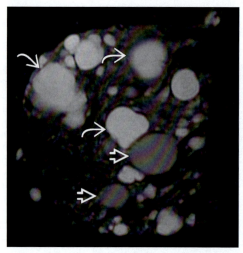

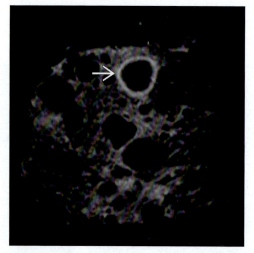

Sagittal STIR MR shows multiple cysts ➡ and proteinaceous cysts ➡ throughout the breast in this 52 y/o seen for high-risk screening due to prior atypical lobular hyperplasia.

Sagittal T1 C+ subtraction MR (same patient as previous image) shows smooth rim-enhancement of one of the cysts ➡, typical of a ruptured/inflamed cyst. This resolved on 6 month follow-up.

TERMINOLOGY

Definitions
- Histopathologic diagnosis: Inflammatory cells surrounding cyst wall and/or cyst contents
- Fibrocystic changes (FCC): Pathologic term, constellation of fibrosis, micro- or macroscopic cysts and adenosis

IMAGING FINDINGS

General Features
- Best diagnostic clue
  - Rim-enhancing cyst on MR in setting of simple cysts
  - Indistinct cyst wall on US in context of multiple simple cysts
    - Biopsy (or aspiration) often still required
- Location: Terminal duct lobular unit
- Morphology: Round or oval, occasionally lobulated mass

Mammographic Findings
- Oval, round, or rarely lobulated mass

  - Partially circumscribed, partially obscured margins
  - May be indistinctly marginated
  - Usually less dense or equal in density to surrounding parenchyma
- Most often seen in company of other (bilateral) cysts and complicated cysts: Multiple bilateral rounded masses
- Can have dependent milk-of-calcium
- Can show calcification in wall (peripheral, curvilinear) of cysts

Ultrasonographic Findings
- Grayscale Ultrasound
  - Thick-walled cystic mass, i.e., a "complex" cystic lesion
    - Contents range from anechoic fluid to hypoechoic tumefactive debris
    - Can be difficult to distinguish from solid mass, especially when < 8 mm
  - Posterior enhancement usually present
    - May be absent or difficult to perceive, especially small, e.g., < 8 mm
  - Indistinct margins most common
  - May see fluid-debris level

DDx: Lesions Mimicking Ruptured/Inflamed Cysts

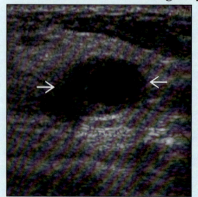

High Grade IDC

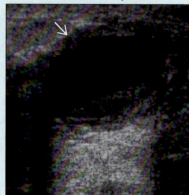

Abscess

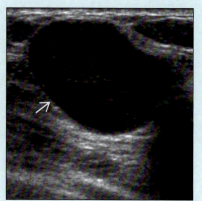

Invasive Papillary Cancer

CYSTS, RUPTURED/INFLAMED

Key Facts

Terminology
- Histopathologic diagnosis: Inflammatory cells surrounding cyst wall and/or cyst contents

Imaging Findings
- Rim-enhancing cyst on MR in setting of simple cysts
- Indistinct cyst wall on US in context of multiple simple cysts
- Usually hyperintense on T2WI due to central fluid
- Protein content of fluid can reduce signal intensity
- May see fluid-debris level
- Usually multiple other cysts and/or complicated cysts
- Rim-enhancement is usually smooth, thin, typically < 2 mm
- Thick-walled cystic mass, i.e., a "complex" cystic lesion

- US appearance nonspecific, often requires aspiration ± biopsy
- Commonly, other cysts, complicated cysts, clustered microcysts present

Top Differential Diagnoses
- Abscess
- Central necrosis in high grade IDC can mimic
- Internal vascularity suggests malignancy
- Papillary carcinoma
- Bland Cyst or Complicated Cyst Without Inflammation
- Epidermal Inclusion Cyst or Sebaceous Cyst

Pathology
- Etiology: Thought to be due to leakage of irritating cyst contents which incites inflammatory response

---

  - Debris can be adherent, mimic intracystic mass
- Internal septations can be seen
- Echogenic areas: Cholesterol crystals rarely evident
  - Can present as irregular mass with linear echogenic cholesterol crystals
  - Inflammatory mass around what had been cyst contents
- Rarely: Echogenic Ca++ in wall
- US appearance nonspecific, often requires aspiration ± biopsy
- Commonly, other cysts, complicated cysts, clustered microcysts present
- Color Doppler: Can be highly vascular, mimics malignancy

MR Findings
- T1WI
  - Hypointense fluid-filled round or oval mass
  - Protein content (or blood) in fluid can increase signal
  - May see fluid-debris level
- T2WI FS
  - Usually hyperintense on T2WI due to central fluid
  - Protein content of fluid can reduce signal intensity
  - May see fluid-debris level
  - Rarely internal septations
  - Usually multiple other cysts and/or complicated cysts
  - Can rarely appear solid or be unseen, especially if small (e.g., ≤ 5 mm)
- T1 C+ FS
  - Rim-enhancing oval or round mass with central nonenhancement
  - Rim-enhancement is usually smooth, thin, typically < 2 mm
  - Slow initial enhancement, progressive (persistent) increase in delayed phase
  - Rare enhancing internal septations
- Second-look US after MR usually successful in identifying, can be used to guide biopsy as needed

Biopsy
- Approaches vary

- Initial aspiration of contents under US guidance
- Sample residual mass (if any) with 14-g core needle biopsy (CNB) technique
- Direct 14-g CNB
  - Favored for very small lesions
- Place clip if concern for malignancy, lesion gone or inconspicuous after biopsy
  - Facilitates correlation with mammography, MR if needed
- Cyst contents variable
  - Thick, cloudy yellow fluid typical of benign cyst contents: Discard
  - Greenish-black, typical of FCC: Discard
  - Brownish, old blood: Send for cytology
- When core biopsy performed, may note gelatinous yellow-green contents in center of core
- Lesion typically decreases during core biopsy, usually gone at follow-up

Imaging Recommendations
- Best imaging tool
  - US readily depicts, can be used to guide biopsy
  - When typical in appearance on MR, may be able to be dismissed as benign or probably benign: Further study warranted

DIFFERENTIAL DIAGNOSIS

Abscess
- Erythema, tender, skin thickening, edema
- Usually close to nipple
- Typically a thick-walled cystic lesion
- May show fluid-debris level; contents often echogenic

Malignancy
- Infiltrating ductal carcinoma (IDC), NOS
  - Central necrosis in high grade IDC can mimic
  - May show posterior enhancement
  - Rim-enhancing mass on MR, but rim is usually thick (> 2 mm), irregular
  - May be hyperintense on T2WI, but has internal structure, usually solid

- o Internal vascularity suggests malignancy
- Papillary carcinoma
  - o Papillary ductal carcinoma in situ ± invasive papillary carcinoma
  - o Intracystic mass; can appear solid
  - o Papillary DCIS typically mostly circumscribed
  - o Indistinct or spiculated margin suggests invasive component
  - o May show hypervascular stalk ± internal vascularity

Bland Cyst or Complicated Cyst Without Inflammation

- Imperceptible wall
- Anechoic
- Posterior enhancement
- Complicated cyst may contain homogeneous low-level echoes or fluid-debris level

Epidermal Inclusion Cyst or Sebaceous Cyst

- Within the skin
- May demonstrate "claw sign" at interface with adjacent skin
- May show increased vascularity
- Mixed internal echogenicity: Hyper- and hypoechoic

PATHOLOGY

General Features

- General path comments: Seen with other fibrocystic changes
- Etiology: Thought to be due to leakage of irritating cyst contents which incites inflammatory response
- Epidemiology
  - o Parallels FCC in general
  - o ↑ In women who are nulliparous, never taken oral contraceptives
  - o Thick-walled cystic lesions represent 6% of all cystic lesions (one series)
    - ▪ 89% successfully aspirated; 11% with residual solid component (one series)
- Associated abnormalities
  - o Often mammographically dense tissue due to fibrosis
  - o Simple ± complicated cysts either macroscopically or microscopically elsewhere in breast(s)
  - o Apocrine metaplasia within ruptured cyst or other cysts, clustered microcysts
  - o Other evidence of FCC, sclerosing adenosis

Microscopic Features

- Cyst contents: Proteinaceous fluid, macrophages
  - o May show epithelial cells, apocrine metaplastic cells
- Cyst wall with inflammatory infiltrate
- Cholesterol crystals with surrounding inflammatory infiltrate (e.g., macrophages)
- Multinucleated giant cells: "Foreign body giant cell reaction"

CLINICAL ISSUES

Presentation

- Most common signs/symptoms

- o Asymptomatic, incidental finding on US performed for other reasons
- o Incidental finding on MR performed for other reasons
- Other signs/symptoms
  - o Can be palpable, tender mass
  - o Rarely, axillary tenderness ± enlarged nodes
  - o Diffuse or focal mastalgia with incidental imaging findings

Demographics

- Age
  - o Parallels other fibrocystic changes
  - o Peak in mid-40s, early 50s
  - o Uncommon in post-menopausal women in absence of hormone replacement therapy

Natural History & Prognosis

- After cyst aspiration showing inflammatory changes, 15% risk of cyst recurrence (one series)

Treatment

- Close surveillance reasonable if typical appearance on MR
- When core biopsy performed, patient can resume routine screening once diagnosis established
- Risk of recurrence after US-guided aspiration may be reduced by instilling air

DIAGNOSTIC CHECKLIST

Consider

- Often seen as thick-walled cystic lesion on US
  - o Suspicious, requires biopsy: 30% of thick-walled cystic masses malignant (one series)

Image Interpretation Pearls

- Oval or round mass, uniformly hyperintense on T2WI (or STIR) with thin, smooth rim of enhancement on C+ MR
  - o In company of multiple simple cysts may be able to be dismissed as benign or probably benign and followed: Further study warranted
  - o Thick or irregular rim-enhancement suspicious for malignancy: 40-84% malignant

SELECTED REFERENCES

1. Vargas HI et al: Outcomes of sonography-based management of breast cysts. Am J Surg. 188:443-7, 2004
2. Berg WA et al: Cystic lesions of the breast: sonographic-pathologic correlation. Radiology. 227:183-91, 2003
3. Gizienski TA et al: Breast cyst recurrence after postaspiration injection of air. Breast J. 8:34-7, 2002
4. Liberman L et al: Breast lesions detected on MR imaging: features and positive predictive value. AJR. 179:171-8, 2002
5. Leung JW et al: Multiple bilateral masses detected on screening mammography: assessment of need for recall imaging. AJR. 175:23-9, 2000
6. Venta LA et al: Management of complex breast cysts. AJR. 173:1331-6, 1999

CYSTS, RUPTURED/INFLAMED

IMAGE GALLERY

Typical

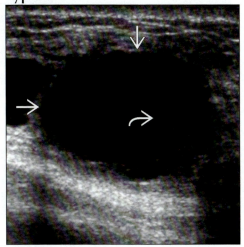

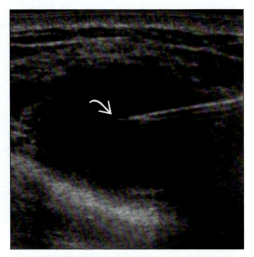

(Left) Ultrasound shows thick-walled ➡ cystic mass with possible intracystic mass ➜ in this 50 y/o with a palpable lump. (Right) Ultrasound (same patient as previous image) shows 20-g needle tip ➜ within mass during US-guided aspiration. Brownish, cloudy fluid suggestive of old blood was withdrawn.

Typical

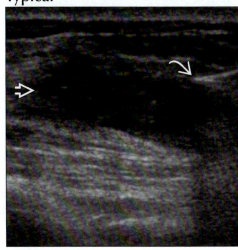

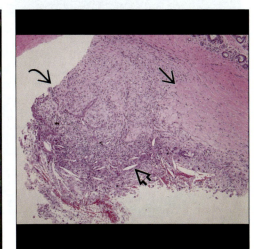

(Left) Ultrasound after aspiration (same patient as previous image) shows residual mass ➡. US-guided 14-g core biopsy was then performed (➜: Needle tip) showing ruptured cyst with acute and chronic inflammation. (Right) Micropathology, low power, H&E shows focal mass due to inflammation ➜ and fibrosis ➜ along wall of ruptured cyst in another patient. Cholesterol clefts/crystals are also seen ➜.

Typical

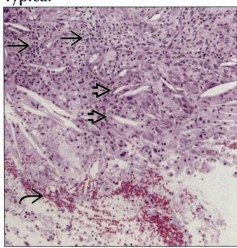

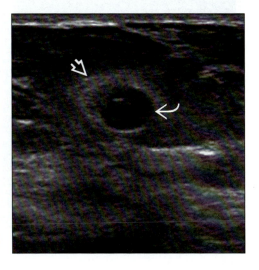

(Left) Micropathology, high power (same as prior image) better shows cholesterol clefts ➜, inflammatory infiltrate ➜. Acute blood ➜ was felt to be due to procedure, though old blood and macrophages are common contents of ruptured cysts (courtesy DWM). (Right) shows thick-walled complex cystic and solid mass ➜ with surrounding echogenic halo ➡, suspicious for malignancy in this 38 y/o. US-guided 14-g core biopsy showed ruptured cyst.

Variant

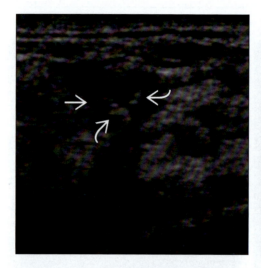

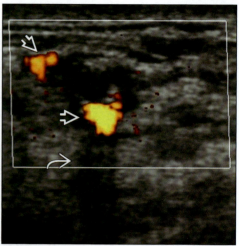

(Left) US shows incidental irregular, hypoechoic mass ➡ with central echogenic foci ➡ in this 58 y/o with dense breasts and multiple prior cyst aspirations. *(Right)* Power Doppler US (same as left) shows marked increased vascularity ➡. Posterior shadowing is also evident ➡. US-guided core biopsy showed ruptured cyst with cholesterol crystals (which corresponded to the echogenic foci).

Typical

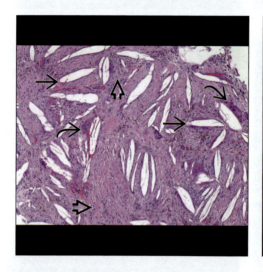

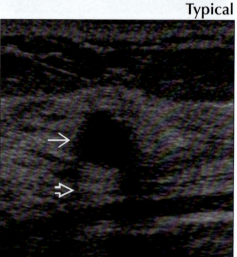

(Left) Micropathology, medium power, H&E, from another patient shows cholesterol crystals ➡ with surrounding inflammatory infiltrate ➡, including multinucleated giant cells ➡, compatible with reaction to ruptured cyst. *(Right)* US shows irregular, thick-walled cystic mass ➡ with posterior enhancement ➡ in a 56 y/o. This resolved on US-guided aspiration, yielding cloudy yellow fluid typical of cyst contents, compatible with inflamed cyst.

Typical

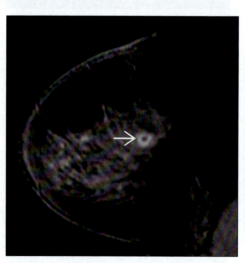

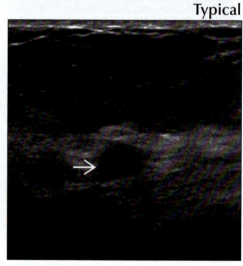

(Left) Sagittal T1 C+ FS MR shows 9 mm rim-enhancing mass ➡ which was slightly hyperintense on STIR images in this 54 y/o for high-risk screening. The mass showed persistent kinetics. *(Right)* Targeted US (same as left) shows hypoechoic, indistinctly-marginated mass ➡ of intermediate suspicion, BI-RADS 4B. US-guided 14-g core biopsy showed scar with old hemorrhage and giant cell reaction around cholesterol clefts consistent with reaction to ruptured cyst.

Typical

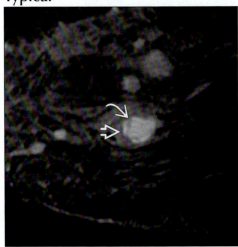 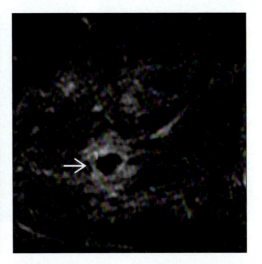

(Left) Sagittal STIR MR shows hyperintense cystic mass ⇨ with few hypointense septations ⇨ in this 45 y/o with multiple cysts and ipsilateral invasive ductal cancer. *(Right)* Sagittal T1 C+ subtraction MR shows rim-enhancement of this mass ⇨ (same as left), suspicious for malignancy.

Typical

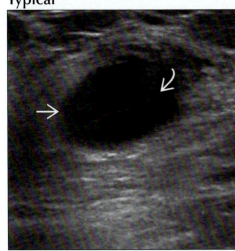 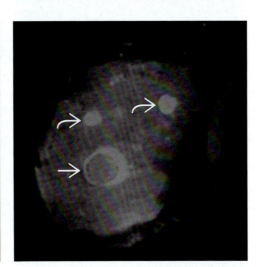

(Left) Targeted US (same as prior 2 images) shows thick-walled cystic mass ⇨ with thick internal septations ⇨, felt to correspond to the MR-depicted mass. US-guided biopsy showed ruptured/inflamed cyst, concordant. *(Right)* Sagittal T1 C+ FS MR shows rim-enhancing mass ⇨ in this 45 y/o with contralateral breast cancer one year earlier. Other enhancing masses ⇨ are known fibroadenomas.

IV

2

21

Typical

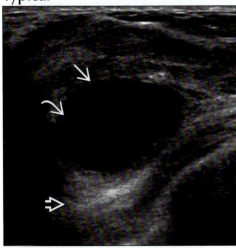 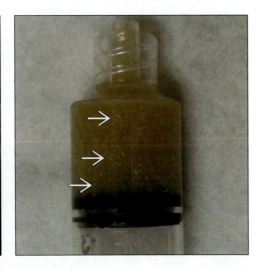

(Left) Ultrasound (same patient as previous image) targeted to the MR-abnormality shows thick-walled cystic mass ⇨ with posterior enhancement ⇨ and intracystic mass vs. debris ⇨. US-guided aspiration was performed. *(Right)* Clinical photograph (same as prior 2 images) shows cloudy yellow fluid with floating cholesterol crystals ⇨, typical of benign cyst contents, discarded.

FAT NECROSIS

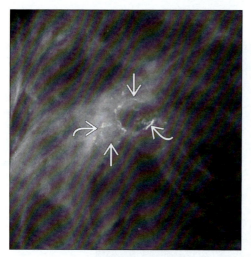

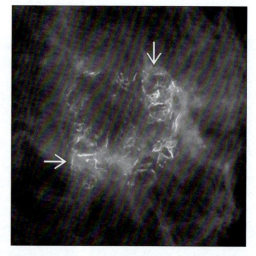

MLO mammography with magnification shows a bilobed lucent mass ⮕ with curvilinear rim Ca++ ⮕, typical of fat necrosis in the right breast in this 43 y/o s/p bilateral reduction mammoplasty 5 years ago.

CC mammography with magnification (same patient as on left) shows the typical curvilinear calcifications ⮕ seen with fat necrosis. This corresponded to a palpable mass left breast.

TERMINOLOGY

Definitions

- Result of injury to breast fat
- Benign nonsuppurative process related to breast trauma/surgery
- May have other etiologies such as ischemia
  - Post-radiation vasculitis
  - Extensive surgery: Quadrantectomy, multiple re-excisions for margins
  - After autologous reconstruction, e.g., transverse rectus abdominis myocutaneous (TRAM) flap
    - Entire blood supply to flap dependent on microvascular anastomosis
    - Fat necrosis most common in upper outer portion of flap where blood supply most tenuous
- Chemical irritation
  - Ruptured cyst or ectatic ducts: Cholesterol crystals
  - Plasma cell mastitis

IMAGING FINDINGS

General Features

- Best diagnostic clue: Oil cyst(s) ± rim calcifications (Ca++) on mammography
- Location
  - Most common in subareolar and superficial areas near skin
    - More vulnerable to trauma
- Size: Few millimeters to several centimeters

Mammographic Findings

- Round, oval, or lobulated lucent mass
  - Oil cyst(s) when round, oval
  - Develop peripheral rim Ca++
  - Inner aspect of mass appears circumscribed
  - Indistinct interface with breast tissue
    - Surrounding increased density due to edema, fibrosis, inflammatory infiltrate
- Isolated calcifications
  - Fine linear or pleomorphic Ca++
    - Early manifestation
    - May be confused with ductal carcinoma in situ (DCIS)

DDx: Other Fat-Containing Masses

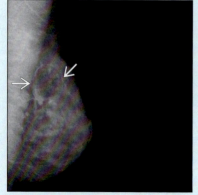

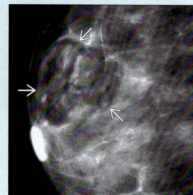

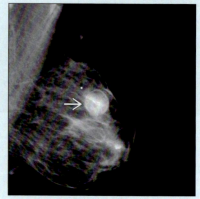

Lipoma

Fibroadenolipoma

Galactocele

FAT NECROSIS

Key Facts

Terminology
- Benign nonsuppurative process related to breast trauma/surgery

Imaging Findings
- Round, oval, or lobulated lucent mass
- Develop peripheral rim Ca++
- Fine linear or pleomorphic Ca++
- Fat necrosis Ca++ coarsen over time → dystrophic
- Spiculated or irregular mass/asymmetry
- Band-like density

Top Differential Diagnoses
- Infiltrating Ductal (IDC) or Lobular Carcinoma (ILC)
- Ductal Carcinoma in Situ (DCIS)
- Encapsulated Fat-Containing Lesions

Pathology
- Accidental injury
- Iatrogenic injury
- No history of prior trauma or surgery in 35-50%

Clinical Issues
- No malignant potential
- No treatment usually necessary

Diagnostic Checklist
- Imaging findings overlap with malignancy
- Proper clinical history helpful: Trauma, surgery
- Fat necrosis mass(es) should decrease over time
- Ca++ develop 1.5-5 yrs (or later) post trauma, coarsen over time
- Ca++ at lumpectomy site within first 1.5 years more likely residual carcinoma

---

- o Fat necrosis Ca++ coarsen over time → dystrophic
- o Lucent-centered, eggshell, at edge of oil cyst(s)
- o Ca++ unusual before at least 18 months post trauma, coarsen over time
- Spiculated or irregular mass/asymmetry
  - o Due to fibrosis/desmoplastic reaction
- Band-like density
  - o Ask patient about prior seatbelt injury
- Asymmetry/mass should decrease over time

Ultrasonographic Findings
- Sonographic appearances evolve over time
  - o Acute phase: Within days of event
    - ▪ Edema of breast fat → increased echogenicity
    - ▪ Compare to unaffected side if large area
  - o Subacute: Complex cystic phase
    - ▪ Ill-defined complex cystic areas within edematous fat: Mixed hyper- and hypo- to anechoic mass
    - ▪ Thin echogenic cyst wall develops: May be multi-loculated
    - ▪ Diffuse low level internal echoes
    - ▪ Posterior enhancement
  - o Late phase: 18 months or more from event
    - ▪ Wall calcifies: Posterior enhancement changes to intense shadowing
    - ▪ May well look thick-walled or even solid
    - ▪ If post-surgical, may have angular margins
- Sonographic spectrum therefore includes anechoic mass, irregular hypoechoic mass, complex cystic and solid mass, architectural distortion
- Posterior features change with time: Enhancement to shadowing once fibrosis ± Ca++ develop
- Color Doppler
  - o Internal flow increases concern for recurrent tumor in lumpectomy patient
    - ▪ May see flow in granulation tissue within 6 months of surgery
    - ▪ Hyperemia post-radiation therapy persists longer; generally settles within a year

MR Findings
- T1WI: High signal central fat
- T2WI FS

- o Low signal with fat suppression
- o May see surrounding ↑ signal due to edema
- T1 C+ FS
  - o Thin rim of peripheral enhancement may persist up to 18 months post trauma/surgery
    - ▪ Rarely, fat necrosis will enhance years later

Imaging Recommendations
- Best imaging tool: Mammography, magnification views for subtle Ca++
- Protocol advice: US helpful if mammography negative or shows asymmetry, ill-defined mass

DIFFERENTIAL DIAGNOSIS

Infiltrating Ductal (IDC) or Lobular Carcinoma (ILC)
- Some fat necrosis can mimic if densely fibrotic, inflammatory mass
- Review old films for evolution of fat necrosis changes
- No history of trauma
- If in doubt → biopsy

Ductal Carcinoma in Situ (DCIS)
- Fine linear, pleomorphic Ca++, can be similar to fat necrosis
- Only associated with a mass in about 10% of cases
  - o Associated mass not lucent

Encapsulated Fat-Containing Lesions
- Lipoma
  - o No history of trauma, no Ca++
- Fibroadenolipoma
  - o Encapsulated fat and glandular elements
  - o "Breast-within-a-breast" mammographic appearance
- Galactocele
  - o Typically associated with lactation
  - o Echogenic, usually with fluid-debris layer (nondependent debris due to fat content)
  - o Aspiration yields milky fluid or creamy inspissated secretions

FAT NECROSIS

PATHOLOGY

General Features
- General path comments
  - Inflammation/hemorrhage into fat → damage to adipocytes
  - Damaged cells leak fat → breakdown to fatty acids → more inflammation
  - Fibrous capsule forms to encapsulate process
  - Saponification of fatty acids in capsule → calcium deposition
  - Non-encapsulated fatty acids incite granulomatous foreign body-like reaction
  - Chronic foreign body-like reaction → fibrosis, skin retraction
    - Can be hard to differentiate from desmoplastic reaction in cancer
- Etiology
  - Accidental injury
    - Blunt trauma: Direct blow to the thorax, seatbelt injury
    - Penetrating trauma: Stab wound, gunshot wound
  - Iatrogenic injury
    - Surgery: Biopsy, lumpectomy, flap reconstruction, reduction, augmentation, explantation
    - Post lumpectomy adjuvant radiation therapy
    - Direct silicone injection
  - Spontaneous development reported in patients with diabetes or collagen vascular disease
  - No history of prior trauma or surgery in 35-50%

Gross Pathologic & Surgical Features
- Firm or hard nodular mass
- Yellowish-white color
- May be associated with recent or old hemorrhage

Microscopic Features
- Loss of nuclei, fusion of adipocytes
  - Damaged cells coalesce
  - Creation of expanded fatty spaces
- Accumulation of foamy histiocytes
  - Fuse into multinucleated giant cells
- Inflammatory reaction
  - Accumulation of lymphocytes, polymorphonucleocytes, plasma cells
- Peripheral fibrosis
- Central necrosis

CLINICAL ISSUES

Presentation
- Highly variable clinical presentation
  - May be asymptomatic on screening
  - Tender or non-tender, palpable mass or masses
  - Firm, fixed mass
  - Occasional skin thickening, retraction
- Imaging findings may be preceded by ecchymosis ± erythema

Natural History & Prognosis
- Excellent
  - No malignant potential

Treatment
- No treatment usually necessary
- Rarely requires excision for painful mass

DIAGNOSTIC CHECKLIST

Consider
- Differentiation of fat necrosis from tumor recurrence in patients treated with breast conservation may be difficult
- All phases of fat necrosis may be present simultaneously in the same breast
- Fat necrosis findings are complicated by those of the underlying process, e.g., seroma/hematoma, ischemia
- Imaging findings overlap with malignancy
  - Biopsy required if diagnosis unclear

Image Interpretation Pearls
- Proper clinical history helpful: Trauma, surgery
- Spot compression mammography may be very helpful
  - Demonstration of oil cysts within a spiculated mass reassuring for diagnosis of fat necrosis
  - Invasive tumor invades fat, does not engulf it
- Fat necrosis mass(es) should decrease over time
  - Rarely inflammatory mass due to fat necrosis will increase: Biopsy appropriate
- Ca++ develop 1.5-5 yrs (or later) post trauma, coarsen over time
- Ca++ at lumpectomy site within first 1.5 years more likely residual carcinoma
  - Particularly if original tumor had Ca++
- Ultrasound technique
  - Scan plane parallel to scar
    - Mass-like appearance due to orientation along surgical dissection planes
  - Scan plane perpendicular to scar
    - Linear appearance, less mass-like
    - Track to skin scar usually evident

SELECTED REFERENCES

1. Gatta G et al: Clinical, mammographic and ultrasonographic features of blunt breast trauma. Eur J Radiol. 2006
2. Crystal P et al: Sonographic findings of palpable isoechoic breast fat necrosis: look for skin integrity. J Ultrasound Med. 24(1):105-7, 2005
3. Kang BJ et al: Breast MRI findings after modified radical mastectomy and transverse rectus abdominis myocutaneous flap in patients with breast cancer. J Magn Reson Imaging. 21(6):784-91, 2005
4. Chala LF et al: Fat necrosis of the breast: mammographic, sonographic, computed tomography, and magnetic resonance imaging findings. Curr Probl Diagn Radiol. 33(3):106-26, 2004
5. Williams HJ et al: Imaging features of breast trauma: a pictorial review. Breast. 11(2):107-15, 2002
6. Soo MS et al: Fat necrosis in the breast: sonographic features. Radiology. 206(1):261-9, 1998
7. Gluck BS et al: Microcalcifications on postoperative mammograms as an indicator of adequacy of tumor excision. Radiology. 188(2):469-72, 1993
8. Mendelson EB: Evaluation of the postoperative breast. Radiol Clin North Am. 30(1):107-38, 1992

FAT NECROSIS

IMAGE GALLERY

Variant

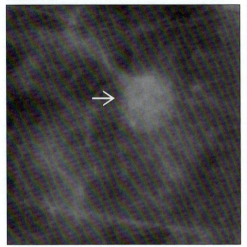
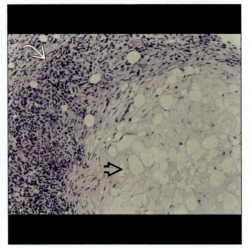

(Left) CC mammography spot compression shows new spiculated round mass ➡ near surgical bed, 18 months post lumpectomy in this 65 y/o. Stereotactic biopsy showed fat necrosis. *(Right)* Micropathology, high power of 14-g core biopsy specimen (another patient) shows rounded mass composed of fat ⤷, with peripheral inflammatory infiltrate ➡, i.e., fat necrosis. The inflammatory infiltrate can create spiculated or indistinct margins as in the case on left.

Typical

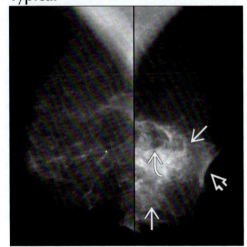
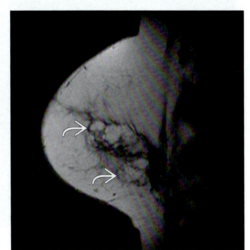

(Left) MLO mammography 7 months post reduction mammoplasty in this 68 y/o with left breast lump shows a geographic area of increased density ➡ containing oval and round lucencies ➡ due to fat necrosis. Note the overlying skin retraction ➡. *(Right)* Sagittal T1WI MR (performed due to incidental atypical lobular hyperplasia in the reduction specimen, same patient as left) shows central hyperintensity of fat ➡ within the lobulated mass.

Typical

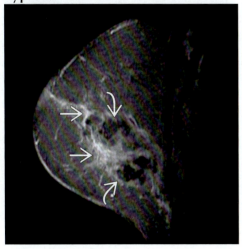
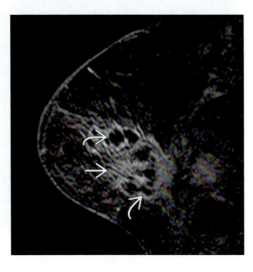

(Left) Sagittal STIR MR (same as prior 2 images) confirms hypointense fat ➡ within the lobulated mass due to fat necrosis. Surrounding hyperintense edema is noted ➡. *(Right)* Sagittal T1 C+ subtraction MR (same as left) shows minimal rim-enhancement ➡ around the fatty masses and mild enhancement in a region of edema ➡. Persistent MR enhancement within the first 18 months after surgery is common.

FAT NECROSIS

(Left) CC mammography of the right breast performed 9 months after reduction mammoplasty in this 55 y/o demonstrates a lobulated, lucent mass ➡ typical of fat necrosis. (Right) CC mammography 4 years later (same case as left) shows reduction in size of the mass ➡, with interval development of peripheral round Ca++ ➡, as well as a dystrophic Ca++ ➡, compatible with fat necrosis. Ca++ due to fat necrosis are uncommon < 18 months post event.

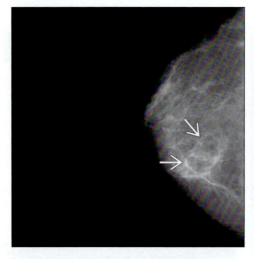 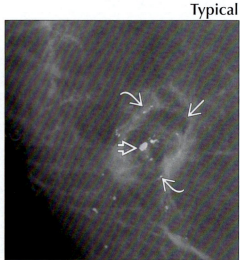

Variant

(Left) MLO mammography magnification shows coarse, dystrophic Ca++ ➡ typical of fat necrosis at site of benign stereotactic core biopsy 3 years earlier in this 52 y/o (clip denoted by ➡). Fat necrosis is unusual after core biopsy. (Right) Densely calcified oil cysts have become dystrophic Ca++ ➡ as seen on this MLO mammogram in a 60 y/o who developed fat necrosis following a car accident 8 yrs earlier.

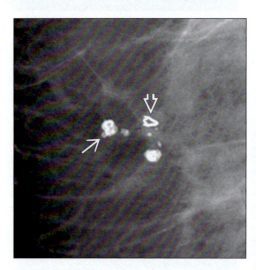 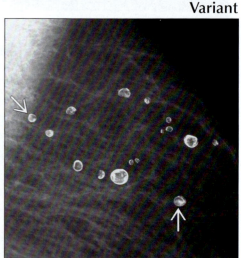

Variant

(Left) CC mammography one yr following lumpectomy in this 50 y/o shows lucent oil cyst ➡, with surrounding increased density ➡. (Right) CC mammography spot compression 4 years later (same as left) shows dense rim Ca++ in the oil cyst ➡, with ↓ density anteriorly ➡ and new ill-defined mass medially ➡ with ↑ skin thickening and nipple retraction ➡. Biopsy showed recurrent IDC. Fat necrosis and scar should decrease in size over time.

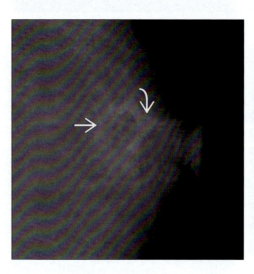 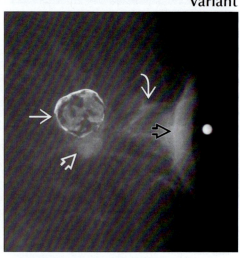

IV

2

26

FAT NECROSIS

Typical

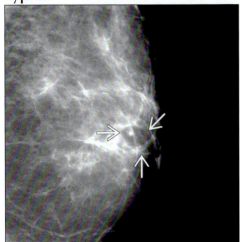

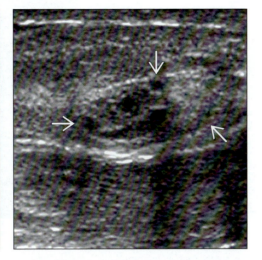

(Left) CC mammography spot compression view of a palpable mass in a 65 y/o show circumscribed lucent mass ➡. *(Right)* Ultrasound (same as left), performed electively, demonstrates oval, mixed echogenicity mass ➡. Concern regarding palpable findings prompted biopsy despite the benign imaging features. Fat necrosis was confirmed.

Typical

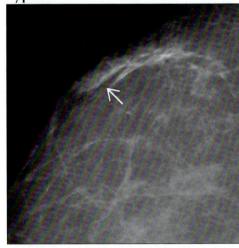

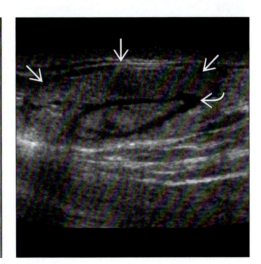

(Left) CC mammography shows a band-like asymmetry ➡ in an area of clinical concern in a 62 y/o woman who sustained blunt trauma (fall) to the breast a few weeks earlier. *(Right)* Ultrasound of the palpable mass (same as left) shows an ovoid area of increased echogenicity ➡ with some anechoic fluid components ➡ and minimal posterior enhancement. In this case, findings resolved on follow-up.

Typical

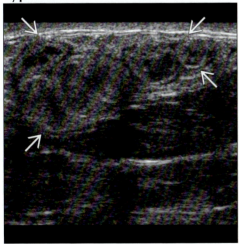

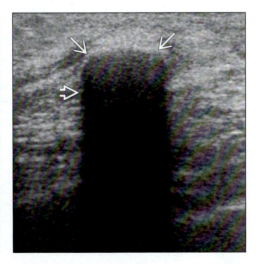

(Left) Ultrasound with a stand-off pad shows a mixed echogenicity mass ➡ at the site of a mammographically suspicious asymmetry. This 69 y/o had sustained breast trauma one year earlier. Biopsy (for concerning mammographic mass) showed fat necrosis. *(Right)* Ultrasound shows palpable, intensely shadowing ➡ mass with anterior echogenic rim ➡ at site of lumpectomy in a 38 y/o. Patient requested excision which showed fat necrosis.

FIBROADENOLIPOMA

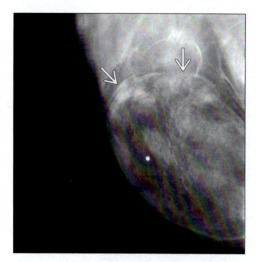

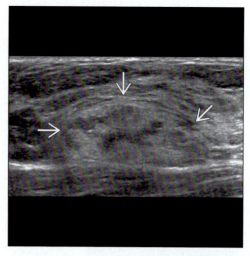

CC mammography magnification shows a classic large fibroadenolipoma of the right lower inner quadrant, marked by a BB. The compressed pseudocapsule is clearly evident superiorly ➡.

Sagittal ultrasound shows large circumscribed ovoid mass with mixed internal echogenicity, compressing and displacing surrounding parenchyma and producing a mainly echogenic rim or pseudocapsule ➡.

TERMINOLOGY

Abbreviations and Synonyms
- Fibroadenolipoma (FAL), hamartoma, lipofibroadenoma, adenolipofibroma

Definitions
- Encapsulated fat and glandular element proliferation
- Focal developmental pseudotumor composed of normal breast tissues

IMAGING FINDINGS

General Features
- Best diagnostic clue: "Breast-within-a-breast" appearance on mammogram
- Location
  - Anywhere in the breast
    - May be multiple
  - May occur in ectopic breast tissue
    - Axillary, inguinal
- Size: Any size, typically 3-6 cm at diagnosis

- Morphology: Circumscribed, mass-like lesion with mixture of glandular tissue and fat

Mammographic Findings
- Round or oval circumscribed lesion
- Varying mixtures of prominent fat and fibroglandular tissue elements
  - May be uniformly dense if minimal fat present
- Pseudocapsule, a rim of compressed parenchyma, often visible
- Benign appearing calcifications may be present

Ultrasonographic Findings
- Grayscale Ultrasound
  - Mixture of sonolucent fat and echogenic glandular elements on US
    - Heterogeneous internal echogenicity
    - May be uniformly hyperechoic if minimal fat present
  - Usually circumscribed
    - Oval shape almost universal
  - Pseudocapsule has variable echogenicity
  - Posterior enhancement variable
  - Compressible, deformable with pressure
  - Rarely, may contain small cysts

DDx: Lesions Containing Fat

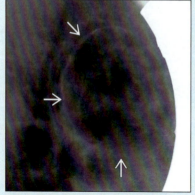

Lipoma

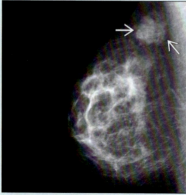

Glandular Island

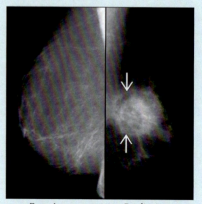

Post Lumpectomy, Radiation

FIBROADENOLIPOMA

Key Facts

Terminology
- Fibroadenolipoma (FAL), hamartoma, lipofibroadenoma, adenolipofibroma
- Encapsulated fat and glandular element proliferation

Imaging Findings
- Best diagnostic clue: "Breast-within-a-breast" appearance on mammogram
- Varying mixtures of prominent fat and fibroglandular tissue elements
- Pseudocapsule, a rim of compressed parenchyma, often visible
- Mixture of sonolucent fat and echogenic glandular elements on US

Top Differential Diagnoses
- Asymmetries

- Fibroadenoma
- Galactocele
- Fat Necrosis
- Lipoma

Pathology
- Focal developmental malformation that resembles a neoplasm
- Genetics: No genetic predisposition or inheritance
- Etiology: Developmental

Clinical Issues
- Usually asymptomatic
- Age: Range 20-80 years, mean 45 years
- FAL itself is benign
- Extremely rarely, malignancy may arise within contained tissue elements

---

- Color Doppler: No hypervascularity evident

MR Findings
- T1WI: Variable amounts of fat within an encapsulated otherwise nonspecific collection of glandular tissue
- T1 C+ FS: Enhances similarly with breast tissue

Imaging Recommendations
- Best imaging tool: Mammography, including spot compression views
- Protocol advice
  - Routine mammographic views usually characteristic
  - Spot mammograms and ultrasound usually confirm
  - No further imaging when typical mammographic appearance is present
  - Biopsy if atypical features (e.g., suspicious microcalcifications, spiculated area)

DIFFERENTIAL DIAGNOSIS

Asymmetries
- Glandular asymmetry or glandular island
- Entrapped fat interspersed with glandular tissue
- Thins on spot compression, no encapsulation; not as discrete as FAL
- Developing asymmetry merits further evaluation

Fibroadenoma
- May be mistaken for hamartoma
  - If margin is not clearly defined on mammogram
  - When fat projected onto lesion, or adipose metaplasia present
  - No lobular elements on histology

Galactocele
- Most are radiolucent, smoothly margined masses
- Lesions contain fat and inspissated secretions
- May demonstrate fat-fluid level on lateral mammogram

Fat Necrosis
- History of trauma or surgery

- Mixed fatty and tissue density, surrounding edema (echogenic)

Lipoma
- Uniformly fatty

Hibernoma
- Indistinguishable from glandular island on imaging
- Located in axillary tail or axilla
- Contain brown fat only, not parenchyma

Fibrolipoma
- Very rare
- Mature adipose tissue and collagenous stroma
- Slightly prominent fibroblasts

Chondrolipoma
- Extremely rare
- Mature adipose tissue and hyaline cartilage
- Benign; have been treated with excisional biopsy

Muscular or Myoid Hamartoma
- Extremely rare
- Well-defined tumor with smooth muscle and fat

Non-Fatty Hamartoma
- Some hamartomas do not contain fat
  - Muscular or myoid
  - Vascular

PATHOLOGY

General Features
- General path comments
  - Hamartoma definition
    - Focal developmental malformation that resembles a neoplasm
    - Abnormal mixture of tissue elements, or an abnormal proportion of a single element normally present at that site
  - Size range up to 13 cm
  - Type of biphasic breast lesion

FIBROADENOLIPOMA

- Contain integral epithelial and stromal components
- Mixture of nonspecialized and specialized stroma
  - Adenolipoma is most common variant
  - Core needle biopsy will show nonspecific benign breast tissue, insufficient for specific histopathologic diagnosis
- Genetics: No genetic predisposition or inheritance
- Etiology: Developmental
- Epidemiology
  - Any age
  - About 4% of all breast tumors

Gross Pathologic & Surgical Features

- Cut surface has a variegated mix of fat and fibrous parenchyma
  - May appear white, rubbery & firm: Predominantly glandular and stromal elements
  - May appear yellow, soft: Predominantly fatty elements
- Cysts may be present within lesion, arising from glandular elements

Microscopic Features

- Fat mixed in varying proportions with mammary parenchyma
  - Epithelial and mesenchymal components
- Pseudocapsule = compressed breast tissue
- Lobules & ducts appear normal
  - Both lobules and ducts present, unlike fibroadenoma
  - Little or no proliferative change
  - No cytologic atypia, unlike that seen in phyllodes tumors with adipose stroma
- Other features may be present
  - Benign epithelial hyperplasia
  - Pseudo-angiomatous stromal hyperplasia
  - Apocrine metaplasia, cystic ducts
  - Calcification
  - Stromal giant cells
  - Adenosis
- Immunohistochemistry
  - Strong positivity for cytokeratin and epithelial membrane antigen in epithelial cells
  - Vimentin and muscle-specific actin positive in stromal and myoepithelial cells
  - S-100 protein positive in myoepithelial cells
  - Estrogen and progesterone receptors positive in most cases

CLINICAL ISSUES

Presentation

- Most common signs/symptoms
  - Usually asymptomatic
  - May present as a vague soft breast mass or thickening
  - When palpable, mass is painless

Demographics

- Age: Range 20-80 years, mean 45 years
- Gender
  - Almost exclusively female

- Fewer than 5 male cases reported

Natural History & Prognosis

- FAL itself is benign
- Extremely rarely, malignancy may arise within contained tissue elements
  - Infiltrating ductal and/or lobular ductal carcinoma in situ (DCIS)

Treatment

- No treatment necessary unless appearance is atypical (e.g., suspicious calcifications or intrinsic mass lesion)
- Complete surgical excision only if extremely large
  - May require mammoplasty and reconstruction

DIAGNOSTIC CHECKLIST

Consider

- Distinguish from asymmetric glandular tissue

Image Interpretation Pearls

- Circumscribed mixed density mass with "breast-within-a-breast" appearance on mammography

SELECTED REFERENCES

1. Borges da Silva B et al: Large mammary hamartoma of axillary supernumerary breast tissue. Breast. 2005
2. Lerwill MF: Biphasic lesions of the breast. Semin Diagn Pathol. 21(1):48-56, 2004
3. Baron M et al: Invasive lobular carcinoma in a breast hamartoma. Breast J. 9(3):246-8, 2003
4. Gomez-Aracil V et al: Fine needle aspiration cytology of mammary hamartoma: a review of nine cases with histological correlation. Cytopathology. 14(4):195-200, 2003
5. Lee EH et al: Invasive ductal carcinoma arising in a breast hamartoma: two case reports and a review of the literature. Clin Radiol. 58(1):80-3, 2003
6. Park SY et al: Sonographic findings of breast hamartoma: emphasis on compressibility. Yonsei Med J. 44(5):847-54, 2003
7. Herbert M et al: Breast hamartomas: clinicopathological and immunohistochemical studies of 24 cases. Histopathology. 41(1):30-4, 2002
8. Tse GM et al: Ductal carcinoma in situ arising in mammary hamartoma. J Clin Pathol. 55(7):541-2, 2002
9. Ravakhah K et al: Hamartoma of the breast in a man: first case report. Breast J. 7(4):266-8, 2001
10. Rosen PP: Rosen's Breast Pathology. Philadelphia, Lippincott Williams & Wilkins. Chapter 40, 779-81, 2001
11. Wahner-Roedler DL et al: Hamartomas of the breast: clinical, radiologic, and pathologic manifestations. Breast J. 7(2):101-5, 2001
12. Weinzweig N et al: Giant hamartoma of the breast. Plast Reconstr Surg. 107(5):1216-20, 2001
13. Chiacchio R et al: Mammary hamartomas: an immunohistochemical study of ten cases. Pathol Res Pract. 195(4):231-6, 1999
14. Khunamornpong S et al: Muscular hamartoma of the breast: a rare breast lesion containing smooth muscle. J Med Assoc Thai. 80(10):675-9, 1997
15. Dworak O et al: Hamartoma of an ectopic breast arising in the inguinal region. Histopathology. 24(2):169-71, 1994
16. Altermatt HJ et al: Multiple hamartomas of the breast. Appl Pathol. 7:145-8, 1989

FIBROADENOLIPOMA

IMAGE GALLERY

Typical

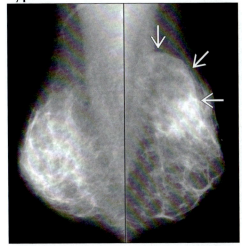
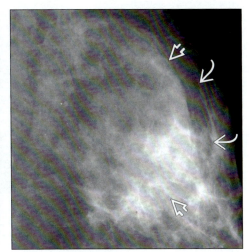

(Left) MLO mammography shows a prominent asymmetric mass in the left upper outer quadrant ➡ composed of a mixture of fat and glandular density, with a very well-defined border superiorly. *(Right)* MLO mammography magnification view shows the smooth border ➡ with a halo of compressed fat ➡. The internal mixture of fat and glandular density is well seen.

Typical

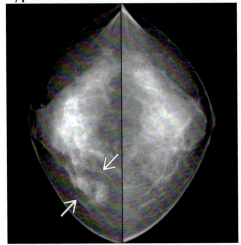
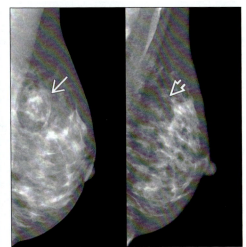

(Left) CC mammography shows a non-palpable encapsulated fat-containing mass ➡ in the inner right breast diagnostic of a fibroadenolipoma, BI-RADS 2, benign. *(Right)* MLO mammography shows an encapsulated fat containing 4.5 cm mass ➡ in the upper breast unchanged (but better imaged) from three years earlier ➡.

Typical

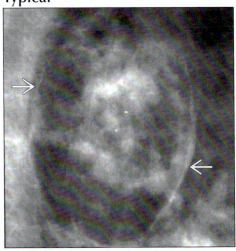
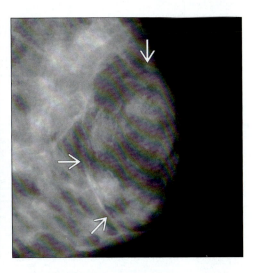

(Left) MLO close-up (same as above right) shows to better advantage the capsule ➡ and the classic appearance of "breast-within-a-breast" nature of this fibroadenolipoma. *(Right)* Close-up MLO mammogram shows 8 cm encapsulated mass ➡ containing fat and parenchymal density compatible with FAL in this 39 year old. Despite its size, the mass was not palpable.

FIBROADENOMA

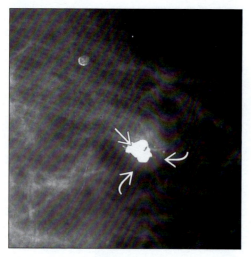
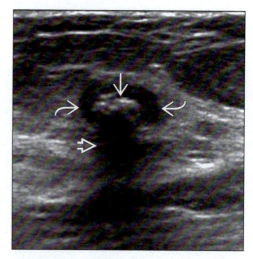

CC mammography magnification in 62 y/o woman shows a partially circumscribed mass ➔ with dense central "popcorn" calcification ➔, typical of a benign, degenerating fibroadenoma.

Radial ultrasound (same lesion as left) shows an oval circumscribed hypoechoic mass ➔. Coarse, echogenic macrocalcifications ➔ cause posterior shadowing ➔.

TERMINOLOGY

Abbreviations and Synonyms
- Fibroadenoma (FA)
- Adenofibroma (historical)
- Degenerating FA = sclerosed FA = involuting FA

Definitions
- Benign fibroepithelial tumor with mixed stromal and epithelial elements
- Major types: Adult-type and juvenile ("cellular")
- Complex FA: FA with cysts > 3 mm, sclerosing adenosis, epithelial calcifications, papillary apocrine metaplasia
- Giant FA: > 500 g or disproportionately large relative to breast
- Sclerosed FA: FA with paucicellular, hyalinized, fibrotic stroma, and sparse, atrophic epithelial elements
  - Natural history of FA to become sclerosed
  - Can occur at any age, tends to be post-menopausal

IMAGING FINDINGS

General Features
- Best diagnostic clue
  - Most common solid mass in women of all ages
  - Mammogram: Oval or lobulated circumscribed mass with dense coarse calcifications (Ca++)
  - Ultrasound: Hypoechoic circumscribed oval mass with homogeneous internal echoes
  - MRI: Smooth, moderately enhancing lobulated mass ± nonenhancing internal septations
- Location
  - Anywhere in breast parenchyma
  - Rarely in ectopic glandular tissue, e.g., axilla, accessory breast
- Size
  - Adult-type: 0.5-5 cm
  - Juvenile-type and giant FA: Up to 15 cm
- Morphology: Typically oval or 2-3 gentle lobulations

Mammographic Findings
- Oval, macrolobulated, or rounded mass
  - Low density or isodense to breast parenchyma
  - Often partly obscured margins

DDx: Hypoechoic Circumscribed Masses

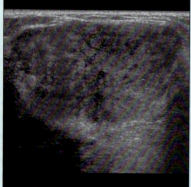
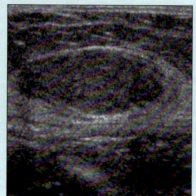
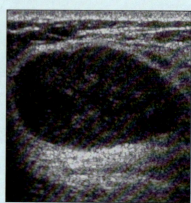

Phyllodes Tumor

Focal (Stromal) Fibrosis

PASH

FIBROADENOMA

Key Facts

Terminology
- Benign fibroepithelial tumor with mixed stromal and epithelial elements
- Major types: Adult-type and juvenile ("cellular")
- Giant FA: > 500 g or disproportionately large relative to breast

Imaging Findings
- Most common solid mass in women of all ages
- Mammogram: Oval or lobulated circumscribed mass with dense coarse calcifications (Ca++)
- Ultrasound: Hypoechoic circumscribed oval mass with homogeneous internal echoes
- MRI: Smooth, moderately enhancing lobulated mass ± nonenhancing internal septations
- "Popcorn" shaped, very dense large Ca++
- Clustered coarse heterogeneous Ca++

- Circumscribed oval or gently lobulated hypo- to isoechoic mass
- Long axis parallel to skin surface
- Posterior enhancement variable

Top Differential Diagnoses
- Other Benign Lesions
- Phyllodes tumor: 23% show cysts, esp. if malignant
- Malignant Neoplasm

Pathology
- Multiple tumors in 15% of adult-type FA

Diagnostic Checklist
- Growth > 20% in diameter in 6 months suggests possible phyllodes, recommend excision
- "Cellular" FA on core biopsy in woman > 45 yrs suspect for phyllodes, recommend excision

---

- Involuting FA often calcified
  - "Popcorn" shaped, very dense large Ca++
  - Clustered coarse heterogeneous Ca++
  - When very small, only Ca++, no mass visible
- May mimic malignancy (indistinctly marginated mass, suspicious Ca++)

Ultrasonographic Findings
- Grayscale Ultrasound
  - Circumscribed oval or gently lobulated hypo- to isoechoic mass
    - Long axis parallel to skin surface
    - Length (L) to depth (D) ratio typically > 1.4 (range 0.9-4.1, mean 1.84)
  - Homogeneous, low-level, internal echogenicity
    - Can be isoechoic with fat (minimize by restricting dynamic range to 60-65 dB)
  - Adjacent tissue may be compressed ⇒ hyperechoic "pseudocapsule"
  - Associated Ca++ may be seen: Echogenic
  - May show echogenic septations
  - Approximately 2-4% contain small cystic foci; favors phyllodes tumor
  - Posterior enhancement variable
    - Posterior shadowing if hyalinized or large Ca++
- Color Doppler
  - Peripheral and feeding vessels often visible
  - Larger lesions may show internal septal vessels
  - Ultrasound contrast agents show vessels in 68%

MR Findings
- T2WI FS
  - Typically isointense with parenchyma
  - Myxoid FAs, FAs in young women may be moderately hyperintense
- T1 C+ FS
  - Oval or macrolobulated smooth enhancing mass
  - Variable enhancement
    - Usually moderately rapid, homogeneous, moderately intense enhancement
    - Intense, very rapid enhancement may occur
    - Weak to no enhancement if densely hyalinized
  - May have nonenhancing internal septations

Nuclear Medicine Findings
- PET: Can show FDG uptake

Imaging Recommendations
- Best imaging tool: Ultrasound

DIFFERENTIAL DIAGNOSIS

Other Benign Lesions
- Focal (stromal) fibrosis
- Fat lobule
- Complicated cyst (may appear solid)
- Pseudoangiomatous stromal hyperplasia (PASH)
- Lactating adenoma
- Tubular adenoma
- Intraductal papilloma
- Fibroadenomatoid change

Locally Aggressive Lesions
- Phyllodes tumor: 23% show cysts, esp. if malignant

Malignant Neoplasm
- Invasive ductal carcinoma NOS
- Ductal carcinoma in situ (DCIS), esp. solid or papillary
- Mucinous, medullary carcinoma
- Metastases (rare): To intramammary node(s); melanoma

PATHOLOGY

General Features
- General path comments
  - Solid tumor with mixture of stromal and epithelial components
  - Cellular FA can be difficult to distinguish from phyllodes tumor on needle biopsy
  - Multiple tumors in 15% of adult-type FA
  - Juvenile type usually solitary
- Etiology
  - Hormonally influenced growth and involution

FIBROADENOMA

- o Develop on chronic cyclosporine A (CsA) therapy after renal transplantation
  - ~ 2% of women, may be multiple and/or large
- Epidemiology
  - o Most common breast mass in women under 35 yrs
  - o 10% of breast masses in post-menopausal women
- Associated abnormalities
  - o Fibrocystic changes in up to 50% of cases
  - o Fibroadenomatoid change (sclerosing lobular hyperplasia) common in surrounding stroma
  - o Atypical ductal hyperplasia can be present in FA

Gross Pathologic & Surgical Features
- Firm, rubbery circumscribed mass

Microscopic Features
- Pseudocapsule of compressed connective tissue
- Adult FA: Bland fibroblastic stroma, hypocellular to variably hypercellular
  - o No stromal mitoses, atypia uncommon
  - o Frequently hyalinized or calcified
  - o Myxoid FA: Mucinous stromal component, may be sporadic or (rarely) in Carney complex
    - Carney complex: Familial cardiac, stromal and cutaneous myxomas, endocrine overactivity, melanotic schwannomas
  - o Rarely, stromal differentiation into fat, cartilage, bone or smooth muscle
- Elongated, compressed ducts lined by epithelial and myoepithelial cells
- Juvenile: "Cellular" fibroadenoma
  - o No leaf-like growth pattern (distinguishes from phyllodes tumor)
  - o Uniform stromal hypercellularity, no atypia
  - o Frequent epithelial and myoepithelial hyperplasia, mimics gynecomastia

Staging, Grading or Classification Criteria
- Pericanalicular: Stroma surrounds round ducts
- Intracanalicular: Stroma compresses ducts into slit-like spaces
- May be complex (see "Definitions")
- Rarely, foci of in situ or invasive ductal or lobular carcinoma within FA

CLINICAL ISSUES

Presentation
- Most common signs/symptoms: Highly mobile palpable painless firm mass
- Other signs/symptoms: Juvenile or giant FA: Rapidly growing mass in a very young woman
- Clinical Profile
  - o Usually palpable or detected at screening
  - o Often multiple & bilateral, esp. adult-type

Demographics
- Age
  - o Any after 10 yrs, mean at diagnosis 30 yrs, median 25 yrs
  - o Juvenile FA: Usually 10-20 years old, rare > 45 yrs
    - Most FA in teenagers are of adult-type
- Gender: Almost exclusively female

- Ethnicity: Giant FA more common in African-American women

Natural History & Prognosis
- Vast majority self-limited, involute spontaneously following menopause
- Slight increase in size may occur on followup US
  - o Mean diameter change ≤ 20% in 6 months (95th percentile < 50 y/o, 90th percentile ≥ 50 y/o)
- Relative risk (RR) increase for carcinoma, either breast
  - o RR ~ 2.0 overall, 1.0 when family history and adjacent proliferative changes removed
  - o RR ~ 3.0 if complex FA, ~ 1.0 if atypia confined to FA
  - o Increased risk persists for 20 years or longer after diagnosis

Treatment
- Clinical and sonographic follow-up adequate for many
  - o Possible even if palpable: Further study warranted
- Biopsy if new, enlarging, or suspicious features
- Complete excision curative
  - o Vacuum-assisted core biopsy can completely remove lesions < 1.5 cm
- Cryoablation therapy (no long-term data)
  - o < 2 cm, ~ 75% become impalpable in 12 months; > 2 cm, majority remain palpable

DIAGNOSTIC CHECKLIST

Consider
- Annual follow-up after core biopsy showed FA
  - o Growth > 20% in diameter in 6 months suggests possible phyllodes, recommend excision
- "Cellular" FA on core biopsy in woman > 45 yrs suspect for phyllodes, recommend excision

SELECTED REFERENCES

1. Binokay F et al: Risk of developing fibroadenoma with the use of cyclosporine A in renal transplant recipients. Ren Fail. 27:721-5, 2005
2. Nurko J et al: Interim results from the fibroadenoma Cryoablation Treatment Registry. Am J Surg. 190:647-51; discussion 651-2, 2005
3. Graf O et al: Follow-up of palpable circumscribed noncalcified solid breast masses at mammography and US: can biopsy be averted? Radiology. 233:850-6, 2004
4. Strano S et al: Color Doppler imaging of fibroadenomas of the breast with histopathologic correlation. J Clin Ultrasound. 32:317-22, 2004
5. El-Wakeel H et al: Systematic review of fibroadenoma as a risk factor for breast cancer. Breast. 12:302-7, 2003
6. Gordon PB et al: Solid breast masses diagnosed as fibroadenoma at fine-needle aspiration biopsy: acceptable rates of growth at long-term follow-up. Radiology. 229:233-8, 2003
7. Sperber F et al: Diagnosis and treatment of breast fibroadenomas by ultrasound-guided vacuum-assisted biopsy. Arch Surg. 138:796-800, 2003
8. Carter BA et al: No elevation in long-term breast carcinoma risk for women with fibroadenomas that contain atypical hyperplasia. Cancer. 92:30-6, 2001

FIBROADENOMA

IMAGE GALLERY

Typical

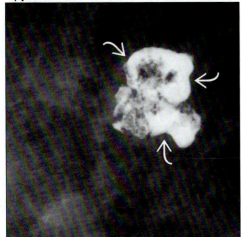

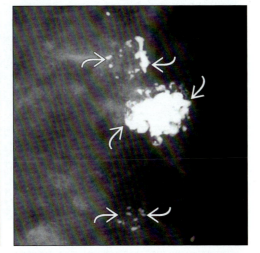

(Left) MLO mammography magnification shows FA with typically benign "popcorn" Ca++ ➡ in a 55 y/o woman. (Right) MLO mammography magnification shows multiple groups of dense, large, irregular Ca++ ➡ in a 52 y/o woman representing hyalinized fibroadenomas. The largest lesion shows coalescence of the Ca++.

Variant

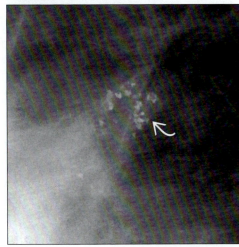

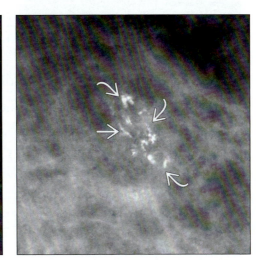

(Left) Lateral mammography magnification shows clustered coarse heterogeneous Ca++ ➡ in this 57 y/o woman. 11-g vacuum-assisted biopsy showed a sclerosed fibroadenoma with extensive Ca++. (Right) MLO mammography magnification shows multiple clustered pleomorphic heterogeneous Ca++ ➡ with some branching forms ➡ in this 53 y/o woman, BI-RADS 4. Excision biopsy showed a benign fibroadenoma with Ca++.

Variant

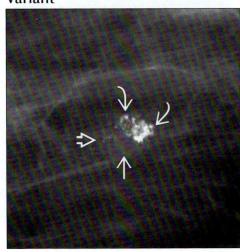

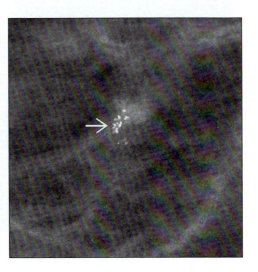

(Left) Lateral mammography magnification shows clustered coarse heterogeneous Ca++ ➡, in a faint low-density mass ➡ with amorphous Ca++ ➡ in a 64 y/o woman. Stereotactic core biopsy showed hyalinized fibroadenoma with Ca++. (Right) CC mammography magnification in a 60 y/o shows cluster of pleomorphic Ca++ ➡ with minimal associated density. Fibroadenoma on 14-g stereotactic core biopsy.

Typical

(Left) CC mammography magnification shows partially circumscribed ➔, partially obscured ➔ oval mass, isodense to parenchyma in this 43 y/o woman. *(Right)* Transverse spatial compounding ultrasound of the same lesion shows an oval, hypoechoic circumscribed mass ➔ with homogeneous internal echoes and a rim of compressed echogenic tissue ➔. Biopsy proven fibroadenoma.

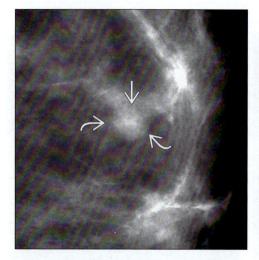
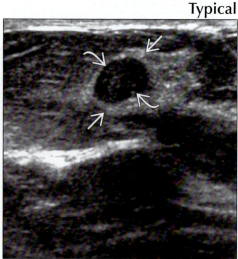

Typical

(Left) Radial ultrasound in a 56 y/o woman shows circumscribed, hypoechoic, oval mass ➔ with long axis parallel to the skin, homogeneous internal echoes, and no posterior features. Biopsy proven fibroadenoma. *(Right)* Axial T1 C+ FS MR shows solitary smooth, oval, homogeneously enhancing mass ➔ in the posterior right breast of this 38 y/o woman. Biopsy proven fibroadenoma.

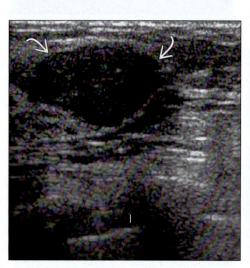

Typical

(Left) Axial T1 C+ FS MR in a 42 y/o woman shows a large, lobulated, smooth enhancing mass in the right breast ➔ with nonenhancing internal septations ➔. Biopsy proven fibroadenoma. *(Right)* Sagittal T1 C+ subtraction MR shows an enhancing lobulated mass ➔ with typical nonenhancing internal septations ➔ in a 54 y/o woman with a known FA in the axillary tail of the breast.

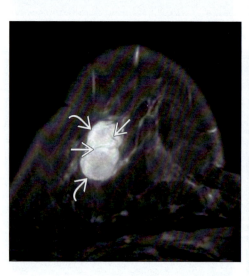
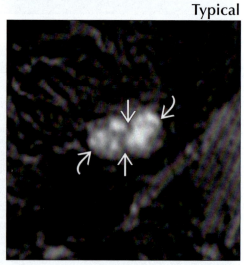

IV

2

36

FIBROADENOMA

Variant

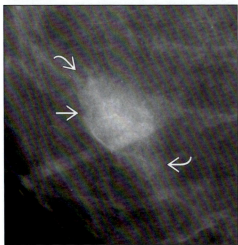 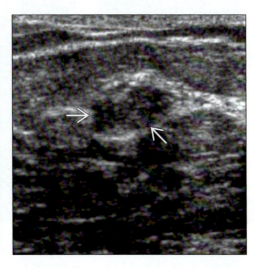

(Left) CC mammography spot compression shows a partially circumscribed ➡, partially indistinctly-marginated ➡ asymmetric density in a 30 y/o woman. *(Right)* Ultrasound (same case as previous image) shows a microlobulated, hypoechoic oval mass ➡ with no posterior features. US-guided core biopsy showed FA.

Variant

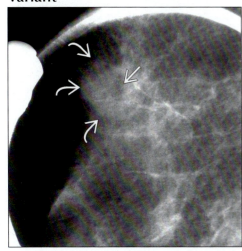 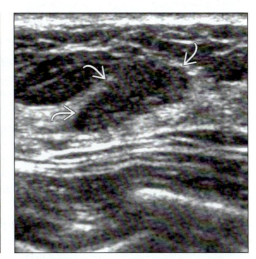

(Left) MLO mammography spot compression shows a partly circumscribed ➡ nodular asymmetry with apparently mixed fatty density ➡ in this 47 y/o woman. *(Right)* Radial ultrasound (same lesion as previous image) shows obliquely oriented hypoechoic oval mass ➡ with indistinct margins, isoechoic with fat, with no posterior features. Fibroadenoma on 14-g core biopsy.

Variant

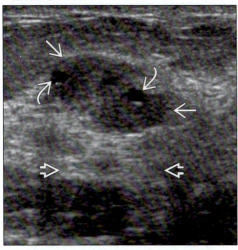 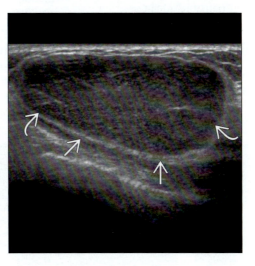

(Left) Ultrasound shows microlobulated mass ➡, isoechoic with fat, with minimal posterior enhancement ➡ and small cystic areas ➡. Core biopsy in this 41 y/o showed FA with apocrine metaplasia. *(Right)* Ultrasound shows a large, circumscribed oval hypoechoic solid mass ➡ with a hyperechoic pseudocapsule ➡ in a 22 y/o woman with a rapidly growing tumor. Juvenile fibroadenoma with no evidence of phyllodes tumor at excisional biopsy.

FIBROADENOMATOID CHANGE

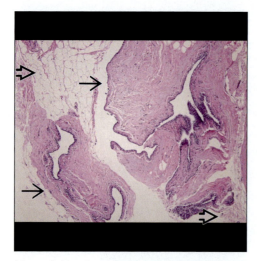

Histopathology, low power, H&E shows focal areas resembling fibroadenoma ➡, with areas of interspersed fat ▷. The overall lesion is not very discrete, compatible with FAC (Courtesy DWM).

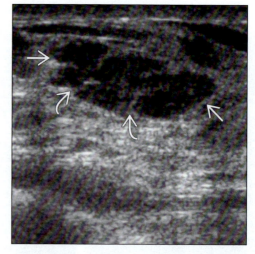

Radial ultrasound shows a circumscribed, lobulated mass ➡ with echogenic septations ➡ in a 34 y/o with a palpable mass. US-guided core biopsy showed FAC; concordant.

TERMINOLOGY

Abbreviations and Synonyms
- Fibroadenomatoid change (FAC)
- Fibroadenomatous hyperplasia
- Fibroadenomatoid mastopathy

Definitions
- Benign proliferative lesion
- Differs from fibroadenoma (FA) as the stromal hyperplasia may not have well-defined borders and usually involves several lobules

IMAGING FINDINGS

General Features
- Size: Often microscopic; when palpable, mean diameter = 4 cm

Mammographic Findings
- Mammography: Mostly circumscribed, lobulated mass ± calcifications (Ca++), less discrete than FA
  - Coarse, amorphous, pleomorphic Ca++

- May be occult, esp. in dense breast tissue

Ultrasonographic Findings
- US: Circumscribed lobulated mass with internal echogenic septations
  - Mixed hypo- and hyperechoic mass

MR Findings
- T1 C+ FS
  - Variable enhancement patterns: Focus of enhancement, mass, non-enhancing septations
  - Ductal enhancement reported (one series)

DIFFERENTIAL DIAGNOSIS

Fibroadenoma
- Includes all proliferations of intralobular stroma, most with well-defined borders
- Circumscribed oval or gently lobulated mass ± Ca++

Fibrocystic Change
- Amorphous, punctate, pleomorphic Ca++
- Low-density mammographic mass ± Ca++

DDx: Similar Imaging or Histologic Features

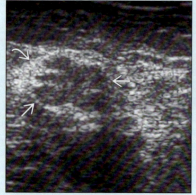

PASH

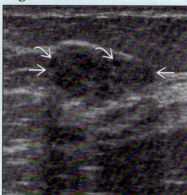

FA with Apocrine Metaplasia

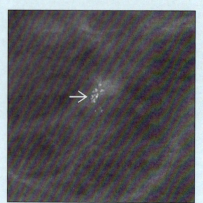

Fibroadenoma with Ca++

FIBROADENOMATOID CHANGE

Key Facts

Terminology
- Differs from fibroadenoma (FA) as the stromal hyperplasia may not have well-defined borders and usually involves several lobules

Imaging Findings
- Mammography: Mostly circumscribed, lobulated mass ± calcifications (Ca++), less discrete than FA
- US: Circumscribed lobulated mass with internal echogenic septations

Top Differential Diagnoses
- Fibroadenoma
- Fibrocystic Change

Clinical Issues
- No reported malignant potential

Diagnostic Checklist
- FAC at core biopsy for a mass requires radiologic confirmation that the mass was biopsied

---

Tubular Adenoma
- Proliferation of ductules with sparse stroma

PATHOLOGY

General Features
- General path comments
  - FAC may represent intermediate step (or arrested development at intermediate stage) during histogenesis of fibroadenoma
    - Initial process: Proliferation of both epithelial and stromal components of multiple lobules; occurs either spontaneously or due to hormonal alterations
    - Gradual confluence of nodules occurs
    - Formation of fibroadenomatoid nodules
    - Fibroadenomatoid nodules coalesce to form a fully developed fibroadenoma
- Associated abnormalities
  - Found in breast tissue surrounding FAs in ~ 50%
    - FAC may be overlooked

CLINICAL ISSUES

Demographics
- Age: Mean = 32
- Gender: Rare in males; possible relation to spironolactone, cyclosporine A (case reports)

Natural History & Prognosis
- No reported malignant potential

DIAGNOSTIC CHECKLIST

Consider
- FAC at core biopsy for a mass requires radiologic confirmation that the mass was biopsied

SELECTED REFERENCES

1. Langer SA et al: Pathologic correlates of false positive breast magnetic resonance imaging findings: which lesions warrant biopsy? Am J Surg. 190:633-40, 2005
2. Woodhams R et al: ADC mapping of benign and malignant breast tumors. Magn Reson Med Sci. 4:35-42, 2005
3. Liberman L et al: Ductal enhancement on MR imaging of the breast. AJR. 181:519-25, 2003
4. Kamal M et al: Fibroadenomatoid hyperplasia: a cause of suspicious microcalcification on mammographic screening. AJR. 171:1331-4, 1998
5. Tan PE et al: Fibroadenomatoid mastopathy: another distractive breast lesion? Malays J Pathol. 13:101-4, 1991
6. Nielsen BB. Fibroadenomatoid hyperplasia of the male breast. Am J Surg Pathol. 14:774-7, 1990
7. Hanson CA et al: Fibroadenomatosis (fibroadenomatoid mastopathy): a benign breast lesion with composite pathologic features. Pathology. 19:393-6, 1987
8. Ofcel L et al: Histogenetic study of mammary gland fibroadenomas. Ann Anat Pathol (Paris). 18:255-76, 1973

IMAGE GALLERY

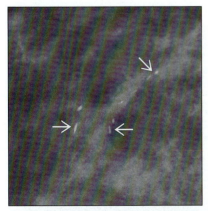
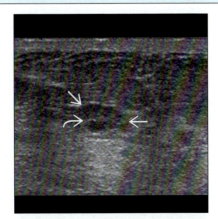
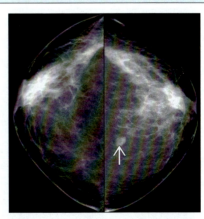

(Left) CC mammography magnification in a 68 y/o shows smooth, rather coarse, linear Ca++ in a linear distribution ➡ limited to one segment. Biopsy showed FAC with Ca++. *(Center)* Ultrasound in a 38 y/o with contralateral fibroadenoma shows an oval circumscribed hypoechoic mass ➡ with internal echogenic septations ➡. Biopsy showed FAC. *(Right)* CC mammography shows an oval, circumscribed 8 mm mass ➡ in the inner left breast in a 54 y/o. Biopsy at patient request showed FAC. Imaging surveillance stable at 3 years.

FIBROCYSTIC CHANGES

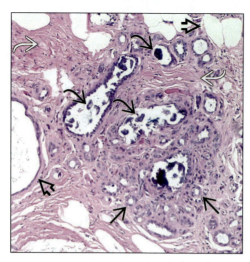

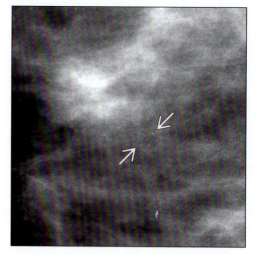

Specimen micropathology, low power, H&E from 11-g stereotactic biopsy shows typical FCC with cysts ⊡, fibrosis ➡, and adenosis ➡. Numerous calcifications are evident in microcysts ➡.

CC mammography magnification (same case as previous image) shows subtle cluster of amorphous Ca++ ➡, seen on baseline screening in this 41 y/o, prompting biopsy.

TERMINOLOGY

Abbreviations and Synonyms
- Fibrocystic changes (FCC)

Definitions
- FCC: Histopathologic diagnosis: Constellation of cysts, fibrosis, and adenosis
  - Cysts can be gross or microscopic
  - Usual intraductal hyperplasia (IDH) often present
  - Apocrine metaplasia (AM) frequently found in areas of cystic change, but not required
- Term "fibrocystic disease" to be avoided as FCC is considered in spectrum of normal variation

IMAGING FINDINGS

General Features
- Best diagnostic clue
  - Mammographically dense breasts with scattered punctate calcifications (Ca++, in adenosis) and fluctuating cysts
  - Findings can be focal, regional, or diffuse

Mammographic Findings
- Changing pattern of bilateral, partially circumscribed, partially obscured masses due to cysts developing and regressing
  - Carefully examine each mass to assure margins are no worse than partially obscured
  - At least 75% of margin is visualized and circumscribed
  - Any suspicious, dominant or discretely symptomatic mass merits US
- Other masses
  - Fibrosis: Focal or global asymmetry, oval, or irregular mass
    - Can be indistinguishable from malignancy, may require biopsy
  - Nodular adenosis: Typically oval, mostly circumscribed
    - May contain punctate, amorphous Ca++
- Diffuse, scattered, bilateral Ca++
  - Mostly punctate
  - Some coarse, heterogeneous and amorphous Ca++ admixed
  - Occasional random loose groupings expected

DDx: Malignancies Admixed with FCC

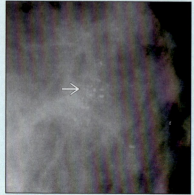

Milk-of-calcium, DCIS

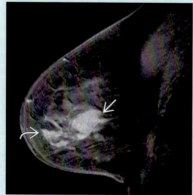

Fibrosis, IDC (Posteriorly)

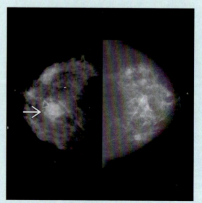

Cysts and IDC

FIBROCYSTIC CHANGES

Key Facts

Terminology
- FCC: Histopathologic diagnosis: Constellation of cysts, fibrosis, and adenosis
- Usual intraductal hyperplasia (IDH) often present
- Term "fibrocystic disease" to be avoided as FCC is considered in spectrum of normal variation

Imaging Findings
- Mammographically dense breasts with scattered punctate calcifications (Ca++, in adenosis) and fluctuating cysts
- Findings can be focal, regional, or diffuse
- Scattered cysts
- Scattered foci of enhancement on MR, ≤ 5 mm, diffuse, bilateral

Top Differential Diagnoses
- Atypical Ductal Hyperplasia (ADH)
- Lobular Neoplasia
- Ductal Carcinoma in Situ (DCIS)

Clinical Issues
- "Proliferative changes" carry slight, ~ 1.3-1.9x, ↑ risk of developing breast cancer in either breast
- Proliferative changes: IDH, sclerosing adenosis, fibroadenomas, radial scar, papillomas
- Nonproliferative: Cysts, apocrine metaplasia

Diagnostic Checklist
- Not an indication for diagnostic mammography per se in absence of focal symptoms or abnormalities on screening

---

- ○ Baseline magnification views can be helpful
- ○ Can usually be dismissed as benign
- New clustered Ca++: Pleomorphic, amorphous, punctate
  - ○ Merit work-up with magnification views
  - ○ Unless can be shown to layer on 90° lateral view (i.e., due to milk-of-calcium), often require biopsy
  - ○ Sclerosing adenosis, apocrine metaplasia most common causes
- Other
  - ○ Clustered coarse heterogeneous Ca++ due to fibrosis
  - ○ Coarse and occasionally finer linear Ca++ can be seen in fibrosis (rare)
  - ○ Architectural distortion: Very uncommon
    - ▪ Usually requires biopsy: Co-existent radial scar/radial sclerosing lesion
  - ○ Regional Ca++: May require biopsy if not shown to be milk-of-calcium

Ultrasonographic Findings
- Grayscale Ultrasound
  - ○ Scattered echogenic foci due to Ca++
    - ▪ May occasionally be seen in cysts (i.e., milk-of-calcium)
  - ○ Simple cysts
  - ○ Complicated cysts
  - ○ Clustered microcysts
  - ○ Complex cystic and solid masses
    - ▪ Mixture of fibrosis and cystic changes
    - ▪ Ruptured or inflamed cysts
    - ▪ Often difficult to distinguish from malignancy: Often require biopsy
  - ○ Echogenic tissue due to ↑ fibrosis
    - ▪ Heterogeneous echotexture when mixed with residual fat
  - ○ Discrete masses due to fibrosis
    - ▪ Mixed hyper- and hypoechoic ovoid mass
    - ▪ Uniformly echogenic mass
    - ▪ Can appear irregular with shadowing, often requiring biopsy

MR Findings
- T1WI

- ○ Cysts typically isointense to parenchyma
- ○ Variable signal when hemorrhagic or proteinaceous
- ○ May show fluid-debris levels
- T2WI FS
  - ○ Scattered cysts
    - ▪ Variable signal content: Proteinaceous cysts relatively hypointense
    - ▪ Fluid-debris levels may be seen
  - ○ Occasionally clustered microcysts observed though resolution can be limiting
- T1 C+ FS
  - ○ Inflamed cysts: Smooth rim-enhancement of cyst wall 2 mm or less in thickness
  - ○ Scattered foci of enhancement on MR, ≤ 5 mm, diffuse, bilateral
  - ○ Fibrosis: Can present as diffuse, regional, or focal enhancement
    - ▪ Fibrosis may show suspicious kinetics
    - ▪ Irregular masses, often requiring biopsy

Biopsy
- Indeterminate Ca++ on standard CC and 90° magnification views will occasionally layer on prone stereotactic table
  - ○ Benign milk-of-calcium, biopsy not needed
  - ○ Milk-of-calcium can co-exist with malignant Ca++: Proceed with biopsy if uncertain

Imaging Recommendations
- Best imaging tool
  - ○ Annual mammography
    - ▪ CC and 90° magnification views may be needed for adequate characterization of Ca++
  - ○ Ultrasound helpful in characterizing masses
- Protocol advice: Perform MR in days 7-14 after onset of menses when possible to diminish false positives

---

DIFFERENTIAL DIAGNOSIS

Atypical Ductal Hyperplasia (ADH)
- Frequently seen on core biopsy of clustered or regional amorphous Ca++; may be incidental at pathology

FIBROCYSTIC CHANGES

- Overlap in appearance with FCC

Lobular Neoplasia

- Atypical lobular hyperplasia (ALH) and lobular carcinoma in situ (LCIS) typically occult on mammography
- May be seen adjacent to amorphous Ca++: Rarely contain Ca++
- Can cause indistinct, irregular masses on US, MR

Ductal Carcinoma in Situ (DCIS)

- Clustered pleomorphic or amorphous Ca++ overlap in appearance with FCC
- Ca++ in linear or segmental distribution favor DCIS
- Clumped, linear or segmental enhancement on MR most common

Invasive Carcinoma, Ductal (IDC) and/or Lobular (ILC)

- Most often an irregular, often spiculated mass
- IDC can show associated Ca++

PATHOLOGY

General Features

- Epidemiology
  - Higher socioeconomic status, fewer pregnancies, less lactation than controls
  - Trend to ↑ nulliparity, later menopause relative to controls
  - ↑ Cyst formation in post-menopausal women on hormone replacement, especially estrogen alone
- Associated abnormalities
  - Apocrine metaplasia (AM)
  - Sclerosing adenosis
  - Columnar cell changes
  - Focal or diffuse FCC may be seen with any breast pathology

Microscopic Features

- Gland proliferation, i.e., adenosis
- Stromal fibrosis
- Microscopic and macroscopic cyst formation
- Frequently associated Ca++ in stroma, cysts, adenosis
  - Ca++ oxalate in microcysts seen with polarized light

CLINICAL ISSUES

Presentation

- Most common signs/symptoms: Mastalgia: Focal or diffuse, particularly in outer portions of breasts
- Other signs/symptoms
  - Palpable lump
  - Benign findings on mammography
  - Suspicious findings on mammography ± US ± MR
  - Rare: Greenish or black nipple discharge
    - Cysts can communicate with ducts → nipple

Demographics

- Age: More common in pre-menopausal women; changes usually lessen in post-menopausal women

Natural History & Prognosis

- "Proliferative changes" carry slight, ~ 1.3-1.9x, ↑ risk of developing breast cancer in either breast
  - Proliferative changes: IDH, sclerosing adenosis, fibroadenomas, radial scar, papillomas
  - Nonproliferative: Cysts, apocrine metaplasia

Treatment

- Residual Ca++ similar to those biopsied with result of FCC can be followed, usually at 6 months initially
  - Increase in Ca++ should still be viewed as suspicious

DIAGNOSTIC CHECKLIST

Consider

- FCC is within spectrum of normal breast physiology
- Not an indication for diagnostic mammography per se in absence of focal symptoms or abnormalities on screening
  - Focal pain not a sign of malignancy though US can be performed for reassurance
- Ca++ are frequently (~ 16%) present in both adjacent benign and malignant areas
  - Assure adequate sampling of suspicious Ca++
- Random sampling of benign dense breast tissue will often yield fibrosis
  - Assure correlation of imaging and histopathologic findings: Discordant result should be rebiopsied
  - MR-guided biopsy yielding fibrosis is particularly problematic: Further study warranted

Image Interpretation Pearls

- True lateral mammogram helpful in depicting benign milk-of-calcium
- Diffuse, scattered, bilateral similar findings favor benign etiology

SELECTED REFERENCES

1. Collins LC et al: The influence of family history on breast cancer risk in women with biopsy-confirmed benign breast disease: results from the Nurses' Health Study. Cancer, in press, 2006
2. Liberman L et al: Does size matter? Positive predictive value of MRI-detected breast lesions as a function of lesion size. AJR. 186:426-30, 2006
3. Berg WA et al: Sonographically depicted breast clustered microcysts: is follow-up appropriate? AJR. 185:952-9, 2005
4. Berg WA et al: Cystic lesions of the breast: sonographic-pathologic correlation. Radiology. 227:183-91, 2003
5. Leung JW et al: Utility of targeted sonography in the evaluation of focal breast pain. J Ultrasound Med. 21:521-6, quiz 528-9, 2002
6. Shetty MK et al: Sonographic findings in focal fibrocystic changes of the breast. Ultrasound Q. 18:35-40, 2002
7. Leung JW et al: Multiple bilateral masses detected on screening mammography: assessment of need for recall imaging. AJR. 175:23-9, 2000
8. Dupont WD et al: Breast cancer risk associated with proliferative breast disease and atypical hyperplasia. Cancer. 71:1258-65, 1993
9. Nomura A et al: Epidemiologic characteristics of benign breast disease. Am J Epidemiol. 105:505-12, 1977

FIBROCYSTIC CHANGES

IMAGE GALLERY

Typical

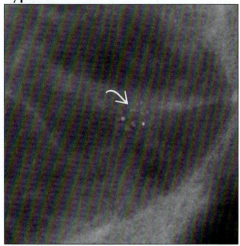

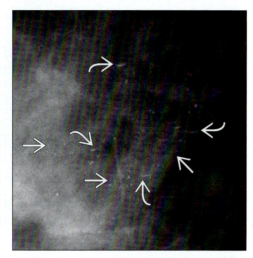

(Left) Lateral mammography magnification shows clustered pleomorphic Ca++ ➔ identified on baseline screening in this 45 y/o. Stereotactic 11-g biopsy showed FCC with IDH and sclerosing adenosis. *(Right)* Lateral mammography magnification shows layering of some of these regional Ca++ ➔ compatible with milk-of-calcium in this 50 y/o. Others do not layer ➔, prompting stereotactic 11-g biopsy yielding FCC with sclerosing adenosis.

Variant

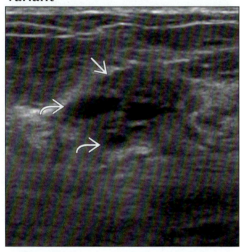

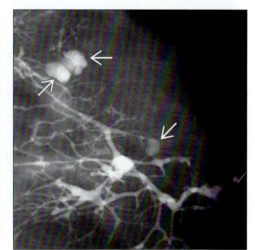

(Left) US shows oval hypoechoic mass ➔ with multiple small cysts ➔ in this 49 y/o with mass on mammography. Because this was a complex cystic and solid mass, US-guided 14-g core biopsy was performed; showing FCC, concordant. *(Right)* Galactogram in this 33 y/o with greenish nipple discharge shows filling of normal appearing ducts which terminate in several small cysts ➔, typical of FCC.

Typical

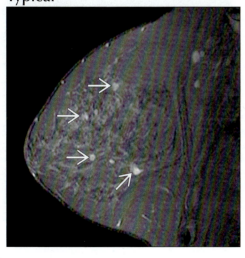

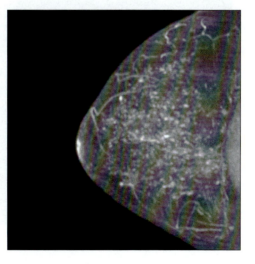

(Left) Sagittal T2WI FS MR shows multiple small cysts ➔ in this 46 y/o for high-risk screening. *(Right)* Sagittal MIP of T1 C+ subtraction MR (same patient as previous image) shows diffuse, scattered foci of enhancement throughout the breast, typical of FCC, BI-RADS 2, benign. Similar findings were seen in the contralateral breast.

IV

2

44

(Left) MLO mammography shows lower left asymmetry ➡ in a background of heterogeneously dense parenchyma in this 51 y/o. *(Right)* Antiradial US targeted to the mammographic abnormality (same case as left) shows circumscribed, oval, complex cystic and solid mass ➡ with posterior enhancement, and adjacent clustered microcysts ➡. US-guided 14-g core biopsy showed FCC including AM, IDH, duct ectasia, and stromal fibrosis.

(Left) MLO mammography shows dense parenchyma in this 38 y/o with left breast lump (skin marker ➡). US was unrevealing and MR was performed for more complete evaluation. *(Right)* Sagittal MIP of T1 C+ subtraction MR (same as left) shows triangular segment of persistent enhancement ➡ in the right breast. The left breast was unremarkable.

(Left) Sagittal T2WI FS MR (same as prior 2 images) shows triangular segment of multiple tiny cysts ➡ corresponding to the area of enhancement. *(Right)* US right breast targeted to the segment of enhancement (same as prior 3 images) shows multiple small cysts ➡, isolated to this region of the breast. At the patient's request, US-guided biopsy was performed, confirming FCC.

Variant

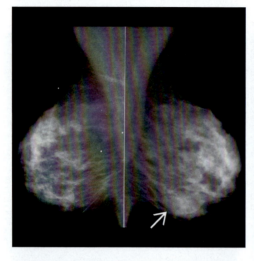
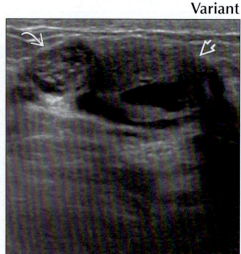

Variant

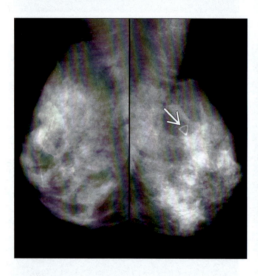
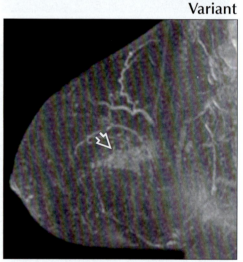

Variant

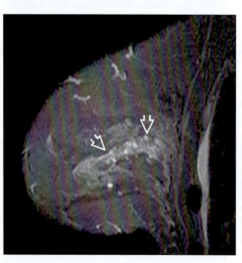
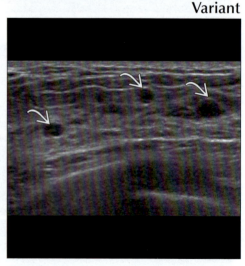

FIBROCYSTIC CHANGES

Typical

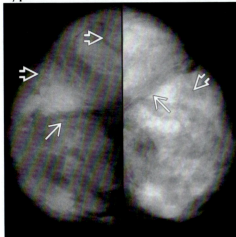

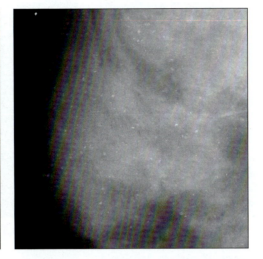

(Left) CC mammography in this 45 y/o shows dense parenchyma with diffuse bilateral scattered punctate and coarse heterogeneous Ca++ ➡. The patient had reduction mammoplasties, with associated deformity noted ➡. Diffuse FCC were found in the reduction specimens. *(Right)* Close-up of right CC mammogram (same as left) better shows diffuse scattered punctate and coarse heterogeneous Ca++.

Typical

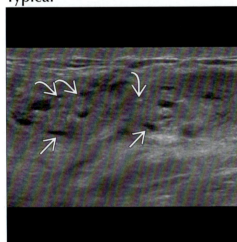

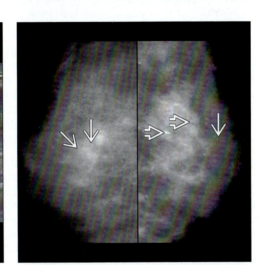

(Left) Representative US image (same case as prior 2 images) of the inner right breast shows multiple small cysts ➡ and scattered echogenic foci due to Ca++ ➡ as seen mammographically, typical of FCC. BI-RADS 2 benign. *(Right)* Bilateral lateral mammograms in this 48 y/o shows dense parenchyma with bilateral regional punctate and coarse heterogeneous Ca++ ➡. A few Ca++ layer ➡: Milk-of-calcium.

Typical

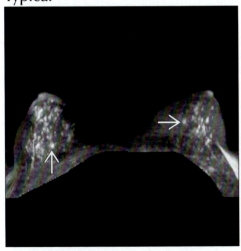

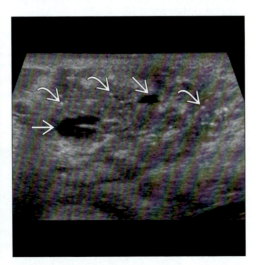

(Left) Axial MIP of T1 C+ subtraction MR (same case as prior image) shows scattered bilateral foci of enhancement ➡ with no one discrete suspicious area. *(Right)* Representative US image (same as left) shows diffusely heterogeneous echotexture with multiple small cysts ➡ and diffuse scattered echogenic foci: Ca++ ➡, typical of FCC. BI-RADS 2 benign.

FIBROSIS

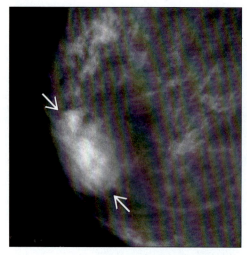

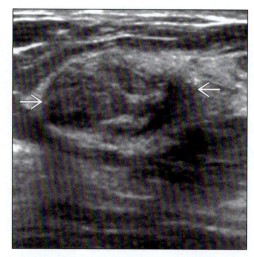

MLO mammography close-up view of a 68 y/o with palpable lump shows an indistinctly marginated, dense mass ➡ corresponding to palpable lump. Appearance was similar on CC view (not shown).

Ultrasound of this area shows mixed echogenicity mass ➡. Due to palpable finding, 14-g core biopsy was performed, revealing focal fibrosis. It has been stable on 3 year follow-up.

TERMINOLOGY

Abbreviations and Synonyms
- Focal fibrosis, stromal fibrosis, fibrosis associated with fibrocystic change (FCC)
- Terminal duct lobular unit (TDLU)

Definitions
- Prominence of fibrous tissue; may be global in extent
- Frequent incidental finding at histopathology
- Focal fibrosis: Synonymous with fibrous tumor in some classifications; also known as fibrous mastopathy
  - Benign mesenchymal tumor
  - Discrete often palpable growth composed of collagenized stroma
- Stromal fibrosis: Nonspecific term reflecting densely collagenized stroma between TDLUs
  - Causes ↑ mammographic density, either focal or diffuse
- Fibrocystic change (FCC): Constellation of cysts, fibrosis and adenosis

IMAGING FINDINGS

General Features
- Best diagnostic clue: Range of mammographic findings: Ill-defined to occasional circumscribed mass
- Location: Upper outer quadrant most common
- Size: 0.5-6 cm; mean ~ 2 cm

Mammographic Findings
- Mammographic asymmetry: 34%
- Ill-defined mass: 25%
- Circumscribed mass: 14%
- Architectural distortion: 5%
  - May be discordant result: Excision recommended
- Lobulated mass: 5%
- Associated calcifications (Ca++) uncommon: Coarse, heterogeneous
  - May represent sclerosed fibroadenoma (FA)

Ultrasonographic Findings
- Grayscale Ultrasound
  - Visible on ultrasound ~ 72-75% cases
  - Hypoechoic mass ~ 60%
  - Mixed hyper- and hypoechoic mass ~ 30%

DDx: Other Fibrous Breast Lesions

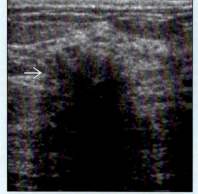

Diabetic Mastopathy

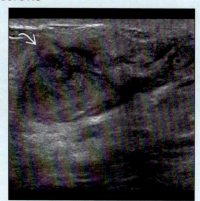

Chronic Inflammation, Fibrosis

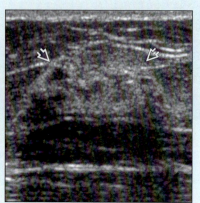

PASH

FIBROSIS

Key Facts

Terminology
- Focal fibrosis, stromal fibrosis, fibrosis associated with fibrocystic change (FCC)
- Prominence of fibrous tissue; may be global in extent
- Frequent incidental finding at histopathology
- Fibrocystic change (FCC): Constellation of cysts, fibrosis and adenosis

Imaging Findings
- Best diagnostic clue: Range of mammographic findings: Ill-defined to occasional circumscribed mass
- May show some interspersed fat
- Visible on ultrasound ~ 72-75% cases
- Circumscribed in ~ 55%: May mimic FA
- Relatively discrete ovoid area of ↑ echogenicity
- Concordance on MR-guided biopsy is an area of investigation

Top Differential Diagnoses
- Invasive Ductal (IDC) or Lobular Carcinoma (ILC)
- Fibroadenoma
- Post-Surgical Scar
- Diabetic Mastopathy
- Pseudoangiomatous Stromal Hyperplasia

Pathology
- 2-8% of core breast biopsies

Clinical Issues
- Peri-menopausal most common

Diagnostic Checklist
- Random sampling of dense breast tissue ⇒ fibrosis: May have missed the lesion on core biopsy

---

- ○ Isoechoic mass ~ 8%
- ○ May show dense posterior shadowing, suspicious
  - ■ With or without identifiable mass
- ○ Margins characteristics vary
  - ■ Circumscribed in ~ 55%: May mimic FA
  - ■ Lobulated in ~ 25%
  - ■ Ill-defined in ~ 15%: May mimic malignancy
- ○ Fibrous tumor
  - ■ Relatively discrete ovoid area of ↑ echogenicity
  - ■ Essentially a normal variant: Dense fibroglandular tissue

MR Findings
- T1WI
  - ○ Localized area isointense with dense parenchyma
  - ○ May show some interspersed fat
- T2WI FS: Similar to breast parenchyma, can be edematous
- T1 C+ FS
  - ○ Source of false positive suspicious findings on MR
  - ○ Regional, focal areas most common
  - ○ Irregular mass, requiring biopsy
  - ○ Most often persistent kinetics but can show plateau

Biopsy
- Percutaneous core biopsy with imaging-pathologic concordance adequate in many cases
  - ○ 6 month follow-up to confirm stability
  - ○ False negative rate with 14-g core biopsy: ~ 3%
- Assess concordance
  - ○ Discrete mass on imaging should be discrete mass at histopathology
    - ■ "Benign breast tissue" is not concordant with a mass-forming lesion
    - ■ When discrete process present, pathologists encouraged to describe this process, e.g., focal fibrosis
  - ○ Repeat biopsy or excision for discordance
  - ○ Spiculated mass discordant, lesion likely missed
  - ○ Random sampling of dense breast tissue can be perceived as "fibrosis" by pathologist
  - ○ Concordance on MR-guided biopsy is an area of investigation

Imaging Recommendations
- Best imaging tool
  - ○ Combination of mammography and US
  - ○ Correlate with clinical setting

DIFFERENTIAL DIAGNOSIS

Invasive Ductal (IDC) or Lobular Carcinoma (ILC)
- Findings may be indistinguishable: Asymmetry, distortion, posterior shadowing on ultrasound
- ILC: Focal asymmetry, irregular hypoechoic mass
- IDC: May present as dense shadowing on US

Fibroadenoma
- Circumscribed oval or gently lobulated, homogeneously slightly hypoechoic
- May have associated usually coarse Ca++; "popcorn" Ca++ typical as scleroses
- When sclerosed or "hyalinized", little epithelium

Fibroadenolipoma
- Encapsulated fat-containing mass

Post-Surgical Scar
- Clinical history of prior intervention

Diabetic Mastopathy
- Presentation of very firm, nontender 2-10 cm mass(es) and thickening
- Long-standing history of type I insulin-dependent diabetes

Pseudoangiomatous Stromal Hyperplasia
- Benign mesenchymal tumor composed of myofibroblasts
- Distinctive feature: Empty, anastomosing slit-like spaces

Fibromatosis
- Locally aggressive benign proliferation of fibroblasts and collagen

FIBROSIS

- Mammographic findings: Irregular dense spiculated mass
  - Usually close to or arising from pectoralis muscle
  - Associated Ca++ rare

PATHOLOGY

General Features
- Etiology
  - Unclear: Several theories postulated
    - Due to selective hormonal stimulation of fibroelastic tissue
    - Variant of normal breast involution
    - End result of chronic inflammatory process
  - Diabetic mastopathy
    - Usually in patients with type I insulin-dependent diabetes
    - Average interval between diagnosis and mastopathy: 20 years
    - More common in pre-menopausal women; reported in males
  - Secondary to radiation treatment
    - Diffuse with whole breast irradiation (WBI)
    - Fibrosis is more focally prominent, geographic to treated area with accelerated partial breast irradiation (APBI)
    - Fibrosis and retraction may progress over 2-3 years
    - Generally stabilizes after about 3 years
- Epidemiology
  - ↑ Incidence with screening mammography
    - 2-8% of core breast biopsies
  - May develop in peri-menopausal women: Hormonal influences
- Associated abnormalities
  - Dense breast parenchyma
  - Typically a part of fibrocystic changes, along with cysts, adenosis

Gross Pathologic & Surgical Features
- Fibrous tumor: Firm, hard mass; cut surface white, rubbery

Microscopic Features
- Normal loose connective tissue replaced by dense collagenous fibrous tissue
  - Surrounding atrophic ducts and acini
- Mild inflammatory infiltrate may be present
- Fibrous tumor
  - Hypocellular, collagenous stroma
  - Few or absent atrophic ductal and lobular elements
  - Sparse capillaries, vessels, lymphatic channels
  - No inflammatory infiltrate

CLINICAL ISSUES

Presentation
- Most common signs/symptoms
  - Incidental on screening mammogram or US performed for other reasons
  - May present as painless, firm, palpable mass

Demographics
- Age
  - Peri-menopausal most common
  - If post-menopausal, likely on hormonal therapy

Natural History & Prognosis
- Excellent prognosis
- No associated risk of malignancy

Treatment
- No treatment necessary

DIAGNOSTIC CHECKLIST

Consider
- Relatively common incidental suspicious finding on US and MR, often requiring biopsy
- Random sampling of dense breast tissue ⇒ fibrosis: May have missed the lesion on core biopsy
  - Discordant with spiculated mass or fine linear Ca++: Excise
  - Equivocal concordance with focal shadowing on US: 6 month follow-up recommended
  - Concordance with MR findings often ambiguous: 4-6 month follow-up MR recommended

Image Interpretation Pearls
- Most common: Developing global asymmetry in axillary tail in peri-menopausal woman, echogenic on US
  - When typical in appearance, can be followed
  - Contains interspersed fat
  - If clinically suspicious, biopsy

SELECTED REFERENCES

1. Goel NB et al: Fibrous lesions of the breast: imaging-pathologic correlation. Radiographics. 25(6):1547-59, 2005
2. You JK et al: Focal fibrosis of the breast diagnosed by a sonographically guided core biopsy of nonpalpable lesions: imaging findings and clinical relevance. J Ultrasound Med. 24(10):1377-84, 2005
3. Shetty MK et al: Sonographic findings in focal fibrocystic changes of the breast. Ultrasound Q. 18(1):35-40, 2002
4. Sklair-Levy M et al: Stromal fibrosis of the breast. AJR Am J Roentgenol. 177(3):573-7, 2001
5. Revelon G et al: Focal fibrosis of the breast: imaging characteristics and histopathologic correlation. Radiology. 216(1):255-9, 2000
6. Rosen EL et al: Focal fibrosis: a common breast lesion diagnosed at imaging-guided core biopsy. AJR. 173(6):1657-62, 1999
7. Venta LA et al: Imaging features of focal breast fibrosis: mammographic-pathologic correlation of noncalcified breast lesions. AJR. 173(2):309-16, 1999
8. Berg WA et al: Predictive value of specimen radiography for core needle biopsy of noncalcified breast masses. AJR. 171(6):1671-8, 1998
9. Berg WA et al: Lessons from mammographic-histopathologic correlation of large-core needle breast biopsy. Radiographics. 16(5):1111-30, 1996

FIBROSIS

IMAGE GALLERY

Typical

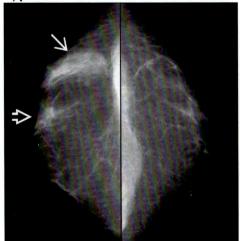
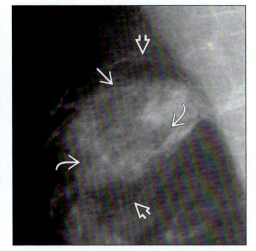

(Left) CC mammography of a 48 y/o shows focal asymmetry laterally ➡ at palpable site, new compared to prior mammograms. A focal asymmetry ➡ in the retroareolar right breast was unchanged. *(Right)* MLO mammography close-up (same patient as left), shows interspersed fat ➡ within the asymmetry ➡. There is surrounding fat and a subtle capsule ➡, suggesting fibroadenolipoma.

Typical

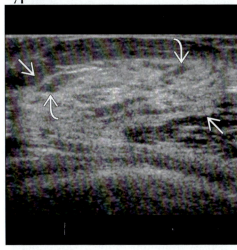
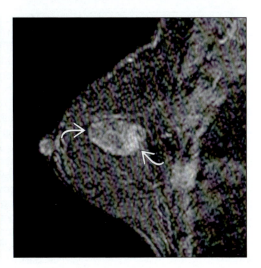

(Left) Radial ultrasound (same as prior 2 images) shows ovoid hyperechoic mass ➡ corresponding to palpable & mammographic abnormality. Interspersed fat ➡ is visible. *(Right)* Sagittal T1 C+ subtraction MR (same as prior 3 images) shows persistent heterogeneous enhancement in oval mass ➡. Due to clinical concern, US-guided biopsy was performed, showing benign tissue & stromal fibrosis, concordant with imaging findings.

Typical

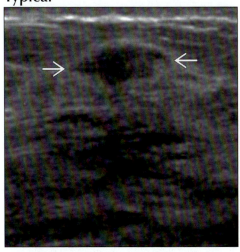
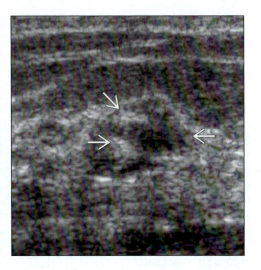

(Left) Anti-radial ultrasound of a 45 y/o shows an irregular, hypoechoic mass ➡ with no posterior features, intermediate suspicion, BI-RADS 4B. Core biopsy showed benign breast tissue and stromal fibrosis. *(Right)* Anti-radial ultrasound shows a mixed echogenicity mass ➡ with minimal posterior enhancement, of intermediate suspicion, BI-ARDS 4B. Core biopsy yielded stromal fibrosis, concordant with imaging findings. It was stable for two years.

HEMATOMA

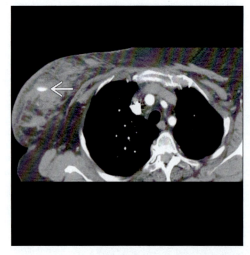

Axial CECT in a "trauma 1" 74 y/o involved in a motor vehicle collision shows extravasation of contrast material ➡ into the right breast indicating active arterial bleeding.

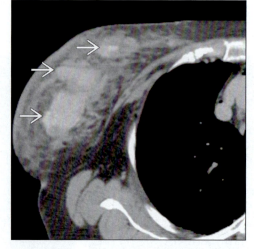

Axial CECT (same patient as previous image) shows extensive high density hematoma ➡ throughout breast parenchyma. The patient had severe head and facial trauma requiring immediate management.

TERMINOLOGY

Definitions
- Localized collection of extravasated blood
  - Mixed fluid/solid components: Serum and clot

IMAGING FINDINGS

General Features
- Best diagnostic clue: Clinical history of trauma or intervention
- Location
  - Occupies either a surgical cavity or traumatic tear
  - May spread into parenchyma, connective tissue, or adipose tissue

Mammographic Findings
- Findings often mimic malignancy
  - History vital to avoid unnecessary intervention in post-operative patient
- Early changes (days to weeks)
  - Round or oval mass
    - Margins ill-defined at first, especially if pain limits compression during mammography
    - Margins better defined as hematoma organizes
  - Air-fluid levels occasionally observed in post-operative collections
  - ↑ Density in adjacent parenchyma
    - Due to associated interstitial edema
  - Skin thickening
- Late changes (months to years)
  - Decrease in size
  - Spiculated mass; architectural distortion
  - Residual skin thickening in some patients
  - Fat necrosis may occur as end result
    - Oil cysts; rim, dystrophic calcifications
- Seatbelt injury
  - Characteristic distribution (upper inner right, driver side; upper inner left, passenger side)
    - Band-like density from upper inner to lower outer quadrant

Ultrasonographic Findings
- Grayscale Ultrasound
  - Hyperacute (hours)
    - Often completely anechoic collection

DDx: Complex Cystic Mass

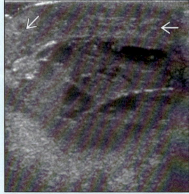

Abscess

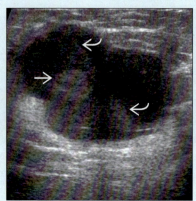

Intracystic Papillary DCIS

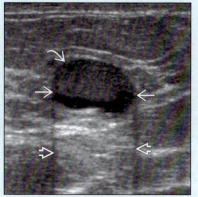

Galactocele

HEMATOMA

Key Facts

Terminology
- Localized collection of extravasated blood

Imaging Findings
- Findings often mimic malignancy
- History vital to avoid unnecessary intervention in post-operative patient
- Use Doppler to look for internal flow
- Hematoma is avascular
- Any internal flow should increase suspicion for mass
- Imaging not required if diagnosis is clinically obvious
- Consider performance of mammography as soon as can be tolerated in patient with breast trauma
- Most hematomas resolve rapidly
- 60% patients had visible hematoma on immediate post-biopsy films (14-g vacuum-assisted)

- 5% in same group had residual hematoma at subsequent wire localization

Top Differential Diagnoses
- Seroma
- Hemorrhagic Cyst
- Intracystic Carcinoma
- Galactocele
- Fibroadenolipoma (Hamartoma)
- Contusion

Clinical Issues
- Should resolve spontaneously without intervention
- May evolve into fat necrosis with oil cyst formation

Diagnostic Checklist
- Exclude intracystic mass if cyst aspiration yields bloody fluid

---

- ○ Acute (days)
  - ▪ Hypoechoic interior
  - ▪ Low-level internal echoes, increasingly echogenic as clot develops
  - ▪ Whorled appearance common as clot solidifies
  - ▪ Fluid-debris level
  - ▪ May see fibrin strands traversing the cavity
  - ▪ Edema (increased echogenicity) of surrounding tissue
- ○ Subacute (weeks)
  - ▪ Irregular margin
  - ▪ Thick hyperechoic walls with mural nodules
  - ▪ Avascular thick internal septations
- ○ Chronic (months to years)
  - ▪ Highly variable appearance
  - ▪ May be confused with neoplasm
- Color Doppler
  - ○ Use Doppler to look for internal flow
    - ▪ Hematoma is avascular
    - ▪ Any internal flow should increase suspicion for mass
- Ultrasound-guided aspiration
  - ○ May be difficult to aspirate if primarily solid clot
  - ○ Use "cine-loop" function to document needle is movable within interstices of lesion
    - ▪ Needle moves through clot, seroma, pus
    - ▪ Solid mass will move with the needle

MR Findings
- T1WI: Hyperintense acutely (days to weeks); hypointense hemosiderin (months to years)
- T2WI FS
  - ○ Heterogeneous signal, varies over time
  - ○ May show fluid-fluid levels
  - ○ Hyperintense rim acutely due to surrounding edema and serum
  - ○ Chronic: Hypointense rim due to susceptibility artifacts, hemosiderin
- T1 C+
  - ○ No internal enhancement
  - ○ Uniform peripheral rim enhancement ≤ 4 mm may be seen in post-operative hematoma
    - ▪ Progressive enhancement, i.e., not washout

CT Findings
- NECT
  - ○ May be seen in post-operative patients
    - ▪ High density acutely; margins may be irregular
  - ○ History and clinical correlation important to avoid unnecessary intervention for "mass" due to hematoma

Imaging Recommendations
- Best imaging tool
  - ○ Ultrasound
    - ▪ Better tolerated than mammography
    - ▪ Better ability to differentiate hematoma from solid mass
- Protocol advice
  - ○ Imaging not required if diagnosis is clinically obvious
    - ▪ Patients may request US for reassurance if "lump" develops after biopsy
  - ○ Consider performance of mammography as soon as can be tolerated in patient with breast trauma
    - ▪ Establishes size and location of hematoma
    - ▪ Allows mammographic follow-up
    - ▪ Increases confidence in diagnosis of post-traumatic fat necrosis on later mammograms
- After aspiration or biopsy wait at least two weeks before mammography (other than post-clip mammogram)
  - ○ Most hematomas resolve rapidly
    - ▪ 60% patients had visible hematoma on immediate post-biopsy films (14-g vacuum-assisted)
    - ▪ 5% in same group had residual hematoma at subsequent wire localization

DIFFERENTIAL DIAGNOSIS

Seroma
- Cannot distinguish from hematoma on mammography
- Occupies post-operative cavity

HEMATOMA

- US: Simple fluid collection, may have floating fibrin strands

Hemorrhagic Cyst
- Typically circumscribed
- No history of trauma
- Fluid-debris level
- Exclude intracystic mass as cause

Intracystic Carcinoma
- Carcinomas are solid
- Look for internal vascularity
  - Blood flow implies fibrovascular stalk, neoplasm

Galactocele
- Associated with breastfeeding
- Circumscribed
- Can be echogenic due to high fat content

Fibroadenolipoma (Hamartoma)
- "Breast within a breast" appearance
- Circumscribed, no fluid levels

Contusion
- Subtle diffuse infiltration of tissues by blood or edema
- Mild architectural distortion and trabecular thickening

PATHOLOGY

General Features
- Etiology
  - Iatrogenic
    - Core or vacuum-assisted biopsy
    - Cyst aspiration
    - Fine needle aspiration/biopsy
  - Surgery
    - Lumpectomy/excisional biopsy
    - Breast augmentation/mastopexy
    - Reduction mammoplasty
  - Occasionally occurs spontaneously
    - Anticoagulant therapy
    - Bleeding diathesis
    - Underlying carcinoma

CLINICAL ISSUES

Presentation
- Painful, palpable mass after known trauma or intervention
- Ecchymosis, skin discoloration
- Bleeding may occur spontaneously into inflamed cyst or degenerating neoplasm
  - With over anticoagulation or other bleeding diathesis
- May be fluctuant on palpation
  - Distinguishes fluid-filled from solid lesion
- Clinical symptoms usually completely resolve
  - Post-traumatic: Up to six weeks
  - Post-lumpectomy: Up to one year

Natural History & Prognosis
- Should resolve spontaneously without intervention
- May evolve into fat necrosis with oil cyst formation

Treatment
- Prevention
  - Aggressive use of lidocaine with epinephrine if bleeding encountered during stereotactic biopsy
  - Vacuum out cavity prior to placing clip
  - Post-procedural compression to ensure hemostasis
  - Use of support garments after plastic surgery
- Small
  - Supportive care: Ice pack (acute), warm compresses, analgesia
- Large, painful
  - Aspiration or surgical drainage

DIAGNOSTIC CHECKLIST

Consider
- Hematoma is the most common problem resulting from breast trauma
- Suggest early mammography after significant breast trauma to establish baseline findings

Image Interpretation Pearls
- History of prior intervention or trauma vital
- Exclude intracystic mass if cyst aspiration yields bloody fluid
  - Blood not felt to be due to trauma of procedure itself
- If apparent fluid-debris level, move patient during ultrasound
  - Proves debris non-adherent therefore not mass
  - Allows evaluation of all parts of wall
- Negative Doppler assessment less helpful than positive
  - Positive flow implies perfusion → neoplasm more likely
  - Lack of flow seen with debris, adherent clot, infarcted neoplasm

SELECTED REFERENCES

1. Mauro S et al: Late recurrent capsular hematoma after augmentation mammaplasty: case report. Aesthetic Plast Surg. 29(1):10-2, 2005
2. Veiga DF et al: Late hematoma after aesthetic breast augmentation with textured silicone prosthesis: a case report. Aesthetic Plast Surg. 29(5):431-3; discussion 434, 2005
3. Nahabedian MY et al: Factors associated with anastomotic failure after microvascular reconstruction of the breast. Plast Reconstr Surg. 114(1):74-82, 2004
4. Myhre A et al: Hemorrhage into the breast in a restrained driver after a motor vehicle collision. AJR. 179:690, 2002
5. Kanegusuku MS et al: Recurrent spontaneous breast hematoma: report of a case and review of the literature. Rev Hosp Clin Fac Med Sao Paulo. 56(6):179-82, 2001
6. Majeski J: Shoulder restraint injury to the female breast: a crush injury with long-lasting consequences. J Trauma. 50(2):336-8, 2001
7. Nagasawa M et al: Sudden hemorrhage of the breast caused by breast cancer: a case report and review of the literature. Breast Cancer. 7(2):176-8, 2000
8. Deutch BM et al: Stereotactic core breast biopsy of a minimal carcinoma complicated by a large hematoma: a management dilemma. Radiology. 202(2):431-3, 1997

HEMATOMA

IMAGE GALLERY

Typical

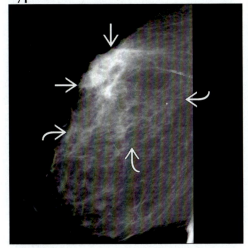
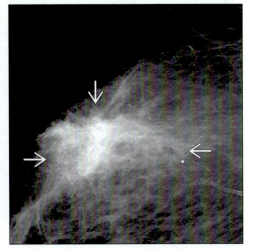

(Left) Lateral mammography in a 46 y/o one year following a car accident shows a new dense mass ➡ in the right upper outer quadrant with surrounding diffuse increased density and trabecular thickening ➡. *(Right)* MLO mammography spot compression confirms a dense irregular mass ➡ with indistinct margins. The patient had very little memory of the accident but her daughter recalled her having a "huge bruise". Biopsy confirmed chronic hematoma and fat necrosis.

Typical

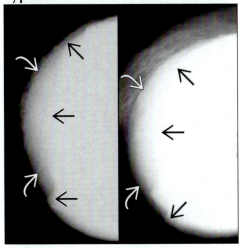
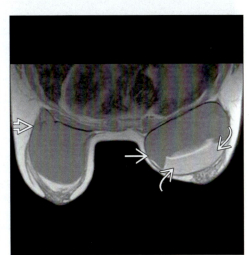

(Left) This woman noted enlarging right breast soon after implant placement. CC (left) and MLO (right) mammograms show a dense, undulating implant contour ➡, with additional dense material anterior to the implant ➡. MR was suggested for further evaluation. *(Right)* Axial T1WI MR shows a normal-appearing left implant ➡. On the right there is a hyperintense, intracapsular fluid collection ➡ anterior to the implant ➡.

Typical

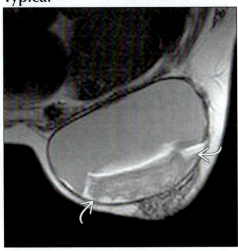
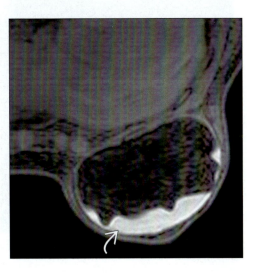

(Left) Axial T2WI FS MR confirms the intracapsular fluid collection ➡. On this sequence the fluid is hypointense. *(Right)* Axial T2WI FS MR with silicone suppression shows high signal intensity fluid ➡, compatible with acute blood, i.e., intracapsular hematoma. This was surgically evacuated. There are case reports of delayed peri-implant hematoma attributed to erosion of capsular arteries (Courtesy DAL).

Typical

(Left) CC mammography in 48 y/o one year post-lumpectomy and XRT shows dense, indistinctly-marginated mass ➡ with skin ➡ and trabecular thickening ➡. *(Right)* US of the lumpectomy site (same patient as previous image) shows a thick-walled complex cystic mass ➡ with internal septations and debris. The track to the overlying skin scar is visible in this plane ➡.

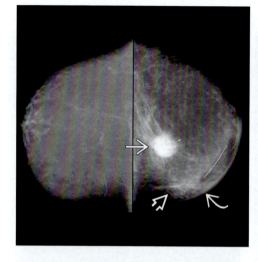 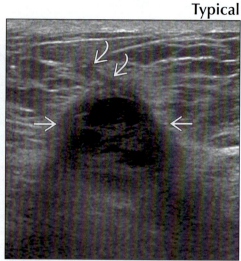

Typical

(Left) CC mammography magnification shows pleomorphic calcifications (Ca++) ➡ associated with an area of architectural distortion. Stereotactic biopsy showed DCIS. The patient was scheduled for lumpectomy. *(Right)* CC mammography performed as the scout view for wire localization (same patient as prior image) shows small post-biopsy hematoma ➡ adjacent to marker clip ➡ placed at the time of stereotactic biopsy.

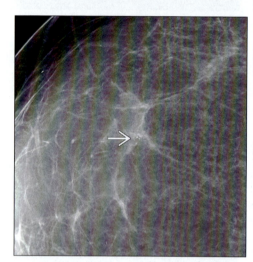 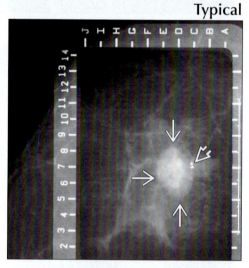

Typical

(Left) Specimen radiograph (same patient as prior 2 images) confirms excision of residual Ca++ ➡ and the marker clip ➡. The hematoma ➡ has also been excised. *(Right)* US in this 51 y/o 3 weeks post excision of IDC with positive margins shows thick-walled collection ➡ with thick septations and debris ➡, compatible with hematoma. Seromas tend to be thin-walled and simple. At re-excision, there was no residual tumor.

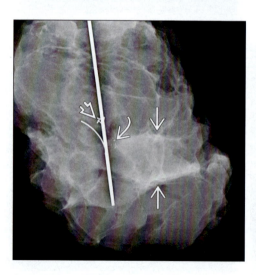 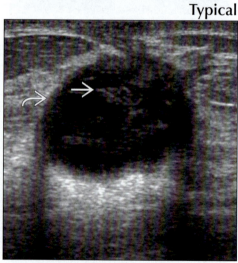

IV

2

54

HEMATOMA

Typical

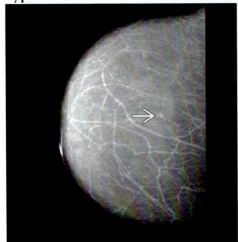

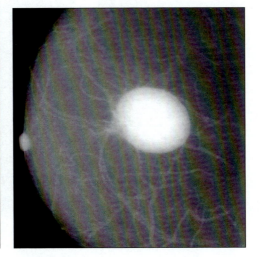

(Left) CC mammography shows a new mass ➡ in the central breast in a 61 y/o. The patient insisted upon excision: Wire-localized biopsy was performed with benign result. *(Right)* CC mammography (same patient as prior image) performed for evaluation of a palpable mass post-operatively confirms a dense, oval, partly circumscribed mass at the site of the excision. This is typical of a hematoma.

Typical

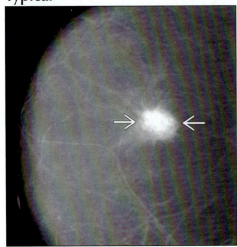

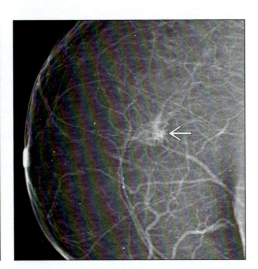

(Left) CC mammography two years later (same patient as prior two images) shows a smaller, dense, irregular mass ➡ with spiculated margins in the same area. Without prior films, this would have been very concerning for invasive cancer. With the old films, the true etiology was apparent. *(Right)* CC mammography (same as prior 3 images) seven years after excisional biopsy shows small residual scar ➡ ± fat necrosis.

Typical

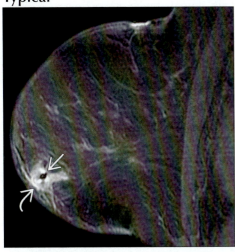

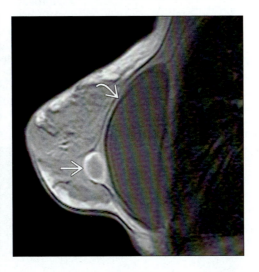

(Left) Sagittal T1 C+ FS MR shows clip artifact ➡ in hyperintense collection ➡ due to hematoma at time of MR-guided biopsy in this 63 y/o. Hematomas may obscure any residual enhancing lesion at time of MR biopsy. *(Right)* Sagittal T1WI MR shows peripherally hyperintense mass ➡ due to hematoma adjacent to implant ➡ in this 43 y/o status post stereotactic biopsy for colloid carcinoma one week earlier. At excision, 3 mm residual cancer was found.

LIPOMA

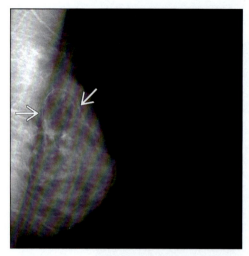

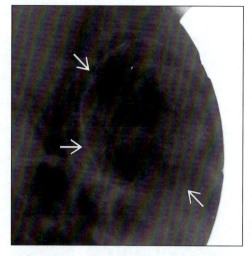

Left MLO mammogram in this 40 year old woman shows a lucent mass in the upper outer posterior left breast ➡.

MLO spot compression view (same case as left-hand image) shows circumscribed fatty mass ➡ = lipoma, a benign finding. Pseudocapsule is due to compressed normal tissue.

TERMINOLOGY

Definitions
- A benign tumor composed of mature adipose cells

IMAGING FINDINGS

General Features
- Best diagnostic clue: Radiolucent circumscribed oval or round mass
- Location: Breast, axilla, intramuscular in chest wall

Mammographic Findings
- Oval, round, gently lobulated
- Contains only fat, completely radiolucent
- Subject to fat necrosis, as any fat-containing lesion
  - May exhibit typical spherical calcifications
  - Usually circumscribed; fat necrosis can → indistinct
- Mass effect on surrounding tissue

Ultrasonographic Findings
- Grayscale Ultrasound
  - Ovoid or round, circumscribed mass
  - Nearly isoechoic or slightly hyperechoic to subcutaneous fat

MR Findings
- Not indicated in the diagnostic work-up of lipoma
- T1 ± C: Bright, nonenhancing: Composed of fat

Imaging Recommendations
- Best imaging tool: Mammography if parenchymal; US if palpable and cannot be included on mammogram

DIFFERENTIAL DIAGNOSIS

Benign Fat-Containing Lesions
- Lipomatous pseudomass
  - Increasing incidence with advancing age
- Fibroadenolipoma and variants (hamartoma)
  - Typically have fibroglandular component
- Fat necrosis, oil cysts
  - Round, lucent mass(es), often calcified rim
- Galactocele
  - Typically radiolucent, smoothly-margined masses
  - May show fat-fluid level on lateral view, US
- Steatocystoma

DDx: Lipoma within Different Tissue Compositions

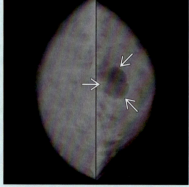

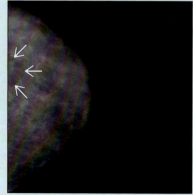

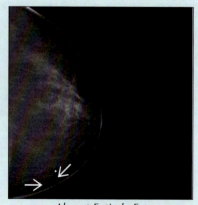

Extremely Dense

Heterogeneously Dense

Almost Entirely Fat

LIPOMA

Key Facts

Terminology
- A benign tumor composed of mature adipose cells

Imaging Findings
- Best diagnostic clue: Radiolucent circumscribed oval or round mass

Top Differential Diagnoses
- Lipomatous pseudomass
- Fibroadenolipoma and variants (hamartoma)

- Fat necrosis, oil cysts
- Galactocele
- Steatocystoma
- Liposarcoma and Atypical Lipoma

Clinical Issues
- Most common soft tissue tumor in adults

Diagnostic Checklist
- Definitively benign on mammography

  ○ Sebum-containing dermal cyst(s)
- Hibernoma
  ○ Usually in the axillary tail or axilla
  ○ Brown fat, resembles fat in hibernating animals

Liposarcoma and Atypical Lipoma
- Usually contain radiodense areas; rare

PATHOLOGY

Gross Pathologic & Surgical Features
- Well-circumscribed, round or discoid, yellow mass

Microscopic Features
- Benign tumor of mature adipose tissue without atypia
- Pseudocapsule due to compressed normal tissue
- Lipoma variants have been described in the breast
  ○ Spindle cell lipoma, hibernoma, adenolipoma, angiolipoma
  ○ Pleomorphic lipoma: May be confused histologically with variants of liposarcoma

CLINICAL ISSUES

Presentation
- Most common signs/symptoms
  ○ Slow growing freely movable, soft mass
    ▪ May be somewhat firm secondary to fat necrosis
  ○ Usually painless and asymptomatic
  ○ Multiple lipomas may occur; bilateral in 3%

- Other signs/symptoms
  ○ Dercum disease (lipomatosis dolorosa): Multiple painful lipomas usually in middle aged women
  ○ Benign symmetric lipomatosis (Madelung disease): Fatty masses symmetrically around the body
- Clinical Profile
  ○ Most common soft tissue tumor in adults
  ○ Solitary most common in women; multiple in men

Treatment
- No treatment necessary; may be removed electively

DIAGNOSTIC CHECKLIST

Image Interpretation Pearls
- Definitively benign on mammography

SELECTED REFERENCES

1. Pant R et al: An unusual case of an intramuscular lipoma of the pectoralis major muscle simulating a malignant breast mass. Ann Acad Med Singapore. 34:275-6, 2005
2. Rosen PP: Rosen's Breast Pathology. Philadelphia, Lippincott Williams & Wikins. Chapter 40, 786, 2001
3. Kopans D: Breast Imaging. 2nd ed. Philadelphia, Lippincott-Raven. Chapter 19, 551-8, 1998
4. Hall FM et al: Lipomatous pseudomass of the breast: diagnosis suggested by discordant palpatory and mammographic findings. Radiology. Vol 164, 463-4, 1987

IMAGE GALLERY

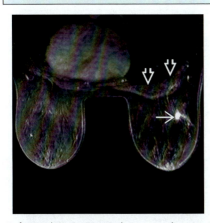
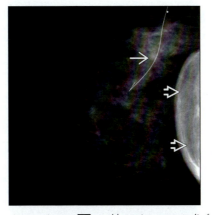
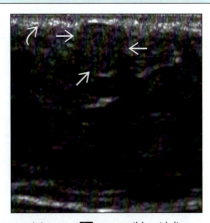

(Left) Axial T1 C+ FS MR shows an enhancing invasive carcinoma ➡, and large intrapectoralis fat-containing mass ➤, compatible with lipoma. *(Center)* CC mammography at wire localization (same case as left-hand image) shows known carcinoma ➡ as well as lipoma ➡ within the pectoral muscle. *(Right)* US of the axilla in this 61 year old, with history of prior lipomas resected in this area, shows a palpable superficial oval, circumscribed mass ➡ slightly hyperechoic to surrounding fat, just deep to the skin ➤, compatible with a benign lipoma.

MYOEPITHELIAL NEOPLASMS

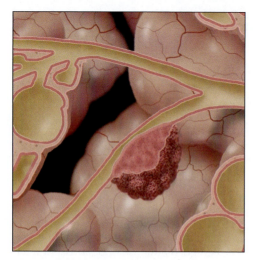

Drawing shows the characteristic location of a myoepithelial tumor between the endothelium and the basement membrane of a duct, distinguishing it from an epithelial or stromal mass.

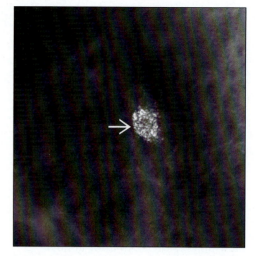

MLO mammography magnification shows an unusual small mass with densely packed, variable sized microcalcifications in the axillary tail ➡. Stereotactic core biopsy confirmed a benign adenomyoepithelioma.

TERMINOLOGY

Definitions
- Benign or malignant neoplasms arising from myoepithelial cells

IMAGING FINDINGS

General Features
- Best diagnostic clue: Focal, often circumscribed mass with clustered dense microcalcifications (Ca++)
- Location: Adenomyoepitheliomas tend to be central
- Size
  - 1-7 cm (adenomyoepithelioma)
  - 1-20 cm (malignant myoepithelioma)
- Morphology: Lobulated, fairly well-defined mass(es)

Mammographic Findings
- Nonspecific, circumscribed mass or asymmetry
- Amorphous to coarse heterogeneous Ca++, esp. adenomyoepithelioma

Ultrasonographic Findings
- Grayscale Ultrasound
  - Circumscribed mass, usually hypoechoic
  - May show echogenic Ca++
  - May appear as intracystic mass(es)
- Color Doppler: Usually hypovascular unless malignant

Imaging Recommendations
- Protocol advice: Image-guided core biopsy usually diagnostic

DIFFERENTIAL DIAGNOSIS

Fibroadenoma
- Calcifications coarser, peripheral

Papilloma, Peripheral
- Cannot reliably distinguish without biopsy

Intracystic Papilloma or Papillary Carcinoma
- Cannot reliably distinguish without biopsy

Invasive or Intraductal Carcinoma
- Cannot reliably distinguish without biopsy

DDx: Mimics of Adenomyoepithelioma

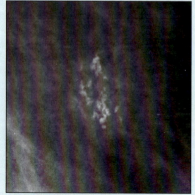

Fibroadenoma, Atypical Ca++

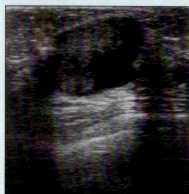

Intracystic Papilloma

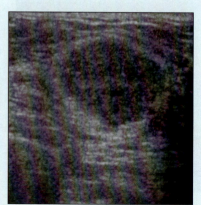

Focal (Stromal) Fibrosis

MYOEPITHELIAL NEOPLASMS

Terminology
- Benign or malignant neoplasms arising from myoepithelial cells

Top Differential Diagnoses
- Fibroadenoma
- Papilloma, Peripheral
- Intracystic Papilloma or Papillary Carcinoma
- Invasive or Intraductal Carcinoma
- Phyllodes Tumor

Key Facts
- Focal (Stromal) Fibrosis
- Pseudoangiomatous Stromal Hyperplasia (PASH)

Pathology
- Adenomyoepithelioma, benign or malignant
- Myoepithelioma (extremely rare)
- Pleomorphic adenoma (extremely rare)
- Adenoid cystic carcinoma (extremely rare)

Phyllodes Tumor
- Calcifications uncommon

Focal (Stromal) Fibrosis
- Indeterminate mass, sometimes with Ca++

Pseudoangiomatous Stromal Hyperplasia (PASH)
- Indeterminate mass, no Ca++

PATHOLOGY

Gross Pathologic & Surgical Features
- Firm rubbery masses with areas of cystic, hyaline or hemorrhagic degeneration

Microscopic Features
- Myoepithelial cells between epithelium and basement membrane
- Proliferative hyperplastic myoepithelial cells
- Adenomyoepithelioma: Spindle, tubular or lobulated
  - May show marked atypia even when benign

Staging, Grading or Classification Criteria
- Adenomyoepithelioma, benign or malignant
- Myoepitheliosis (no imaging findings)
- Myoepithelioma (extremely rare)
- Pleomorphic adenoma (extremely rare)
- Adenoid cystic carcinoma (extremely rare)

CLINICAL ISSUES

Presentation
- Most common signs/symptoms: Often palpable, focal mass, may be tender
- Clinical Profile: Often detected at screening (calcifications)

Demographics
- Age: Range 25-85, median 50-70

Natural History & Prognosis
- Adenomyoepithelioma may be unchanged for years
- Malignant adenomyoepithelioma
  - No metastases if < 2 cm at excision

Treatment
- Complete excision of adenomyoepithelioma curative
- Malignant lesions: No evidence for treatment other than complete excision

SELECTED REFERENCES
1. Howlett DC et al: Adenomyoepithelioma of the breast: spectrum of disease with associated imaging and pathology. AJR. 180:799-803, 2003
2. Doyle AJ et al: Myoepithelial lesions of the breast: imaging characteristics and diagnosis with large-core needle biopsy in two cases. Radiology. 193:787-8, 1994
3. Tavassoli FA: Myoepithelial lesions of the breast. Myoepitheliosis, adenomyoepithelioma, and myoepithelial carcinoma. Am J Surg Pathol. 15:554-68, 1991

IMAGE GALLERY

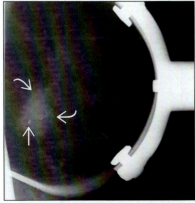 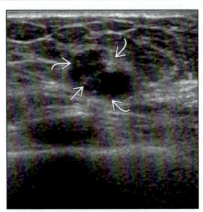 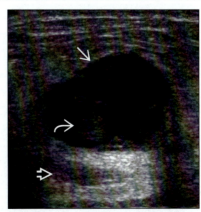

(Left) Mammography spot compression shows an indistinctly-marginated mass ➡ with a few Ca++ ➡. *(Center)* Ultrasound (same as left) shows an unusual hypoechoic mass ➡ with heterogeneous internal echoes ➡, possibly the mammographic Ca++. 14-g core biopsy showed benign adenomyoepithelioma. *(Right)* Ultrasound in another patient shows a complex thick-walled cystic lesion ➡ with intracystic masses ➡ & posterior enhancement ➡ suggestive of intracystic papillary carcinoma. Excision showed benign adenomyoepithelioma.

PAPILLOMA

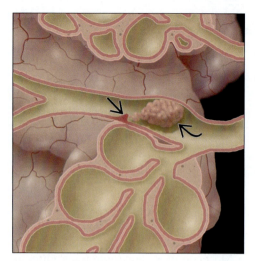

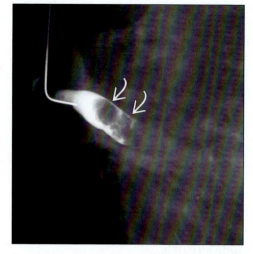

Sagittal graphic shows the typical location of a central papilloma ➔ within a dilated duct close to the nipple. Note the delicate stalk ➔ within which vessels may be seen using color Doppler.

Lateral galactography with magnification shows multiple lobulated filling defects ➔ within the duct in this typical case of benign papilloma presenting with bloody nipple discharge.

TERMINOLOGY

Abbreviations and Synonyms
- Intraductal papilloma
- Large duct papilloma = central papilloma
- Intracystic papilloma = papilloma with surrounding duct distension

Definitions
- Benign ductal neoplasm with proliferation of epithelial and myoepithelial cells supported by a frond-forming fibrovascular stalk
- Distinguish from papillomatosis: Form of epithelial hyperplasia
- Atypical papilloma: Papilloma with focal atypical epithelial proliferation with low-grade nuclei

IMAGING FINDINGS

General Features
- Best diagnostic clue
  - Periareolar intraductal soft-tissue mass
    - Often mammographically occult

- Size: 0.5-3 cm
- Morphology: Oval or round
- Central, periareolar (70-90%)
  - Usually solitary
  - Usually in large ducts
  - May be intracystic (in dilated duct)
  - Most present with nipple discharge
- Peripheral (10-30%)
  - Any quadrant; usually multiple
  - Arise in terminal ductal lobular unit (TDLU)
  - Usually a mammographic or microscopic finding
  - Compared to central papillomas, more often associated with radial sclerosing lesions, atypical ductal hyperplasia (ADH), ductal carcinoma in situ (DCIS), invasive carcinoma

Radiographic Findings
- Galactography
  - Intraluminal filling defect(s)
  - Duct dilatation leading up to lesion
    - Fluid secretions/blood distend duct over time
  - Abrupt duct "cutoff"

Mammographic Findings
- Usually not visible

DDx: Intraductal Filling Defects

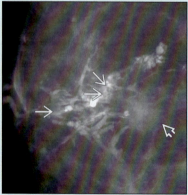

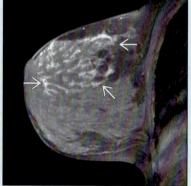

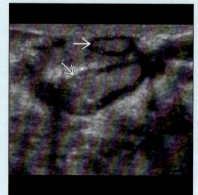

IDC (Dominant Mass) with EIC

Extensive DCIS

Dilated Ducts with Debris

PAPILLOMA

Key Facts

Terminology
- Benign ductal neoplasm with proliferation of epithelial and myoepithelial cells supported by a frond-forming fibrovascular stalk
- Distinguish from papillomatosis: Form of epithelial hyperplasia

Imaging Findings
- Central, periareolar (70-90%)
- Intraductal mass near nipple most common
- May see internal vascularity in stalk
- Ultrasound has higher yield than galactography

Top Differential Diagnoses
- Papillary Carcinoma
- Atypical Papilloma
- Intraductal Epithelial Proliferations
- Duct Ectasia with Debris
- Nipple Adenoma

Clinical Issues
- Majority present with bloody nipple discharge
- Excision recommended when benign papilloma diagnosed by CNB or VAB
- 12-14% upgrade to carcinoma on excision
- 17-22% upgrade to ADH or other high-risk lesion
- More frequent upgrade with peripheral papillomas

Diagnostic Checklist
- Papilloma is most common cause of bloody nipple discharge
- Variability within papillary lesions: Can be focally involved by ADH, DCIS

- Dilated duct
- Round or oval circumscribed or indistinctly-marginated mass ± clustered amorphous and/or punctate calcifications (Ca++)
  - Can be large, irregular, dense Ca++
- Sclerosing papilloma may be spiculated
  - Especially if associated with radial scar

Ultrasonographic Findings
- Grayscale Ultrasound
  - Intraductal mass near nipple most common
  - Dilated ducts around lesion common
    - Ducts may contain echogenic fluid if bleeding has occurred
  - Complex cystic and solid lesion: Intracystic mass
  - Focal hypoechoic solid mass
    - Circumscribed or indistinct margins
    - Usually lobulated
- Power Doppler
  - May see internal vascularity in stalk
    - Proves echogenic intraductal material = mass, not debris

MR Findings
- T2WI FS: May see hyperintense duct with intraductal hypointense mass
- T1 C+ FS: Variable weak enhancement to malignant enhancement profile
- MR can be used to evaluate nipple discharge
  - Series of 15 pathologically proven papillomas
    - 27% not seen on MR
    - 27% smooth mass in dilated duct
    - 46% irregular mass with washout kinetics

Biopsy
- FNA not reliable: Sensitivity as low as 44%
- Current literature indicates excision appropriate for papillomas, even if benign on initial core needle (CNB) or vacuum-assisted biopsy (VAB)
  - Consider direct excision for typical intraductal masses
  - Initial CNB for nonspecific masses ± Ca++
  - Initial CNB can be helpful for irregular intracystic masses: Can be due to invasive cancer

Imaging Recommendations
- Best imaging tool
  - Ultrasound has higher yield than galactography
    - Less discomfort, easier for staff and patient
  - Galactography can help map extent of multiple papillomas
- Protocol advice
  - Retroareolar angled US allows assessment of nipple areolar complex without shadowing from the nipple
  - "Rolled nipple" imaging technique
    - Nipple "rolled" over examiner's finger
    - Transducer applied to elongated superficial surface
    - Allows visualization of distal intraductal lesions
  - Identify often eccentric orifice of discharging duct in nipple, direct US to that axis
  - Confirm apparent lesion in two scan planes
    - Ducts are tortuous
    - Branch points may simulate filling defect in one scan plane
  - Use "standoff" pad or generous gel
    - Better near-field resolution of superficial masses

DIFFERENTIAL DIAGNOSIS

Papillary Carcinoma
- Usually intracystic, synonymous with papillary DCIS
- More likely to be irregular in shape
- Lacks myoepithelial layer
- When invasive, usually focally so along margin of distended duct

Atypical Papilloma
- Subtle distinction at histopathology
- 30-38% upgrade to carcinoma at excision after core biopsy

Intraductal Epithelial Proliferations
- No fibrovascular core-not true papillary lesion
  - Atypical ductal hyperplasia

PAPILLOMA

- ○ Ductal carcinoma in situ

Duct Ectasia with Debris
- No flow seen with Doppler

Nipple Adenoma
- Benign proliferation of ductules in nipple

PATHOLOGY

General Features
- General path comments
  - ○ Frozen section may misdiagnose as carcinoma
    - ■ May have cellular atypia
  - ○ May be found adjacent to or be focally involved by papillary carcinoma
- Epidemiology
  - ○ Peak incidence in 40s and 50s
  - ○ < 10% of benign breast neoplasms
  - ○ Rare in adolescents, young adults

Gross Pathologic & Surgical Features
- Dilated duct with mural soft-tissue cauliflower-like mass

Microscopic Features
- Dilated ducts around mass
- Epithelial fronds with fibrovascular stroma
  - ○ Central core of connective tissue
  - ○ Covered with cuboidal or columnar epithelial cells
  - ○ Intervening myoepithelial cell layer
- Hemorrhagic infarction of fronds common
  - ○ May simulate invasive cancer

CLINICAL ISSUES

Presentation
- Most common signs/symptoms
  - ○ Majority present with bloody nipple discharge
    - ■ Spontaneous
    - ■ Single orifice in nipple
    - ■ Often have trigger point: Pressure on one part of breast causes discharge
  - ○ Discharge may also be clear or serous
  - ○ Occasionally clinically palpable mass
    - ■ "Intracystic" papilloma: Within hugely dilated duct; cyst is palpable
    - ■ If cyst aspiration yields bloody fluid, consider excisional biopsy

Natural History & Prognosis
- Slight ↑ risk of developing breast cancer
  - ○ Same breast in area of papilloma
  - ○ Similar to risk with ADH
- May undergo spontaneous infarction
- Cured if completely excised
- < 10% recurrence rate

Treatment
- Breast endoscopy
  - ○ Direct visualization of intraluminal lesions
  - ○ Direct intraluminal biopsy can be performed
  - ○ Useful as a prelude to surgery

- ■ Typical "blind" ductal resection extends 2-3 cm
- ■ Deeper lesions will be missed
- ■ Duct resection → bleeding "cured" but pathology not adequately treated
- Excision recommended when benign papilloma diagnosed by CNB or VAB
  - ○ Sampling error on core biopsy
    - ■ 12-14% upgrade to carcinoma on excision
    - ■ 17-22% upgrade to ADH or other high-risk lesion
    - ■ Independent of vacuum-assisted or core biopsy technique
    - ■ More frequent upgrade with peripheral papillomas
- When suggested with galactography
  - ○ Localize lesion(s) and surgically excise
- When found by ultrasound
  - ○ US-guided VAB "excision" can be performed, but role unclear
    - ■ Can eliminate nipple discharge
    - ■ Potential sampling error persists
  - ○ Ultrasound-guided localization and excision

DIAGNOSTIC CHECKLIST

Consider
- Papilloma is most common cause of bloody nipple discharge
- Variability within papillary lesions: Can be focally involved by ADH, DCIS
  - ○ Excision prudent after result of benign papilloma on CNB, VAB

Image Interpretation Pearls
- Use "rolled nipple" technique in ultrasound
- When performing galactography
  - ○ Early filling views important to avoid obscuring a small distal mass with contrast
  - ○ Use magnification mammography

SELECTED REFERENCES

1. Bhattarai N et al: Intraductal papilloma: features on MR ductography using a microscopic coil. AJR Am J Roentgenol. 186(1):44-7, 2006
2. Lewis JT et al: An analysis of breast cancer risk in women with single, multiple, and atypical papilloma. Am J Surg Pathol. 30(6):665-72, 2006
3. Liberman L et al: Is surgical excision warranted after benign, concordant diagnosis of papilloma at percutaneous breast biopsy? AJR Am J Roentgenol. 186(5):1328-34, 2006
4. Mercado CL et al: Papillary lesions of the breast at percutaneous core-needle biopsy. Radiology. 238(3):801-8, 2006
5. Nelson RS et al: Twenty-year outcome following central duct resection for bloody nipple discharge. Ann Surg. 243(4):522-4, 2006
6. Dooley WC et al: Office-based breast ductoscopy for diagnosis. Am J Surg. 188(4):415-8, 2004
7. Daniel BL et al: Magnetic resonance imaging of intraductal papilloma of the breast. Magn Reson Imaging. 21(8):887-92, 2003
8. Hild F et al: Ductal orientated sonography improves the diagnosis of pathological nipple discharge of the female breast compared with galactography. Eur J Cancer Prev. 7 Suppl 1:S57-62, 1998

PAPILLOMA

IMAGE GALLERY

Typical

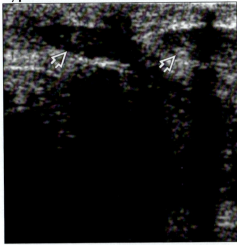
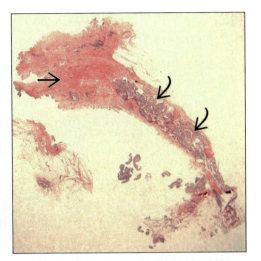

(Left) Radial ultrasound in 67 y/o presenting with bloody nipple discharge shows multiple hypoechoic masses ➡ within dilated ducts approximately 1 cm from the nipple. The patient underwent duct excision. *(Right)* Micropathology, low power, H&E of the resected duct ➡ (same as left) shows multiple benign intraductal papillomas ➡. Complete resection of the papillomas is considered curative. The patient can return to screening mammography.

Typical

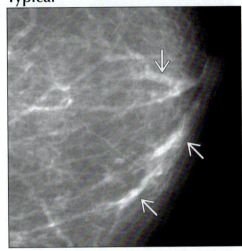
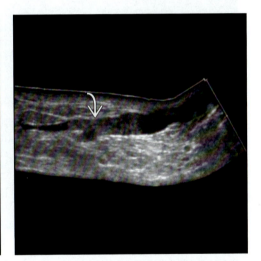

(Left) CC mammography demonstrates several dilated ducts ➡ in the retroareolar left breast in this 50 y/o with spontaneous clear nipple discharge. There are neither discrete masses nor Ca++. *(Right)* Radial US (same patient as previous image) utilizing extended-field-of-view imaging demonstrates a mass ➡ within a dilated duct. Several other dilated ducts and masses were seen in real time. Excision confirmed multiple benign papillomas.

Typical

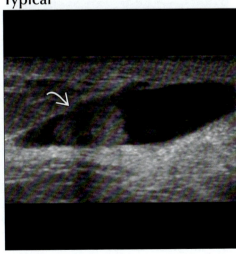
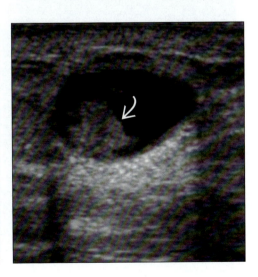

(Left) Radial ultrasound was performed to evaluate bloody nipple discharge in this 41 y/o with palpable mass near the nipple, demonstrating an intraductal mass ➡ in a large dilated duct. *(Right)* Anti-radial US (same patient as previous image) confirms a true intraluminal mass ➡. Doppler interrogation (not shown) revealed internal vascularity. This is typical for an intraductal papilloma, confirmed at excision.

PAPILLOMA

Typical

(Left) CC mammography spot compression shows two, indistinctly-marginated masses in this 73 y/o woman. Remote US core biopsy of the larger mass ➡ showed fibrocystic changes. The smaller mass ➡ was new. *(Right)* Ultrasound (same as left) confirms two masses ➡, ➡: Sclerosed papillomas on US core biopsy, confirmed at excision. A diagnosis of benign papilloma on core biopsy carries a 14-22% risk of unsampled malignancy or atypia.

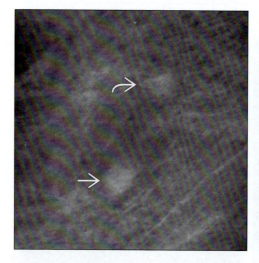

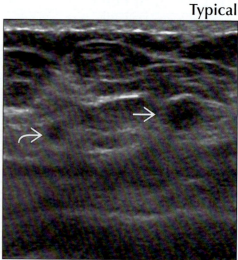

Typical

(Left) Sagittal T1 C+ SPGR MIP MR shows a dominant enhancing lobulated mass ➡ in the lower central breast in this 69 y/o with prior atypical lobular hyperplasia. *(Right)* MLO mammography (same patient as previous image) reveals a lobulated mass ➡ containing amorphous Ca++. The mass is just posterior to a clip ➡ in expected location of the MR-depicted mass. Stereotactic 11-g VAB and excision showed benign papilloma.

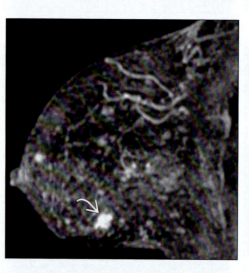

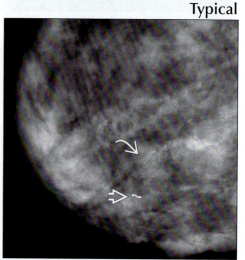

Variant

(Left) CC mammography magnification shows punctate Ca++ ➡ within a low-density circumscribed mass ➡, an incidental finding on screening in this 58 y/o woman. 11-g VAB showed benign papilloma. Five years later, the patient developed DCIS nearby. *(Right)* CC mammography shows coarse linear Ca++ ➡ in a tubular mass ➡ in this asymptomatic 68 y/o. Excision showed sclerosed papilloma with Ca++.

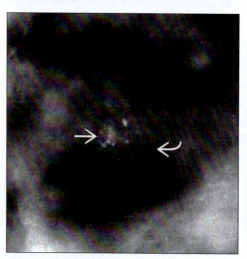

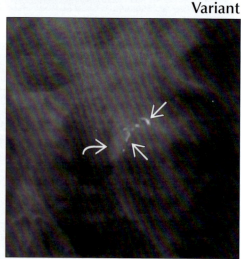

PAPILLOMA

Variant

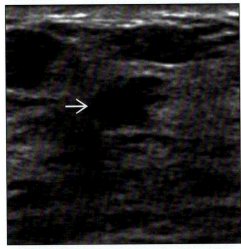
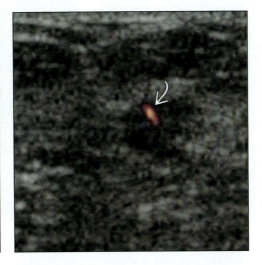

(Left) Radial spatial compounding ultrasound shows an irregular 5 mm mass ➡ incidentally found on ultrasound for nodular densities seen elsewhere on mammography in this 48 y/o. *(Right)* Radial power Doppler ultrasound (same as left) shows flow ➡ in this sclerosed papilloma. Diagnosis by 14-g US-guided core biopsy was confirmed by excision as the mass was irregular, an unusual appearance for a benign papilloma.

Variant

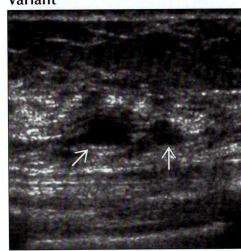
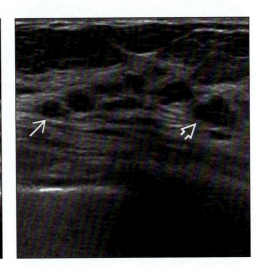

(Left) US shows two adjacent hypoechoic oval masses ➡ in this 37 y/o with clear nipple discharge. US-guided 14-g CNB showed papillomas. Patient had surveillance. *(Right)* Two years later she developed bloody nipple discharge (same as left). US shows multiple masses, with US-guided 14-g CNB of one ➡ yielding atypical papilloma and the other ➡ showing benign papilloma. At excision, DCIS and ADH were found admixed with multiple papillomas.

Variant

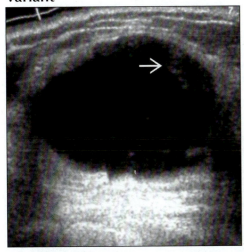
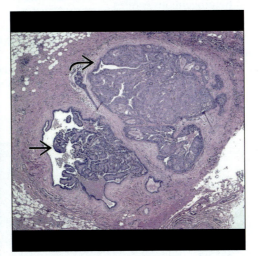

(Left) US shows small mural mass ➡ within this predominantly cystic, palpable mass in a 45 y/o woman. Initial US-guided aspiration yielded blood. A single 14-g core was then obtained showing papilloma, benign to one pathologist and possibly atypical to another. *(Right)* Micropathology, low power, H&E shows excisional histopathology (same as left). A portion of the mass was indeed a benign papilloma ➡, with adjacent papillary DCIS ➡.

PASH

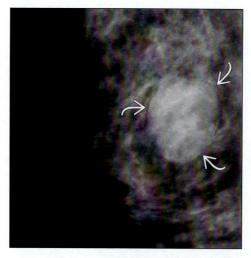

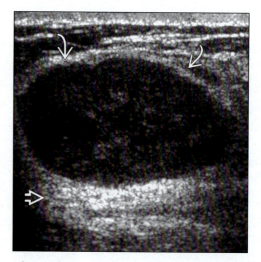

MLO mammography of the right breast in a patient with biopsy-proven pseudoangiomatous stromal hyperplasia (PASH) shows circumscribed mass with prominent lucent halo ➡.

Ultrasound (same patient as previous image) shows a smooth oval solid mass with a hyperechoic rim ➡, *heterogeneous internal echoes and posterior enhancement* ➡.

TERMINOLOGY

Abbreviations and Synonyms
- Pseudoangiomatous stromal hyperplasia (PASH)
- Pseudoangiomatous hyperplasia of the mammary stroma

Definitions
- Benign myofibroblastic hyperplastic process
- Contains extensive anastomosing slit-like spaces lined by fibroblasts, mimicking vascular channels

IMAGING FINDINGS

General Features
- Best diagnostic clue: Large solid oval mass with well-defined borders, internal heterogeneous echoes
- Size: Range 1-10 cm, mean 4-6 cm
- Morphology: Rounded or oval shape

Mammographic Findings
- Round or oval isodense mass
  - 1-10 cm
  - Margins circumscribed; may be partly indistinct, obscured, or show halo of compressed fat
  - Almost never calcify
- Often occult, incidental finding at biopsy

Ultrasonographic Findings
- Grayscale Ultrasound
  - Round or oval solid mass
    - Variable margin characteristics, usually circumscribed, macrolobulated
  - Usually mixed internal echogenicity
    - Predominantly hypoechoic with patchy heterogeneous internal echoes
    - Rarely hyperechoic
  - Sound transmission variable
- Color Doppler: Minimal vascularity evident

MR Findings
- T1WI: Intermediate signal mass with interspersed hypointense signal
- T2WI FS: Mixed high and low signal in a smooth mass
- T1 C+ FS
  - May show clumped enhancement, focal areas of enhancement or irregular enhancing mass on MR

DDx: Lesions Mimicking PASH

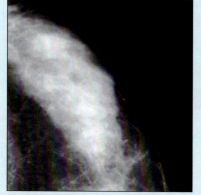

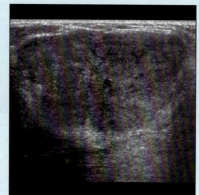

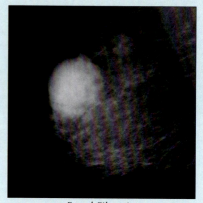

Asymmetric Parenchyma

Phyllodes Tumor

Focal Fibrosis

PASH

Key Facts

Terminology
- Pseudoangiomatous stromal hyperplasia (PASH)
- Benign myofibroblastic hyperplastic process
- Contains extensive anastomosing slit-like spaces lined by fibroblasts, mimicking vascular channels

Imaging Findings
- Best diagnostic clue: Large solid oval mass with well-defined borders, internal heterogeneous echoes
- Size: Range 1-10 cm, mean 4-6 cm
- Core biopsy usually diagnostic
- Best imaging tool: Ultrasound

Top Differential Diagnoses
- Asymmetric Glandular Parenchyma
- Fibroadenoma
- Phyllodes Tumor

- Fibroadenolipoma (Hamartoma)
- Focal (Stromal) Fibrosis
- Low Grade Angiosarcoma

Pathology
- Benign mesenchymal process which may form a mass
- Striking stromal hyperplastic changes

Clinical Issues
- Most commonly diagnosed microscopically as an incidental finding
- Screen-detected mass
- Premenopausal women, 18-50 usually
- Excellent prognosis without treatment in most cases
- Wide local excision usually curative when indicated

- Usually benign-type slowly increasing enhancement, similar to normal parenchyma

Biopsy
- Fine needle aspiration (FNA) can be inconclusive
  - May mimic phyllodes tumor or mucinous carcinoma
  - FNA may yield mucicarmine-positive intracystic material
- Core biopsy usually diagnostic
- Surgical excision rarely required for definitive diagnosis

Imaging Recommendations
- Best imaging tool: Ultrasound
- Protocol advice
  - Workup as for all palpable masses
  - Usually requires core needle biopsy to differentiate from other pathologies

DIFFERENTIAL DIAGNOSIS

Asymmetric Glandular Parenchyma
- Lacks discrete margin
- No focal lesion on additional mammographic views or ultrasound

Fibroadenoma
- Usually smaller, 2-3 cm typically
- Cellular findings may be similar on fine needle aspiration
- Frequently typical coarse calcifications

Phyllodes Tumor
- More common, usually first differential for larger PASH lesions
- Cellular aspirates on FNA may limit correct diagnosis

Fibroadenolipoma (Hamartoma)
- Fat-containing on imaging, usually readily distinguished on mammography
- PASH cases reportedly misdiagnosed as hamartomas at pathology
- No myofibroblastic-lined stromal spaces

Focal (Stromal) Fibrosis
- Can present as oval hypoechoic solid mass on ultrasound
- May be indistinguishable from PASH on conventional imaging
- Core biopsy usually diagnostic

Low Grade Angiosarcoma
- Vasoformative neoplastic tumor containing anastomosing epithelial-lined vascular spaces

PATHOLOGY

General Features
- General path comments
  - Benign mesenchymal process which may form a mass
    - Diffuse or focal stromal changes
    - Prominent proliferation of myofibroblasts
    - Nonspecific proliferative epithelial changes
    - May be an incidental finding at surgical pathology
  - Most PASH diagnosed as subclinical microscopic changes
    - At least one microscopic focus in 23% of breast specimens reported in one series
- Etiology: Likely related to a hormonal stimulus
- Epidemiology: If in a post-menopausal patient, hormone replacement therapy is likely
- Associated abnormalities
  - Microscopic PASH commonly found with or in other pathologies
    - Normal breast tissue
    - Gynecomastia
    - Fibrocystic changes
    - Fibroadenomatoid changes
    - Fibroadenomas

Gross Pathologic & Surgical Features
- No macroscopic lesion may be evident
- Focal solid firm mass
  - Smooth, well-demarcated surface

PASH

- May contain cysts, < 1 cm diameter

Microscopic Features

- Striking stromal hyperplastic changes
  - Separation of wavy, dense stromal collagen fibers
- Complex anastomosing pattern of pseudovascular slit-like spaces
  - Mimics vascular channels of an angiomatous neoplasm
  - Lining cells not endothelial
    - Fibroblasts & myofibroblasts, confirmed by immunohistochemistry: Factor VIII negative; CD34, actin, calponin positive
- Epithelial elements
  - Lobular and ductal structures
  - May show proliferative changes
- Progesterone receptor antibody positivity
  - Patchy, intense labeling of stromal cells
  - Distinct from normal stroma, juvenile hyperplasia and hamartomas
    - Note: Myoid hamartomas have similar patchy progestogenic staining
- Immunohistochemistry
  - CD34 positive spindle cell staining
  - Marker bcl-2 frequently positive
  - These suggest long-lived bcl-2-positive mesenchymal cell origin for PASH

CLINICAL ISSUES

Presentation

- Most common signs/symptoms
  - Most commonly diagnosed microscopically as an incidental finding
  - Screen-detected mass
- Other signs/symptoms
  - Rarely palpable
  - Rarely, large mass with peau d'orange
    - May mimic inflammatory carcinoma clinically
- Clinical Profile
  - Palpable, unilateral, painless, firm or rubbery mass
  - Frequently associated in gynecomastia
  - Post-menopausal
    - Mammographic mass in woman taking hormone replacement
  - Reported in axillary tissue

Demographics

- Age
  - Premenopausal women, 18-50 usually
    - Mean age: 40
- Gender
  - Usually, but not exclusively, female
  - In males, almost always in gynecomastia

Natural History & Prognosis

- Typically stable with slow or no growth
  - May show very rapid growth
  - Requires biopsy for differentiation from neoplasm, esp. phyllodes
- No malignant potential
- Excellent prognosis without treatment in most cases

Treatment

- Wide local excision usually curative when indicated
  - If clinical or patient concerns over symptomatic mass
  - If mass is enlarging
  - If imaging features are atypical or suspicious for malignancy
- Local recurrence common if excision is incomplete
- For smaller stable lesions, conservative expectant management is feasible option

DIAGNOSTIC CHECKLIST

Consider

- Unusual cause of asymmetric large solid mass
- May be diagnosed incidentally in other pathologies
- > 50% of cases have multiple foci, at least microscopically

Image Interpretation Pearls

- Can cause large asymmetric circumscribed mass
- Heterogeneous mammographic density
- Hypoechoic with patchy heterogeneous internal echoes

SELECTED REFERENCES

1. Zúbor P et al: Rapidly growing nodular pseudoangiomatous stromal hyperplasia of the breast in an 18-year-old girl. APMIS. 114:389-92, 2006
2. Moore T et al: Expression of CD34 and bcl-2 in phyllodes tumours, fibroadenomas and spindle cell lesions of the breast. Histopathology. 38:62-7, 2001
3. Kirkpatrick UJ et al: Imaging appearance of pseudoangiomatous hyperplasia of mammary stroma. Clin Radiol. 55:576-8, 2000
4. Piccoli CW et al: Developing asymmetric breast tissue. Radiology. 211:111-7, 1999
5. Simsir A et al: Additional mimics of mucinous mammary carcinoma: fibroepithelial lesions. Am J Clin Pathol. 109:169-72, 1998
6. Vicandi B et al: Nodular pseudoangiomatous stromal hyperplasia of the breast: cytologic features. Acta Cytol. 42:335-41, 1998
7. Zanella M et al: Pseudoangiomatous hyperplasia of the mammary stroma: true entity or phenotype? Pathol Res Pract. 194:535-40, 1998
8. Badve S et al: Pseudoangiomatous hyperplasia of male breast. Histopathology. 26:463-6, 1995
9. Anderson C et al: Immunocytochemical analysis of estrogen and progesterone receptors in benign stromal lesions of the breast. Evidence for hormonal etiology in pseudoangiomatous hyperplasia of mammary stroma. Am J Surg Pathol. 15:145-9, 1991
10. Ibrahim RE et al: Pseudoangiomatous hyperplasia of mammary stroma. Some observations regarding its clinicopathologic spectrum. Cancer. 63:1154-60, 1989
11. Vuitch MF et al: Pseudoangiomatous hyperplasia of mammary stroma. Hum Pathol. 17:185-91, 1986

PASH

IMAGE GALLERY

Typical

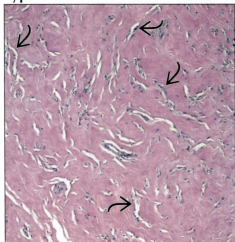
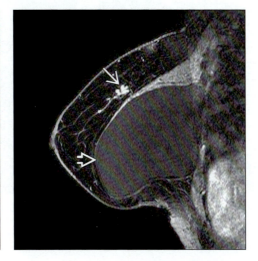

(Left) Micropathology (H&E, high power) in a woman with PASH shows typical dense wavy collagenous stroma with irregular, slit-like spaces ➡ lined by spindle cells. *(Right)* Sagittal T1 C+ FS MR shows clumped enhancement ➡ in the upper breast, above a subpectoral saline implant ➡, in a 39 y/o woman. MR findings of PASH include clumped enhancement, focal areas of enhancement and irregular enhancing masses.

Typical

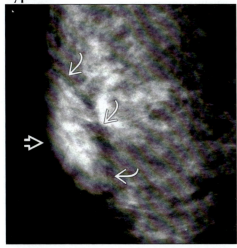
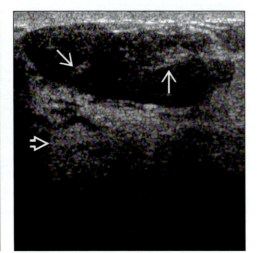

(Left) MLO mammography shows an oval soft tissue mass ➡ with mixed internal density and a clearly visible halo of compressed fat ➡. *(Right)* Longitudinal ultrasound (same patient as previous image) shows a circumscribed, hypoechoic oval mass with patchy heterogeneous internal echoes ➡, and mild posterior acoustic enhancement ➡. Multiple core needle biopsy specimens showed PASH.

Variant

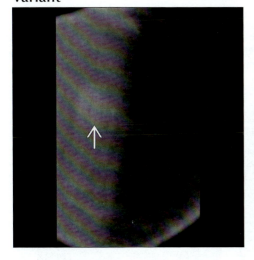
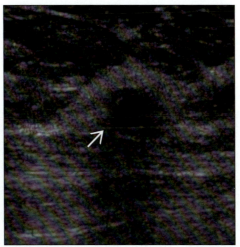

(Left) MLO mammography spot compression shows an indistinct focal asymmetry in the upper posterior breast ➡ of a 48 y/o woman, which remained poorly defined on spot compression views. *(Right)* Sagittal ultrasound (same patient as previous image) shows an irregular 1.8 cm hypoechoic mass ➡ with indistinct margins. Excisional biopsy showed PASH and fibrocystic changes (case courtesy EAR).

ATYPICAL DUCTAL HYPERPLASIA

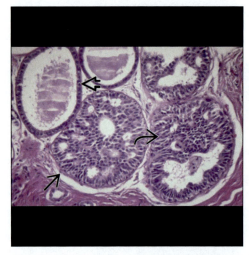

ADH (high power H&E) with 3 duct profiles: Normal ⇨. Center ➡: Uniform cells and lumina ~ DCIS, but diagnosis requires ≥ 2 duct profiles. Third ↗, has variable secondary spaces: ADH (Courtesy OBI).

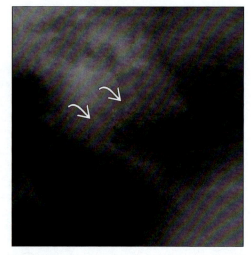

Lateral mammography magnification shows clustered amorphous Ca++ ⇲ noted on screening in this 51 y/o. Stereotactic 11-g biopsy and excision showed ADH. 20% of biopsies for amorphous Ca++ show ADH.

TERMINOLOGY

Abbreviations and Synonyms
- Atypical ductal hyperplasia (ADH)
- Atypical intraductal hyperplasia (AIDH)

Definitions
- Intraductal epithelial proliferative lesion of monomorphic cells
  - Criteria vary for diagnosis of ADH
  - Architectural and/or cytologic features nearly meet criteria for low-grade ductal carcinoma in situ (DCIS)

IMAGING FINDINGS

General Features
- Location: Terminal duct lobular unit (TDLU) and terminal ducts
- Considered a high-risk lesion
- Both breasts at risk

Mammographic Findings
- Amorphous calcifications (Ca++) most common
  - Clustered distribution > regional
- Other Ca++ morphologies: Punctate, pleomorphic
  - Fine linear Ca++ favor DCIS
- ADH can be incidental finding at histopathology
  - Within a fibroadenoma (FA) or papilloma
  - Within fibrosis, other fibrocystic changes (FCC)
  - Along spicules of radial scar or radial sclerosing lesion (RSL)
    - RSL may be manifest as architectural distortion
  - Adjacent to or admixed with carcinoma

Ultrasonographic Findings
- Grayscale Ultrasound: Usually incidental to biopsy for other reasons, e.g., FA

MR Findings
- T1 C+ FS
  - Linear, focal, regional enhancement
  - Evaluate remainder of both breasts for additional suspicious lesions

Biopsy
- Goal is adequate sampling of imaging target
  - At least 10 samples, at least 11-g vacuum-assisted stereotactic biopsy (VAB) of Ca++

DDx: Associated Abnormalities

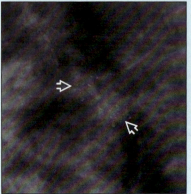

ADH Mixed with ALH

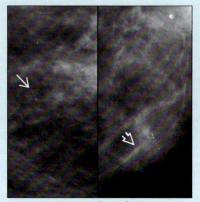

ADH, Ipsilateral IDC

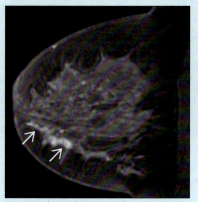

Ipsilateral DCIS only on MR

ATYPICAL DUCTAL HYPERPLASIA

Key Facts

Terminology
- Atypical ductal hyperplasia (ADH)
- Intraductal epithelial proliferative lesion of monomorphic cells
- Architectural and/or cytologic features nearly meet criteria for low-grade ductal carcinoma in situ (DCIS)

Imaging Findings
- Considered a high-risk lesion
- Both breasts at risk

Top Differential Diagnoses
- Usual Intraductal Hyperplasia (IDH)
- Flat Epithelial Atypia (FEA)
- Low-Grade Ductal Carcinoma In Situ (DCIS)
- Fibrocystic changes (FCC)

Pathology
- 4-13% of all breast biopsies
- 20% of all biopsies for amorphous Ca++
- 13% of malignant biopsies also have ADH
- Variable criteria to distinguish from low grade DCIS
- Features: DCIS but insufficient quantity ⇒ ADH
- To diagnose lesion as DCIS, at least 2 duct profiles must meet the criteria for DCIS

Clinical Issues
- ↑ Risk for developing invasive breast cancer: 4-5x
- 2.4-4x general population if no family history
- 7-13x if concomitant first-degree family history
- ADH on core biopsy should be excised
- 18% upgrade to malignancy after 11-g VAB
- Consider chemoprevention: Tamoxifen (TAM), raloxifene

- ○ VAB may also be appropriate for US-guided biopsy when sampling Ca++ visible under US
- ○ Document Ca++ retrieval with specimen radiography
- FNA insufficient: May show atypia, requires biopsy

DIFFERENTIAL DIAGNOSIS

Usual Intraductal Hyperplasia (IDH)
- Proliferation of heterogeneous cell population, often both epithelial and myoepithelial
- Streaming and overlapping of cells in areas of bridging
- Irregular, variable secondary spaces

Flat Epithelial Atypia (FEA)
- Single layer of columnar cell change with nuclei turned, flat

Low-Grade Ductal Carcinoma In Situ (DCIS)
- Quantitative ± qualitative differences
- Complete overlap in imaging findings

Other Amorphous Ca++
- Fibrocystic changes (FCC)
- Atypical lobular hyperplasia (ALH), lobular carcinoma in situ (LCIS), usually adjacent to Ca++

PATHOLOGY

General Features
- General path comments
  - ○ Some, but not all, features of low-grade DCIS
  - ○ Variability in pathologists' interpretations
- Genetics
  - ○ ADH regarded as nonobligate precursor to DCIS and invasive carcinoma
    - ■ Shares loss of heterozygosity (LOH) patterns with invasive carcinoma in same breast
    - ■ LOH at chromosomes 16q, 17p, 11q13
- Epidemiology
  - ○ 4-13% of all breast biopsies

- ○ 20% of all biopsies for amorphous Ca++
- ○ Frequent in prophylactic mastectomies of women at high risk
  - ■ 42% of non BRCA-mutation carriers, more often than the 17% of BRCA-1 or -2 mutation carriers
  - ■ ADH more common over age 40
- Associated abnormalities
  - ○ 13% of malignant biopsies also have ADH
  - ○ Frequent coexistence with IDH, FCC, ALH, RSL
  - ○ Common in women with newly diagnosed cancer elsewhere in either breast
    - ■ ADH does not affect risk of recurrence, prognosis
  - ○ Can exist within fibroadenomas (FA)
    - ■ No significant ↑ risk of subsequent malignancy
    - ■ Management, upgrade rates not well documented
  - ○ Can exist within papillomas
    - ■ < 3 mm area qualitatively resembling DCIS
    - ■ ↑ Risk of breast cancer > 4x in such patients
    - ■ Risk of breast cancer is at that site
    - ■ "Atypical papilloma" includes cellular atypia as well as frank ADH
    - ■ Atypical papilloma on CNB → excise

Microscopic Features
- Variable criteria to distinguish from low grade DCIS
  - ○ Proliferation of monomorphic epithelial cells in both ADH and DCIS
    - ■ Acinus partially (ADH) or completely filled (ADH or DCIS)
  - ○ Uniform (round or oval) secondary lumina (ADH or DCIS); variable secondary lumina: Crescentic, serpiginous (ADH)
  - ○ Features: DCIS but insufficient quantity ⇒ ADH
- Cribriform, solid, or micropapillary architecture
- Ca++ phosphate crystals in areas of ADH
- 90% of ADH have lost high molecular weight cytokeratins
  - ○ IDH shows diffusely + or mosaic staining

Staging, Grading or Classification Criteria
- Low-grade DCIS: Monomorphic, low nuclear grade cells with uniform secondary spaces and no necrosis

ATYPICAL DUCTAL HYPERPLASIA

- To diagnose lesion as DCIS, at least 2 duct profiles must meet the criteria for DCIS
- Total cross-sectional diameter > 2 mm (variable)
- Additional recuts may distinguish DCIS from ADH

CLINICAL ISSUES

Presentation
- Most common signs/symptoms: Amorphous Ca++ on screening mammography
- Other signs/symptoms
  - Uncommonly a mass lesion on imaging
  - Rarely palpable

Demographics
- Age: Peak in mid 40s
- Gender
  - Women; 4-13% of gynecomastia specimens
  - 22% of male breast cancer (DCIS ± associated invasive carcinoma) has associated ADH

Natural History & Prognosis
- Nonobligate precursor to malignancy
  - Average of 8.2 yrs to development of invasive cancer
- ↑ Risk for developing invasive breast cancer: 4-5x
  - 2.4-4x general population if no family history
  - 7-13x if concomitant first-degree family history

Treatment
- ADH on core biopsy should be excised
  - Upgrade to malignancy most commonly DCIS
    - 10-25% of upgrades show invasive carcinoma
  - 45% upgrade to malignancy after 14-g CNB
    - Rates similar after US or stereotactic biopsy
  - 25% upgrade to malignancy after 14-g VAB
  - 18% upgrade to malignancy after 11-g VAB
  - Upgrades persist even if all imaging evidence of lesion (e.g., Ca++) removed
    - 8-19% upgrade; no advantage to complete removal of imaging target in most series
  - Upgrade more common when ≥ 4 ducts or TDLUs of ADH on CNB
    - More common with micropapillary architecture
- Following surgical excision
  - Clinical and imaging follow-up
  - Not an indication for re-excision when present at margins
  - Consider chemoprevention: Tamoxifen (TAM), raloxifene
    - 49-72% ↓ risk of developing invasive breast cancer, TAM = raloxifene
    - Fewer cases DCIS with TAM but ↑ risk endometrial cancer, pulmonary embolism, deep vein thrombosis
  - High-risk screening
    - Possible supplemental screening with US or MR, esp. if also family history: Studies ongoing

DIAGNOSTIC CHECKLIST

Consider
- Frequent upgrade to malignancy after CNB diagnosis

Image Interpretation Pearls
- Clustered amorphous Ca++ suspicious, merit biopsy
- Patient is at high risk for developing cancer
  - Careful evaluation of both breasts at time of diagnosis of ADH
  - High-risk surveillance: Strategies evolving

SELECTED REFERENCES

1. Hoogerbrugge N et al: Numerous high-risk epithelial lesions in familial breast cancer. Eur J Cancer. 2006
2. Vogel VG et al: Effects of tamoxifen vs raloxifene on the risk of developing invasive breast cancer and other disease outcomes: the NSABP Study of Tamoxifen and Raloxifene (STAR) P-2 trial. JAMA. 295(23):2727-41, 2006
3. Grady I et al: Ultrasound-guided, vacuum-assisted, percutaneous excision of breast lesions: an accurate technique in the diagnosis of atypical ductal hyperplasia. J Am Coll Surg. 201(1):14-7, 2005
4. Ho BC et al: Flat epithelial atypia: concepts and controversies of an intraductal lesion of the breast. Pathology. 37(2):105-11, 2005
5. Prasad V et al: Bilateral atypical ductal hyperplasia, an incidental finding in gynaecomastia--case report and literature review. Breast. 14(4):317-21, 2005
6. Berg WA: Image-guided breast biopsy and management of high-risk lesions. Radiol Clin North Am. 42(5):935-46, vii, 2004
7. Jackman RJ et al: Atypical ductal hyperplasia: can some lesions be defined as probably benign after stereotactic 11-gauge vacuum-assisted biopsy, eliminating the recommendation for surgical excision? Radiology. 224:548-54, 2002
8. Liberman L et al: To excise or to sample the mammographic target: what is the goal of stereotactic 11-gauge vacuum-assisted breast biopsy? AJR. 179:679-83, 2002
9. Berg WA et al: Biopsy of amorphous breast calcifications: pathologic outcome and yield at stereotactic biopsy. Radiology. 221:495-503, 2001
10. Carter BA et al: No elevation in long-term breast carcinoma risk for women with fibroadenomas that contain atypical hyperplasia. Cancer. 92:30-6, 2001
11. Ely KA et al: Core biopsy of the breast with atypical ductal hyperplasia: a probabilistic approach to reporting. Am J Surg Pathol. 25:1017-21, 2001
12. Page DL et al: Premalignant and malignant disease of the breast; the roles of the pathologist. Mod Pathol. 11:120-8, 1998
13. Page DL et al: Subsequent breast carcinoma risk after biopsy with atypia in a breast papilloma. Cancer. 78:258-66, 1996
14. Dupont WD et al: Breast cancer risk associated with proliferative breast disease and atypical hyperplasia. Cancer. 71:1258-65, 1993
15. Stomper PC et al: Atypical hyperplasia: frequency and mammographic and pathologic relationships in excisional biopsies guided with mammography and clinical examination. Radiology. 189:667-71, 1993
16. Schnitt SJ et al: Interobserver reproducibility in the diagnosis of ductal proliferative breast lesions using standardized criteria. Am J Surg Pathol. 16:1133-43, 1992
17. Page DL et al: Atypical hyperplastic lesions of the female breast. A long-term follow-up study. Cancer. 55:2698-708, 1985

ATYPICAL DUCTAL HYPERPLASIA

IMAGE GALLERY

Typical

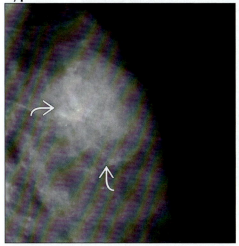
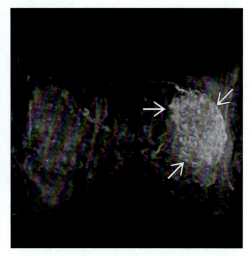

(Left) MLO mammography close-up shows regional asymmetry and associated punctate and amorphous Ca++ ➡ in a 53 y/o woman. Initial stereotactic 11-g biopsy showed atypical ductal hyperplasia. (Right) Coronal MIP of T1 C+ subtraction MR (same patient as previous image) shows regional enhancement upper outer left breast ➡. Excision showed additional atypical ductal hyperplasia. The patient was placed on Tamoxifen.

Variant

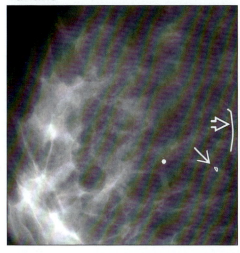
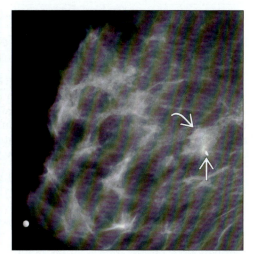

(Left) Lateral mammography magnification shows clip ➡ at site of stereotactic biopsy for Ca++ = ADH in this 55 y/o. Excision was recommended, but the patient did not pursue this initially. One year earlier she had had excision of ADH bordering on DCIS at the same site (scar marked ➡). (Right) MLO mammography one year later (same case as on left) shows development of an indistinctly marginated mass ➡ at the biopsy site/clip ➡.

Variant

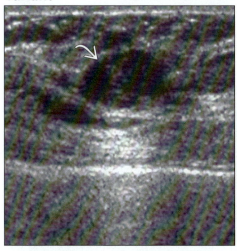
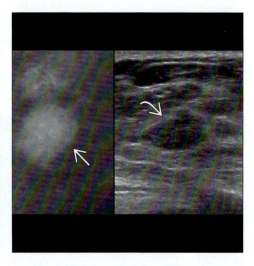

(Left) US (same as prior image) shows intracystic mass ➡ at prior biopsy site. Excision showed papillary DCIS. Excision is recommended after core biopsy diagnosis of ADH due to potential sampling error. (Right) Spot compression mammogram (left) shows indistinctly-marginated mass ➡ found on screening in a 37 y/o. US (right) shows lobulated hypoechoic mass ➡. US-guided core and excision showed FA with ADH.

ATYPICAL LOBULAR HYPERPLASIA

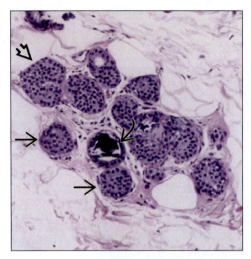

Micropathology, high-power (H&E) of 11-g biopsy shows ALH: Most acini in this TDLU are filled with monomorphic cells ➡ with little distention of the acini ⮞. Targeted Ca++ ➡ was in a benign ductule.

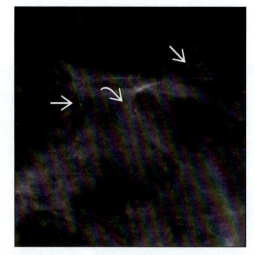

Lateral mammography magnification (same patient as previous image) shows targeted amorphous Ca++ ➡ as well as adjacent clustered Ca++ ➡. Excision showed DCIS adjacent to clip from 11-g biopsy (see ref. 4).

TERMINOLOGY

Abbreviations and Synonyms
- Atypical lobular hyperplasia (ALH)
- Lobular carcinoma in situ (LCIS)

Definitions
- ALH: Atypical proliferation of monomorphic epithelial cells in acini of terminal duct lobular unit (TDLU) where some acini are filled and others are not
- In LCIS, acini in TDLU are filled and > 50% are distended with monomorphic atypical epithelial cells
  - If ≤ 50% of acini are distended, same lesion is termed ALH
- Lobular neoplasia (LN): Spectrum encompassing both ALH and LCIS
- Pagetoid spread: Intraepithelial nests of ALH and/or LCIS extending to involve terminal ducts, proliferating beneath the native epithelial layer
  - Can be difficult to distinguish from ductal carcinoma in situ (DCIS)

IMAGING FINDINGS

General Features
- Location: TDLU

Mammographic Findings
- Usually an incidental finding at biopsy of amorphous calcifications (Ca++)
  - Ca++ can be directly in the ALH: 7-34% of cases
  - Adjacent to fibrocystic changes (FCC), atypical ductal hyperplasia (ADH)

Ultrasonographic Findings
- Grayscale Ultrasound
  - Typically occult on US
  - Can be seen at US-guided biopsy of a variety of other lesions

MR Findings
- T1 C+ FS: Can show enhancement

Biopsy
- When ALH ± LCIS is the most severe finding at core biopsy, excision generally recommended

DDx: Adjacent Abnormalities

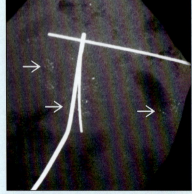

1.1 cm Grade I IDC + ALH (Ca++)

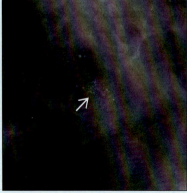

Fibrocystic Changes with Ca++, ALH

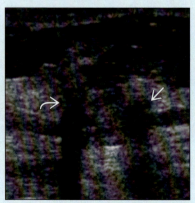

ILC (left), ALH (right)

ATYPICAL LOBULAR HYPERPLASIA

Key Facts

Terminology
- ALH: Atypical proliferation of monomorphic epithelial cells in acini of terminal duct lobular unit (TDLU) where some acini are filled and others are not
- In LCIS, acini in TDLU are filled and > 50% are distended with monomorphic atypical epithelial cells

Imaging Findings
- Usually an incidental finding at biopsy of amorphous calcifications (Ca++)

- When ALH ± LCIS is the most severe finding at core biopsy, excision generally recommended

Top Differential Diagnoses
- Lobular Carcinoma in Situ (LCIS)
- Atypical Ductal Hyperplasia (ADH)
- Ductal Carcinoma in Situ (DCIS)

Pathology
- E-cadherin expression weak or absent

DIFFERENTIAL DIAGNOSIS

Lobular Carcinoma in Situ (LCIS)
- Qualitative and quantitative histologic differences

Atypical Ductal Hyperplasia (ADH)
- Variable cells and secondary spaces

Ductal Carcinoma in Situ (DCIS)
- Cancerization of lobules mimics LN
- E-cadherin expression retained

PATHOLOGY

General Features
- Epidemiology: 1-2% of all biopsies
- Associated abnormalities: LCIS, ADH, DCIS, FCC, columnar cell changes (CCC), invasive (usually lobular) carcinoma often admixed

Microscopic Features
- Monomorphic cells fill some but not all acini of TDLU
- Moderate clear cytoplasm with rounded nuclei
- E-cadherin expression weak or absent

CLINICAL ISSUES

Presentation
- Asymptomatic, incidental finding at biopsy

Demographics
- Age: Peak incidence mid 40s

Natural History & Prognosis
- Relative risk (RR) for developing cancer: 3-4x
  - 3x as likely ipsilateral as contralateral
- ALH + first-degree family history breast cancer RR: 8x
- Risk higher with pagetoid spread into ducts

Treatment
- Following percutaneous biopsy findings of ALH
  - Treatment controversial: Usually excision
  - 0-23% malignant at excision, average 14%
    - Not all lesions excised; incomplete follow-up
  - Upgrade more common when associated mass lesion or residual suspicious Ca++
  - Malignancy often adjacent to area of LN
- High-risk lesion: High-risk surveillance, possibly MR

SELECTED REFERENCES

1. Arpino G et al: Lobular neoplasia on core-needle biopsy--clinical significance. Cancer. 101:242-50, 2004
2. Foster MC et al: Lobular carcinoma in situ or atypical lobular hyperplasia at core-needle biopsy: is excisional biopsy necessary? Radiology. 231:813-9, 2004
3. Dmytrasz K et al: The significance of atypical lobular hyperplasia at percutaneous breast biopsy. Breast J. 9:10-2, 2003
4. Berg WA et al: Atypical lobular hyperplasia or lobular carcinoma in situ at core-needle breast biopsy. Radiology. 218:503-9, 2001

IMAGE GALLERY

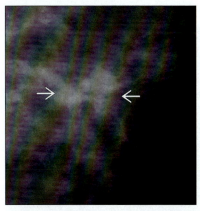
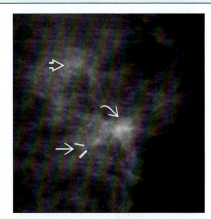
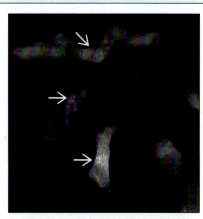

(Left) CC mammography spot compression shows asymmetry & distortion ➡ in a 54 y/o. Needle-localized excision showed FCC & ALH. *(Center)* CC mammography (9 yrs later, same patient as left) shows clips at site of remote excision: ALH ➡, with new adjacent spiculated mass & Ca++ ➡. Core biopsy showed IDC with ILC. Second asymmetry with Ca++ more lateral ➡: DCIS. ALH is a marker of high risk. *(Right)* Specimen radiograph shows clustered amorphous Ca++ ➡. Histopathology: CCC with atypia, Ca++ & adjacent ALH. Excision showed FCC.

LOBULAR CARCINOMA IN SITU

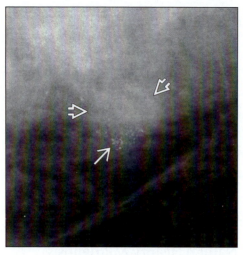

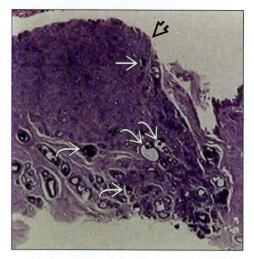

CC mammography magnification shows clustered amorphous Ca++ ➡ along the edge of an obscured oval mass ⊳. Findings suspicious, BI-RADS 4. Stereotactic biopsy showed retrieval of Ca++ & a mass.

Micropathology, low power of 11-g core specimen (same patient as previous) shows Ca++ ➡ in FCC adjacent to the mass ⊳ of LCIS. A few Ca++ are within the LCIS ➡. Excision = FCC. (from ref. 8)

TERMINOLOGY

Abbreviations and Synonyms
- Lobular carcinoma in situ (LCIS)
- Atypical lobular hyperplasia (ALH)

Definitions
- LCIS: Atypical monomorphic epithelial proliferation filling, and often distending, acini of the terminal duct lobular unit (TDLU)
- ALH: Similar to LCIS, less extensive, some acini only partially filled, little or no distention of acini
- Lobular neoplasia (LN): Spectrum of LCIS and ALH, including spread of LCIS and ALH into terminal ducts
  - Some literature uses LN as synonymous with LCIS only
- Pagetoid spread: Intraepithelial nests of monomorphic cells of LN in terminal ducts, proliferating beneath the native epithelial layer
  - Overlaps in appearance with ductal carcinoma in situ (DCIS)

IMAGING FINDINGS

Mammographic Findings
- Usually an incidental finding on biopsy for amorphous calcifications (Ca++)
  - Ca++ are usually not in the LCIS itself
- Rarely: Mass ± Ca++

Ultrasonographic Findings
- Grayscale Ultrasound: Irregular hypo- to anechoic mass

MR Findings
- T1 C+ FS
  - Non-mass ductal enhancement pattern reported in LCIS in 10% of MR-detected biopsied lesions (one series)
  - May be seen as an irregular enhancing mass

Biopsy
- LCIS at core biopsy: Incidence 0.24-1.2%
- Excision recommended after core biopsy result of LCIS: Upgrade to carcinoma in ~ 27%
- Upgrade rates not affected by number of samples, gauge of needle (small series)

DDx: Examples of Amorphous and Punctate Calcifications Prompting Biopsy

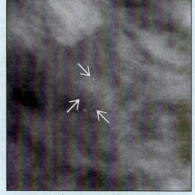

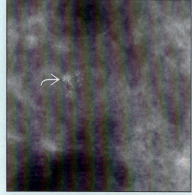

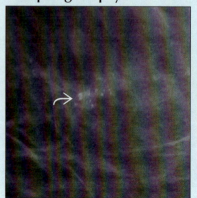

Fibrocystic Change

Columnar Cell Changes

Ductal Carcinoma in Situ

LOBULAR CARCINOMA IN SITU

Key Facts

Terminology
- LCIS: Atypical monomorphic epithelial proliferation filling, and often distending, acini of the terminal duct lobular unit (TDLU)

Imaging Findings
- Usually an incidental finding on biopsy for amorphous calcifications (Ca++)
- LCIS at core biopsy: Incidence 0.24-1.2%
- Excision recommended after core biopsy result of LCIS: Upgrade to carcinoma in ~ 27%

Top Differential Diagnoses
- Associated Benign Entities that May Prompt Biopsy by Presence of Ca++
- Atypical Lobular Hyperplasia (ALH)

- Cancerization of Lobules by Ductal Carcinoma in Situ (DCIS)

Pathology
- Multicentric in 85%, bilateral in 30-67%
- Frequently associated with invasive lobular carcinoma (ILC), ALH and ADH

Clinical Issues
- Relative risk for developing cancer: 8-12x
- Both breasts at equal risk; lesion often multifocal
- LCIS present at margins of resection not an indication for reexcision

Diagnostic Checklist
- Lower threshold for further evaluation of lesions both ipsilateral and contralateral to diagnosed LCIS

Imaging Recommendations
- Best imaging tool: Mammography with CC and 90° lateral magnification views for Ca++; US for masses

DIFFERENTIAL DIAGNOSIS

Associated Benign Entities that May Prompt Biopsy by Presence of Ca++
- Sclerosing adenosis
  - Combination of stromal sclerosis and adenosis
  - Ca++ (often punctate or amorphous) ± mass on mammogram
- Fibrocystic change (FCC)
  - Most common result at biopsy of amorphous Ca++
  - Typically in areas of usual duct hyperplasia, adenosis, apocrine metaplasia
- Proliferative changes affecting terminal ducts and lobules
  - "Pseudolactational" hyperplasia
  - Differentiating microscopic findings
    - Clear cell changes
    - Apocrine metaplasia
- Atypical ductal hyperplasia (ADH)
  - Amorphous Ca++ most common mammographic appearance for ADH
  - 20% amorphous Ca++ yield ADH, ALH, or LCIS

Atypical Lobular Hyperplasia (ALH)
- Fewer than half of acini filled with monomorphic epithelial cells
- Some acini partially filled
- Typically occult on mammography
  - Incidental finding on biopsy of amorphous Ca++: Up to 34% may have Ca++ within ALH
- Upgrade to carcinoma at excision after initial diagnosis on core biopsy: Average 14%
- Marker of ↑ risk of cancer: 3-4x relative risk compared to general population
- Subsequent cancers are 3x more common in breast ipsilateral to breast showing ALH

  - ALH may be intermediate between local precursor and bilateral risk indicator for future development of breast cancer

Cancerization of Lobules by Ductal Carcinoma in Situ (DCIS)
- Differentiate with E-cadherin (immunostain)
  - E-cadherin is lost in lobular lesions (LCIS, ILC) and retained in DCIS

PATHOLOGY

General Features
- General path comments
  - First described in 1941: "A disease of small lobular ducts and lobules"
  - Multicentric in 85%, bilateral in 30-67%
- Genetics: Loss of material from 16p, 16q, 17p, 22q; gain from 6q
- Epidemiology: Autopsy reports incident range 0-3.6%
- Associated abnormalities
  - Frequently associated with invasive lobular carcinoma (ILC), ALH and ADH
  - Often coexists with other benign entities
    - Sclerosing adenosis, columnar cell hyperplasia
  - Coexists with 21% of DCIS
    - E-cadherin expression lost in lobular lesions; retained in ductal lesions

Gross Pathologic & Surgical Features
- No specific features: Microscopic finding

Microscopic Features
- Distention of > 50% of lobular acini with uniform monomorphic cells
- Associated pagetoid spread in up to 75% of cases
- Classic type
  - Small round nuclei and scant cytoplasm
  - No nucleoli
  - Associated Ca++ uncommon
- Pleomorphic type
  - Larger nuclei; some with nucleoli

- o Cytoplasm heterogeneity; may contain vacuoles
- o Central necrosis; Ca++ may be present

CLINICAL ISSUES

Presentation
- Most common signs/symptoms: Asymptomatic: Incidental finding at biopsy for other reasons
- Clinical Profile
  - o High-risk marker for development of invasive carcinoma
  - o Both breasts likely at equal risk of developing invasive cancer
  - o Often an incidental pathologic finding
  - o Frequently multifocal and bilateral

Demographics
- Age
  - o More common in pre-menopausal women; mean age 44-47
    - ▪ May regress following cessation of estrogen stimulation
- Ethnicity: 12x more frequent in whites than blacks

Natural History & Prognosis
- Considered a nonobligate precursor of invasive lobular carcinoma (ILC)
  - o Morphologic similarity to cells of ILC
  - o Development of tumors ↑ in regions of ALH/LCIS
  - o Concordant chromosomal abnormalities in paired ILC and LCIS from the same patients
- Relative risk for developing cancer: 8-12x
  - o Both breasts at equal risk; lesion often multifocal
  - o Risk of breast cancer: 1-2% per year over 30-40 years
  - o Invasive cancer may be ductal or lobular; ILC overrepresented
- Relative risk not affected by family history of breast cancer
- May be different based on histologic type of LCIS
  - o Classic form may be incidental
  - o Pleomorphic form may have greater tendency to develop (into) invasive carcinoma

Treatment
- Surgical excision following LCIS diagnosed with percutaneous core biopsy
  - o Controversial: Earlier literature stated LCIS need not be excised unless
    - ▪ Ambiguity of findings with overlap of histologic characteristics of LCIS and DCIS
    - ▪ LCIS co-existed with another high-risk lesion (ADH, ALH, radial scar)
    - ▪ Imaging-histologic discordance existed
  - o More recent literature recommends that LCIS (and all lobular neoplasia) found at core biopsy should be excised
    - ▪ Histologic upgrade to DCIS or invasive cancer at excision in 27%
    - ▪ Studies confounded by possibility that the original core biopsy was actually DCIS with cancerization of lobules; e-cadherin staining had not been performed

- ▪ Overall rate of upgrade for all lobular neoplasia at 17%, within the range of upgrades reported for ADH
- o All studies are based on small numbers of cases, without excision of all lesions
- LCIS present at margins of resection not an indication for reexcision
- Recommendations following final diagnosis
  - o Recent survey series where surgeons gave primary counseling found women's perception of lifetime risk for invasive cancer was variable
    - ▪ 35% placed on selective estrogen-receptor modulator, e.g., tamoxifen
    - ▪ 28% had bilateral mastectomy
    - ▪ Screening recommendations: 64% annual mammography

DIAGNOSTIC CHECKLIST

Consider
- Consider high-risk screening, possible supplemental US or MR, for surveillance
- May be appropriate to perform MR for further evaluation prior to excision after core biopsy diagnosis, particularly if parenchyma dense

Image Interpretation Pearls
- Lower threshold for further evaluation of lesions both ipsilateral and contralateral to diagnosed LCIS

SELECTED REFERENCES

1. Bassett LW et al: Breast core needle biopsy: imaging-pathology assessment of results. Breast Imaging: RSNA Categorical Course in Diagnostic Radiology. 55-65, 2005
2. Garreau JR, et al: Risk counseling and management in patients with lobular carcinoma in situ. Am J Surg. 189:614-5, 2005
3. Berg WA: Imaging-guided breast biopsy and management of high-risk lesions. Radiol Clin North Am. 42:935-46, 2004
4. Foster MC et al: Lobular carcinoma in situ or atypical lobular hyperplasia at core-needle biopsy: is excisional biopsy necessary? Radiology. 231:813-9, 2004
5. Liberman L et al: Ductal enhancement on MR imaging of the Breast. AJR. 181:519-25, 2003
6. Middleton LP et al: Lobular carcinoma in situ diagnosed by core needle biopsy: when should it be excised? Mod Pathol. 16:120-9, 2003
7. Page DL et al: Atypical lobular hyperplasia as a unilateral predictor of breast cancer risk: a retrospective cohort study. Lancet. 361:125-9, 2003
8. Berg WA et al: Atypical lobular hyperplasia or lobular carcinoma in situ at core-needle breast biopsy. Radiology. 218:503-9, 2001
9. Georgian-Smith D: Calcifications of lobular carcinoma in situ of the breast radiologic-pathologic correlation. AJR. 176:1255-9, 2001
10. Rosen PP: Rosen's Breast Pathology. Philadelphia, Lippincott Williams & Wilkins. Chapter 33, 581-610, 2001
11. Foote F et al: Lobular carcinoma in situ: a rare from of mammary cancer. Am J Pathol. 17:491-95, 1941

LOBULAR CARCINOMA IN SITU

IMAGE GALLERY

Typical

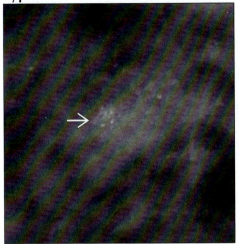

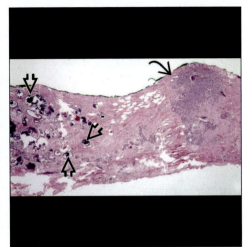

(Left) Lateral mammography magnification shows tightly clustered amorphous Ca++ ➡ of intermediate suspicion, BI-RADS 4B. This 63 year-old woman underwent stereotactic biopsy. *(Right)* Micropathology, low power (same patient as previous image) shows numerous Ca++ ➡ within FCC on the left-hand portion of the field, while in the right-hand portion of the field ➡ there is ALH and LCIS.

Typical

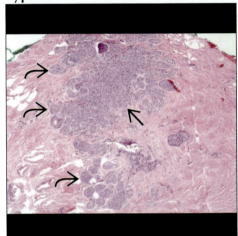

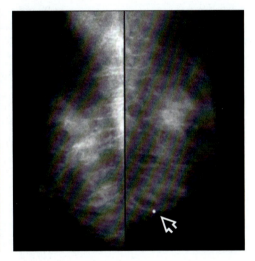

(Left) Micropathology, high power (same patient as prior 2 images) shows the lobular neoplasia with numerous lobules filled with monomorphic cells. LCIS ➡, and ALH ➡. Excision showed residual LCIS only. *(Right)* MLO mammography shows dense parenchyma with no discrete abnormality in the area indicated as palpable by a skin BB ➡ in this 41 year-old woman. US was performed (see following image).

Typical

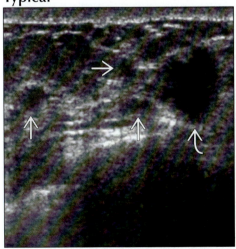

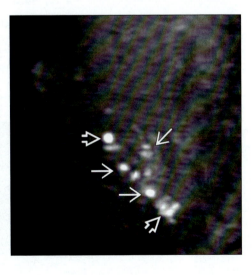

(Left) Radial ultrasound shows multiple, irregular, nearly anechoic masses ➡ with dominant mass ➡ = palpable abnormality with biopsy = ILC. MR was performed (on right). *(Right)* Sagittal T1 C+ SPGR MIP MR shows multiple enhancing masses, 2 of which ➡ were biopsy proven ILC (more inferior one = palpable mass). At mastectomy, other enhancing lesions ➡ were shown to be LCIS and FCC (from Berg WA et al: Radiology 233:830-49, 2004).

MUCOCELE-LIKE LESIONS

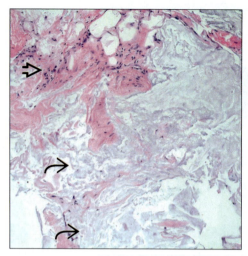

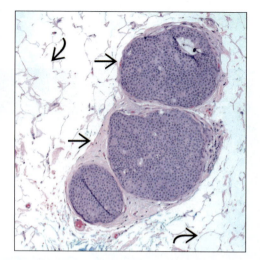

Micropathology, low power, H&E of 11-g core biopsy specimen shows extensive extracellular mucin ⊅ and minimal adjacent bland fibrosis ⊳. Excision was recommended (right).

Micropathology, low power, H&E of excision (same patient as previous image) shows solid-type DCIS ⊅ surrounded by extensive extracellular mucin ⊅ (Courtesy OBI).

TERMINOLOGY

Abbreviations and Synonyms
- Mucocele-like lesions (MLL)

Definitions
- "Cele" = sac
- Mucocele = sac containing mucin
- MLL: Uncommon lesion composed of mucin-containing cysts that may rupture → extracellular mucin
  ○ Can be isolated benign condition
  ○ Can coexist with atypical ductal hyperplasia (ADH) and ductal carcinoma in situ (DCIS)
- Mucin is produced in mucinous (colloid) carcinoma
  ○ Mucin-filled ducts commonly coexist with mucinous carcinoma

IMAGING FINDINGS

Mammographic Findings
- In 85%, calcifications (Ca++) dominant finding
- Coarse heterogeneous Ca++ ± lobulated mass

○ Pleomorphic ± amorphous Ca++ ± mass
- Isolated lobulated dense mass, mostly circumscribed
  ○ Can be indistinctly marginated due to rupture of mucocele

Ultrasonographic Findings
- Grayscale Ultrasound
  ○ Hypoechoic round, oval, or lobulated mass ± Ca++
  ○ Intracystic mass, mural nodule(s) reported

MR Findings
- T1WI FS: Hyperintense lobulated mass
- T1 C+ FS: Enhancement varies

Biopsy
- Result of MLL on core biopsy should prompt excision
  ○ MLL + ADH on core: ~ 85% upgrade to malignancy
  ○ Risk of adjacent unsampled malignancy even if no atypia: ~ 20-30%
- Diagnosis particularly problematic on FNAB

Imaging Recommendations
- Best imaging tool
  ○ Mammography with magnification views for Ca++
  ○ US to further characterize masses, guide biopsy

DDx: Mimics of Mucocele-Like Lesions

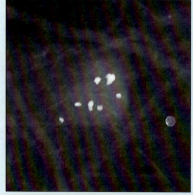

Myxoid Fibroadenoma

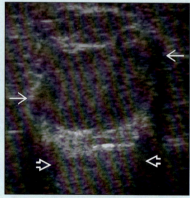

Mucinous Carcinoma

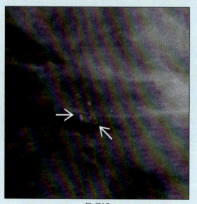

DCIS

MUCOCELE-LIKE LESIONS

Key Facts

Terminology
- Mucocele = sac containing mucin
- MLL: Uncommon lesion composed of mucin-containing cysts that may rupture → extracellular mucin
- Can be isolated benign condition

Imaging Findings
- Coarse heterogeneous Ca++ ± lobulated mass
- Pleomorphic ± amorphous Ca++ ± mass

Top Differential Diagnoses
- Mucinous Carcinoma
- Ductal Carcinoma in Situ

Pathology
- > 50% of all MLL have associated ADH or malignancy

Diagnostic Checklist
- Excision recommended if core biopsy shows MLL

DIFFERENTIAL DIAGNOSIS

Mucinous Carcinoma
- Dense, partially circumscribed mass ± Ca++
- Isoechoic mass with enhancement on US

Ductal Carcinoma in Situ
- Fine pleomorphic or fine linear Ca++ most common

Benign Lesions
- Myxoid fibroadenoma, fibrocystic changes (FCC), papilloma

PATHOLOGY

General Features
- > 50% of all MLL have associated ADH or malignancy

CLINICAL ISSUES

Presentation
- Most common signs/symptoms
  - Usually found on mammographic screening
  - Incidental on breast biopsy for other reasons

Demographics
- Age: Range 24-79 years, mean age 50

Treatment
- Excision for all MLL

- Depends on final pathology

DIAGNOSTIC CHECKLIST

Consider
- Excision recommended if core biopsy shows MLL

SELECTED REFERENCES

1. Leibman AJ et al: Mucocelelike lesions of the breast: mammographic findings with pathologic correlation. AJR Am J Roentgenol. 186(5):1356-60, 2006
2. Farshid G et al: Mucocele-like lesions of the breast: a benign cause for indeterminate or suspicious mammographic microcalcifications. Breast J. 11(1):15-22, 2005
3. Kim JY et al: Benign and malignant mucocele-like tumors of the breast: mammographic and sonographic appearances. AJR Am J Roentgenol. 185(5):1310-6, 2005
4. Ramsaroop R et al: Mucocele-like lesions of the breast: an audit of 2 years at BreastScreen Auckland (New Zealand). Breast J. 11(5):321-5, 2005
5. Glazebrook K et al: Original report. Mucocele-like tumors of the breast: mammographic and sonographic appearances. AJR Am J Roentgenol. 180(4):949-54, 2003
6. Jacobs TW et al: Nonmalignant lesions in breast core needle biopsies: to excise or not to excise? Am J Surg Pathol. 26(9):1095-110, 2002
7. Hamele-Bena D et al: Mammary mucocele-like lesions. Benign and malignant. Am J Surg Pathol. 20(9):1081-5, 1996
8. Rosen PP: Mucocele-like tumors of the breast. Am J Surg Pathol. 10(7):464-9, 1986

IMAGE GALLERY

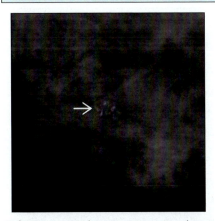 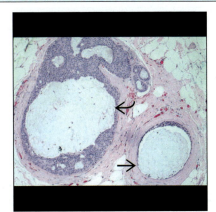 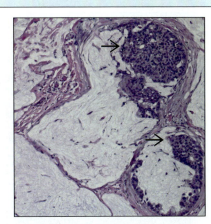

(Left) Mammography spot compression shows clustered coarse, heterogeneous Ca++ ➡. 11-g stereotactic biopsy showed benign breast tissue w/focal mucin extravasation and Ca++. Excision showed only benign tissue and FCC. *(Center)* Micropathology, low power, H&E shows DCIS w/extensive mucin in duct lumen with DCIS ➡, adjacent normal duct lumen ➡. Initial stereotactic biopsy showed only extracellular mucin. *(Right)* Micropathology, low power, H&E shows two duct profiles with ADH ➡, bordering on DCIS, w/extensive associated mucin production.

PAPILLOMA, ATYPICAL

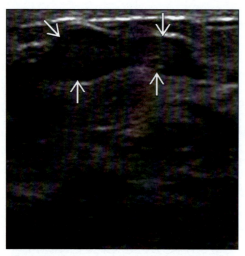

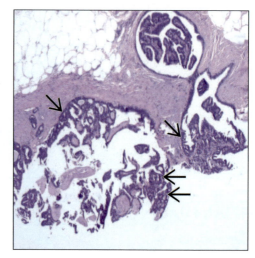

Ultrasound in this 47 year old woman with bloody nipple discharge and negative mammography shows a lobulated solid mass ➡ within a dilated retroareolar duct. Excision showed papilloma with focal atypia.

Histopathology (different case than left-hand image) shows proliferating epithelial cells forming complex papillary structures with focal atypia ➡ (H&E x 40).

TERMINOLOGY

Abbreviations and Synonyms
- Intraductal papillary neoplasm with atypia

Definitions
- Papilloma with atypical epithelial proliferation [e.g. atypical ductal hyperplasia (ADH)], or cellular atypia

IMAGING FINDINGS

General Features
- Best diagnostic clue
  - There are no specific imaging findings to distinguish benign from atypical or malignant
  - Usually small solid or complex cystic mass, subareolar or peripheral
  - Mammography is of limited utility
- Location
  - Peripheral: More often multiple, more often contain atypia; increased risk of subsequent cancer
  - Central: Usually solitary, subareolar, and more frequently presents with nipple discharge

Mammographic Findings
- Circumscribed or obscured mass ± amorphous, punctate calcifications (Ca++)
- Solitary dilated duct
- Frequently non-revealing
- Galactography: May show filling defect(s) or cut-off

Ultrasonographic Findings
- Grayscale Ultrasound
  - Intraductal or intracystic mass
  - Solid ovoid or lobulated mass
- Color Doppler: May see flow in fibrovascular stalk

MR Findings
- T1 & T2WI FS: Nonspecific soft tissue mass ± (solitary) dilated duct
- T1 C+ FS: Linear or ductal enhancement; enhancing smooth, or microlobulated mass(es)

Biopsy
- Atypical papilloma on core needle biopsy (CNB): 36-38% upgraded to malignancy at excision
- Can be difficult to distinguish benign from atypical papilloma on CNB

DDx: Atypical Papilloma Manifestations

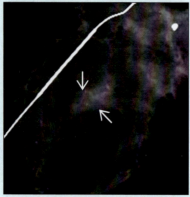

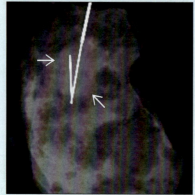

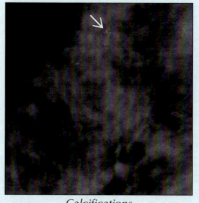

Calcifications within Mass

Mass

Calcifications

PAPILLOMA, ATYPICAL

Key Facts

Terminology
- Papilloma with atypical epithelial proliferation [e.g. atypical ductal hyperplasia (ADH)], or cellular atypia

Imaging Findings
- There are no specific imaging findings to distinguish benign from atypical or malignant
- Usually small solid or complex cystic mass, subareolar or peripheral

Top Differential Diagnoses
- Complicated Cyst, Abscess, Galactocele
- Benign papilloma, papilloma with foci of carcinoma in situ, and "carcinoma arising in a papilloma"
- Non-invasive or invasive papillary carcinoma

Diagnostic Checklist
- Any atypical papilloma at CNB should be excised

DIFFERENTIAL DIAGNOSIS

Complicated Cyst, Abscess, Galactocele
- May appear complex cystic; benign

Intraductal Epithelial Proliferations
- Usual hyperplasia, including papillomatosis; ADH or ductal carcinoma in situ (DCIS)
- Lack of fibrovascular core: Not true papillary lesion

Sclerosing Adenosis Nodule
- May be associated with peripheral papilloma

Fibroadenoma
- Circumscribed, gently lobulated mass ± Ca++

Papillary Neoplasms
- Benign papilloma, papilloma with foci of carcinoma in situ, and "carcinoma arising in a papilloma"
- Sclerosing papilloma: Pseudoinvasive growth pattern, frequently mistaken for carcinoma
- Non-invasive or invasive papillary carcinoma

PATHOLOGY

Microscopic Features
- Papillary neoplasm: Proliferation of epithelial cells overlying fibrovascular stalks
- Atypia or ADH within papilloma; < 3mm area resembling low grade DCIS; often concurrent atypia in surrounding breast parenchyma

CLINICAL ISSUES

Presentation
- Most common signs/symptoms: Nipple discharge

DIAGNOSTIC CHECKLIST

Consider
- Multiple, peripheral papillomas more often atypical than solitary
- Any atypical papilloma at CNB should be excised

SELECTED REFERENCES

1. Liberman L et al: Is surgical excision warranted after benign, concordant diagnosis of papilloma at percutaneous breast biopsy? AJR. 186:1328-34, 2006
2. Mercado CL et al: Papillary lesions of the breast at percutaneous core-needle biopsy. Radiology. 238:801-8, 2006
3. Orel SG et al: MR imaging in patients with nipple discharge: initial experience. Radiology. 216:248-54, 2000
4. Hild F et al: Ductal oriented sonography improves the diagnosis of pathological nipple discharge of the female breast compared with galactography. Eur J Cancer Prev. 7 Suppl 1:S57-62, 1998
5. Tavassoli FA: Papillary lesions. In: Tavassoli FA, 2nd ed. Pathology of the Breast. Norwalk, Appleton & Lange. 325-71, 1992

IMAGE GALLERY

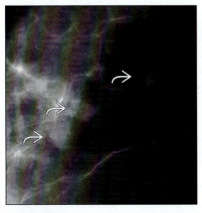 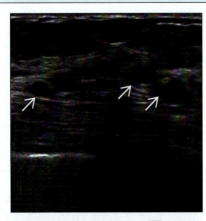 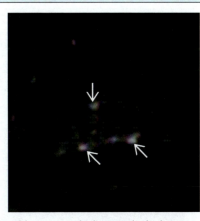

(Left) Mammography close-up CC view shows multiple partially obscured masses ➤ in this 39 year old woman with clear nipple discharge. (Center) Ultrasound (same patient as left-hand image) shows multiple hypoechoic masses ➤. US-guided core biopsy revealed sclerosed papillomas with ADH. (Right) Sagittal T1 C+ subtraction MR confirms multiple enhancing masses in the central right breast ➤ (same patient as left-hand image). Subsequent excision showed papillomas with focal ADH and DCIS.

RADIAL SCAR

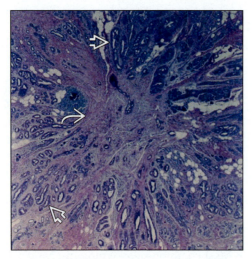

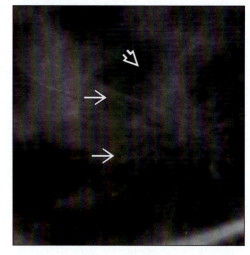

Micropathology, low power, H&E shows RSL with central fibroelastosis ➔ and epithelial proliferation (adenosis, ➤) along spicules radiating into the adjacent fat (Courtesy RHH).

CC mammography magnification view shows spiculated mass ➤ with lucency between spicules ➔. Excision (previous image) showed radial scar.

TERMINOLOGY

Abbreviations and Synonyms
- Complex sclerosing lesion (CSL, when over 1-2 cm)
- Radial sclerosing lesion (RSL) refers to both radial scars and larger complex sclerosing lesions
- Sclerosing duct hyperplasia or proliferation
- Nonencapsulated sclerosing lesion

Definitions
- Benign proliferative lesion with central fibroelastosis and a spiculated appearance radiographically and histologically

IMAGING FINDINGS

General Features
- Best diagnostic clue
  - Classic imaging appearance: Spiculated mass or area of architectural distortion with central lucency on mammography
    - Not specific
    - Same appearance may = invasive carcinoma

Mammographic Findings
- Long radiating spicules with intervening lucency
- No central mass (lucency at center)
- Architectural distortion
- Variable appearance on different projections
- May have associated calcifications (33-50%)
  - Calcifications usually in associated adenosis or atypical ductal hyperplasia (ADH)
- Absence of overlying skin thickening or retraction

Ultrasonographic Findings
- Grayscale Ultrasound
  - Irregular, hypoechoic mass when visible on US
    - RSL itself often quite subtle on US
    - When associated with malignancy, often more conspicuous on US
  - Architectural distortion: Tethering of Cooper ligaments
  - Posterior shadowing can be seen
  - Features indistinguishable from carcinoma

MR Findings
- T1WI: Can be seen as spiculated mass if surrounded by fat

DDx: Lesions Mimicking Radial Scar

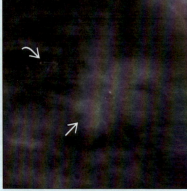

IDC, DCIS

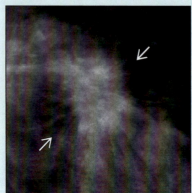

IDC, Grade I

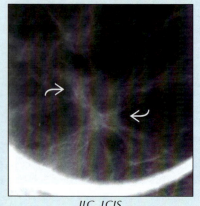

ILC, LCIS

RADIAL SCAR

Key Facts

Terminology
- Radial sclerosing lesion (RSL) refers to both radial scars and larger complex sclerosing lesions
- Benign proliferative lesion with central fibroelastosis and a spiculated appearance radiographically and histologically

Imaging Findings
- Classic imaging appearance: Spiculated mass or area of architectural distortion with central lucency on mammography
- Calcifications usually in associated adenosis or atypical ductal hyperplasia (ADH)
- Spiculated enhancing mass on MR
- Irregular, hypoechoic mass when visible on US

- Associated ADH, atypical lobular hyperplasia (ALH) or lobular carcinoma in situ (LCIS) should prompt excision
- RSL without atypia on 14-g core biopsy, 4-12% rate of malignancy at excision

Top Differential Diagnoses
- Tubular Carcinoma
- Infiltrating Ductal Carcinoma not Otherwise Specified (NOS)
- Infiltrating Lobular Carcinoma (ILC)
- Post-Surgical Scar

Clinical Issues
- Usually an incidental finding at mammography or histopathology

---

- T2WI FS: Typically occult
- T1 C+ FS
  - Spiculated enhancing mass on MR
  - Indistinguishable from carcinoma

Biopsy
- Stereotactic biopsy
  - Associated ADH, atypical lobular hyperplasia (ALH) or lobular carcinoma in situ (LCIS) should prompt excision
    - 28-54% risk of malignancy
  - When RSL is incidental adjacent to targeted calcifications, < 2% malignancy rate at excision
    - Requires at least 12 samples with at least 11-g system
  - RSL manifest as a mass or architectural distortion, without atypia
    - May not require excision if at least 12 samples with at least 11-g system (controversial)
    - 4-12% rate of malignancy if < 12 samples, < 11-g biopsy device
- US-guided biopsy
  - RSL without atypia on 14-g core biopsy, 4-12% rate of malignancy at excision

Imaging Recommendations
- Best imaging tool: Mammography with spot magnification views

---

DIFFERENTIAL DIAGNOSIS

Tubular Carcinoma
- Indistinguishable radiographically
- Spiculated mass most common, more likely to be dense centrally

Infiltrating Ductal Carcinoma not Otherwise Specified (NOS)
- Indistinguishable, usually central mass
- May show associated calcifications

Infiltrating Lobular Carcinoma (ILC)
- Indistinguishable, usually central mass

Post-Surgical Scar
- History, markers on skin scar may be helpful for mammography

---

PATHOLOGY

General Features
- General path comments: Similar appearance to small invasive carcinomas on gross
- Etiology
  - Unknown
  - Not related to surgery or prior trauma
- Epidemiology
  - Most common 40-60 years
  - 1% prevalence on mammography
  - 7-28% prevalence in autopsy series
    - Most are mammographically and clinically occult
  - 2x risk of subsequent breast cancer in either breast
  - 4-5x risk of breast cancer if associated ADH
- Associated abnormalities
  - 22% of excised RSL show infiltrating carcinoma or less often ductal carcinoma in situ (DCIS)
    - Tubular carcinoma most common
    - Loss of myoepithelial cell layer in tubular carcinoma: Actin or p63 staining negative in tubular carcinoma but retained in adenosis
    - Actin stain may be required to confirm tubular carcinoma
    - DCIS will usually show associated calcifications
    - Carcinoma more common with RSL > 2 cm or palpable
    - No malignancies reported when RSL < 6 mm in size
    - Associated carcinoma more common in women > 50 years of age; rare < 40 years
    - Associated carcinoma more common when RSL manifest as spiculated mass mammographically

RADIAL SCAR

- More common when ADH, ALH, or LCIS found at core biopsy
- 1-2% malignancy rate when an incidental finding on biopsy of an adjacent finding
  - 18% of excised RSL show ADH or LCIS
    - ADH will often show associated calcifications
  - Sclerosing adenosis (SA)
    - Can mimic tubular carcinoma
    - Actin or p63 staining to confirm retained myoepithelial cell layer in SA

Gross Pathologic & Surgical Features
- Irregular firm mass, gray-white, indurated with central retraction
- Bands of pale stroma extend radially into surrounding fat

Microscopic Features
- Hypertrophic fibroelastic core
  - Surrounded by stellate projections of ducts
    - Varying degrees of hyperplasia
    - Peripheral ducts may be dilated cystically
  - Contains trapped glandular elements
    - May be confused with tubular carcinoma
- Various proliferative components in RSL
  - Sclerosing adenosis
  - Duct hyperplasia
  - Papillomatosis
  - Cysts

CLINICAL ISSUES

Presentation
- Most common signs/symptoms
  - Usually an incidental finding at mammography or histopathology
  - Rarely palpable
    - A palpable lesion with similar imaging characteristics should suggest carcinoma
  - Absent skin thickening or retraction
    - Associated skin thickening or retraction suggests invasive carcinoma

Natural History & Prognosis
- 2x risk of developing invasive breast carcinoma in either breast

Treatment
- When diagnosed on percutaneous biopsy (controversial)
  - Surgical excision
    - Required if associated malignancy or atypical hyperplasia on core
    - 4-12% malignant at excision if RSL seen as mass or architectural distortion on imaging and no atypia on core
  - If no associated atypical hyperplasia (ADH or ALH) or (LCIS)
    - RSL must be incidental, e.g., adjacent to targeted calcifications
    - Lesion must have been well sampled (≥ 12 specimens, 11-g at least)
    - Imaging follow-up may suffice

DIAGNOSTIC CHECKLIST

Consider
- If presents as a spiculated mass with architectural distortion, excision will be needed
  - Initial core biopsy can help distinguish invasive carcinoma from RSL
  - If invasive carcinoma found on core biopsy, allows attempt at clear margins and sentinel node biopsy at initial surgery

Image Interpretation Pearls
- Long radiating spicules with intervening lucency and absent central mass suggest diagnosis of radial scar

SELECTED REFERENCES

1. Cawson JN: Fourteen-gauge needle core biopsy of mammographically evident radial scars. Is excision necessary? Cancer. 97:345-51, 2003
2. Brenner RJ et al: Percutaneous core needle biopsy of radial scars of the breast: when is excision necessary? AJR. 179:1179-84, 2002
3. Tabar L et al: Teaching Atlas of Mammography. 3rd ed. Stuttgart, Thieme. 93-6, 102-6, 2001
4. Cohen MA et al: Role of sonography in evaluation of radial scars of the breast. AJR. 174:1075-8, 2000
5. Reynolds HE: Core needle biopsy of challenging benign breast conditions: a comprehensive literature review. AJR. 174:1245-50, 2000
6. Hassell P et al: Radial sclerosing lesions of the breast: mammographic and pathologic correlation. Can Assoc Radiol J. 50:370-75, 1999
7. Jacobs TW et al: Radial scars in benign breast-biopsy specimens and the risk of breast cancer. NEJM. 340:430-6, 1999
8. Frouge C et al: Mammographic lesions suggestive of radial scars: microscopic findings in 40 cases. Radiology. 195:623-5, 1995
9. Sloane JP et al: Carcinoma and atypical hyperplasia in radial scars and complex sclerosing lesions: importance of lesion size and patient age. Histopathology. 23:225-31, 1993
10. Orel SG et al: Radial scar with microcalcifications: radiologic-pathologic correlation. Radiology. 183:479-82, 1992

RADIAL SCAR

IMAGE GALLERY

Typical

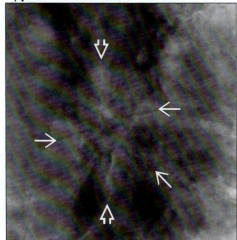

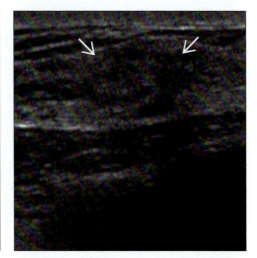

(Left) MLO mammography, magnification shows spiculated lesion ⮞ with lucency between spicules ➡ and no central mass, typical of a RSL. US was performed (next image). *(Right)* Radial ultrasound shows subtle mixed hyper- and hypoechoic mass ➡. US-guided core biopsy and excision showed radial scar with LCIS.

Typical

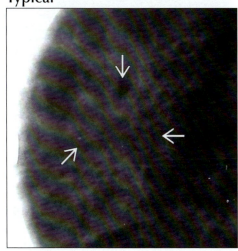

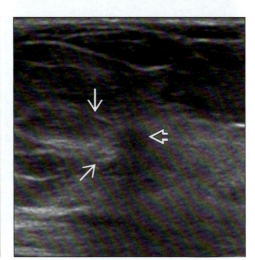

(Left) CC mammography spot compression shows subtle architectural distortion ➡ without a central mass. US was performed (next image). *(Right)* Radial ultrasound shows 4 mm hypoechoic mass ⮞ with associated architectural distortion ➡. Additional imaging follows.

Typical

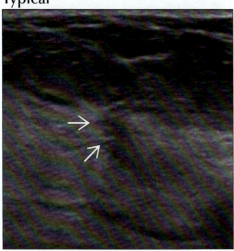

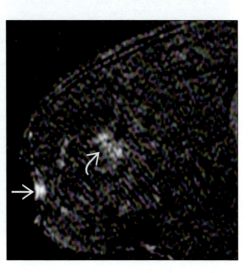

(Left) Anti-radial ultrasound shows spiculated margins to the mass (➡, same lesion as previous image). MR was performed (next image). *(Right)* Sagittal T1 C+ subtraction MR shows spiculated enhancing lesion ⮞ at site of mammographic and US lesion. Excision showed radial scar and LCIS. Recent nipple surgery site also enhances ➡.

Typical

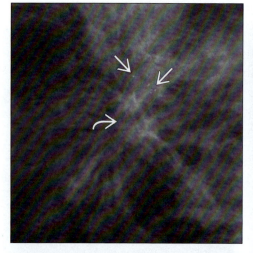
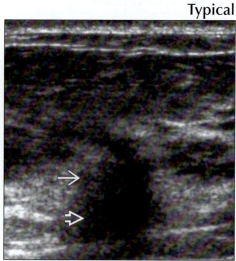

(Left) CC mammography magnification shows architectural distortion with central lucency ⇗ and associated pleomorphic calcifications ⇨. US was performed (next image). (Right) Radial ultrasound shows irregular, hypoechoic mass ⇨ with posterior shadowing ⇨. Excisional biopsy showed CSL with three small associated foci of invasive lobular cancer. Calcifications were in CSL and associated sclerosing adenosis.

Typical

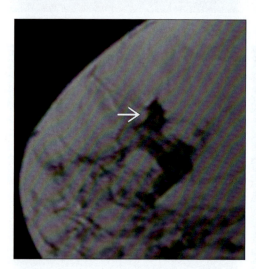
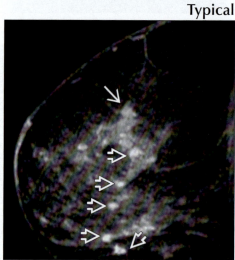

(Left) Sagittal T1WI MR shows a spiculated mass ⇨ in a 50 year old with prior ADH and strong family history of breast cancer. (Right) Sagittal T2WI FS MR (same as previous image) shows the spiculated mass ⇨, isointense to parenchyma, and multiple cysts ⇨.

Typical

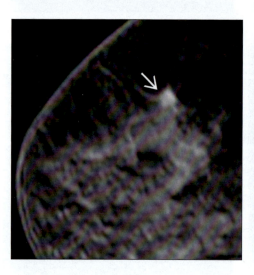
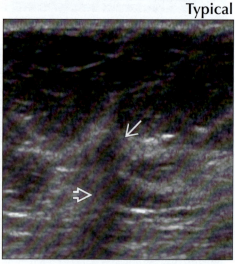

(Left) Sagittal T1 C+ FS MR (same case as prior two images) shows enhancement in the spiculated mass ⇨, suspicious for malignancy. US was performed for biopsy guidance. (Right) Anti-radial ultrasound targeted to MR finding (previous image) shows an irregular mass ⇨ with posterior shadowing ⇨. US core biopsy showed benign breast tissue, which was discordant with the MRI findings. Excision was then performed, showing radial scar and florid ductal hyperplasia.

RADIAL SCAR

Variant

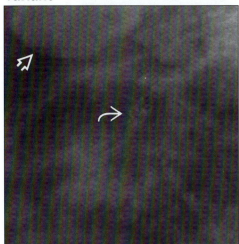
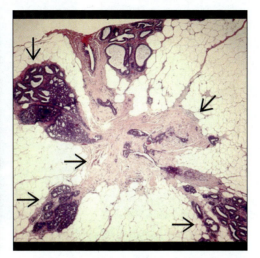

(Left) CC mammography magnification shows cluster of heterogeneous calcifications ➔ and adjacent cyst ➔. Stereotactic biopsy was performed (next image). **(Right)** Micropathology, low power, H&E shows incidental RSL ➔ entirely contained in an 11-g core specimen. The targeted calcifications were in adjacent fibrocystic changes. Excision may not be needed in such cases.

Typical

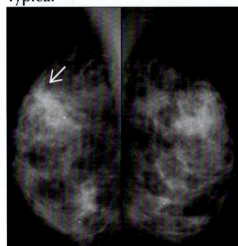
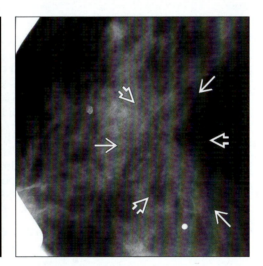

(Left) MLO mammography shows subtle focal asymmetry and distortion ➔ in the upper right breast of a 56 year old. **(Right)** CC mammography spot compression (same as left) shows this to be a spiculated mass ➔ with lucency between the spicules ➔. US was performed (below left).

Typical

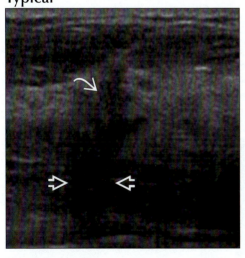
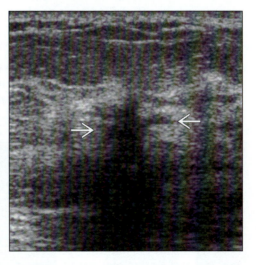

(Left) Radial ultrasound (same as above) shows an irregular, hypoechoic mass ➔ with posterior shadowing ➔. US-guided 14-g core biopsy showed RSL. Excision was performed, showing 11 mm of low grade DCIS with RSL. MRI was performed. **(Right)** Radial harmonic ultrasound of left breast (same patient as above and left) targeted to enhancing lesion seen only on MR, shows a spiculated mass ➔. Excision showed radial scar with multiple small foci of low grade DCIS.

FIBROMATOSIS

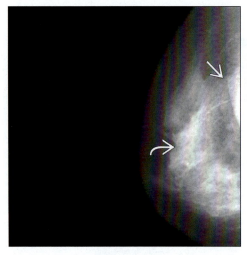

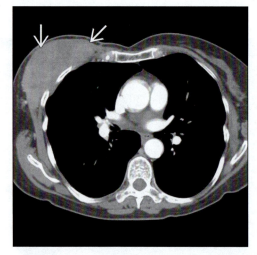

CC mammography shows architectural distortion ⮕ which was biopsied with a result of DCIS. Mastectomy was performed. The subtle posterior density ⮕ was not further investigated initially.

Axial CECT (same as left) shows a mass involving the right pectoralis muscle ⮕. Biopsy revealed aggressive fibromatosis. Wide excision was performed.

TERMINOLOGY

Abbreviations and Synonyms

- Aggressive fibromatosis, extra-abdominal desmoid tumor

Definitions

- Locally aggressive proliferation of fibroblasts and myofibroblasts without metastatic potential
  - Usually arises from the pectoralis fascia
  - Intramammary origin less common

IMAGING FINDINGS

General Features

- Best diagnostic clue: Irregular mass on mammography, US, or MR
- Location: Intraparenchymal or posteriorly when arises from pectoralis fascia
- Size: 1-12 cm; average 2.5-3 cm

Mammographic Findings

- Irregular, dense mass with spiculated margins

- Typically close to or arising from pectoralis muscle
- Rare associated calcifications
- Associated findings (occasional)
  - Skin thickening, dimpling, nipple retraction
  - Reduction in breast size, increased density
- Absence of lymphadenopathy

Ultrasonographic Findings

- Grayscale Ultrasound
  - Hypoechoic, irregular or indistinctly marginated mass ± posterior shadowing
    - Occasional echogenic rim
    - Rarely oval, circumscribed

MR Findings

- T1WI: Generally hypo- or isointense spiculated mass
- T2WI FS
  - Variable signal intensities reported
    - Hypointense fibrous tissue
    - Hyperintense myxoid tissue
- T1 C+ FS
  - Irregular spiculated mass
  - Variable enhancement characteristics reported
    - Slow, progressive enhancement
    - Rapid enhancement, plateau ± washout curves

DDx: Spiculated Lesions Mimicking Fibromatosis

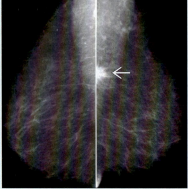

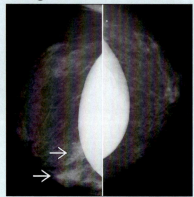

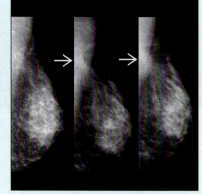

Mixed IDC-ILC Invading Pectoralis

IDC and Implant

Recurrent IDC

FIBROMATOSIS

Key Facts

Terminology
- Aggressive fibromatosis, extra-abdominal desmoid tumor
- Locally aggressive proliferation of fibroblasts and myofibroblasts without metastatic potential
- Usually arises from the pectoralis fascia

Imaging Findings
- Best diagnostic clue: Irregular mass on mammography, US, or MR
- MR may define extent for pre-operative planning

Top Differential Diagnoses
- Invasive Ductal Carcinoma (IDC) NOS or Invasive Lobular Carcinoma (ILC)
- Post-Operative Scar
- Spindle cell carcinoma

- Fibrosis

Pathology
- Trauma: Anecdotal reports of direct blow to chest
- Prior surgery: Liposuction reduction
- Association with silicone implants reported
- In spectrum between non-aggressive fibrous tumors and low grade fibrosarcomas

Clinical Issues
- Painless, palpable, firm mass
- Local recurrence rates 21-27%
- Initial core needle biopsy facilitates one-step surgical planning; no need for lymph node sampling
- Wide local excision is standard

Nuclear Medicine Findings
- No standard role for nuclear medicine evaluation
- Uptake of Tc-99m dimercaptosuccinic acid (DMSA) reported
  - DMSA structurally similar to phosphate anion; uptake in rapidly proliferating cells

CT Findings
- Soft-tissue density mass within breast, chest wall
- Offers large field of view to evaluate findings outside breast

Biopsy
- Core biopsy shows spindle cell proliferation (excludes primary breast cancer)
  - Can be difficult to distinguish benign from malignant with limited sampling
  - May be misinterpreted as bland stromal fibrosis

Imaging Recommendations
- Best imaging tool
  - MR may define extent for pre-operative planning
    - Characterize chest wall invasion if present

DIFFERENTIAL DIAGNOSIS

Invasive Ductal Carcinoma (IDC) NOS or Invasive Lobular Carcinoma (ILC)
- Spiculated or indistinct mass, indistinguishable
- Calcifications more common in IDC

Post-Operative Scar
- Should decrease over time

Fat Necrosis
- Usually centrally fat-containing mass
- Peripheral curvilinear calcifications over several years

Diabetic Mastopathy
- Unclear if manifestation of inflammation
- Longstanding type I diabetes

Histopathologic Mimics
- Spindle cell carcinoma
  - Usually has a recognizable carcinoma component
  - Stain with epithelial markers
    - Most of the neoplasm assumes a pseudosarcomatous growth pattern
    - Resembles fibromatosis or fibrosarcoma
- Fibrosarcoma
  - More cellular, nuclear pleomorphism, many mitotic figures
- Fibrous histiocytoma
- Nodular fasciitis
  - Circumscribed, many mitotic figures, myxoid component
- Fibrosis
  - Dense collagen, paucicellular relative to fibromatosis

PATHOLOGY

General Features
- Etiology
  - Multiple postulated etiologies
    - Trauma: Anecdotal reports of direct blow to chest
    - Prior surgery: Liposuction reduction
    - Exogenous hormone treatment
  - Association with silicone implants reported
    - No proven causal relationship
    - May arise from fibrous capsule or along surgical incision sites
- Epidemiology
  - Extremely rare
  - Incidence: 0.2% of breast neoplasms
  - Up to 4% bilateral, synchronous
- Types of fibromatosis
  - Superficial (e.g. palmar, plantar, penile)
  - Deep-seated fibromatosis
    - In spectrum between non-aggressive fibrous tumors and low grade fibrosarcomas
    - Extra-abdominal: Within axial musculature or rarely within breast parenchyma

FIBROMATOSIS

- Abdominal: In anterior abdominal wall musculoaponeurosis, most often pregnancy related
- Intraabdominal: In mesentery or pelvic walls, associated with Gardner syndrome (autosomal dominant variant of familial adenomatous polyposis with gastrointestinal (GI) polyps, multiple osteomas, epidermoid cysts, desmoid tumors)

Gross Pathologic & Surgical Features
- Ill-defined mass
- Tan, white or gray firm fibrous tissue
- Cut surface may have whorled appearance

Microscopic Features
- Homogeneous spindle cell proliferation
  - Cells (fibroblasts) form bundles and fascicles
  - Variable degree of cellularity or collagen content
    - Chest wall lesions more cellular than breast origin lesions
- Infiltrates adjacent fat and parenchyma, may entrap ductal or lobular units
  - May mimic malignancy, except
    - Little cellular or nuclear pleomorphism
    - Mitotic figures typically undetectable

CLINICAL ISSUES

Presentation
- Most common signs/symptoms
  - Painless, palpable, firm mass
    - May enlarge over time
    - Usually mobile
    - May be fixed to pectoralis muscle, especially if chest wall origin
- Other signs/symptoms
  - Skin and/or nipple retraction (mimics IDC, ILC)
  - "Shrinking breast," mimics invasive ILC

Demographics
- Age
  - Usually reproductive-age women
    - Age range 13-80 years, average 37
- Gender: Has been reported in men

Natural History & Prognosis
- Local recurrence rates 21-27%
  - Usually within 3 years
    - Higher risk recurrence with chest wall lesions than breast parenchyma origin
  - Higher risk recurrence with positive surgical margins
    - Reported recurrence 57-89% for chest wall origin masses with positive surgical margins
- No metastatic potential
- Spontaneous regression has rarely been reported

Treatment
- Initial core needle biopsy facilitates one-step surgical planning; no need for lymph node sampling
- Wide local excision is standard
  - May remove less tissue if significant deformity would result

- Wide clear margins needed to reduce risk of local recurrence
- Radiation therapy controversial
  - May be useful for large lesions, invasion of vital structures
  - Reduced risk of post-operative recurrence reported
    - With or without positive surgical margins
- Hormonal therapy controversial
  - Most lack estrogen ± progesterone receptors
  - May decrease recurrence via other mechanisms
- Chemotherapy
  - May decrease recurrence, not generally recommended

DIAGNOSTIC CHECKLIST

Consider
- Imaging appearance indistinguishable from primary breast malignancy

Image Interpretation Pearls
- Cross-sectional imaging evaluation (CT, MR) may be helpful
  - Larger field of view
  - Assess for invasion of
    - Chest wall
    - Heart, great vessels
    - Brachial plexus

SELECTED REFERENCES

1. Schwartz GS et al: Fibromatosis of the breast: case report and current concepts in the management of an uncommon lesion. Breast J. 12:66-71, 2006
2. Erguvan-Dogan B et al: Primary desmoid tumor (extraabdominal fibromatosis) of the breast. AJR. 185:488-9, 2005
3. Goel NB et al: Fibrous lesions of the breast: imaging-pathologic correlation. Radiographics. 25:1547-59, 2005
4. Mesurolle B et al: Dynamic breast MR in recurrent fibromatosis. AJR. 184:696-7; author reply 697, 2005
5. Papantoniou V et al: Recurrent bilateral mammary fibromatosis (desmoid tumor) imaged with technetium-99m pentavalent dimercaptosuccinic acid [99mTc-(V)DMSA] scintimammography. Gynecol Oncol. 97:964-9, 2005
6. Privette A et al: Desmoid tumor: a case of mistaken identity. Breast J. 11:60-4, 2005
7. Nakazono T et al: Dynamic MR of fibromatosis of the breast. AJR. 181:1718-9, 2003
8. Greenberg D et al: Aggressive fibromatosis of the breast: a case report and literature review. Breast J. 8:55-7, 2002
9. Rosen PP: Rosen's Breast Pathology. Philadelphia, Lippincott Williams & Wilkins. Chapter 40, 749-57, 2001
10. Kopans D: Breast Imaging. 2nd ed. Philadelphia, Lippincott-Raven. Chapter 19, 563-5, 1998

FIBROMATOSIS

IMAGE GALLERY

Typical

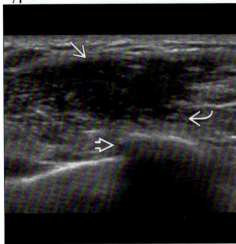

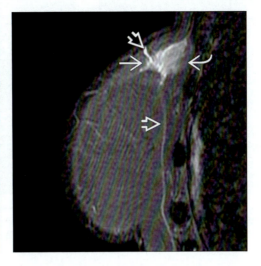

(Left) Sagittal ultrasound of a palpable mass that developed after a cat scratch injury, demonstrates a hypoechoic mass with anterior circumscribed ➡ & posterior angular margins ⬈, extending almost to the rib ➡. US-guided core biopsy = fibrosis. MR done for discordance (on right). *(Right)* Sagittal T2WI FS MR (same case as on left) demonstrates T2-hyperintensity of the mass ➡ & underlying pectoralis muscle ⬈ & demonstrates feeding vessel ➡.

Typical

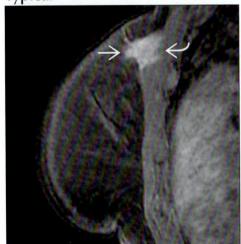

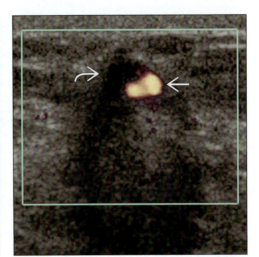

(Left) Sagittal T1 C+ FS MR (same case as previous two images) shows rapid, intense enhancement ➡ and involvement of underlying pectoralis muscle ⬈. Excision = fibromatosis with pectoralis muscle invasion, and multiple positive margins. *(Right)* This 20 year old underwent liposuction reduction 14 months earlier. A palpable, indistinct mass was noted as well as this irregular, hypoechoic, shadowing mass ⬈, hypervascular ➡ on power Doppler US.

Typical

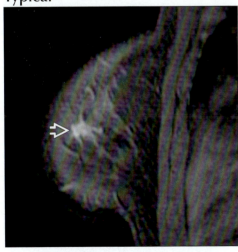

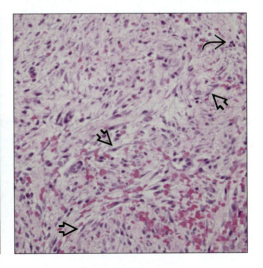

(Left) Sagittal T1 C+ FS MR (same case as previous image), shows rapid enhancement of the irregular mass ➡. Both masses had similar characteristics. US-guided core biopsy performed of both. *(Right)* Micropathology, medium power, H&E (same as on left) shows spindle cell proliferation ➡ with a solitary mitotic figure ➡. Consensus of pathologists = fibromatosis both lesions. Wide excision recommended.

GRANULAR CELL TUMOR

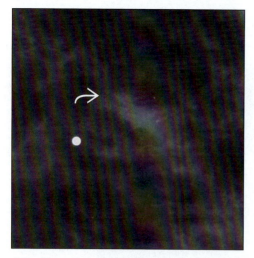

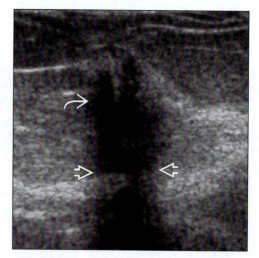

CC mammography spot compression shows an ill-defined mass ➡ corresponding to a palpable abnormality as marked with a BB in this 46 year old woman.

Ultrasound of the palpable area (same patient as left-hand image) reveals a nearly anechoic, irregular, angular mass ➡ with marked posterior shadowing ⬇. Both 14-gauge core biopsy and excision showed GCT.

TERMINOLOGY

Definitions
- Granular cell tumor (GCT) is composed of nests or sheets of cells that contain eosinophilic cytoplasmic granules
  - Usually benign; malignant in approximately 2%

IMAGING FINDINGS

General Features
- Best diagnostic clue: Irregular, hypoechoic, shadowing mass on US
- Location
  - Any site of the body; most frequently found in the head and neck area, particularly in the oral cavity
  - Breast GCTs represent 6-8% of total GCTs
  - More frequent in upper and inner breast
- Morphology: Round, oval or irregular discrete mass

Mammographic Findings
- Usually high density mass without calcifications
- Spiculated, lobulated or circumscribed margins

Ultrasonographic Findings
- Grayscale Ultrasound
  - Hypoechoic mass with irregular, angular margins
  - Heterogeneous internal echo pattern or anechoic
  - Marked posterior shadowing is frequent

DIFFERENTIAL DIAGNOSIS

Invasive Carcinoma
- Irregular mass, may have calcifications
- Breast cancer 1000x more common

Benign: Fat necrosis; Fibromatosis
- May have irregular margins; may have history of trauma, surgery

PATHOLOGY

General Features
- General path comments
  - Tumor of putative schwannian origin
  - Multiple in 5-10% of cases

DDx: Mimics of Granular Cell Tumor

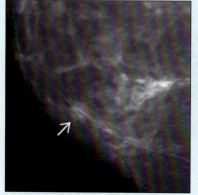

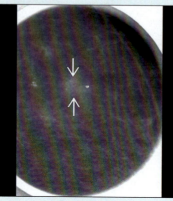

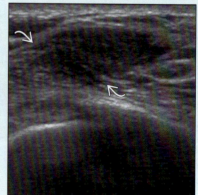

Invasive Ductal Carcinoma

Fat Necrosis

Fibromatosis

GRANULAR CELL TUMOR

Key Facts

Terminology
- Granular cell tumor (GCT) is composed of nests or sheets of cells that contain eosinophilic cytoplasmic granules
- Usually benign; malignant in approximately 2%

Imaging Findings
- Best diagnostic clue: Irregular, hypoechoic, shadowing mass on US
- Usually high density mass without calcifications
- Spiculated, lobulated or circumscribed margins

Top Differential Diagnoses
- Invasive Carcinoma
- Breast cancer 1000x more common
- Benign: Fat necrosis; Fibromatosis

Clinical Issues
- Mimics breast cancer: Firm, painless mass; may cause skin retraction and nipple inversion

---

- Genetics: Predisposition in African-Americans

Gross Pathologic & Surgical Features
- Usually ill-defined infiltrative margins
- Cut surface is white, gray or yellow-tan in color

Microscopic Features
- Infiltrative growth pattern resembling carcinoma
- Granular eosinophilic cytoplasm due to abundant intracytoplasmic lysosomes
  - Granules are PAS positive and diastase resistant
  - Nuclei are prominent, round or oval
- Typically positive stains for S-100 and CD68
  - Negative stains for cytokeratin, ER and PR
- Malignant GCT: Nuclear pleomorphism, mitotic activity and necrosis

CLINICAL ISSUES

Presentation
- Most common signs/symptoms
  - Mimics breast cancer: Firm, painless mass; may cause skin retraction and nipple inversion
  - Asymmetric firm lump with slow growth; may see skin fixation, and/or ulceration
- Other signs/symptoms: If deep, may involve pectoralis fascia

Demographics
- Age: Wide range: 17-75 years (average in the 30's)
- More frequent in females (but at least 10% in males)

Natural History & Prognosis
- Clinical behavior usually benign; rare local recurrence, extremely rare lymph node metastases, reported

Treatment
- Excise after core biopsy; can be locally aggressive
- Surgical excision is curative for benign tumors
  - Wide excision for malignant tumors

DIAGNOSTIC CHECKLIST

Consider
- While usually benign, excision recommended

Image Interpretation Pearls
- GCT must be included in the differential diagnosis of a breast mass with spiculated or lobulated margins

SELECTED REFERENCES

1. Yang WT et al: Sonographic and mammographic appearances of granular cell tumors of the breast with pathological correlation. J Clin Ultrasound. 34:153-60, 2006
2. Capobianco G et al: Granular cell tumor of the breast. Breast J. 11:519-20, 2005
3. Adeniran A et al: Granular cell tumor of the breast: a series of 17 cases and review of the literature. Breast J. 10:528-31, 2004
4. Page DL et al: Diagnostic Histopathology of the Breast. UK, Longman Group. Limited. Chapter 18. 312-3, 1987

IMAGE GALLERY

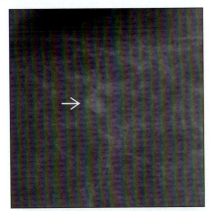 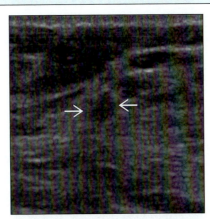 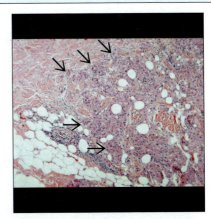

(Left) CC mammography spot compression shows a subtle, 5 mm partially circumscribed, partially indistinct mass ➡, which was new compared to earlier exams. *(Center)* Ultrasound (same case as left) shows an irregular, isoechoic mass corresponding to the mammographic mass ➡. Histopathology at US-guided core biopsy showed GCT, concordant with the imaging findings. *(Right)* Micropathology, low power, H&E shows 42 year old patient with GCT (different patient than left-hand images). Histology shows granular cells infiltrating ➡ the fibrofatty breast stroma.

PHYLLODES TUMOR

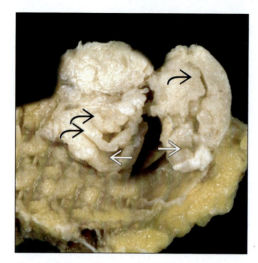

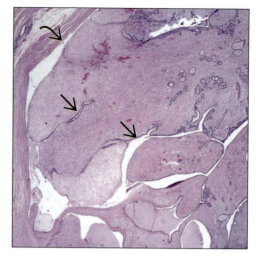

Gross pathology of a resected palpable mass shows the typical appearance of a phyllodes tumor with leaf-like excrescences ⊟ and cystic spaces ➡ between the protuberances.

Micropathology (medium power, H&E) (different patient) shows pushing margins ⊟ and slit-like spaces ⊟ between leaf-like epithelial-lined stromal projections in this benign phyllodes tumor.

TERMINOLOGY

Abbreviations and Synonyms
- Cystosarcoma phyllodes (term out of favor as most phyllodes tumors are benign)
- Periductal stromal tumor

Definitions
- Phyllodes tumor (PT): Biphasic neoplasm with double-layered epithelial component surrounded by overgrowing stroma
  - Arise from periductal stroma
  - Papillary growths of epithelial-lined stroma protrude as leaf-like masses (phyllodes: "Leaf-like" in Greek)
    - Clefts between leaf-like masses form "cystic" spaces
  - Spectrum from benign to borderline to malignant
  - Even benign PT treated as locally aggressive

IMAGING FINDINGS

General Features
- Best diagnostic clue: Large, rapidly growing circumscribed mass without calcifications (Ca++)

- Size
  - Size range: 1-45 cm; mean size 4-5 cm
    - May occupy entire breast

Mammographic Findings
- Mass: Dense, round or oval shape
- Circumscribed or lobulated margins
  - Partially indistinct margins favor malignant PT
- Ca++ rare, can be large, chunky

Ultrasonographic Findings
- Grayscale Ultrasound
  - Oval, round, or lobulated circumscribed, hypoechoic mass
  - Can be partially indistinctly marginated
  - Variable posterior features
  - May have intramural cystic spaces, favoring malignant phyllodes
- Color Doppler: ↑ Vascularity common

MR Findings
- T1WI
  - Heterogeneous low signal intensity
    - May see hemorrhage as high signal areas
- T2WI FS

DDx: Large Circumscribed Mass

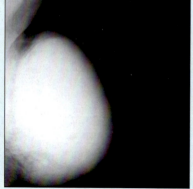

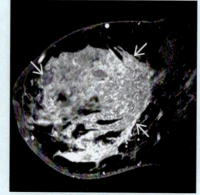

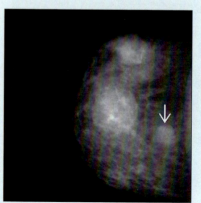

Giant Fibroadenoma

Angiosarcoma

Circumscribed Cancer, Cysts

PHYLLODES TUMOR

Key Facts

Terminology

- Phyllodes tumor (PT): Biphasic neoplasm with double-layered epithelial component surrounded by overgrowing stroma
- Papillary growths of epithelial-lined stroma protrude as leaf-like masses (phyllodes: "Leaf-like" in Greek)
- Spectrum from benign to borderline to malignant
- Even benign PT treated as locally aggressive

Imaging Findings

- Best diagnostic clue: Large, rapidly growing circumscribed mass without calcifications (Ca++)
- Excision recommended if possible PT
- Rapidly enlarging "fibroadenoma" (> 20% ↑ in diameter in 6 months)
- "Cellular fibroadenoma" in post-menopausal woman

Top Differential Diagnoses

- Fibroadenoma
- Invasive Cancer

Pathology

- Distinguishing benign, borderline, malignant phyllodes tumors is challenging

Clinical Issues

- Lump may show rapid growth over few weeks
- Overlying skin may be stretched or ulcerated
- Median age 45-49
- 21% risk recurrence, most within 2 yrs
- 5-year survival for malignant phyllodes: 55-75%
- Complete surgical excision often curative
- Axillary node dissection unnecessary
- Radiation therapy reduces local recurrence

- ○ Lobulated mass with hyperintense fluid in slit-like spaces
- ○ ↑ Signal in surrounding tissues in 21%
  - Only 1.2% of fibroadenomas (FAs) show this sign
- T1 C+ FS
  - ○ Rapidly-enhancing, lobulated mass
  - ○ Suspicious contrast dynamics observed in 33%
  - ○ Non-enhancing internal septations in 45%
  - ○ Cystic spaces common, favor malignant PT
- MR helpful for surgical planning

CT Findings

- CECT: Useful to determine extent of metastatic disease in abdomen, central nervous system
- NECT: Useful to determine extent of metastatic disease in lungs

Biopsy

- On core biopsy, difficult to distinguish fibroadenoma (FA) with highly cellular stroma from PT
  - ○ FA can show cellular stroma in young women, usually < age 40
  - ○ Excision recommended if possible PT
    - Rapidly enlarging "fibroadenoma" (> 20% ↑ in diameter in 6 months)
    - "Cellular fibroadenoma" in post-menopausal woman

DIFFERENTIAL DIAGNOSIS

Fibroadenoma

- Typically occurs in younger women, peak age 25-30
- Commonly have Ca++
- Less cellular stroma, no leaf-like proliferation
  - ○ "Giant" FA ~ "juvenile" FA; quite large, ↑ stromal cellularity, epithelial hyperplasia, usually adolescents
- 2-4% have cystic component

Invasive Cancer

- More likely to have indistinct margins
- More likely to have associated pleomorphic Ca++

Periductal Stromal Sarcoma, Low Grade

- Related, malignant tumor, locally invasive
- Lack of epithelial component: Absent leaf-like processes
- Spindle cell proliferation around tubules that retain open lumina

Primary Sarcoma of Breast

- Absence of epithelial component distinguishes from malignant PT
- Clinical course similar to malignant PT

PATHOLOGY

General Features

- Genetics: No hereditary factors
- Etiology: Unknown
- Epidemiology
  - ○ < 1% of all breast neoplasms
  - ○ 2.5% of all fibroepithelial tumors (FA far more common)
  - ○ Series of 335 phyllodes tumors at one institution
    - 75% benign; 16% borderline; 9% malignant
- Associated abnormalities
  - ○ Epithelial component may have associated lobular carcinoma in situ (LCIS), ductal carcinoma in situ (DCIS), invasive cancer
  - ○ Stromal component may have liposarcoma, rhabdomyosarcoma, osteosarcoma (1% of cases)
  - ○ Presence of associated pseudoangiomatous stromal hyperplasia (PASH) is favorable

Gross Pathologic & Surgical Features

- Solid, fleshy leaf-like mass with bulging surface, cystic areas
- Circumscribed, nonencapsulated
- Gray to yellow foci of necrosis and hemorrhage

Microscopic Features

- Benign epithelial component (unless associated DCIS or invasive cancer)
- Cellular spindle cell fibroblastic stroma

PHYLLODES TUMOR

- ○ Stromal overgrowth: Epithelial elements absent in at least one 40x field
- Leaf-like stromal protuberances
- Highly atypical or multinucleated giant cells may occur
- Metaplasia (lipoid, chondroid, osteoid) may occur
- Immunohistochemistry
  - ○ p53+: Correlates with malignancy but not local recurrence
  - ○ ↑ CD117 (c-kit): Predicts ↑ risk local recurrence
- Histology may vary within a given mass
  - ○ FA ↔ benign phyllodes ↔ borderline PT

Staging, Grading or Classification Criteria
- Distinguishing benign, borderline, malignant phyllodes tumors is challenging
  - ○ Malignant
    - Marked stromal hypercellularity
    - > 10 mitoses per high power (40x) field (hpf)
    - Invasive margins
    - Marked stromal overgrowth, little epithelial component
    - Diffuse p53+ staining, ↑ Ki-67
    - Epidermal growth factor (EGFR) receptor overexpression in 75%
    - Vascular endothelial growth factor (VEGF) overexpression in stroma → angiogenesis
  - ○ Benign
    - Few mitoses per hpf (< 4)
    - Uniform stromal distribution
    - Pushing margin

CLINICAL ISSUES

Presentation
- Woman in middle age with firm, mobile, palpable lump
  - ○ Lump may show rapid growth over few weeks
  - ○ Overlying skin may be stretched or ulcerated

Demographics
- Age
  - ○ Older age group than fibroadenoma
  - ○ Age range 10-80, rare < 30 or > 60
    - Median age 45-49
- Gender: Predominately women; case reports in men

Natural History & Prognosis
- 21% risk recurrence, most within 2 yrs
  - ○ 10-17% in benign, 25-29% in borderline, 27-36% in malignant
- 5-year survival for malignant phyllodes: 55-75%
- Metastases to lung and bone most common, chest wall invasion
  - ○ 10% rate of metastases overall: 0% with benign, 4% with borderline, 22% with malignant
- Axillary node metastases uncommon: 10-15% with systemic disease

Treatment
- Complete surgical excision often curative
  - ○ Wide local excision required
    - Margin ≥ 1 cm: ↓ Recurrence risk by 52%

- ○ Mastectomy for very large tumors
- ○ Axillary node dissection unnecessary
- Adjuvant therapy
  - ○ Radiation therapy reduces local recurrence
  - ○ No benefit from chemotherapy

DIAGNOSTIC CHECKLIST

Consider
- Imaging cannot reliably distinguish FA from PT
- Frozen section accuracy as low as 38%
- Core needle biopsy (CNB) usually accurate
  - ○ 83% correct differentiation of PT from FA and 93% correct identification of FA (one series)
  - ○ Subtle distinction of PT from cellular FA on CNB
- Accurate pre-operative diagnosis
  - ○ Wide local resection as initial treatment
  - ○ Axillary node sampling avoided

Image Interpretation Pearls
- Consider PT if rapidly enlarging circumscribed mass or "cellular" fibroadenoma, especially > age 40

SELECTED REFERENCES

1. Kersting C et al: Amplifications of the epidermal growth factor receptor gene (egfr) are common in phyllodes tumors of the breast and are associated with tumor progression. Lab Invest. 86(1):54-61, 2006
2. Chen WH et al: Surgical treatment of phyllodes tumors of the breast: retrospective review of 172 cases. J Surg Oncol. 91(3):185-94, 2005
3. Franceschini G et al: Phyllodes tumor of the breast: magnetic resonance imaging findings and surgical treatment. Breast J. 11(2):144-5, 2005
4. Franceschini G et al: Surgical treatment and MRI in phyllodes tumors of the breast: our experience and review of the literature. Ann Ital Chir. 76(2):127-40, 2005
5. Tan PH et al: p53 and c-kit (CD117) protein expression as prognostic indicators in breast phyllodes tumors: a tissue microarray study. Mod Pathol. 18(12):1527-34, 2005
6. Tse GM et al: Stromal nitric oxide synthase (NOS) expression correlates with the grade of mammary phyllodes tumour. J Clin Pathol. 58(6):600-4, 2005
7. Tse GM et al: Stromal expression of vascular endothelial growth factor correlates with tumor grade and microvessel density in mammary phyllodes tumors: a multicenter study of 185 cases. Hum Pathol. 35(9):1053-7, 2004
8. Gordon PB et al: Solid breast masses diagnosed as fibroadenoma at fine-needle aspiration biopsy: acceptable rates of growth at long-term follow-up. Radiology. 229(1):233-8, 2003
9. Komenaka IK et al: Core needle biopsy as a diagnostic tool to differentiate phyllodes tumor from fibroadenoma. Arch Surg. 138(9):987-90, 2003
10. Tse GM et al: Tumour angiogenesis and p53 protein expression in mammary phyllodes tumors. Mod Pathol. 16(10):1007-13, 2003
11. Liberman L et al: Benign and malignant phyllodes tumors: mammographic and sonographic findings. Radiology. 198:121-4, 1996

PHYLLODES TUMOR

IMAGE GALLERY

Typical

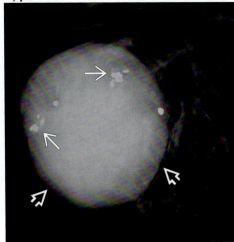

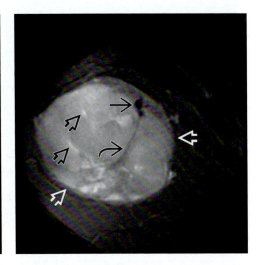

(Left) CC mammography shows a large, circumscribed, dense mass ⮕ corresponding to a palpable abnormality in this 34 y/o. Chunky, coarse, "popcorn" calcifications are noted within the mass ➡. *(Right)* Sagittal T2WI FS MR (same as left) shows a hyperintense mass ⮕ with signal voids at the sites of calcification ➡. Hypointense septations ➡ and hyperintense fluid-filled slit-like spaces ⮕ are seen within the mass.

Typical

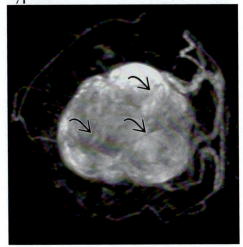

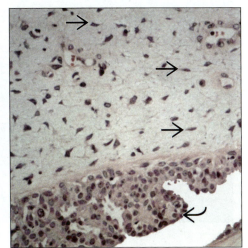

(Left) Coronal MIP of T1 C+ subtraction MR (same as prior 2 images) shows intense enhancement of the hypervascular mass. Note nonenhancing internal septations ➡. 14-g core biopsy showed benign phyllodes, confirmed at wide excision. *(Right)* Micropathology, low power, H&E in a different patient shows the typical low grade phyllodes tumor with bland stroma, occasional spindle cells ➡ & well differentiated epithelium forming papillary projections ➡.

Typical

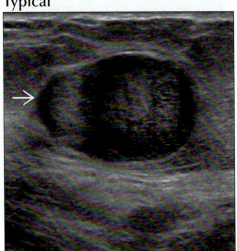

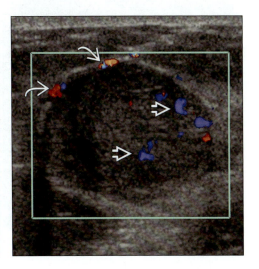

(Left) US shows circumscribed, oval, hypoechoic mass ➡ corresponding to palpable abnormality in a 32 y/o. *(Right)* Color Doppler US (same as left) shows internal vascularity ⮕ as well as marginal vessels ➡. Excision showed benign phyllodes tumor.

PHYLLODES TUMOR

(Left) MLO mammography shows dense, round, circumscribed mass ➡ at the site of a palpable finding in the inferior breast of a 47 y/o. Biopsy showed benign phyllodes tumor. *(Right)* CC mammography in a 32 y/o presenting with a right-sided palpable breast mass shows an extremely large mass ➡ occupying most of the breast. The size of the mass prevented adequate exposure.

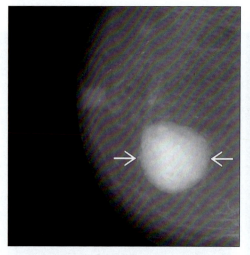
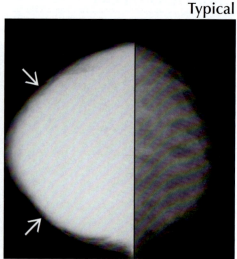

Typical

(Left) US (same as prior image) shows a circumscribed mass with deep margin beyond transducer penetration. Anechoic tubular areas ➡ likely represent slit-like fluid spaces. Fine needle aspiration showed a proliferative epithelial lesion without atypia. *(Right)* Sagittal T2WI FS MR (same as prior two images) confirms fluid-filled clefts ➡. Most of the mass is hyperintense, though inferior portion ➡ is hypointense on this sequence.

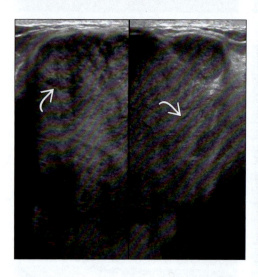
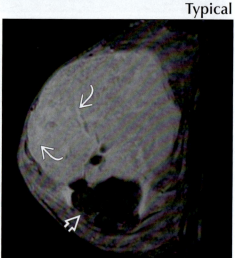

Typical

(Left) Sagittal T1WI MR (same as prior 3 images) shows a smooth mass ➡ with heterogeneous signal inferiorly ➡. Note the fat ➡ trapped centrally. At resection, invasive growth into fat was noted. *(Right)* Sagittal T1 C+ subtraction MR (same as prior 4 images) shows intense enhancement within upper portion of the mass ➡ except for central fatty area ➡ and inferior portion of tumor ➡. This illustrates the heterogeneity of phyllodes tumors.

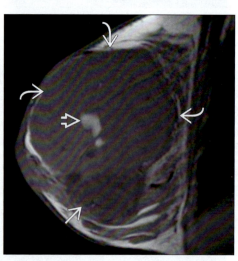
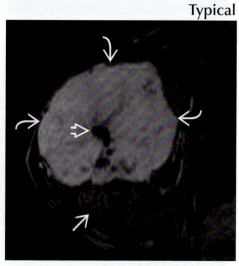

Typical

PHYLLODES TUMOR

Variant

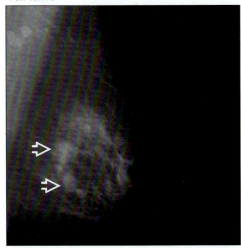 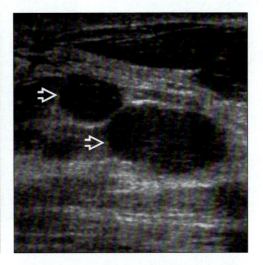

(Left) MLO mammography of the left breast shows multiple partially circumscribed, partially obscured new unilateral masses ➡ in this 57 y/o. **(Right)** Ultrasound (same case as left) confirms two circumscribed masses ➡; other similar masses were present in the same breast. Core biopsy of three masses showed benign phyllodes tumors. Because wide excision is needed, and there were multiple proven phyllodes tumors, the patient underwent mastectomy.

Typical

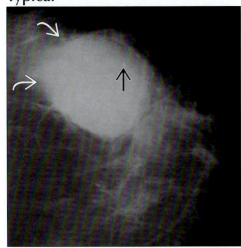 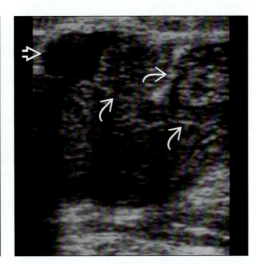

(Left) CC mammography shows partially circumscribed, partially indistinct margins ➡ to this palpable mass (marked by a BB ➡) in a 33 y/o. **(Right)** Ultrasound (same patient as previous image) shows hyperechoic internal septations ➡ and eccentric cystic space ➡. Biopsy showed low grade malignant phyllodes tumor. Cystic spaces ± microlobulated margins in a mass resembling FA suggests the possibility of phyllodes tumor.

Variant

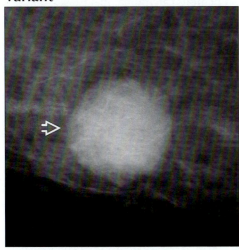 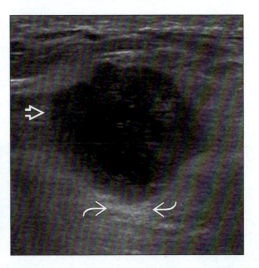

(Left) CC mammography close-up shows dense, microlobulated mass ➡ corresponding to palpable lump in a 43 y/o, new compared to prior mammogram 2 years earlier. **(Right)** US (same patient as previous image) shows complex cystic and solid microlobulated mass ➡ with posterior enhancement ➡. Biopsy showed high-grade DCIS involving a phyllodes tumor. This was highly vascular on Doppler.

ADENOID CYSTIC CARCINOMA

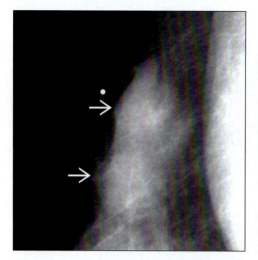

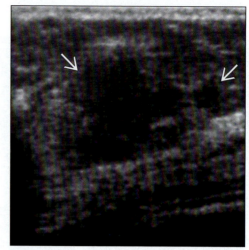

CC mammography magnification reveals a subtle, partially obscured bilobed ➡ palpable mass in the right upper outer quadrant. The patient noted the mass one week after a normal screening mammogram.

US (same patient as previous image) shows irregular, hypoechoic mass ➡ with microlobulated margins. US-guided core biopsy revealed adenoid cystic carcinoma.

TERMINOLOGY

Abbreviations and Synonyms
- Cylindroma, adenocystic basal cell carcinoma

Definitions
- Rare malignant breast tumor, indistinguishable from adenoid cystic carcinoma (ACC) found in other parts of the body, especially major and minor salivary glands
  - Entwined cylinders of stroma (± acellular basement membrane material) and epithelial cells (proliferating glands) = adenoid component

IMAGING FINDINGS

General Features
- Best diagnostic clue: Circumscribed, lobular mass
- Location: Can occur anywhere; subareolar/central region most common
- Size: Median: 2 cm; range: 0.2-12 cm

Mammographic Findings
- Slowly growing mostly circumscribed lobular mass
- Less common: Irregular mass, asymmetry ± architectural distortion

Ultrasonographic Findings
- Grayscale Ultrasound: Irregular hypoechoic mass

MR Findings
- T1 C+ FS: Irregular or smooth enhancing mass

DIFFERENTIAL DIAGNOSIS

Imaging
- Circumscribed or indistinctly marginated mass
  - Invasive ductal carcinoma (NOS), papillary, medullary, mucinous carcinoma, metastases
  - Fibroadenoma, papilloma

Pathology
- Intraductal and invasive cribriform carcinoma
- Collagenous spherulosis (benign)

DDx: Adenoid Cystic Carcinoma Mimics

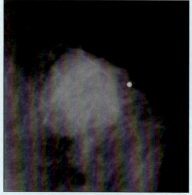

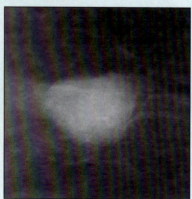

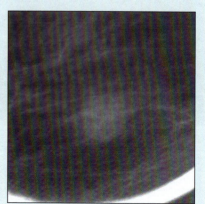

Medullary Carcinoma

Mucinous Carcinoma

Metastasis to Breast

ADENOID CYSTIC CARCINOMA

Key Facts

Terminology
- Rare malignant breast tumor, indistinguishable from adenoid cystic carcinoma (ACC) found in other parts of the body, especially major and minor salivary glands

Imaging Findings
- Best diagnostic clue: Circumscribed, lobular mass

Top Differential Diagnoses
- Intraductal and invasive cribriform carcinoma

Pathology
- 0.1% of all breast cancers
- Low incidence of axillary node metastasis (≤ 5%)

Clinical Issues
- Excellent prognosis; death rare

PATHOLOGY

General Features
- General path comments
  - 0.1% of all breast cancers
  - Low incidence of axillary node metastasis (≤ 5%)
  - Distant metastasis uncommon
    - Lung most common site
    - Other sites: Bone, liver, brain and kidney
    - Can occur without prior lymph node involvement
  - ER/PR previously reported to be negative
    - Recent large series: 45% ER positive, 35% PR positive
- Etiology
  - Cell of origin controversial
    - Possibly derived from ductal, myoepithelial or stem cells

Gross Pathologic & Surgical Features
- Circumscribed or grossly nodular firm mass
- Gross cystic degeneration noted in larger tumors

Microscopic Features
- Characterized by glandular and stromal elements
  - Microscopic cystic areas not uncommon
  - Cribriform architecture common
- Two main cell components: Modified fusiform myoepithelial cells and glandular cuboid cells
- 50% demonstrate invasive growth pattern
- Perineural invasion and lymphatic tumor emboli rare

CLINICAL ISSUES

Presentation
- Most common signs/symptoms
  - Firm, palpable, discrete subareolar or central mass
    - Often painful
    - Not associated with nipple discharge
- Clinical Profile: Slow growth

Demographics
- Age
  - 25-80 years: Mean age at diagnosis 50-66 years
    - Rarely described in children
- Gender: Isolated reports in men

Natural History & Prognosis
- Excellent prognosis; death rare

Treatment
- Lumpectomy, followed by radiation for local control
- Adjuvant chemotherapy thought to be of no benefit

SELECTED REFERENCES

1. Arpino G et al: Adenoid cystic carcinoma of the breast: molecular markers, treatment, and clinical outcome. Cancer. 94(8):2119-27, 2002
2. Santamaria G et al: Adenoid cystic carcinoma of the breast: mammographic appearance and pathologic correlation. AJR Am J Roentgenol. 171(6):1679-83, 1998

IMAGE GALLERY

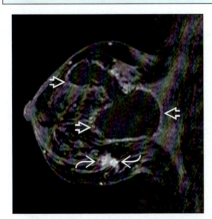
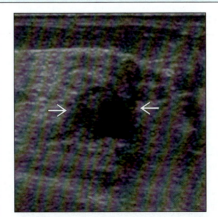
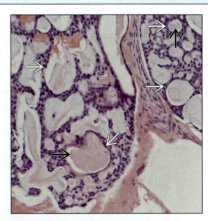

(Left) Sagittal T1 C+ FS MR shows large seroma ⇒ in patient who underwent excisional biopsy for adenoid cystic carcinoma. A second unsuspected enhancing spiculated mass ⇒ was noted. *(Center)* Second-look US after MR (same patient as previous) revealed an irregular, hypoechoic mass ⇒. US-guided core biopsy showed this to be a second adenoid cystic carcinoma. *(Right)* Micropathology, low power shows classic example of adenoid cystic carcinoma. Note multiple cribriform-type spaces ⇒ containing eosinophilic basement-membrane material ⇒.

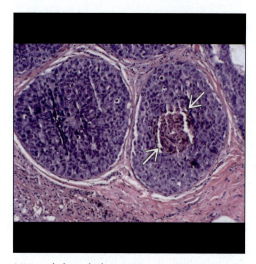

Micropathology, high power H&E stain shows the typical "blue" appearance of ductal carcinoma in situ, high nuclear grade with central necrosis ➡.

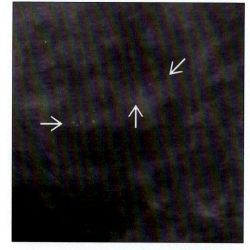

MLO mammography magnification shows pleomorphic microcalcifications in a linear (ductal) distribution ➡ on screening mammogram of a 55 y/o woman. Core biopsy and excision showed DCIS.

TERMINOLOGY

Abbreviations and Synonyms
- Ductal carcinoma in situ (DCIS); intraductal carcinoma; preinvasive, or noninvasive cancer

Definitions
- Clonal proliferation of malignant epithelial cells originating in terminal duct lobular unit (TDLU) without invasion of the basement membrane
- Multifocal: > 1 site within one quadrant or same duct system or within 4 or 5 cm
- Multicentric: Tumor foci in > 1 quadrant or different duct systems or separated by at least 4 or 5 cm

IMAGING FINDINGS

General Features
- Best diagnostic clue: Mammographic calcifications (Ca++); sensitivity 70-80%

Mammographic Findings
- Ca++ most common finding
- Fine linear or branching Ca++ highly suggestive of DCIS, usually high-grade
  - Due to casting of necrotic debris within ducts
- Pleomorphic Ca++: 25-40% due to DCIS, any grade
- Amorphous Ca++: 20% malignant, of which 90% are DCIS, usually low-grade
- Clustered distribution most common
- Linear or segmental distribution of any Ca++ morphology suggests DCIS
  - Excludes smooth ≥ 1 mm rod-like secretory Ca++
- Regional distribution of Ca++: Intermediate suspicion
- Appearance does not reliably predict grade
- Mass with Ca++ 10%; mass alone 10%
  - Mass more common with papillary DCIS
  - Mass/asymmetry favors invasive component

Ultrasonographic Findings
- Grayscale Ultrasound
  - Sensitivity ~ 50%
    - Dilated ducts, indistinct walls ± echogenic Ca++
    - May be visible as hypoechoic mass ± Ca++
    - Isolated Ca++: Mimic speckle artifact, subtle
    - Papillary DCIS: Intracystic or circumscribed mass
- Power Doppler: Increased vascularity common

DDx: Suspicious Calcifications Due to Benign Etiologies

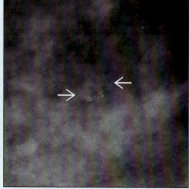

Calcifying Fibroadenoma

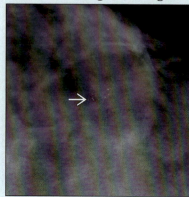

Apocrine Metaplasia

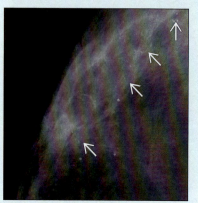

Fat Necrosis

DCIS, GENERAL

Key Facts

Terminology
- Ductal carcinoma in situ (DCIS); intraductal carcinoma; preinvasive, or noninvasive cancer
- Clonal proliferation of malignant epithelial cells originating in terminal duct lobular unit (TDLU) without invasion of the basement membrane

Imaging Findings
- Best diagnostic clue: Mammographic calcifications (Ca++); sensitivity 70-80%
- MR 88-95% sensitivity with high morphologic resolution (1 mm in-plane)
- Linear or segmental clumped enhancement

Top Differential Diagnoses
- Invasive carcinoma
- Fibrocystic changes, sclerosing adenosis

- Fat necrosis with early Ca++
- Fibroadenoma
- ADH: Fulfills some, but not all, criteria for low grade DCIS
- Microinvasive carcinoma
- Columnar cell lesion with atypia
- Lobular carcinoma in situ (LCIS)
- Ductal extension of LCIS mimics DCIS
- E-cadherin lost in lobular lesions, retained in DCIS

Pathology
- Multifocality more frequent if > 2-2.5 cm, especially common with micropapillary subtype

Diagnostic Checklist
- Biopsy suspicious Ca++ regardless of stability
- Magnification views to characterize extent of Ca++

MR Findings
- T1 C+ FS
  - MR 88-95% sensitivity with high morphologic resolution (1 mm in-plane)
  - Detection rates of low grade DCIS ~ high grade
  - Kinetics unreliable: Often slow, persistent
  - Linear or segmental clumped enhancement
    - Focal area(s), regional clumped enhancement

Biopsy
- Core needle biopsy (CNB): 11-g or larger device, ≥ 10 specimens for Ca++
  - Difficult to distinguish atypical ductal hyperplasia (ADH) from low grade DCIS
    - ADH upgraded to DCIS at excision: 18% of 11-g biopsies
  - 14-g CNB sufficient for masses: 3-5 specimens
- DCIS at CNB upgraded to invasive carcinoma at excision: 11% across multiple series
- Needle-localized excision when nonpalpable
  - Bracket localization for area of Ca++ > 2 cm
- Follow-up & management
  - Specimen radiography standard for CNB of Ca++ and needle-localized excisions
  - Post-operative mammogram if breast conserved and close or positive margins or multifocal Ca++
  - Residual Ca++ highly predictive of residual tumor: 67%; up to 90% when number > 5
  - Residual disease at re-excision in up to 31% with "negative" margin of 1-2 mm
    - Uncommon with > 2 mm negative margins

Imaging Recommendations
- Best imaging tool
  - Mammography and MR
    - Extent may be underestimated on mammography, especially micropapillary and cribriform types
- Protocol advice
  - Orthogonal CC and 90° lateral magnification views
  - Extent of Ca++ predicts extent of DCIS to within 2 cm in 80-85% of cases
  - Bilateral MR to determine extent in selected cases

DIFFERENTIAL DIAGNOSIS

Imaging
- Invasive carcinoma
- Atypical ductal hyperplasia (ADH)
- Fibrocystic changes, sclerosing adenosis
- Fat necrosis with early Ca++
- Columnar cell lesions
- Fibroadenoma

Pathologic
- ADH: Fulfills some, but not all, criteria for low grade DCIS
  - Qualitative and quantitative differences
- Microinvasive carcinoma
- Columnar cell lesion with atypia
- Lobular carcinoma in situ (LCIS)
  - Ductal extension of LCIS mimics DCIS
  - E-cadherin lost in lobular lesions, retained in DCIS

PATHOLOGY

General Features
- General path comments
  - Nuclear grade: Degree of pleomorphism
    - Low, intermediate, high grade
  - Histologic types based on architecture: Variable, often mixed
    - Comedo: Pleomorphic cells with high grade nuclei and necrosis in duct lumens
    - Noncomedo: Solid, cribriform, micropapillary; with or without necrosis
    - Other rare types: Papillary, apocrine, clear cell, signet ring, spindle cell, cystic hypersecretory
  - Arises in terminal duct lobular unit growing toward nipple
    - High-grade more likely to show contiguous growth (90%) than low grade (30%)
    - Discontinuous (multifocal): Skip areas usually < 1 mm; 70% of low-grade DCIS has skip areas

- ■ Multifocality more frequent if > 2-2.5 cm, especially common with micropapillary subtype
  - ○ Microinvasion: Carcinoma cells extend beyond basement membrane, no focus > 1 mm
    - ■ ↑ Likely with ↑ size, especially > 2.5 cm
    - ■ 63% of comedo DCIS vs. 11% of non-comedo
    - ■ May show associated mass or asymmetry
- • Epidemiology
  - ○ Detection increased by mammographic screening
  - ○ 25-33% of all screen-detected malignancies; 5% of symptomatic cancers
  - ○ ~ 80% are high nuclear grade
  - ○ 30-67% DCIS patients eventually develop invasive carcinoma in same region

Gross Pathologic & Surgical Features
- • Usually not grossly evident
- • Necrotic debris may extrude from cut surface: "Comedones" in comedo type

Microscopic Features
- • Monomorphic cells within lumen of involved TDLU
- • Size & extent of DCIS has significant prognostic implications
  - ○ Histologic assessment often inaccurate & unreliable
  - ○ Various proposed methods include
    - ■ Number of slides with DCIS, multiplied by separation of sections (~ 2 mm)
    - ■ Distance between farthest involved ducts
    - ■ Volume based on number of involved sections
  - ○ Pathology report should include method of measurement
- • Immunohistochemistry
  - ○ Estrogen receptor (ER) positivity: 70-80%; more frequent in noncomedo DCIS, women > 55 years old
  - ○ Her-2/neu positivity 42-61%; more frequent in comedo DCIS
  - ○ p53 expression variable
  - ○ Confirm non-invasion by retained myoepithelial cell layer: Smooth muscle actin, p63; occasionally smooth muscle myosin heavy chain, calponin, H-caldesmon
    - ■ Retained basement membrane: Laminin, collagen type IV; limited by high background staining

Staging, Grading or Classification Criteria
- • Stage 0: DCIS
- • DCIS with microinvasion (≤ 1 mm): T1mic → stage 1

CLINICAL ISSUES

Presentation
- • Asymptomatic in majority
- • Lump, bloody nipple discharge, Paget disease

Demographics
- • Age: Mean age at detection ~ 50 years

Natural History & Prognosis
- • 2.5% recurrence/year without XRT
  - ○ Higher with close or positive margins
- • XRT decreases recurrence by 50%
- • Tamoxifen reduces recurrence risk another 50%

- • 50% recurrences = invasive disease, worse prognosis
  - ○ 19% distant metastases; 13% mortality at 4 years
- • > 95% 20-year adjusted survival if properly treated

Treatment
- • Lumpectomy with negative margins
- • Mastectomy may be recommended for
  - ○ Multicentric disease or > 5 cm area
  - ○ Need to achieve clear margins; poor cosmesis
- • Sentinel lymph node biopsy (SNB): When mastectomy will be performed; may consider with > 2.5 cm of high-grade DCIS
  - ○ 2-4% of lymph nodes metastatic on H&E
  - ○ Lymph node metastasis implies occult invasive component
  - ○ Additional yield with immunohistochemistry: Isolated tumor cells of uncertain significance
- • XRT following lumpectomy; selected patients post mastectomy
- • Tamoxifen for ER positive cases
  - ○ Aromatase inhibitors in post-menopausal women

DIAGNOSTIC CHECKLIST

Consider
- • Biopsy suspicious Ca++ regardless of stability

Image Interpretation Pearls
- • Magnification views to characterize extent of Ca++

SELECTED REFERENCES

1. Al-Attar MA et al: The impact of image guided needle biopsy on the outcome of mammographically detected indeterminate microcalcification. Breast. 2006
2. Weaver DL et al: Pathologic findings from the Breast Cancer Surveillance Consortium: population-based outcomes in women undergoing biopsy after screening mammography. Cancer. 106:732-42, 2006
3. Groves AM et al: Characterization of pure high-grade DCIS on magnetic resonance imaging using the evolving breast MR lexicon terminology: can it be differentiated from pure invasive disease? Magn Reson Imaging. 23:733-8, 2005
4. Harms SE: The use of breast magnetic resonance imaging in ductal carcinoma in situ. Breast J. 11:379-81, 2005
5. Menell JH et al: Determination of the presence and extent of pure ductal carcinoma in situ by mammography and magnetic resonance imaging. Breast J. 11:382-90, 2005
6. Harris JR et al: Diseases of the Breast. Philadelphia, Lippincott Williams & Wilkins. 521-38, 2004
7. Moon WK et al: US of ductal carcinoma in situ. Radiographics. 22:269-80; discussion 280-1, 2002
8. Ioffe OB: Local extent of disease: a pathology perspective. Semin Breast Dis. 4:179-90, 2001
9. Stomper PC et al: Mammographic detection and staging of ductal carcinoma in situ: mammographic-pathological correlation. Semin Breast Dis. 3:26-41, 2000
10. Rosen PP: Rosen's Breast Pathology. Philadelphia, Lippincott-Raven. 209-74, 1997
11. Lev-Toaff AS et al: Stability of malignant breast microcalcifications. Radiology. 192:153-6, 1994
12. Dershaw DD et al: Ductal carcinoma in situ: mammographic findings and clinical implications. Radiology. 170:411-5, 1989

DCIS, GENERAL

IMAGE GALLERY

Typical

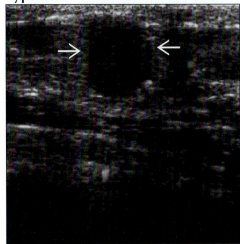

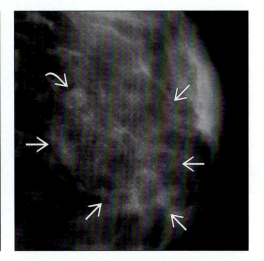

(Left) Transverse ultrasound of a palpable lump in a 38 y/o lactating woman shows a small hypoechoic mass ➡ with vertical orientation. Mammogram was also obtained (following image). *(Right)* CC mammography magnification shows extensive pleomorphic calcifications ➡. The mass ➡ corresponds to US lesion & palpable lump. On biopsy the mass was invasive ductal carcinoma; calcifications were DCIS.

Typical

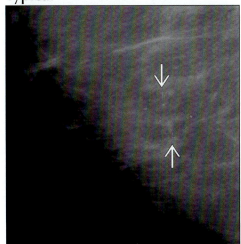

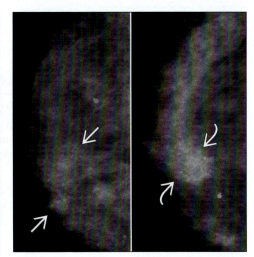

(Left) MLO mammography close-up from screening mammogram of this 44 y/o shows clustered pleomorphic calcifications ➡ without associated mass or density. Core needle biopsy, then excision revealed DCIS, intermediate grade. *(Right)* Mammography of a 59 y/o woman shows increasing focal density and calcifications on MLO ➡ and CC ➡ views. Biopsy and subsequent excision showed DCIS, high nuclear grade, with microinvasion.

Typical

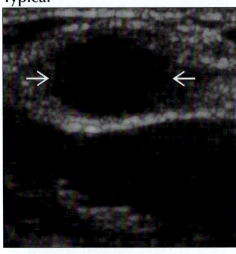

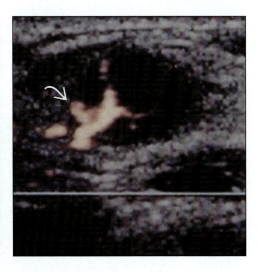

(Left) Longitudinal ultrasound of a palpable lump in a 31 y/o with positive family history shows a hypoechoic mass ➡ with microlobulated margins, parallel orientation, no posterior shadowing. *(Right)* Power Doppler ultrasound (same patient as previous image), shows penetrating prominent tumor vessels ➡. Core needle biopsy revealed DCIS only. No calcifications were seen on mammography. ~ 10% of DCIS presents as a mass only.

DCIS, LOW GRADE

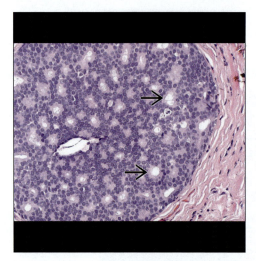

Micropathology, high power illustrates the typical uniform "punched out" secondary spaces ➡ of cribriform DCIS, low nuclear grade, without necrosis.

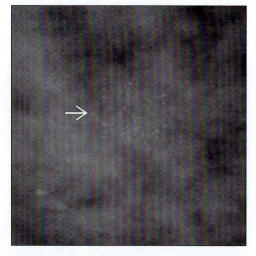

Lateral mammography close-up shows clustered amorphous Ca++ ➡ on screening exam of a 52 y/o. Stereotactically guided 11-g biopsy revealed cribriform and micropapillary DCIS, low grade.

TERMINOLOGY

Abbreviations and Synonyms
- Ductal carcinoma in situ (DCIS)

Definitions
- DCIS: Clonal proliferation of malignant epithelial cells with intact basement membrane
  - Single myoepithelial cell layer is retained, but can be discontinuous or focally absent
- "Low grade" DCIS refers to low nuclear grade and includes absence of necrosis
  - Monomorphous, small nuclei, no or very few mitoses
  - No or few apoptotic bodies, nuclei usually diploid
- Central necrosis: Cell death with nuclear fragments and necrotic debris in duct lumen
  - Comedocarcinoma: DCIS with central necrosis
  - Low grade DCIS lacks central necrosis = non-comedocarcinoma
- Nuclear grade may vary within any given DCIS lesion: Use highest grade
- Architectural subtypes: Cribriform, micropapillary, papillary, and solid

- Not of prognostic value
- Each can be seen in low, intermediate, and high grade DCIS

IMAGING FINDINGS

General Features
- Best diagnostic clue: Amorphous, granular, or indistinct microcalcifications (Ca++) on mammography
- Location: Terminal duct lobular unit (TDLU)

Mammographic Findings
- Microcalcifications in majority of low grade DCIS
  - Amorphous morphology most common: 20% malignant; 90% DCIS, usually low grade
  - Punctate morphology favors cribriform subtype
  - Fine linear Ca++: 18% in one series; favors high-grade DCIS
  - Clustered distribution most common
  - Regional distribution occasionally
  - Linear or segmental distribution most suspicious
- Circumscribed or slightly indistinctly-marginated oval mass ± Ca++ (uncommon)

DDx: Calcifications of Other Etiology

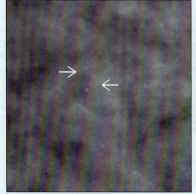

Fibrocystic Changes

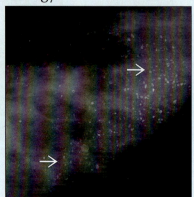

Sclerosing Adenosis

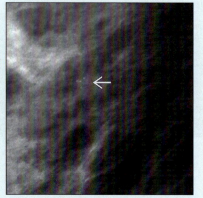

Lobular Neoplasia

DCIS, LOW GRADE

Key Facts

Terminology
- "Low grade" DCIS refers to low nuclear grade and includes absence of necrosis
- Architectural subtypes: Cribriform, micropapillary, papillary, and solid

Imaging Findings
- Best diagnostic clue: Amorphous, granular, or indistinct microcalcifications (Ca++) on mammography
- Magnification CC and 90° lateral views to characterize Ca++ morphology and extent

Top Differential Diagnoses
- Fibrocystic Changes (FCC)
- Atypical Ductal Hyperplasia (ADH)

- Atypical Lobular Hyperplasia (ALH) or Lobular Carcinoma in Situ (LCIS)
- High and Intermediate Grade DCIS
- Benign or Atypical Papilloma

Pathology
- 70-100% estrogen and progesterone receptor positive
- Pure micropapillary type frequently multifocal and multicentric
- ~ 13-20% of screen-detected DCIS is low grade

Clinical Issues
- Excellent cure rate if adequately treated

Diagnostic Checklist
- Stability of indeterminate or suspicious Ca++ should not dissuade from biopsy
- Review entire breast to determine extent of disease

- ○ Favors papillary DCIS
- Focal asymmetry ± Ca++ (uncommon)
- Galactography
  - ○ Used to evaluate nipple discharge
  - ○ Irregular filling defects
  - ○ Narrowing or abrupt cut-off of duct(s)

Ultrasonographic Findings
- Grayscale Ultrasound
  - ○ Usually occult on US
    - ■ Circumscribed or ill-defined hypoechoic mass, no posterior features ± echogenic Ca++
    - ■ Papillary DCIS can be intracystic or intraductal mass, rarely microlobulated with cystic areas
    - ■ Subtle Ca++ in duct(s) may be visible: Rare with low grade DCIS

MR Findings
- T2WI FS: Usually occult but may be hyperintense in ductal distribution
- T1 C+ FS
  - ○ Linear or ductal clumped enhancement most common; rarely mass
  - ○ May show delayed, persistent kinetics: Morphology helpful
  - ○ 88-90% accuracy for residual, multicentric disease
  - ○ Sensitivity for high-grade = that for low grade DCIS

Biopsy
- Diagnosis usually requires at least 2 duct profiles to meet criteria
- Undersampling problematic
  - ○ At least 10 samples of at least 11-g vacuum-biopsy for Ca++
  - ○ Specimen radiography to confirm Ca++ retrieval
  - ○ 18% of ADH on 11-g vacuum-assisted biopsy upgraded to malignancy, usually DCIS
  - ○ DCIS upgraded to invasive carcinoma: 11%

Imaging Recommendations
- Best imaging tool: Mammography
- Protocol advice

- ○ Magnification CC and 90° lateral views to characterize Ca++ morphology and extent
- ○ Entire breast should be carefully imaged
  - ■ Determine maximal span of suspicious Ca++
  - ■ Look for multifocal and multicentric disease

DIFFERENTIAL DIAGNOSIS

Fibrocystic Changes (FCC)
- Apocrine metaplasia, sclerosing adenosis: Amorphous, punctate Ca++
- Milk of calcium will layer on 90° lateral view
- Nodular adenosis can be circumscribed mass ± Ca++

Atypical Ductal Hyperplasia (ADH)
- Most often clustered amorphous Ca++
- Can be difficult to distinguish from DCIS at histopathology
  - ○ Nuclei & secondary spaces variable in size and shape, streaming of cells
  - ○ Often admixed with DCIS

Atypical Lobular Hyperplasia (ALH) or Lobular Carcinoma in Situ (LCIS)
- Amorphous Ca++ adjacent to or within
- Associated mass favors LCIS
- Both ALH & LCIS usually mammographically occult
- Cancerization of lobules by DCIS can mimic LCIS
  - ○ E-cadherin lost in lobular lesions

High and Intermediate Grade DCIS
- Fine linear or branching Ca++ favor high-grade DCIS
- Appearances frequently indistinguishable

Benign or Atypical Papilloma
- Circumscribed or indistinctly marginated mass
- May be intraductal
- Frequent cause of bloody or clear nipple discharge

DCIS, LOW GRADE

PATHOLOGY

General Features
- General path comments
  - Arises in TDLU and grows toward nipple in discontinuous (non-comedo) pattern
  - 70-100% estrogen and progesterone receptor positive
  - Pure micropapillary type frequently multifocal and multicentric
- Genetics: Often associated with 16q loss
- Epidemiology
  - ~ 13-20% of screen-detected DCIS is low grade
  - DCIS peak 40s-50s; low grade more variable
- Associated abnormalities
  - Invasive ductal carcinoma, usually low grade
    - Frequency increases with size of DCIS lesion
    - 10% risk with 10 mm area of punctate or amorphous Ca++; 20% when 11 mm or larger area
  - Frequently coexists with ADH, ALH

Microscopic Features
- Ca++ in duct lumen: Usually psammomatous type (calcium phosphate)
  - Excess production by tumor cells or from cell death
  - Ca++ frequently in both DCIS and FCC admixed
- Tends to form gland-like or papillary structures
- Subtypes based on architecture
  - Cribriform: Ca++ in punched out "cookie cutter" spaces in duct lumen
  - Micropapillary: Ca++ and mucin in lumen; papillary fronds
    - Cystic hypersecretory: Subtype, usually presents as large palpable mass
  - Papillary: In larger ducts; may present as circumscribed mass
  - Solid: May coexist with comedo-type DCIS
- Microinvasion uncommon

Staging, Grading or Classification Criteria
- Stage 0 when pure DCIS
- Stage 1 (T1mic): Associated microinvasion ≤ 1 mm

CLINICAL ISSUES

Presentation
- Most common signs/symptoms: Asymptomatic, screen-detected
- Other signs/symptoms
  - Spontaneous bloody or clear nipple discharge
  - Rare: Palpable lump
  - Rare: Paget disease of nipple

Natural History & Prognosis
- Excellent cure rate if adequately treated
- If untreated, 30-60% progress to invasive cancer over 10-30 years

Treatment
- Lumpectomy (breast-conserving surgery, BCS): Wide local excision with negative margins (at least 2 mm recommended, perhaps up to 1 cm or more)
- Radiation (XRT)

- No subcategory of patients in whom recurrence rates are not reduced by XRT
  - Even < 3 mm size lesion
  - Even with wide negative margins > 1 cm
- Mastectomy if patient not a candidate for BCS + XRT
  - Post-mastectomy XRT if margins close or positive
- Tamoxifen for estrogen receptor (ER)+ cases
  - Decreases risk of developing subsequent invasive or intraductal carcinoma
  - ± Aromatase inhibitors for post-menopausal women

DIAGNOSTIC CHECKLIST

Consider
- Stability of indeterminate or suspicious Ca++ should not dissuade from biopsy
- Histologic extent of disease underestimated on mammography by ≥ 2 cm in 15-20%, more likely in larger lesions and with micropapillary subtype

Image Interpretation Pearls
- Review entire breast to determine extent of disease

SELECTED REFERENCES

1. Wong JS et al: Prospective study of wide excision alone for ductal carcinoma in situ of the breast. J Clin Oncol. 24:1031-6, 2006
2. Menell JH et al: Determination of the presence and extent of pure ductal carcinoma in situ by mammography and magnetic resonance imaging. Breast J. 11(6):382-90, 2005
3. Khan A et al: Diagnosis and management of ductal carcinoma in situ. Curr Treat Options Oncol. 5(2):131-44, 2004
4. Kricker A et al: Ductal carcinoma in situ of the breast, a population-based study of epidemiology and pathology. Br J Cancer. 90(7):1382-5, 2004
5. Jaffer S et al: Histologic classification of ductal carcinoma in situ. Microsc Res Tech. 59(2):92-101, 2002
6. Kessar P et al: How significant is detection of ductal carcinoma in situ in a breast screening programme? Clin Radiol. 57(9):807-14, 2002
7. Berg WA et al: Biopsy of amorphous breast calcifications: pathologic outcome and yield at stereotactic biopsy. Radiology. 221:495-503, 2001
8. Feig SA: Ductal carcinoma in situ: implications for screening mammography. Radiol Clin N Amer. 38: 653-68, vii, 2000
9. Bonzanini M et al: Cytologic features of 22 radial scar/complex sclerosing lesions of the breast, three of which associated with carcinoma: clinical, mammographic, and histologic correlation. Diagn Cytopathol. 17(5):353-62, 1997
10. Holland R et al: Microcalcifications associated with ductal carcinoma in situ: mammographic-pathologic correlation. Semin Diagn Pathol. 11(3):181-92, 1994
11. Lev-Toaff AS et al: Stability of malignant breast microcalcifications. Radiology. 192:153-6, 1994
12. Bassett LW: Mammographic analysis of calcifications. Radiol Clin North Am. 30(1):93-105, 1992
13. Stomper PC et al: Ductal carcinoma in situ of the breast: Correlation between mammographic calcification and tumor subtype. AJR. 159:483-5, 1992

DCIS, LOW GRADE

IMAGE GALLERY

Typical

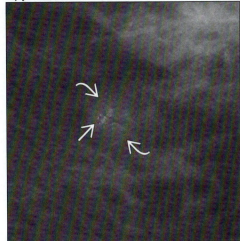 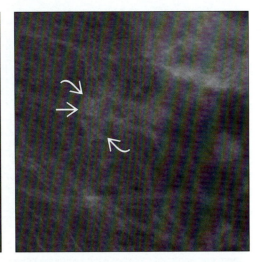

(Left) Lateral mammography magnification on a 78 y/o shows clustered amorphous calcifications ➜ with ill-defined associated soft tissue density ➜. (Right) MLO mammography from 5 years earlier (same patient as previous image), also shows asymmetry ➜ with associated amorphous Ca++ ➜. Despite the relative stability at 5 years, the findings were indeterminate. Stereotactically guided 11-g biopsy revealed low grade DCIS with Ca++.

Typical

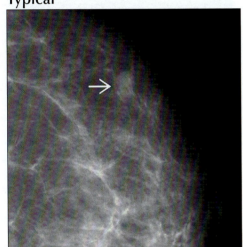 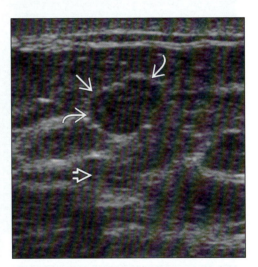

(Left) CC mammography of a 79 y/o shows a bilobed nodule ➜, enlarged compared to 2 years earlier; despite its benign appearance, additional evaluation is needed. (Right) Ultrasound (same patient as previous image) shows a bilobed mass ➜, with microlobulated margins ➜ and minimal posterior enhancement ➜. Biopsy showed solid and cribriform DCIS, low grade.

Typical

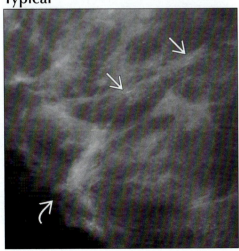 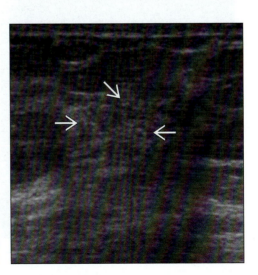

(Left) Lateral mammography magnification shows a spiculated mass ➜, and amorphous Ca++ ➜ in linear distribution over a 7 cm segment in this 74 y/o. US-guided biopsy of the primary mass revealed grade I invasive ductal carcinoma. (Right) Anti-radial ultrasound (same patient as previous image) directed to area of Ca++ shows subtle echogenic foci ➜, representing Ca++. Mastectomy revealed extensive micropapillary DCIS associated with Ca++.

DCIS, LOW GRADE

(Left) CC mammography magnification shows a subtle cluster of amorphous and pleomorphic Ca++ ➡, without associated mass, in a 50 y/o. **(Right)** Lateral mammography magnification (same patient as previous image) again shows subtle Ca++ ➡, without evidence of layering. These are of intermediate concern for malignancy, BI-RADS 4B. Core needle biopsy showed low grade, cribriform DCIS with Ca++.

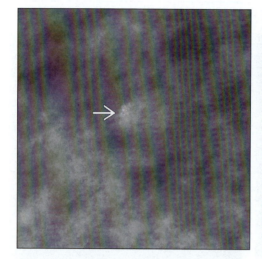
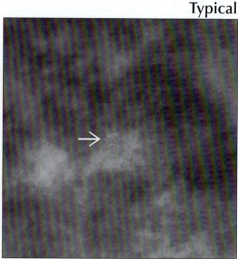

(Left) CC mammography close-up view of inner right breast in a 64 y/o shows heterogeneously dense parenchyma with diffuse, scattered, mostly punctate Ca++ ➡, unchanged from prior exams. **(Right)** CC mammography magnification of the outer right breast (same patient as previous image) shows a new cluster of suspicious fine linear calcifications and associated density ➡. Biopsy showed micropapillary DCIS, multiple positive margins.

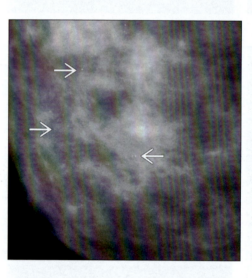
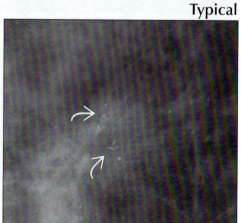

(Left) Axial MIP of T1 C+ subtraction MR (same patient as prior two images) to assess disease extent prior to definitive surgery, shows segmental clumped enhancement over 11 cm ➡, compatible with DCIS. **(Right)** Radial ultrasound (same case as prior 3 images) shows small hypoechoic masses ➡ with Ca++ ➡ and posterior shadowing ➡ in corresponding distribution. Mastectomy confirmed extensive micropapillary DCIS.

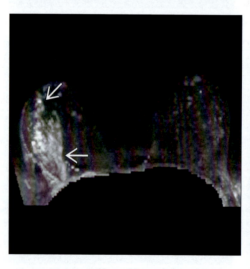
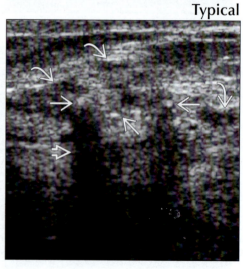

IV

2

112

DCIS, LOW GRADE

Typical

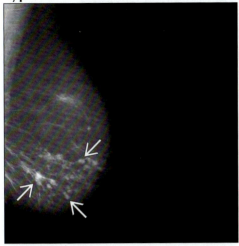

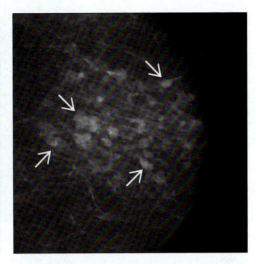

(Left) MLO mammography of a 75 y/o illustrates an unusual manifestation of DCIS. Compared to older studies, there was gradual increase in segmentally arranged small masses ➡. *(Right)* CC mammography (same patient as previous image) better demonstrates these masses ➡, which proved to be ductal dilatation secondary to extensive DCIS, low grade, cribriform, solid and micropapillary types. Patient is disease free 6 years after total mastectomy.

Typical

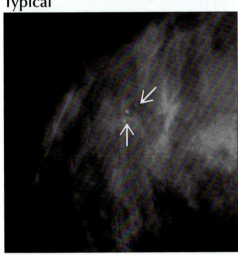

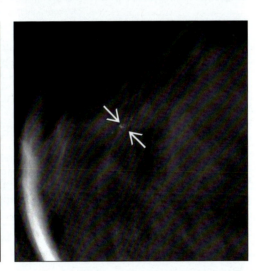

(Left) CC mammography magnification on a 49 y/o shows clustered punctate and amorphous Ca++ ➡ without associated mass. Core biopsy revealed invasive ductal carcinoma and low grade cribriform & solid DCIS. *(Right)* Lateral mammography spot compression (same patient as previous image) confirms Ca++ ➡ without visible mass. This case illustrates the frequent association of low grade DCIS with invasive carcinoma.

Typical

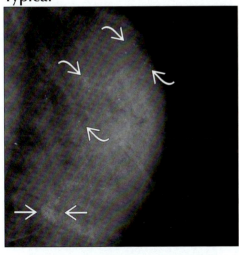

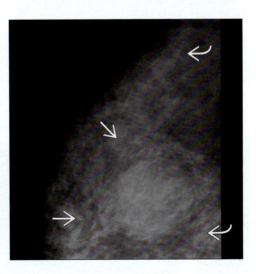

(Left) MLO mammography magnification of a 41 y/o shows clustered amorphous Ca++ ➡ at site of lump, & scattered punctate Ca++ ➡. Invasive carcinoma with positive margins found at lumpectomy. Mastectomy showed low grade cribriform & solid DCIS. *(Right)* CC mammography screening of a 48 y/o shows importance of assessing extent of disease. Clustered Ca++ span lateral half of breast ➡ ➡. Core biopsy of two disparate groups ➡ showed low grade DCIS.

DCIS, INTERMEDIATE GRADE

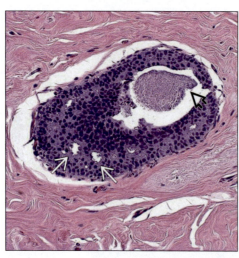

Micropathology, low power, H&E shows intermediate nuclear grade DCIS, predominantly solid type with a few punched out areas ➡ of cribriform type, and focal necrosis ⇥.

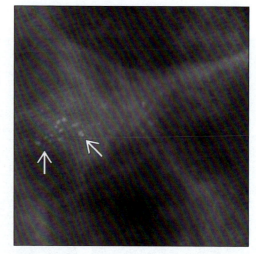

Lateral mammography magnification shows new clustered pleomorphic Ca++ ➡ with associated density, BI-RADS 5. Core biopsy and excision revealed intermediate grade DCIS, concordant with imaging.

TERMINOLOGY

Definitions
- Intraductal carcinoma composed of low nuclear grade cells, with focal areas of necrosis (not central necrosis)
- Low- and intermediate-grade DCIS are both noncomedocarcinoma

IMAGING FINDINGS

General Features
- Best diagnostic clue: Microcalcifications (Ca++) on mammography

Mammographic Findings
- Ca++: Amorphous, pleomorphic
  ○ Fine linear morphology favors high-grade DCIS
- Ca++ may be present in only part of the DCIS
- ± Associated mass or asymmetry uncommon, suggests invasive component

Ultrasonographic Findings
- Grayscale Ultrasound

○ Low-, intermediate-grade DCIS often occult on US
○ Less likely to see Ca++ than with high-grade DCIS
○ Occasionally manifests as hypoechoic mass

MR Findings
- T1 C+
  ○ MRI most sensitive imaging tool for diagnosing DCIS
    ▪ Linear or ductal clumped enhancement in majority
    ▪ Morphology more reliable than kinetics
    ▪ May appear as irregular mass (uncommon)

Biopsy
- For Ca++, favor initial diagnosis by stereotactic biopsy
  ○ ≥ 10 specimens, ≥ 11-g vacuum-assisted most reliable
  ○ 11% of such biopsies showing DCIS upgraded to invasive carcinoma at excision
  ○ Few upgrades if all mammographic evidence of lesion removed
- US-guided core biopsy if visible under US
- Needle localization and excision of suspicious Ca++ or after percutaneous biopsy

DDx: Similar Calcifications, Varied Etiology

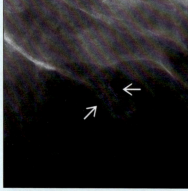

Severe Atypical Duct Hyperplasia

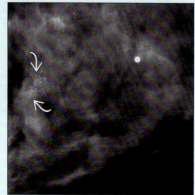

High-Grade DCIS

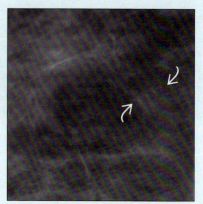

Flat Epithelial Atypia

DCIS, INTERMEDIATE GRADE

Key Facts

Terminology
- Intraductal carcinoma composed of low nuclear grade cells, with focal areas of necrosis (not central necrosis)

Imaging Findings
- Best diagnostic clue: Microcalcifications (Ca++) on mammography
- Ca++ may be present in only part of the DCIS
- MRI most sensitive imaging tool for diagnosing DCIS

Top Differential Diagnoses
- High-Grade and Low-Grade DCIS
- Invasive Ductal Carcinoma (NOS)
- Atypical Duct Hyperplasia (ADH)
- Atypical Lobular Hyperplasia (ALH), Lobular Carcinoma in Situ (LCIS)

- Fibrocystic Changes (FCC)
- Fibroadenoma
- Columnar Cell Lesions

Pathology
- Often admixed with other grades of DCIS: Default to highest grade present

Clinical Issues
- DCIS progresses to invasive cancer in 30-50%
- Van Nuys Prognostic Index: Nuclear grade and necrosis, extent of disease, surgical margins
- Excellent cure rate if adequately treated

Diagnostic Checklist
- Biopsy indeterminate or suspicious Ca++ despite stability
- Magnification views to determine extent of disease

- Bracket needle localization if lumpectomy planned, malignant Ca++ > 2 cm span
- Specimen radiography routinely used for all biopsies of Ca++
  - Confirm sampling ± excision of Ca++

Imaging Recommendations
- Best imaging tool
  - Mammography with CC and 90° lateral magnification views
    - Maximal span of the Ca++ should be reported
    - Entire breast should be examined for multifocality, multicentricity
- Protocol advice: Biopsy suspicious Ca++ regardless of stability
- Extent of Ca++ may underestimate extent of DCIS
  - Low- and intermediate-grade DCIS extent underestimated by ≥ 2 cm: 50% of cases
  - ↑ Underestimation with ↑ lesion size
- Post-operative mammogram post lumpectomy if large area malignant Ca++ resected
  - Assess for residual suspicious Ca++

DIFFERENTIAL DIAGNOSIS

High-Grade and Low-Grade DCIS
- Ca++ morphology and distribution not specific
  - Cannot reliably differentiate histologic findings of DCIS subtypes

Invasive Ductal Carcinoma (NOS)
- More often irregular mass ± Ca++
- Ca++ uncommon in lobular carcinoma

Atypical Duct Hyperplasia (ADH)
- Quantitative and qualitative microscopic differences

Atypical Lobular Hyperplasia (ALH), Lobular Carcinoma in Situ (LCIS)
- Typically mammographically occult
  - May be adjacent to or demonstrate amorphous Ca++
- Duct extension of LCIS can mimic DCIS

- Cancerization of lobules by DCIS can mimic LCIS
- E-cadherin lost in lobular lesions; retained in DCIS

Fibrocystic Changes (FCC)
- Amorphous or pleomorphic Ca++

Fibroadenoma
- Indeterminate Ca++ ± mass
- Early: Pleomorphic or amorphous Ca++

Columnar Cell Lesions
- Round or punctate Ca++
- Flat epithelial atypia likely a precursor of DCIS

PATHOLOGY

General Features
- General path comments
  - Pathologic classification of DCIS evolving
  - Considered intermediate grade
    - Cribriform, solid or papillary with necrosis
    - Lacks nuclear anaplasia of comedocarcinoma
  - Micropapillary subtype often multicentric
  - Embryology-anatomy
    - Arises in terminal duct lobular unit (TDLU)
    - Grows in ducts toward nipple in a discontinuous (noncomedo) pattern: Skip areas typically < 1 mm
- Epidemiology: Diagnosed more frequently due to mammographic screening
- Associated abnormalities
  - Often admixed with other grades of DCIS: Default to highest grade present
  - Microinvasion: Disruption of basement membrane by nest(s) of tumor cells
    - No nest > 1 mm
  - Often coexists with invasive carcinoma, usually invasive ductal NOS grade II
    - More common with ↑ size area of DCIS
  - Can be admixed with LCIS

Microscopic Features
- Intermediate nuclear grade usually with focal necrosis
- Often a mixture of architectural types

- ○ Solid: Small foci of necrosis
- ○ Cribriform: Proliferation with fenestrated pattern
- ○ Papillary: May present as palpable mass
- ○ Rare subtypes of low- to intermediate-nuclear grade
  - ▪ Spindle cell; clear cell
- ○ Rare subtypes of intermediate- to high-nuclear grade
  - ▪ Apocrine; signet ring
- ○ 80-88% estrogen receptor (ER)+

Staging, Grading or Classification Criteria

- Tis: Stage 0, DCIS
- T1mic: ≤ 1 mm microinvasion, stage I

CLINICAL ISSUES

Presentation

- Asymptomatic in majority: Ca++ on mammography most common
- Palpable breast lump rare: Micropapillary most common
- Paget disease or (bloody) nipple discharge

Demographics

- Age: Peak age late 40s

Natural History & Prognosis

- DCIS progresses to invasive cancer in 30-50%
- DCIS may persist for years before becoming invasive
- Van Nuys Prognostic Index: Nuclear grade and necrosis, extent of disease, surgical margins
  - ○ Higher score predicts ↑ recurrence risk with or without radiation therapy (XRT)
  - ○ ↑ Risk recurrence with close (< 2mm) or positive margins
- Post-conservation surveillance is important
  - ○ ~ 50% recurrences are invasive

Treatment

- Lumpectomy: Wide local excision with clear margins
  - ○ Clear margins: At least 2 mm, possibly up to 10 mm for DCIS
- XRT following surgical treatment
  - ○ No subgroup for which risk of recurrence not reduced post lumpectomy
  - ○ No survival benefit demonstrated
  - ○ > Age 70, low risk, mortality from other causes may render small ↓ risk of recurrence irrelevant
  - ○ Post-mastectomy XRT for close or positive margins
- Mastectomy
  - ○ > 5 cm DCIS ± poor cosmesis anticipated from lumpectomy
  - ○ Multicentric disease
- Sentinel lymph node biopsy in select cases
  - ○ Consider when extent > 2.5 cm
  - ○ Suspected or proven microinvasion
  - ○ Mastectomy being performed due to extent of disease
- Tamoxifen (TAM) if ER+
  - ○ 50% ↓ risk of subsequent invasive cancer
  - ○ Aromatase inhibitors for post-menopausal women
    - ▪ Often used sequentially after 2-3 years TAM
- Excellent cure rate if adequately treated
- Less favorable prognosis when

- ○ Positive surgical margin(s)
- ○ Large lesion size

DIAGNOSTIC CHECKLIST

Consider

- Biopsy indeterminate or suspicious Ca++ despite stability

Image Interpretation Pearls

- Magnification views to determine extent of disease

SELECTED REFERENCES

1. Collins LC et al: Outcome of patients with ductal carcinoma in situ untreated after diagnostic biopsy: results from the Nurses' Health Study. Cancer. 103(9):1778-84, 2005
2. Hwang ES et al: Patterns of chromosomal alterations in breast ductal carcinoma in situ. Clin Cancer Res. 10(15):5160-7, 2004
3. Silverstein MJ et al: Ductal carcinoma in situ: USC/Van Nuys Prognostic Index and the impact of margin status. Breast. 12(6):457-71, 2003
4. Bonnett M et al: Histologic and radiographic analysis of ductal carcinoma in situ diagnosed using stereotactic incisional core breast biopsy. Mod Pathol. 15(2):95-101, 2002
5. Cserni G: Sentinel lymph node biopsy as a tool for the staging of ductal carcinoma in situ in patients with breast carcinoma. Surg Today. 32(2):99-103, 2002
6. Jaffer S et al: Histologic classification of ductal carcinoma in situ. Microsc Res Tech. 59(2):92-101, 2002
7. Kessar P et al: How significant is detection of ductal carcinoma in situ in a breast screening programme? Clin Radiol. 57(9):807-14, 2002
8. Morrow M et al: Standard for the management of ductal carcinoma in situ of the breast (DCIS). CA Cancer J Clin. 52(5):256-76, 2002
9. Evans AJ et al: Screen detected ductal carcinoma in situ (DCIS): overdiagnosis or an obligate precursor of invasive disease? J Med Screen. 8(3):149-51, 2001
10. Farshid G et al: Spindle cell ductal carcinoma in situ. An unusual variant of ductal intra-epithelial neoplasia that simulates ductal hyperplasia or a myoepithelial proliferation. Virchows Arch. 439(1):70-7, 2001
11. Leal C et al: Apocrine ductal carcinoma in situ of the breast: histologic classification and expression of biologic markers. Hum Pathol. 32(5):487-93, 2001
12. Renshaw AA et al: Atypical ductal hyperplasia in breast core needle biopsies. Correlation of size of the lesion, complete removal of the lesion, and the incidence of carcinoma in follow-up biopsies. Am J Clin Pathol. 116(1):92-6, 2001
13. Slanetz PJ et al: Mammographic appearance of ductal carcinoma in situ does not reliably predict histologic subtype. Breast J. 7(6):417-21, 2001
14. Wahedna Y et al: Mammographic size of ductal carcinoma in situ does not predict the presence of an invasive focus. Eur J Cancer. 37(4):459-62, 2001
15. Goldstein NS et al: Differences in the pathologic features of ductal carcinoma in situ of the breast based on patient age. Cancer. 88(11):2553-60, 2000
16. Stomper PC et al: Flow cytometric DNA analysis of specimen mammography-guided fine-needle aspirates of ductal carcinoma in situ. J Exp Clin Cancer Res. 19(3):309-15, 2000

DCIS, INTERMEDIATE GRADE

IMAGE GALLERY

Typical

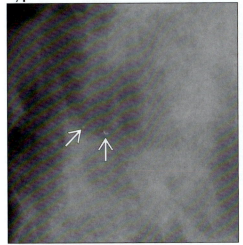
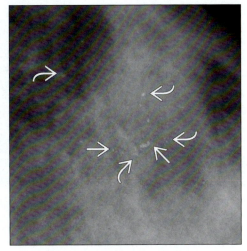

(Left) CC mammography magnification shows a few punctate and coarse Ca++ in a linear distribution ➡ in a 56 y/o. *(Right)* Lateral mammography magnification 6 months later (same patient as previous image) shows the original group ➡ as well as scattered new punctate and linear Ca++ ➡. Core biopsy (and mastectomy) showed intermediate grade DCIS with central necrosis and Ca++.

Typical

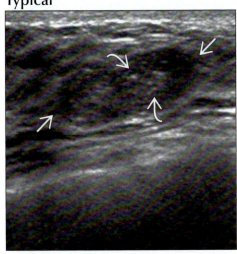
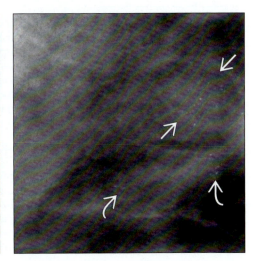

(Left) Ultrasound in an area of palpable lump in a 33 y/o shows circumscribed hypoechoic mass ➡ containing echogenic foci ➡ representing Ca++, seen on mammogram in next image. *(Right)* MLO mammography close-up (same patient as previous image) shows clustered, mildly pleomorphic Ca++ in area of mass ➡, and in adjacent tissue ➡. Core needle biopsy of the mass showed intermediate-grade DCIS.

Typical

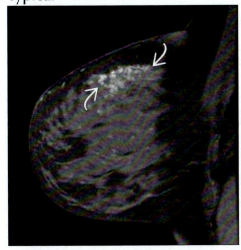
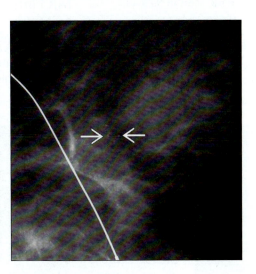

(Left) Sagittal T1 C+ FS MR in a high-risk 50 y/o shows clumped enhancement in a 6 cm area ➡. There were no corresponding Ca++ on mammography. MR-directed excisional biopsy showed intermediate-grade DCIS. *(Right)* CC mammography (same patient as previous image) shows a cluster of punctate Ca++ ➡ in lower outer ipsilateral breast. Wire localization & excision showed benign columnar cell change, adjacent LCIS & ALH.

DCIS, HIGH GRADE

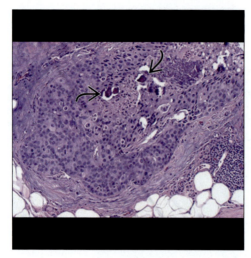

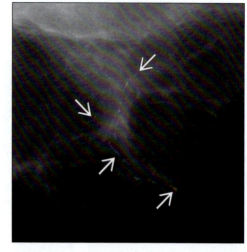

Micropathology, high power, illustrates the typical appearance of high nuclear grade DCIS, with associated calcifications ⇗ in areas of necrosis.

CC mammography magnification of a 70 y/o shows fine linear Ca++ in a linear distribution ➜ suggesting filling of a duct and its branches. Biopsy showed high-grade DCIS with comedonecrosis.

TERMINOLOGY

Abbreviations and Synonyms
- Poorly differentiated ductal carcinoma in situ, high-grade DCIS, comedocarcinoma

Definitions
- Pathologic diagnosis based on cytologic criteria
  - Pleomorphic nuclei 2.5-3x the size of a red blood cell (> 15 microns)
  - Central necrosis in duct lumens (comedonecrosis) almost universal, not required

IMAGING FINDINGS

General Features
- Best diagnostic clue
  - Calcifications (Ca++): Hallmark, seen in 94% of comedo DCIS
    - Classic: Exuberant fine linear & branching Ca++
  - Accounts for 75-80% DCIS detected as Ca++ on mammography

Mammographic Findings
- Fine linear-branching = casting Ca++
- Other morphologies: Pleomorphic, coarse heterogeneous, uncommonly amorphous
- Distribution often reflects duct (linear) or ductal segment (segmental)
- Associated irregular mass or asymmetry: Suspicious for invasive component

Ultrasonographic Findings
- Grayscale Ultrasound
  - Echogenic intraductal Ca++ may be visible
    - Thick, hypoechoic duct walls
  - Generalized hypoechoic irregular tissue
  - Identification of associated mass favors invasive component
  - Visualization allows US-guided core biopsy

MR Findings
- T1 C+
  - MR sensitivity ~ 88%, including non-calcified DCIS
  - Clumped linear or ductal enhancement
  - Mass enhancement less common
  - Morphology more reliable than kinetics

DDx: Calcifications of Other Etiologies

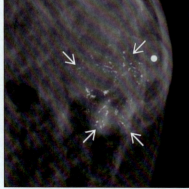

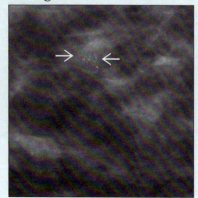

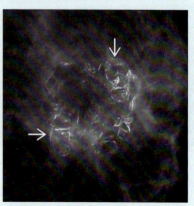

Invasive Ductal Carcinoma

Lobular Carcinoma In Situ

Fat Necrosis

DCIS, HIGH GRADE

Key Facts

Terminology
- Poorly differentiated ductal carcinoma in situ, high-grade DCIS, comedocarcinoma

Imaging Findings
- Calcifications (Ca++): Hallmark, seen in 94% of comedo DCIS
- Fine linear-branching = casting Ca++
- Distribution often reflects duct (linear) or ductal segment (segmental)
- Associated irregular mass or asymmetry: Suspicious for invasive component
- MR sensitivity ~ 88%, including non-calcified DCIS
- Mammography with CC and 90° lateral magnification views for suspicious Ca++
- Mammography estimates lesion size more reliably than for intermediate or low grade DCIS

Top Differential Diagnoses
- Invasive Carcinoma
- Low and Intermediate Grade DCIS
- Atypical Duct Hyperplasia
- Sclerosing Adenosis
- Columnar Cell Lesions
- Fibroadenoma

Clinical Issues
- < 10%: Palpable mass or bloody nipple discharge
- Van Nuys prognostic index: Probability of recurrence with & without XRT, based on 3 features

---

  - No more or less likely to exhibit enhancement than low or intermediate grade DCIS

Biopsy
- US: Target mass component, more likely invasive
  - Automated core biopsy sufficient for masses
- Stereotactic: ≥ 11-g vacuum-assisted biopsy, ≥ 10 samples, more accurate for Ca++
  - Can be sampled under US guidance if visible
  - Specimen radiograph to confirm Ca++ retrieval
  - 11% of DCIS upgraded to invasive carcinoma
- If multiple areas of suspicious Ca++, sample areas farthest apart to prove extent pre-operatively
- Bracket needle localization if lumpectomy planned, > 2 cm span of nonpalpable disease

Imaging Recommendations
- Best imaging tool
  - Mammography with CC and 90° lateral magnification views for suspicious Ca++
    - Maximal extent of Ca++ should be reported
- Mammography estimates lesion size more reliably than for intermediate or low grade DCIS
- Post-operative mammogram if large area of malignant Ca++ resected: Assess for residual suspicious Ca++ prior to radiation therapy (XRT)

DIFFERENTIAL DIAGNOSIS

Invasive Carcinoma
- Ca++ most often associated with ductal carcinoma

Low and Intermediate Grade DCIS
- Ca++ morphology and distribution not specific, cannot reliably distinguish histologic DCIS subtypes

Atypical Duct Hyperplasia
- Quantitative and qualitative microscopic differences

Sclerosing Adenosis
- Punctate, amorphous Ca++ ± oval mass

Columnar Cell Lesions
- Punctate or round Ca++; often incidental at pathology

Fibroadenoma
- Early: Pleomorphic or amorphous Ca++ ± mass

PATHOLOGY

General Features
- General path comments
  - Pathologic classification of DCIS evolving; based on architecture and nuclear cytology
  - Presence or absence of necrosis & architecture can be considered
    - Comedocarcinoma usually high grade
    - Papillary infrequently high grade
    - Cribriform and micropapillary rarely high grade
    - Apocrine DCIS: Cytoplasm maybe granular, eosinophilic or vacuolated and clear
    - Signet ring DCIS: Eccentric nuclei pushed aside by mucin vacuole
- Genetics
  - Associated with loss on 8p chromosome
  - Allelic imbalance on BRCA-1 gene, chromosome 17q12-23
  - Allelic loss at FHIT and ATM genes
- Epidemiology
  - ↑ Detection due to mammographic screening
  - Age: 5-10 years younger than for invasive carcinoma
  - High grade, necrosis, & microinvasion favor younger age
- Associated abnormalities: Coexisting invasive carcinoma in ~ 50% cases of DCIS > 2.5 cm

Gross Pathologic & Surgical Features
- Extensive comedo type DCIS: Granular character, pale yellow foci of necrotic debris exuding from ducts = "comedones"

Microscopic Features
- Luminal necrosis almost universal

DCIS, HIGH GRADE

- Tumor cells have high nuclear grade & extensive necrosis
- Large pleomorphic nuclei with clumped chromatin
- Enlarged nucleoli
- Abnormal mitotic figures common
- Can → cancerization lobules, mimic lobular carcinoma in situ (LCIS)
  - E-cadherin retained in DCIS, lost in LCIS
- Immunohistochemistry: 57-64% estrogen receptor (ER)+

Staging, Grading or Classification Criteria
- Stage 0 when pure DCIS
- Stage 1 (T1mic): Associated microinvasion ≤ 1 mm

CLINICAL ISSUES

Presentation
- Asymptomatic: Ca++ on mammography most common
- < 10%: Palpable mass or bloody nipple discharge
- Uncommon: Paget disease of nipple

Demographics
- Age: Younger than invasive carcinoma and low grade DCIS

Natural History & Prognosis
- Majority of high-grade DCIS progresses to invasion
- Excellent cure rate if adequately treated
- Axillary metastases seen in ~ 2% cases of pure DCIS
- Distant metastases develop in ~ 2% cases, despite appropriate treatment
- Most likely type of DCIS to recur
  - Close (< 2 mm) or positive margins ↑ risk of recurrence
  - Time to recurrence directly related to nuclear grade
  - > 50% of recurrence is invasive carcinoma
- Other factors which lead to less favorable prognosis
  - Degree of necrosis
  - Age < 50 years, positive family history
- Van Nuys prognostic index: Probability of recurrence with & without XRT, based on 3 features
  - Histology (nuclear grade & necrosis), tumor size, and margin status; higher score → worse prognosis

Treatment
- Treatment based on assessment of
  - Histologic grade
  - Margin status
  - Extent of disease
- Lumpectomy: Wide local excision with negative margins
- Radiation therapy (XRT)
- Mastectomy may be recommended in case of
  - Multicentric disease
  - Extensive high grade DCIS
- Tamoxifen for ER+ tumors
- Sentinel lymph node biopsy
  - Consider if disease > 2.5 cm or mastectomy planned

DIAGNOSTIC CHECKLIST

Consider
- Tends to have contiguous growth pattern: Mammographically separated areas of Ca++ often prove to be contiguous disease

Image Interpretation Pearls
- Fine linear, branching Ca++ typically high grade DCIS
- Search for associated mass, suggests invasive component: US can be helpful, guide biopsy

SELECTED REFERENCES

1. Collins LC et al: Outcome of patients with ductal carcinoma in situ untreated after diagnostic biopsy: results from the Nurses' Health Study. Cancer. 103(9):1778-84, 2005
2. Groves AM et al: Characterization of pure high-grade DCIS on magnetic resonance imaging using the evolving breast MR lexicon terminology: can it be differentiated from pure invasive disease? Magn Reson Imaging. 23(6):733-8, 2005
3. Burstein HJ et al: Ductal carcinoma in situ of the breast. N Engl J Med. 350(14):1430-41, 2004
4. De Roos MA et al: Correlation between imaging and pathology in ductal carcinoma in situ of the breast. World J Surg Oncol. 2(1):4, 2004
5. Kricker A et al: Ductal carcinoma in situ of the breast, a population-based study of epidemiology and pathology. Br J Cancer. 90(7):1382-5, 2004
6. Neubauer H et al: High grade and non-high grade ductal carcinoma in situ on dynamic MR mammography: characteristic findings for signal increase and morphological pattern of enhancement. Br J Radiol. 76(901):3-12, 2003
7. Silverstein MJ et al: Ductal carcinoma in situ: USC/Van Nuys Prognostic Index and the impact of margin status. Breast. 12(6):457-71, 2003
8. Jaffer S et al: Histologic classification of ductal carcinoma in situ. Microsc Res Tech. 59(2):92-101, 2002
9. Kessar P et al: How significant is detection of ductal carcinoma in situ in a breast screening programme? Clin Radiol. 57(9):807-14, 2002
10. Kothari AS et al: Paget disease of the nipple: a multifocal manifestation of higher-risk disease. Cancer. 95(1):1-7, 2002
11. Moon WK et al: Multifocal, multicentric, and contralateral breast cancers: Bilateral whole-breast US in the preoperative evaluation of patients. Radiology 224(2):569-76, 2002
12. Evans AJ et al: Screen detected ductal carcinoma in situ (DCIS): overdiagnosis or an obligate precursor of invasive disease? J Med Screen. 8(3):149-51, 2001
13. Viehweg P et al: In situ and minimally invasive breast cancer: morphologic and kinetic features on contrast-enhanced MR imaging. MAGMA. 11(3):129-37, 2000
14. Hetelekidis S et al: Predictors of local recurrence following excision alone for ductal carcinoma in situ. Cancer. 85(2):427-31, 1999
15. Lagios MD et al: Ductal carcinoma in situ. The success of breast conservation therapy: a shared experience of two single institutional nonrandomized prospective studies. Surg Oncol Clin N Am. 6(2):385-92, 1997
16. Holland et al: Extent, distribution and mammographic/histological correlations of breast ductal carcinoma in situ. Lancet 335:519-22, 1990

DCIS, HIGH GRADE

IMAGE GALLERY

Typical

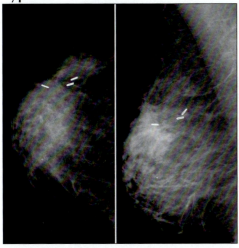
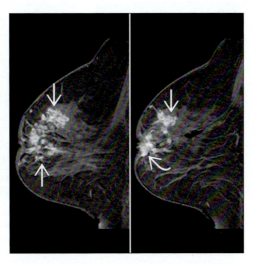

(Left) CC (left) and MLO (right) mammographic views of this 53 y/o with history of high-grade DCIS 5 years previously, showed no change or new abnormality. Patient reported new nipple retraction. *(Right)* Sagittal T1 C+ FS MR (same patient as previous image), shows large irregular region of clumped and mass-like enhancement ➜ on two contiguous slices, also involving the nipple and subareolar tissues ➜. Biopsy revealed recurrence as invasive ductal carcinoma.

Typical

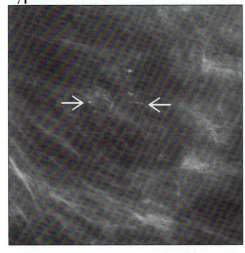
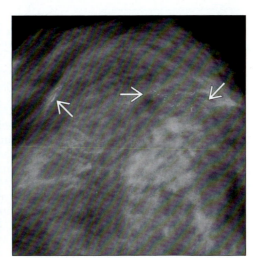

(Left) Lateral mammography magnification shows new fine linear, casting Ca++ ➜ in 58 y/o who had lumpectomy & XRT for ipsilateral invasive and in situ carcinoma 4 years ago. Biopsy showed high-grade DCIS with microinvasion. *(Right)* Mammography close-up view of a 46 y/o patient shows new pleomorphic Ca++ in linear branching distribution ➜. Stereotactic 11-g biopsy showed high-grade DCIS, cribriform & solid, confirmed on excision.

Typical

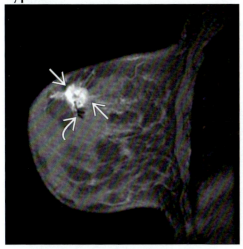
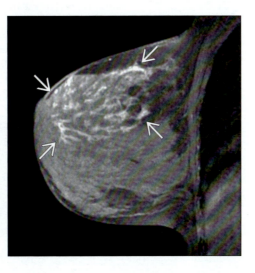

(Left) Sagittal T1 C+ FS MR on a 31 y/o with lump shows a corresponding 2 cm spiculated, rapidly enhancing mass ➜. Core biopsy, performed before MR (clip artifact: ➜) showed invasive carcinoma. *(Right)* Another image of the same patient, same series, same breast, shows extensive linear branching enhancement ➜ over a 10 cm area. On mastectomy this was high grade DCIS, comedo, cribriform, solid & micropapillary types.

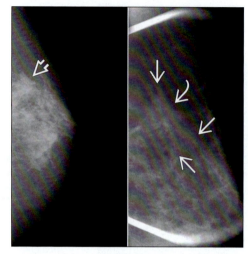

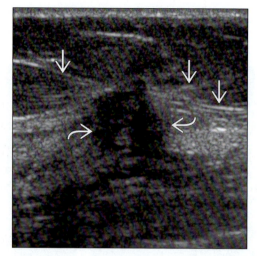

CC mammography (left side) in a 60 y/o woman shows an area of focal distortion laterally ➵, which on spot compression (right side) shows a central mass ➵ with spiculated margins ➵.

US (same case as left image) shows a highly suspicious irregular, hypoechoic mass ➵ with tethering of Cooper ligaments (distortion) ➵. IDC NOS at core biopsy.

TERMINOLOGY

Abbreviations and Synonyms
- Not otherwise specified (NOS): No special type (NST)
- Invasive ductal carcinoma (IDC), scirrhous carcinoma
- Ductal carcinoma in situ (DCIS): Intraduct carcinoma

Definitions
- Invasive (infiltrating): Extension of tumor cells through basement membrane
- "Ductal": Implies cellular origin from ductal epithelium, vs. "lobular" from breast lobules
  - Current concept: All breast carcinomas arise from terminal ductal lobular unit (TDLU)
- When IDC does not fit any defined subtype
  - Special types: Medullary, mucinous, tubular etc. should comprise ≥ 90% of tumor

IMAGING FINDINGS

General Features
- Best diagnostic clue: Spiculated mass
- Location

  - Anywhere in breast parenchyma
  - Also rarely in axilla, ectopic, supernumerary or accessory breast
- Size: 0.5-5 cm usually; range 0.3-15 cm
- Morphology: Typically irregular mass with spiculated or microlobulated margins

Mammographic Findings
- Classic: Dense mass with spiculated margins
- Focal asymmetric density ± distortion
- ± Associated calcifications (Ca++): Benign, indeterminate or malignant-appearing
- Less common findings
  - New or enlarging density or mass and/or Ca++
  - Diffuse increased density, thickening of Cooper ligaments ± skin thickening
  - Circumscribed oval or rounded mass (rare)

Ultrasonographic Findings
- Grayscale Ultrasound
  - Irregular hypoechoic shadowing mass
  - Taller-than-wide or (more often) parallel to skin
  - Architectural distortion; may have echogenic halo
  - Rarely: Circumscribed, rounded, hypo- to anechoic with posterior enhancement

---

DDx: Irregular Masses Mimicking IDC

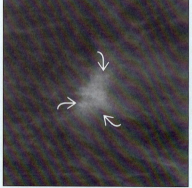

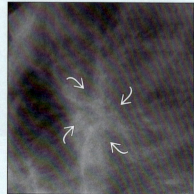

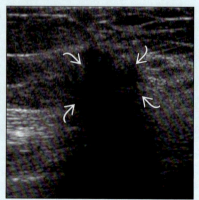

Invasive Lobular Carcinoma

Radial Scar

Paraffin Granuloma

INFILTRATING DUCTAL NOS, GENERAL

Key Facts

Terminology
- Not otherwise specified (NOS): No special type (NST)
- When IDC does not fit any defined subtype

Imaging Findings
- Anywhere in breast parenchyma
- Classic: Dense mass with spiculated margins
- Focal asymmetric density ± distortion
- Perform presurgical core biopsy for histologic confirmation

Top Differential Diagnoses
- Fibroadenoma, fat necrosis, scar
- Abscess, granuloma, or inflammatory lesion
- Radial scar/radial sclerosing lesion
- Special types of invasive ductal carcinoma
- Invasive lobular carcinoma

Pathology
- 65-80% of all breast cancers
- Genetics: ~ 90% sporadic, ~ 10% genetic (BRCA)
- Most common in women over 40 y/o

Clinical Issues
- Palpable thickening or firm lump
- Abnormality on screening mammogram
- < 40 y/o, suspect familial cancer ± BRCA mutation
- Rare < age 30, ↑ incidence with ↑ age in Western industrialized countries
- Staging & 5 yr survival: I: 90%, II: 70%, III: 50%, IV: 20%
- Breast conservation surgery (lumpectomy) with adjuvant radiation standard for most cases
- Mastectomy for large tumor, multicentric or extensive (> 1 quadrant) disease

---

- Color Doppler: Hypervascular with penetrating vessels

MR Findings
- T2WI FS: Usually hypointense focal mass if visible
- T1 C+ FS
  - ~ 90% Of IDC NOS enhance rapidly and intensely
    - May have rim-enhancement, internal enhancing septations, washout after 5-10 minutes
    - Densely fibrotic IDC may enhance slowly, weakly
- MRS: Elevated choline peak may be present

Nuclear Medicine Findings
- PET
  - Whole body FDG PET: Insensitive to tumors < 2 cm
    - Assess metastases, local recurrence, treatment response
  - Dedicated FDG PET devices with compression: 89% sensitivity for IDC, median size 21 mm
- Tc-99m-sestamibi or tetrofosmin scintimammography
  - Results similar to PET; dedicated devices available

Imaging Recommendations
- Best imaging tool
  - Mammography mainstay of screening
    - Of IDC in dense breasts, > 50% occult
  - Ultrasound for masses, guide biopsy
- Protocol advice
  - Perform presurgical core biopsy for histologic confirmation
  - Perform mammography for overview
    - Extent of Ca++ important for surgical planning, esp. extensive intraductal component (EIC): Magnification views
    - Detection of multifocal and bilateral disease
  - US for lesion characterization, biopsy guidance
    - High yield: Scan quadrant for multifocal disease
    - Identify, guide aspiration/biopsy of suspicious axillary node(s): Known metastatic node pre-operatively → direct axillary node dissection
    - Can scan bilateral breasts for extent (esp. if dense)
  - T1 C+ FS MR ideal for mapping disease extent; risk of false positives

DIFFERENTIAL DIAGNOSIS

Benign Lesions
- Fibroadenoma, fat necrosis, scar
- Abscess, granuloma, or inflammatory lesion

High-Risk Lesions
- Radial scar/radial sclerosing lesion
- Lobular carcinoma in situ (LCIS) on MR, US

Other Malignancies
- Special types of invasive ductal carcinoma
- Invasive lobular carcinoma
- Metastases

PATHOLOGY

General Features
- General path comments
  - 65-80% of all breast cancers
  - Marked fibrosis and cicatrization common
- Genetics: ~ 90% sporadic, ~ 10% genetic (BRCA)
- Etiology
  - Unknown in most cases
  - Radiation exposure (esp. mantle radiation for Hodgkin lymphoma)
  - Strong family history, BRCA mutation
- Epidemiology
  - Most common in women over 40 y/o
  - Incidence varies between countries, races

Gross Pathologic & Surgical Features
- Gritty, hard whitish irregular shaped mass

Microscopic Features
- About one-third contain small foci of specific IDC subtypes, e.g., tubular, medullary, papillary, mucinous
- 6% combined with infiltrating lobular carcinoma

Staging, Grading or Classification Criteria
- TNM staging
  - T (tumor size): Applies to largest mass if > 1 tumor

- TX: Primary tumor cannot be assessed
- T0: No evidence of primary tumor
- T1: Tumor ≤ 2 cm diameter; T1a: 0.1-0.5 cm, T1b: 0.6-1.0 cm, T1c: 1.1-2.0 cm
- T2: Tumor 2.1-5.0 cm diameter
- T3: Tumor > 5 cm diameter
- T4: Tumor any size with extension to chest wall or skin, **or** inflammatory carcinoma
- N (regional lymph nodes)
  - NX: Nodes cannot be assessed
  - N0: No regional node metastasis
  - N1: Involved mobile ipsilateral axillary nodes; pN1mi: Micrometastasis ≤ 0.2 cm
  - N2: Fixed or matted ipsilateral axillary nodes or clinically evident ipsilateral internal mammary nodes (IMNs)
  - N3: Involved ipsilateral IMNs or other local node(s)
- M (metastasis)
  - MX: Distant metastasis cannot be assessed
  - M0: No distant metastasis
  - M1: Distant metastasis
- **Classic staging, based on largest invasive tumor**
  - Stage I: Tumor ≤ 2 cm, no metastases
  - Stage II: Tumor 2.1-5 cm, or positive axillary nodes but no distant metastases
  - Stage IIIA: Tumor any size, matted axillary nodes
  - Stage IIIB: Tumor any size, with skin and/or chest wall involvement
  - Stage IV: Distant metastatic disease
- **Pathologic grading (nuclear or histologic)**
  - Modified Bloom & Richardson (B&R) score: Tubule formation (1-3), nuclear size (1-3), mitoses per 10 high power fields (1-3)
  - GX: Grade cannot be assessed
  - G1: Well-differentiated (B&R score 3-5)
  - G2: Moderately differentiated (B&R score 6-7)
  - G3: Poorly differentiated (B&R score 8-9)
  - G4: Undifferentiated
- **Extensive intraductal component (EIC)**
  - DCIS forms ≥ 25% of main tumor mass, with foci of DCIS outside main tumor mass
  - Increased risk for positive margins
- Other factors: Necrosis, angiogenesis, neural invasion, lymphatic invasion, vascular invasion
- Immunohistochemistry staining for specific receptors
  - Estrogen receptor (ER), progesterone receptor (PR)
    - Tamoxifen or aromatase inhibitors if positive
  - Human epidermal growth factor receptor status: Her-2/neu or c-erb B-2 staining
    - Consider trastuzumab (Herceptin) therapy if +

CLINICAL ISSUES

Presentation

- Most common signs/symptoms
  - Palpable thickening or firm lump
  - Abnormality on screening mammogram
- Other signs/symptoms
  - Nipple and/or skin retraction/tethering common
  - Paget disease of nipple may be present

- May be fixed to chest wall **or** directly involve skin with "peau d'orange", ulceration, nodules **or** inflammatory carcinoma (T4)
- Clinical Profile
  - Most women present with a palpable mass unless routinely screened
  - < 40 y/o, suspect familial cancer ± BRCA mutation
  - Older women, esp. with low socioeconomic status, may have locally advanced tumors at presentation

Demographics

- Age
  - Rare < age 30, ↑ incidence with ↑ age in Western industrialized countries
  - Plateau or decline in incidence after age 50 in most non-Western countries
- Gender
  - > 99% occur in women
  - < 1% occur in men; investigate BRCA carrier status
- Ethnicity
  - Caucasian women: Highest incidence worldwide
  - African-American women: Similar incidence to Caucasians in USA, lower incidence elsewhere
  - Asian women have lowest incidence overall

Natural History & Prognosis

- If untreated: Local and nodal invasion, hematogenous distant metastases
- Staging & 5 yr survival: I: 90%, II: 70%, III: 50%, IV: 20%
- Nottingham Prognostic Index (NPI): Validated, simple, widely used internationally
  - NPI = size points + grade points + node points
    - Size: Maximum diameter in cm x 0.2 = size points
    - Nuclear grade 1-3 = 1 to 3 points
    - Nodes: Negative = 1 point; 1-3 positive = 2 points; ≥ 4 nodes positive = 3 points
  - Good prognosis: NPI < 3.4; 80% survival at 15 years; adjuvant chemotherapy of doubtful benefit
  - Moderate prognosis: NPI 3.4-5.4; 42% survival at 15 years; adjuvant chemotherapy may be beneficial
  - Poor prognosis: NPI > 5.4; 13% survival at 15 years; adjuvant chemotherapy highly advisable

Treatment

- Breast conservation surgery (lumpectomy) with adjuvant radiation standard for most cases
  - Tumor ~ < 5 cm, within 1 quadrant
- Mastectomy for large tumor, multicentric or extensive (> 1 quadrant) disease
- Adjuvant chemotherapy for lymph node involvement
- Adjuvant chemotherapy for ER+, node-negative IDC can be tailored to gene expression arrays
- Consider neoadjuvant chemotherapy for stage III (± II)

SELECTED REFERENCES

1. Kopans DB: Breast Imaging. Philadelphia: Lippincott-Raven. 107-34, 576-82, 1998
2. Rosen PP: Rosen's Breast Pathology. Philadelphia: Lippincott-Raven. 253-6, 325-64, 1997
3. Galea MH et al: The Nottingham prognostic index in primary breast cancer. Breast Cancer Res Treat. 22:207-19, 1992

IMAGE GALLERY

Typical

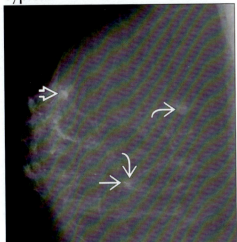

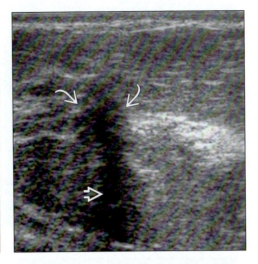

(Left) MLO mammography in a 61 y/o woman shows two screen-detected small irregular densities ➡; the lower lesion has focal Ca++ ➡. A third lesion ➡ was only recognized after MR. (Right) Transverse ultrasound (same as left) shows the MR-detected lesion is an irregular mass ➡ with posterior shadowing ➡. The other 2 lesions appeared similar. Multicentric IDC NOS confirmed in all 3 lesions at excision.

Typical

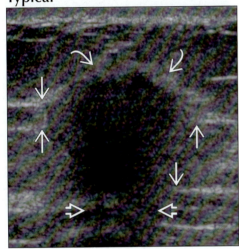

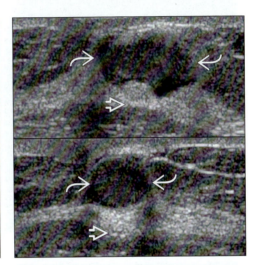

(Left) Anti-radial ultrasound in a 64 y/o woman shows a large irregular hypoechoic mass with an echogenic rim (halo) ➡ & posterior shadowing ➡. Note Cooper ligaments ➡ interrupted at lesion edge. IDC NOS on core biopsy. (Right) Ultrasound in radial (upper) and antiradial (lower) planes of a palpable lump in a 45 y/o shows a hypoechoic mass ➡ which appears rounded in one plane, with posterior enhancement ➡. Grade 3 IDC NOS on biopsy.

Typical

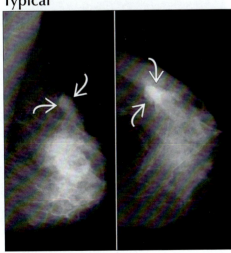

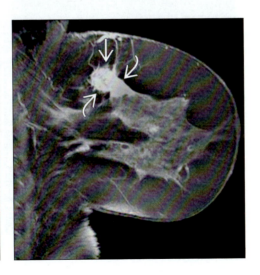

(Left) Mammography in the MLO and CC projections in another patient shows a dense mass with indistinct margins ➡ and associated architectural distortion. US (not shown) showed hypoechoic mass with shadowing. (Right) Sagittal T1 C+ FS MR (same as left) shows the tumor as an intensely enhancing irregular mass ➡ with spiculated margins ➡. IDC NOS on biopsy.

IV

2

125

INFILTRATING DUCTAL NOS, GENERAL

(Left) MLO mammography shows subtle area of distortion ⇒ and asymmetry, confirmed at spot compression ⇒ *(right image)* in this 49 y/o woman with dense glandular tissue. *(Right)* Anti-radial color Doppler ultrasound *(same as left)* shows hypervascular ⇒, hypoechoic, irregular mass ⇒ without posterior features. IDC NOS at biopsy.

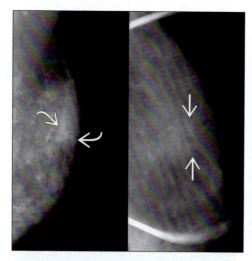

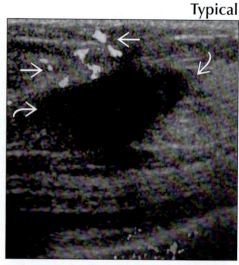

(Left) MLO mammography shows focal asymmetry and distortion ⇒ in the axillary tail right breast in this 43 y/o woman with dense breasts and a previous benign biopsy at this site. This was initially considered to be a scar. *(Right)* Sagittal T1 C+ FS MR *(same as left)* shows intensely enhancing mass ⇒ with spiculated margins ⇒ corresponding to the mammographic abnormality. Grade 2 IDC NOS at biopsy.

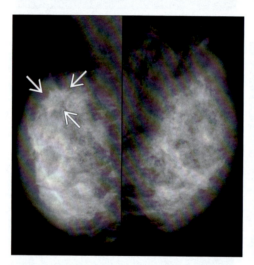

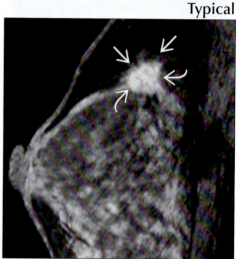

(Left) Specimen mammography magnification shows a classic spiculated small carcinoma ⇒ which was screen-detected in this 63 y/o woman. *(Right)* Sagittal T1 C+ SPGR MIP MR in a 50 y/o woman with a palpable UIQ lump shows spiculated enhancing highly suspicious mass ⇒. The lower mass has rim-enhancement ⇒ and heterogeneous internal enhancement ⇒. Both were IDC NOS at mastectomy.

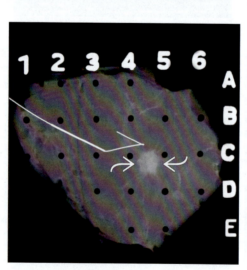

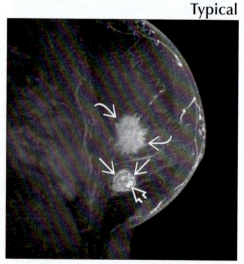

Variant

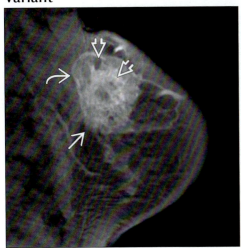

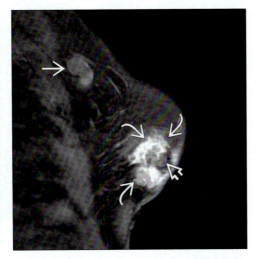

(Left) Sagittal T1 C+ FS MR in a woman with locally advanced IDC NOS prior to neoadjuvant chemotherapy shows a large partially circumscribed ➔, partially spiculated ➔, rim-enhancing mass, with heterogeneous internal enhancement ➔. *(Right)* Sagittal T1 C+ FS MR in another woman shows a large, heterogeneously intensely enhancing IDC ➔ with hypoenhancing central necrosis ➔ and an enlarged metastatic axillary lymph node ➔.

Variant

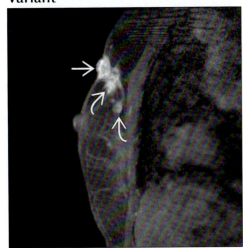

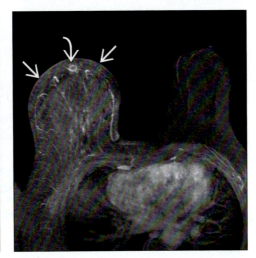

(Left) Sagittal T1 C+ FS MR in a woman presenting with an ulcerating IDC shows a spiculated heterogeneously enhancing mass ➔ with skin retraction and direct skin invasion ➔. T4 IDC NOS. *(Right)* Axial T1 C+ SPGR MIP MR in another woman presenting with a right inflammatory carcinoma shows a grossly enlarged right breast with subcutaneous thickening ➔ and small rim-enhancing IDC NOS ➔.

Variant

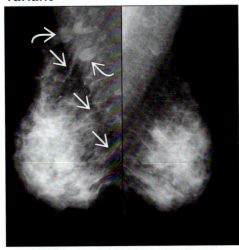

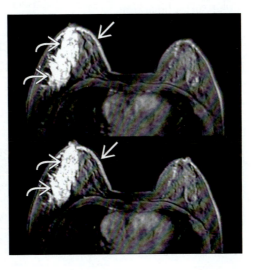

(Left) MLO mammography in this 52 y/o woman with right breast swelling shows diffuse increase in density with thickening of Cooper ligaments ➔ and axillary lymphadenopathy ➔. Freehand blind core biopsy showed IDC NOS. *(Right)* Axial T1 C+ subtraction MR (same as left) shows enlargement, skin thickening ➔ and intense irregular segmental enhancement in most of the right breast ➔. Multifocal IDC with EIC found at mastectomy.

INFILTRATING DUCTAL NOS, GRADE I, II, III

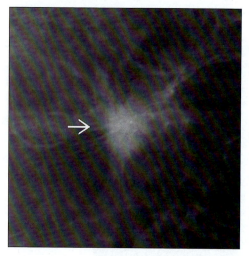
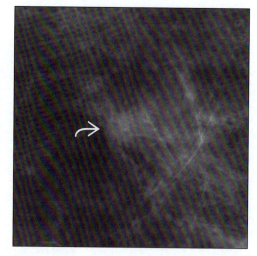

Mammography spot compression shows spiculated, dense mass ➔ with few central amorphous Ca++ right breast noted on screening in this 71 y/o. Biopsy showed grade I IDC NOS and low-grade DCIS.

Mammography spot compression (same patient as left) shows subtle spiculated mass ➔ in the contralateral breast. Biopsy showed tubular carcinoma, a special type of IDC.

TERMINOLOGY

Abbreviations and Synonyms
- Invasive ductal carcinoma (IDC), scirrhous carcinoma
- Not otherwise specified (NOS): No specific (or no "special") type (NST)
- No specific (or no "special") type (NST)
- Grade I: Well-differentiated; grade II: Moderately differentiated; grade III: Poorly differentiated
- Estrogen receptor (ER); progesterone receptor (PR)

Definitions
- Infiltrating (invasive): Extension of tumor cells through duct basement membrane
- "Ductal" implies tumors derived from ductal epithelium and "lobular" carcinomas from lobules
  - Current concept: Both ductal and lobular carcinomas arise from terminal duct lobular unit (TDLU)
- IDC NOS: Does not meet criteria for special type
  - Special types of IDC: Mucinous, medullary, tubular, etc., must comprise ≥ 90% of tumor
- Minimal carcinoma: < 1 cm, invasive

- Microinvasion: Ductal carcinoma in situ (DCIS) with no focus of invasion > 0.1 cm

IMAGING FINDINGS

General Features
- Best diagnostic clue: Irregular mass ± calcifications (Ca++)

Mammographic Findings
- Irregular mass, spiculated margins in 70%
  - 72% of low-grade IDC NOS vs. 24% of high-grade IDC NOS
- Architectural distortion
- Focal or global asymmetry, esp. new or ↑
- Mass or asymmetry ± pleomorphic ± fine linear Ca++
  - Ca++ more common with grade III IDC: 31% vs. 6% of low-grade IDC
  - Ca++ often seen in associated ductal carcinoma in situ (DCIS) component
- Uncommon: Skin or nipple retraction
- Isolated Ca++ rare: Mass may be occult in dense breast tissue

---

DDx: Benign Conditions that Mimic IDC

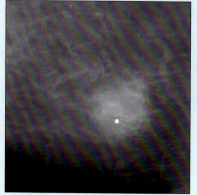
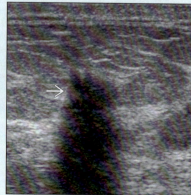
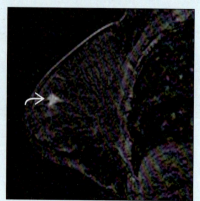

Abscess

Focal Fibrosis

Fibrocystic Changes

INFILTRATING DUCTAL NOS, GRADE I, II, III

Key Facts

Terminology
- Grade I: Well-differentiated; grade II: Moderately differentiated; grade III: Poorly differentiated
- Infiltrating (invasive): Extension of tumor cells through duct basement membrane
- Special types of IDC: Mucinous, medullary, tubular, etc., must comprise ≥ 90% of tumor

Imaging Findings
- Best diagnostic clue: Irregular mass ± calcifications (Ca++)
- Circumscribed margin in 11-16% of grade III IDC, may be thick-walled cystic mass
- Mammography mainstay of screening
- Of IDC in dense breast tissue, over half is occult
- US and MR both show > 90% sensitivity to IDC

Pathology
- 60-70% of all invasive breast cancer is IDC NOS
- DCIS thought to be a nonobligate precursor
- Grade of DCIS usually parallels grade of IDC, i.e., low-grade DCIS seen with grade I IDC, etc.
- More likely Her-2/neu 3+ with ↑ grade
- More likely ER, PR negative with ↑ grade

Clinical Issues
- Special types, esp. tubular carcinoma and grade I IDC more common in screened population
- Prognosis: Lymph node status > tumor size >> grade
- Grade II, III more often larger size, + nodes at detection than grade I
- Tumor grade predicts time to recurrence
- Distant failure fastest for grade III IDC
- Higher grade ⇒ better response to chemotherapy

Ultrasonographic Findings
- Grayscale Ultrasound
  - Irregular or lobulated hypoechoic mass
  - Circumscribed margin in 11-16% of grade III IDC, may be thick-walled cystic mass
  - Thick echogenic rim or halo
    - Do not include in measurement of tumor size
  - Posterior shadowing common
    - 71% of grade I IDC vs. 28% of grade III IDC
    - Posterior enhancement: 36% of grade III IDC vs. 9% of grade I-II tumors
  - Parallel; vertical orientation highly suspicious, uncommon in lesions > 1 cm

MR Findings
- T2WI FS: Usually hypointense; central necrosis can be hyperintense, more common in grade III IDC
- T1 C+ FS
  - Spiculated or lobulated heterogeneous mass
  - Rim-enhancement present in < 50% of IDC
    - More common in grade II and grade III IDC
  - Early intense enhancement
  - Washout more common than plateau kinetics

Biopsy
- US-guided 14-g core needle biopsy (CNB) preferred
- Grade on CNB predicts grade at excision: More accurate with more material obtained
  - 32% with 1 core; 68% for 3 passes; 74% with 4

Imaging Recommendations
- Best imaging tool
  - Mammography mainstay of screening
    - Of IDC in dense breast tissue, over half is occult
  - US for palpable masses, guide biopsy
  - US and MR both show > 90% sensitivity to IDC
    - Selected supplemental screening (evolving area)

DIFFERENTIAL DIAGNOSIS

Malignancies
- Infiltrating lobular carcinoma
  - Focal asymmetry or irregular mass without Ca++
- Ductal carcinoma in situ (DCIS)
  - Suspicious Ca++ most common
- Metastases to breast

Risk Lesions
- Lobular neoplasia
  - Typically mammographically occult
  - May be irregular mass on MR, US
- Radial scar/radial sclerosing lesion
  - Architectural distortion

Benign Lesions
- Fat necrosis, fibrosis, scar, abscess, fibroadenoma, granulomatous mastitis, fibromatosis

PATHOLOGY

General Features
- General path comments
  - 60-70% of all invasive breast cancer is IDC NOS
  - ~ 28% mixed, 50-89% component special type
  - ~ 15-20% grade I; 35-40% grade II; 40-45% grade III
- Genetics
  - ↑ Risk IDC if known or suspected BRCA-1 or -2 carrier
    - > 50% are grade III histology
  - Suspected BRCA-1 or 2 carrier
    - ≥ 2 cases of breast cancer same side of family < age 50 yrs
    - Breast and ovarian cancer same side of family
    - ≥ 3 cases of breast cancer same side of family
    - Family history of breast cancer < age 35
    - Family history of male breast cancer
- Etiology
  - DCIS thought to be a nonobligate precursor
    - IDC often develops at site of DCIS
    - Similar genetic abnormalities
- Epidemiology
  - Grade III histology more common in interval cancers
    - Clinically evident between screening intervals

INFILTRATING DUCTAL NOS, GRADE I, II, III

○ Other markers of high risk
  ▪ Personal history of breast cancer
  ▪ Prior DCIS: > 50% of recurrences are invasive
  ▪ Prior lobular neoplasia
  ▪ Prior atypical ductal hyperplasia
  ▪ Prior chest or axillary radiation
• Associated abnormalities
  ○ DCIS component present in > 75% of IDC
  ○ Grade of DCIS usually parallels grade of IDC, i.e., low-grade DCIS seen with grade I IDC, etc.

Gross Pathologic & Surgical Features
• Gritty, hard mass

Microscopic Features
• If no distinct features, classified as NOS
• More likely Her-2/neu 3+ with ↑ grade
• More likely ER, PR negative with ↑ grade

Staging, Grading or Classification Criteria
• Grading: Nottingham combined histologic grade
  ○ Elston-Ellis modification of Scarff-Bloom-Richardson
  ○ Tubule/gland formation score: Count only structures with central lumina
    ▪ More gland formation indicates more well-differentiated tumor
    ▪ 1: Tubules in majority of tumor (> 75%)
    ▪ 2: Moderate degree (10-75%)
    ▪ 3: Little or none (< 10%)
  ○ Nuclear pleomorphism score
    ▪ 1: Small, regular, uniform cells
    ▪ 2: Moderate increase in size, vascularity
    ▪ 3: Marked variation
  ○ Mitotic activity
    ▪ Score 1-3 depending on # mitoses per field area
  ○ Grade I: Well differentiated, 3-5 points
  ○ Grade II: Moderately differentiated, 6-7 points
  ○ Grade III: Poorly differentiated, 8-9 points
• Staging applies to size of largest invasive cancer
  ○ Stage I: Tumor ≤ 2 cm
  ○ Stage II: Tumor > 2 cm but not > 5 cm, or positive axillary nodes
  ○ Stage III: Tumor > 5 cm or matted nodes
    ▪ IIIB: Skin or chest wall involvement
  ○ Stage IV: Distant metastatic disease

CLINICAL ISSUES

Presentation
• Most common signs/symptoms
  ○ Asymptomatic, screen detected
    ▪ Special types, esp. tubular carcinoma and grade I IDC more common in screened population
• Other signs/symptoms
  ○ Firm, palpable mass
    ▪ Grade III IDC more likely palpable, larger
  ○ Skin and/or nipple retraction
  ○ Rare: Bloody nipple discharge (more often DCIS)
  ○ Rare: Paget disease of nipple

Demographics
• Age: Peak: Mid to late 50s
• Gender: Women; most male breast cancer is IDC

• Ethnicity: Compared to caucasian women with similar mammography history
  ○ ↑ Rate grade III histology in African Americans
  ○ ↓ Rate of advanced stage in Asian, Native American women

Natural History & Prognosis
• Prognosis: Lymph node status > tumor size >> grade
  ○ Clinical stage, distant metastases also important
  ○ Grade II, III more often larger size, + nodes at detection than grade I
• Tumor grade predicts time to recurrence
  ○ Distant failure fastest for grade III IDC
• Higher grade ⇒ better response to chemotherapy

Treatment
• Primary surgical treatment stage I, II disease
  ○ "Clear margin" for IDC has no minimum
• ± Radiation (XRT), ± chemo-, ± hormonal therapy
• Consider neoadjuvant chemotherapy for stage III (± II)

DIAGNOSTIC CHECKLIST

Consider
• Multifocal and multicentric disease common
  ○ Use of supplemental US ± MR will identify additional tumor foci occult on mammography
  ○ XRT and chemotherapy may treat many occult foci

SELECTED REFERENCES

1. Jinguji M et al: Rim enhancement of breast cancers on contrast-enhanced MR imaging: relationship with prognostic factors. Breast Cancer. 13:64-73, 2006
2. Smith-Bindman R et al: Does utilization of screening mammography explain racial and ethnic differences in breast cancer? Ann Intern Med. 144:541-53, 2006
3. Rotstein AH et al: Ultrasound characteristics of histologically proven grade 3 invasive ductal breast carcinoma. Australas Radiol. 49:476-9, 2005
4. McIlhenny C et al: Optimum number of core biopsies for accurate assessment of histological grade in breast cancer. Br J Surg. 89:84-5, 2002
5. Lamb PA et al: Correlation between ultrasound characteristics, mammographic findings and histological grade in patients with invasive ductal carcinoma of the breast. Clin Radiol. 55:40-4, 2000
6. Pinder SE et al: The importance of the histologic grade of invasive breast carcinoma and response to chemotherapy. Cancer. 83:1529-39, 1998
7. Nixon AJ et al: Relationship of tumor grade to other pathologic features and to treatment outcome of patients with early stage breast carcinoma treated with breast-conserving therapy. Cancer. 78:1426-31, 1996
8. Lampejo OT et al: Evaluation of infiltrating ductal carcinomas with a DCIS component: correlation of the histologic type of the in situ component with grade of the infiltrating component. Semin Diagn Pathol. 11:215-22, 1994
9. Elston CW et al: Pathological prognostic factors in breast cancer. I. The value of histological grade in breast cancer: experience from a large study with long-term follow-up. Histopathology. 19:403-10, 1991
10. Bloom HJ et al: Histological grading and prognosis in breast cancer; a study of 1409 cases of which 359 have been followed for 15 years. Br J Cancer. 11:359-77, 1957

INFILTRATING DUCTAL NOS, GRADE I, II, III

IMAGE GALLERY

Variant

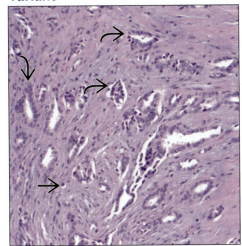

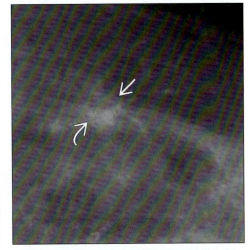

(Left) Micropathology (medium power H&E) shows > 75% of tumor composed of tubules ➘ (1 point); small, uniform nuclei (1 point), and 1 mitotic figure in this field ➘ (1 point), for a total of 3 points, compatible with grade I IDC. *(Right)* CC mammography spot compression shows spiculated mass ➘ with associated amorphous Ca++ ➘ noted on screening in this 64 y/o. Stereotactic 11-g biopsy showed grade I IDC NOS with Ca++ in the IDC.

Typical

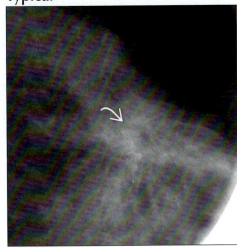

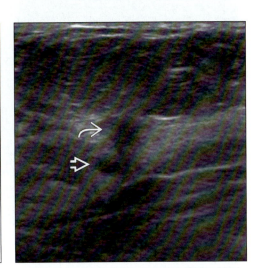

(Left) CC mammography spot compression shows subtle architectural distortion ➘ noted on screening in this 55 y/o. *(Right)* US (same as left) shows spiculated 4 mm hypoechoic, vertical mass ➘ with incidental adjacent cyst ➘. US-guided core biopsy and excision showed grade I IDC NOS with minor cribriform DCIS component.

Typical

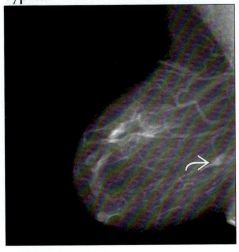

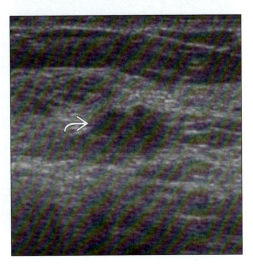

(Left) MLO mammography shows subtle focal asymmetry ➘ seen on only one view in this 74 y/o with contralateral breast cancer and no prior mammograms. *(Right)* US (same as left) shows vague isoechoic mass ➘ felt to correspond to the mammographic abnormality. US-guided core biopsy and excision showed grade I IDC NOS.

Typical

(Left) Micropathology *(medium power H&E) shows < 10% of tumor composed of tubules* ➔ *(3 points); moderate variation in nuclear size and shape (2 points); and few mitotic figures* ➔ *(1 point). Total score = 6 points, grade II IDC.* **(Right)** *MLO mammography spot compression shows irregular mass* ➔ *at edge of parenchyma noted on screening in this 55 y/o.*

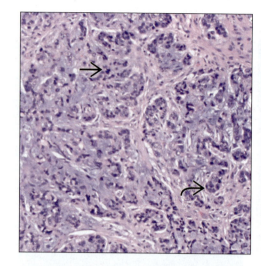

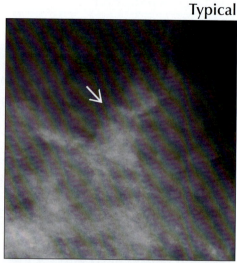

Typical

(Left) US *(same as prior image) shows angular, vertical isoechoic mass* ➔ *with a thick echogenic halo* ➔ *. US-guided biopsy showed grade II IDC NOS with intermediate grade DCIS.* **(Right)** *Sagittal T1 C+ FS MR (same as prior 2 images) shows irregular, heterogeneous enhancing mass* ➔ *corresponding to the known cancer.*

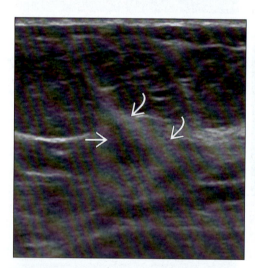

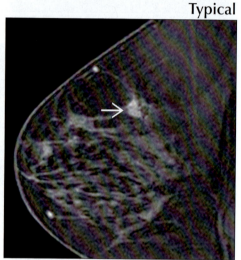

Typical

(Left) MLO mammography *spot compression shows spiculated mass* ➔ *noted on screening mammogram in this 60 y/o.* **(Right)** *US (same as left) shows markedly hypoechoic, spiculated mass* ➔ *with marked posterior shadowing* ➔ *. US-guided biopsy and excision showed grade II IDC NOS with 5 metastatic axillary nodes, stage II.*

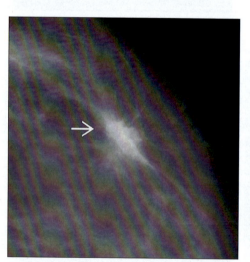

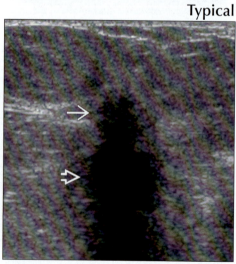

IV

2

132

Typical

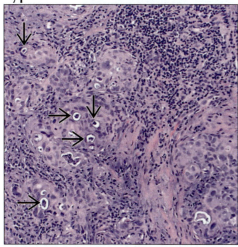

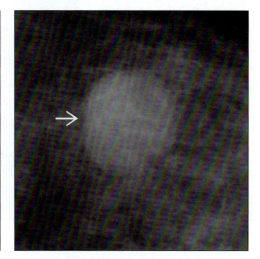

(Left) Micropathology (medium power H&E) shows lack of tubule formation (3 points); marked nuclear pleomorphism (3 points); and intermediate mitotic figure ➔ count (2 points). Total score = 8 points, grade III IDC. *(Right)* Lateral mammography magnification shows partially circumscribed, partially indistinctly marginated round mass ➔ noted on screening in this 55 y/o.

Typical

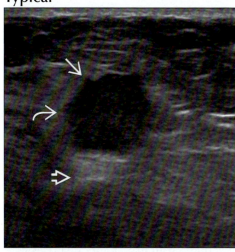

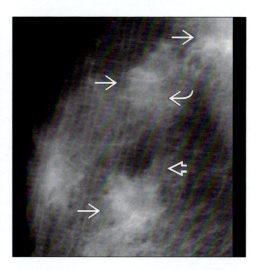

(Left) US (same as previous) shows subtly microlobulated ➔ & indistinct margins ➔ to the mass, as well as posterior enhancement ➔. Biopsy showed grade III IDC NOS. *(Right)* Lateral mammography magnification shows multiple irregular, spiculated masses ➔ in this 54 y/o with palpable masses. Associated pleomorphic Ca++ are evident within largest mass ➔ & at edge of a second mass ➔. Biopsies showed multicentric grade III IDC NOS with high-grade DCIS in areas of Ca++.

IV

2

133

Typical

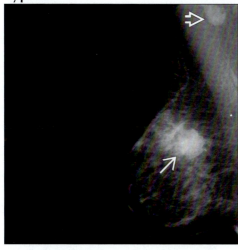

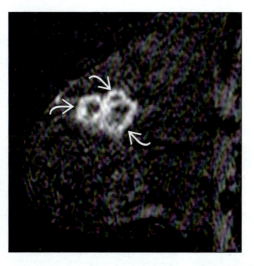

(Left) MLO mammography shows irregular, indistinctly marginated mass ➔ corresponding to palpable mass in this 71 y/o. Dense, large node suspicious for metastasis is noted in left axilla ➔. *(Right)* Sagittal T1 C+ subtraction MR (same as left) shows lobulated rim-enhancing mass ➔ corresponding to proven grade III IDC NOS (with axillary nodal metastasis).

INFLAMMATORY BREAST CANCER

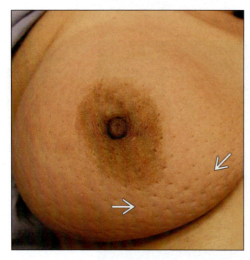

Clinical photograph of a hard, tender, erythematous right breast with peau d'orange best seen in the lower inner quadrant ➡. This 53 year old had been treated with antibiotics without response.

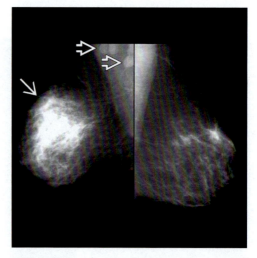

MLO mammography (same as previous) shows marked increased density and trabecular thickening right breast ➡ and dense axillary nodes ➡. Biopsies confirmed inflammatory carcinoma and metastatic nodes.

TERMINOLOGY

Abbreviations and Synonyms
- Inflammatory breast cancer (IBC)

Definitions
- IBC: Locally advanced breast cancer with inflammatory skin changes
  - Diffuse breast erythema
  - Warmth, enlargement, pain, induration
  - Peau d'orange (skin like an orange peel)
  - Edema of more than 2/3 of the breast
- Punch biopsy → tumor emboli in dermal lymphatics; not required for or unique to diagnosis of IBC
- Primary (neoadjuvant) chemotherapy: Chemotherapy prior to surgery
- Adjuvant chemotherapy: Chemotherapy following surgery
- cCR or pCR: Complete response (CR) to primary chemotherapy, i.e. no clinical (c) or no pathologic (p) evidence of disease
- PR: Partial response, clinical ↓ tumor size by > 50%

IMAGING FINDINGS

General Features
- Best diagnostic clue
  - Clinical findings: Peau d'orange, erythema
  - Lack of response to brief course of antibiotics

Mammographic Findings
- Common features
  - Skin thickening
  - Diffuse increased in breast density: Global asymmetry with respect to normal breast
  - Trabecular thickening
- Other findings may be present
  - Axillary adenopathy
    - Dense, large nodes with loss of fatty hila typical
  - Irregular mass(es), focal asymmetry
  - Architectural distortion
  - Nipple retraction
  - Calcifications (Ca++) uncommon

Ultrasonographic Findings
- Grayscale Ultrasound
  - Skin thickening (> 2 mm), usually dramatic

DDx: Mimics of Inflammatory Carcinoma

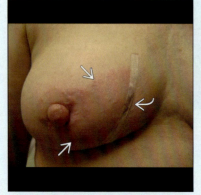

Cellulitis Post Core Biopsy

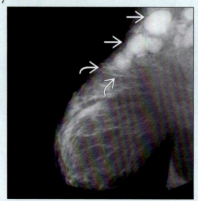

Mastitis

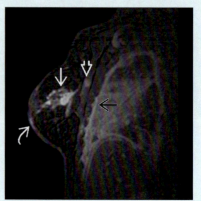

Metastatic Lung Cancer

INFLAMMATORY BREAST CANCER

Key Facts

Terminology
- IBC: Locally advanced breast cancer with inflammatory skin changes
- Diffuse breast erythema
- Warmth, enlargement, pain, induration
- Peau d'orange (skin like an orange peel)

Imaging Findings
- 18FDG PET-CT helpful in whole body staging at diagnosis

Top Differential Diagnoses
- Secondary Skin Invasion by Breast Cancer
- Leukemia, uncommonly lung cancer metastases
- Mastitis ± Abscess
- Post Lumpectomy and Radiation Therapy

Pathology
- 1-6% of breast cancers
- Poorly differentiated IDC NOS
- Tumor emboli in dermal lymphatics typical

Clinical Issues
- May be misdiagnosed as benign inflammatory process
- Multimodality treatment: 5 year survival up to 50%
- Lymph node metastases common, adverse prognosis
- Early systemic metastases
- Risk of false negative sentinel node biopsy

Diagnostic Checklist
- Skin punch biopsy preferred to breast core biopsy
- Targeted US-guided core biopsy if punch biopsy nondiagnostic

---

- ○ Diffuse increased echogenicity and dilated lymphatics: Edema
- ○ May identify mammographically occult mass
  - ▪ Irregular, hypoechoic, often posterior shadowing
  - ▪ May be subtle, diffuse
- ○ May distinguish abscess, guide drainage
- Color Doppler: Tends to be highly vascular

MR Findings
- T1WI
  - ○ Skin thickening, adenopathy
  - ○ Tumor mass not well seen, isointense with parenchyma
  - ○ Distortion may be evident
- T1WI FS: Edema evident in parenchyma and skin
- T1 C+ FS
  - ○ Intense rapid enhancement, usually washout
    - ▪ Irregular masses, may be contiguous
    - ▪ Poorly defined regional or diffuse
    - ▪ Reticular/dendritic enhancement: Tumor in lymphatic channels
  - ○ Skin enhancement often seen
    - ▪ Usually focal areas
    - ▪ Usually not in direct contiguity with mass
- MR used to document tumor size prior to neoadjuvant chemotherapy
  - ○ Helps exclude chest wall invasion
  - ○ Follow-up MR to assess response to treatment
    - ▪ MR spectroscopy may show treatment effect (↓ choline peak) earlier than ↓ tumor size
    - ▪ Size of tumor on MR accurately predicts response

Nuclear Medicine Findings
- PET
  - ○ 18FDG PET-CT helpful in whole body staging at diagnosis
    - ▪ More accurate than bone scan at depicting bone metastases

Biopsy
- Punch biopsy of skin: Dermal lymphatics involved by tumor

- ○ Can be nondiagnostic as skin diffusely erythematous and thickened, but not all involved by tumor
- US-guided core biopsy of suspicious mass(es)
  - ○ If punch biopsy of skin nondiagnostic
  - ○ Make skin incision in normal skin at periphery
  - ○ Clip placement recommended
    - ▪ Rare profound response to primary chemotherapy
    - ▪ Facilitates identification of biopsy site if tumor shrinks
- US-guided fine needle aspiration biopsy (FNAB) or core biopsy of suspicious axillary node(s)
  - ○ Document axillary status prior to primary chemotherapy
  - ○ Sentinel node biopsy sometimes performed pre-treatment
  - ○ Nodes can be cleared of tumor by chemotherapy, falsely negative after treatment

DIFFERENTIAL DIAGNOSIS

Secondary Skin Invasion by Breast Cancer
- A separate entity, locally advanced
- Usually invasive ductal carcinoma (IDC) NOS
- Progression of infiltrating carcinoma to directly involve overlying skin
- Breast masses and malignant Ca++ more common
- Slightly better overall 5 year survival

Metastatic Disease Involving the Breast
- History of nonbreast primary malignancy
- Leukemia, uncommonly lung cancer metastases

Mastitis ± Abscess
- Most common in lactating women
- Should improve within 2 weeks on antibiotics
  - ○ Surgical excision of non-responsive/recurrent abscesses

Post Lumpectomy and Radiation Therapy
- Swelling, hardening worst on first post-treatment exam; should decrease over time

INFLAMMATORY BREAST CANCER

Radiation Dermatitis
- Diffuse erythema, edema
- During or immediately after treatment

Edema
- Lacks erythema
- Clinical history usually helpful
- Asymmetric congestive heart failure
  - No adenopathy
- Metastatic adenopathy with lymphatic obstruction

Paget Disease of the Nipple
- Localized eczematoid change of the nipple
- May have nipple retraction
- Underlying carcinoma often mammographically occult

PATHOLOGY

General Features
- General path comments
  - 1-6% of breast cancers
  - 24-40% of locally advanced breast cancer
- Genetics
  - LIBC gene: "Lost in inflammatory breast cancer" expression lost in 80% of IBC vs. 21% of non-IBC
  - RhoC GTPase, involved in cytoskeletal reorganization, overexpressed in 90% of IBC vs. 38% of non-IBC

Gross Pathologic & Surgical Features
- Breast skin changes: Erythema, peau d'orange
  - Palpable mass variable

Microscopic Features
- Diffuse infiltration without well-defined tumor mass
- Poorly differentiated IDC NOS
  - Majority are ER, PR negative
  - Majority overexpress p53
  - Variable Her-2/neu expression
- Tumor emboli in dermal lymphatics typical
  - Diffuse lymphovascular invasion (LVI) common

Staging, Grading or Classification Criteria
- T4d; subcategory of stage IIIB
- Distant metastases: Stage IV

CLINICAL ISSUES

Presentation
- Most common signs/symptoms
  - Breast erythema, warmth, skin thickening, peau d'orange, pain, mass
  - Rapidly progressive over weeks to few months
  - May be misdiagnosed as benign inflammatory process
- Other signs/symptoms
  - Discrete palpable mass: 50%
  - Palpable or matted axillary nodes

Demographics
- Age

  - Slightly younger than IDC: Mean age 55 years
    - Age-specific incidence levels off > age 50
- Ethnicity: More common in African-American women

Natural History & Prognosis
- Worse than noninflammatory breast cancer of same size, node status
- Best when CR to primary chemotherapy
- Multimodality treatment: 5 year survival up to 50%
- Without multimodality treatment: 5 year survival < 5%
- Lymph node metastases common, adverse prognosis
- Early systemic metastases

Treatment
- Multimodality
  - Induction chemotherapy (anthracycline, taxanes)
    - Goal: Reduce tumor size
    - Facilitates clear margins
    - CR or PR to treatment predict better outcome
  - Mastectomy if at least PR to initial chemotherapy
    - Require clear margins; ± improved outcome
  - Axillary lymph node sampling
    - Usually full axillary dissection performed
    - Risk of false negative sentinel node biopsy
  - Whole breast radiation therapy (XRT) even without mastectomy
    - Improves local control
    - Possible survival benefit
  - Adjuvant chemotherapy
- Initial surgery often contraindicated by diffuse skin involvement
  - High risk of positive margins, failed wound closure
  - Lumpectomy not appropriate: Mastectomy standard

DIAGNOSTIC CHECKLIST

Consider
- Skin punch biopsy preferred to breast core biopsy
- Targeted US-guided core biopsy if punch biopsy nondiagnostic
- May show slight improvement briefly on antibiotics
  - Can be difficult to distinguish from mastitis initially
  - If likely mastitis, close follow-up in 2-4 weeks with low threshold for biopsy
- Recurrent carcinoma can present as IBC

Image Interpretation Pearls
- Early signs: Focal trabecular thickening, subtle masses
- Rapidly progressive: Low threshold for biopsy

SELECTED REFERENCES

1. Merajver SD et al: Inflammatory breast cancer. In: Harris JR et al eds: Diseases of the Breast. 3rd ed. Philadelphia, Lippincott Williams & Wilkins. 971-82, 2004
2. Cristofanilli M et al: Update on the management of inflammatory breast cancer. Oncologist. 8:141-8, 2003
3. Giordano SH et al: Inflammatory breast cancer: clinical progress and the main problems that must be addressed. Breast Cancer Res. 5:284-8, 2003
4. Kushwaha AC: Primary inflammatory carcinoma of the breast: retrospective review of mammographic findings. AJR. 174:535-48, 2000

INFLAMMATORY BREAST CANCER

IMAGE GALLERY

Typical

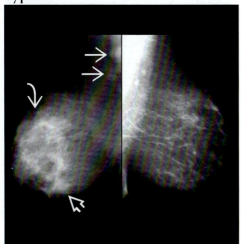

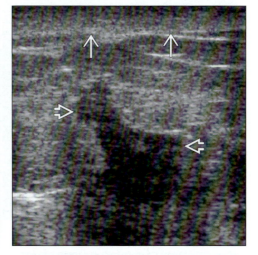

(Left) MLO mammography shows diffuse trabecular thickening right breast ➡, with indistinct mass inferiorly ➡ and dense, prominent axillary nodes ➡ in this 44 year old with right breast swelling, erythema, and peau d'orange. *(Right)* US (same patient as previous image) shows irregular, hypoechoic shadowing mass ➡ inferiorly, with overlying skin thickening ➡.

Typical

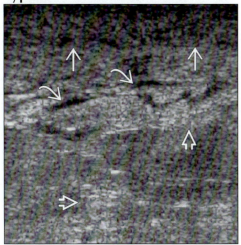

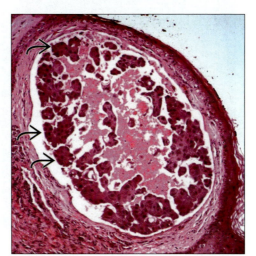

(Left) US in another portion of the breast (same as prior two images) shows dilated lymphatics ➡, diffuse increased echogenicity ➡, and overlying skin thickening ➡. *(Right)* Micropathology, high power of punch skin biopsy (same patient as previous image) shows dermal lymphatic distended with adenocarcinoma cells ➡, pathognomonic of IBC.

Variant

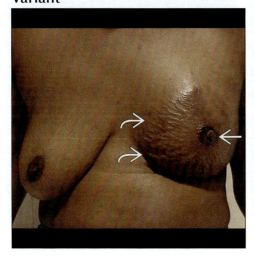

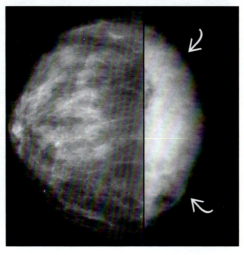

(Left) Clinical photograph shows shrunken left breast with nipple retraction ➡, skin thickening ➡ and erythema in this 43 year old. *(Right)* CC mammography (same patient as previous image) shows shrunken, dense left breast ➡. Initial punch biopsy was negative. US-guided biopsy → poorly-differentiated infiltrating carcinoma with LVI. While the breast is usually swollen with IBC, diffuse tumor mass can cause shrinking.

INFLAMMATORY BREAST CANCER

(Left) This 49 year old had lumpectomy and XRT 2 years earlier for IDC and noted 2-3 months of progressive swelling and hardening of her left breast. MLO mammogram shows diffuse increased density, new compared to prior exam 4 months earlier. *(Right)* US *(same patient as previous image)* shows marked skin thickening ➡, diffuse irregular, hypoechoic mass ➡ with shadowing, and increased echogenicity of the parenchyma ➡. MR was requested.

Variant

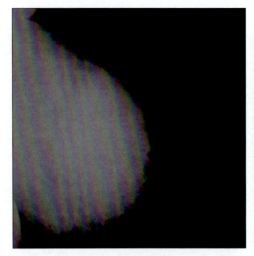
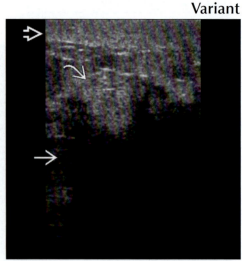

(Left) Sagittal T1WI MR *(same as prior 2 images)* shows marked skin thickening ➡. There is architectural distortion at the lumpectomy scar ➡. *(Right)* Sagittal T2WI FS MR *(same as previous image)* shows hyperintensity due to edema in thickened skin ➡ and scattered areas ➡. The scar is again seen ➡.

Variant

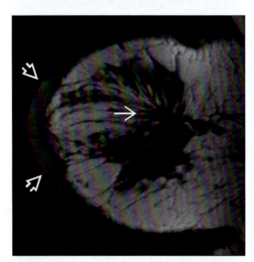
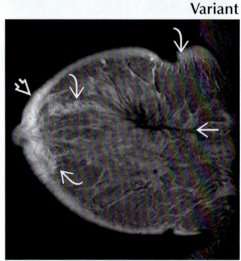

(Left) Sagittal T1 C+ FS MR *(same as prior 4 images)* shows multiple rim-enhancing masses ➡ as well as reticular/dendritic enhancement inferiorly ➡ & patchy areas of skin enhancement ➡. *(Right)* T1 C+ subtraction MR *(same patient as left)* better depicts extensive nature of rim-enhancing masses ➡ & reticular enhancement ➡. Biopsy showed grade II infiltrating ductal carcinoma. With her history of prior breast cancer, this is considered "secondary" IBC.

Variant

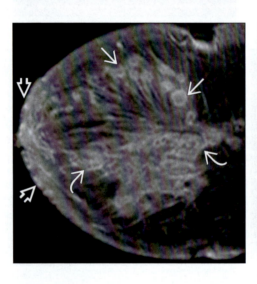
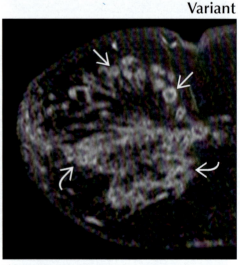

INFLAMMATORY BREAST CANCER

Variant

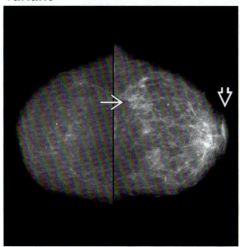 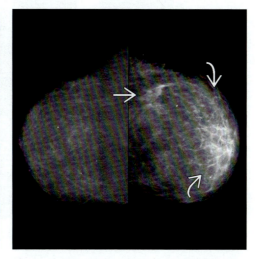

(Left) CC mammography shows skin thickening ⮕ and stable focal asymmetry ➜ in 76 year old with left breast swelling. Punch biopsy was negative. She was treated with antibiotics. *(Right)* CC mammography (same as previous image) 12 months later shows new, diffuse trabecular thickening ⮕. Vague distortion is now present with the asymmetry ⮕. US-guided biopsy → grade II IDC (3 cm in size at MR). Lymph node and lung metastases were found at diagnosis of this IBC.

Typical

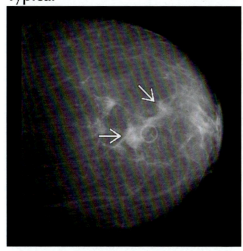 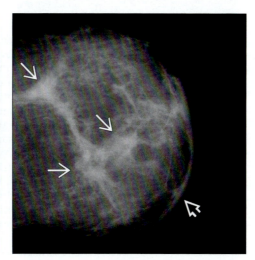

(Left) This 35 year old was treated with mantle radiation for Hodgkin lymphoma 17 years earlier. A palpable, irregular mass was noted ⮕ on CC mammogram. *(Right)* The patient (same as previous image) was next seen 7 months later with new swelling, hardening, & erythema of left breast. Current CC mammogram shows enlargement of now more diffuse irregular mass ⮕ with new skin thickening ⮕. US-guided core biopsy showed poorly differentiated IDC.

IV
2
139

Typical

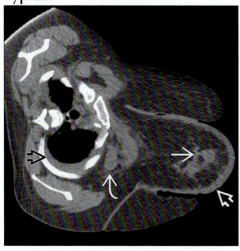 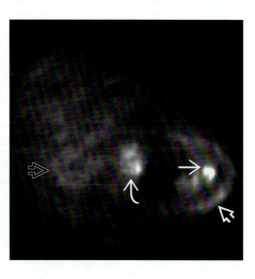

(Left) Staging FDG PET-CT (same as prior two images) shows the left breast mass ⮕, skin thickening ⮕, chest wall mass ⮕ and pleural effusion ⮕. *(Right)* PET at the same level (as previous image) shows increased metabolic activity in the known cancer ⮕, the involved skin ⮕, the chest wall metastasis ⮕, and lymphangitic spread of tumor in the left lung ⮕. Bone metastases were also found (not shown). IBC is often rapidly progressive, with early metastases.

INTERVAL CANCERS

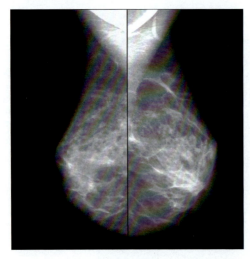

MLO mammography in a 56 y/o asymptomatic woman shows heterogeneously dense breasts with no focal abnormality. Interpreted as BI-RADS 1, negative.

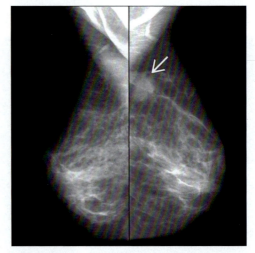

MLO mammography (same case as left image) 12 months later shows a mass ➡ (palpable) seen only on the MLO view. Biopsy showed grade III 1.9 cm infiltrating ductal carcinoma (IDC).

TERMINOLOGY

Abbreviations and Synonyms
- Breast Imaging Reporting and Data System (BI-RADS®)
- Odds ratio (OR)

Definitions
- Breast cancers presenting with clinical findings during the interval between recommended screenings
  - Screening interval varies: Range 12-36 months
    - American College of Radiology (ACR), American Cancer Society (ACS): Every year
    - Dutch, Scandinavian, Canadian, Australian, New Zealand Screening Programs: Every 2 years
    - UK NHS National Breast Screening Program: Every 3 years
  - Longer interval between screenings → higher rate of interval cancers
  - USA performs two view (MLO and CC) mammography; variable use of CC views in other programs
  - ± Suspicious finding on retrospective review of prior screening or recall study

- May be within area or breast different from a prospective "suspicious" assessment (if any)
  - May be mammographically occult
  - ± Attributable to inferior quality prior study
    - Suboptimal positioning, artifacts
- Interval cancers can be mammographically occult, missed on prior mammography, or a new mammographic finding
- Screening mammogram: Testing to detect cancer in women with no signs or symptoms of breast cancer
- Diagnostic mammogram: Examination performed with monitoring by an on-site radiologist
  - Symptoms: Lump, nipple discharge or retraction, change in breast size or shape, skin thickening, etc.
  - Recall from screening for additional imaging following perception of an abnormality
  - Short-interval follow-up of findings deemed probably benign on prior workup
- Screen-detected cancers: Regular interval mammographic examination reveals breast cancer with prior mammogram prospectively having been interpreted as negative, benign, probably benign
  - Additional scenarios with screen-detected cancers
    - Prior biopsy for other benign lesions

DDx: Variations in Cancer Presentation at Mammography

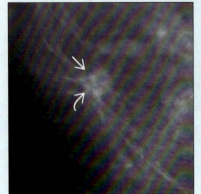

Screen-Detected

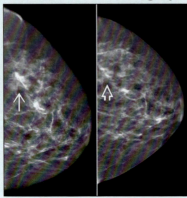

Screen-Detected, Prior was Missed

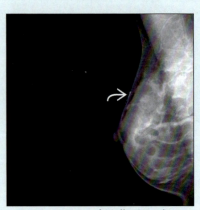

Mammographically Occult

INTERVAL CANCERS

Key Facts

Terminology
- Breast cancers presenting with clinical findings during the interval between recommended screenings
- Screening interval varies: Range 12-36 months
- Longer interval between screenings → higher rate of interval cancers
- Interval cancers can be mammographically occult, missed on prior mammography, or a new mammographic finding

Imaging Findings
- Best diagnostic clue: New clinical findings presenting between regular interval screening examinations
- Typical malignant features often evident at presentation

Top Differential Diagnoses
- Screen-Detected Cancer
- Mammographically Occult Asymptomatic Cancer

Pathology
- Interval cancers ⇒ 53% ↑ risk of death from breast cancer vs. screen-detected cancers
- Women with very dense breasts (OR 6.1) (as compared with fatty breasts)
- ↑ Lobular (OR = 1.9), mucinous (OR = 5.5) histology

Diagnostic Checklist
- As interpreting physician, you are responsible for the quality of interpreted images

---

- Annual contralateral screening in women with history of lumpectomy and radiation for breast cancer
- Missed cancer: Retrospective assessment of prior mammogram (prospectively interpreted as negative, benign or probably benign) in the setting of a routine interval asymptomatic mammogram revealing breast cancer
  - Presence and nature of a finding at the site where cancer develops
    - May be judged as suspicious for cancer
    - Perceptible finding without characteristics judged as having required further work-up at that time

IMAGING FINDINGS

General Features
- Best diagnostic clue: New clinical findings presenting between regular interval screening examinations

Mammographic Findings
- Typical malignant features often evident at presentation
- Features associated with subsequent interval carcinoma
  - Nonspecific asymmetry most common finding in cases reviewed with "subtle signs of malignancy" in retrospect
- Occult: Common in dense breast tissue

Ultrasonographic Findings
- US may be primary imaging modality when suspicious lesion mammographically occult
- Technique critical to avoid false negatives
  - Too low a gain ⇒ solid masses appear anechoic
    - Internal vascularity can improve recognition as solid

MR Findings
- T1 C+ FS
  - May depict multifocal, multicentric, or bilateral cancer

- Upstaging may affect surgical planning
  - Biopsy additional abnormalities

Imaging Recommendations
- Methods to improve performance detecting breast cancer
  - Initial training, continuing medical education
  - Rigorous insistence on images of excellent quality
  - Careful review of previous imaging
  - Standardized reporting; understanding and use of BI-RADS lexicon
  - Careful attention to subtle findings, changes over time
  - Double reading: Human-human; human-CAD (computer-aided detection)

DIFFERENTIAL DIAGNOSIS

Screen-Detected Cancer
- Patient without clinical signs of breast cancer
- New malignancy seen on screening mammogram
  - ± Suspicious finding present on prior mammogram (retrospective review)
- Alternative setting includes clinical finding unknown to interpreting radiologist; palpable finding in retrospect

Mammographically Occult Asymptomatic Cancer
- Despite optimal imaging techniques, clinically apparent neoplasm not visible on mammography
  - Typical for infiltrating lobular carcinoma (ILC)
- May comprise 11-15% of all breast cancers or more
- MR, US depicts 4-6% synchronous contralateral breast cancers occult on mammography
- Up to 2% rate of cancers only on screening MR in high-risk women
- Screening US can double detection rate of nonpalpable cancers in dense breast tissue (studies ongoing)

INTERVAL CANCERS

PATHOLOGY

General Features

- General path comments
  - Interval cancers ⇒ 53% ↑ risk of death from breast cancer vs. screen-detected cancers
    - Data assessed based on the Health Insurance Plan (HIP) and Canadian National Breast Cancer Screening Studies (CNBSS) randomized screening mammogram trial evaluations
    - ↑ Risk found after adjusting for tumor size, stage, and lymph node status
- Genetics
  - No specific genetic factors known to predispose
  - Evidence suggests family history contributes to higher interval cancer risk
    - Possible role of BRCA, other genetic mutations: More frequent grade III histology
- Epidemiology
  - With 3-year screening interval, incidence of interval cancers ↑ with ↑ time elapsed between screenings
    - First year: 2-6 per 10,000 screens
    - 2nd & 3rd years: ~ 10-18 per 10,000 screens
  - Factors associated with ↑ incidence of interval cancers
    - Women with very dense breasts (OR 6.1) (as compared with fatty breasts)
    - Women recalled from screening with additional imaging evaluation assessed (erroneously) as benign (OR 2.2-3.2)
    - Improperly positioned mammograms (OR 2.6)
  - Some populations may have greater age-adjusted cancer incidence
    - Awareness of high-risk groups may improve sensitivity
  - Data may be confounded by patients presenting at recommended screening intervals > 12 months

Microscopic Features

- Typical features of malignancy
  - Varies with histologic subtype
- Compared to screen-detected cancers
  - ↑ Lobular (OR = 1.9), mucinous (OR = 5.5) histology
  - Higher proportion of proliferating cells (OR = 2-4)
  - Lower rate of ductal carcinoma in situ (DCIS)

Staging, Grading or Classification Criteria

- More aggressive than screen-detected cancers
  - Higher histologic grade (OR = 2.1)
  - Negative estrogen receptor (ER) status (OR = 1.8)
  - Her-2/neu oncogene amplification and protein over-expression (OR = 14.1)
  - Axillary lymph nodes more likely to show metastasis than with screen-detected cancers

CLINICAL ISSUES

Presentation

- Most common signs/symptoms
  - Usually palpable new lump
  - Occasionally present with signs of locally advanced disease

- Skin dimpling, erythema, nipple retraction
- Uncommon: Bloody nipple discharge
  - May present with metastases: Axillary lymph nodes, distant

Demographics

- Age: Slight predilection for pre-menopausal women

Natural History & Prognosis

- Prognosis for interval cancers similar to symptomatic, unscreened breast cancers
  - Significantly worse than that in screening-detected cancers

DIAGNOSTIC CHECKLIST

Consider

- Maintain & review facility and practitioner performance statistics (i.e., recall rate, missed cancers)
  - Statistics should not influence action appropriate for imaging findings
  - Increased recall rate not advised
    - Estimated additional 100-400 recalls to detect one additional interval cancer

Image Interpretation Pearls

- As interpreting physician, you are responsible for the quality of interpreted images

SELECTED REFERENCES

1. Shen Y et al: Role of detection method in predicting breast cancer survival: analysis of randomized screening trials. J Natl Cancer Inst. 97:1195-203, 2005
2. Buist DS et al: Factors contributing to mammography failure in women aged 40-49 years. J Natl Cancer Inst. 96:1432-40, 2004
3. Anttinen J et al: Her-2/neu oncogene amplification and protein over-expression in interval and screen-detected breast cancers. Anticancer Res. 23:4213-8, 2003
4. Ikeda DM et al: Analysis of 172 subtle findings on prior normal mammograms in women with breast cancer detected at follow-up screening. Radiology. 226:494-503, 2003
5. Wang SC: The Singapore National Breast Screening Programme: principles and implementation. Ann Acad Med Singapore. 32:466-76, 2003
6. Warren RM et al: Radiology review of the UKCCCR breast screening frequency trial: potential improvements in sensitivity and lead time of radiological signs. Clin Radiol. 58:128-32, 2003
7. Gilliland FD et al: Biologic characteristics of interval and screen-detected breast cancers. J Natl Cancer Inst. 92:743-9, 2000
8. Mandelson MT et al: Breast density as a predictor of mammographic detection: Comparison of interval-and screen-detected cancers. J Natl Cancer Inst. 92:1081-7, 2000
9. Porter PL et al: Breast tumor characteristics as predictors of mammographic detection: comparison of interval-and screen-detected cancers. J Natl Cancer Inst. 91:2020-7, 1999
10. Burrell HC et al: Screening interval breast cancers: mammographic features and prognosis factors. Radiology 199:811-7, 1996

INTERVAL CANCERS

IMAGE GALLERY

Typical

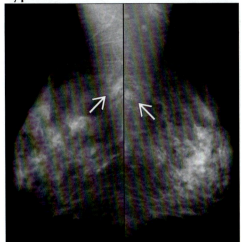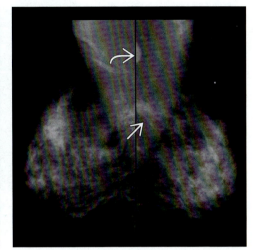

(Left) MLO mammography in an asymptomatic 43 y/o shows bilateral areas of minor asymmetry ➡, BI-RADS 2. *(Right)* MLO mammography of the same patient, performed 8 months later for a palpable left breast mass, shows a mass in the left axillary tail ➡ and another in the left axilla ➡. US-guided core biopsy of the breast mass showed grade II IDC. Two metastatic nodes were confirmed.

Typical

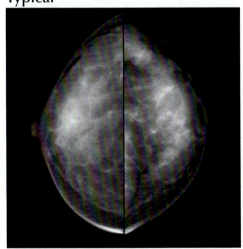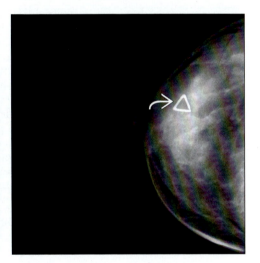

(Left) CC mammography of a screening mammogram in a 49 y/o shows heterogeneously dense parenchyma with no suspicious findings. *(Right)* CC mammography in the same patient four months later, shows a marker ➡ on a new palpable mass. Direct excision showed mammographically occult 9 mm ILC and multiple associated foci of lobular carcinoma in situ (LCIS).

Typical

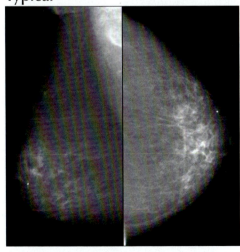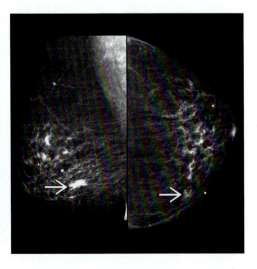

(Left) MLO (left side) and CC (right side) screening mammogram in a 60 y/o woman status post right mastectomy 4 yrs earlier for DCIS shows no abnormality. *(Right)* MLO (left side) & CC (right side) in same patient < 8 months later with a palpable medial mass was shown on mammogram to be an indistinct mass with associated suspicious calcifications ➡. Biopsy followed by mastectomy showed high nuclear grade DCIS.

INFILTRATING LOBULAR CARCINOMA

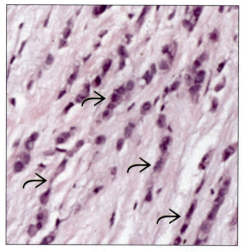

Micropathology, high power shows single file columns of invasive lobular carcinoma ➾, with intervening stroma.

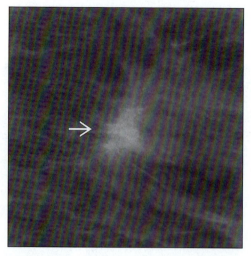

MLO mammography spot compression view (same patient as left) shows spiculated dense mass ➡ with associated architectural distortion. US-guided core biopsy showed ILC.

TERMINOLOGY

Abbreviations and Synonyms
- ILC
- Invasive lobular carcinoma

Definitions
- Invades as single file columns of cells

IMAGING FINDINGS

General Features
- Best diagnostic clue: Developing focal asymmetry with distortion, palpable thickening
- Size
  - Size underestimated on mammography and US
  - Size best determined by MR

Mammographic Findings
- Spiculated mass (most common) on mammography
- Isolated architectural distortion
- New focal asymmetry, often seen only on CC view
  - Spot compression views, US

- Calcifications rare (1-11%)
- 52% sensitivity on mammography (range 34-72%)
- 15-20% mammographically subtle
- Difficult to detect mammographically due to insidious growth pattern
  - Commonly multifocal or multicentric
  - Increased rate of contralateral cancer
  - Size underestimated on mammography in > 2/3 patients
  - Larger at diagnosis than infiltrating ductal carcinoma (IDC)
  - More likely positive lymph nodes than IDC
- Overrepresented among missed or delayed diagnoses of cancer

Ultrasonographic Findings
- Grayscale Ultrasound
  - 88% sensitivity on US (range 82-94% better than mammography)
  - Irregular mass, intense posterior shadowing
  - May show architectural distortion
  - Can be nearly anechoic with posterior enhancement
    - Indistinct or angular margins distinguish from cyst

DDx: Infiltrating Lobular Carcinoma Mimics

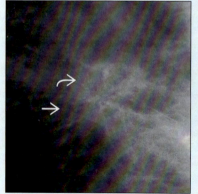

Infiltrating Ductal Carcinoma

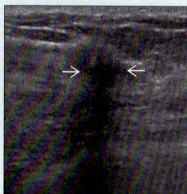

Scar Post Core

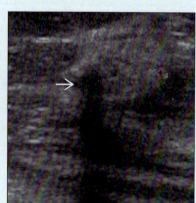

Fibrosis

INFILTRATING LOBULAR CARCINOMA

Key Facts

Imaging Findings
- Size underestimated on mammography and US
- Spiculated mass (most common) on mammography
- Isolated architectural distortion
- New focal asymmetry, often seen only on CC view
- Calcifications rare (1-11%)
- 52% sensitivity on mammography (range 34-72%)
- Difficult to detect mammographically due to insidious growth pattern
- Commonly multifocal or multicentric
- Increased rate of contralateral cancer
- Overrepresented among missed or delayed diagnoses of cancer
- 88% sensitivity on US (range 82-94% better than mammography)
- Irregular mass, intense posterior shadowing

- Up to 65% false negative on PET
- Best imaging tool: MRI useful for accurately sizing and determining extent in both breasts

Top Differential Diagnoses
- Infiltrating Ductal Carcinoma (IDC)
- LCIS appearances overlap with ILC on US, MR
- Fibrosis
- Scar
- Diabetic Mastopathy

Pathology
- 10% of all breast cancer
- Associated abnormalities: Often coexists with LCIS and ALH
- High rate of positive margins at excision (> 50%) in absence of MR

- ○ US often underestimates size of tumor
- ○ US helps depict mammographically subtle or occult ILC
- ○ US-guided FNAB of suspicious axillary node(s)

MR Findings
- T1 C+
  - ○ Spiculated mass with architectural distortion
  - ○ Can present as multiple small foci +/- interconnecting septal enhancement
  - ○ Isolated enhancing septae
  - ○ Associated lobular carcinoma in situ (LCIS) can be source of false positive US, MR
  - ○ Can be a source of false negative MR examination

Nuclear Medicine Findings
- PET
  - ○ Up to 65% false negative on PET
  - ○ Lymph node metastases can be false negative on PET

Imaging Recommendations
- Best imaging tool: MRI useful for accurately sizing and determining extent in both breasts

DIFFERENTIAL DIAGNOSIS

Infiltrating Ductal Carcinoma (IDC)
- Large overlap in appearances
- Associated suspicious calcifications suggest IDC

Lobular Carcinoma In Situ (LCIS)
- Usually mammographically occult, nonpalpable
- LCIS appearances overlap with ILC on US, MR

Fibrosis
- No associated architectural distortion, rarely palpable
- Can be irregular, shadowing mass on US, indistinguishable
- Mixed hypo- and hyperechoic mass on US more common
- Enhancement on MR less common, can be indistinguishable

Scar
- Architectural distortion
- Extends to overlying skin
- Irregular, hypoechoic on US (indistinguishable)
- Generally will not enhance on MR > 18 months post-operatively

Diabetic Mastopathy
- Long-standing type I diabetes
- Dense, fibrotic, shadowing mass
- Indistinguishable on mammography, US
- Usually little enhancement on MR

PATHOLOGY

General Features
- General path comments
  - ○ Grows as "single file" linear columns of tumor cells with intervening stroma
    - ■ Subtle change in architecture, often not a discrete mass
    - ■ Does not incite intense desmoplastic response
  - ○ Lacks e-cadherin on immunohistochemistry
    - ■ IDC and DCIS will stain positive for e-cadherin
    - ■ E-cadherin also lost in LCIS
- Etiology
  - ○ LCIS may be a precursor lesion
    - ■ Ipsilateral invasive cancers after LCIS at that site
    - ■ Vast majority of invasive cancer after LCIS is ILC
    - ■ Clonality of genetic alterations in most ILC with LCIS
- Epidemiology
  - ○ 10% of all breast cancer
  - ○ More common in patients with prior LCIS or atypical lobular hyperplasia (ALH)
- Associated abnormalities: Often coexists with LCIS and ALH

Gross Pathologic & Surgical Features
- High rate of positive margins at excision (> 50%) in absence of MR

INFILTRATING LOBULAR CARCINOMA

- Firm hard tumor, scirrhous appearance

Microscopic Features
- Variants
  - Classical
    - Linear columns of small cells (1-2 thick) with uniform nuclei infiltrating fibrous stroma
  - Solid (cellular) pattern
    - Cells arranged as sheets or large, irregularly-shaped nests
  - Pleomorphic = histiocytoid cell type
    - Abundant, eosinophilic cytoplasm (apocrine)
  - Signet-ring cell type
    - Eccentric semilunar nuclei, prominent cytoplasmic vacuoles
  - Alveolar pattern
    - Circumscribed globular nests of cells, simulates LCIS
  - Tubulolobular carcinoma
    - Small tubules grow in targetoid pattern in a background of classic invasive lobular carcinoma
  - Mixed
- Lymphocytic reaction rare

Staging, Grading or Classification Criteria
- No stage 0 (LCIS is not treated as cancer)
- Stage I: Primary tumor 2 cm or smaller, negative nodes
- Stage IIA: Primary tumor 2.1-5.0 cm with negative axillary nodes, or primary tumor ≤ 2 cm with movable axillary node metastasis(es)
- Stage IIB: Primary tumor 2.1-5.0 cm with movable axillary node metastases, or primary tumor 5.1 cm or larger with negative nodes
- Stage IIIA: Primary tumor 5.1 cm or larger, positive node(s) or smaller primary tumor and fixed axillary nodal metastases
- Stage IIIB: Invasion of skin or chest wall or inflammatory carcinoma
- Stage IV: Distant metastases

CLINICAL ISSUES

Presentation
- Most common signs/symptoms: Palpable thickening
- Other signs/symptoms
  - Shrinking breast
  - Skin retraction

Natural History & Prognosis
- Compared to IDC, ILC has higher incidence of bilaterality, multicentricity, multifocality
- Metastasizes frequently to bone, peritoneum, adrenals, gastrointestinal tract, ovary and leptomeninges
- Stage for stage, prognosis equal to IDC NOS
- Classic pattern may have better prognosis
- Tubulolobular carcinoma has better prognosis
  - Lower incidence of positive nodes, distant metastases, recurrence
- Solid pattern may have worse prognosis
- Pleomorphic cell type has poor prognosis

Treatment
- Same as for IDC

- Surgical excision with clear margins
- Axillary lymph node sampling (sentinel node)
- Ipsilateral radiation to breast following conservative surgery or post mastectomy for extensive tumor
- Neoadjuvant chemotherapy for locally advanced breast cancer (stage III, some larger stage II tumors)
- Chemotherapy for stage II-IV disease

DIAGNOSTIC CHECKLIST

Consider
- Can be seen in only one mammographic projection (more often CC)
- Developing focal asymmetry and/or subtle architectural distortion merits work-up
- MR recommended for evaluating disease extent

Image Interpretation Pearls
- Do not dismiss subtle neodensities or architectural distortion
- Encourage use of US

SELECTED REFERENCES

1. Berg WA et al: Diagnostic accuracy of mammography, clinical examination, US, and MR imaging in preoperative assessment of breast cancer. Radiology. 233:830-49, 2004
2. Fisher ER et al: Pathologic findings from the National Adjuvant Breast and Bowel Project: 12 year observations concerning lobular carcinoma in situ. Cancer. 100:238-44, 2004
3. Evans III WP et al: Invasive lobular carcinoma of the breast: mammographic characteristics and computer-aided detection. Radiology. 225:182-9, 2002
4. Qayyum A et al: MR imaging features of infiltrating lobular carcinoma of the breast: histopathologic correlation. AJR. 178:1227-32, 2002
5. Weinstein SP et al: MR imaging of the breast in patients with invasive lobular carcinoma. AJR. 176:399-406, 2001
6. Avril N et al: Breast imaging with positron emission tomography and fluorine-18 fluorodeoxyglucose: use and limitations. J Clin Oncol 18:3495-502, 2000
7. Harvey JA et al: Apparent ipsilateral decrease in breast size at mammography: s sign of infiltrating lobular carcinoma. Radiology. 214:883-9, 2000
8. Butler RS et al: Sonographic evaluation of infiltrating lobular carcinoma. AJR. 172:325-30, 1999
9. Rodenko GN et al: MR imaging in the management before surgery of lobular carcinoma of the breast: correlation with pathology. AJR. 167:1415-19, 1996
10. Hilleren DJ et al: Invasive lobular carcinoma: mammographic findings in a 10-year experience. Radiology. 178:149-54, 1992
11. LeGal M et al: Mammographic features of 455 invasive lobular carcinomas. Radiology. 185:705-8, 1992
12. Sickles EA et al: Subtle and atypical mammographic features of invasive lobular carcinoma. Radiology. 178:25-6, 1991
13. Mendelson EB et al: Infiltrating lobular carcinoma: mammographic patterns with pathologic correlation. AJR. 153:265-71, 1989
14. Dixon JM et al: Infiltrating lobular carcinoma of the breast: an evaluation of the incidence and consequence of bilateral disease. Br J Surg. 70:513-6, 1983

INFILTRATING LOBULAR CARCINOMA

IMAGE GALLERY

Typical

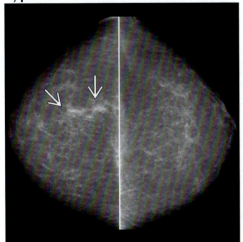
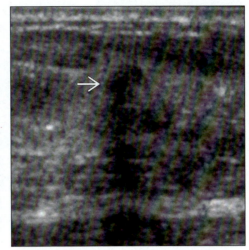

(Left) CC mammography shows focal asymmetry central and posterior right breast ➔, visible only on CC view. US was performed (next image). *(Right)* Transverse ultrasound of right breast 12:00 shows markedly hypoechoic mass ➔ with posterior shadowing. US-guided core biopsy and excision revealed a 6 mm invasive lobular carcinoma (Courtesy HKG).

Typical

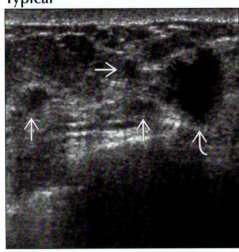
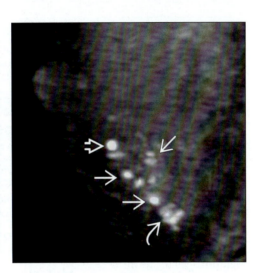

(Left) Radial ultrasound of mammographically-occult, palpable mass shows dominant irregular anechoic ➔ as well as multiple smaller similar masses ➔. The two largest were ILC, with the smaller masses LCIS. *(Right)* Sagittal T1 C+ SPGR MIP MR of patient in previous image shows multiple enhancing masses: Two (➔ and ➔) were ILC, and multiple smaller masses ➔ were LCIS (Case from reference 1).

Typical

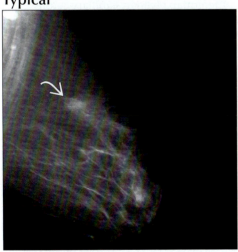
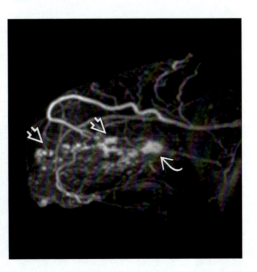

(Left) MLO mammography shows focal asymmetry upper left breast ➔. US-guided biopsy showed ILC, and MR (next image) was recommended to evaluate disease extent. *(Right)* Sagittal T1 C+ SPGR MIP MR shows the mammographically-depicted mass ➔ as well as multiple additional masses in a segmental distribution ➔, which proved to be extensive ILC.

INVASIVE MICROPAPILLARY CARCINOMA

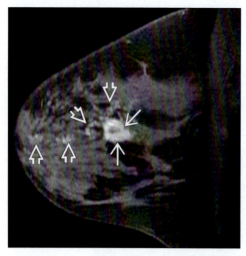

Sagittal T1 C+ FS MR shows enhancing mass in a 34 y/o woman with a palpable mass. Core biopsy showed IMPC ➡. Clumped linear enhancement ➡ around the tumor was DCIS.

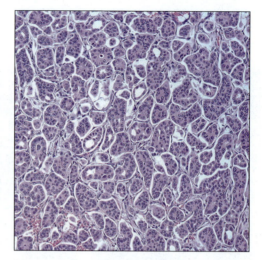

Histology of invasive micropapillary carcinoma. Low-power view shows papillary cell clusters surrounded by clear empty spaces (H&E) (Courtesy SJS).

TERMINOLOGY

Definitions

- Invasive micropapillary carcinoma (IMPC) is an aggressive and distinctive variant of breast cancer
  - Aggregates of carcinoma cells lying in clear spaces
- Unrelated to micropapillary subtype of DCIS

IMAGING FINDINGS

General Features

- Best diagnostic clue: No described distinguishing features; same as invasive ductal carcinoma (IDC)

Mammographic Findings

- Irregular or circumscribed mass; same as IDC
- One case reported as mammographic calcifications

Ultrasonographic Findings

- Grayscale Ultrasound: Solid mass; same as IDC

MR Findings

- Irregular mass; indistinguishable from IDC
- T1 C+ FS: Mass with rapid wash-in & wash-out

Imaging Recommendations

- Best imaging tool: Mammography is usually unrevealing; MR is the most sensitive tool

DIFFERENTIAL DIAGNOSIS

Other Types of Invasive Breast Carcinoma

- IDC or invasive lobular carcinoma (ILC)

Benign Lesions

- Fat necrosis (history of surgery or trauma)
- Diabetic mastopathy
- Fibroadenoma

Fibromatosis

- Spiculated mammographic density

Metastatic Micropapillary Tumors

- Histological differential: Ovarian papillary serous adenocarcinoma, micropapillary variant of transitional cell carcinoma of the urinary bladder, micropapillary carcinomas of other organs (e.g., lung, salivary gland)

DDx: Lymph Node Metastases at Presentation in Other Types of Breast Cancer

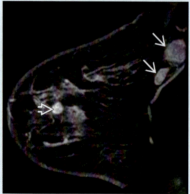

IDC (High Grade)

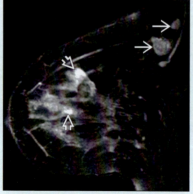

ILC (Mammographically Occult)

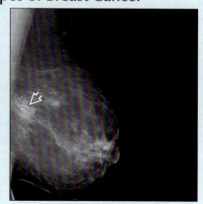

Basal-Like Cancer

INVASIVE MICROPAPILLARY CARCINOMA

Key Facts

Terminology
- Invasive micropapillary carcinoma (IMPC) is an aggressive and distinctive variant of breast cancer
- Aggregates of carcinoma cells lying in clear spaces
- Unrelated to micropapillary subtype of DCIS

Imaging Findings
- Best diagnostic clue: No described distinguishing features; same as invasive ductal carcinoma (IDC)

Top Differential Diagnoses
- IDC or invasive lobular carcinoma (ILC)
- Metastatic Micropapillary Tumors

Pathology
- Peritumoral angioinvasion in 33-67% of cases

Clinical Issues
- Axillary lymph node metastases in 72-77% at first presentation

PATHOLOGY

General Features
- Pure form: Less than 2% of all invasive cancers
- Focal micropapillary growth areas in 3-6% of IDCs

Gross Pathologic & Surgical Features
- Mass with lobulated outline
- High incidence of lymph node metastasis with extranodal extension

Microscopic Features
- Clusters of infiltrating micropapillae without a fibrovascular core within clear spaces separated by a fine reticular stroma lacking desmoplasia
- Peritumoral angioinvasion in 33-67% of cases
- Associated DCIS component 67-70% of cases
- Rates of ER and PR+ and Her-2/neu overexpression similar to those of IDC

Staging, Grading or Classification Criteria
- Criteria are the same for all invasive cancers

CLINICAL ISSUES

Natural History & Prognosis
- Presentation: Breast mass ± enlarged axillary nodes
- Invasive micropapillary component has been described in tumors of several organs and is usually associated with aggressive biologic behavior
- Striking propensity for lymphatic and nodal spread
  - Axillary lymph node metastases in 72-77% at first presentation
  - Extranodal extension is frequent; marker for increased regional recurrence
- Poor prognosis: High incidence of local recurrence, distant metastases

Treatment
- Same as for IDC

DIAGNOSTIC CHECKLIST

Image Interpretation Pearls
- Scanning of axilla may reveal large metastatic axillary lymph nodes

SELECTED REFERENCES

1. Nagi C et al: N-cadherin expression in breast cancer: correlation with an aggressive histologic variant--invasive micropapillary carcinoma. Breast Cancer Res Treat. 94(3):225-35, 2005
2. Kuroda H et al: Clinical and pathologic features of invasive micropapillary carcinoma. Breast Cancer. 11:169-74, 2004
3. Pettinato G et al: Invasive micropapillary carcinoma of the breast: clinicopathologic study of 62 cases of a poorly recognized variant with highly aggressive behavior. Am J Clin Pathol. 121:857-66, 2004
4. Jaffer S et al: Infiltrating micropapillary carcinoma of the breast. Cytologic findings. Acta Cytol. 46:1081-7, 2002
5. Siriaunkgul S et al: Invasive micropapillary carcinoma of the breast. Mod Pathol. 6(6):660-2, 1993

IMAGE GALLERY

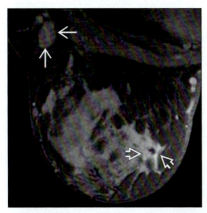 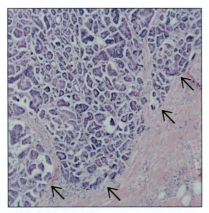 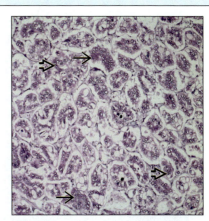

(Left) Palpable axillary mass in a 39 y/o with prior reduction mammoplasty. Axial T1 C+ FS MR shows an enlarged lymph node ➡ and an enhancing irregular mass ➡. Biopsy showed IMPC and lymph node metastasis. *(Center)* Micropathology, low power, H&E of IMPC shows lobulated margins ➡ (Courtesy KK). *(Right)* Histology, mid power, H&E of another case shows papillary growth of tumor cells with eosinophilic cytoplasm ➡ and high-grade nuclei ➡ without true fibrovascular cores (Courtesy OBI).

MEDULLARY CARCINOMA

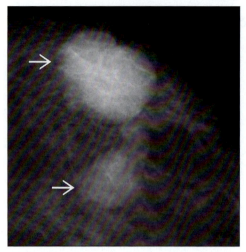

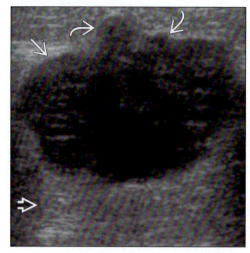

CC mammography shows two adjacent mostly circumscribed, partially indistinctly marginated masses ➡ in this 40 year old woman with a lump.

Ultrasound of the larger mass (same as on left) shows mostly circumscribed ➡, partially microlobulated ➡ markedly hypoechoic mass with posterior enhancement ➡. Biopsy and excision showed medullary carcinoma.

TERMINOLOGY

Definitions
- A special type of invasive ductal carcinoma (IDC)
- Well-circumscribed carcinoma with poorly-differentiated cells, little stroma, and lymphoid infiltration
- Five key features must be present in ≥ 90% of tumors; if only some, then = "atypical medullary carcinoma"
  - Lymphoplasmacytic reaction: Must involve periphery and diffusely involve the tumor itself
  - Microscopic circumscription: Edge of tumor pushes rather than infiltrating breast; no islands of glandular or fatty tissue within the tumor
  - Syncytial growth: 75% or more of tumor in sheets or islands of cells difficult to individually distinguish
  - High nuclear grade
  - High mitotic rate
- Atypical medullary carcinoma = IDC NOS with medullary features; distinguish from "medullary carcinoma"
- Distinction of atypical medullary carcinoma from IDC NOS has no clinical import

IMAGING FINDINGS

General Features
- Best diagnostic clue
  - Partially circumscribed mass on mammogram
    - Lymphoplasmacytic infiltration of fat can cause indistinct margin
- Location: Upper outer quadrant most common

Mammographic Findings
- Oval, round or lobular mass
  - Partially circumscribed margins
  - Often at least partially indistinct margin
- Calcifications uncommon
- Satellite nodules common, can be in situ component
  - Can be contiguous → microlobulated margin
- Enlarged axillary nodes common
  - Can be reactive, not metastatic

Ultrasonographic Findings
- Grayscale Ultrasound
  - Round, oval, or lobulated, hypoechoic mass
  - Mostly circumscribed, partially indistinct margins

DDx: Other Mostly Circumscribed Neoplasms

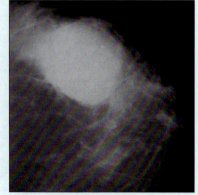

Phyllodes Tumor

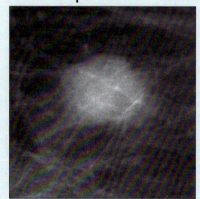

Mucinous Carcinoma

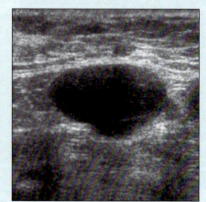

Non-Hodgkin Lymphoma Node

MEDULLARY CARCINOMA

Key Facts

Terminology
- Well-circumscribed carcinoma with poorly-differentiated cells, little stroma, and lymphoid infiltration
- Distinction of atypical medullary carcinoma from IDC NOS has no clinical import

Imaging Findings
- Partially circumscribed mass on mammogram
- Large lesions may show cystic component due to necrosis

Top Differential Diagnoses
- Fibroadenoma
- Phyllodes
- Circumscribed Non-Medullary Breast Cancer

Pathology
- 5-7% of all breast cancers
- 10% of breast cancers in patients < 35 years
- Rapid growth, locally aggressive
- Typically ER, PR, Her-2/neu negative
- Strict histologic diagnostic criteria important for management

Clinical Issues
- Enlarging, palpable mass: Soft, mobile
- Survival better than IDC NOS: 5 year survival 89-95%

Diagnostic Checklist
- Axillary lymph nodes may be large even in absence of nodal metastases

---

- ○ Occasionally see microlobulated margins, can be secondary to DCIS
- ○ Thick echogenic halo of peritumoral edema
- ○ Large lesions may show cystic component due to necrosis
- ○ Posterior enhancement common → pseudocystic appearance; may confuse with lymphoma

MR Findings
- T2WI FS: May show cystic component in necrotic areas
- T1 C+ FS: Oval or lobulated enhancing mass

Biopsy
- Core biopsy sampling may allow suggestion of diagnosis
- For definitive diagnosis, complete excision required

Imaging Recommendations
- Best imaging tool: Mammography and US
- MR can be used to define disease extent

DIFFERENTIAL DIAGNOSIS

Fibroadenoma
- Most common mass in women under 35 years
  - ○ Peak age 20-30 years
- Well-circumscribed, oval mass on mammography, US
- Cystic changes rare

Phyllodes
- Median age 45-49 years
- Large, mostly circumscribed round, oval or lobulated mass on mammography
- Hypoechoic mass on ultrasound
  - ○ Often see inhomogeneous internal echoes and peripheral cystic spaces

Circumscribed Non-Medullary Breast Cancer
- Infiltrating ductal carcinoma NOS or mucinous carcinoma

- Uncommonly ductal carcinoma in situ (DCIS), e.g. papillary DCIS
- Indistinguishable on imaging

Non-Hodgkin Lymphoma
- Mostly circumscribed mass on mammography
  - ○ Often multiple
- Mixed echogenicity on US, posterior enhancement

PATHOLOGY

General Features
- General path comments
  - ○ 5-7% of all breast cancers
    - ■ 10% of breast cancers in patients < 35 years
  - ○ Rapid growth, locally aggressive
  - ○ DCIS often found at periphery
  - ○ Bilateral 3-18%
  - ○ Axillary metastases 20-45%
  - ○ Multicentric 8-10%
  - ○ Typically ER, PR, Her-2/neu negative
  - ○ High rate p53 protein accumulation
  - ○ Strict histologic diagnostic criteria important for management
- Genetics: Possible association with BRCA-1
  - ○ Not an indication for genetic testing absent other family history

Gross Pathologic & Surgical Features
- Ovoid or lobulated mass
- Median size 2-3 cm
- Multilobulated or microlobulated surface
  - ○ Cut edge reveals nodular internal architecture
- Easily mistaken for fibroadenoma
- Not as firm as most IDC NOS carcinomas (necrosis → soft)
- Less frequently attached to surrounding tissues than IDC NOS
- Necrosis, sometimes hemorrhage
  - ○ Extent of necrosis related to tumor size
  - ○ Necrotic tissue can appear grossly caseous or granular

○ Increasing necrosis → cystic foci (prominent in tumors ≥ 5 cm)
  ▪ Similar in gross appearance to cystic papillary carcinoma

Microscopic Features

- Moderate to severe lymphoplasmacytic reaction
  ○ May be composed entirely of either lymphocytes or plasma cells, but usually a combination of both
  ○ Must involve ≥ 75% of periphery of lesion, as well as within the tumor
  ○ If extensive, germinal centers form → difficult to differentiate from metastatic lymph nodes
- Margins histologically circumscribed
  ○ Thin capsule of compressed breast tissue around most of lesion
  ○ Pushing margins
  ○ Lymphoplasmacytic infiltrate can mix with adjacent fat
- At least 75% syncytial growth
  ○ Only small part of tumor composed of tubules, cords or papillary growth
- Malignant cells high or intermediate nuclear grade
  ○ Large pleomorphic nuclei with coarse chromatin; prominent nucleoli
- High mitotic rate; 85% aneuploid
- Focal squamous metaplasia in 10-16% of cases
- Minimal desmoplastic stromal reaction
- No glandular elements or fat incorporated into tumor
- Infiltration into surrounding tissues present in only one location
  ○ Two or more areas of direct invasion → atypical type (NOS with medullary features)

Staging, Grading or Classification Criteria

- Histologic grading not used for medullary carcinoma
- Staging otherwise as for IDC NOS

CLINICAL ISSUES

Presentation

- Most common signs/symptoms
  ○ Enlarging, palpable mass: Soft, mobile
    ▪ May be perceived by patient and/or clinician as benign
- Other signs/symptoms
  ○ Axillary adenopathy at presentation common
    ▪ Often benign reactive changes, not metastases

Demographics

- Gender: Rarely found in the male breast
- Ethnicity: More common in Japanese and African-American women
- Typically occurs in younger patients than IDC NOS
  ○ Mean age 46-54

Natural History & Prognosis

- Survival better than IDC NOS: 5 year survival 89-95%
- Recurrences tend to occur early
  ○ Rare after five years
  ○ Usually systemic, survival brief

Treatment

- Standard surgical cancer treatment
  ○ Lumpectomy and radiation therapy; mastectomy when needed
  ○ Sentinel lymph node biopsy
  ○ Chemotherapy based on size and nodal status

DIAGNOSTIC CHECKLIST

Consider

- Often overdiagnosed absent strict adherence to all diagnostic criteria
  ○ May lead to inappropriate conservative therapy
- Axillary lymph nodes may be large even in absence of nodal metastases

Image Interpretation Pearls

- Irregular or spiculated border unusual for typical medullary carcinoma
  ○ Thorough pathologic review of entire tumor recommended to rule out atypical form

SELECTED REFERENCES

1. Vu-Nishino H et al: Clinicopathologic features and long-term outcome of patients with medullary breast carcinoma managed with breast-conserving therapy (BCT). Int J Radiat Oncol Biol Phys. 62(4):1040-7, 2005
2. Eichhorn JH: Medullary carcinoma, provocative now as then. Semin Diagn Pathol. 21(1):65-73, 2004
3. Gombos EC et al: Infiltrating carcinoma with medullary features in the male breast: imaging and pathologic findings. Breast J. 10(6):548-9, 2004
4. Iau PT et al: Are medullary breast cancers an indication for BRCA1 mutation screening? A mutation analysis of 42 cases of medullary breast cancer. Breast Cancer Res Treat. 85:81-8, 2004
5. Osin P et al: Distinct genetic and epigenetic changes in medullary breast cancer. Int J Surg Pathol. 11(3):153-8, 2003
6. Yilmaz E et al: Comparison of mammographic and sonographic findings in typical and atypical medullary carcinomas of the breast. Clin Radiol. 57(7):640-5, 2002
7. Rosen P: Rosen's Breast Pathology. 2nd ed. Philadelphia, Lippincott Williams&Wilkins. Chapter 17, 405-22, 2001
8. Cheung YL et al: Sonographic and pathological findings in typical and atypical medullary carcinomas of the breast. J Clin Ultrasound. 28:325-31, 2000
9. Jensen ML et al: Prognostic comparison of three classifications for medullary carcinomas of the breast. Histopathology. 30(6):523-32, 1997
10. Liberman L et al: Overdiagnosis of medullary carcinoma: a mammographic-pathologic correlative study. Radiology. 201:443-6, 1996
11. Cook DL et al: Comparison of DNA content, S-Phase fraction, and medullary and ductal carcinoma of the breast. J Clin Path. 104:17-22, 1995
12. Moore Jr OS et al: The relatively favorable prognosis of medullary carcinoma of the breast. Cancer. 2:635-42, 1949
13. Foote Jr FW et al: A histologic classification of carcinoma of the breast. Surgery. 19:74-99, 1946

MEDULLARY CARCINOMA

IMAGE GALLERY

Typical

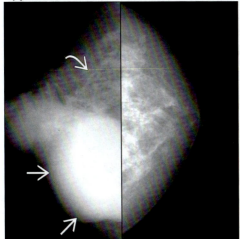

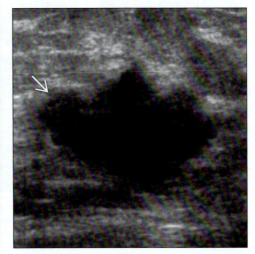

(Left) CC mammography shows a large mass ➡ occupying most of the right breast. Associated trabecular coarsening is suggested ➡, but it is possible that this is normal under-compressed tissue. Core biopsy revealed medullary carcinoma. *(Right)* Ultrasound in a 47 year old woman reveals an irregular, markedly hypoechoic left upper outer quadrant mass ➡ which was palpable. 14-g US-guided core biopsy showed medullary carcinoma.

Typical

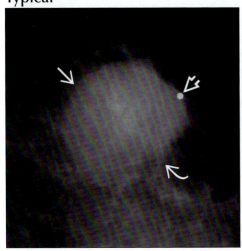

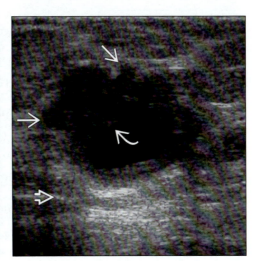

(Left) MLO mammography spot compression shows a palpable, partially circumscribed mass ➡ in the left upper outer quadrant, marked with a BB ➡. The inferior margins are somewhat indistinct ➡. *(Right)* Ultrasound of preceding case, directed to palpable mass, shows an irregular, thick-walled complex cystic mass ➡ with internal septations ➡ and posterior enhancement ➡. US-guided core biopsy revealed medullary carcinoma.

Typical

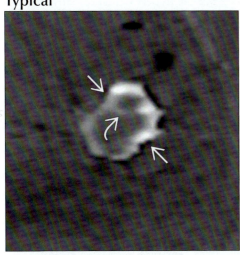

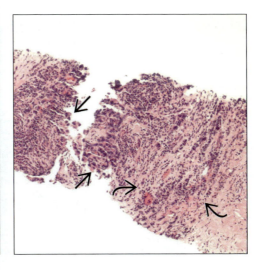

(Left) Coronal T1 C+ subtraction MR (same case as prior 2 images) performed to confirm disease extent demonstrated the known medullary cancer, which was seen as a rim-enhancing mass ➡ with enhancing internal septations ➡. *(Right)* Micropathology, low power, H&E of core biopsy (same as on left-hand image) shows syncytial growth of tumor cells ➡, with dense lymphoplasmacytic infiltrate ➡ in this medullary carcinoma.

METAPLASTIC CARCINOMA

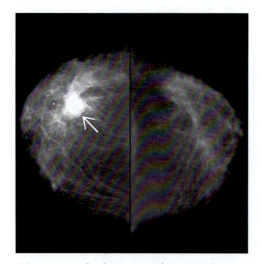

CC mammography shows a very dense, irregular, mass in the right breast ➡. Poorly differentiated metaplastic carcinoma with spindle cell differentiation at biopsy.

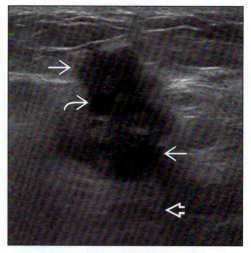

Radial spatial compounding ultrasound (same as prior) shows a vertically-oriented, hypoechoic, microlobulated mass ➡ with posterior enhancement ➡. Cystic area ➡ is due to prior vacuum-assisted biopsy.

TERMINOLOGY

Abbreviations and Synonyms
- Dedifferentiated carcinoma
- Adenosquamous carcinoma
- Squamous carcinoma
- Carcinosarcoma
- Carcinoma with sarcomatous metaplasia
- Sarcomatoid carcinoma
- Adenoacanthoma sarcomatoides

Definitions
- Coexistence of invasive ductal carcinoma with areas of matrix-producing, spindle cell, sarcomatous, or squamous differentiation

IMAGING FINDINGS

General Features
- Best diagnostic clue: Large breast mass, usually partially circumscribed; may have ossification
- Location: Anywhere in breast cone
- Size

- ○ Typically large (3-5 cm) at diagnosis
- ○ Size range: 1-20 cm
  - ■ Mean 2.5-4.5 cm
- Morphology: Rounded, lobulated or irregular

Mammographic Findings
- Lobulated or irregular rounded mass
  - ○ May be partially circumscribed, partially indistinct
- Absent, subtle or (rarely) prominent calcification (Ca++) or ossification
- May be too large to study by mammogram

Ultrasonographic Findings
- Grayscale Ultrasound
  - ○ Hypoechoic, partially circumscribed mass
  - ○ Unusual internal echotexture on ultrasound
    - ■ Densely calcified (marked posterior shadowing)
    - ■ Heterogeneous echogenicity
    - ■ Areas of cystic degeneration may be present
- Power Doppler: May be hypervascular (usually rim)

MR Findings
- T1WI
  - ○ Large nonspecific hypointense mass
  - ○ Usually isointense with glandular parenchyma

DDx: Other Large, Partially Circumscribed Tumors

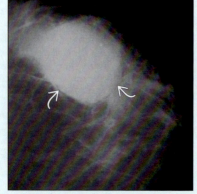

Malignant Phyllodes Tumor

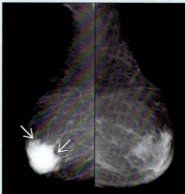

Mucinous Carcinoma

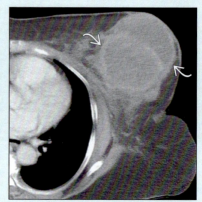

Multicystic Sarcoma

METAPLASTIC CARCINOMA

Key Facts

Terminology
- Coexistence of invasive ductal carcinoma with areas of matrix-producing, spindle cell, sarcomatous, or squamous differentiation

Imaging Findings
- Best diagnostic clue: Large breast mass, usually partially circumscribed; may have ossification
- Typically large (3-5 cm) at diagnosis
- Best imaging tool: Contrast-enhanced MR

Top Differential Diagnoses
- Infiltrating Ductal Carcinoma (IDC) NOS Without Metaplasia
- Malignant Phyllodes Tumor
- Breast Metastasis from Remote Malignancy
- Primary Breast Sarcoma

Pathology
- Special uncommon carcinoma variants
- May be confused with true sarcomas
- Variable cell composition; named by dominant cell type
- < 1% of ductal carcinomas
- Two major types: Squamous and pseudosarcomatous
- Majority are of intermediate or high nuclear grade
- Majority are p63 positive; highly specific for metaplastic carcinoma

Clinical Issues
- No significant difference in outcome if matched by stage and grade against NOS carcinomas
- 5-year overall survival 71% (95% CI: 46-96%)
- Limited chemotherapy and tamoxifen response

- T2WI FS
  - Nonspecific mass, hyperintense, isointense or hypointense to breast tissue
  - High signal intensity on T2WI MR related to necrotic component
- T1 C+ FS
  - Markedly hyperintense rapid enhancement
  - Large lobulated rounded mass
  - Rim-enhancement may be prominent
  - Central necrosis or hypoperfusion not uncommon

Nuclear Medicine Findings
- Bone Scan
  - Uptake of bone scan isotope (e.g., Tc-99m MDP) in breast mass
    - Chondro-osseous and osteosarcomatous types

CT Findings
- CECT: Enhancing large rounded mass(es)
- NECT: May show incidental Ca++ if osteosarcomatous

Imaging Recommendations
- Best imaging tool: Contrast-enhanced MR
- Protocol advice
  - Role of imaging: Usually intramammary staging
  - Bone scan useful for staging in chondro-osseous, osteosarcomatous type
  - MR shows internal architecture, size and shape best

DIFFERENTIAL DIAGNOSIS

Infiltrating Ductal Carcinoma (IDC) NOS Without Metaplasia
- Imaging overlap in appearances

Mucinous Carcinoma
- May appear similar on imaging
- Dense unilateral rounded mass on mammography
- Areas of cystic necrosis on US and MR

Malignant Phyllodes Tumor
- Also large rapidly growing mass

- May have sarcomatous elements
- Distinct microscopic growth pattern

Papilloma with Squamous Metaplasia
- Presentation & imaging usually differ
- Primarily pathological differential diagnosis

Breast Metastasis from Remote Malignancy
- Squamous carcinoma or sarcoma

Primary Breast Sarcoma
- Pure sarcomatous stromal tumor without adenocarcinoma
- Arises from mesenchymal elements only
- Spindle cell metaplasia difficult to distinguish from fibrosarcoma, malignant fibrous histiocytoma: Cytokeratin-positive squamous nests in metaplasia
- Immunohistochemistry differs

PATHOLOGY

General Features
- General path comments
  - Special uncommon carcinoma variants
  - May be confused with true sarcomas
  - Epithelial and/or myoepithelial cell origins
  - Variable cell composition; named by dominant cell type
  - Suspect if mixed malignant cells in fine needle aspirate or core biopsy
- Etiology: Unknown
- Epidemiology
  - Usually women > 50, age range 20-90
  - < 1% of ductal carcinomas
  - 16% of medullary carcinomas
  - Pseudosarcomatous metaplasia in 0.2% of adenocarcinomas

Gross Pathologic & Surgical Features
- Solid firm to hard nodular mass +/- cystic degeneration (squamous)

METAPLASTIC CARCINOMA

Microscopic Features
- Two major types: Squamous and pseudosarcomatous
- Squamous types (all cytokeratin positive)
  - Purely squamous carcinoma
  - Intermixed adenosquamous carcinoma
    - Focal squamous large cell nests in adenocarcinoma
  - Pseudoangiosarcomatous/angiomatoid
    - Large spaces lined by cytokeratin positive cells (vs. factor VIII or CD34 in angiosarcoma)
  - Spindle cell
    - Extensive spindle cell component; may appear purely spindle cell
    - Cytokeratin rarely positive in true fibrosarcoma
- Pseudosarcomatous
  - Poorly-differentiated adenocarcinoma with areas of matrix-producing differentiation
  - Chondrosarcomatous, chondro-osseous or osteosarcomatous
  - Very rarely rhabdomyosarcomatous, liposarcomatous, angiosarcomatous
- Low grade fibromatosis-like
  - Rare, good prognosis subtype

Staging, Grading or Classification Criteria
- Majority are of intermediate or high nuclear grade
- Nodal and distant metastases usually absent at diagnosis
- Genetic features
  - Majority are p63 positive; highly specific for metaplastic carcinoma
- Immunohistochemistry quite distinct
  - Estrogen receptor (ER) usually negative
  - Progestogen receptor (PR) usually negative
  - Her-2/neu usually negative
  - Epidermal growth factor receptor (EGFR) negative
  - Cytokeratin positive in squamous types

CLINICAL ISSUES

Presentation
- Most common signs/symptoms: Large palpable mass

Demographics
- Age: Peak incidence > 55 years
- Gender: Almost exclusively female

Natural History & Prognosis
- May grow very rapidly or be stable and low grade for years
- Low grade fibromatosis-like type does not metastasize
  - Has good prognosis and survival
- Nodal metastases are common at diagnosis
  - Major influence on overall outcome
- No significant difference in outcome if matched by stage and grade against NOS carcinomas
  - May appear more aggressive as often larger, higher grade with distant spread at diagnosis
  - Adjuvant therapy or extent of surgery does not influence outcome
- 5-year overall survival 71% (95% CI: 46-96%)
- 5-year disease-free survival 42% (95% CI: 20-65%)

- 5-year stage-specific overall survival
  - Stage I: 100%
  - Stage II: 83%
  - Stage III: 53%

Treatment
- Primary surgical excision as for ductal carcinoma
  - Adjuvant radiation therapy (XRT) if breast conserved or positive or close margins at mastectomy
- Limited chemotherapy and tamoxifen response
- May benefit from pre-operative XRT

DIAGNOSTIC CHECKLIST

Consider
- Actually a type of dedifferentiated carcinoma
- Most "sarcomas" of the breast are actually metaplastic carcinomas
- MR is best method for accurate evaluation of extent
- Accurate final histopathologic diagnosis cannot be made without complete excision
  - Dependent on dominant histological component of tumor
  - Requires evaluation of entire lesion

SELECTED REFERENCES

1. Beatty JD et al: Metaplastic breast cancer: clinical significance. Am J Surg. 191:657-64, 2006
2. Carter MR et al: Spindle cell (sarcomatoid) carcinoma of the breast: a clinicopathologic and immunohistochemical analysis of 29 cases. Am J Surg Pathol. 30:300-9, 2006
3. Dave G et al: Metaplastic carcinoma of the breast: a retrospective review. Int J Radiat Oncol Biol Phys. 64:771-5, 2006
4. Kim YJ et al: Metaplastic carcinoma with extensive chondroid differentiation in the breast (chondroid carcinoma). Yonsei Med. J 47:259-63, 2006
5. Tse GM et al: Metaplastic carcinoma of the breast: a clinico-pathological review. J Clin Pathol. 2006
6. Tse GM et al: p63 is useful in the diagnosis of mammary metaplastic carcinomas. Pathology. 38:16-20, 2006
7. Gibson GR et al: Metaplastic breast cancer: clinical features and outcomes. Am Surg. 71:725-30, 2005
8. Velasco M et al: MRI of metaplastic carcinoma of the breast. AJR. 184:1274-8, 2005
9. Kurian KM et al: Sarcomatoid/metaplastic carcinoma of the breast: a clinicopathological study of 12 cases. Histopathology. 40:58-64, 2002
10. Park JM et al: Metaplastic carcinoma of the breast: mammographic and sonographic findings. J Clin Ultrasound. 28:179-86, 2000
11. Rayson D et al: Metaplastic breast cancer: prognosis and response to systemic therapy. Ann Oncol. 10:413-9, 1999

METAPLASTIC CARCINOMA

IMAGE GALLERY

Typical

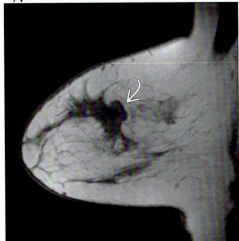

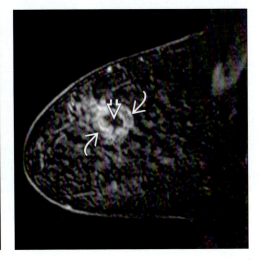

(Left) Sagittal T1WI MR of the right breast shows an irregular hypointense mass ➘. Metaplastic carcinoma with spindle cell differentiation on biopsy. *(Right)* Sagittal T1 C+ subtraction MR in the same patient shows a rim-enhancing lesion with a thick irregular rim ➘ and central nonenhancing necrosis ➘. Nonenhancing necrosis is not uncommon in this entity.

Typical

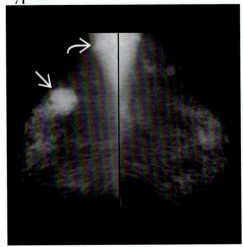

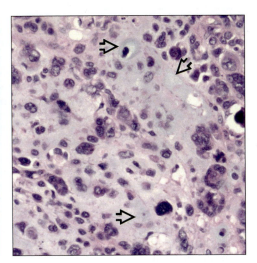

(Left) MLO mammography shows a dense, lobulated palpable mass in the upper outer right breast ➘. A dense, enlarged metastatic node is also seen in the right axilla ➘. Metaplastic carcinoma at biopsy. *(Right)* Specimen micropathology, high power (same patient as left) shows areas of light blue chondroid matrix ➘. Other areas (not included in this image) showed squamous differentiation with keratin pearls.

Typical

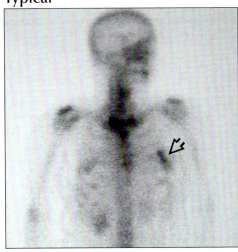

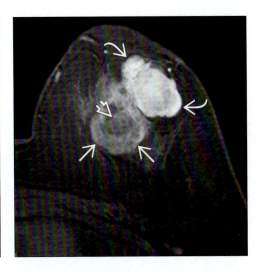

(Left) Frontal Tc-99m MDP bone scan shows extra-osseous radiotracer uptake ➘ corresponding to a large palpable left breast mass in a 49 y/o woman. Metaplastic carcinoma with osteosarcomatous differentiation at biopsy. *(Right)* Axial T1 C+ SPGR MIP MR with fat suppression (same case as left) shows the lesion to be complex with a large solid component anteriorly ➘ and a rim-enhancing ➘ component with central necrosis ➘ posteriorly.

MISSED CANCERS

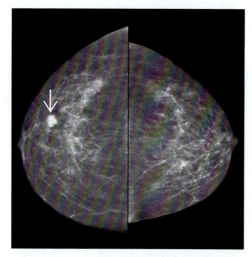

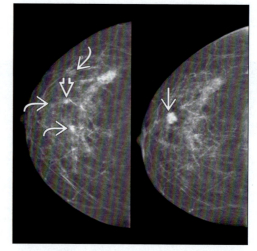

CC mammography in an asymptomatic 57 y/o woman shows a dense lobulated mass ➡ with indistinct margins. Pathology: 1.3 invasive ductal, ER/PR+, DCIS. Prior mammogram was reviewed (next image).

CC mammograms 2 yrs apart show non-actionable nonspecific tissue density ➡ where cancer later developed (right) ➡. Other (benign) asymmetries are scattered elsewhere on earlier study ➡.

TERMINOLOGY

Abbreviations and Synonyms
- Breast Imaging Reporting and Data System (BI-RADS)®

Definitions
- Patient with newly diagnosed breast cancer
  - Any of the following scenarios may result in a finding that could be deemed as "missed" when prior mammograms prospectively classified as negative, benign or probably benign are reviewed
    - Asymptomatic screening mammogram
    - Patient with a clinically suspicious finding presenting between regular interval screening mammograms
    - Patient presenting for scheduled interval screening mammogram with a clinically suspicious finding
  - Academic use of this term: Routine interval screening mammogram where cancer is detected & prior mammogram is re-evaluated with particular attention to area where cancer developed
    - Examine site where cancer developed as to the presence and nature of any finding in retrospect

- Judged as suspicious for cancer; may be termed "true miss"
- Perceptible finding without characteristics judged as having required further work-up at that time
- Cases may be included as false negatives on practice audits
- Screening mammogram: Testing to detect cancer in women with no signs or symptoms of breast cancer
- Diagnostic mammogram: Examination performed with monitoring by an on-site radiologist
  - Symptoms: Lump, nipple discharge or retraction, change in breast size or shape, skin thickening or retraction
  - Recall from screening for additional imaging
- "Actionable": Retrospective determination that a finding was present on the prior mammogram that should have prompted further evaluation
  - Six published retrospective blinded screening mammogram studies found actionable findings in 25-41%
    - Two of these 6 studies had study sets including multiple normal cases and found actionable cases in 27-29%

DDx: Non-Actionable Cancer Developing 15 Months after Negative Mammogram

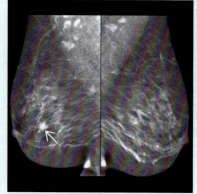

MLO Current

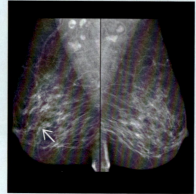

MLO Prior

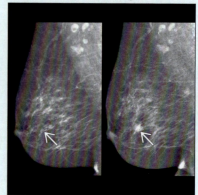

MLO Prior and Current

MISSED CANCERS

Key Facts

Terminology
- Academic use of this term: Routine interval screening mammogram where cancer is detected & prior mammogram is re-evaluated with particular attention to area where cancer developed
- Interval cancer: Cancers detected clinically during the interval between recommended screenings

Imaging Findings
- Often found at edge of fibroglandular tissue
- Edge of film/image
- Error of perception
- Error of interpretation
- May minimize errors with attention to practice habits
- Careful review of prior imaging studies
- Judicious use of BI-RADS 3, probably benign
- Rigorous insistence on images of excellent quality
- Review facility and individual performance statistics
- Double reading

Top Differential Diagnoses
- Interval Cancer
- Mammographically-Occult Cancer

Pathology
- Invasive tumors 68-75%
- DCIS 25-30%

Diagnostic Checklist
- Few benign-appearing Ca++: 18%
- Certain subset of screen-detected asymptomatic cancers display, in retrospect, perceptible findings (area of tissue-density, few benign-appearing Ca++) that do not warrant recall as judged by blinded panels

---

- Nine retrospective non-blinded studies of screening mammograms found actionable findings in 23-77%
- Interval cancer: Cancers detected clinically during the interval between recommended screenings
  - Time interval variable based on screening recommendations: 12-36 months
  - Account for mean 7-13% of breast cancers in women ≥ 40 undergoing annual screening
  - Tend to be larger, higher grade & lymph node metastases more likely compared to screen-detected cancers

IMAGING FINDINGS

General Features
- Best diagnostic clue: Mammographic mass and/or calcifications (Ca++), architectural distortion, developing asymmetry
- Location
  - Often found at edge of fibroglandular tissue
  - Edge of film/image
- Morphology
  - Mass: 19-64%
    - Asymmetries reported as high as 53% (one study, 1993); included lesions seen on only one view and lesions without discrete borders; prior to BI-RADS lexicon
  - Calcifications: 18-34%
  - Architectural distortion: 4-12%
  - Mass and calcifications: 2%

Mammographic Findings
- Reader error may account for failure to diagnose cancer
- Error of perception
  - Abnormality not seen: Incomplete search pattern, satisfaction of search due to distracting feature(s) elsewhere
  - Finding obscured by overlying tissue
  - Finding seen on only one view
  - Dense or large breasts
  - Poor positioning/technique

- Subtle lesion growth
  - No prior films for comparison
- Error of interpretation
  - Finding was perceptible but without characteristics prompting action
    - Area looked like normal tissue
    - Calcifications looked benign or obscured by vessel
  - Finding stable over time but with suspicious characteristics
  - Finding had characteristics suggestive of breast cancer, interpretation was incorrect

Imaging Recommendations
- Cannot eliminate regardless of screening modality(ies)
- May minimize errors with attention to practice habits
  - Training, experience, continuing medical education
  - Interpret both screening and diagnostic mammograms
  - Careful review of prior imaging studies
  - Judicious use of BI-RADS 3, probably benign
  - Rigorous insistence on images of excellent quality
    - Observer error and technical problems responsible for delayed detection in 22% (one series)
    - Technical factors judged as affecting diagnosis of breast cancer in 17% (one series)
    - Lesions in retroglandular regions may be more often overlooked because of poor exposure
    - Interpreted mammograms are assumed to be technically adequate; interpreting radiologist ultimately responsible for image quality
  - Review facility and individual performance statistics
    - Audit should not influence action appropriate for individual case imaging findings
    - Should not attempt to lower false positive rate by artificially reducing recalls
  - Double reading
    - Human/human or human/computer-aided detection (CAD)
    - Not presently standard of care
    - Increase sensitivity: No consensus; all abnormal findings recalled
    - Increase specificity: Employ consensus; limit number of recalls

MISSED CANCERS

- Human-human double reading increases cancer detection by 5-15%
- CAD sensitivity greater for Ca++ than masses; may help improve Ca++ detection
- CAD breast cancer detection increase 7-20%; validated for use with screening and diagnostic mammograms
  - Digital mammography suggests some improvement in cancer detection in specific groups
    - No overall difference film vs. digital performance
    - Improved detection with digital mammography in subgroups: Women with dense breasts, women < 50 years of age, and pre-menopausal women
  - Screening US for dense breasts: Ongoing multicenter trial (ACRIN 6666)
  - Evolving role of MR screening of high-risk women
    - Known or suspected BRCA-1 or BRCA-2 mutation
    - Personal history of breast cancer (controversial)
    - Prior mantle irradiation treatment for Hodgkin disease

DIFFERENTIAL DIAGNOSIS

Interval Cancer
- Malignancy presenting clinically during interval between screenings
- ± Suspicious findings on prior study and/or recall assessment
- Excludes cancers found at regular screening round
- May be mammographically-occult

Mammographically-Occult Cancer
- Statistics vary, may comprise 11-14% of all cancers; up to 30-62% of cancers in dense breasts

PATHOLOGY

General Features
- General path comments
  - Invasive tumors 68-75%
    - Size range 3-55 mm
    - 21% with lymph node metastases
  - DCIS 25-30%
    - Size range 2-90 mm

CLINICAL ISSUES

Presentation
- Most common signs/symptoms: Asymptomatic screening mammogram

DIAGNOSTIC CHECKLIST

Consider
- Radiologists determined whether prior mammograms actionable in 173 screen-detected cancers
  - 5-radiologist panel assessment of case sets enriched with other cancer cases and normal mammograms

- Panels determined whether prior mammograms were BI-RADS 1, 2 (non-actionable) or BI-RADS 3, 4, 5 (actionable)
  - No case was judged actionable by a majority (3/5) of radiologists
- Retrospective subjective assessment by 2 radiologists specializing in breast imaging: 137 non-action and 35 actionable findings
  - Not blinded to the areas where cancer later developed
  - Categorization of common findings where cancer later developed for 137 non-actionable findings
  - Focal asymmetry ("normal appearing tissue"): 47%
  - Few benign-appearing Ca++: 18%
  - Benign-appearing Ca++ cluster: 17%
- Certain subset of screen-detected asymptomatic cancers display, in retrospect, perceptible findings (area of tissue-density, few benign-appearing Ca++) that do not warrant recall as judged by blinded panels
  - Failure to act on these nonspecific findings does not indicate interpretation below standard of care

Image Interpretation Pearls
- Volunteers looking for common tools (e.g., a hammer) within a busy background of 2400 images
  - Findings differed based on prevalence
  - When tool present 1/2 the time, 7% were missed
  - When tool present in only 10:1000 (1% prevalence, similar to the 0.3-0.6% cancer rate on screening mammography), 30% missed

SELECTED REFERENCES

1. Bassett LW et al: Diagnosis of Diseases of the Breast. 2nd ed. Philadelphia, Elsevier Saunders. Chapter 13, 193-223, 2005
2. Wolfe JM et al: Cognitive psychology: rare items often missed. Nature. 435:439-40, 2005
3. Roubidoux MA et al: Invasive cancers detected after breast cancer screening yielded a negative result: relationship of mammographic density to tumor prognostic factors. Radiology. 230:42-8, 2004
4. Ikeda DM et al: Analysis of 172 subtle findings on prior normal mammograms in women with breast cancer detected at follow-up screening. Radiology. 226:494-503, 2003
5. Majid AS et al: Missed breast carcinoma: pitfalls and pearls. RadioGraphics. 23:881-95, 2003
6. Birdwell RL et al: Mammographic characteristics of 115 missed cancers later detected with screening mammography and the potential utility of computer-aided detection. Radiology. 219:192-202, 2001
7. Siegle RL et al: Rates of disagreement in imaging interpretation in a group of community hospitals. Acad Radiol. 5:148-54, 1998
8. Nodine CF et al: Nature of expertise in searching mammograms for breast masses. Acad Radiol. 3:1000-6, 1996
9. Harvey JA et al: Previous mammograms in patients with impalpable breast carcinoma: retrospective vs. blinded interpretation. AJR. 161:1167-72, 1993
10. Bird RE et al: Analysis of cancers missed at screening mammography. Radiology. 184:613-7, 1992

MISSED CANCERS

IMAGE GALLERY

Typical

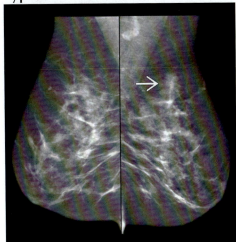 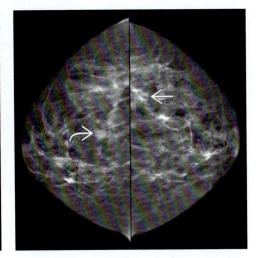

(Left) MLO mammography of a screen-detected left invasive carcinoma seen as an irregular asymmetry ➡. *(Right)* CC mammography on the same patient as previous image does not show the grade II invasive tumor well ➡. In the right breast is an oval density ➡ found at US to be a hypoechoic mass. Right breast biopsy showed fibroadenoma with DCIS away from the mass. The DCIS was serendipitous, not a missed cancer.

Typical

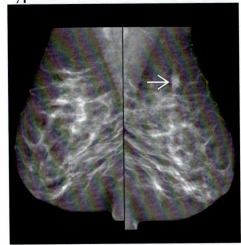 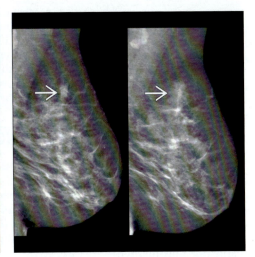

(Left) Earlier MLO mammograms (same case as prior 2 images) show vertical left breast asymmetry ➡. Right mass was not visible on the prior, not considered actionable. *(Right)* Side-by-side MLO mammograms (previous on left, current on right, same as prior 3 images) highlight upper breast finding ➡. This is a case of a lesion seen only on one view at the edge of tissue with findings retrospectively judged as actionable.

Typical

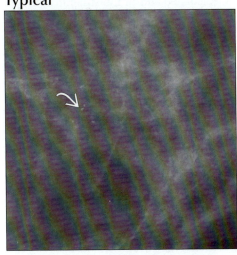 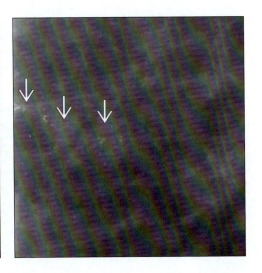

(Left) CC mammography close-up shows loose group of heterogeneous Ca++ ➡ in this 56 y/o. These were new compared to prior but were considered probably benign. *(Right)* CC mammography magnification (same as left) 8 months later shows dramatic increase in Ca++ ➡ which are pleomorphic in a linear distribution, highly suggestive of malignancy. Stereotactic biopsy and excision showed high-grade DCIS. Prior image may have been actionable.

MIXED INVASIVE DUCTAL AND LOBULAR

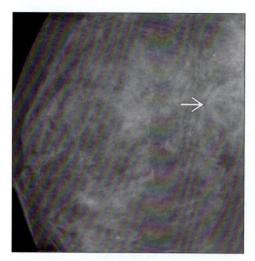

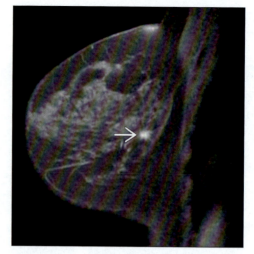

Mammography spot compression shows architectural distortion ➡ *in the posterior right breast on the MLO view only in an asymptomatic 51 year old woman. Sonogram was negative.*

Sagittal T1 C+ FS MR (same patient as on left) shows a spiculated enhancing mass ➡. *Excision showed invasive carcinoma, duct cell type with lobular features.*

TERMINOLOGY

Abbreviations and Synonyms
- Invasive (infiltrating) carcinoma with ductal and lobular features
- Invasive (infiltrating) carcinoma, duct cell type with lobular features
- Invasive (infiltrating) carcinoma with lobular features

Definitions
- Heterogeneous group of invasive carcinomas having both ductal and lobular elements
  - Clinically does not appear to have distinctive features
- Invasive ductal carcinoma (IDC) with no specialized pattern, comprises between 10-49% of the tumor, with the rest of lobular type
  - Descriptive statement, probably not a distinct type of invasive cancer
    - Invasive lobular pattern may be present within IDC to variable degree
    - Variant types of invasive cancer should each be graded

  - Most of mixed invasive ductal and lobular cancers are intermediate combined grade
- Distinguish from IDC NOS: ≥ 50% of the tumor is not a special type
- Distinguish from special types of invasive carcinoma: At least 90% is lobular, tubular, cribriform, mucinous, or medullary

IMAGING FINDINGS

General Features
- Best diagnostic clue: Irregular mass
- Heterogeneous group
  - Imaging findings overlap with findings of other types of invasive cancer
  - Wide range of appearances

Mammographic Findings
- Irregular mass, spiculated and/or indistinct margins ± pleomorphic calcifications
- New focal asymmetry
  - May be mammographically subtle or occult, similar to invasive lobular carcinoma (ILC)

DDx: Mixed Invasive Ductal and Lobular Cancer: Sonographic Appearances

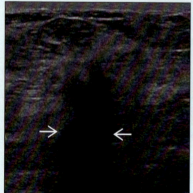

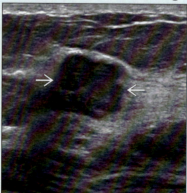

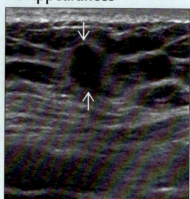

Posterior Shadowing

Microlobulated Mass

Vertical Orientation

MIXED INVASIVE DUCTAL AND LOBULAR

Key Facts

Terminology
- Heterogeneous group of invasive carcinomas having both ductal and lobular elements
- Clinically does not appear to have distinctive features
- Invasive ductal carcinoma (IDC) with no specialized pattern, comprises between 10-49% of the tumor, with the rest of lobular type

Top Differential Diagnoses
- Invasive ductal carcinoma (IDC) NOS
- Invasive lobular carcinoma (ILC)
- Post-Surgical Scar, Fat Necrosis
- Radial Scar
- Fibromatosis (rare)
- Granular Cell Tumor
- Focal Fibrosis, granulomatous mastitis, diabetic mastopathy, sarcoid

Pathology
- May have an association with combined estrogen and progesterone hormone replacement therapy (HRT)
- HRT use is more strongly associated with increased risk of ILC and mixed lobular-ductal breast carcinoma than with IDC

Clinical Issues
- Similar outcome to ductal histology stage for stage

Diagnostic Checklist
- May present as subtle neodensity ± distortion; similar to ILC
- US may identify mammographically occult lesions
- MR useful in evaluation of disease extent

- ○ Mammographic underestimation of multifocality, multicentricity or size may occur
- Architectural distortion

Ultrasonographic Findings
- Grayscale Ultrasound
  - ○ Irregular hypoechoic mass ± posterior shadowing
    - ■ Heterogeneous or homogeneous echotexture
    - ■ Vertical or parallel orientation
    - ■ Thick, irregular echogenic rim
  - ○ Architectural distortion
  - ○ Useful in detecting mammographically subtle or occult cancer and in guiding core biopsy

MR Findings
- T1WI: May show spiculated mass ± architectural distortion
- T2WI FS: May show spiculated mass ± architectural distortion, variable signal intensity
- T1 C+ FS
  - ○ Range of appearances
    - ■ Rapid wash-in and wash-out
    - ■ Rim-enhancing, heterogeneous mass
    - ■ Multiple small foci ± interconnecting reticular enhancement

Imaging Recommendations
- Best imaging tool
  - ○ Careful comparison with previous mammograms to detect developing asymmetries
  - ○ MR most sensitive in determining extent
- Protocol advice: Second-look or targeted US may help guide biopsy of additional lesions seen on MR

DIFFERENTIAL DIAGNOSIS

Other Malignancy
- Invasive ductal carcinoma (IDC) NOS
  - ○ Imaging features indistinguishable
  - ○ Histology: Forms glandular structures
- Invasive lobular carcinoma (ILC)

- ○ May appear as focal asymmetry ± distortion on routine views
- ○ Histology: Less cohesive than IDC, tends to invade in single file
- ○ Loss of E-cadherin expression
- Ductal carcinoma in situ (DCIS)
  - ○ Most commonly suspicious calcifications

Post-Surgical Scar, Fat Necrosis
- History of surgical biopsy or trauma

Radial Scar
- Spiculated area of distortion, may lack central mass; overlap of imaging features with malignancy

Fibromatosis (rare)
- Can be irregular, shadowing mass on US

Granular Cell Tumor
- Mimics malignancy clinically and at imaging
- Irregular mass with spiculated, lobulated or circumscribed margins

Other Benign Causes
- Focal Fibrosis, granulomatous mastitis, diabetic mastopathy, sarcoid

PATHOLOGY

General Features
- Genetics
  - ○ ER-α A908G mutation
    - ■ Present at a low frequency in invasive breast tumors and may occur more frequently in higher grade cancers
    - ■ Mutation may be associated with mixed ductal-lobular tumor type
  - ○ Loss of E-cadherin gene expression in lobular areas: Deletion of 16q correlates with loss of E-cadherin
- Etiology
  - ○ May have an association with combined estrogen and progesterone hormone replacement therapy (HRT)

MIXED INVASIVE DUCTAL AND LOBULAR

- From 1987 through 1999, USA incidence rates of lobular tumors increased 1.52-fold, mixed ductal-lobular increased 1.96-fold, and ductal carcinoma rates remained constant
  - HRT use is more strongly associated with increased risk of ILC and mixed lobular-ductal breast carcinoma than with IDC
- Epidemiology: Approximately 2.2-6% of invasive carcinomas
- For a tumor to be typed as IDC NOS it must have a non-specialized pattern in over 50% of its mass
- If ductal NOS pattern comprises between 10 and 49% of the tumor, then it is one of the mixed groups: Mixed ductal and special type carcinoma
  - Special type invasive carcinomas: Lobular, tubular, cribriform, medullary and mucinous
- If the ductal NOS pattern comprises less than 10% of the tumor, it is recognized as special type

Microscopic Features
- A portion of invasive breast cancers are not readily classifiable as either ductal or lobular
- Mixed invasive ductal and lobular cancer is a heterogeneous group
  - May have ductal and lobular areas or have foci transitional between the two patterns
    - Cytologically may have variable component with ductal characteristics or show round, low grade nuclei characteristic of classic invasive lobular cancer
    - Architecturally may have variable component of single-file pattern or ductal characteristics

Staging, Grading or Classification Criteria
- Criteria are the same for all invasive cancers
  - Elston and Ellis modification of Bloom and Richardson grading system
    - Tubule formation (more gets lower score), nuclear pleomorphism and mitotic activity each scored on a scale of 1-3
    - Sum of scores is 3-5: Histologic grade 1 (well differentiated)
    - Sum of scores is 6-7: Histologic grade 2 (moderately differentiated)
    - Sum of scores is 8-9: Histologic grade 3 (poorly differentiated)
  - Most invasive carcinomas with lobular features are intermediate combined grade, however more frequently poorly differentiated (grade 3) than ILC
  - Nuclear grade of lobular carcinoma component increases as percentage of the carcinoma that is ductal type increases

CLINICAL ISSUES

Presentation
- Most common signs/symptoms
  - Asymptomatic
  - Hard palpable mass or focal breast thickening
- Other signs/symptoms
  - Nipple and/or skin retraction
  - Shrinking breast

Natural History & Prognosis
- Similar outcome to ductal histology stage for stage

Treatment
- Same as for IDC
  - Mixed lobular-ductal or lobular histology should not influence decisions regarding therapy

DIAGNOSTIC CHECKLIST

Consider
- May present as subtle neodensity ± distortion; similar to ILC
- US may identify mammographically occult lesions
- MR useful in evaluation of disease extent

Image Interpretation Pearls
- Focal developing asymmetry requires explanation

SELECTED REFERENCES

1. Bartella L et al: Nonpalpable mammographically occult invasive breast cancers detected by MRI. AJR. 186:865-70, 2006
2. Bane AL et al: Invasive lobular carcinoma: To grade or not to grade. Mod Pathol. 18:621-8, 2005
3. Harigopal M et al: Aberrant E-cadherin staining patterns in invasive mammary carcinoma. World J Surg Oncol. 3:73, 2005
4. Berg WA et al: Diagnostic accuracy of mammography, clinical examination, US, and MR imaging in preoperative assessment of breast cancer. Radiology. 233:830-49, 2004
5. Buist DS et al: Factors contributing to mammography failure in women aged 40-49 years. J Natl Cancer Inst. 96:1432-40, 2004
6. Korkola JE et al: Differentiation of lobular versus ductal breast carcinomas by expression microarray analysis. Cancer Research. 63:7167-75, 2003
7. Li CI et al: Trends in incidence rates of invasive lobular and ductal breast carcinoma. JAMA. 289:1421-24, 2003
8. Evans, III WP et al: Invasive lobular carcinoma of the breast: mammographic characteristics and computer-aided detection. Radiology. 225:182-9, 2002
9. Goldstein NS: Does the level of E-cadherin expression correlate with the primary breast carcinoma infiltration pattern and type of systemic metastases? Am J Clin Pathol. 118:425-34, 2002
10. Peiro G et al: The influence of infiltrating lobular carcinoma on the outcome of patients treated with breast-conserving surgery and radiation therapy. Breast Cancer Res Treat. 59:49-54, 2000
11. Schnitt SJ et al: Pathology of invasive breast cancer. In: Harris JR et al: Diseases of the Breast. 2nd ed. Philadelphia, Lippincott Williams & Wilkins. 431, 2000
12. Rodenko GN et al: MR imaging in the management before surgery of lobular carcinoma of the breast: correlation with pathology. AJR. 167:1415-19, 1996
13. Le Gal M et al: Mammographic features of 455 invasive lobular carcinomas. Radiology. 185:705-8, 1992
14. Sickles EA et al: Subtle and atypical mammographic features of invasive lobular carcinoma. Radiology. 178:25-6, 1991

MIXED INVASIVE DUCTAL AND LOBULAR

IMAGE GALLERY

Typical

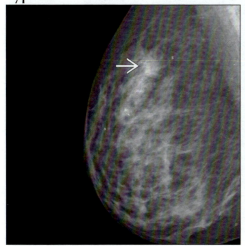
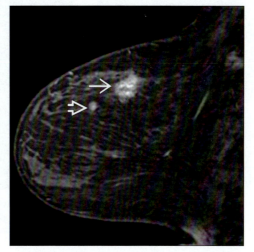

(Left) 51 year old woman with history of Hodgkin disease 30 years ago, treated with radiation. MLO mammography shows an irregular mass in the upper breast ➡. US-guided core biopsy revealed invasive carcinoma, duct cell type with lobular features. *(Right)* Sagittal T1 C+ FS MR (same patient as on left) shows the known cancer ➡ and another small enhancing nodule ⇨ more anteriorly. The latter proved to be a papilloma.

Typical

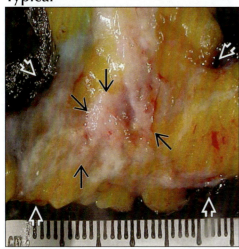
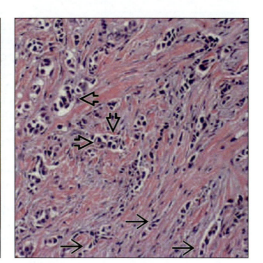

(Left) Gross pathology of an invasive carcinoma with mixed ductal and lobular features shows ill-defined mass ➡. Margins inked black ⇨. *(Right)* Corresponding histopathology image (same patient as on left) shows ductal pattern ⇨ on the upper left and linear strands of infiltrating cancer cells of lobular type ➡ on the lower right.

Typical

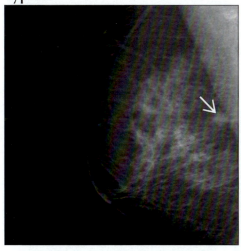
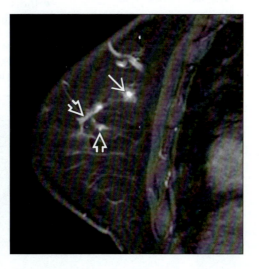

(Left) MLO mammography shows an irregular mass ➡ in the posterior breast, detected on screening mammogram of this 48 year old woman. No other lesion was seen at mammography or sonography. US-guided core biopsy showed mixed invasive ductal and lobular cancer. *(Right)* Sagittal T1 C+ FS MR (same patient as on left) shows the known cancer ➡, and additional enhancing areas ⇨. All proved to be carcinoma at excision.

MUCINOUS CARCINOMA

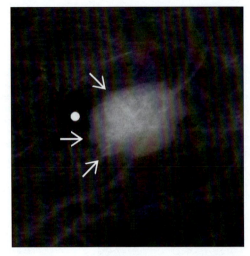

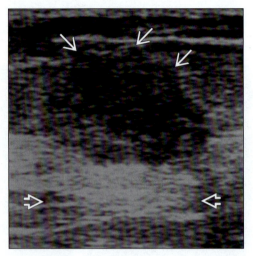

CC mammography shows a dense, microlobulated mass ➡ marked as palpable with a skin BB. While fairly well-defined, this is not a circumscribed lesion and is dense. Ultrasound (right image) was performed.

Ultrasound shows hypoechoic, microlobulated mass ➡ with posterior enhancement ➡. US-guided 14-g core biopsy and excision showed mucinous carcinoma.

TERMINOLOGY

Abbreviations and Synonyms
- Colloid carcinoma, gelatinous carcinoma or mucous carcinoma

Definitions
- An uncommon special type of infiltrating ductal carcinoma characterized by large amounts of extracellular mucin
  - Pure type: ≥ 90% of tumor shows mucin production
  - Mixed type: 75-89% has mucinous features

IMAGING FINDINGS

General Features
- Best diagnostic clue
  - Partially circumscribed round, oval, or lobulated, dense mass on mammography
  - Isoechoic, microlobulated mass with posterior enhancement on US
- Location: No particular predilection
- Size: Range: Less than 1 cm to 20 cm

Mammographic Findings
- Round, oval or lobulated, dense mass
  - Partially circumscribed margins, microlobulated in 39%
  - At least a portion of the margin is typically indistinct, particularly in mixed type
- Irregular shape, spiculated margins may be seen with mixed type
- Calcifications not characteristic: Amorphous, punctate, rarely pleomorphic
  - More common in mixed type
- Approximately 20% not detected by mammography

Ultrasonographic Findings
- Grayscale Ultrasound
  - Variable shape: Round, oval or irregular
  - Partially circumscribed or microlobulated margins
    - Mixed type may have angular, spiculated margins
    - Indistinct margins favor mixed type
  - Isoechoic to fat, especially when small, ≤ 1.5 cm
    - Larger lesions, mixed type, usually hypoechoic
    - Can be overlooked
  - Posterior enhancement in > 50%
    - Posterior shadowing rare

DDx: Mimics of Mucinous Carcinoma

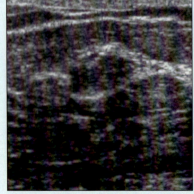

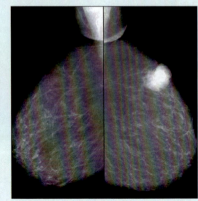

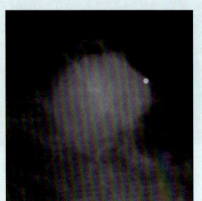

| Fibroadenoma | Infiltrating Ductal Carcinoma, NOS | Medullary Carcinoma |

MUCINOUS CARCINOMA

Key Facts

Terminology
- Colloid carcinoma, gelatinous carcinoma or mucous carcinoma
- An uncommon special type of infiltrating ductal carcinoma characterized by large amounts of extracellular mucin
- Pure type: ≥ 90% of tumor shows mucin production
- Mixed type: 75-89% has mucinous features

Imaging Findings
- Partially circumscribed round, oval, or lobulated, dense mass on mammography
- Isoechoic, microlobulated mass with posterior enhancement on US
- Irregular shape, spiculated margins may be seen with mixed type

- T2WI FS: High signal intensity due to large mucin component

Top Differential Diagnoses
- Fibroadenoma (FA)
- Infiltrating Ductal Carcinoma (IDC), NOS
- Mucocele-Like Lesion

Pathology
- 2% of all breast carcinomas

Clinical Issues
- Palpable in 50% of patients
- Soft to firm on clinical exam
- Pure type more common in postmenopausal women
- Slow growing
- More favorable prognosis than IDC NOS

- ○ Homogeneity usually associated with pure lesions
  - ▪ Mixed type may have mixed cystic, solid components
- ○ Most have parallel orientation; can be vertical when < 1 cm in size
- ○ Less compressible than lipoma or fibroadenoma
- Power Doppler
  - ○ Vascularity noted in ~ one third of tumors
    - ▪ Reported in both the center and periphery

MR Findings
- T1WI
  - ○ Smooth or indistinct, round, oval, or microlobulated mass
  - ○ Variable signal intensity: Low to high
- T2WI FS: High signal intensity due to large mucin component
- T1 C+ FS
  - ○ Reports vary: Slow to rapid initial enhancement
  - ○ Post-initial phase: Persistent or plateau kinetics

Imaging Recommendations
- Best imaging tool: Mammography and ultrasound
- Protocol advice: Turn off spatial compounding on US to improve detection of posterior enhancement

DIFFERENTIAL DIAGNOSIS

Fibroadenoma (FA)
- Circumscribed oval or gently lobulated mass
- Usually slightly hypoechoic
- Normal or enhanced through transmission
- Develop coarse calcifications

Infiltrating Ductal Carcinoma (IDC), NOS
- Irregular mass
- Indistinct or spiculated margins
- Pleomorphic calcifications may be present
- Posterior shadowing or no posterior features on US
- High grade IDC can be mostly circumscribed and show posterior enhancement on US
  - ○ May have cystic component (necrosis)

Mucocele-Like Lesion
- Composed of mucin-containing cysts
- Well-circumscribed lobulated lesions on mammography; hypoechoic on US
- Most have indeterminate calcifications

PATHOLOGY

General Features
- General path comments
  - ○ 2% of all breast carcinomas
    - ▪ 1% in women ≤ 35 years of age
    - ▪ 7% in women ≥ 75 years of age
  - ○ Associated DCIS in 75% of cases
    - ▪ Cribriform, papillary, micropapillary and/or comedo
    - ▪ Generally found at the periphery of the lesion
    - ▪ May also exhibit extracellular mucin production
  - ○ Axillary metastases
    - ▪ Pure form 6%
    - ▪ Mixed form 30-40%
    - ▪ Usually demonstrate histologic characteristics of primary tumor, but nonmucinous metastases can occur

Gross Pathologic & Surgical Features
- Cut surface moist and glistening; semitransparent
- Pure type
  - ○ Circumscribed, smooth lobulated mass
  - ○ Firm to soft: Greater % of mucin, softer to palpation
  - ○ Borders: Pushing, rather than infiltrating
- Mixed type
  - ○ Ill-defined
  - ○ Grossly appears to be attached to, or infiltrating surrounding tissue
  - ○ Increased fibrous stromal reaction → firmer to palpation

Microscopic Features
- Aggregates of tumor cells surrounded by abundant extracellular mucin

MUCINOUS CARCINOMA

- Cellular arrangement
  - Slender strands
  - Alveolar nests
  - Papillary clusters
  - Compartmentalized by fibrovascular bands
- Tumor cells tend to be small and uniform
  - Low or intermediate nuclear grade
- Tubule and gland formation uncommon
- Neuroendocrine differentiation
  - 25-50% cases
  - Argyrophilic and dense-core secretory granules
  - No prognostic significance
- ER positive 90% on immunohistochemical studies
- PR positive 50-68%
- Her-2/neu immunoreactivity ≤ 5%
- Low S-phase
- Increased MUC2 and MUC5 expression; decreased MUCU1
- Fewer chromosomal abnormalities than IDC NOS

CLINICAL ISSUES

Presentation
- Most common signs/symptoms
  - Palpable in 50% of patients
    - Soft to firm on clinical exam
    - May be confused clinically with cyst or FA
  - When large, can be fixed to skin or chest wall
  - Pain, nipple discharge uncommon
  - May be asymptomatic
    - Initially detected on imaging
- Core biopsy more reliable than fine needle aspiration

Demographics
- Age
  - Pure type more common in postmenopausal women
    - Average age 63
    - Range: 21-95
  - Mixed type more common in younger women
- Gender
  - Predominantly female
    - Rare cases reported in males

Natural History & Prognosis
- Slow growing
- More favorable prognosis than IDC NOS
  - 10 year survival for pure form 90%
  - Survival for mixed form similar to IDC NOS
- Tumor size does not appear to impact survival
  - Large mucin volume → overestimate tumor burden
- Systemic recurrences after 10 years not unusual
- Unusual complications
  - Mucin embolism → cerebral infarction
  - Pseudomyxoma peritonei

Treatment
- Standard surgical treatment
  - Lumpectomy
    - Mastectomy reserved for large tumors or multicentric disease
  - Sentinel node biopsy
  - Radiation therapy after lumpectomy [breast-conserving treatment (BCT)]

- Chemotherapy based on size and nodal status

DIAGNOSTIC CHECKLIST

Consider
- Mucinous carcinoma for a circumscribed dense mammographic mass, isoechoic on ultrasound

Image Interpretation Pearls
- Can be easily overlooked on US: Look for posterior enhancement, isoechoic mass

SELECTED REFERENCES

1. Lam WW et al: Role of fine needle aspiration and tru cut biopsy in diagnosis of mucinous carcinoma of breast--from a radiologist's perspective. Clin Imaging. 30(1):6-10, 2006
2. Bassett L et al: Diagnosis of Diseases of the Breast. Philadelphia, Elsevier Saunders. Chapter 27, 504-6, 2005
3. Farshid G et al: Mucocele-like lesions of the breast: a benign cause for indeterminate or suspicious mammographic microcalcifications. Breast J. 11(1):15-22, 2005
4. Mizuta Y et al: A case of non-metastatic giant mucinous carcinoma of the breast. Breast Cancer. 12(4):337-40, 2005
5. Rakha EA et al: Expression of mucins (MUC1, MUC2, MUC3, MUC4, MUC5AC and MUC6) and their prognostic significance in human breast cancer. Mod Pathol. 18(10):1295-304, 2005
6. Harris J et al: Diseases of the Breast. 3rd ed. Philadelphia, Lippincott Williams & Wilkins. Chapter 34, 549-41, 2004
7. Komenaka IK et al: Pure mucinous carcinoma of the breast. Am J Surg. 187(4):528-32, 2004
8. Lam WW et al: Sonographic appearance of mucinous carcinoma of the breast. AJR Am J Roentgenol. 182(4):1069-74, 2004
9. Stavros AT: Breast Ultrasound. Philadelphia, Lippincott Williams & Wilkins. Chapter 14, 645-8, 2004
10. Gupta RK et al: Needle aspiration cytodiagnosis of mucinous (colloid) carcinoma of male breast. Pathology. 35(6):539-40, 2003
11. Rosen P: Rosen's Breast Pathology. 2nd ed. Philadelphia, Lippincott Williams & Wilkins. Chapter 20, 463-81, 2001
12. Matsuda M et al: Mammographic and clinicopathological features of mucinous carcinoma of the breast. Breast Cancer. 7(1):65-70, 2000
13. Memis A et al: Mucinous (colloid) breast cancer: mammographic and US features with histologic correlation. Eur J Radiol. 35(1):39-43, 2000
14. Georgiev Ch et al: [Mucinous breast carcinomas with neuroendocrine differentiation] Khirurgiia (Sofiia). 55(5):22-4, 1999
15. Avisar E et al: Pure mucinous carcinoma of the breast: a clinicopathologic correlation study. Ann Surg Oncol. 5(5):447-51, 1998
16. Fujikawa T et al: A case of Mucinous Carcinoma of the Male Breast with Unusual Ultrasonographic Findings Mimicking Phyllodes Tumor. Breast Cancer. 5(1):83-86, 1998
17. Simsir A et al: Additional mimics of mucinous mammary carcinoma: fibroepithelial lesions. Am J Clin Pathol. 109(2):169-72, 1998

MUCINOUS CARCINOMA

IMAGE GALLERY

Typical

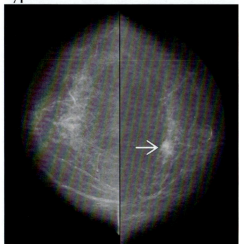

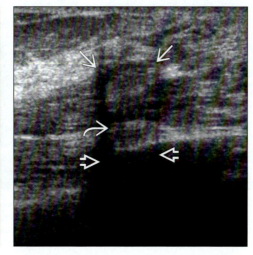

(Left) CC mammography from a screening exam shows an oval, partially obscured high density mass ➡ in the left inner breast. This was even more subtle on the MLO view (not shown). *(Right)* Longitudinal ultrasound (same mass as left) shows an irregular isoechoic mass ➡ with indistinct margins, edge refraction ➡, and minimal posterior enhancement ➡. Biopsy = mucinous carcinoma.

Typical

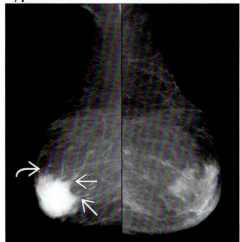

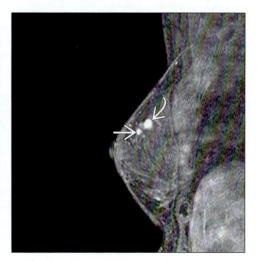

(Left) MLO mammography shows a very dense round mass ➡ with indistinct margins and associated microcalcifications ➡. Core biopsy = grade I mucinous carcinoma with low nuclear grade DCIS. *(Right)* Sagittal T1WI MR in another woman with a negative mammogram shows two enhancing masses, one 5 mm ➡ and the other 9 mm ➡ in size. MR-guided biopsy showed both to be mucinous carcinoma.

Typical

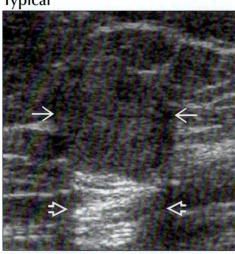

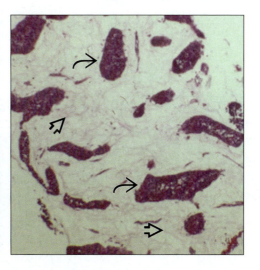

(Left) Sagittal ultrasound shows a subtle, isoechoic mass ➡ with posterior acoustic enhancement ➡ which on mammogram was dense and indistinctly marginated. US-guided biopsy showed mucinous carcinoma. *(Right)* Micropathology, low power, H&E of a mucinous carcinoma (same mass as left) is characterized by nests of uniform round tumor cells ➡ surrounded by extensive extracellular mucin ➡.

PAPILLARY CARCINOMA, INVASIVE

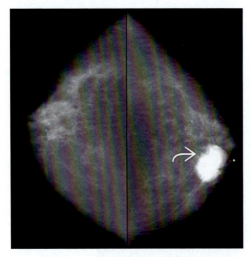

CC mammography of this 55 year old woman shows a breast mass immediately behind the left nipple with indistinct and microlobulated margins ➔.

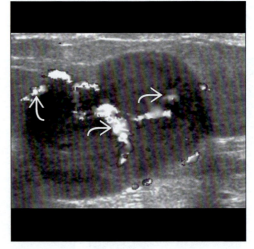

Color Doppler ultrasound (same case as left-hand image) demonstrates exuberant vascularity ➔. Excisional biopsy revealed a 3 cm moderately differentiated invasive papillary carcinoma.

TERMINOLOGY

Abbreviations and Synonyms
- Infiltrating papillary carcinoma

Definitions
- Invasive carcinoma with a papillary architecture
  - Stromal invasion is present; different from (the more frequent) non-invasive papillary carcinoma
  - Invasive papillary carcinoma frequently has (papillary) ductal carcinoma in situ (DCIS) in the surrounding breast
  - Focal invasion is typically present at the periphery of intracystic papillary carcinoma
    - Non-invasive papillary carcinoma = papillary DCIS; intracystic papillary carcinoma is papillary DCIS within a dilated duct

IMAGING FINDINGS

General Features
- Best diagnostic clue

  - Mostly circumscribed complex cystic and solid mass in an elderly patient
  - Partially indistinct margin suggests invasive component
  - Imaging findings cannot distinguish invasive from in situ papillary carcinoma in most cases
- Morphology
  - Two types
    - Solid: Has higher tendency to invade
    - Cystic: May develop in a dilated lobule or duct
  - May be solitary or multiple

Mammographic Findings
- Round, oval or lobulated, mostly circumscribed, partially indistinctly marginated dense mass
- Multiple masses may occur, often within one quadrant
- Calcifications, if present, are amorphous or pleomorphic
- Spiculations are rare: Minimal fibrotic reaction
- Galactographic findings
  - May be helpful in evaluation of nipple discharge
  - Ductal obstruction, wall irregularity, filling defects

Ultrasonographic Findings
- Grayscale Ultrasound

DDx: Invasive Papillary Carcinoma: Typical Sonographic Appearances

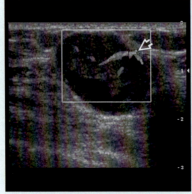

Increased Vascularity

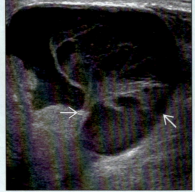

Complex Cystic Mass

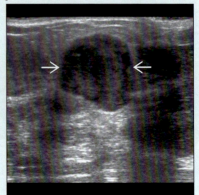

Heterogeneous Solid Mass

PAPILLARY CARCINOMA, INVASIVE

Key Facts

Terminology
- Infiltrating papillary carcinoma
- Invasive carcinoma with a papillary architecture
- Stromal invasion is present; different from (the more frequent) non-invasive papillary carcinoma

Imaging Findings
- Mostly circumscribed complex cystic and solid mass in an elderly patient
- Solid: Has higher tendency to invade
- Cystic: May develop in a dilated lobule or duct
- May be solitary or multiple
- Round, oval or lobulated, mostly circumscribed, partially indistinctly marginated dense mass
- Solid or complex cystic and solid mass(es)

Top Differential Diagnoses
- Simple Cyst or Complicated Cyst
- Fibroadenoma
- Hematoma, Infection, Abscess
- Galactocele
- Intraductal papillary proliferations
- Sclerosing papilloma
- Invasive Ductal Carcinoma (IDC)
- Phyllodes Tumor

Diagnostic Checklist
- US-guided core biopsy helps establish diagnosis of malignancy
- Frequent underestimation of presence of invasion (invasive component generally focally present at periphery)

- ○ Solid or complex cystic and solid mass(es)
- ○ Intracystic mass or mural nodules
  - ▪ Intracystic portion is usually due to DCIS
- ○ Papillary projections and septae
- ○ Sequelae of hemorrhage may be seen
- ○ Posterior enhancement or normal sound transmission
- Color Doppler: Frequently shows increased vascularity within solid areas

MR Findings
- T1 C+ FS
  - ○ Heterogeneous enhancing smooth mass if solid
  - ○ Mural/nodular enhancement of intracystic mass (± hemorrhage)

Biopsy
- Aspiration may yield bloody fluid: Send for cytology
- US-guided core biopsy of solid component
  - ○ May sample only the (frequently associated) in situ component

Imaging Recommendations
- Best imaging tool: Mammography and US: Mostly circumscribed, solid or complex cystic mass
- Protocol advice: Direct core biopsy to indistinctly marginated, solid portion(s) of mass to facilitate sampling of invasive component

DIFFERENTIAL DIAGNOSIS

Simple Cyst or Complicated Cyst
- Lobulated simple cyst with adjacent parenchyma projecting into cyst
- Tumefactive debris adherent to wall, mimicking intracystic mass

Fibroadenoma
- Occurs in younger age group
- Circumscribed, oval, hypoechoic mass

Hematoma, Infection, Abscess
- History of trauma, biopsy or infection is suggestive

- Hemorrhagic debris can mimic mass

Galactocele
- Lactating or pregnant younger patient
- Relatively echogenic fluid due to fat content

Spectrum of Papillary Neoplasms
- Intraductal papillary proliferations
  - ○ Benign papilloma, papilloma with foci of carcinoma in situ, non-invasive papillary carcinoma (papillary DCIS)
  - ○ Usually smaller size
  - ○ Similar mammographic and US findings
  - ○ Indistinct margin suggests invasive component
  - ○ May present as single or multiple circumscribed masses
- Sclerosing papilloma
  - ○ Pseudoinvasive growth pattern, can be mistaken for carcinoma

Invasive Ductal Carcinoma (IDC)
- IDC NOS most common; medullary, mucinous types
- Usually solid mass; may be complex cystic and solid mass, may appear mostly circumscribed
- Centrally necrotic mass may appear partially anechoic, thick-walled cyst

Phyllodes Tumor
- Dense mammographic mass, usually circumscribed
- Circumscribed hypoechoic mass ± cystic foci on US

Lymphoma or Metastatic Disease
- Dense, mostly circumscribed mass on mammography
- Often multiple

PATHOLOGY

General Features
- Epidemiology
  - ○ 1-2% of all invasive breast cancers
  - ○ Older women (mean age 65 years)
  - ○ Slow growth rate

PAPILLARY CARCINOMA, INVASIVE

Gross Pathologic & Surgical Features
- Circumscribed in 2/3 of cases
- Frequently indistinguishable from IDC
- Often contain hemorrhagic and cystic areas

Microscopic Features
- Hallmark of all papillary neoplasms (benign or malignant)
  - Proliferating epithelium in villous-like projections
- Histologic diagnosis of papillary lesions known to be challenging
  - Complete absence of myoepithelial layer indicates carcinoma
  - Presence of myoepithelial cells does not exclude intraductal cancer
- Invasion is usually at the periphery of papillary DCIS
  - Invasive component is not papillary in most cases; has IDC pattern
  - Invasive cancer may have a papillary pattern (rare)
- Concomitant DCIS frequently present in surrounding breast tissue
- Papillary structure fragile, may become fragmented and tends to bleed
  - Following needling procedures, displaced papillary epithelium along needle track may mimic invasion
- Often ER +, PR +, and Her-2/neu not amplified
- Lymphovascular invasion (LVI) in one third of cases

Staging, Grading or Classification Criteria
- Staging same as for all invasive carcinoma staging
- Most of the tumors are histologic grade 2

CLINICAL ISSUES

Presentation
- Firm but not hard, mobile mass
- Mass may be large owing to cystic component
- Nipple discharge in up to one third of cases
  - Usually bloody or serosanguineous

Demographics
- Age: Typically postmenopausal patients
- Gender
  - Women: Approximately 1-2% of invasive cancers
  - Men: Approximately 2-3% of invasive cancers
    - Second most frequent invasive cancer in men after IDC NOS
- Ethnicity: Disproportionate number of cases in non-Caucasian women

Natural History & Prognosis
- Size of invasive component small in relation to lesion size
- Axillary metastases infrequent
- Relatively good prognosis
- NSABP-BO4 trial: One of "favorable" histology tumors (along with pure tubular and mucinous carcinomas); better survival per univariate analysis

Treatment
- Excision, lymph node sampling

- As most of tumor is usually in situ, large tumor on imaging (> 5 cm) does not usually indicate locally advanced breast cancer
  - Not usually appropriate for neoadjuvant chemotherapy

DIAGNOSTIC CHECKLIST

Consider
- US-guided core biopsy helps establish diagnosis of malignancy
  - Frequent underestimation of presence of invasion (invasive component generally focally present at periphery)

Image Interpretation Pearls
- Focally indistinct margins and usually complex cystic/solid appearance on US dictate need for biopsy

SELECTED REFERENCES

1. Mercado CL et al: Papillary lesions of the breast at percutaneous core-needle biopsy. Radiology. 238:801-8, 2006
2. Carder PJ et al: Needle core biopsy can reliably distinguish between benign and malignant papillary lesions of the breast. Histopathology. 46:320-7, 2005
3. Hill CB et al: Myoepithelial cell staining patterns of papillary breast lesions: from intraductal papillomas to invasive papillary carcinomas. Am J Clin Pathol. 123:36-44, 2005
4. Nagi C et al: Epithelial displacement in breast lesions: a papillary phenomenon. Arch Pathol Lab Med. 129:1465-9, 2005
5. Putti TC et al: Breast pathology practice: most common problems in a consultation service. Histopathology. 7:445-57, 2005
6. Yang WT et al: Sonographic, mammographic, and histopathologic correlation of symptomatic ductal carcinoma in situ. AJR. 182:101-10, 2004
7. Blaumeiser B et al: Invasive papillary carcinoma of the male breast. Eur Radiol. 12:2207-10, 2002
8. Hoda SA et al: Practical considerations in the pathologic diagnosis of needle core biopsies of breast. Am J Clin Pathol. 118:101-8, 2002
9. Renshaw AA: Predicting invasion in the excision specimen from breast core needle biopsy specimens with only ductal carcinoma in situ. Arch Pathol Lab Med. 126:39-41, 2002
10. Liberman L et al: Intracystic papillary carcinoma with invasion. Radiology. 219:781-4, 2001
11. Orel SG et al: MR imaging in patients with nipple discharge: initial experience. Radiology. 216:248-54, 2000
12. Philpotts LE et al: Uncommon high-risk lesions of the breast diagnosed at stereotactic core-needle biopsy: clinical importance. Radiology. 216:831-7, 2000
13. Liberman L et al: Percutaneous large-core biopsy of papillary breast lesions. AJR. 172:331-7, 1999
14. McCulloch GL et al: Radiological features of papillary carcinoma of the breast. Clin Radiol. 52:865-8, 1997
15. Soo MS et al: Papillary carcinoma of the breast: Imaging findings. AJR. 164:321-6, 1995
16. Mitnick JS et al: Invasive papillary carcinoma of the breast: mammographic appearance. Radiology. 177:803-6, 1990
17. Tabar L et al: Galactography: the diagnostic procedure of choice for nipple discharge. Radiology. 149:31-8, 1983
18. Kraus FT et al: The differential diagnosis of papillary tumors of the breast. Cancer. 15:444-55, 1962

PAPILLARY CARCINOMA, INVASIVE

IMAGE GALLERY

Typical

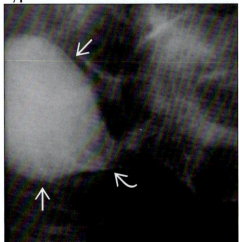

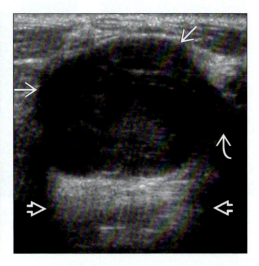

(Left) Close-up of MLO mammogram shows a mostly circumscribed mass ➡ in the posterior left breast. The anterior margin of the mass is focally indistinctly marginated ➡. *(Right)* Ultrasound (same patient as left-hand image) shows a complex cystic mass ➡ with posterior enhancement ➡. The margins are partially indistinct ➡. Excision showed papillary DCIS and microscopic invasive component along the anterior margin.

Typical

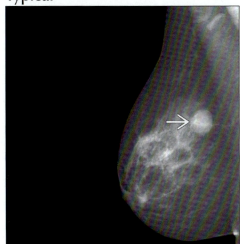

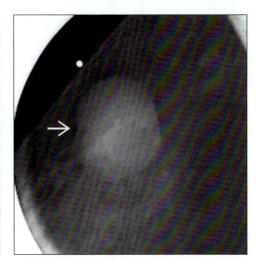

(Left) MLO mammography shows a round, circumscribed mass ➡ in a 63 year-old woman with a palpable mass in the right breast. *(Right)* MLO spot compression (same patient as left-hand image) again shows the dense circumscribed mass ➡. Excisional biopsy showed intracystic papillary carcinoma with invasion. (Courtesy EAR)

Typical

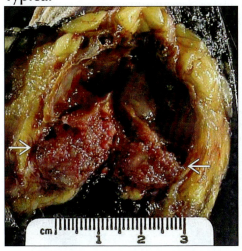

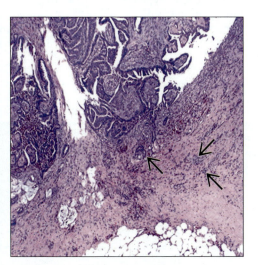

(Left) Gross appearance of an intracystic papillary carcinoma with invasion ➡ in a 75 year old woman. Macroscopically it is indistinguishable from papilloma or intracystic papillary carcinoma; the large size and patient age favor malignancy. *(Right)* Histology reveals (same patient as left-hand image) intraductal papillary carcinoma and invasive component at the periphery ➡ (H&E x 40).

PLEOMORPHIC LOBULAR CARCINOMA

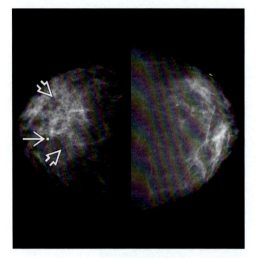

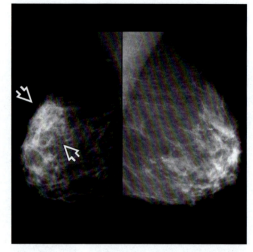

CC mammography shows the right breast to be smaller than the left in this 56 year old woman with palpable thickening ➡ *(marked with a BB). Increased density and calcifications are seen* ➡.

MLO mammography again shows the "shrinking" right breast ➡ *(same patient as left-hand image). US-guided 14-g core biopsy showed pleomorphic lobular carcinoma, with associated calcifications.*

TERMINOLOGY

Abbreviations and Synonyms
- Pleomorphic lobular carcinoma (PLC)
- Poorly differentiated/high grade infiltrating lobular carcinoma (ILC)

Definitions
- PLC: A variant histopathologic pattern of ILC exhibiting cellular atypia

IMAGING FINDINGS

Radiographic Findings
- Mammography
  - Fine linear/pleomorphic calcifications
    - Frequently extensive, segmental or regional
    - Calcifications usually absent in classic type ILC
  - Mass, architectural distortion, asymmetry, or "shrinking breast"
  - Can be diffuse, often subtle

Ultrasonographic Findings
- Mass, shadowing, architectural distortion, ± Ca++

MR Findings
- T1 C+ FS: Irregular mass with rapid wash-in & wash-out ± rim-enhancement, may be reticular/dendritic

Imaging Recommendations
- Best imaging tool: MR most sensitive, best depicts extent
- Protocol advice: Magnification mammographic views of calcifications

DIFFERENTIAL DIAGNOSIS

Malignancy
- Invasive carcinoma: Invasive ductal carcinoma (IDC), ILC or special types: Irregular mass
  - Appearances indistinguishable
- Ductal carcinoma in situ: Fine-linear calcifications

DDx: Pleomorphic Lobular Carcinoma Appearances

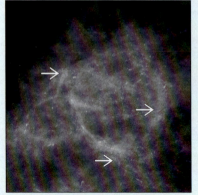

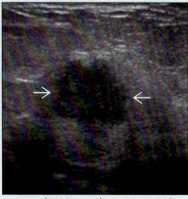

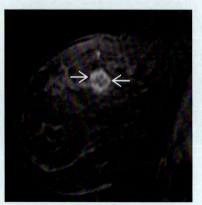

Pleomorphic Calcifications

Irregular Hypoechoic Mass (US)

Rim Enhancing Mass (MR)

PLEOMORPHIC LOBULAR CARCINOMA

Key Facts

Terminology

- Poorly differentiated/high grade infiltrating lobular carcinoma (ILC)
- PLC: A variant histopathologic pattern of ILC exhibiting cellular atypia

Imaging Findings

- Fine linear/pleomorphic calcifications
- Mass, architectural distortion, asymmetry, or "shrinking breast"

Top Differential Diagnoses

- Invasive carcinoma: Invasive ductal carcinoma (IDC), ILC or special types: Irregular mass
- Ductal carcinoma in situ: Fine-linear calcifications

Clinical Issues

- Aggressive biologic behavior; worse prognosis than classical ILC

Other Entities Mimicking Malignancy

- Benign: Post-Surgical scar, fat necrosis, radial scar, focal fibrosis, diabetic mastopathy, sarcoid
- Fibromatosis, granular cell tumor

PATHOLOGY

General Features

- Genetics
  - Often aneuploid
  - Loss of 16q and gain of 1q, associated with lack of E-cadherin expression, as in classic ILC
  - Some PLCs show additional molecular genetic changes analogous to high grade DCIS: E.g., gain of c-myc and Her-2/neu
- Metastatic patterns of PLC are similar to classic ILC
  - Propensity to metastasize to the leptomeninges, peritoneum, retroperitoneum, gastrointestinal tract and reproductive organs
  - Metastatic infiltration in lymph nodes in a single cell pattern; may be difficult to identify

Microscopic Features

- Growth pattern of ILC retained: Non-cohesive cells infiltrate in single-file linear pattern
- Abundant eosinophilic cytoplasm, eccentric nuclei
- Nuclear pleomorphism is characteristic (in contrast to the monomorphous nuclei typical of ILC)
- Most PLCs lack ER, PR
- May have apocrine differentiation

- May have associated "pleomorphic lobular carcinoma in situ", cytologically similar to invasive component
- E-cadherin staining usually negative as with other ILC

CLINICAL ISSUES

Presentation

- Most common: Breast mass ± enlarged axillary nodes

Natural History & Prognosis

- Incidence rate of PLC is increasing (together with ILC)
- Aggressive biologic behavior; worse prognosis than classical ILC

SELECTED REFERENCES

1. Maly B et al: Pleomorphic variant of invasive lobular carcinoma of the male breast. Virchows Arch. 446:344-5, 2005
2. Moe RE et al: Distinctive biology of pleomorphic lobular carcinoma of the breast. J Surg Oncol. 90:47-50, 2005
3. Reis-Filho JS et al: Pleomorphic lobular carcinoma of the breast: role of comprehensive molecular pathology in characterization of an entity. J Pathol. 207(1):1-13, 2005
4. Varga Z et al: Preferential HER-2/neu overexpression and/or amplification in aggressive histological subtypes of invasive breast cancer. Histopathology. 44:332-8, 2004
5. Tot T: The diffuse type of invasive lobular carcinoma of the breast: morphology and prognosis. Virchows Arch. 443:718-24, 2003

IMAGE GALLERY

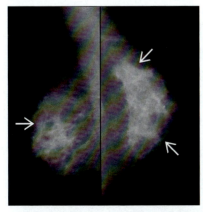
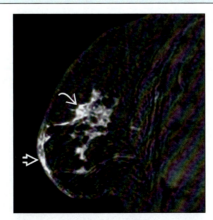
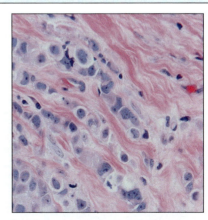

(Left) Left MLO and CC mammography views show diffuse increased density ➡, more evident on the left CC view. *(Center)* Sagittal T1 C+ FS MR shows diffuse irregular mass ➡ and skin enhancement inferiorly ➡ (same case as left-hand images). Mastectomy revealed pleomorphic lobular carcinoma and involvement of the dermal lymphatics. *(Right)* Micropathology, high power H&E (different patient than left-hand images) shows PLC. The cancer cells infiltrate in linear files and there is prominent nuclear pleomorphism. (Courtesy of KK).

SARCOMAS

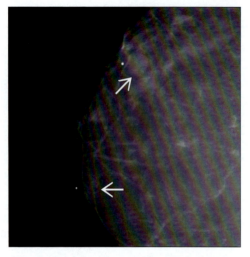

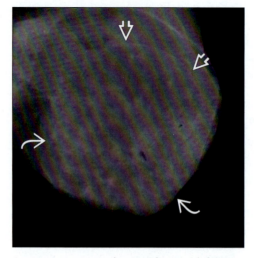

CC mammography shows two circumscribed masses ➔, both of which were palpable. Both masses show internal lucency. Both were low grade angiosarcomas.

Specimen mammography magnification of the more medial mass in the prior image. The mass ➔ is well-circumscribed, partially encapsulated ➔ and has internal fat.

TERMINOLOGY

Definitions
- Malignant stromal breast neoplasms

IMAGING FINDINGS

Mammographic Findings
- Angiosarcoma
  - Mammography: Lobulated or ill-defined mass
  - May have associated coarse calcifications
  - Average size = 5 cm; very few < 2 cm
- Others reported
  - Malignant fibrous histiocytoma, osteogenic sarcoma, liposarcoma, fibrosarcoma, leiomyosarcoma, rhabdomyosarcoma

Ultrasonographic Findings
- Grayscale Ultrasound
  - US: Circumscribed or spiculated mass; most with suspicious features; require biopsy
  - Variable internal echogenicity, can have hyperechoic areas
  - May or may not have posterior acoustic enhancement
- Color Doppler: May be very vascular

MR Findings
- T1 C+ FS: Nonspecific enhancing lobulated or spiculated mass; +/- internal enhancement

DIFFERENTIAL DIAGNOSIS

Benign Lesions
- Fibroadenomas, phyllodes
- Fat necrosis
- Fibroadenolipoma

Invasive Ductal Carcinoma
- Imaging characteristics are indistinguishable

Metaplastic Carcinoma
- Mammary carcinomas with metaplasia

Locally-Aggressive Lesions
- Phyllodes tumor

DDx: Other Examples of Angiosarcomas

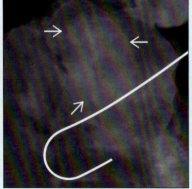

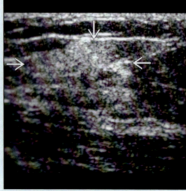

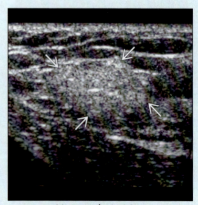

Circumscribed

Hyperechoic Mass

Hyperechoic Mass

SARCOMAS

Key Facts

Terminology
- Malignant stromal breast neoplasms

Imaging Findings
- Mammography: Lobulated or ill-defined mass
- US: Circumscribed or spiculated mass; most with suspicious features; require biopsy

Top Differential Diagnoses
- Fibroadenomas, phyllodes
- Fat necrosis
- Fibroadenolipoma
- Invasive Ductal Carcinoma
- Metaplastic Carcinoma

Pathology
- Angiosarcoma most common; arises de novo in breast more than in any other organ
- Relationship to radiation exposure

PATHOLOGY

General Features
- General path comments
  - Large core needle or excisional biopsy needed to provide sufficient tissue for diagnosis
    - Metaplastic carcinoma must be excluded
  - Angiosarcoma most common; arises de novo in breast more than in any other organ
- Etiology
  - Relationship to radiation exposure
    - Angiosarcoma, malignant fibrous histiocytoma, fibrosarcoma
  - Lymphedema-associated lymphangiosarcoma (Stewart-Treves syndrome)
    - Chronic lymphedema following treatment for breast and other cancers; usually fatal
- Epidemiology: < 1% of malignant breast lesions

Microscopic Features
- Angiosarcoma; types I-III (low - high grade)
  - Anastomosing vascular channels, I: Cellular proliferations, II: Mitoses and III: Necrosis
- Osteogenic sarcoma
  - Multinucleated osteoclastic giant cells
- Malignant fibrous histiocytoma
  - Spindle cells arranged in a pinwheel pattern

Staging, Grading or Classification Criteria
- American Joint Committee on Cancer staging system for soft tissue sarcomas
  - Includes histologic grade, tumor size, regional nodal status, distant metastases

CLINICAL ISSUES

Presentation
- Most common signs/symptoms: Palpable, often rapidly enlarging, unilateral mass
- Other signs/symptoms: Angiosarcoma associated with overlying bluish skin discoloration

Demographics
- Age: Angiosarcoma mean age at diagnosis = 35

Natural History & Prognosis
- Based on tissue type and grade; hematogenous metastases to lungs, bone marrow, liver most common

Treatment
- Mastectomy most common
- No axillary dissection; axillary metastases rare

SELECTED REFERENCES

1. Stavros AT: Breast Ultrasound. Philadelphia, Lippincott Williams & Wilkins. Chapter 14, 666-7, 2004
2. Harris JR et al: Diseases of the breast. Philadelphia, Lippincott Williams & Wilkins. Chapter 43, 685-6, 2000
3. Rosen PP: Breast Pathology: Diagnosis by needle core biopsy. Philadelphia, Lippincott Williams & Wilkins. Chapter 23, 234-40, 1999

IMAGE GALLERY

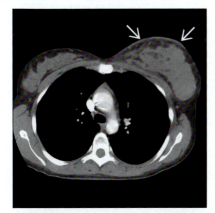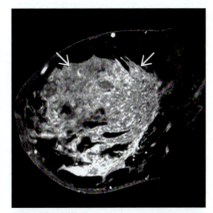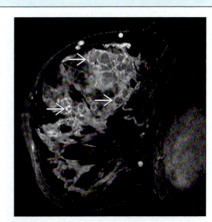

(Left) Axial CECT shows the left breast to be much larger than the right with visible skin thickening ➡ on the left. (Center) Sagittal T1 C+ FS MR (same case as left image) shows a portion of the more homogeneously enhancing ➡ 9 cm high grade angiosarcoma occupying most of the upper left breast. (Right) Sagittal T1 C+ FS MR (same case as prior 2 images) shows the more medial portion of the large 9 cm high grade angiosarcoma where multiple areas of rim-enhancement ➡ are apparent.

TUBULAR CARCINOMA

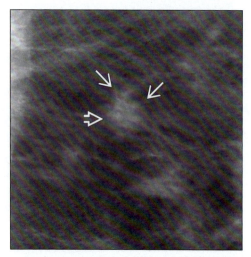

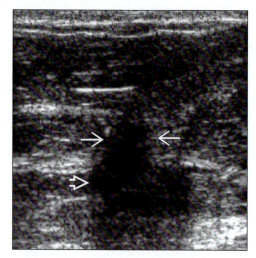

CC mammography spot compression shows a spiculated mass ➡ in the left breast of this asymptomatic patient. Note spicules ➡ extending into fatty tissue, a characteristic of tubular carcinoma.

Radial ultrasound of patient in previous image demonstrates a corresponding irregular, hypoechoic mass ➡ with posterior shadowing ➡. US-guided 14-g core biopsy showed tubular carcinoma.

TERMINOLOGY

Definitions

- Special type of well differentiated invasive ductal carcinoma (IDC) composed of well differentiated tubular structures with open lumina lined by a single layer of epithelial cells
  - Ductules are surrounded by abundant reactive fibroblastic stroma
- Pure: Proportion of tubular structures ≥ 90%
- Mixed: 50-89% tubular pattern

IMAGING FINDINGS

General Features

- Best diagnostic clue: Small spiculated mass on mammogram, can be stable for years
- Location
  - Usually occurs in peripheral portions of breast
    - Areas of breast where fibroglandular elements have involuted
- Size
  - One of the smallest infiltrating cancers

- Rarely > 2 cm
  - Mean size 8 mm when nonpalpable; 12 mm when palpable

Mammographic Findings

- Small, irregular mass surrounded by fat
  - Spiculated margins common
  - Usually centrally dense (unlike many radial scars)
    - Can have long spicules
  - Associated amorphous or pleomorphic microcalcifications (Ca++) in up to 50%
- Architectural distortion, asymmetry ± Ca++
- Rarely isolated Ca++
- Round, oval, or gently lobulated masses uncommon
- Most lesions detected by mammography

Ultrasonographic Findings

- Grayscale Ultrasound
  - Irregular mass with spiculated or indistinct margins
  - Associated distortion with tethering of Cooper ligaments
  - Hypoechoic to markedly hypoechoic
  - Posterior shadowing typical; may be absent
  - Echogenic foci due to Ca++ may be seen
  - Vertical orientation common; can be parallel

DDx: Tubular Carcinoma Mimics

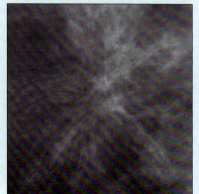

Radial Scar

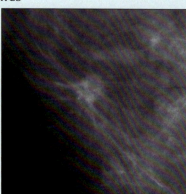

Invasive Ductal Carcinoma, NOS

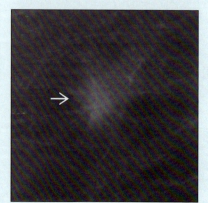

Invasive Lobular Carcinoma

TUBULAR CARCINOMA

Key Facts

Terminology
- Special type of well differentiated invasive ductal carcinoma (IDC) composed of well differentiated tubular structures with open lumina lined by a single layer of epithelial cells

Imaging Findings
- Best diagnostic clue: Small spiculated mass on mammogram, can be stable for years
- One of the smallest infiltrating cancers
- Associated amorphous or pleomorphic microcalcifications (Ca++) in up to 50%
- Can be source of false negative MR
- Typically highly conspicuous on US

Top Differential Diagnoses
- Radial Scar or Radial Sclerosing Lesion (RSL)

- Tubular carcinoma may co-exist with radial scar/RSL
- Invasive Ductal Carcinoma (IDC), NOS
- Infiltrating Lobular Carcinoma (ILC)
- Sclerosing Adenosis

Pathology
- 2% of female breast cancers
- ↑ Incidence of contralateral carcinoma: 10-15%
- Myoepithelial cell layer absent: Lacks actin or p63 staining (sometimes performed to distinguish from sclerosing adenosis)

Clinical Issues
- Most lesions detected on screening mammography
- Mean: 50 years
- Slow growing, favorable prognosis
- 95-98% five-year survival

○ Rarely circumscribed, oval, lobulated

MR Findings
- T2WI FS: Iso- to slightly hypointense to parenchyma
- T1 C+ FS
  ○ Irregular, spiculated enhancing mass
    ▪ Usually rapid initial then washout or plateau kinetics
    ▪ Inhomogeneous enhancement
    ▪ Rim-enhancement rare
  ○ Can be source of false negative MR
    ▪ Slow, mild enhancement if hypovascular

Imaging Recommendations
- Best imaging tool
  ○ Spot compression or spot magnification mammography
  ○ Typically highly conspicuous on US
- Protocol advice: Turn off spatial compounding on US to see shadowing

DIFFERENTIAL DIAGNOSIS

Radial Scar or Radial Sclerosing Lesion (RSL)
- Indistinguishable on imaging
- Tubular carcinoma may co-exist with radial scar/RSL
- Spiculated mass on mammography
  ○ May contain central lucent area, long spicules
  ○ Associated punctate or amorphous Ca++
- Architectural distortion
- Histology
  ○ Distorted ducts with adenosis, epithelial proliferations
  ○ Surrounding fibrosis and elastosis
  ○ Two cell-layer ductules

Invasive Ductal Carcinoma (IDC), NOS
- Imaging characteristics indistinguishable

Infiltrating Lobular Carcinoma (ILC)
- Similar imaging characteristics, lacks Ca++
- May present as architectural distortion
- False negative mammograms not uncommon

Ductal Carcinoma in Situ (DCIS)
- Clustered amorphous, pleomorphic, or fine linear Ca++ ± asymmetry
- Occasional intracystic or indistinct mass
- Rarely: Spiculated mass

Sclerosing Adenosis
- Circumscribed or indistinct mass ± punctate or amorphous Ca++
- Can be difficult to distinguish at histopathology
  ○ Isolated ductule can resemble invasion
  ○ Distinguish by retained myoepithelial layer in benign lesions
    ▪ Actin or p63 stain used to confirm when necessary

Post-Surgical Scar, Fat Necrosis
- Appropriate history of surgery, trauma
- Spiculated asymmetry
- May develop dystrophic or peripheral curvilinear Ca++

PATHOLOGY

General Features
- General path comments
  ○ 2% of female breast cancers
  ○ 1% of male breast cancers
  ○ Low incidence of axillary lymph node metastasis: 7-15%
    ▪ Lymph node involvement may not affect survival
  ○ Associated with (low-grade) DCIS: 52-65%
    ▪ Typically papillary and/or cribriform patterns
    ▪ Usually located in center of lesion
  ○ Associated lobular neoplasia 15%
  ○ ↑ Incidence of contralateral carcinoma: 10-15%
  ○ Multifocality: 20%
  ○ ER+ 80-90%, PR+ 68-75%
  ○ Lower S-phase fraction compared to IDC NOS
  ○ Her-2/neu and epidermal growth factor receptor-negative
  ○ Rare mucin secretion
    ▪ Stains pink with mucicarmine stain

TUBULAR CARCINOMA

- Associated abnormalities
  - Most frequent carcinoma found with radial scars
  - Associated benign columnar cell change (CCC) and flat epithelial atypia (FEA) common
    - FEA may be precursor lesion of low-grade DCIS and tubular carcinoma (controversial)

Gross Pathologic & Surgical Features
- Ill-defined firm or hard mass
- Gray to white in color
  - Tan or pale yellow: Suggests extensive elastosis
- When bisected appears stellate, surface may retract

Microscopic Features
- Composed of small glands or tubules of relatively uniform caliber
  - Glands may demonstrate irregular shapes and angular contours
  - Haphazardly arranged in stroma
  - Single layer of neoplastic epithelial cells arranged in tubules
    - Homogeneous in a given lesion: Cuboidal or columnar epithelium
    - Intraluminal projections: CCC may be present
  - Myoepithelial cell layer absent: Lacks actin or p63 staining (sometimes performed to distinguish from sclerosing adenosis)
  - Basement membrane incomplete or absent
- Cell characteristics
  - Round or oval hyperchromatic nuclei
    - Basally oriented
  - Low mitotic rate
  - Abundant cytoplasm
- Stroma: Increased cellularity, collagenization and abundant elastic tissue
- Ca++ microscopically evident 50% cases
- Lymphovascular and perineural invasion rare

CLINICAL ISSUES

Presentation
- Most common signs/symptoms
  - Most lesions detected on screening mammography
  - 30-40% of patients present with a palpable mass

Demographics
- Age
  - Mean: 50 years
    - Slightly younger than IDC NOS

Natural History & Prognosis
- Slow growing, favorable prognosis
- 95-98% five-year survival

Treatment
- Breast conserving surgery with clear margins
  - Adequate except for multicentric disease
- Sentinel node biopsy
- Radiation and chemotherapy controversial
  - Low risk of local recurrence without radiation, 4% at median 5 year follow-up (one series)

- Adjuvant therapy may not provide significant benefit, even with node-positive disease, especially in older patients
  - Further study warranted

DIAGNOSTIC CHECKLIST

Consider
- Can be mammographically stable or slowly-growing for years
- Can be false negative on MR or PET imaging

Image Interpretation Pearls
- Subtle distortion or spiculated mass, may be visible as one-view-only finding

SELECTED REFERENCES

1. Bassett LW et al: Diagnosis of diseases of the breast. Philadelphia, WB Saunders Co. Chapter 27, 506-7, 2005
2. Fernandez-Aguilar S et al: Is complete axillary lymph node dissection neccessary in T1 stage invasive pure tubular carcinomas of the breast? Breast. 14(4):325-8, 2005
3. Khirwadkar N et al: Fine needle aspiration cytology of tubular carcinoma of the breast. Acta Cytol. 49(3):344-5, 2005
4. Leonard CE et al: Excision only for tubular carcinoma of the breast. Breast J. 11(2):129-33, 2005
5. Livi L et al: Tubular carcinoma of the breast: outcome and loco-regional recurrence in 307 patients. Eur J Surg Oncol. 31(1):9-12, 2005
6. Sullivan T et al: Tubular carcinoma of the breast: a retrospective analysis and review of the literature. Breast Cancer Res Treat. 93(3):199-205, 2005
7. Goldstein NS et al: Refined morphologic criteria for tubular carcinoma to retain its favorable outcome status in contemporary breast carcinoma patients. Am J Clin Pathol. 122(5):728-39, 2004
8. Stavros AT: Breast Ultrasound. Philadelphia, Lippincott Williams & Wilkins. Chapter 14, 650-3, 2004
9. Cabral AH et al: Tubular carcinoma of the breast: an institutional experience and review of the literature. Breast J. 9(4):298-301, 2003
10. Holland DW et al: Tubular breast cancer experience at Washington University: a review of the literature. Clin Breast Cancer. 2(3):210-4, 2001
11. Kader HA et al: Tubular carcinoma of the breast: a population-based study of nodal metastases at presentation and of patterns of relapse. Breast J. 7(1):8-13, 2001
12. Rosen P: Rosen's Breast Pathology. 2nd edition. Philadelphia, Lippincott Williams &Wilkins. Chapter 14, 365-80, 2001
13. Wurdinger S et al: False-negative findings of malignant breast lesions on preoperative magnetic resonance mammography. Breast. 10: 131-9, 2001
14. Sheppard DG et al: Tubular carcinoma of the breast: mammographic and sonographic features. AJR Am J Roentgenol. 174(1):253-7, 2000
15. Mitnick JS et al: Tubular carcinoma of the breast: sensitivity of diagnostic techniques and correlation with histopathology. AJR Am J Roentgenol. 172(2):319-23, 1999
16. Gupta RK et al: Fine needle aspiration cytology of tubular carcinoma of the breast. Acta Cytol. 41(4):1139-43, 1997
17. McBoyle MF et al: Tubular carcinoma of the breast: an institutional review. Am Surg. 63(7):639-44; discussion 644-5, 1997

TUBULAR CARCINOMA

IMAGE GALLERY

Typical

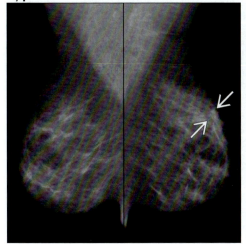

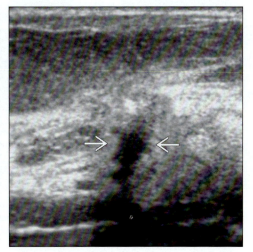

(Left) MLO mammography shows architectural distortion ➡ in the left upper outer quadrant of a 75 year-old woman who presented for screening. (Right) Transverse ultrasound (same patient as previous image) shows markedly hypoechoic, taller-than-wide mass ➡. Needle-localized excision showed tubular carcinoma.

Typical

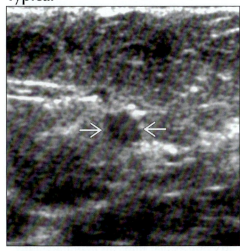

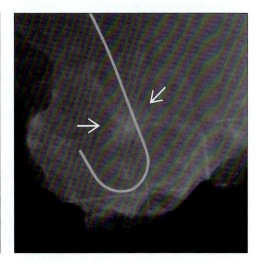

(Left) Ultrasound in a 60-year old with spiculated mass on screening reveals irregular hypoechoic mass ➡ with no posterior features. Core biopsy demonstrated tubular carcinoma. (Right) Magnification specimen mammography of needle-localized specimen in a 53 y/o depicts a spiculated mass ➡ due to a 4 mm tubular carcinoma. The mass was quite subtle on screening mammography.

Variant

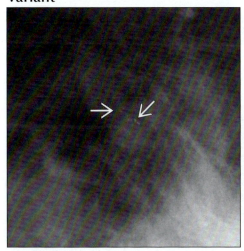

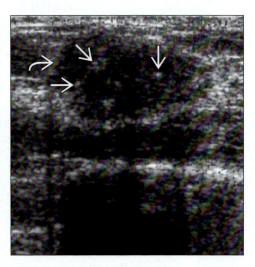

(Left) Lateral mammography magnification shows pleomorphic Ca++ ➡ with associated asymmetry in a 58 y/o. Stereotactic 11-g vacuum biopsy showed tubular carcinoma with Ca++. (Right) Ultrasound in a 53 y/o with new regional amorphous Ca++ on mammography (not shown) demonstrates an indistinctly-marginated oval mass ➡ with Ca++ ➡. US-guided core biopsy and excision showed tubular carcinoma.

TUBULOLOBULAR CARCINOMA

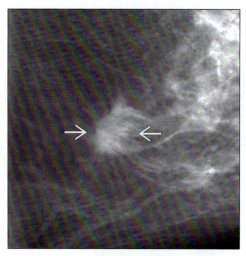

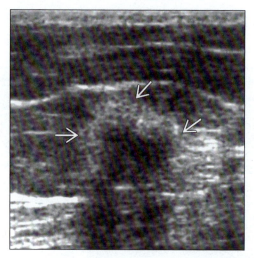

CC mammography shows spiculated mass ➡ at the fat-mammary interface, medial left breast, in an asymptomatic 70 year-old woman.

Ultrasound (same patient as left) shows hypoechoic mass with echogenic rim ➡. Pathology at excision demonstrated tubulolobular carcinoma.

TERMINOLOGY

Abbreviations and Synonyms
- Tubulolobular carcinoma (TLC)

Definitions
- Rare type of infiltrating breast cancer
  - Histologic features of both tubular and lobular carcinoma
  - Initially described as a tubular variant of lobular carcinoma
  - Now thought to be a variant of well-differentiated ductal carcinoma demonstrating a lobular growth pattern

IMAGING FINDINGS

General Features
- Size: Median 1.3 cm

Mammographic Findings
- Small, spiculated, dense mass
- Similar to tubular carcinoma

Ultrasonographic Findings
- Grayscale Ultrasound
  - Irregular, hypoechoic mass with posterior shadowing
    - Angular or spiculated margins
    - Echogenic halo

Imaging Recommendations
- Best imaging tool: Mammography and ultrasound

DIFFERENTIAL DIAGNOSIS

Tubular Carcinoma
- Small irregular mass, often surrounded by fat

Invasive Lobular Carcinoma
- Focal asymmetry or irregular mass on mammography

Radial Scar
- Architectural distortion with spiculations radiating from lucent center

DDx: Small Spiculated Masses

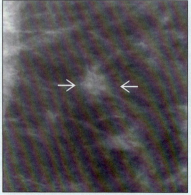

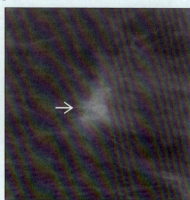

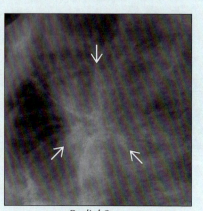

Tubular Carcinoma

Invasive Lobular Carcinoma

Radial Scar

TUBULOLOBULAR CARCINOMA

Key Facts

Terminology

- Rare type of infiltrating breast cancer
- Histologic features of both tubular and lobular carcinoma

Top Differential Diagnoses

- Tubular Carcinoma
- Invasive Lobular Carcinoma
- Radial Scar

Pathology

- Tubulolobular pattern requisite in ≥ 75% of tumor
- Mixture of single-file cord cells and small, round-to-angulated tubules
- Lobular pattern of infiltration

Clinical Issues

- Intermediate prognosis between pure tubular and invasive lobular carcinoma

---

PATHOLOGY

General Features

- General path comments
  - Tubulolobular pattern requisite in ≥ 75% of tumor
  - Multifocal: 19%
  - Axillary lymph node metastasis: 17%
  - Estrogen and progesterone receptor positive
  - Hybrid immunophenotype
    - E-cadherin and 34BetaE12 positive

Gross Pathologic & Surgical Features

- Small, indurated gray-tan mass
- Stellate appearance of cut surface

Microscopic Features

- Mixture of single-file cord cells and small, round-to-angulated tubules
- Lobular pattern of infiltration
- Small, round nuclei
  - Mild hyperchromasia and inconspicuous nucleoli
- Stroma dense and collagenous
- Lymphovascular invasion rare
- Associated with both ductal carcinoma in situ and lobular carcinoma in situ

CLINICAL ISSUES

Presentation

- Usually detected on screening mammogram

Demographics

- Age
  - Range: 32-79 years
  - Median (reports vary): 51-60 years
- Gender: Reported in males

Natural History & Prognosis

- Intermediate prognosis between pure tubular and invasive lobular carcinoma
  - 91% 10-year survival

Treatment

- Standard surgical cancer treatment based on size and nodal status
- Axillary node sampling
- Chemotherapy based on size and nodal status
- Hormonal therapy when hormonally sensitive

SELECTED REFERENCES

1. Kuroda H et al: Expression of E-cadherin, alpha-catenin, and beta-catenin in tubulolobular carcinoma of the breast. Virchows Arch. 448:500-5, 2006
2. Wheeler DT et al: Tubulolobular carcinoma of the breast. Am J Surg Pathol. 28:1587-93, 2004
3. Green I et al: A comparative study of pure tubular and tubulolobular carcinoma of the breast. Am J Surg Pathol. 21:653-7, 1997
4. Boppana S et al: Cytologic characteristics of tubulolobular carcinoma of the breast. Acta Cytologica. 40:465-71, 1996

IMAGE GALLERY

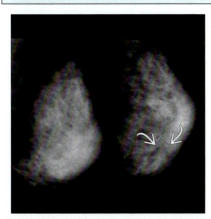 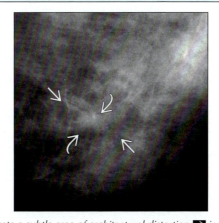 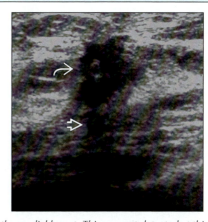

(Left) MLO (left) and CC (right) views demonstrate a subtle area of architectural distortion ➔ in the medial breast. This was not detected at this time. *(Center)* CC mammography magnification (same case as left) reveals ill-defined mass ➔ with associated architectural distortion ➔, recalled from screening the following year. *(Right)* Ultrasound (same case as prior 2 images) shows an irregular solid mass ➔ with shadowing ➔. 14-g core biopsy suggested tubular carcinoma; excision confirmed tubulolobular carcinoma.

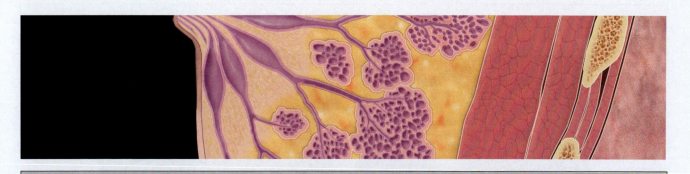

SECTION 3: Anatomic Considerations

NIPPLE DISCHARGE

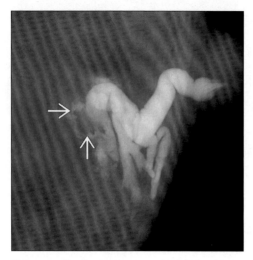

Galactography demonstrates a microlobulated mass within a dilated duct ➡ in this 34 year old with bloody nipple discharge. The patient underwent duct excision showing benign papilloma.

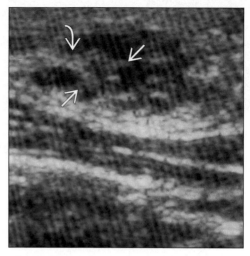

Ultrasound 4 yrs later (same patient), bloody nipple discharge recurred with a palpable mass near nipple. US showed an intracystic microlobulated mass ➡ on a stalk ➡. Excision again showed benign papilloma.

TERMINOLOGY

Definitions
- Pathologic nipple discharge (clinically significant)
  - Unilateral, uniductal, or originates from a few ducts
  - Usually persistent and non-lactational, spontaneous
  - Suspicious types (even these are most often due to benign etiology)
    - Bloody: Requires further evaluation
    - Serosanguineous or serous: Less concerning if only with stimulation
    - Watery (clear); rare reports of single duct spontaneous discharge related to ductal carcinoma in situ (DCIS)
- Galactorrhea: Discharge of milk from the breast
  - Physiologic: Associated with pregnancy and breastfeeding or induced by manipulation
  - Non-physiologic: Due to underlying anatomic abnormality or exposure to some drugs
  - Benign, usually bilateral either spontaneous or stimulated
- Greenish or blackish clear discharge typical of fibrocystic changes

IMAGING FINDINGS

General Features
- Best diagnostic clue
  - Pathologic discharge: Tissue diagnosis necessary in most spontaneous clear or any bloody unilateral uniductal case
    - Imaging evaluation is essential to localize the underlying cause, extent, and plan appropriate treatment

Radiographic Findings
- Mammography
  - Required in patients with pathologic discharge
  - May identify dilated ducts, calcifications, mass or architectural distortion
  - Frequently false negative (10-50% or higher)
  - Negative mammography & pathologic discharge requires further evaluation (US, MR, galactography)
- Galactography: Sensitive in detecting intraductal lesions
  - Depicts extent when multiple intraductal lesions, even peripheral lesions

DDx: Galactographic Appearances with Bloody Nipple Discharge

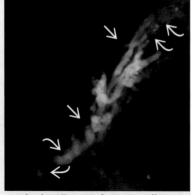

Multiple Filling Defects (Papillomas)

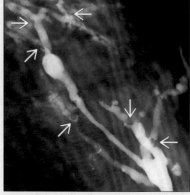

Irregular Wall, Filling Defects (DCIS)

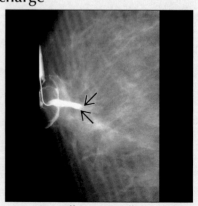

Cut-Off Sign (Papilloma)

NIPPLE DISCHARGE

Key Facts

Terminology
- Pathologic nipple discharge (clinically significant)
- Unilateral, uniductal, or originates from a few ducts
- Usually persistent and non-lactational, spontaneous
- Suspicious types (even these are most often due to benign etiology)
- Bloody: Requires further evaluation
- Serosanguineous or serous: Less concerning if only with stimulation

Imaging Findings
- Pathologic discharge: Tissue diagnosis necessary in most spontaneous clear or any bloody unilateral uniductal case
- US 93% sensitivity to source of nipple discharge vs. 68% for galactography in one series

Top Differential Diagnoses
- Papilloma(s)
- Duct Ectasia
- DCIS, most frequent malignancy causing nipple discharge
- Ductal Hyperplasia ± Atypia (ADH)
- Nipple Adenoma

Diagnostic Checklist
- Any bloody nipple discharge merits evaluation: Papillomas most common; ~ 13% due to malignancy (most often DCIS)
- Spontaneous uniductal clear discharge merits evaluation: < 1% malignant

---

- Pre-operative galactography can guide excision; increases probability of surgical removal
  - With no pre-operative galactographic localization a more distal lesion may be left in the breast with central duct excision
- Requires presence of discharge at time of procedure; cannulation may not be technically possible
- Typical positive galactographic findings
  - Filling defect(s) that may represent masses (benign or malignant) or inspissated ductal material
  - Cut-off sign: Duct completely obstructed by an intraluminal mass (usually papilloma)
  - Duct wall irregularity suggests DCIS

Ultrasonographic Findings
- Grayscale Ultrasound
  - Good complementary tool to detect duct ectasia, mass(es)
  - Intraductal position of mass when surrounded by fluid
  - May be used in lieu of galactography; central lesions more common, often visible
    - US 93% sensitivity to source of nipple discharge vs. 68% for galactography in one series
  - Sonographic "trigger-point sign": Nipple discharge elicited by pressure by the transducer over a sonographically localized intraductal lesion
  - "Second-look" ultrasound after galactography or MR may show lesion and direct biopsy
    - US-guided vacuum-assisted core biopsy a reliable diagnostic and potentially therapeutic tool
  - Peripheral small papillomas are frequently missed by sonography
  - DCIS often not detected by sonography
    - Symptomatic DCIS more readily detected: 92% in one series
- Color Doppler: Papillomas have (fibro) vascular cores and may show increased color Doppler flow
- Ultrasound-guided percutaneous galactography
  - Proposed alternative technique when galactography is not successful

MR Findings
- T2WI FS: May show intraductal location of a mass and the duct filled with bright signal of fluid
- T1 C+: May reveal lesion(s) when conventional methods unsuccessful

Imaging Recommendations
- Best imaging tool: US for intraductal mass near nipple
- Protocol advice: Determine orientation of discharging duct within nipple: Duct-oriented US

DIFFERENTIAL DIAGNOSIS

Papilloma(s)
- 35-70% of pathologic nipple discharge cases
- May appear as a mass ± associated calcifications
- MR: Mass indistinguishable from invasive tumor
  - Small luminal mass: Small, smooth enhancing masses connected to the nipple by an enlarged duct
- Central papilloma (large duct papilloma)
  - Serosanguineous or sanguinous nipple discharge in 64-88% of cases
  - Retroareolar mass; usually intraductal or intracystic hypoechoic mass on US
- Peripheral papilloma; nipple discharge less frequent
  - Multiple well-circumscribed peripheral masses, nodular prominent ducts or clustered calcifications
  - More frequent association with radial scar, sclerosing adenosis, ADH, DCIS or invasive ductal carcinoma (IDC) than is central papilloma
  - Relative risk of subsequent invasive carcinoma may be higher compared to central papilloma

Duct Ectasia
- 17-36% of pathologic nipple discharge cases
- Dilated fluid-filled ducts at sonography

Carcinoma
- 5-21% of pathologic nipple discharge cases
- DCIS, most frequent malignancy causing nipple discharge
  - Variant of DCIS: Intracystic papillary carcinoma

○ Hypoechoic or isoechoic, often microlobulated mass; may have suspicious calcifications
• Invasive cancer: Nipple discharge is rare

Ductal Hyperplasia ± Atypia (ADH)
• Frequent finding at duct excision
  ○ Proliferation may resemble papillary structures but no fibrovascular core
    ▪ The term "papillomatosis" should be avoided: Variably used for usual ductal hyperplasia as well as for multiple papillomas

Nipple Adenoma
• Also known as papillary adenoma, erosive adenomatosis
• Proliferation of small tubules around nipple ducts
• Most frequent presenting symptom is bloody or serous nipple discharge

Fibrocystic Changes
• Cyst(s) communicating with duct
• Cloudy yellow, greenish or blackish discharge

PATHOLOGY

General Features
• General path comments
  ○ Hemoccult test detects occult blood
  ○ Breast specimen recommendations
    ▪ Inked and oriented margins with suture at distal duct end for orientation
    ▪ Preferably, entire specimen submitted for microscopic examination
• Etiology: Benign papilloma most common cause
• Epidemiology
  ○ In 1-5% of breast cancers nipple discharge is principal symptom
  ○ Non-pathologic, benign discharge: Occurs in 10-50% of women

Microscopic Features
• True papillary lesions have a fibrovascular core
• Intraductal "micropapillary" proliferations have no fibrovascular stalk = epithelial hyperplasia ± atypia
• Cytology information from nipple aspiration or ductal lavage
  ○ Papanicolaou or Giemsa stains; read as negative, atypical, suspicious, or cancer cells present; may also reveal papillary formation of the exfoliated cells
    ▪ Overlap of cytological appearance of lesions with atypia and low grade malignancy
    ▪ Negative cytology does not exclude malignancy
  ○ Does not localize the causative lesion(s)

CLINICAL ISSUES

Demographics
• Age: At older age, higher percent of patients with nipple discharge have underlying cancer

Treatment
• Pathologic bloody discharge: Tissue diagnosis is necessary in most of the cases

○ Ductal excision: Success depends on identifying correct origin of discharge
○ When a specific duct cannot be identified, blind excision of retroareolar ductal system may be performed
  ▪ This may "cure" nipple discharge because duct no longer communicates with the nipple, but an undiagnosed lesion could still be present
• Non-bloody discharge: If US negative, monitor, avoid stimulation
• Galactorrhea: Physiologic (lactating); consider blood tests
  ○ Human HCG, Prolactin and TSH levels, renal function chemistry
• Consider ductoscopy: Fiberoptics 0.9-1.2 mm in external diameter, under local anesthesia
  ○ Examines only 1-2 ducts and obtains only cytologic material

DIAGNOSTIC CHECKLIST

Consider
• Any bloody nipple discharge merits evaluation: Papillomas most common; ~ 13% due to malignancy (most often DCIS)
• Spontaneous uniductal clear discharge merits evaluation: < 1% malignant
• The secretion of serous or bloody nipple discharge does not distinguish benign etiology from cancer
• Papillary lesions can develop associated atypia or malignancy over time

Image Interpretation Pearls
• Intraductal mass is suspicious and merits biopsy
• Consider direct excision

SELECTED REFERENCES
1. Escobar PF et al: The clinical applications of mammary ductoscopy. Am J Surg. 191:211-5, 2006
2. Yang WT et al: Sonographic, mammographic, and histopathologic correlation of symptomatic ductal carcinoma in situ. AJR. 182:101-10, 2004
3. Daniel BL et al: Magnetic resonance imaging of intraductal papilloma of the breast. Magn Reson Imaging. 21:887-92, 2003
4. Dennis MA at al: Incidental treatment of nipple discharge caused by benign intraductal papilloma through diagnostic Mammotome biopsy. AJR. 174:1263-8, 2000
5. Orel SG et al: MR imaging in patients with nipple discharge: initial experience. Radiology. 216:248-54, 2000
6. Sickles EA: Galactography and other imaging investigations of nipple discharge. Lancet.11;356:1622-3, 2000
7. Hild F et al: Ductal oriented sonography improves the diagnosis of pathological nipple discharge of the female breast compared with galactography. Eur J Cancer. Prev 7 Suppl 1:S57-62, 1998
8. Cardenosa G et al: Ductography of the breast: technique and findings. AJR. 162:1081-7, 1994
9. Tabar L et al: Galactography: the diagnostic procedure of choice for nipple discharge. Radiology. 149:31-8, 1983

NIPPLE DISCHARGE

IMAGE GALLERY

Typical

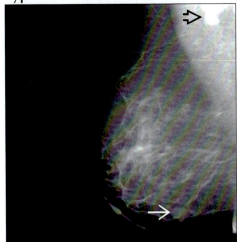 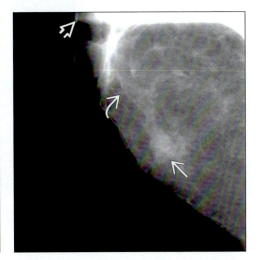

(Left) MLO mammography in this 39 year old woman with bloody nipple discharge shows an irregular mass with indistinct margins ➡ in the lower breast with visible axillary adenopathy ⮞. (Right) CC spot compression view (same patient as left-hand image), shows suspicious faint pleomorphic calcifications ➡ between the mass ➡ and nipple ➡. Bx = IDC and DCIS; axillary nodal bx was positive.

Typical

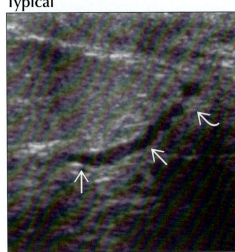 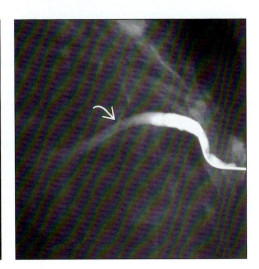

(Left) Ultrasound shows a dilated duct ➡ with a possible tiny intraductal mass ➡ in this 54 year old woman with spontaneous bloody nipple discharge. (Right) Galactography (same patient as left-hand image) shows a 2 mm intraductal mass ➡ at the same site as seen by US. Duct excision revealed a benign papilloma.

Typical

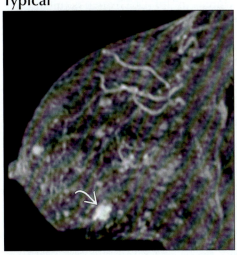 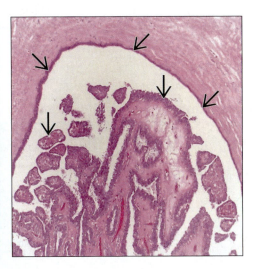

(Left) Sagittal T1 C+ SPGR MIP MR shows a dominant enhancing lobulated mass in the lower breast ➡ distant from the nipple in a woman without nipple discharge. Biopsy showed a benign papilloma. (Right) Low power histopathology (different patient with serosanguineous discharge) shows benign intraductal papilloma (H&E) ➡.

NIPPLE RETRACTION

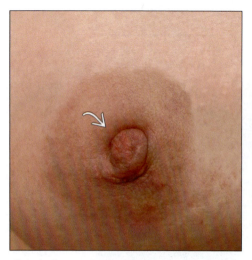

Clinical photograph shows subtle retraction of the superior portion of the nipple ➽ in this 44 year old. MR was performed (right-hand image).

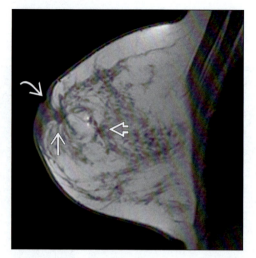

Sagittal T1WI MR shows skin thickening and retraction at the nipple ➽ due to spiculated mass ➞. A second spiculated mass was seen centrally ➞. Both masses were in situ and infiltrating carcinoma, mostly lobular.

TERMINOLOGY

Abbreviations and Synonyms
- Flattening or tethering of nipple

Definitions
- Nipple retraction = pulling in of the nipple, partial or complete, may or may not involve the areola
  - "Nipple retraction" preferentially used to describe finding when thought to be pathologic
- Nipple inversion = entire nipple retracted, with apex deep to level of breast itself
  - "Nipple inversion" preferentially used when describing normal variant

IMAGING FINDINGS

Mammographic Findings
- Nipple retraction more readily visualized on digital mammography than film due to tissue equalization algorithms for subcutaneous tissues and skin
- Assure nipple(s) in profile: Exclude pseudoinversion due to malpositioned mammograms

- Bilateral, long-standing nipple inversion does not require further evaluation
- New nipple retraction requires additional work-up
  - Spot compression views with nipple in profile help reveal and characterize underlying mass
  - Spot magnification views (CC and true lateral) to assess calcifications if any
  - US if mammogram unrevealing

Ultrasonographic Findings
- Grayscale Ultrasound
  - Normal nipple can cause shadowing
  - Duct ectasia readily demonstrated
  - Highly successful at demonstrating associated invasive carcinoma if present
    - Irregular, hypoechoic mass, often shadowing
    - Associated architectural distortion common in this setting
    - Guide biopsy
  - Ductal carcinoma in situ (DCIS) often occult at US
    - Isoechoic tubular mass(es), often hypervascular
    - May show echogenic calcifications
  - Abscess collections readily demonstrated and can be drained under US guidance

DDx: Benign Nipple Inversion

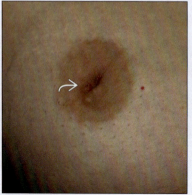

Entire Nipple Inverted

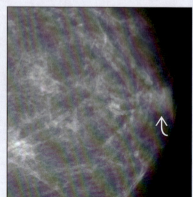

Nipple Mimics Mass

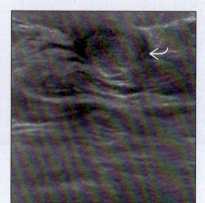

Nipple Mimics Mass

NIPPLE RETRACTION

Key Facts

Terminology
- Nipple retraction = pulling in of the nipple, partial or complete, may or may not involve the areola
- Nipple inversion = entire nipple retracted, with apex deep to level of breast itself

Imaging Findings
- Isolated enhancement of the nipple is a common normal variant on MR and is not sufficient to call nipple involvement

Top Differential Diagnoses
- Normal Variant Nipple Inversion
- Benign nipple inversion usually reversible by applying manual pressure at margins of nipple
- Invasive ductal carcinoma (IDC) NOS
- Invasive lobular carcinoma (ILC)

- DCIS
- Inflammatory carcinoma
- Duct Ectasia
- Secretory Changes (Plasma Cell Mastitis)
- Post-Surgical Change
- Fat Necrosis
- Abscess
- Mastitis

Clinical Issues
- Paget disease of the nipple (eczematoid changes) can be seen, usually due to underlying DCIS

Diagnostic Checklist
- Distinguish rapid (several months), progressive onset (suspicious), from congenital or long-standing nipple inversion (benign)

MR Findings
- T1WI
  - Nipple retraction often best appreciated on T1WI
  - Architectural distortion and skin thickening often seen
  - May visualize mass isointense to parenchyma
- T2WI FS
  - DCIS can be hyperintense
  - Abscess collections hyperintense as are post-operative seromas
- T1 C+
  - Isolated enhancement of the nipple is a common normal variant on MR and is not sufficient to call nipple involvement
  - Direct extension of tumor with contiguous enhancement of the nipple and often adjacent skin implies involvement
  - Mastitis can have identical appearance to malignancy

Imaging Recommendations
- Best imaging tool
  - Mammography (ideally digital) with spot compression, followed by US
  - MR if above unrevealing
- Protocol advice
  - Spot compression mammographic views may reveal underlying mass
  - Nipple itself can cause shadowing on US
    - Scan adjacent to nipple and angle under the nipple to facilitate evaluation
    - Use glob of gel or standoff pad to facilitate focusing in the most superficial tissues
  - Clinical examination at time of US
    - Is the nipple retraction reversible?
    - Palpable mass?
    - Associated Paget disease of the nipple

DIFFERENTIAL DIAGNOSIS

Normal Variant Nipple Inversion
- Benign nipple inversion usually reversible by applying manual pressure at margins of nipple
- Often congenital, first noted at puberty
- As a response to touch or cold stimuli
- Often bilateral
- Can interfere with lactation

Malignancy
- Usually within close proximity of nipple
- Invasive ductal carcinoma (IDC) NOS
  - Spiculated mass with or without calcifications
  - Indistinctly marginated mass with or without calcifications
  - Tethering of skin and nipple or less often direct extension of tumor
- Invasive lobular carcinoma (ILC)
  - Spiculated mass or focal asymmetry
  - Often associated architectural distortion
  - Nipple retraction in 26% in one series (vs. 17% of other breast cancers)
- DCIS
  - May have associated Paget disease of nipple
  - May have associated IDC [possibly with extensive intraductal component, (EIC)]
  - May or may not show suspicious calcifications mammographically, often occult on mammography in this context
- Inflammatory carcinoma
  - Associated peau d'orange, erythema
  - Large area of breast involved
  - Diffuse edema
  - Often metastatic adenopathy
  - Diagnosis by punch biopsy of skin showing tumor emboli in dermal lymphatics
  - Nipple retraction in 38-43%
- Leukemia (rare)
  - Patient with systemic disease, can involve breast
  - Diffusely infiltrative, irregular mass(es)
  - Diffuse edema

NIPPLE RETRACTION

- Other malignancy (rare)
  - Lymphoma, primary or secondary
  - Other metastases to breast

Duct Ectasia
- Dilated subareolar ducts
- Often bilateral
- Thought to be post inflammatory, periductal mastitis, in some cases
  - Anaerobic organisms sometimes implicated
  - Can be painful when infectious etiology
- Involutional in some women, often asymptomatic

Secretory Changes (Plasma Cell Mastitis)
- Uncommon before age 60
- Usually bilateral
- Associated smooth, rod-like calcifications > 1 mm in diameter: Wall of duct or intraluminal

Post-Surgical Change
- History and clinical correlation should suffice
- Density at scar should decrease after initial mammogram
- May have associated collection seen best on US or MR, with track to overlying skin incision

Fat Necrosis
- History of trauma or surgery
- Associated fibrosis can cause nipple retraction over time
- Lucencies in mass on mammography, may develop peripheral curvilinear calcifications over several years
- Mixed hyper- and anechoic mass on US
- Surrounding edema

Abscess
- Usually due to crack in skin of nipple
- Palpable, tender mass
- US: Mixed echogenicity collection, often thick wall

Mastitis
- Erythema, mastalgia
- Often palpable mass
- Edema
- Associated adenopathy
- Difficult to distinguish from inflammatory carcinoma clinically
  - Mastitis will usually respond to two week course of antibiotics directed to skin organisms
- Rare: Granulomatous mastitis including TB

Fibromatosis (Rare)
- Suspicious mass, often with skin and/or nipple retraction
- Can be quite extensive, rapidly growing

PATHOLOGY

General Features
- Etiology
  - Several potential causes
    - Weakening of muscle or erectile tissue in nipple, can be congenital

- Muscle contraction in response to touch or cold temperature
- Fibrous tissue underlying nipple as a response to inflammatory conditions or surgery
- Tethering of Cooper ligaments by malignancy, causing overlying skin and nipple retraction

Staging, Grading or Classification Criteria
- In and of itself, nipple retraction does not necessarily imply skin involvement
- Fixation, induration, and thickening of skin due to underlying cancer suggests skin involvement: Stage IIIb

CLINICAL ISSUES

Presentation
- Most common signs/symptoms: Skin thickening and retraction near and involving nipple
- Other signs/symptoms
  - Paget disease of the nipple (eczematoid changes) can be seen, usually due to underlying DCIS
  - Palpable mass may be present
  - Erythema suggests mastitis or inflammatory carcinoma
  - Uncommonly, clear or bloody nipple discharge may be present

Demographics
- Gender: Skin or nipple retraction present in 36% of male breast cancer

DIAGNOSTIC CHECKLIST

Image Interpretation Pearls
- Distinguish rapid (several months), progressive onset (suspicious), from congenital or long-standing nipple inversion (benign)
- Bilateral favors benign inversion

SELECTED REFERENCES

1. Gunhan-Bilgen I et al: Inflammatory breast carcinoma: mammographic, ultrasonographic, clinical, and pathologic findings in 142 cases. Radiology. 223:829-38, 2002
2. Magro G et al: Fibromatosis of the breast: a clinical, radiological and pathological study of 6 cases. Pathologica. 94:238-46, 2002
3. Singletary SE: Revision of the American Joint Committee on Cancer staging system for breast cancer. J Clin Oncol. 20:3628-36, 2002
4. Kushwaha AC et al: Primary inflammatory carcinoma of the breast: Retrospective review of mammographic findings. AJR. 174:535-8, 2000
5. Burke ET et al: Paget disease of the breast: a pictorial essay. Radiographics. 18:1459-64, 1998
6. Gough DB et al: A 50-year experience of male breast cancer: is outcome changing? Surg Oncol. 2:325-33, 1993
7. LeGal M et al: Mammographic features of 455 invasive lobular carcinomas. Radiology. 185:705-8, 1992
8. Rees BI et al: Nipple retraction in duct ectasia. Br J Surg. 64:577-80, 1977

NIPPLE RETRACTION

IMAGE GALLERY

Typical

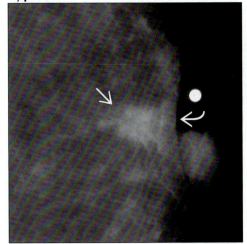 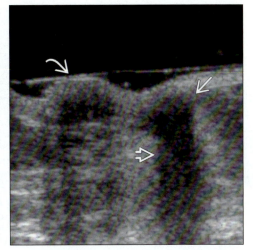

(Left) CC mammography spot compression shows a spiculated mass ➡ with overlying skin thickening and skin retraction ➡ in this 50 year old with new nipple retraction. (Right) US (same patient as left-hand image) shows irregular, hypoechoic mass ➡ with posterior shadowing ➡ adjacent to the retracting nipple ➡. Biopsy showed ILC + LCIS.

Variant

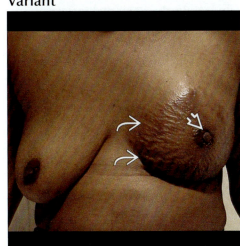 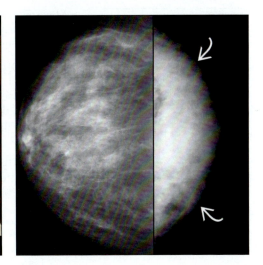

(Left) Clinical photograph shows shrunken left breast with flattening of the nipple ➡ and diffuse skin thickening ➡ in this 43 year old. (Right) CC mammography (same patient as left-hand image) shows marked diffuse increased density in the shrunken left breast ➡. Biopsy showed poorly differentiated carcinoma with angiolymphatic invasion.

Typical

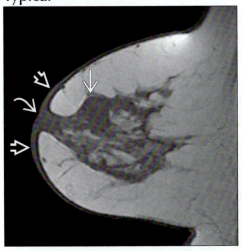 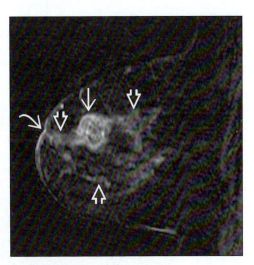

(Left) Sagittal T1WI MR in this 56 year old with Paget disease of nipple shows nipple retraction ➡, adjacent skin thickening ➡, and a lobulated mass ➡. (Right) Sagittal T1 C+ subtraction MR (same as left-hand image) shows irregular enhancing mass ➡ = high grade IDC with DCIS at biopsy. Segmental enhancement ➡ due to DCIS extends to involve nipple, and there is enhancement of nipple ➡ and adjacent skin anteriorly.

PAGET DISEASE OF THE NIPPLE

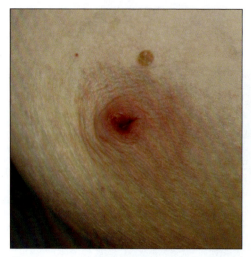

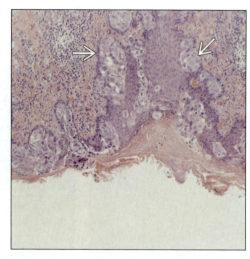

Clinical photograph shows typical case of Paget disease. Note eczematous changes and ulceration of the nipple.

Micropathology, low power, H&E illustrates typical case of Paget disease of the nipple. Note nests of Paget cells ➡ infiltrating the epidermis. The cells have prominent nuclei and pale cytoplasm.

TERMINOLOGY

Definitions

- Carcinoma in situ involving the nipple epidermis; associated with a local inflammatory response, pruritus and excoriation
  ○ Malignant cells extend to nipple surface through lactiferous ducts
  ○ Characteristic eczematoid skin changes of nipple

IMAGING FINDINGS

General Features

- Best diagnostic clue: Clinical: Erythema, flaking of skin of nipple
- Location: Usually confined to the nipple-areolar complex

Mammographic Findings

- Nipple and areolar thickening, nipple retraction
- Subareolar mass and/or calcifications
- Mass and/or calcifications away from nipple
  ○ Indicates separate, distant carcinoma
- May severely underestimate extent of disease
- Often falsely negative in absence of palpable mass: 71% one series

Ultrasonographic Findings

- Grayscale Ultrasound
  ○ Paget disease per se not identified on ultrasound
  ○ May see dilated, irregular subareolar ducts
  ○ Underlying DCIS often occult; invasive cancer well seen

MR Findings

- T1WI: Flattening, thickening and/or retraction of nipple/areolar region
- T1 C+
  ○ Abnormal nipple enhancement
    ■ Ill-defined, thickened nipple-areolar complex
    ■ Strong initial contrast-enhancement
    ■ Plateau or wash-out
  ○ May play important role in selecting patients for breast-conserving surgery
    ■ Identify underlying malignancy
    ■ Increasing importance in defining extent of disease

DDx: Other Conditions Affecting Skin of Nipple-Areolar Complex

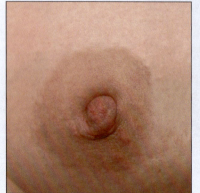

Retraction, IDC-ILC

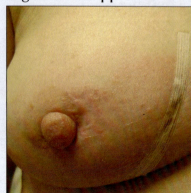

Cellulitis (Courtesy DNS)

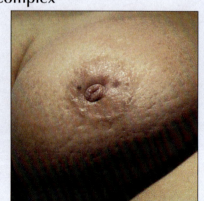

Inflammatory Breast Cancer

PAGET DISEASE OF THE NIPPLE

Key Facts

Terminology
- Carcinoma in situ involving the nipple epidermis; associated with a local inflammatory response, pruritus and excoriation
- Malignant cells extend to nipple surface through lactiferous ducts
- Characteristic eczematoid skin changes of nipple

Imaging Findings
- Best diagnostic clue: Clinical: Erythema, flaking of skin of nipple

Top Differential Diagnoses
- Dermatological conditions
- Subareolar abscess

Pathology
- General path comments: 1-3% of all breast cancers
- Underlying associated malignancy, 95-98%
- Absent a palpable mass, 66-93% due to DCIS
- With palpable mass, vast majority due to IDC

Clinical Issues
- Mimics benign dermatological conditions
- Age: Median age 56-62 years

Diagnostic Checklist
- Biopsy of any skin lesion of nipple-areolar complex that does not resolve promptly with topical therapy: Wedge biopsy
- MR can help depict underlying malignancy and extent

Imaging Recommendations
- Mammography in all patients
  - Magnification views behind nipple
- Ultrasound selected patients
  - Palpable or nonpalpable mass, guide biopsy
- MR
  - Increasing role to identify underlying malignancy and extent

DIFFERENTIAL DIAGNOSIS

Clinical
- Dermatological conditions
  - Eczema, psoriasis, melanoma
- Nipple adenoma
  - Erosion, ulceration and nipple enlargement
- Protruding intraductal papilloma
  - Weeping, red lesion
- Subareolar abscess
  - Skin thickening, erythema, tender
  - Retroareolar mass
- Cellulitis
  - Not typically centered at nipple; broad area
- Breast cancer directly invading skin
  - Uncommon at nipple
  - Invasive ductal carcinoma (IDC) or invasive lobular carcinoma (ILC)
- Inflammatory breast cancer
  - Skin involvement: Erythema, warmth, edema
  - Usually involves whole breast

Pathological
- Malignant melanoma
  - Arises in the areola; nipple origin rare
  - Excluded by demonstration of estrogen receptor
- Florid ductal papillomatosis
- Squamous or basal cell carcinoma
- Nipple adenoma

PATHOLOGY

General Features
- General path comments: 1-3% of all breast cancers
- Etiology
  - Underlying associated malignancy, 95-98%
    - Absent a palpable mass, 66-93% due to DCIS
    - With palpable mass, vast majority due to IDC
    - Rare case reports: Invasive and/or in situ lobular carcinoma
    - C-erb B2 overexpression 79-83%
  - Most DCIS high grade, comedo, or solid type
    - May be associated with invasion or exist alone
  - Associated invasive lesions
    - High grade, often poorly differentiated
  - Axillary lymph node involvement
    - With palpable mass 44-60%
  - Rare cases reported without underlying DCIS or invasive carcinoma
    - DCIS arises from ductal epithelium at squamocolumnar duct junction

Gross Pathologic & Surgical Features
- Duplicate those seen clinically
- Occasionally enlarged lactiferous ducts
- Underlying palpable tumors have no specific features

Microscopic Features
- Paget cells (adenocarcinoma) in keratinizing epithelium of nipple epidermis
- Hyperplasia and hyperkeratosis of epidermis may occur
- Superficial dermal stroma of nipple infiltrated by lymphocytic reaction
- Large nuclei with prominent nucleoli
- Abundant pale or clear cytoplasm
  - Mucin detected with periodic acid-Schiff stain after diastase digestion
- Her-2/neu expression
- Melanin pigment may be present
- Low-molecular weight cytokeratins detected using CAM 5.2

PAGET DISEASE OF THE NIPPLE

CLINICAL ISSUES

Presentation
- Most common signs/symptoms
  - Skin changes involving nipple
  - 50% have underlying palpable mass
- Initial
  - Erythema and/or scaling of nipple and areola
  - Pruritus
- Advanced
  - Moist, scaling, eczematous changes
  - Ulceration, crusting and erosion of nipple
  - Serous or bloody nipple discharge
- Mimics benign dermatological conditions
  - Inflammatory component can be improved with topical treatment
  - May result in delay in diagnosis
- Diagnosis
  - Wedge biopsy
  - Shave and punch biopsy less reliable
  - If no epidermis in specimen → rebiopsy
    - Can occur with ulceration and denuding of epithelium

Demographics
- Age: Median age 56-62 years
- Gender
  - Extremely rare in males
    - Up to 12% of male breast cancer

Natural History & Prognosis
- Excellent when DCIS only
- Determined by stage of invasive cancer
  - More advanced in Paget disease
- 10 year survival rates
  - Pure intraductal disease, mastectomy 100%
  - Invasive disease, node negative 70%
  - Worse prognosis with C-erb B-2 amplification

Treatment
- Standard
  - Mastectomy with axillary node dissection or sentinel node biopsy
    - Extensive DCIS
    - Invasive tumor or DCIS separate from Paget
    - Close margins in nipple-areolar biopsy specimen
- Selected cases
  - Breast conservation and radiation therapy
    - Limited extent of underlying DCIS
    - No associated palpable mass or imaging abnormality beyond surgical field
- Radiation therapy
  - Mandatory after breast conserving surgery (must have histologically negative margins)
  - Local control
  - Stand-alone therapy: Controversial
- Chemotherapy
  - Invasive tumors only
    - Same treatment criteria as for other IDC

DIAGNOSTIC CHECKLIST

Consider
- Biopsy of any skin lesion of nipple-areolar complex that does not resolve promptly with topical therapy: Wedge biopsy

Image Interpretation Pearls
- Thickening of nipple and areola may be only clue on mammogram
  - Skin changes seen to better advantage on digital mammography
  - MR can help depict underlying malignancy and extent

SELECTED REFERENCES

1. Amano G et al: MRI accurately depicts underlying DCIS in a patient with Paget's disease of the breast without palpable mass and mammography findings. Jpn J Clin Oncol. 35(3):149-53, 2005
2. Fox LP et al: Images in clinical medicine. Paget's disease of the breast. N Engl J Med. 353(3):e3, 2005
3. Frei KA et al: Paget disease of the breast: findings at magnetic resonance imaging and histopathologic correlation. Invest Radiol. 40(6):363-7, 2005
4. Kawase K et al: Paget's disease of the breast: there is a role for breast-conserving therapy. Ann Surg Oncol. 12(5):391-7, 2005
5. Echevarria JJ et al: Usefulness of MRI in detecting occult breast cancer associated with Paget's disease of the nipple-areolar complex. Br J Radiol. 77(924):1036-9, 2004
6. Hanna W et al: The role of HER-2/neu oncogene and vimentin filaments in the production of the Paget's phenotype. Breast J. 9(6):485-90, 2003
7. Marshall JK et al: Conservative management of Paget disease of the breast with radiotherapy: 10- and 15-year results. Cancer. 97(9):2142-9, 2003
8. Kothari AS et al: Paget disease of the nipple: a multifocal manifestation of higher-risk disease. Cancer. 95(1):1-7, 2002
9. Polgar C et al: Breast-conserving therapy for Paget disease of the nipple: a prospective European Organization for Research and Treatment of Cancer study of 61 patients. Cancer. 94(6):1904-5, 2002
10. Bijker N et al: Breast-conserving therapy for Paget disease of the nipple: a prospective European Organization for Research and Treatment of Cancer study of 61 patients. Cancer. 91(3):472-7, 2001
11. Fu W et al: Paget disease of the breast: analysis of 41 patients. Am J Clin Oncol. 24(4):397-400, 2001
12. Singh A et al: Is mastectomy overtreatment for Paget's disease of the nipple? Breast. 8(4):191-4, 1999
13. Burke ET et al: Paget disease of the breast: a pictorial essay. Radiographics. 18(6):1459-64, 1998
14. Kollmorgen DR et al: Paget's disease of the breast: a 33-year experience. J Am Coll Surg. 187(2):171-7, 1998
15. Yim JH et al: Underlying pathology in mammary Paget's disease. Ann Surg Oncol. 4(4):287-92, 1997
16. Desai DC et al: Paget's disease of the male breast. Am Surg. 62(12):1068-72, 1996
17. Gupta RK et al: The role of cytology in the diagnosis of Paget's disease of the nipple. Pathology. 28(3):248-50, 1996
18. Jamali FR et al: Paget's disease of the nipple-areola complex. Surg Clin North Am. 76(2):365-81, 1996
19. Ikeda DM: Paget's disease of the nipple: Radiologic-pathologic correlation. Radiology. 189:89-94, 1993

PAGET DISEASE OF THE NIPPLE

IMAGE GALLERY

Typical

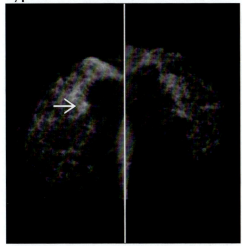

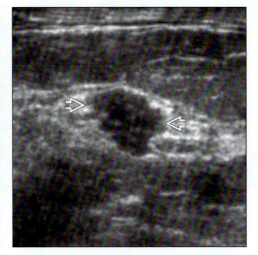

(Left) CC mammography shows subtle mass ➡ in the right upper outer quadrant in this 44 year old woman with Paget disease. The nipple appeared normal on this mammogram. *(Right)* US (same patient as left-hand image) demonstrates a microlobulated, hypoechoic mass ➡ with no posterior features. Biopsy showed invasive ductal carcinoma.

Typical

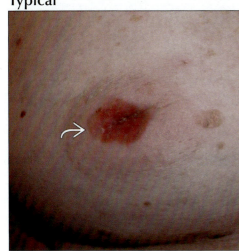

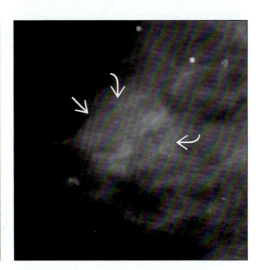

(Left) Clinical photograph shows eczematoid changes of nipple and central areola ➡ in this 56 year old woman. *(Right)* CC mammography magnification (same patient as left-hand image) shows lobulated 3 cm mass ➡ with calcifications ➡ centered 4 cm deep to the nipple. US-guided biopsy showed grade III IDC with DCIS. An extensive intraductal component extended to the nipple.

Typical

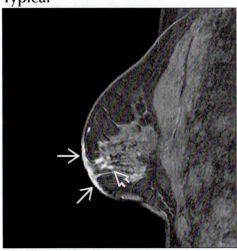

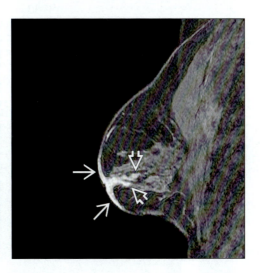

(Left) Sagittal T1 C+ FS MR demonstrates enhancement and skin thickening ➡ in the area of the areola in this 52 year old woman. In addition, there is clumped linear enhancement ➡ deep to the nipple, suggesting extent of disease. *(Right)* Sagittal T1 C+ FS MR (same patient as left-hand image) shows enhancement ➡ of the areola. On this slice, the clumped linear enhancement ➡ is more conspicuous. At surgery, there was a 1.5 cm segment of high grade DCIS and 3 mm IDC.

DERMAL CALCIFICATIONS

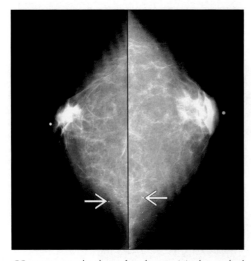

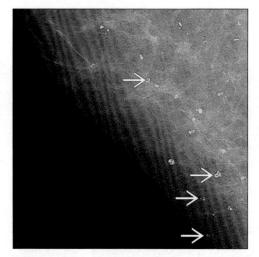

CC mammography shows fatty breasts (nipples marked with BBs). Medial dermal calcifications ➡ are present. Morphology is better shown on photomagnification image (on right-hand image).

CC mammography (photomagnification) shows small round and polygonal calcifications ➡, many with lucent centers, in small groups within the medial skin. BI-RADS 2, benign.

TERMINOLOGY

Abbreviations and Synonyms
- Skin calcifications

Definitions
- Calcifications within sebaceous glands

IMAGING FINDINGS

General Features
- Best diagnostic clue: Multiple, fairly dense, rounded/spherical or polygonal calcifications with lucent or umbilicated centers
- Location
  - Usually medial and inferior skin
  - Also common in axilla
- Size: 1-2 mm
- Morphology
  - Centrally lucent or solid, round or polygonal
  - Often clustered and scattered

Mammographic Findings
- Spherical or polygonal calcifications some with lucent or umbilicated centers; may be single, multiple; one or both breasts
- Full field digital imaging highlights the skin and may allow verification of dermal location without further work-up
- Indeterminate morphology may require skin localization to confirm dermal location

Imaging Recommendations
- Suspect on mammography when cluster of polygonal small calcifications seen near a skin surface
  - Dismiss when typical or characteristic
  - May require additional work-up to confirm presence within skin rather than breast parenchyma
    - Magnification mammography; skin localization
- Skin localization work-up
  - Grid coordinates as with needle localization, with appropriate skin surface exposed
  - Place BB on skin at coordinates of calcifications
  - Confirm proper BB placement while in grid
  - Orthogonal magnification view tangential to skin surface covered with BB

DDx: Other Dermal, Subcutaneous, or Artifactual Calcifications

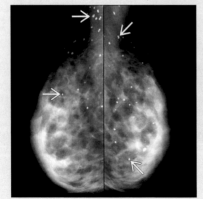

Cystic Acne

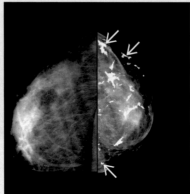

Post Irradiation

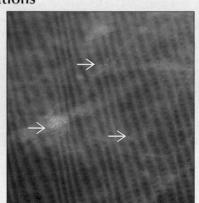

Talc in Moles

DERMAL CALCIFICATIONS

Key Facts

Terminology
- Skin calcifications
- Calcifications within sebaceous glands

Imaging Findings
- Best diagnostic clue: Multiple, fairly dense, rounded/spherical or polygonal calcifications with lucent or umbilicated centers
- Dismiss when typical or characteristic

- May require additional work-up to confirm presence within skin rather than breast parenchyma

Top Differential Diagnoses
- Talc in Skin Pores or Moles
- Subcutaneous Calcifications
- Skin Scar Calcifications

Clinical Issues
- No clinical significance

- Stereotactic localization
  - Needle tip at skin edge when targeted

DIFFERENTIAL DIAGNOSIS

Talc in Skin Pores or Moles
- Particles denser, smaller, without lucent centers
- Appropriate distribution
- Can be cleaned off and mammogram repeated

Subcutaneous Calcifications
- Subcutaneous, typically dystrophic, with coarse irregular forms, some with internal lucency
- Usually secondary to prior radiotherapy; seen in dermatomyositis; no prognostic significance

Skin Scar Calcifications
- Periareolar after reduction mammoplasty
- History of prior breast surgery

Tattoos
- Pigments may have similar density to calcifications
- Usually neither lucent-centered nor polygonal

Dermal Foreign Body Giant Cell Reaction
- May have indeterminate calcifications
- Location in skin on tangential views

Intramammary Calcifications
- Variable shapes and distributions within glandular tissue

PATHOLOGY

General Features
- General path comments: Very common; calcifications within sweat glands

CLINICAL ISSUES

Presentation
- Asymptomatic screening mammographic findings
- May be palpable if of significant size (uncommon)

Natural History & Prognosis
- No clinical significance

Treatment
- No treatment necessary: Reassurance

SELECTED REFERENCES

1. Bassett LW et al: Diagnosis of Diseases of the Breast. 2nd ed. Philadelphia, Elsevier. Chapter 25, 402-5, 2005
2. Linden SS et al: Breast skin calcifications: localization with a stereotactic device. Radiology. 171:570-1, 1989
3. Berkowitz JE et al: Dermal breast calcifications: localization with template-guided placement of skin marker. Radiology. 163:282, 1987

IMAGE GALLERY

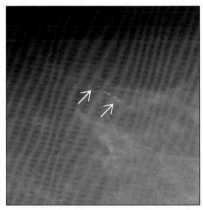 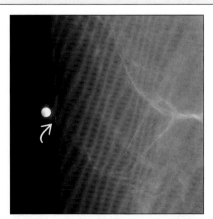 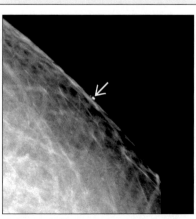

(Left) CC mammography magnification shows round and oval calcifications in a (suspicious) linear distribution ➜ near a skin surface. Skin localization was performed (next image). *(Center)* CC mammography magnification tangential view over the BB placed using a grid coordinate confirms the calcifications to be within the skin ➜. BI-RADS 2, benign. *(Right)* CC mammography shows a small group of round smooth calcifications ➜ in the upper outer left breast. Non-magnified digital image clearly demonstrates the dermal location. BI-RADS 2, benign.

EPIDERMAL INCLUSION CYST

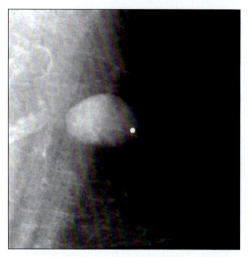

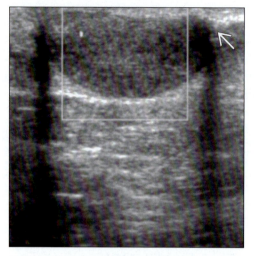

MLO mammography magnification shows a palpable, inflamed superficial mass in the left axilla, consistent with a benign epithelial skin cyst. This is a typical example of an epidermal inclusion cyst.

Radial ultrasound demonstrates superficial, hypoechoic mass of previous case. Note hyperechoic skin wrapping around the anterior edge of the lesion ➡ *, known as the "claw" sign.*

TERMINOLOGY

Definitions
- A benign cutaneous or subcutaneous epithelial cyst arising from obstructed hair follicle

IMAGING FINDINGS

General Features
- Best diagnostic clue
  - Superficial mass involving the skin
  - Astute technologist marking skin lesion prior to mammogram
- Location
  - Anywhere in skin of breast or axilla
    - Occasionally found in parenchyma, away from skin
  - Most often around areola, inframammary fold, axilla
- Size: Few mm up to 10 cm

Mammographic Findings
- Well-circumscribed round to oval mass
  - Iso- to hyperdense

  - Superficial
    - May project over breast parenchyma on any view
    - Tangential view helpful in determining skin location
  - Often burned out by appropriate exposure to denser areas
    - Use bright light
    - Digital mammography with tissue equalization improves visualization of superficial tissues
  - Portion of border may be ill-defined
  - Overlying skin often thickened
- Heterogeneous calcifications 20%
- Mammogram may be normal

Ultrasonographic Findings
- Grayscale Ultrasound
  - Well-defined, round to oval-shaped mass
  - Acoustic properties variable: Hypoechoic, isoechoic or hyperechoic
    - Hypoechoic or mixed echogenicity most common
    - Heterogeneous internal echoes due to thickened intralesional material
  - Superficial location
  - Posterior enhancement common

DDx: Other Examples of Epidermal Inclusion Cyst

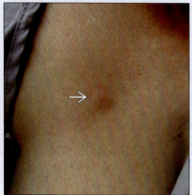

Photograph of Cyst

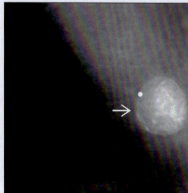

Calcified

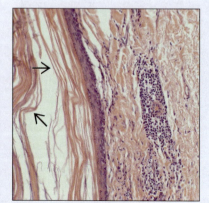

Keratin in Cyst

EPIDERMAL INCLUSION CYST

Key Facts

Terminology
- A benign cutaneous or subcutaneous epithelial cyst arising from obstructed hair follicle

Imaging Findings
- Anywhere in skin of breast or axilla
- Well-circumscribed round to oval mass
- Iso- to hyperdense
- Avoid fine needle aspiration (FNA) or core biopsy of epidermal inclusion cysts or sebaceous cysts
- Standoff pad or glob of gel may be necessary for optimal US

Top Differential Diagnoses
- Sebaceous Cyst
- Cyst

Pathology
- Arises from skin
- Often erroneously referred to as sebaceous cyst
- More common in other parts of the body: Face, scalp, neck and trunk
- Arises from obstructed hair follicle
- May occur along embryonic lines of closure
- Squamous metaplasia of sweat duct
- May arise in preexisting sebaceous cyst
- Thick contents: White, flaky, waxy

Clinical Issues
- Elevated, round, firm mass in breast skin
- Avoid biopsy when clinical, imaging criteria met
- Age: No age predilection
- Reported in males with same frequency as females

- ○ Often see hypoechoic line extending from mass to skin
  - ■ Represents thickened or obstructed hair follicle
- ○ US best modality for determining precise relationship to skin
  - ■ Lesion entirely within skin
  - ■ Most of lesion in subcutaneous tissue, but "claw" of skin surrounds anterior portion
  - ■ Lesion entirely within subcutaneous tissue, hair follicle seen coursing toward skin
- ○ Differentiating features from sebaceous cyst
  - ■ Squamous cells produce keratin → hyperechoic multilaminar appearance, like "onion skin"
  - ■ Multiple layers represent the sloughed keratin within cyst
  - ■ Keratin may calcify
- Power Doppler: Vascular when inflamed

MR Findings
- T1 C+: Often enhances after administration of contrast material

Biopsy
- Avoid fine needle aspiration (FNA) or core biopsy of epidermal inclusion cysts or sebaceous cysts
  - ○ Contents often irritating to surrounding tissue
  - ○ Inflammatory response, even abscess may occur
- Use of skin incision during core biopsy: Helps avoid epithelial (skin) displacement which can cause epidermal inclusion cyst within breast parenchyma

Imaging Recommendations
- Best imaging tool: Ultrasound
- Ultrasound
  - ○ Standoff pad or glob of gel may be necessary for optimal US
    - ■ Even current high frequency (≥ 12 MHz) transducers not optimally focused in most superficial 7 mm of tissue
- Mammography
  - ○ Mark lesion with BB prior to exam
    - ■ Tangential view helpful
    - ■ Demonstrates cutaneous/subcutaneous location

DIFFERENTIAL DIAGNOSIS

Sebaceous Cyst
- Arises from obstructed sebaceous gland
- Imaging and clinical features often indistinguishable from epidermal inclusion cyst

Cyst
- Parenchymal location distinguishing feature
- Anechoic

Montgomery Gland Cyst
- Confined to areola

Breast Neoplasm
- Parenchymal location
- Squamous metaplasia of benign or malignant breast epithelium can mimic epidermal inclusion cyst

PATHOLOGY

General Features
- General path comments
  - ○ Arises from skin
    - ■ Cutaneous or subcutaneous
  - ○ Often erroneously referred to as sebaceous cyst
    - ■ Imaging and clinical findings indistinguishable
  - ○ Most common epithelial skin cyst of breast
    - ■ 80% of skin cysts
  - ○ More common in other parts of the body: Face, scalp, neck and trunk
- Genetics: Multiple cysts of the scalp and back may be seen as part of Gardner syndrome: Autosomal dominant
- Etiology
  - ○ Arises from obstructed hair follicle
    - ■ Most common
  - ○ May occur along embryonic lines of closure
  - ○ Squamous metaplasia of sweat duct
    - ■ Not connected to skin
  - ○ Traumatic downward implantation of epidermal fragments

- Reduction mammoplasty
- Following FNA or core biopsy
○ May arise in preexisting sebaceous cyst
  - Squamous epithelium grows down fundus of sebaceous gland

Gross Pathologic & Surgical Features
- Firm, gray-to-white encapsulated nodule
- Thick contents: White, flaky, waxy
- Small, blackened pore may be seen at dome of lesion

Microscopic Features
- Wall composed of true epidermis
  ○ Stratified squamous epithelium
- Filled with keratin, often lamellated, "onion skin"
- Calcifications
- No sebaceous glands
- Young cyst: Several layers of squamous and granular cells
- Old cyst: Atrophic wall, only one or two layers of flattened cells
- H&E stain
  ○ Melanocytes identified in African-American patients, rarely in Caucasians

CLINICAL ISSUES

Presentation
- Most common signs/symptoms
  ○ Elevated, round, firm mass in breast skin
  ○ Slow growing
    - Patients often report lesion present for months to years
  ○ Usually palpable ± blackhead or whitehead
  ○ Occasionally painful
  ○ Often visually evident on clinical breast exam
  ○ May be moveable or fixed to skin
- Other signs/symptoms
  ○ Superficial, inflamed mass may be presenting symptom
  ○ May give history of spontaneous white discharge
- Diagnosis
  ○ Clinical
    - Avoid biopsy when clinical, imaging criteria met
  ○ Excisional biopsy
    - Reserved for cases to rule out malignancy (rare)
    - Symptomatic relief for large or painful lesions
  ○ Avoid needle biopsy
    - Complication: Rupture → cyst contents released into dermis → inflammation, abscess

Demographics
- Age: No age predilection
- Gender
  ○ Reported in males with same frequency as females
    - Skin, not a parenchymal breast lesion

Natural History & Prognosis
- Excellent
  ○ Malignant transformation extremely rare

Treatment
- No treatment usually necessary

○ Unless painful or inflamed
○ Usually resolves on its own
- Older literature recommended complete resection
  ○ Remote possibility of malignant transformation

DIAGNOSTIC CHECKLIST

Consider
- Avoid intervention except to rule out malignancy, treat infection or alleviate pain

Image Interpretation Pearls
- Hypoechoic line from superficial mass to skin confirms diagnosis

SELECTED REFERENCES

1. Bergmann-Koester CU et al: Epidermal cyst of the breast mimicking malignancy: clinical, radiological, and histological correlation. Arch Gynecol Obstet. 273(5):312-4, 2006
2. Crystal P et al: Concentric rings within a breast mass on sonography: lamellated keratin in an epidermal inclusion cyst. AJR Am J Roentgenol. 184(3 Suppl):S47-8, 2005
3. Kim HS et al: Spectrum of sonographic findings in superficial breast masses. J Ultrasound Med. 24(5):663-80, 2005
4. Celik V et al: Epidermal inclusion cyst of the breast: clinical, radiologic, and pathologic correlation. Breast J. 10(1):57, 2004
5. Kwak JY et al: Imaging findings in a case of epidermal inclusion cyst arising within the breast parenchyma. J Clin Ultrasound. 32(3):141-3, 2004
6. Kapila K et al: Fine needle aspiration cytology of epidermal inclusion cysts in the male breast. Acta Cytol. 47(2):315-7, 2003
7. Morris PC et al: Epidermal cyst of the breast: detection in a screening programme. Australas Radiol. 43(1):12-5, 1999
8. Davies JD et al: Mammary epidermoid inclusion cysts after wide-core needle biopsies. Histopathology. 31(6):549-51, 1997
9. Denison CM: Epidermal inclusion cysts of the breast: three Lesions with calcifications. Radiology. 204:493-96, 1997
10. Cooper RA et al: Epidermal inclusion cysts in the male breast. Can Assoc Radiol J. 47(2):92-3, 1996
11. Chantra PK: Circumscribed fibrocystic mastopathy with formation of epidermal cyst. AJR. 163: 831-32, 1994
12. Fajardo LL: Epidermal inclusion cyst after reduction mammoplasty. Radiology. 186(1):103-06, 1993
13. Shousha S et al: Recurrent epidermal cysts of the breast. Histopathology. 21(3):299-300, 1992

EPIDERMAL INCLUSION CYST

IMAGE GALLERY

Typical

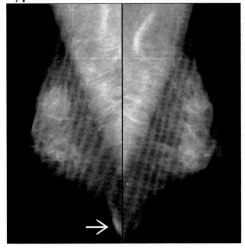
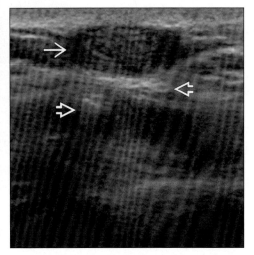

(Left) MLO mammography demonstrates a circumscribed, superficial mass ➡ in the inframammary fold of the right breast. The inferior breast is a common location of epidermal inclusion cysts. *(Right)* Ultrasound (same mass as left-hand image) shows circumscribed, oval mostly hypoechoic, though peripherally anechoic mass ➡, with minimal posterior enhancement ➡. US-guided 14-g core biopsy confirmed diagnosis of epidermal inclusion cyst.

Typical

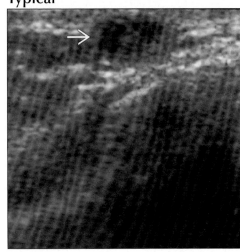
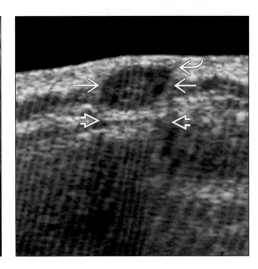

(Left) US demonstrates a hypoechoic mass within the skin ➡ which is difficult to adequately characterize, due to its superficial location in the near field. *(Right)* US shows (same mass as on left), except with a standoff pad. Lesion characteristics, including margins ➡ and posterior enhancement ➡, seen to better advantage. Note hypoechoic line extending to surface ➡, representing obstructed hair follicle of this epidermal inclusion cyst.

Typical

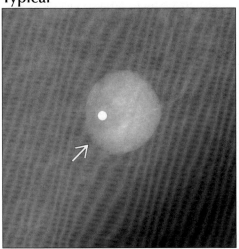
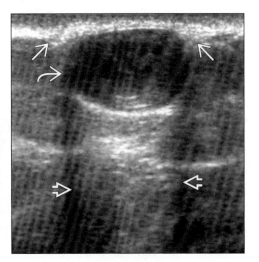

(Left) CC mammography spot compression shows well-circumscribed hyperdense, palpable mass ➡ in the medial right breast. Although it is in the skin, it projects over parenchyma. *(Right)* US (same mass as left-hand image) shows a heterogeneously hypoechoic, circumscribed mass ➡ with posterior enhancement ➡, corresponding to palpable lump of preceding case. Note "claw sign," ➡ indicating its intradermal location.

SEBACEOUS CYST

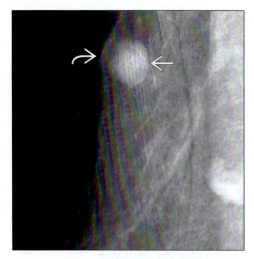

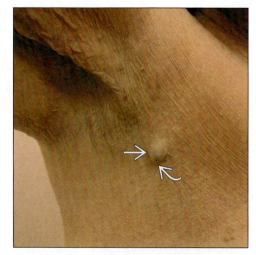

MLO mammography spot compression shows a round, circumscribed mass in the right axilla ➡. The overlying skin is bulging ➤. This is the typical appearance of a sebaceous cyst.

Clinical photograph shows the lesion ➡ of the previous case, evident as a smooth, rounded superficial mass. Note blackhead ➤ at its apex.

TERMINOLOGY

Abbreviations and Synonyms
- Pilar or trichilemmal cyst

Definitions
- A benign cutaneous or subcutaneous epithelial skin cyst that contains sebaceous glands

IMAGING FINDINGS

General Features
- Best diagnostic clue
  - Superficial, palpable mass arising from the skin
  - Clinically and on imaging: Indistinguishable from epidermal inclusion cyst
- Location
  - Anywhere on the skin of the breast or axilla
    - Most common in areas of redundant skin folds: Inframammary fold, parasternal, axilla
  - Unlike epidermal inclusion cysts: Always originate in skin
- Size: Few mm up to 10 cm; usually ≤ 1 cm

Mammographic Findings
- Superficial circumscribed round or oval mass

Ultrasonographic Findings
- Grayscale Ultrasound
  - Circumscribed oval or round mass within skin
  - Hypoechoic line from mass to skin represents dilated or obstructed sebaceous gland; seen only with scan plane parallel to gland
  - Variable echogenicity: Hypoechoic, but can be isoechoic; occasionally hyperechoic, mixed
  - Often hypervascular

Imaging Recommendations
- Best imaging tool: Ultrasound: Use standoff pad or glob of gel
- Protocol advice
  - Begin with mammography
    - Place BB on skin overlying mass
    - Tangential view to verify location in skin
    - Bright light or digital mammography to visualize skin

DDx: Epidermal Inclusion Cyst

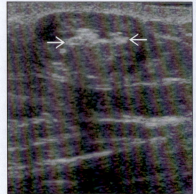

Partially Calcified

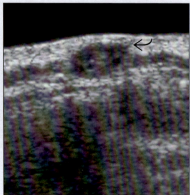

Hair Follicle

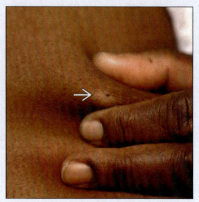

Blackhead

SEBACEOUS CYST

Key Facts

Terminology
- A benign cutaneous or subcutaneous epithelial skin cyst that contains sebaceous glands

Imaging Findings
- Clinically and on imaging: Indistinguishable from epidermal inclusion cyst
- Place BB on skin overlying mass
- Tangential view to verify location in skin

Top Differential Diagnoses
- Epidermal Inclusion Cyst
- Montgomery Gland Cyst

Pathology
- Etiology: Arises from obstructed sebaceous gland
- Contents of cyst: Yellow, smooth and buttery

Clinical Issues
- Excellent prognosis: No malignant potential

DIFFERENTIAL DIAGNOSIS

Epidermal Inclusion Cyst
- Does not contain sebaceous glands
- Sloughed keratin within cyst

Montgomery Gland Cyst
- Confined to areola

Breast Neoplasm
- Parenchymal location

PATHOLOGY

General Features
- Genetics: Can be seen as part of Cowden syndrome: Autosomal dominant; multiple
- Etiology: Arises from obstructed sebaceous gland

Gross Pathologic & Surgical Features
- Smooth, firm, white-walled cyst
- Contents of cyst: Yellow, smooth and buttery
- Easily enucleated
- Orifice of gland often visible as blackhead
- Dark color, rancid odor of contents when infected

Microscopic Features
- Cyst wall: Epithelial cells, no clearly visible intercellular bridges
- Cysts contents: Homogeneous eosinophilic material

CLINICAL ISSUES

Presentation
- Most common signs/symptoms: Smooth, round, raised skin lesion ± blackhead

Demographics
- Gender: Equally common in males

Natural History & Prognosis
- Excellent prognosis: No malignant potential
- May become infected
- If ruptures → foreign body reaction → partial or complete disintegration of cyst

Treatment
- Usually requires no treatment
  - Oral antibiotics for infection
  - Excision if persistently painful or enlarges

DIAGNOSTIC CHECKLIST

Consider
- Incites inflammatory response if ruptured: Leave it alone (including no FNA or core)

SELECTED REFERENCES

1. Elder D: Lever's Histopathology of the Skin. 8th Ed. Philadelphia, Lippincott-Raven. Chapter 30, 694-7, 1997

IMAGE GALLERY

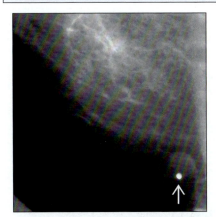 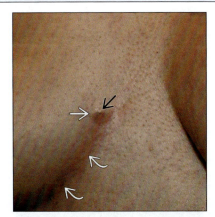 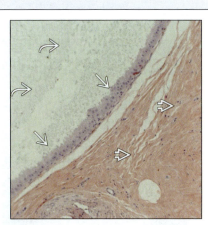

(Left) CC mammography spot compression shows a superficial, circumscribed mass ➡ in the right inframammary fold. *(Center)* Clinical photograph shows nonerythematous skin lesion ➡ with a central blackhead ➡, depicted in mammogram of previous case. Note inframammary fold location ➡ in this case of suspected sebaceous cyst. *(Right)* Micropathology shows example of sebaceous cyst. Note epithelial lining of cyst ➡, normal parenchyma ➡ and amorphous contents of cyst ➡.

SKIN LESIONS, NON-CYSTIC

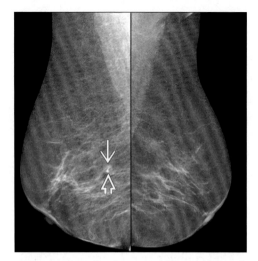

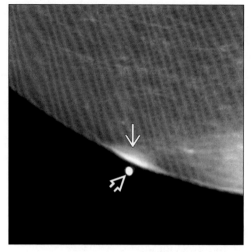

MLO mammography shows a small lesion ➡ nicely identified as a skin lesion with the BB skin marker ➡. This small lesion could have been misinterpreted as parenchymal.

CC mammography (same case as left image) shows the BB skin marker ➡ directly over a slightly raised mole ➡. Full-field digital as compared with analog mammography enhances visualization of the skin.

TERMINOLOGY

Definitions
- Findings related to the skin projecting over breast tissue on mammography
- Entities may be isolated, extensions of diffuse cutaneous abnormalities, manifestation of systemic processes, iatrogenic, traumatic

IMAGING FINDINGS

General Features
- Best diagnostic clue
  - Mammographic mass with sharply outlined borders and crevices outlined by air
  - Lesion(s) may be near skin surface on at least one view
  - Palpable mass in skin

Mammographic Findings
- Skin lesions often project over breast parenchyma on two-view mammography
  - Most of breast skin superimposed over parenchyma
    - Only small amount of skin is tangential to X-ray beam
    - Distinguishing skin from parenchymal lesions may be difficult
    - Full-field digital imaging highlights the skin more than does high-contrast analog imaging
- Raised lesion of significant size should be marked by technologist before exam
  - Small metallic BB or semi-opaque circle marker; alternatively lesion can be annotated on history sheet breast icon
    - BB superimposed over lesion most views; lesion identified directly beneath BB on tangential view
- Single or multiple
  - If too numerous, BBs not helpful
- History and visual inspection of the breast may be necessary; technologist attention to these findings essential
  - Meticulous technique to avoid misdiagnosis
- Shape variable
  - Round
  - Oval
  - Lobulated
  - Irregular

DDx: Additional Non-Cystic Skin Lesions

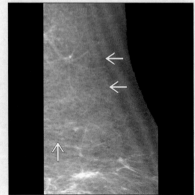

Skin Pores

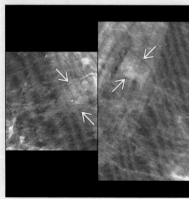

Bilateral Keloids

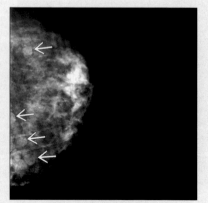

Neurofibromatosis

SKIN LESIONS, NON-CYSTIC

Key Facts

Terminology
- Findings related to the skin projecting over breast tissue on mammography

Imaging Findings
- Mammographic mass with sharply outlined borders and crevices outlined by air
- Skin lesions often project over breast parenchyma on two-view mammography
- Raised lesion of significant size should be marked by technologist before exam
- Single or multiple
- History and visual inspection of the breast may be necessary; technologist attention to these findings essential
- No specific role, per se
- Usually not necessary to make diagnosis

Top Differential Diagnoses
- Skin Pores
- Seborrheic Keratosis
- Verruca
- Benign Nevus (Pigmented Nevus, Mole)
- Skin Tags
- Scar, Keloid
- Inflammatory Processes
- Neurofibromatosis
- Collagen Vascular Disease
- Steatocystoma Multiplex

Clinical Issues
- Findings pertinent to individual lesions/diseases
- Most common skin lesions do not require treatment

- Margins
  - Usually well-circumscribed: Small amounts of air trapped by compression at borders produce excellent contrast
  - Margins may be obscured
- Surface crevices
  - Crenulated surface traps air: Fine linear or reticular lucencies
- Calcifications or particulate matter such as talc may be visible and can confound identification

Ultrasonographic Findings
- Grayscale Ultrasound
  - Usually not necessary to make diagnosis
  - Can help confirm palpable lesion is within the skin
  - Important role in evaluating parenchymal mammographically detected suspicious masses

MR Findings
- T1 C+: Keloids, hemangiomas, malignancies, some other skin lesions will enhance
- No specific role, per se

Imaging Recommendations
- Best imaging tool: Bilateral mammogram

DIFFERENTIAL DIAGNOSIS

Skin Pores
- Mammography demonstrates numerous small round and oval lucencies
- Common; appearance recognizable; should not cause ambiguity as to etiology

Seborrheic Keratosis
- Also known as verruca senilis or pigmented papilloma
- Most commonly imaged skin lesion
- Benign
- Greasy feeling to the touch
  - Abundant, fatty, keratinous nest within lesion
- Dark brown, elevated, sharply demarcated
- Mammography
  - Circumscribed, round, oval or lobulated mass

- May have air in crevices
- Often see halo around mass from air trapped between border and surrounding skin

Verruca
- More commonly known as warts
- Represent thickening or projections of epidermis
- Often demonstrate air within crevices

Benign Nevus (Pigmented Nevus, Mole)
- Shape variable: Round, oval, irregular
- Crevices may be outlined by air
- May develop calcifications
- Flat, pigmented skin moles not visible on mammography

Skin Tags
- May be too small to be visible on mammogram
- Typically a finding of older women
- Medial and inferior location, typical

Scar, Keloid
- May occur after breast biopsy, benign or malignant; reduction mammoplasty; accidental trauma (burns)
- Mammography typically reveals thickened tissue at incisional or trauma sites
- Location related to biopsy site, traumatized region
  - Benign biopsy less likely to develop significant scar
  - Education mammoplasty inferior breast scars variable as to persistent prominence
  - Lumpectomy biopsy site scar often prominent secondary to changes associated with radiation therapy
- Keloid (exuberant scarring) findings on mammography: Irregular, tube-like or mass-like raised structure

Inflammatory Processes
- Focal or diffuse rashes or areas of acne may lead to patient complaint, but small lesions seldom visible on mammogram
- Larger lesions may be visible mammographically; long-standing cystic acne can develop internal calcifications

○ Severe nodulocystic acne may be seen mammographically as multiple circumscribed lucent masses that may demonstrate fat-fluid levels similar to steatocystoma multiplex

Neurofibromatosis

- Multiple cutaneous lesions; vary in size
  ○ Massive neurofibromas reported; predominate in nipple-areolar complexes
- Derived from nerve cell sheaths
- Autosomal dominant; both females and males
  ○ Reported in association with gynecomastia in young males
- May cover entire body
- Mammography
  ○ Multiple, bilateral skin lesions
  ○ Well-defined margins except where lesions attach to skin

Collagen Vascular Disease

- Skin thickening secondary to scleroderma; reported in systemic lupus erythematosus

Steatocystoma Multiplex

- Autosomal dominant inherited disorder (female and male); uncommon; usually on the upper trunk anteriorly
  ○ May also be found in the axilla and groin
- Hamartomatous malformations of pilosebaceous duct junction composed of small keratin-filled intradermal cysts containing vellus hair shafts
- Often inherited as an autosomal dominant trait of keratinization, pachyonychia-congenita type II, or a variation of Jackson-Sertoli syndrome
- Mammographic findings are those of multiple lucent (fat-containing) masses with peripheral high density rims
  ○ Size range from 0.2-2.0 cm
  ○ Larger lesions may demonstrate fat-fluid levels
  ○ No associated increased risk of malignancy
- Ultrasound: Oval hypoechoic masses with posterior enhancement

Malignant Melanoma

- Usually preceded by flat, hairless mole; light to dark brown pigment
  ○ Not seen on mammography
- Later changes
  ○ Increase in size
  ○ Exophytic growth
    ▪ Can be identified on mammography at this point
  ○ Irregular margins, color variable
- Most common types in breast
  ○ Superficial spreading
  ○ Nodular

Non-Melanomatous Mammary Tumors (Malignant and Benign Entities)

- Adnexal gland (sweat-gland) carcinoma
  ○ Large size may limit visualization of skin origin an confound distinguishing from a true breast parenchymal lesion
- Basal cell carcinoma

○ Cleavage area (greater sun exposure) may be predisposed
- Hidradenoma of the axilla (usually benign)
- Sebaceous adenoma of the nipple (benign)

Cutaneous Metastases

- Breast, other primary sites

PATHOLOGY

General Features

- Findings pertinent to individual lesions

CLINICAL ISSUES

Presentation

- Most common signs/symptoms: Asymptomatic screening mammogram
- Other signs/symptoms: Large lesions may be palpable, inflamed
- Findings pertinent to individual lesions/diseases

Demographics

- Gender: Many skin processes may involve males as well as females, but mammograms not typically indicated for male skin lesions, per se

Natural History & Prognosis

- Most common skin lesions have an excellent prognosis

Treatment

- Most common skin lesions do not require treatment
- Skin manifestations of systemic processes require treatment based on underlying disease

DIAGNOSTIC CHECKLIST

Consider

- Skin lesions as etiology of bilateral multiple masses

SELECTED REFERENCES

1. Millman SL et al: An unusual presentation of neurofibromatosis of the breast. Breast J. 10:45-7, 2004
2. Murat A et al: Neurofibroma of the breast in a boy with neurofibromatosis type 1. Clin Imaging. 28:415-7, 2004
3. Wilson CH et al: Gynaecomastia, neurofibromatosis and breast cancer. Breast. 13(1):77-9, 2004
4. Park KY et al: Steatocystoma multiplex: mammographic and sonographic manifestations. AJR. 180:271-4, 2003
5. Opere E et al: Localized scleroderma of the breast. Eur Radiol. 12:1483-5, 2002
6. Rosen PP: Rosen's Breast Pathology. 2nd ed. Philadelphia, Lippincott williams & Wilkins. Chapter 44, 904-12, 2001
7. Shelty MK: Mondor's disease of the breast: sonographic and mammographic findings. AJR. 177:893-96, 2001
8. Bassett LW et al: Diagnosis of Diseases of the Breast. Philadelphia, WB Saunders Co. Chapter 25, 38-364, 1997
9. Denison CM: Epidermal inclusion cysts of the breast: three lesions with calcifications. Radiology. 204:496-96, 1997

SKIN LESIONS, NON-CYSTIC

IMAGE GALLERY

Typical

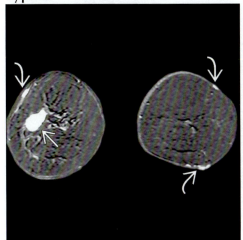

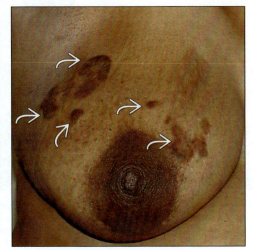

(Left) Coronal T1 C+ subtraction MR shows a known cancer ➜ and multiple enhancing lesions in the skin of both breasts ➜. Clinical examination of the right breast (right image) was correlated. *(Right)* Clinical photograph on correlation with clinical findings on the right breast, the enhancing skin lesions were shown to be due to keloids ➜ (exuberant skin scars).

Typical

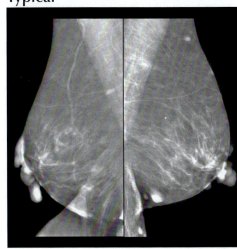

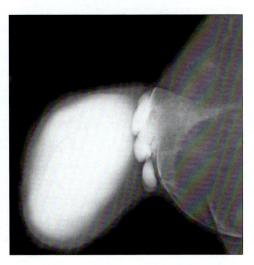

(Left) MLO mammography shows large skin lesions, many near the nipples. The largest lesion on the right could not be fully included on the MLO view (see right image). *(Right)* MLO mammography includes the massive neurofibroma seen in part on the preceding MLO view of the right breast. This patient's mother, brother and son also have type 1 neurofibromatosis.

IV

3

25

Typical

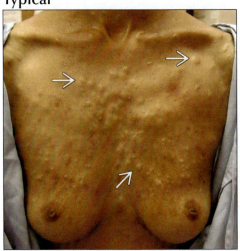

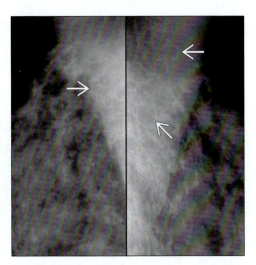

(Left) Clinical photograph shows numerous superficial raised nonerythematous soft lesions involving the chest and neck ➜. MLO mammogram shown in right image. *(Right)* MLO mammography (close-up) show numerous circumscribed lucent masses projecting over both breasts ➜. The patient had prior biopsy of a lesion on her arm, confirming steatocystoma.

SKIN THICKENING AND RETRACTION

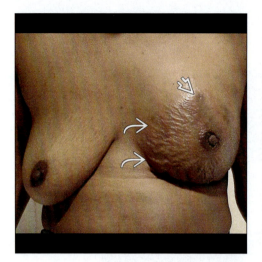

Clinical photograph shows the left breast to be shrunken with marked skin thickening including palpable cord-like masses within the skin ➤. A punch biopsy (12:00 site, ➤) was nondiagnostic.

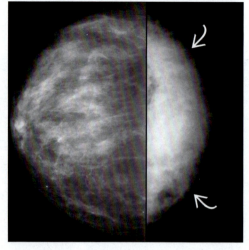

CC mammography (same patient as left-hand image) shows the dense and shrunken left breast ➤. Biopsy = poorly differentiated infiltrating carcinoma with angiolymphatic invasion, c/w inflammatory carcinoma.

TERMINOLOGY

Definitions
- Skin thickening = > 2 mm; can be focal or diffuse
  - Normal skin may be thicker in periareolar region, inframammary fold, parasternally
- Skin retraction = skin is abnormally pulled in, tethered, concave, dimpled
- Skin invasion = tumor extends into skin, usually directly overlying tumor
  - Skin retraction does not necessarily imply skin invasion
  - Usually shows associated skin thickening
- Peau d'orange = skin resembles peel of an orange: Thickened, with prominent skin pores, often also erythematous
  - Implies lymphatic edema, usually seen with inflammatory carcinoma

IMAGING FINDINGS

General Features
- Best diagnostic clue

○ Skin thickness > 2 mm on any modality = skin thickening
○ Clinical appearance most helpful for both skin thickening and retraction
○ Skin invasion seen best on MR: Abnormal enhancement extends to include skin, often directly over tumor

Mammographic Findings
- Standard MLO and CC views may demonstrate findings
- Skin thickening & retraction often overlooked, particularly on high contrast analog images
  - Knowledge of visible or palpable findings indicated by referring physician or attentive technologist often critical for detection
- Digital mammography increases skin visibility: Tissue equalization algorithms for subcutaneous tissues
- Skin retraction: Search for underlying carcinoma
  - Additional imaging often necessary
    - Spot compression views to evaluate mass margins, architectural distortion
    - Magnification views to identify and characterize calcifications (Ca++) if present

DDx: Additional Skin Thickening Examples

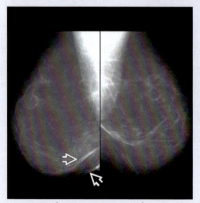

Reduction Mammoplasty

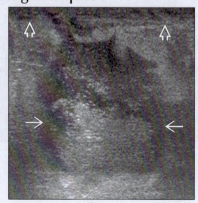

Abscess

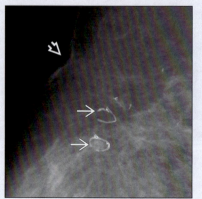

BCT, Suture Calcifications

SKIN THICKENING AND RETRACTION

Key Facts

Terminology
- Skin thickening = > 2 mm; can be focal or diffuse
- Normal skin may be thicker in periareolar region, inframammary fold, parasternally
- Skin retraction = skin is abnormally pulled in, tethered, concave, dimpled
- Skin invasion = tumor extends into skin, usually directly overlying tumor

Imaging Findings
- Mammography (ideally digital) MLO and CC views; additional tangential view(s) may be helpful

Top Differential Diagnoses
- Post-Procedural Skin Thickening
- Unilateral edema, focal or diffuse

- Mastitis: Diffuse skin thickening with erythema, warmth, pain; usually in pregnant or lactating women
- Abscess; focal skin thickening (again with other findings of inflammation/infection); lactating women; post lumpectomy infection (uncommon)
- Inflammatory carcinoma
- Locally advanced breast cancer with overlying skin involvement
- Skin Retraction
- Scarring from prior biopsy
- Fat necrosis
- Underlying malignancy

Pathology
- Skin involvement (extension into skin, fixation) with underlying tumor is T4b, stage IIIB

- Tangential views with or without magnification: Increase conspicuity of subtle skin changes, can improve depiction of underlying mass if present, by displacing mass onto subcutaneous fat
- US for any palpable findings

Ultrasonographic Findings
- Grayscale Ultrasound
  - Verifies clinical impression
  - Can directly measure skin thickening; no distinction malignant vs. benign
    - Underlying pathology may be better evaluated
    - Tumor extension into skin can be suspected/documented; tethering, thickening of Cooper ligaments
    - Ipsilateral axilla may be investigated in cases where a suspicious mass is detected
    - Often used to direct biopsy of parenchymal masses as well as abnormal axillary lymph nodes
  - Dilated lymphatics, increased echogenicity: Edema

MR Findings
- T1WI
  - Skin thickening and retraction readily depicted
  - Post-operative changes: Architectural distortion, skin changes, hemosiderin deposits, signal voids in areas of surgical staples or post-biopsy marker clips
- T2WI
  - Post-surgical seromas, abscess collections, other fluid collections, edema typically hyperintense
  - Ductal carcinoma in situ (DCIS) may be hyperintense
- T1 C+
  - Thickened skin with enhancement can be benign
    - Recent surgery, lumpectomy and irradiation [breast conserving therapy (BCT)]
    - Mastitis, abscess: Appearances indistinguishable from carcinoma
    - Keloids, hemangiomas, other benign skin lesions
  - Thickened skin with enhancement often suspicious
    - Primary underlying lesion may be visible as enhancing mass or ductal enhancement

- Entire breast may enhance, worrisome for inflammatory carcinoma
- Skin enhancement may be only evidence of recurrent carcinoma
- Some cutaneous malignancies may enhance
  - Thickened skin without enhancement
    - Healed biopsy scar
    - Healed post-traumatic scarring (burns, keloids)
    - Post-radiation; may demonstrate ≥ 18 months of associated lumpectomy site enhancement
    - Edema: Congestive heart failure, other

Imaging Recommendations
- Best imaging tool
  - Mammography (ideally digital) MLO and CC views; additional tangential view(s) may be helpful
  - US for clinically and/or mammographically suspicious findings
  - MR if a new finding without antecedent history of recent surgery, and above examinations unrevealing
    - T1WI best to depict skin thickening, retraction

DIFFERENTIAL DIAGNOSIS

Post-Procedural Skin Thickening
- Edema
  - Focal or diffuse
    - Increased density, trabecular thickening (mammography), increased echogenicity, dilated lymphatics (US)
    - Skin thickening and retraction may increase as parenchymal edema decreases
    - Skin changes secondary to radiation or blocked lymphatics from axillary node dissection
    - MR may detect post treatment skin thickening not evident clinically (73%, 11/15 in irradiated breasts, single series)
    - Sign of breast cancer recurrence: Obstructive adenopathy or dermal lymphatic invasion

New Finding
- Unilateral edema, focal or diffuse

- Mastitis: Diffuse skin thickening with erythema, warmth, pain; usually in pregnant or lactating women
- Abscess; focal skin thickening (again with other findings of inflammation/infection); lactating women; post lumpectomy infection (uncommon)
- Inflammatory carcinoma
  - Skin findings often dramatic with large area involved with peau d'orange, erythema; often with metastatic axillary adenopathy
  - May be misdiagnosed as mastitis
  - Shorter clinical symptomatic course than neglected breast carcinoma
  - Focal breast finding such as mass or Ca++ may be absent
  - Skin punch biopsy for diagnosis; US-guided biopsy of mass if punch biopsy non-diagnostic
- Neglected carcinoma
  - Severe denial or illness may lead to frank ulceration of skin from underlying tumor mass
- Trauma
  - Seat-belt injury may lead to focal pain, skin thickening and palpable mass(es)
- Granulomatous diseases; lymphoma; subclavian or innominate vein occlusion; systemic causes of anasarca
- Screening mammographic finding of skin thickening/retraction
  - Locally advanced breast cancer with overlying skin involvement
  - Evaluate for underlying lesion: Mass, Ca++, architectural distortion
    - Invasive ductal carcinoma (IDC) NOS: Irregular mass with or without Ca++
    - Invasive lobular carcinoma (ILC): Spiculated mass or focal asymmetry; often associated architectural distortion

Skin Retraction
- Scarring from prior biopsy
- Fat necrosis
  - History of surgery or trauma
  - Associated fibrosis can cause skin retraction
  - Mammography typically demonstrates central or associated lucencies (fat) and peripheral curvilinear Ca++
  - US shows mixed hyper- and anechoic masses; may show surrounding increased echogenicity secondary to edema
- Underlying malignancy
  - Invasive carcinomas

PATHOLOGY

General Features
- General path comments
  - Post biopsy or traumatic fibrosis associated with scarring
  - Breast cancer may extend to skin via
    - Contiguous spread
    - Through ductal network and lymphatics
  - Lymphangitic congestion of skin

- Associated with trabecular thickening
- Drainage of skin contiguous with breast lymphatics
- Embryology-anatomy
  - Cooper ligaments attach breast to skin: Tethering of Cooper ligaments causes retraction
  - Ductal epithelium in direct contiguity with skin

Staging, Grading or Classification Criteria
- Skin thickening or retraction alone not necessarily indicative of skin involvement by tumor
- Skin involvement (extension into skin, fixation) with underlying tumor is T4b, stage IIIB
  - Includes ipsilateral satellite skin nodules
  - Or ulceration of skin
  - Or edema, peau d'orange
  - Inflammatory carcinoma = T4d

CLINICAL ISSUES

Presentation
- Most common signs/symptoms: Clinically apparent skin changes

Demographics
- Gender
  - Skin changes not typical for presentation of gynecomastia
  - Skin or nipple retraction reported in 36% of male breast cancer

DIAGNOSTIC CHECKLIST

Image Interpretation Pearls
- Correlation with pertinent history important in reporting focal and diffuse findings

SELECTED REFERENCES

1. Kwak JY et al: Unilateral breast edema: spectrum of etiologies and imaging appearances. Yonsei Medical Journal. 46:1-7, 2005
2. D'Orsi CJ et al: Breast Imaging Reporting and Data System: BI-RADS, Mammography, 4th ed. Reston, American College of Radiology, 2003
3. Ikeda DM et al: Breast Imaging Reporting and Data System: BI-RADS, Magnetic Resonance Imaging, 1st ed. Reston, American College of Radiology, 2003
4. Mendelson EB et al: Breast Imaging Reporting and Data System: BI-RADS, Ultrasound, 1st ed. Reston, American College of Radiology, 2003
5. Gunhan-Bilgen I et al: Inflammatory breast carcinoma: mammographic, ultrasonographic, clinical, and pathologic findings in 142 cases. Radiology. 223:829-38, 2002
6. Padhani AR et al: Magnetic resonance imaging of induration in the irradiated breast. Radiother Oncol. 4:157-62, 2002
7. Harris JR et al: Diseases of the Breast. Philadelphia, Lippincott Williams & Wilkins. Chapter 4, 68-9, 1996
8. Sickles EA: Practical solutions to common mammographic problems: Tailoring the examination. AJR. 151:31-9, 1988

SKIN THICKENING AND RETRACTION

IMAGE GALLERY

Typical

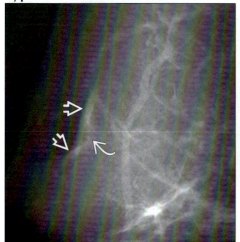
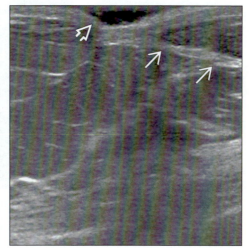

(Left) MLO mammography shows focal skin thickening ⮞ and retraction ➜ at a prior benign biopsy site in the right breast. Some facilities indicate these scar sites with a skin marker. *(Right)* Anti-radial ultrasound (same patient as left-hand image) shows a band-like area of increased echogenicity ➜ extending to overlying skin scar where skin retraction ⮞ is evident. Findings BI-RADS 2, benign.

Typical

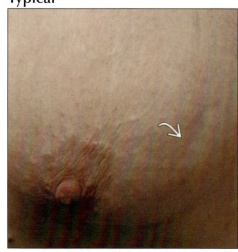
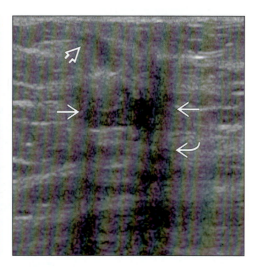

(Left) Clinical photograph shows subtle skin retraction ➜ along the inner right breast. Bilateral mammogram (not shown) showed subtle changes in the area. An US (right image) was performed. *(Right)* Radial ultrasound shows irregular, hypoechoic mass ➜ extending to skin surface ⮞. Posterior shadowing is also noted ➜. 14-g US-guided core biopsy showed infiltrating lobular carcinoma.

Typical

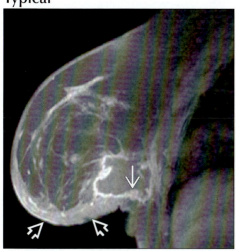
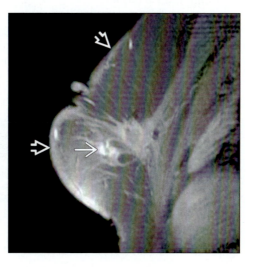

(Left) Sagittal T1 C+ FS MR shows nodular enhancement at the perimeter of a post lumpectomy seroma ➜ and skin thickening ⮞ 18 months out from BCT. US-guided core biopsy = IDC at lumpectomy site. *(Right)* Sagittal T1 C+ FS MR in a 60 yo woman s/p BCT shows nonenhancing skin thickening from radiation ⮞ and unsuspected nodular enhancement ➜ anterior to the lumpectomy site. Biopsy = recurrent IDC.

AXILLARY ADENOPATHY

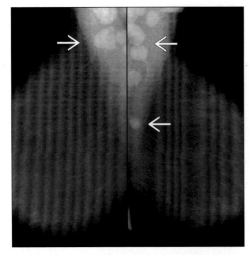

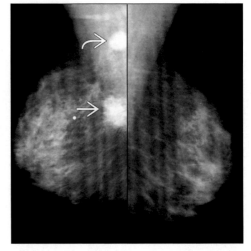

MLO mammography screening shows multiple bilateral axillary lymph nodes of varying size ➡. Fatty hila are visible in some. This 65 year old woman had a history of low grade lymphoma.

MLO mammography shows a 3 cm mass ➡; BI-RADS 5; biopsy = grade III IDC. A dense, round node is seen in the right axilla ➡, highly suspicious for and proven to be a metastatic node.

TERMINOLOGY

Definitions
- Enlarged (usually > 2 cm), not fatty-replaced axillary lymph nodes

IMAGING FINDINGS

General Features
- Best diagnostic clue
  - Dense, rounded or irregular axillary lymph node(s)
    - Diminutive or absent fatty hilum
  - Asymmetric cortical thickening of node
- Location
  - Average total number of nodes: 15-25
    - Level I: Inferior and lateral to pectoralis minor muscle
    - Level II: Beneath pectoralis minor muscle (Rotter nodes)
    - Level III: Superior to pectoralis minor muscle (not typically included in "full axillary dissection")
- Size: Not significant or predictive, range 1.5-5.5 cm
- Morphology
  - Rounded or irregular: Long to short-axis ratio < 1.4 favors malignancy
    - Spiculated margins suggest extranodal extension of breast cancer

Mammographic Findings
- Lower level I nodes visible on routine mammograms
  - Normal: Reniform with relatively thin cortex, radiolucent fatty hilum
  - Abnormal: Dense, obliteration of fatty hilum, thick cortex
- Abnormal nodes seen in 0.3% of screening mammograms

Ultrasonographic Findings
- Grayscale Ultrasound
  - Normal nodes often blend in with surrounding fat
  - Hypoechoic cortex
    - Uniformly thickened cortex favors reactive adenopathy
    - Asymmetrically thickened cortex favors metastatic disease
  - Diminutive echogenic hilum
    - Absence or compression of fatty hilum most specific sign for metastasis

DDx: Variety of Abnormal Axillary Masses

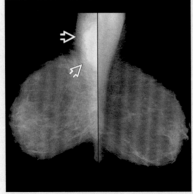

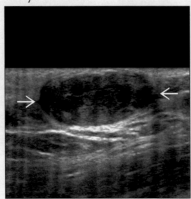

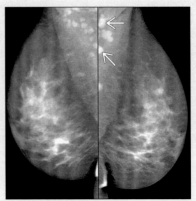

Metastasis, Unknown Primary

Sebaceous Cyst

HIV Adenopathy

AXILLARY ADENOPATHY

Key Facts

Terminology
- Enlarged (usually > 2 cm), not fatty-replaced axillary lymph nodes

Imaging Findings
- Dense, rounded or irregular axillary lymph node(s)
- Diminutive or absent fatty hilum
- Asymmetric cortical thickening of node
- Spiculated margins suggest extranodal extension of breast cancer
- MR test of choice for metastatic axillary adenopathy of unknown source, identify primary: 50-86% cases

Top Differential Diagnoses
- Primary Breast Carcinoma
- Metastases (breast, melanoma, lung)
- Silicone from current or prior rupture, or slow leak

- HIV
- Lymphoproliferative diseases: Lymphoma, leukemia
- Rheumatoid arthritis/collagen vascular diseases

Pathology
- Malignant etiologies 55%

Clinical Issues
- If benign etiology not known, US-guided FNA recommended

Diagnostic Checklist
- History of previously diagnosed malignancy, collagen vascular disease, granulomatous or other infection
- Dense, round or irregular nodes are suspicious regardless of size

---

- o Sensitivity for metastases 56-72%, specificity 70-90%
- o "Snowstorm" appearance pathognomonic for presence of silicone
- Color Doppler
  - o Peripheral flow, transcapsular vessels favor malignancy
    - Peripheral, non-hilar vessels in 47/93 (50.5%) malignant nodes, 3/105 (2.9%) benign in one series

MR Findings
- T1WI: Cortex hypointense; fatty hilum hyperintense
- T2WI
  - o Cortex hyperintense; fatty hilum hypointense
  - o Often adjacent to vessels
- T1 C+: Early enhancement and washout typical
- MR test of choice for metastatic axillary adenopathy of unknown source, identify primary: 50-86% cases

Nuclear Medicine Findings
- Tc-99m Sulfur Colloid
  - o Sentinel lymph node identification, intraoperative gamma probe
    - Alone or in combination with isosulfan blue dye
    - Lymph node replaced by tumor can be falsely negative
- PET
  - o Uptake detectable in malignant nodes > 7-8 mm
    - Sensitivity 61%: 66% for infiltrating ductal carcinoma and 25% for infiltrating lobular carcinoma metastases
  - o Not recommended for routine axillary staging of breast cancer: PPV 62%; NPV 79%

Other Modality Findings
- Clinical examination unreliable: 20% sensitivity to metastatic nodes

Imaging Recommendations
- Best imaging tool: Diagnosis by US-guided fine needle aspiration (FNA) or core needle biopsy

DIFFERENTIAL DIAGNOSIS

Primary Breast Carcinoma
- Primary tumor in axillary breast tissue may mimic adenopathy: Margins usually indistinct or spiculated

Unilateral Enlarged Nodes
- Metastases (breast, melanoma, lung)
- Reactive (inflammation/infection)
- Silicone from current or prior rupture, or slow leak

Bilateral Enlarged Nodes
- HIV
- Lymphoproliferative diseases: Lymphoma, leukemia
- Rheumatoid arthritis/collagen vascular diseases
- Tuberculosis, sarcoidosis

Nodal Calcifications (Ca++)
- Microcalcifications in node
  - o Metastatic breast carcinoma: Ca++ similar to primary tumor
  - o Metastatic ovarian carcinoma: Psammomatous Ca++
- Punctate or amorphous densities mimicking Ca++
  - o Secondary to gold injections for treatment of rheumatoid arthritis
  - o Rarely secondary to tattoo pigment
- Benign, coarse Ca++ in node
  - o Granulomatous disease: Tuberculosis, sarcoidosis

PATHOLOGY

General Features
- General path comments: Tissue/cytology necessary for suspected metastases
- Etiology
  - o Malignant etiologies 55%
  - o Malignant cells travel from breast to axilla in stepwise fashion
    - Level I affected first, followed by II then III; skip metastasis in < 5%
- Epidemiology

AXILLARY ADENOPATHY

○ ~ 50% patients with palpable breast cancer have histologically positive axillary adenopathy
○ Likelihood of axillary nodal involvement in breast cancer varies with location of tumor
  ▪ Most likely with upper outer quadrant cancer, followed by lower outer, upper inner, and lower inner

Gross Pathologic & Surgical Features
• Nodes are usually visible in axillary fat

Microscopic Features
• Malignant cells enter nodes via afferent lymphatics, into marginal sinus, and deposit in cortex
• Quantify size of largest nodal deposit of tumor

Staging, Grading or Classification Criteria
• Breast cancer metastases to axillary nodes
  ○ Stage II: Movable ipsilateral node(s) (N1)
  ○ Stage III: Fixed/matted ipsilateral node(s) (N2)
  ○ Stage IIIc: Ipsilateral supraclavicular node(s) or level III (infraclavicular) node(s) (N3)

CLINICAL ISSUES

Presentation
• Most common signs/symptoms: Palpable axillary nodes in patients with known malignancy prove metastatic in 70% cases

Natural History & Prognosis
• Varies with etiology of adenopathy
• In case of breast cancer axillary adenopathy has high correlation with prognosis
  ○ Prognosis directly correlates with number of nodes involved and the level of axillary involvement
• Five year survival rate from breast cancer is inversely related to number of positive axillary nodes
• Breast cancer recurrence rate is directly related to extent of axillary involvement
• Extranodal extension an adverse prognostic factor: Correlates with increased number of metastatic axillary nodes, reduced survival

Treatment
• In breast cancer patients surgical evaluation of axillary nodes is necessary
  ○ Sentinel lymph node for prognostic information
  ○ Axillary dissection for local control, complete staging
• When sentinel node positive, standard approach is full level I & II axillary dissection
• Internal mammary lymph node dissection not standard at most centers
• Axillary radiation for selected patients at risk for regional nodal failure: ≥ 4 nodal metastases
• If not due to breast cancer, treatment depends on underlying disease
• If no obvious cause of adenopathy such as rheumatoid arthritis, HIV, or known lymphoma, work-up necessary
• Other laboratory tests: Total blood count, chest radiograph, C-reactive protein

• If benign etiology not known, US-guided FNA recommended
• If no identifiable cause on FNA, 3 month follow-up
  ○ If persistent adenopathy, repeat FNA or surgical excision

DIAGNOSTIC CHECKLIST

Consider
• New finding; unilateral or bilateral; associated Ca++
• History of previously diagnosed malignancy, collagen vascular disease, granulomatous or other infection

Image Interpretation Pearls
• Dense, round or irregular nodes are suspicious regardless of size
• US to determine cortical thickness, loss or compression of hilum, guide FNA or biopsy

SELECTED REFERENCES

1. Buchanan CL et al: Utility of breast magnetic resonance imaging in patients with occult primary breast cancer. Ann Surg Oncol. 12(12):1045-53, 2005
2. Esen G et al: Gray scale and power Doppler US in the preoperative evaluation of axillary metastases in breast cancer patients with no palpable lymph nodes. Eur Radiol. 15:1215-23, 2005
3. Lemos S et al: Detection of axillary metastases in breast cancer patients using ultrasound and colour Doppler combined with fine needle aspiration cytology. Eur J Gynaecol Oncol. 26(2):165-6, 2005
4. Patel T et al: The clinical importance of axillary lymphadenopathy detected on screening mammography: revisited. Clin Radiol. 60(1):64-71, 2005
5. Benoit L et al: Concurrent lymphoma and metastatic breast carcinoma in the axillary, confounding sentinel lymph-node biopsy. Eur J Surg Oncol. 30(4):462-3, 2004
6. Brancato B et al: Role of ultrasound-guided fine needle cytology of axillary lymph nodes in breast carcinoma staging. Radiol Med (Torino). 108(4):345-55, 2004
7. Chen C et al: Outcome after treatment of patients with mammographically occult, magnetic resonance imaging-detected breast cancer presenting with axillary lymphadenopathy. Clin Breast Cancer. 5(1):72-7, 2004
8. Muttarak M et al: Role of mammography in diagnosis of axillary abnormalities in women with normal breast examination. Australas Radiol. 48(3):306-10, 2004
9. Said FE et al: Secondary axillary node carcinoma following treatment of Hodgkin's disease. Breast J. 10(2):167-8, 2004
10. Wahl RL et al: Prospective multicenter study of axillary nodal staging by positron emission tomography in breast cancer: a report of the Staging Breast Cancer with PET Study Group. J Clin Oncol. 22:277-85, 2004
11. Muttarak M et al: Mammographic features of tuberculous axillary lymphadenitis. Australas Radiol. 46(3):260-3, 2002
12. Lee CH et al: Clinical importance of unilaterally enlarging lymph nodes on otherwise normal mammograms. Radiology. 203(2):329-34, 1997
13. Murray ME et al: The clinical importance of axillary lymphadenopathy detected on screening mammography. Clin Radiol. 52(6):458-61, 1997
14. Walsh R et al: Axillary lymph nodes: mammographic, pathologic, and clinical correlation. AJR. 168:33-8, 1997
15. Dershaw DD et al: Spiculated axillary adenopathy. Radiology. 201(2):439-42, 1996

AXILLARY ADENOPATHY

IMAGE GALLERY

Typical

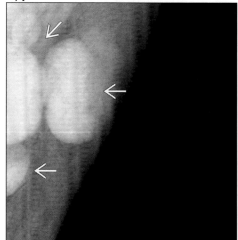

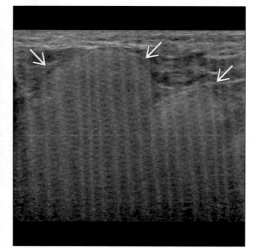

(Left) MLO mammography spot compression of palpable axillary lump in a 54 year old woman, shows dense enlarged nodes ➡; no fatty hila. She had 15 year old silicone implants without perceptible change or other symptoms of leak or rupture. *(Right)* Sagittal ultrasound of the palpable nodes (same patient as left-hand image) shows well-defined echogenic masses ➡ with "snowstorm" appearance and incoherent posterior shadowing, c/w silicone within nodes.

Typical

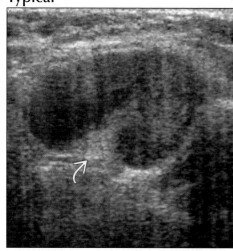

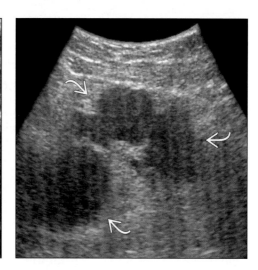

(Left) Longitudinal ultrasound of axilla in patient with newly diagnosed breast cancer shows a plump node with compressed fatty hilum ➡. Core needle biopsy revealed metastatic involvement. *(Right)* Longitudinal ultrasound of palpable axillary lump shows hypoechoic masses with irregular margins ➡. These are nodal metastases from a breast cancer visible only as 2 cm of microcalcifications on mammogram.

Typical

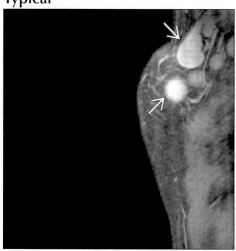

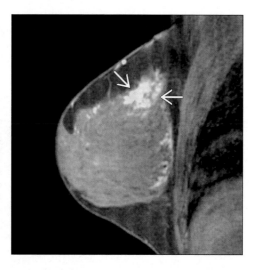

(Left) Sagittal T1 C+ FS MR shows multiple round and oval enhancing axillary masses representing abnormal lymph nodes ➡, in this 44 year old woman at high risk for breast cancer due to family history. *(Right)* Sagittal T1 C+ FS MR (same breast as left image) shows a region of rapid enhancement ➡ in the upper outer breast without mammographic or physical exam correlate. Biopsy showed IDC.

AXILLARY BREAST TISSUE

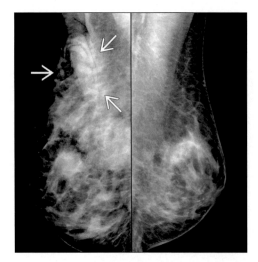

MLO mammography shows the exuberant continuation of the right breast tissue into the right axilla ➡. The woman was asymptomatic and no further work-up was performed.

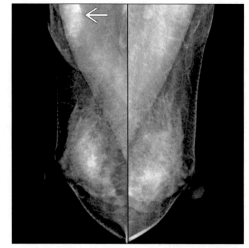

MLO mammography shows the typical appearance of ectopic breast tissue in the right axilla ➡. The patient was asymptomatic and no further evaluation was needed.

TERMINOLOGY

Abbreviations and Synonyms
- Ectopic breast tissue

Definitions
- Supernumerary breast tissue
  - Persistence of mammary ridge tissue
  - May have associated nipple and/or areolar complex
- Aberrant or accessory breast tissue
  - Separate from the mammary glandular parenchyma
  - Close to usual anatomic extent of the breast

IMAGING FINDINGS

General Features
- Best diagnostic clue: MLO mammogram

Mammographic Findings
- Normal appearing breast tissue in the axilla seen on the MLO view
- Aberrant breast tissue more common in left axilla
- Accessory nipples (polythelia) and breasts (polymastia) may be imaged
- Rare reports of cancer development within the accessory breast tissue

Ultrasonographic Findings
- Grayscale Ultrasound
  - Palpable masses warrant ultrasound evaluation
  - Masses may be axillary nodes, hypoechoic masses within the axillary breast tissue or normal appearing tissue

MR Findings
- T1 C+
  - Characteristics of breast tissue
  - Enhancing lesions should be assessed as in the orthoptic breast

Imaging Recommendations
- Best imaging tool: Mammography for asymptomatic axillary breast tissue
- Protocol advice: No further recommendations unless imaging or clinical abnormality is present

IV

3

34

DDx: Axillary Tissue and other "Milk Line" Masses

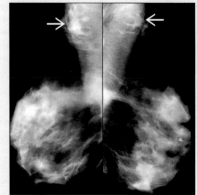

Bilateral Ectopic

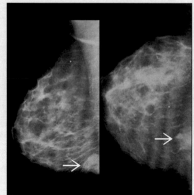

Polymastia

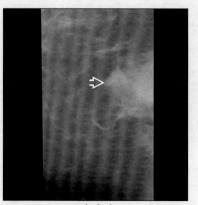

Polythelia

AXILLARY BREAST TISSUE

Key Facts

Terminology
- Ectopic breast tissue

Imaging Findings
- Normal appearing breast tissue in the axilla seen on the MLO view

Top Differential Diagnoses
- Axillary Nodes
- Lipoma

Pathology
- Mammary tissue may persist anywhere long the embryologic "milk line"
- Benign reported tumors: Adenomas and fibroadenomas in axilla and vulva
- Carcinoma most frequent ectopic site = axilla; vulva, other ectopic sites

---

DIFFERENTIAL DIAGNOSIS

Axillary Nodes
- Discrete masses with convex margins and fatty hila
- Margins may be less discrete if enlarged or inflamed

Lipoma
- Circumscribed, well-defined masses of mature adipose tissue
- Axillary glandular tissue may be partly or entirely replaced by fat: May simulate lipoma

PATHOLOGY

General Features
- General path comments: Cytologic findings depend on tissue developmental state
- Etiology
  - Breast tissue same ectodermal origin as skin glands
  - Mammary ridge develops along the "milk line"
    - Base of forelimb bud (primitive axilla) to medial hindlimb base (primitive inguinal area)
    - Mammary tissue may persist anywhere long the embryologic "milk line"
    - Supernumerary nipples or breasts on anterior chest above or below orthotopic breast
    - Benign reported tumors: Adenomas and fibroadenomas in axilla and vulva
    - Carcinoma most frequent ectopic site = axilla; vulva, other ectopic sites

Microscopic Features
- Duct and lobular mammary structures

CLINICAL ISSUES

Presentation
- Most common signs/symptoms: Asymptomatic
- Clinical Profile: Accessory tissue or nipples may be palpable
- Physiologic changes may occur
  - Menstrual cycle
  - Pregnancy
  - Postpartum
    - Swelling
    - Pain
    - Lactation when nipple present

SELECTED REFERENCES
1. Rosen PP: Rosen's breast pathology. Philadelphia, Lippincott Williams & Wilkins. Chapter 2, 25-6, 2001
2. Irvin WP et al: Primary breast carcinoma of the vulva: a case report and literature review. Gynecology Onxol. 73:155-9, 1999
3. Evans DM et al: Carcinoma of the axillary breast. J Surg Oncol. 59:190-5, 1995

IMAGE GALLERY

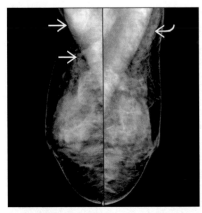 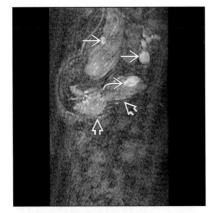 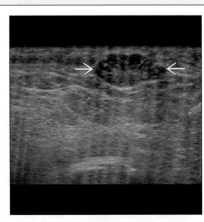

(Left) MLO mammography shows bilateral axillary breast tissue ➔ in a young woman with a palpable left axillary mass ➔. As a part of her evaluation, a breast MR was performed (same patient as next 2 images). *(Center)* Sagittal T1 C+ FS MR shows an oval enhancing axillary mass ➔ within axillary breast tissue ➔. Enhancing normal axillary lymph nodes ➔ are also present. *(Right)* Longitudinal ultrasound shows an oval lobulated hypoechoic mass ➔ correlating with the palpable axillary tissue mass. US-guided core biopsy showed a fibroadenoma.

AXILLARY NODAL CALCIFICATION

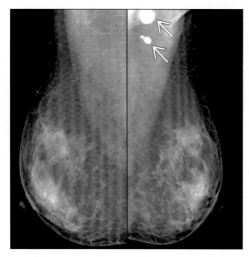

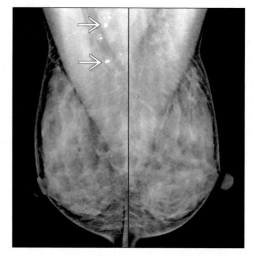

MLO mammography (screening) shows unilateral dense left axillary nodal Ca++ ➡ in a woman from India with non-contributory clinical history. These are likely the sequelae of prior granulomatous infection.

MLO mammography shows unilateral coarse right axillary nodal Ca++ ➡ in a woman from Vietnam with non-contributory clinical history. Likely secondary to prior granulomatous infection.

TERMINOLOGY

Definitions
- Calcifications (Ca++) within axillary lymph nodes

IMAGING FINDINGS

General Features
- Best diagnostic clue
  - Radiodense deposits within either normal or abnormal axillary lymph nodes
    - Normal: Reniform with smooth and relative thin cortex and visible fatty hilum
    - Abnormal: Dense, sometimes round, possibly irregular, normal size or enlarged, with little or no fatty hilum
    - The presence of visible fat within hilum does not rule out tumor involvement
- Location: Lower level I nodes are those typically visible on MLO mammogram
- Size: Axillary nodes may be normal or enlarged; size not predictive as to normal or abnormal; range < 1-5.5 cm

Mammographic Findings
- MLO view often includes level I axillary nodes
- Ca++ or other very bright punctate deposits visible in visualized nodes
- Magnification images for finer detail

Ultrasonographic Findings
- Grayscale Ultrasound
  - Not specific for evaluation of Ca++, per se
  - May suggest findings associated with possible malignancy or other process
    - Thickened cortex possibly with irregular margins; absent or compressed fatty hilum
    - Classic "snowstorm" disruption of ultrasound beam seen with nodal involvement with silicone

MR Findings
- T1WI: Cortex isointense to breast parenchyma and other soft tissue; hilum hyperintense
- T2WI FS
  - Reniform, oval or round hyper- or isointense
  - Microcalcifications without visible finding; large Ca++ may create signal void

---

DDx: Non-Nodal Axillary Densities

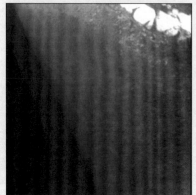

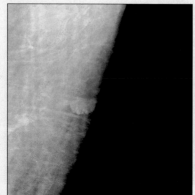

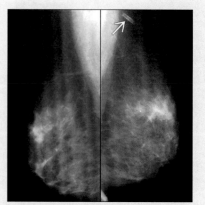

Deodorant Clumps

Talc within Skin Lesion

Retained Catheter Cuff

AXILLARY NODAL CALCIFICATION

Key Facts

Terminology
- Calcifications (Ca++) within axillary lymph nodes

Top Differential Diagnoses
- Granulomatous diseases: Tuberculosis, histoplasmosis; sarcoid; fat necrosis
- Metastatic breast carcinoma; described as amorphous and in a peripheral distribution
- Extramammary metastases (rare); ovarian, thyroid

- Gold deposits in patients with long history of intramuscular gold injections for rheumatoid arthritis (RA) treatment
- Clumped deodorant; talc within crevices of skin lesions; foreign bodies

Clinical Issues
- Treatment required for metastatic or active systemic processes

---

- T1 C+: Lymph nodes typically show early enhancement with washout; nonspecific benign/malignant

Nuclear Medicine Findings
- PET: FDG uptake often detected in enlarged malignant or infectious nodes

Imaging Recommendations
- Best imaging tool: MLO mammography

DIFFERENTIAL DIAGNOSIS

Coarse Calcifications
- Typically indicative of sequelae of prior infection/inflammation
  - Granulomatous diseases: Tuberculosis, histoplasmosis; sarcoid; fat necrosis

Microcalcifications
- Metastatic breast carcinoma; described as amorphous and in a peripheral distribution
- Extramammary metastases (rare); ovarian, thyroid

Punctate or Amorphous Intranodal Particles
- Gold deposits in patients with long history of intramuscular gold injections for rheumatoid arthritis (RA) treatment
- Tattoo pigments (rare)
- Silicone deposits in women with ruptured or leaking silicone breast implants

Bright Densities within Axilla
- Clumped deodorant; talc within crevices of skin lesions; foreign bodies

PATHOLOGY

General Features
- Etiology: Ca++ deposited in areas of necrosis as in granulomatous infectious processes; cytokines and other agents released through inflammation may promote Ca++

CLINICAL ISSUES

Treatment
- Treatment required for metastatic or active systemic processes

SELECTED REFERENCES

1. Ikeda DM: The Requisites: Breast Imaging. Philadelphia,Elsevier Mosby. Chapter 10, 303-05, 2004
2. Singer C et al: Mammographic appearance of axillary lymph node calcification in patients with metastatic ovarian carcinoma. AJR. 176:1437-40, 2001
3. Bruwer A et al: Punctate intranodal gold deposits simulating microcalcifications on mammograms. Radiology. 163:87-88, 1987

IV

3

37

IMAGE GALLERY

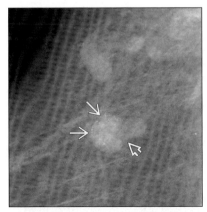 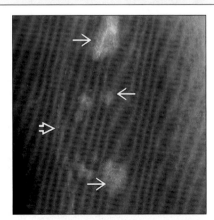 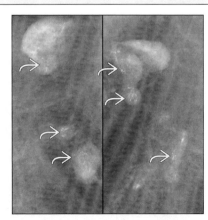

(Left) CC mammography magnification shows rounded lymph node with peripheral fine amorphous Ca++ ➡ and a small fatty hilum ➡. Biopsy = metastatic adenocarcinoma c/w ovarian. *(Center)* MLO mammography close-up of right axilla shows fine amorphous densities ➡ c/w gold particles in this woman with long history of treatment for RA. Note adjacent vascular Ca++ ➡. *(Right)* MLO mammography close-up shows fine particulate radiodensities ➡ within multiple axillary lymph nodes, attributable to uptake of gold particles from long history of treatment for RA.

PECTORALIS MUSCLE VARIANTS

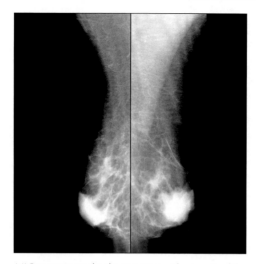

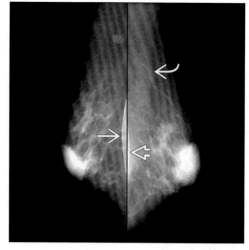

MLO mammography shows patient with agenesis of the right pectoralis muscle who underwent augmentation mammoplasty with subglandular right and subpectoral left implant (right-hand image).

MLO mammography shows calcified right subglandular implant capsule ➡, edge of the subpectoral left implant ➡, and normal left pectoralis major muscle ➡.

TERMINOLOGY

Definitions
- Congenital or developmental variations in pectoralis major muscle (PMM) appearance

IMAGING FINDINGS

General Features
- Best diagnostic clue
  - MLO mammogram
  - Axial imaging helpful in establishing anatomical variations

Mammographic Findings
- Normal: Convex, seen to level of nipple on MLO views
  - Variable contours and densities of normal size PMM
- Variants: Small or absent PMM on MLO views

MR Findings
- T1WI: Axial images of chest wall help to further evaluate confounding mammographic appearances
- T1 C+

- Normal musculature does not enhance; post biopsy enhancement reported
- Suspicious enhancing masses must be further evaluated
- Direct extension of tumor to involve chest wall
  - Obliteration of fat plane alone insufficient
  - Enhancement of PMM and/or intercostal muscles

DIFFERENTIAL DIAGNOSIS

Normal Anatomy/Variants
- Fatty; apparent muscle redundancy and/or compression effect seen with MLO and CC mammography

Poland Anomaly/Poland Syndrome
- Combination of unilateral hypoplasia or absence of the costosternal portion of the PMM (100% of cases); hypoplasia or absence of serratus anterior or external oblique muscles; absence of pectoralis muscle; absence of costal cartilages of some ribs; some cases have hand (esp. syndactyly) and upper limb deformities
- Clinical manifestations vary: Ipsilateral breast may be hypoplastic or absent

DDx: Variable Sizes and Densities of Normal Pectoralis Major Musculature

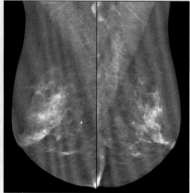

Unremarkable Appearance

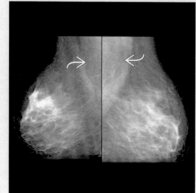

Fatty

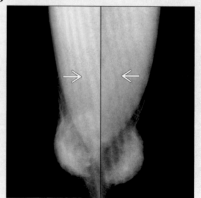

Male, Includes Pectoralis Minor

PECTORALIS MUSCLE VARIANTS

Key Facts

Terminology
- Congenital or developmental variations in pectoralis major muscle (PMM) appearance

Imaging Findings
- Axial imaging helpful in establishing anatomical variations
- Variants: Small or absent PMM on MLO views

Top Differential Diagnoses
- Normal Anatomy/Variants
- Poland Anomaly/Poland Syndrome
- Pectoralis Minor Muscle

Clinical Issues
- History of congenital abnormality with or without augmentation

---

- Defects 2x more common on right side than left
- Males more often affected
- Often not noted until puberty
- Associated malignancies reported
  - Leukemia, non-Hodgkin lymphoma, cervical cancer, leiomyosarcoma, Wilms tumor, lung cancer
- Breast cancer reported in the presence of hypoplasia

Pectoralis Minor Muscle
- In a few women, pectoralis minor muscles may be visualized on MLO mammogram
  - Dense triangles overlying upper portion of PMM on MLO view

Muscle Masses
- Best evaluated with axial imaging: MR, CT

Trauma
- PMM tears rare; reported following bench-pressing weights; may masquerade as breast mass
  - Associated hematomas may become infected (rare)
- Diagnosis made clinically and with musculoskeletal MR evaluation; MR superior to CT
  - Axial T2WI may be most valuable for acute and subacute injuries; axial T1WI more helpful in chronic injuries

CLINICAL ISSUES

Presentation
- Most common signs/symptoms

- Screening mammogram
- History of congenital abnormality with or without augmentation

DIAGNOSTIC CHECKLIST

Consider
- Pneumothorax following fine needle aspiration biopsy reported in patient with Poland syndrome

Image Interpretation Pearls
- If pectoral muscle is straight or concave, or is not seen to level of nipple, posterior breast tissue may not have been fully included on MLO mammograms

SELECTED REFERENCES

1. Kazama T et al: Prospective evaluation of pectoralis muscle invasion of breast cancer by MR imaging. Breast Cancer. 12:312-6, 2005
2. Salhab M et al: Pneumothorax after a clinical breast fine-needle aspiration of a lump in a patient with Poland's syndrome. Int Semin Surg Oncol. 2:14, 2005
3. Morris EA et al: Evaluation of pectoralis major muscle in patients with posterior breast tumors on breast MR images: early experience. Radiology. 214:67-72, 2000
4. Connell DA et al: Injuries of the pectoralis major muscle: evaluation with MR imaging. Radiology. 210:785-91, 1999

IMAGE GALLERY

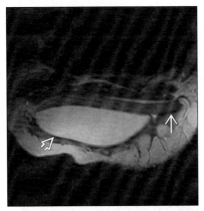
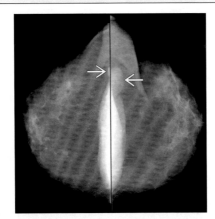
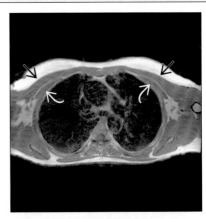

(Left) Axial T2WI shows silicone implant ➡ atop a custom triangular prosthesis ➡ in a woman with Poland syndrome. *(Center)* CC mammography shows lateral posterior densities ➡ adjacent to or parts of the pectoralis muscles. An MR (right-hand image) showed normal anatomy. The appearance is related to compression effect of redundant musculature. *(Right)* Axial T1WI MR demonstrated normal appearance of both pectoralis major ➡ and minor muscles ➡ with no chest wall masses.

STERNALIS MUSCLE

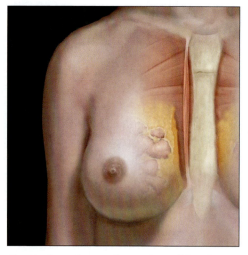

Graphic shows the sternalis muscle paralleling the right side of the sternum. This muscle has no known function, is present in < 8% of the population, and on mammogram is seen only on the CC view.

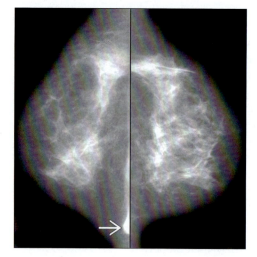

CC mammography shows a rounded density ➡ in the medial posterior right breast consistent with a unilateral sternalis muscle.

TERMINOLOGY

Definitions
- Uncommon anatomic chest wall musculature normal variant

IMAGING FINDINGS

General Features
- Best diagnostic clue: Flame-shaped medial density seen only on CC mammogram
- Location: Parasternal

Mammographic Findings
- Triangular or rounded shape
- 1-2 cm in size
- Smooth or uncommonly ill-defined
- Medial location adjacent to sternum
- Seen only on CC view
- Cleavage view may be helpful to exclude a true mass

Ultrasonographic Findings
- Grayscale Ultrasound: May be helpful to exclude a medial posterior mass

MR Findings
- T1WI
  - T1W1 MR may be helpful in definitive identification
  - Medial soft tissue structure attached to chest wall immediately adjacent to sternum

CT Findings
- NECT
  - NECT may be helpful in definitive identification
  - Medial soft tissue structure attached to chest wall immediately adjacent to sternum

Imaging Recommendations
- Best imaging tool: CC mammogram

DDx: Variable Pectoralis Insertion

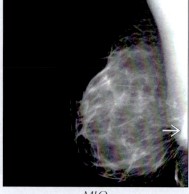

MLO

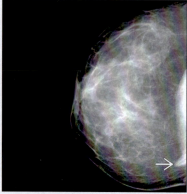

CC View

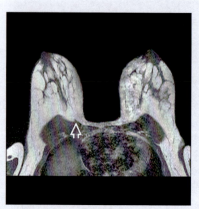

T1 MR

STERNALIS MUSCLE

Key Facts

Terminology
- Uncommon anatomic chest wall musculature normal variant

Imaging Findings
- Best diagnostic clue: Flame-shaped medial density seen only on CC mammogram
- Triangular or rounded shape
- 1-2 cm in size
- Smooth or uncommonly ill-defined

- Medial location adjacent to sternum
- NECT may be helpful in definitive identification
- T1W1 MR may be helpful in definitive identification

Top Differential Diagnoses
- Medially-Located Mass

Pathology
- Normal muscle bundle with unknown function

DIFFERENTIAL DIAGNOSIS

Medially-Located Mass
- Benign and malignant masses may develop in medial posterior breast
- Careful physical examination and additional imaging studies should discriminate

Variable Attachment of the Pectoralis Muscle
- Small free slip of pectoralis muscle adjacent to sternum
- Visualized on both the CC and MLO views
  - Triangular, round, or sometimes flame-shaped
- 1% of women

PATHOLOGY

General Features
- General path comments
  - Normal muscle bundle with unknown function
    - Extends from infraclavicular region to caudal aspect of sternum
    - Superficial to pectoralis major muscle and parallel to the sternum
    - Innervated by pectoral nerves
- Etiology
  - Origin speculated
    - Pectoralis major
    - Rectus abdominis
    - Sternomastoid

- Epidemiology
  - Occurs in < 8% of general population
  - Unilateral in 70%

CLINICAL ISSUES

Presentation
- Clinical Profile
  - An asymptomatic imaging-only finding
  - Many surveyed surgeons unaware of this anatomic chest wall musculature variant

Demographics
- Gender: Present in both females and males

SELECTED REFERENCES
1. Kumar H et al: Bilateral sternalis with unusual left-sided presentation: a clinical perspective. Yonsei Med J. 44(4):719-22, 2003
2. Saeed M et al: Sternalis. An anatomic variant of chest wall musculature. Saudi Med J. 23(10):1214-21, 2002
3. Bailey PM et al: The sternalis muscle: a normal finding encountered during breast surgery. Plast Reconstr Surg. 103:1189-90, 1999
4. Kopans D: Breast imaging. 2nd ed. Philadelphia, Lippincott-Raven. Chapter 2, 9-10, 1998
5. Bradley FM et al: The Sternalis muscle: An unusual normal finding seen on mammography. AJR. 166:33-6, 1996

IMAGE GALLERY

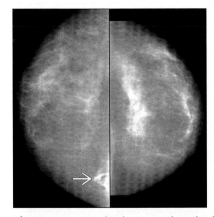 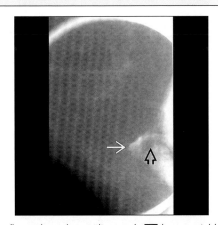 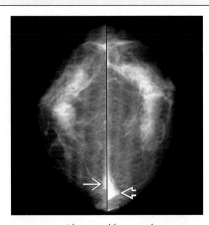

(Left) *CC mammography shows a unilateral right flame-shaped sternalis muscle* ➡ *has a variable appearance with central lucency better seen on the next image.* *(Center)* *CC mammography spot compression shows the somewhat pointed soft tissue portion of the right sternalis muscle* ➡ *which contains fat* ➡. *(Right)* *CC mammography shows bilateral sternalis muscles, demonstrating more of a rounded shape on the right* ➡ *and a triangular shape* ➡ *on the left.*

MONDOR DISEASE

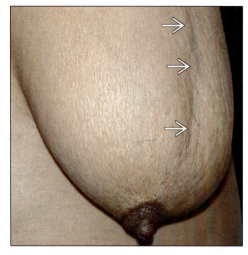

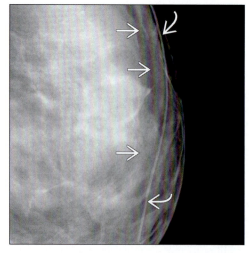

Clinical photograph shows a tender long, palpable linear cord ➡ in a 34 year old woman. Mammogram (right image) was performed. (Courtesy JAW).

MLO mammography (digital) optimized to show the superficial tissues, demonstrates tubular structure ➡ = to the clinical abnormality (skin marker ➤). US (not shown) = thrombosed vein.

TERMINOLOGY

Definitions
- Superficial thrombophlebitis, Mondor phlebitis

IMAGING FINDINGS

General Features
- Best diagnostic clue: Superficial tubular structure, palpable cord

Mammographic Findings
- Superficial tubular or beaded structure; may be negative
- Vessel may undergo calcification in chronic stage

Ultrasonographic Findings
- Grayscale Ultrasound
  - Hypo- or anechoic superficial tubular structure
    - Internal echoes = thrombus
  - Multiple areas of narrowing ⇒ beaded appearance
  - Lack of compressibility of the vein due to clot
- Color Doppler: No flow; or flow if recanalized

DIFFERENTIAL DIAGNOSIS

Dilated Duct
- Retroareolar tubular structure

Normal or Varicose Vein
- Collateral veins with central venous obstruction
  - Dilated veins may present as palpable, soft nodules
- Varicose veins with dialysis shunt graft

Papillomas
- Intraductal masses ± calcifications

Ductal Carcinoma in Situ (DCIS)
- May cause duct distention ± calcifications

Abscess/Mastitis
- Signs of infection such as erythema and warmness
- Mixed echogenicity collection on US

PATHOLOGY

Gross Pathologic & Surgical Features
- Thrombosed, thickened vein

DDx: Other Tubular (Smooth or Beaded) Structures

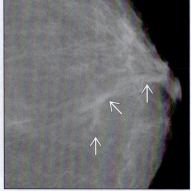

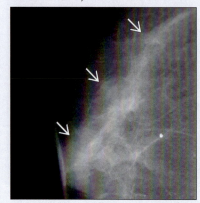

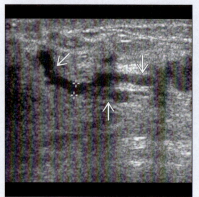

Dilated Duct

Papillomas

DCIS

MONDOR DISEASE

Key Facts

Terminology
- Superficial thrombophlebitis, Mondor phlebitis

Imaging Findings
- Superficial tubular or beaded structure; may be negative
- Vessel may undergo calcification in chronic stage
- Hypo- or anechoic superficial tubular structure
- Internal echoes = thrombus

Clinical Issues
- Most common signs/symptoms: Palpable cord ± pain
- A clinical diagnosis
- Reported association with breast cancer; debated
- Mammography and US indicated primarily for evaluation of the palpable finding
- Benign, self-limited process
- Supportive care, analgesic drugs for pain
- No indication for antibiotics or anticoagulants

- Both breasts equally affected
- Most commonly involves the upper outer or inferior breast and chest wall
  - Thoracoepigastric, lateral thoracic or superior epigastric veins

Microscopic Features
- Venous thrombosis
- Varying stages of organization and recanalization
- Mild inflammation of surrounding tissue

CLINICAL ISSUES

Presentation
- Most common signs/symptoms: Palpable cord ± pain
- Other signs/symptoms: May have associated tender skin retraction/dimpling or discoloration
- Clinical Profile
  - A clinical diagnosis
  - Rarely associated with deep venous thrombosis
- Reported association with breast cancer; debated
  - Mammography and US indicated primarily for evaluation of the palpable finding
- Reported associations: Trauma, biopsy (core or surgical), exercise, injections, jellyfish bites, pregnancy

Demographics
- Age: 20-40 years old
- Gender: Usually women, may occur in men

Natural History & Prognosis
- Benign, self-limited process
  - Most cases resolve over a 2-12 week period
  - Chronic thrombosis may result in vascular calcification

Treatment
- Supportive care, analgesic drugs for pain
- No indication for antibiotics or anticoagulants
- Biopsy avoided with careful clinical and imaging assessment

DIAGNOSTIC CHECKLIST

Consider
- Benign (BI-RADS 2) or probably benign, short interval follow-up (BI-RADS 3), depending on level of certainty

SELECTED REFERENCES
1. Markopoulos C et al: Mondor's disease of the breast: is there any relation to breast cancer? Eur J Gynaecol Oncol. 26:213-4, 2005
2. Jaberi M et al: Stereotactic vacuum-assisted breast biopsy: an unusual cause of Mondor's disease. AJR. 179:185-6, 2002
3. Shetty MK et al: Mondor's disease of the breast; sonographic and mammographic findings. AJR. 177:893-6, 2001
4. Catania S et al: Mondor's disease and breast cancer. Cancer. 69:2267-70, 1992

IV

3

43

IMAGE GALLERY

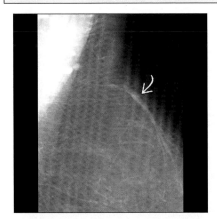 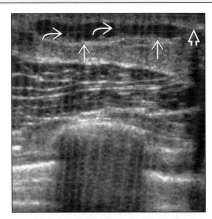 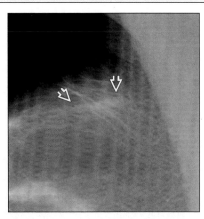

(Left) MLO mammography shows beaded, dilated superficial vein ➦. Clinically, there was a palpable, tender cord in the upper outer left breast. *(Center)* Sagittal ultrasound (same patient as previous image) shows a tubular non-compressible structure ➦, just deep to the skin ➧ with internal echogenic clot ➦. The self-limited thrombophlebitis resolved. *(Right)* MLO mammography shows a tubular structure at the area of a palpable cord ➧ in the upper right breast of this symptomatic woman. US (not shown) revealed a thrombosed vein.

VASCULAR MALFORMATIONS

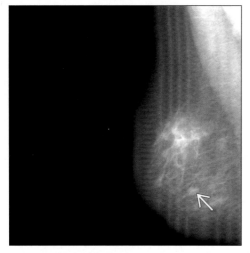

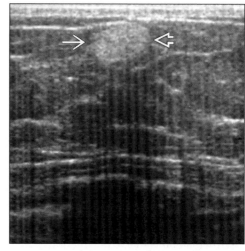

MLO mammography in a 41 year old woman presenting with a superficial palpable lump, shows an oval circumscribed mass ➡, at site of palpable finding. Ultrasound is the appropriate next step.

Ultrasound of this mass shows it to be echogenic, with circumscribed medial margin ➡ and indistinct lateral margin ➡. US-guided core needle biopsy revealed hemangioma.

TERMINOLOGY

Abbreviations and Synonyms
- Benign vascular lesions of the breast

Definitions
- Large spectrum of benign lesions of vascular origin occurring in or near breast tissue
  - Hemangiomas
    - Perilobular (microscopic lesions, incidentally found in up to 5% benign biopsies)
    - Subcutaneous (usually cavernous type, most likely to be clinically encountered)
    - Parenchymal (rare, usually no larger than 2 cm)
    - Hemangioendothelioma (bordering between benign and low grade angiosarcoma)
  - Venous malformations (similar to those in other anatomic locations)
  - Angiolipomas: Benign variant of lipoma, more common in male breast
  - Lymphangiomas or lymphatic malformations, including
    - Acquired lymphangiectasis: Complication of surgery and radiation treatment for malignancy

IMAGING FINDINGS

General Features
- Best diagnostic clue: Superficially located well-defined, lobulated small mass which may contain phleboliths
- Location
  - Hemangiomas and angiolipomas in subcutaneous tissues, superficial to anterior pectoralis fascia, or associated with chest wall
  - Venous malformation and lymphangioma commonly in axillary region
- Size
  - Perilobular hemangiomas microscopic, or less than 2 mm
  - Hemangiomas usually < 2 cm, but can be very large or "giant"
- Morphology
  - Hemangiomas: Circumscribed, macrolobulated mass
  - Angiolipomas can be ill-defined

Radiographic Findings
- Mammography
  - Low to medium density, round or lobulated
    - Angiolipomas may show irregular margins

DDx: More Examples of Vascular Lesions

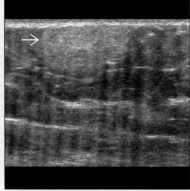

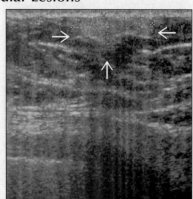

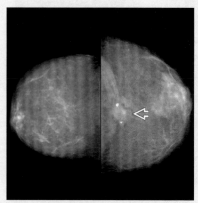

| Angiolipoma | Subcutaneous Hemangioma | Chest Wall Hemangioma |

VASCULAR MALFORMATIONS

Key Facts

Terminology
- Large spectrum of benign lesions of vascular origin occurring in or near breast tissue
- Hemangiomas
- Venous malformations (similar to those in other anatomic locations)
- Angiolipomas: Benign variant of lipoma, more common in male breast
- Lymphangiomas or lymphatic malformations, including
- Acquired lymphangiectasis: Complication of surgery and radiation treatment for malignancy

Imaging Findings
- Best diagnostic clue: Superficially located well-defined, lobulated small mass which may contain phleboliths

Top Differential Diagnoses
- Fibroadenoma
- Complicated cyst
- Blue domed cyst
- Hamartoma
- Pseudoangiomatous stromal hyperplasia (PASH)
- Angiosarcoma

Pathology
- Hemangiomas are usually small and found incidentally on histology; clinical importance lies in distinguishing from angiosarcomas

Diagnostic Checklist
- Skin erythema and palpable superficial mass should raise possibility of vascular lesion

---

   - May contain granular, amorphous, or unusual calcifications; or phleboliths (calcified venous thromboses)
- Superficial location or associated with pectoralis muscle

Ultrasonographic Findings
- Grayscale Ultrasound
   - Circumscribed solid masses usually subcutaneous or dermal
   - Capillary hemangiomas: Often hyperechoic
   - Cavernous hemangiomas: Isoechoic or mildly hyperechoic, heterogeneous echotexture
     - May have appearance of lobulated, complex cyst with thick septations and increased acoustic transmission
     - Degree of echogenicity depends on dominant size of vascular channels
   - Venous malformations: May show large venous channels (up to 1 cm), easily compressible if not thrombosed
   - Angiolipomas: Hyperechoic, circumscribed
   - Lymphangiomas: Appearance similar to cluster of cysts or dilated ducts
- Color Doppler
   - High sensitivity and specificity for distinguishing benign from malignant vascular lesions
     - Hypovascularity with single vascular pole associated with benign lesions
     - Hypervascularity with multiple peripheral poles or internal vessels more common in malignant lesions

MR Findings
- T1WI
   - Isointense relative to soft tissues
   - Hemangiomas of chest wall may show expanded pectoral muscle with fatty proliferation
- T2WI FS: Most are hyperintense
- T1 C+: Slow progressive enhancement indicative of slow flow in vascular lesion with many capillaries

Biopsy
- Diagnosis of superficial hemangiomas and angiolipomas can be made by US-guided 14-gauge core needle biopsy
   - Bleeding complications occur occasionally and are manageable with manual compression

Imaging Recommendations
- Best imaging tool: Mammography and ultrasound

DIFFERENTIAL DIAGNOSIS

Circumscribed Breast Masses
- Fibroadenoma
- Complicated cyst
- Blue domed cyst
- Hamartoma
- Pseudoangiomatous stromal hyperplasia (PASH)
- Mucinous cancer

Angiosarcoma
- Ill-defined low-density, uncalcified, hypoechoic, highly vascular mass, often > 3 cm, may have associated skin discoloration

PATHOLOGY

General Features
- Genetics
   - Vascular malformations are manifestations of many syndromes with variety of inheritance patterns
     - Maffucci, Kasabach-Merritt, Klippel-Trenaunay-Weber, rarely Poland syndrome, Cowden disease, Fabry disease and POEM syndrome
   - Lymphatic vascular malformations may be associated with other syndromes
     - Noonan syndrome, asplenia, Gorham syndrome, tuberous sclerosis
- Etiology: Sporadic, unless associated with a syndrome

VASCULAR MALFORMATIONS

- Epidemiology
  - Hemangiomas are usually small and found incidentally on histology; clinical importance lies in distinguishing from angiosarcomas
  - Account for 7% of all benign soft tissue tumors
- Associated abnormalities: Variable depending on etiology

Gross Pathologic & Surgical Features
- Well-defined, dark, reddish brown, soft and spongy

Microscopic Features
- Thin-walled, blood filled, anastomosing vascular spaces, separated by fibrous septae, with extensive fibrosis and phleboliths
- Atypia, invasion, necrosis usually absent
- Hemangiomas are histologically subdivided into four types
  - Cavernous (most common)
  - Compact capillary
  - Capillary budding
  - Combined cavernous and compact capillary
- Hemangiomas may contain pericytic, smooth muscle, or interstitial components in variable combination
- Hemangioendothelioma is a subtype overlapping with low grade angiosarcoma
- Lymphangiomas: Proliferation of dilated lymphatic vessels forming a mass
- Venous malformations: Disorderly proliferation of venous channels
- PASH: May simulate vascular lesion due to anastomosing slit-like spaces, but distinctly lacks endothelial cells

CLINICAL ISSUES

Presentation
- Most common signs/symptoms: Palpable mass with overlying skin discoloration
- Other signs/symptoms
  - Acquired lymphangiectasis and cutaneous hemangioendotheliomas may be encountered in women who have undergone surgical, radiation and chemotherapy for breast cancer
  - Cutaneous vascular malformations appear as hamartomas in pediatric population
  - Hemangiopericytoma, and cystic lymphangioma seen almost exclusively in the breast
  - Venous malformations have slow flow and therefore prone to thrombosis

Demographics
- Age: Range 5-85 years
- Gender
  - Hemangiomas: F >> M
  - Angiolipomas: M > F

Natural History & Prognosis
- May resolve spontaneously

Treatment
- Complete surgical resection, may sometimes require radical mastectomy

DIAGNOSTIC CHECKLIST

Consider
- Skin erythema and palpable superficial mass should raise possibility of vascular lesion

Image Interpretation Pearls
- Include in differential diagnosis of hypo- or hyperechoic, superficial breast masses

SELECTED REFERENCES

1. Glazebrook KN et al: Vascular tumors of the breast: mammographic, sonographic, and MRI appearances. AJR.184(1):331-338, 2005
2. Lopez-Gutierrez JC et al: Misdiagnosis in hemangiomas and vascular malformations of the breast. Eur J Gynaecol Oncol. 26(6):667; author reply 667-8, 2005
3. Turnbull MM et al: Arteriovenous malformations in Cowden syndrome. J Med Genet. 42(8):e50, 2005
4. Hunt SJ et al: Vascular tumors of the skin: a selective review. Semin Diagn Pathol. 21(3):166-218, 2004
5. Kondis-Pafitis A et al: Clinicopathological study of vascular tumors of the breast: a series of ten patients with a long follow-up. Eur J Gynaecol Oncol. 25(3):324-6, 2004
6. Flis C et al: An unusual case of an enlarging mass on a screening mammogram: a case report and review of the radiology and current literature. Breast. 12(3):220-2, 2003
7. Chung SY et al: Mammographic and sonographic findings of a breast subcutaneous hemangioma. J Ultrasound Med. 21(5):585-8, 2002
8. Mariscal A et al: Breast hemangioma mimicking carcinoma. Breast. 11(4):357-8, 2002
9. Aurello P et al: Hemangioma of the breast: an unusual lesion without univocal diagnostic findings. J Exp Clin Cancer Res. 20(4):611-3, 2001
10. Dener C et al: Haemangiomas of the breast. Eur J Surg. 166(12):977-9, 2000
11. Faul JL et al: Thoracic lymphangiomas, lymphangiectasis, lymphangiomatosis, and lymphatic dysplasia syndrome. Am J Respir Crit Care Med. 161(3 Pt 1):1037-46, 2000
12. Vuorela AL: MRI of breast hemangioma. J Comput Assist Tomogr. 22(6):1009-10, 1998
13. Webb LA et al: Case report: haemangioma of the breast--appearances on mammography and ultrasound. Clin Radiol. 51(7):523-4, 1996
14. Gembala RB et al: Color Doppler detection of a breast perilobular hemangioma. J Ultrasound Med. 12(4):220-2, 1993
15. Yu GH et al: Cellular angiolipoma of the breast. Mod Pathol. 6(4):497-9, 1993
16. Hoda SA et al: Hemangiomas of the breast with atypical histological features. Further analysis of histological subtypes confirming their benign character. Am J Surg Pathol. 16(6):553-60, 1992
17. Nagar H et al: Haemangiomas of the breast in children. Eur J Surg. 158(9):503-5, 1992
18. Shousha S et al: Cavernous haemangioma of breast in a man with contralateral gynaecomastia and a family history of breast carcinoma. Histopathology. 13(2):221-3, 1988
19. Marymont JV et al: Maffucci's syndrome complicated by carcinoma of the breast, pituitary adenoma, and mediastinal hemangioma. South Med J. 80(11):1429-31, 1987
20. Schwartz IS et al: Hemangioma of male breast. Am J Surg Pathol. 11(9):739, 1987

VASCULAR MALFORMATIONS

IMAGE GALLERY

Typical

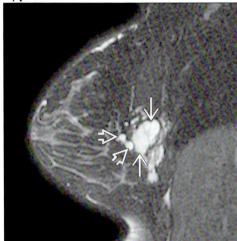

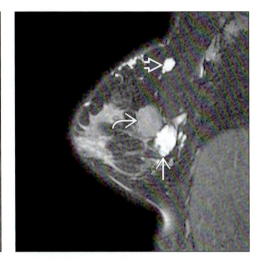

(Left) Sagittal T2WI FS MR shows portions of an extensive chest wall hemangioma as lobulated ➡ and round ➡ high signal masses. These enhanced mildly and were part of an extensive hemangioma. *(Right)* Sagittal T2WI FS MR (same as left image) shows adjacent breast mass ➡, not bright on T2WI FS images. This showed avid enhancement after contrast injection. Biopsy showed a fibroadenoma. MR distinguished this from the hemangioma(s) ➡, ➡.

Typical

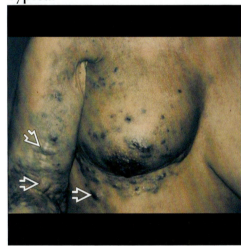

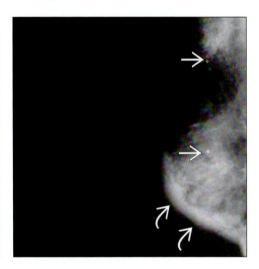

(Left) Clinical photograph shows a large cutaneous capillary hemangioma with associated varicose veins ➡ and hypertrophy of the right arm. *(Right)* MLO mammography shows diffuse increased density, marked skin thickening ➡ and phleboliths ➡. This is an unusual case of Klippel-Trenaunay-Weber syndrome involving the right breast and arm. (Courtesy LG).

Typical

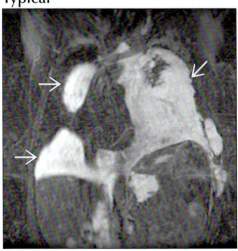

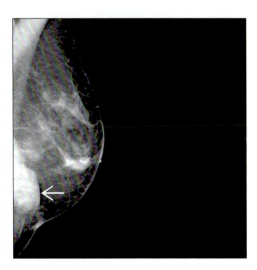

(Left) Coronal T2WI FS MR shows extensive involvement ➡ of the thorax in this 55 year old woman. It is of fluid signal, but has caused mediastinal shift to the right. *(Right)* MLO mammography shows a mass and calcifications within the lower breast ➡. The patient had a long, complicated history of lymphangiomatosis, requiring multiple surgeries.

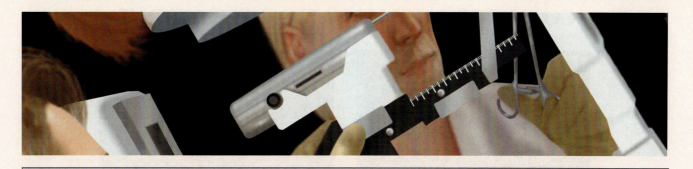

SECTION 4: Post-Operative Imaging Findings

COSMETIC AUGMENTATION INJECTIONS

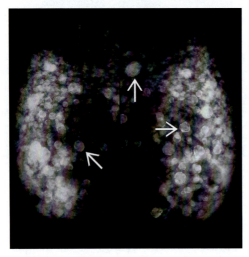

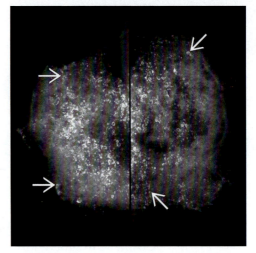

MLO mammography shows diffuse dense, round, peripherally calcifying masses ➡ throughout both breasts, typical of silicone granulomata, in this 53 y/o injected with silicone oil 28 yrs earlier.

MLO mammography shows diffuse, bilateral dystrophic Ca++ ➡ on MLO views in a 70 y/o woman with prior silicone oil injections 40 yrs earlier. The breasts are clinically rock hard.

TERMINOLOGY

Abbreviations and Synonyms
- Paraffinoma; oleogranulomatous mastitis
- Silicone oil injections
- Silicone mastitis
- Polyacrylamide (PAAG) hydrogel augmentation

Definitions
- Injection of liquid oil, wax, or gel into breast parenchyma for cosmetic augmentation
  - Any type of cosmetic injection may result in a foreign body granulomatous reaction
  - "Paraffinoma": Reactive mass surrounding area(s) of injected paraffin
  - "Siliconoma": Reactive mass surrounding area(s) of injected silicone oil
- Paraffin from early 20th century, liquid silicone since 1960s
  - Widespread practice once, now illegal in USA; still used in some parts of Asia
- PAAG since mid-1990s
  - Used for gel electrophoresis, ophthalmic operations, drug treatment, food packaging, water purification

- Jelly-like transparent gel: 95% water and 5% polyacrylamide
- Used in plastic and aesthetic surgery since early 1990s (Soviet Union)
- In China, used for breast augmentation since 1997

IMAGING FINDINGS

General Features
- Best diagnostic clue: Numerous bilateral dense masses ± rim calcifications (Ca++)
- Location
  - Depends on site and plane of injection
  - May be localized (e.g., paraffinoma)
  - Widespread, throughout entire breast (esp. silicone oil)
  - May migrate to chest wall, abdominal wall, esp. silicone
  - May be retromammary (esp. PAAG)
- Size: < 1 up to 5 cm nodules or masses

Mammographic Findings
- Paraffinoma

DDx: Other Prominent Breast Densities

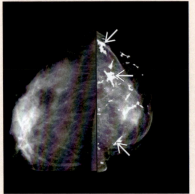

Dystrophic Calcifications

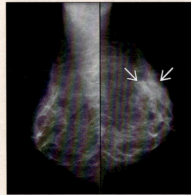

Infiltrating Ductal Carcinoma

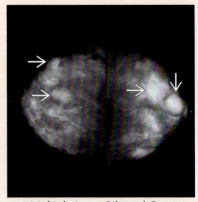

Multiple Large Bilateral Cysts

COSMETIC AUGMENTATION INJECTIONS

Key Facts

Terminology
- Paraffinoma; oleogranulomatous mastitis
- Silicone oil injections
- Polyacrylamide (PAAG) hydrogel augmentation
- Injection of liquid oil, wax, or gel into breast parenchyma for cosmetic augmentation
- Any type of cosmetic injection may result in a foreign body granulomatous reaction
- Paraffin from early 20th century, liquid silicone since 1960s
- PAAG since mid-1990s

Imaging Findings
- Best diagnostic clue: Numerous bilateral dense masses ± rim calcifications (Ca++)
- Mammography and ultrasound usually not useful for cancer detection

- T1 C+ MR may be useful to depict breast cancer

Top Differential Diagnoses
- Infiltrating Ductal (IDC) or Lobular Carcinoma (ILC) for Paraffinoma
- Widespread Dystrophic Calcifications
- Fibrosis, Fibrocystic Changes

Clinical Issues
- May complain of focal or diffuse lumps, hardening or scarring
- Discomfort or pain
- Inflammation or frank infection, esp. with PAAG
- Counseling about risks, inability to detect cancer on standard mammography, US

Diagnostic Checklist
- History of greatest value, often not forthcoming

- ○ Irregular mass(es), droplets, with or without fibrotic distortion
- Silicone granulomas
  - ○ Innumerable round or oval dense masses with rim Ca++
  - ○ Variable-sized, radiodense, silicone droplets
- Silicone oil or PAAG collections
  - ○ Large masses of amorphous moderately dense intraparenchymal foreign material

Ultrasonographic Findings
- Grayscale Ultrasound
  - ○ Granuloma, fibrosis, Ca++: Irregular hypoechoic confluent areas, may have marked shadowing
  - ○ Silicone: "Snowstorm" appearance with highly echogenic noise and shadowing
    - Well-defined, echogenic anteriorly
    - Due to marked acoustic scattering
  - ○ Free silicone collections (rarely): "Cyst-like" globular masses with markedly echogenic interface with parenchyma
  - ○ PAAG: Circumscribed collections with fine hypoechoic granular echogenicity and patchy areas of mixed echoes
- Color Doppler: No abnormal vascularity detectable

MR Findings
- T1WI: Mildly hypointense or isointense mass(es)
- T2WI
  - ○ Paraffinoma: Hypointense, irregular mass
  - ○ Silicone deposits: Mixed intensity areas or hyperintense rounded masses
  - ○ PAAG: Hyperintense masses with internal hypointense foci
- T2WI FS: Similar to T2WI but silicone droplets, PAAG more hyperintense
- STIR: Silicone: Hyperintense rounded masses on water-suppressed STIR
- T1 C+
  - ○ Granulomas show variable enhancement
    - May mimic malignancy, rim-enhancement in surrounding scar

- ○ Silicone oil or PAAG collections: Nonenhancing round masses

Imaging Recommendations
- Best imaging tool
  - ○ MR with and without contrast-enhancement
    - Silicone-specific imaging (e.g., water-suppressed STIR) useful
    - Best in conjunction with mammography (Ca++ poorly seen on MR)
    - Further study warranted
- Protocol advice
  - ○ Mammography and ultrasound helpful to depict extent of injected material
  - ○ Mammography and ultrasound usually not useful for cancer detection
    - Limited by dense material, Ca++, marked image noise and shadowing
  - ○ T1 C+ MR may be useful to depict breast cancer
    - Granulomas may enhance suspiciously, need MR-guided biopsy for diagnosis
  - ○ Tc-99m sestamibi scintimammography can diagnose invasive breast cancer
    - Less useful than MR (poor spatial localization, lower sensitivity for small lesions)

DIFFERENTIAL DIAGNOSIS

Infiltrating Ductal (IDC) or Lobular Carcinoma (ILC) for Paraffinoma
- May be indistinguishable on conventional imaging
- IDC often has associated microcalcifications
- Usually strongly enhancing on MR

Widespread Dystrophic Calcifications
- Usually due to previous radiotherapy

Fibrosis, Fibrocystic Changes
- Fibrosis can cause irregular masses on mammography, US
- May see admixed cysts, scattered Ca++

COSMETIC AUGMENTATION INJECTIONS

PATHOLOGY

General Features
- General path comments: Intense foreign body inflammatory and granulomatous reaction
- Etiology
  - Cosmetic injections, usually performed in beauty parlors in Asia and former Soviet Union
  - PAAG banned for breast augmentation in China in May 2006
- Epidemiology
  - Predominantly Asian patients, esp. from China, Southeast Asia
  - Paraffinomas and silicone injections also reported in male transsexuals

Gross Pathologic & Surgical Features
- Silicone injections
  - Large area of firm, irregular thickening, gritty on bisection
  - Numerous cystic spaces
- Paraffinoma
  - Focal firm fibrous mass lesion
- PAAG
  - Large regions of amorphous gel
  - May have surrounding inflammatory hardening

Microscopic Features
- Diffuse granulomatous reaction with variable fibrosis
- Silicone: Vacuolated spaces with surrounding fibrosis; typically silicone lost in processing
- PAAG injections
  - Rounded deposits and elongated strands, which mimic extracellular matrix
  - Thin layer of fibrous connective tissue occasionally present, not thick fibrous capsule seen after silicone injection
  - Gel collections: Membrane of macrophages and foreign-body giant cells varying with size of gel collection
  - May have acute inflammatory reaction

CLINICAL ISSUES

Presentation
- Most common signs/symptoms
  - May complain of focal or diffuse lumps, hardening or scarring
  - Sometimes focal or global asymmetry
- Other signs/symptoms
  - Discomfort or pain
  - Inflammation or frank infection, esp. with PAAG
- Clinical Profile
  - May be discovered at screening mammography
  - Patient may deny any past procedure
  - Silicone mastitis may have draining sinuses, ulceration, deformity

Demographics
- Age: Most present pre-menopausally
- Gender
  - Female much more common than male
  - Male transsexuals may undergo this procedure

- Ethnicity: Most frequently Asian, esp. Chinese

Natural History & Prognosis
- Paraffinoma: Rarely ulcerates skin
- Silicone oil migrates: Lymph nodes, chest wall, abdomen, groin
- Silicone may cause chronic destructive mastitis
  - Association with scleroderma reported years after silicone oil injection
  - No proven causative link with autoimmune diseases
- No known increase in breast cancer incidence
- PAAG complications usually within 2-3 years of injection

Treatment
- Surgical lavage, drainage or excision
- Mastectomy if ulcerated or destructive mastitis
- Counseling about risks, inability to detect cancer on standard mammography, US

DIAGNOSTIC CHECKLIST

Consider
- Extent and distribution of calcifications
- Density and shape of multiple bilateral masses
- Unusual echogenicity and echotexture masses

Image Interpretation Pearls
- History of greatest value, often not forthcoming

SELECTED REFERENCES

1. Scaranelo AM et al: Sonographic and mammographic findings of breast liquid silicone injection. J Clin Ultrasound. 34:273-7, 2006
2. Qiao Q et al: Management for postoperative complications of breast augmentation by injected polyacrylamide hydrogel. Aesthetic Plast Surg. 29:156-61, 2005
3. Christensen LH et al: Long-term effects of polyacrylamide hydrogel on human breast tissue. Plast Reconstr Surg. 111:1883-90, 2003
4. Cheung YC et al: Lumpy silicone-injected breasts: enhanced MRI and microscopic correlation. Clin Imaging. 26:397-404, 2002
5. Wang J et al.: Silicone migration from silicone-injected breasts: magnetic resonance images. Ann Plast Surg 48:617-21, 2002
6. Han BK et al: Foreign body granulomas of the breast presenting as bilateral spiculated masses. Korean J Radiol. 2:113-6, 2001
7. Lopez H et al: Ultrasound interactions with free silicone in a tissue-mimicking phantom. J Ultrasound Med. 17:163-70, 1998
8. Helbich TH et al: The value of MRI in silicone granuloma of the breast. Eur J Radiol. 24:155-8, 1997
9. Yang WT et al: Paraffinomas of the breast: Mammographic, ultrasonographic and radiographic appearances with clinical and histopathological correlation. Clin Radiol. 51:130-3, 1996
10. Leibman AJ et al: Mammographic and sonographic findings after silicone injection. Ann Plast Surg. 33:412-4, 1994
11. Kumagai Y et al: Clinical spectrum of connective tissue disease after cosmetic surgery. Observations on eighteen patients and a review of the Japanese literature. Arthritis Rheum. 27:1-12, 1984

COSMETIC AUGMENTATION INJECTIONS

IMAGE GALLERY

Variant

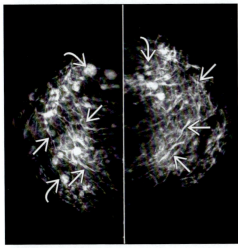
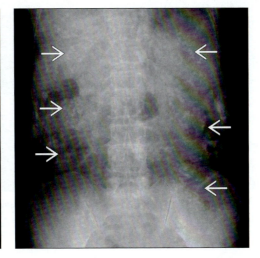

(Left) CC mammography in a 62 y/o woman after silicone oil injections many years earlier shows numerous sharply defined dense rounded deposits of oil bilaterally ➡, with widespread increased density of the Cooper ligaments ➡. *(Right)* Frontal radiograph of the abdomen in a 60 y/o woman shows widespread bizarre calcified foci in the skin and subcutaneous tissues ➡ due to migrated silicone oil from prior breast silicone oil injections many years earlier.

Typical

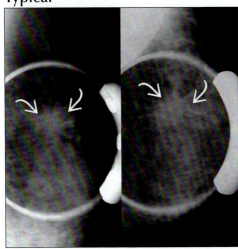
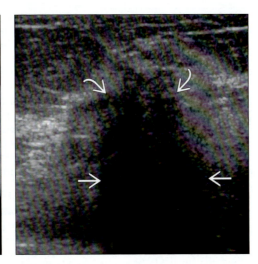

(Left) Mammography spot compression views of the left upper outer breast in the MLO (left) and CC (right) projections show an irregular spiculated mass ➡, highly suspicious for an invasive malignancy. *(Right)* Transverse ultrasound (same case as previous image) shows a hypoechoic irregular mass ➡ with dense shadowing ➡. Core biopsy showed paraffinoma with dense fibrosis. The patient initially denied having any breast injection.

Typical

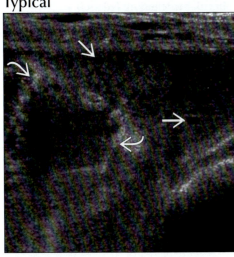
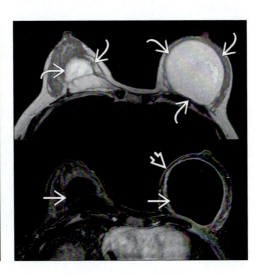

(Left) US of the left breast in a woman with PAAG injections shows characteristic pattern, with prominent echogenic material and tiny innumerable hypoechoic "holes" ➡. There is a heterogeneous region more centrally ➡. *(Right)* Axial MR (same case as left) shows large hyperintense injected gel collections in the upper T2WI ➡ and lack of any enhancement in mass on the lower T1WI C+ FS ➡. Note rim-enhancing scar ➡.

BENIGN SURGICAL BIOPSY, POST-OP IMAGING

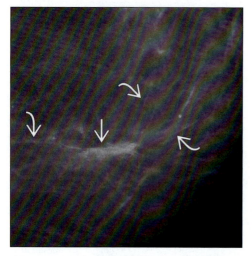

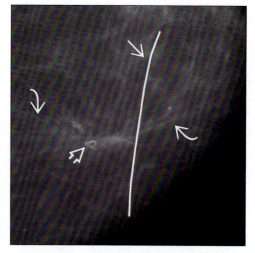

CC mammography shows focal asymmetry ➡ with associated distortion ➡ inner left breast in a 66 y/o with history of prior benign left breast biopsy 9 years earlier.

CC mammography two years later (same as left) now shows dystrophic Ca++ ➡, with tethering of Cooper ligaments ➡ again noted. Scar marker ➡ on skin incision helps confirm this as post-surgical change.

TERMINOLOGY

Definitions
- Imaging findings occurring after surgical biopsy revealing benign histopathology

IMAGING FINDINGS

General Features
- Best diagnostic clue
  - Excisional breast biopsy involves a skin incision and variable degree of tissue interruption and removal
  - Imaging changes occur independent of the nature of the tissue removed
  - Acute changes: Immediate to several weeks and months post-operatively
    - Hematoma, seroma, edema, early fat necrosis
  - Late/chronic: Months to years later
    - Scar: Architectural distortion, focal asymmetry, overlying skin retraction ± skin thickening
    - Scar and edema should decrease over time
    - No visible finding in > 50% of cases
- Fat necrosis
  - Imaging findings are influenced by the degree of development of fibrotic reaction, quantity of liquefied fat and the presence of calcifications (Ca++)
  - Oil cysts ± rim Ca++, dystrophic Ca++
  - Ca++ tend to develop 2-5 years after surgery
  - Irregular mass (uncommon)
  - May mimic malignancy clinically and at imaging
  - Described as more common in obese, usually middle-aged women with fatty, pendulous breasts
    - Most common in superficial and/or periareolar portions of the breast

Mammographic Findings
- Disappearance or reduction of target
- Immediate post-surgery
  - Air in tissues or in hematoma or air-fluid level
- Early/acute changes at mammography
  - Ill-defined mass or focal asymmetry
  - Skin and trabecular thickening (edema)
  - Architectural distortion
- Late changes at mammography
  - No discernible changes in > 50% of cases

DDx: Sonographic Appearances After Benign Surgical Biopsy

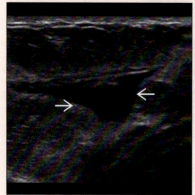

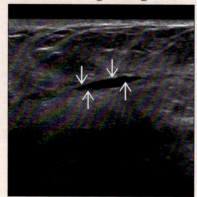

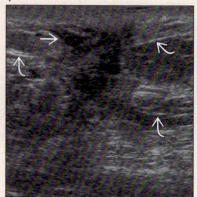

Fluid Collection in Surgical Cavity

Fluid Collection at Dissected Tissue

Hypoechoic Area, Distortion

BENIGN SURGICAL BIOPSY, POST-OP IMAGING

Key Facts

Terminology
- Imaging findings occurring after surgical biopsy revealing benign histopathology

Imaging Findings
- Imaging changes occur independent of the nature of the tissue removed
- Acute changes: Immediate to several weeks and months post-operatively
- Hematoma, seroma, edema, early fat necrosis
- Late/chronic: Months to years later
- Scar: Architectural distortion, focal asymmetry, overlying skin retraction ± skin thickening
- Scar and edema should decrease over time
- No visible finding in > 50% of cases
- Fat necrosis
- Ca++ tend to develop 2-5 years after surgery

- May mimic malignancy clinically and at imaging
- Scars usually do not enhance on MR after 18 months; however, enhancement may occur years later due to fat necrosis with inflammation

Top Differential Diagnoses
- Infiltrating Ductal Carcinoma (IDC) ± Infiltrating Lobular Carcinoma (ILC)
- Radial Scar/Complex Sclerosing Lesion
- Overlapping Normal Breast Tissues
- Focal Fibrosis
- Sclerosing Adenosis (SA)
- Fibromatosis

Diagnostic Checklist
- 2-3% of needle-localized excisions fail to excise the target

---

- ○ "Pseudolesion" at 6 months and later: Asymmetry may be seen in only one view
- ○ Skin retraction, thickening at scar
- ○ Keloid or hypertrophic skin scar: Macrolobulated, circumscribed densities, outlined by a thin halo (surrounding air)
- ○ Parenchymal scar with architectural distortion
- ○ Scar markers (radiopaque skin markers at the site of prior cutaneous incision) facilitate correlation with skin scar
  - Note: Skin incision may be remote from site of excision
- ○ Dystrophic and sutural Ca++; when early, linear and curvilinear, may appear suspicious
- ○ Fat necrosis
  - Coarse Ca++ (when early, may appear fine, linear or pleomorphic)
  - Benign-appearing to indeterminate to malignant-appearing masses
  - May appear as distortion or spiculation
  - Oil cysts: Lucent round mass with thin, well-defined capsule ± benign rim Ca++

Ultrasonographic Findings
- Grayscale Ultrasound
  - ○ Immediate-acute post-surgery
    - Air bubbles may obscure tissue
    - Hypoechoic collection (hematoma/seroma) with surrounding ↑ echogenicity (edema) and associated architectural distortion
    - Hematomas may be ill-defined, contain complex echoes with posterior enhancement ± shadowing
    - Track to overlying skin incision
  - ○ Late changes at sonography
    - Hematoma: Becomes mass-like when organized; fluid becomes more hypoechoic or cystic
    - Fat necrosis: Mixed hyper- and hypo- to anechoic mass(es), may have posterior shadowing ± enhancement
    - Scar: Ill-defined hypoechoic area with architectural distortion ± posterior shadowing, track to overlying skin incision (skin thickening and retraction)

- Echogenic Ca++ may be visible after years
- No visible change, normal tissue

MR Findings
- T1WI
  - ○ Acute hematoma
    - May vary, usually hyperintense
  - ○ Chronic hematoma/seroma: Hypointense
    - Paramagnetic hemosiderin is dark
- T2WI FS
  - ○ Acute hematoma
    - May vary, usually hypointense
  - ○ Chronic hematoma/seroma
    - Hyperintense fluid cavity surrounded by hypointense margin
- T1 C+ FS
  - ○ Acute
    - Early peripheral enhancement of seroma may occur, ≤ 4 mm, smooth
  - ○ Chronic and later
    - Granulation tissue: Usually delayed enhancement
    - Scars usually do not enhance on MR after 18 months; however, enhancement may occur years later due to fat necrosis with inflammation

Imaging Recommendations
- Best imaging tool: Mammography is "gold standard"
- Protocol advice
  - ○ Benign pathology result: Annual screening
  - ○ Biopsy result of high-risk lesion: Annual screening
    - Consider follow-up in 6 months to establish new baseline, especially if Ca++ were target
    - Variable decisions, depending on institution and on a case-by-case basis

DIFFERENTIAL DIAGNOSIS

Infiltrating Ductal Carcinoma (IDC) ± Infiltrating Lobular Carcinoma (ILC)
- May be overlooked initially if in area of prior surgery
- Architectural distortion with or without central mass
- Post-surgical findings can mimic cancer

BENIGN SURGICAL BIOPSY, POST-OP IMAGING

Radial Scar/Complex Sclerosing Lesion
- Often presents as architectural distortion
- Classically without central mass

Overlapping Normal Breast Tissues
- Resolves with spot compression

Focal Fibrosis
- Can be ill-defined hypoechoic mass on US

Sclerosing Adenosis (SA)
- Most common finding is Ca++
- Mass-like appearance is less common (nodular SA)
  - Occasionally irregular and may be indistinguishable from malignancy

Fibromatosis
- May appear as a spiculated mass

Diabetic Mastopathy
- May cause density

Granular Cell Tumor
- Usually a high density, spiculated, lobulated or circumscribed mass without calcifications

PATHOLOGY

General Features
- Pathologic stages of wound healing
  - Inflammatory phase: Immediate to 2-5 days
    - Hemostasis and inflammation
    - Hematoma and seroma occupy surgical cavity or spread along tissue planes and tears
    - Fat and tissue necrosis
    - Leukocytic and histiocytic infiltrate cause resorption and repair along cavity
  - Proliferative phase: 2 days to 3 weeks
    - Angiogenesis, granulation tissue formation and collagen deposition
    - Granulation tissue rich in fibroblasts lay bed of collagen, fills defect and produces new capillaries
  - Remodeling phase: 3 weeks to 2 years and up
    - Contraction: Wound edges pull together and reduce defect
    - Late fat necrosis (years): Ca++ and oil cysts
    - Scar is poorly vascularized dense fibrosis
    - Hypertrophied scar confined at the original skin incision site
    - Keloid continues to enlarge beyond the original size and shape of the wound skin site
- Fat necrosis
  - Nonsuppurative benign inflammatory process
    - Initially there is local adipose cell destruction with hemorrhage and development of vacuoles filled with necrotic lipid material
    - Shortly followed by an influx of inflammatory cell infiltrate with histiocytes that phagocytose necrotic debris within the vacuoles
    - Development of anuclear fat cells surrounded by lipid-laden histiocytes and giant cells
  - Reparative phase: Fibroblasts proliferate at the periphery of the lesion, surrounding areas of necrotic fat
  - Peripheral calcifications may develop
  - Variable degree of fibrotic reaction and quantity of liquefied fat and calcifications

DIAGNOSTIC CHECKLIST

Consider
- Scar can become denser as it contracts
- Increase in size and density of scar is suspicious
- 2-3% of needle-localized excisions fail to excise the target

Image Interpretation Pearls
- Review needle localization films, specimen imaging if there is uncertainty as to excision of target
- It is important to know the site of biopsy
  - Comparison films are very useful
    - Surgical site can be localized by reference to pre- or post-operative mammograms
    - Scar markers may help, however skin incision is often remote from site of excision
    - Technologists recommended to mark the area of scar on history sheet image icon
- Biopsy may be necessary for suspicious lesions
  - Fat necrosis at core biopsy of a suspicious mass is considered a concordant finding as long as targeting is optimal and the fat necrosis is a discrete finding at histopathology

SELECTED REFERENCES

1. Slanetz PJ: Previous breast biopsy for benign disease rarely complicates or alters interpretation on screening mammography. AJR. 170:1539-41, 1998
2. Viehweg P et al: Retrospective analysis for evaluation of the value of contrast-enhanced MR in patients treated with breast conservative therapy. MAGMA. 7:141-52, 1998
3. Jackman RJ et al: Needle-localized breast biopsy: why do we fail? Radiology. 204:677-84, 1997
4. Berg WA et al: Lessons from mammographic-histopathologic correlation of large-core needle breast biopsy. Radiographics. 16:1111-30, 1996
5. Brenner RJ et al: Mammographic changes after excisional breast biopsy for benign disease. AJR. 167:1047-52, 1996
6. Dipiro PJ et al: Seat belt injuries of the breast: findings on mammography and sonography. AJR. 164:317-20, 1995
7. Hogge JP et al: The mammographic spectrum of fat necrosis of the breast. Radiographics. 15:1347-56, 1995
8. Whitehouse GH et al: MR imaging of the breast after surgery for breast cancer. Magn Reson Imaging Clin N Am. 2:591-603, 1994
9. Mendelson EB: Evaluation of the postoperative breast. Radiol Clin North Am. 30:107-38, 1992
10. Leucht WJ et al: Sonographic findings following conservative surgery and irradiation for breast carcinoma. Ultrasound Med Biol. 14 Suppl 1:27-41 1988
11. Sickles EA et al: Mammography of the postsurgical breast. AJR. 136:585-8, 1981
12. Bassett LW et al: Mammographic spectrum of traumatic fat necrosis: the fallibility of "pathognomonic" signs of carcinoma. AJR. 130:119-22, 1978

IMAGE GALLERY

Typical

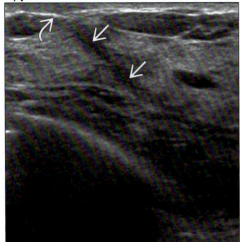 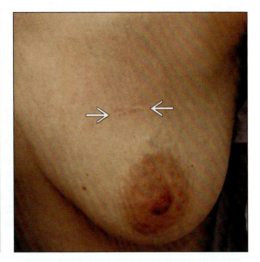

(Left) Anti-radial ultrasound shows hypoechoic track ➡ to area of overlying skin thickening and minimal skin retraction ➡ at site of remote abscess drainage in this 41 y/o woman. *(Right)* Clinical photograph (same as previous image) shows correlating skin incision site ➡. Visual inspection of the area being insonated can help confirm that imaging findings are due to prior surgery.

Typical

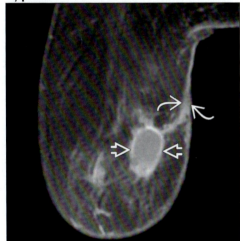 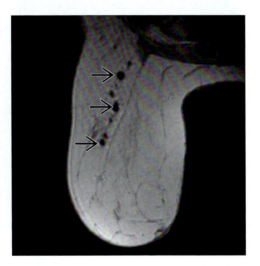

(Left) Axial T1 C+ FS MR shows skin thickening ➡ and hematoma with thin rim of normal enhancement ➡ after recent surgical removal of a benign papilloma in the upper medial left breast. *(Right)* Axial T1WI MR shows ➡ susceptibility artifact, most probably due to hemosiderin deposition from a prior biopsy (same patient as previous image, lower outer aspect of the left breast).

Typical

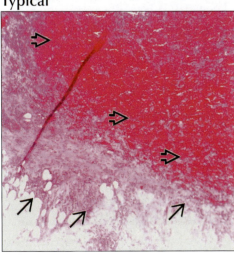 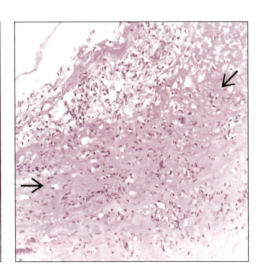

(Left) Biopsy specimen shows fibrosis and granulation tissue ➡, consistent with a recent biopsy cavity containing blood ➡ (H&E; x40). *(Right)* Biopsy specimen shows eosinophilic dense cellular fibrosis ➡ consistent with scar at a recent biopsy site (H&E, x40).

Typical

(Left) Prebiopsy craniocaudal mammogram demonstrates two localization wires, placed in the lateral ⇢ and medial ⇢ left breast. Histology revealed benign findings.
(Right) Postbiopsy craniocaudal mammogram (same patient as previous image) obtained one year after the surgical biopsy. The breast appears to have less parenchyma than before; there are no other visible changes.

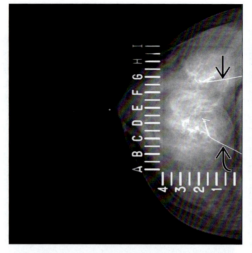 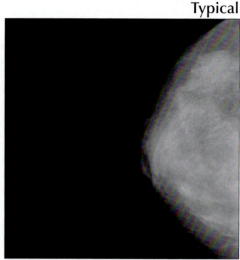

Variant

(Left) CC mammography 3 years after excision of an epidermal inclusion cyst shows very minimal distortion at the excision site ⇢ and focal asymmetry anteriorly ⇢ in this 65 y/o.
(Right) CC mammography 6 years post-operatively (same patient as previous image) shows focal asymmetry ⇢ anterior to scar marker, (incorrectly) attributed to post-surgical change.

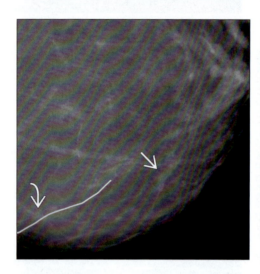 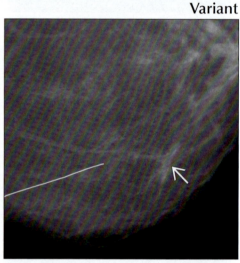

Variant

(Left) CC mammography 7 years post-op (same patient as prior 2 images) shows further increase in focal asymmetry ⇢, now with associated distortion evident ⇢. Again this was misinterpreted as scar. Scars should decrease over time.
(Right) CC mammography spot compression 8 years post-op (same patient as previous image) shows spiculated mass, recognized as suspicious. US-guided biopsy showed invasive lobular carcinoma.

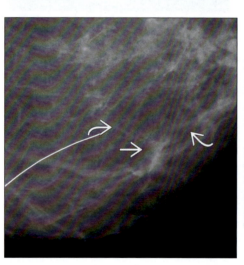 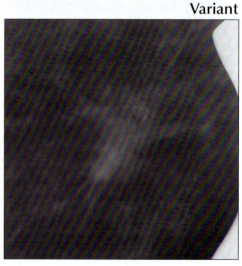

IV
4
10

BENIGN SURGICAL BIOPSY, POST-OP IMAGING

Typical

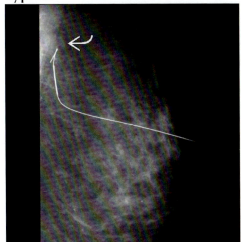

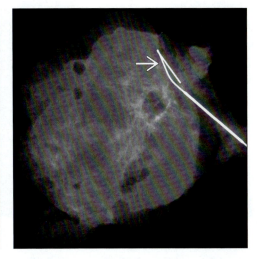

(Left) Lateral mammography obtained after needle localization shows superimposition of hookwire tip on an enlarging 1 cm US-occult mass ➔ in this 61 y/o woman. *(Right)* Specimen radiograph (same patient as previous image) shows hookwire ➔, but no discrete parenchymal abnormality. Histopathology showed only benign breast tissue. There was concern the mass remained in the breast: MR was performed.

Typical

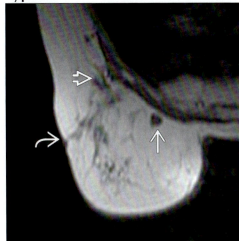

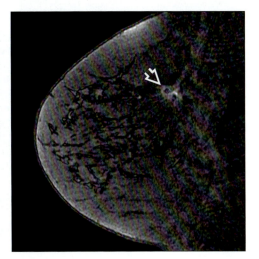

(Left) Axial T1WI MR (same patient as prior 2 images) 6 weeks post-op shows post-surgical scar ➔ with hypointense track extending to overlying skin incision ➔ in outer left breast. The targeted mass ➔ remains in the inner left breast. *(Right)* Sagittal T1 C+ FS MR in the same patient as previous image shows mild enhancement of the surgical biopsy site ➔ outer left breast.

Typical

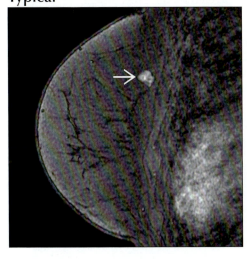

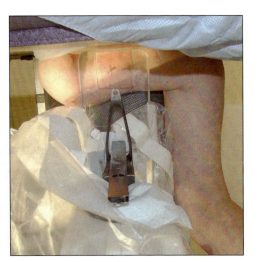

(Left) Sagittal T1 C+ FS MR shows enhancement of the originally targeted mass (remaining in the breast) upper inner left breast ➔. Multiple attempts at second-look US were unsuccessful. *(Right)* Clinical photograph (same patient as prior 5 images) shows special positioning for stereotactic biopsy with arm through the opening in the prone table, allowing successful targeting of this very medial mass (fibroadenoma with sclerosing adenosis).

CLIP PLACEMENT, POST PROCEDURE FINDINGS

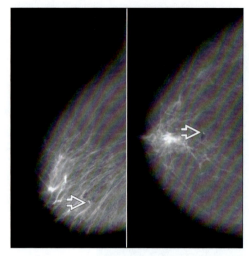

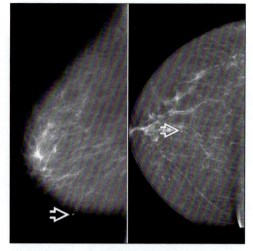

Mammography (ML, CC), after stereotactic biopsy for vague mass, shows clip ➥ to be at the target site. Pathology: Apocrine cysts; routine screening recommended.

MLO and CC mammograms 3 years later (same patient as previous image) shows clip ➥ has migrated superficially to inferior aspect of the breast, within the path of initial inferior biopsy approach.

TERMINOLOGY

Definitions

- Percutaneous biopsy followed by placement of a radiopaque marker clip at the biopsy site
  - Imaging modality used to guide biopsy may be mammographic, US, or MR
- Indications for clip placement
  - Facilitate pre-operative mammographic needle localization
    - Cancer, high risk lesions, or imaging-histopathology discordance require rebiopsy/excision
    - Provide a marker within biopsied area if all imaging evidence of lesion is removed at percutaneous biopsy
    - Reduces challenge of identifying lesion if different facility performs surgery
    - Subtle lesion on US
    - All MR-guided percutaneous biopsies
  - Planned neoadjuvant chemotherapy
    - Complete response to treatment → lesion gone on imaging
    - Clip serves as marker for potential lumpectomy surgery
  - Provide mammographic, US, MR imaging correlation of lesion(s)
    - Confirm biopsy of correct lesion(s)
  - Monitor changes at biopsy site on follow-up mammogram(s)
    - Helps distinguish post-biopsy scar from malignancy
    - Stability of lesion biopsied

IMAGING FINDINGS

General Features

- Best diagnostic clue
  - Radiopaque marker clip at or near biopsy site
    - Residual targeted lesion ± hematoma, air
- Size
  - Clip marker of stainless steel, titanium or carbon particulate
    - Size: 2-3 mm
    - Thickness: 0.13-0.2 mm
    - Volume: 27-512 mm³

DDx: Other Metallic Objects Found Within Breast Tissue

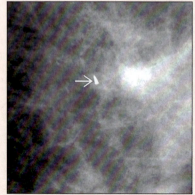

Severed Surgical Needle Tip

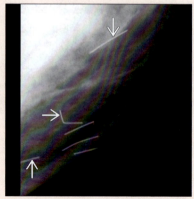

Acupuncture Needles

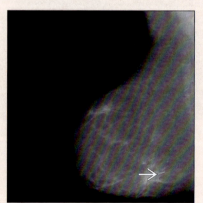

Retained Hookwire

CLIP PLACEMENT, POST PROCEDURE FINDINGS

Key Facts

Terminology
- Indications for clip placement
- Facilitate pre-operative mammographic needle localization
- Subtle lesion on US
- All MR-guided percutaneous biopsies
- Planned neoadjuvant chemotherapy
- Provide mammographic, US, MR imaging correlation of lesion(s)

Imaging Findings
- Same-day post-clip CC and 90° lateral and CC mammograms required
- Report location of clip, relationship to biopsy target
- Current clips produce only a small magnetic susceptibility artifact on T1WI MR

- For lesions seen only with US or MR and biopsy guidance provided by either of these modalities, relationship of clip to biopsy target should be determined by US or MR respectively
- Different clip morphologies available when performing more than one biopsy in same breast

Top Differential Diagnoses
- Retained Needle Localization Wire/Hook
- Surgical Staple
- Other Metallic Foreign Bodies

Clinical Issues
- 10-20% of stereotactically-placed clips are located ≥ 2 cm from biopsy site
- Clip need not be removed if migrated from biopsied lesion site: Controversial

---

- Morphology
  - Two types: Metallic tissue marker alone & US-visible materials
    - One clip is preformed to attach to tissue at time of deployment
    - Some consist of 316 stainless steel formed into different shapes embedded in dehydrated collagen
    - Other clip types include titanium forms embedded within a collagen plug
  - Embedding clips into collagen
    - Thought to be less likely to migrate; cases of delayed migration reported
    - Improves US conspicuity: May allow needle localization with US-guidance
    - May increase hemostasis by expanding within biopsy cavity

Mammographic Findings
- Same-day post-clip CC and 90° lateral and CC mammograms required
  - Include in report of procedure
  - Compare to pre-biopsy imaging
  - Report location of clip, relationship to biopsy target
  - Report hematoma size, other post-biopsy changes if present
  - Assess residual lesion (often limited by post-biopsy air and density)
- Surveillance imaging
  - Post-procedure density in projection parallel to biopsy needle tract on initial follow-up mammogram (one series)
    - 2% for lesions where 11-gauge vacuum-assisted biopsy needle used
    - 0% for lesions where 14-gauge automated biopsy needle used
    - No suspicious findings related specifically to biopsy procedure

Ultrasonographic Findings
- Grayscale Ultrasound
  - Clips echogenic, well seen within masses
  - Clips difficult to see in parenchyma, similar to specular reflectors

- Carbon particulate clip designed to be seen on US
- Track, small seroma, collagen plug may be visualized

MR Findings
- T1WI
  - Current clips produce only a small magnetic susceptibility artifact on T1WI MR
    - Signal void at clip, can be slightly hyperintense adjacent to clip
    - Problematic to adequately visualize clip at time of MR biopsy: Similar to air
    - One outlier (no longer on the market) had a volume of 3042 mm³ which caused a very large susceptibility artifact
    - Older ferromagnetic clips → large artifact
  - Hematoma, fat necrosis hyperintense
- T1 C+
  - Signal void at clip
  - Usually does not interfere with identifying residual lesion or remote suspicious lesions

Imaging Recommendations
- Best imaging tool
  - Same day CC and 90° lateral mammograms
  - For lesions seen only with US or MR and biopsy guidance provided by either of these modalities, relationship of clip to biopsy target should be determined by US or MR respectively
- Protocol advice
  - Suctioning out hematoma at time of biopsy, prior to placing clip, may improve accuracy of clip placement
  - Comparing coordinates on stereoradiographs of target and clip
    - Difficult to assess accuracy in z direction
  - Initial post biopsy mammogram should be obtained in same projection used during core biopsy to limit potential early migration
  - Delayed CC and 90° lateral mammography may be performed immediately prior to needle localization
  - Different clip morphologies available when performing more than one biopsy in same breast

CLIP PLACEMENT, POST PROCEDURE FINDINGS

- Assessment of successful targeting and clip placement of more than one ipsilateral lesion and later follow-up is more accurate utilizing clips of different shapes

DIFFERENTIAL DIAGNOSIS

Benign or Malignant Breast Lesion
- Collagen plug can simulate a semi-opaque foreign body or mass
- Post-biopsy scar: 3% of patients
- Scar should decrease on follow-up

Retained Needle Localization Wire/Hook
- Not completely removed at time of prior needle-localization surgical biopsy procedure

Surgical Staple
- Used for hemostasis and by some surgeons to outline the lumpectomy margin

Other Metallic Foreign Bodies
- Tip of a surgical needle inadvertently left in breast
- Acupuncture needle tips left within tissue following treatment

PATHOLOGY

General Features
- General path comments
  ○ Alerting pathologist to clip within surgical specimen helpful in tissue processing
  ○ Clip displacement from site of deployment is not an uncommon finding

CLINICAL ISSUES

Presentation
- Most common signs/symptoms: Asymptomatic, post-biopsy
- Other signs/symptoms: Mass at site of biopsy (early); mass at skin with clip extrusion (uncommon, delayed)

Natural History & Prognosis
- Majority of clips within 1 cm of targeted lesion
- Early clip migration/erroneous placement
  ○ 10-20% of stereotactically-placed clips are located ≥ 2 cm from biopsy site
  ○ Final clip placement may be at distance from target site (inaccurate) because of procedure-related issues
    ■ Accordion effect: As compressed breast is released, clip may migrate along compression path; best evaluated in projection orthogonal to compression plane used in biopsy
    ■ Migration within fatty tissue
    ■ Hematoma
- Delayed clip migration can occur
  ○ Delayed accordion effect
  ○ Resorption of air at biopsy cavity
  ○ When near skin surface clip may extrude through skin incision

○ Change in tumor size after neoadjuvant chemotherapy and/or radiation therapy
○ Change in clip site after reduction mammaplasty
○ Delayed clip migration is uncommon
  ■ Fatty breasts ↑ risk clip migration

Treatment
- Percutaneous biopsy result of cancer, high-risk lesion and histopathologic/imaging discordance → needle localization and surgical excisional biopsy
- Clip need not be removed if migrated from biopsied lesion site: Controversial

DIAGNOSTIC CHECKLIST

Consider
- When post-core biopsy excision is indicated most beneficial to have available pre-procedure imaging to compare with post-core biopsy clip placement images to ensure that correct area is excised
- Air in breast after a percutaneous biopsy is often remote from biopsy site
  ○ Even when clip placement is within targeted area
  ○ Not a reliable landmark; does not itself indicate inaccurate biopsy

Image Interpretation Pearls
- It should not be assumed that clip is correctly located at biopsy site on subsequent mammograms
  ○ Compare to pre-biopsy mammograms
  ○ For lesions not visible on mammography, US or MR-guided biopsy report should indicate relationship of clip to area biopsied

SELECTED REFERENCES

1. Gombos EC et al: Collagen plug metallic marker clip: mammographic and histopathologic appearance. Breast J. 11(4):292-3, 2005
2. Perlet C et al: [Clip marker placement following MR-guided vacuum biopsy of the breast] Radiologe. 45(3):230-6, 2005
3. Esserman LE et al: Recognizing pitfalls in early and late migration of clip markers after imaging-guided directional vacuum-assisted biopsy. Radiographics. 24(1):147-56, 2004
4. Birdwell RL et al: Clip or marker migration 5-10 weeks after stereotactic 11-gauge vacuum-assisted breast biopsy: report of two cases. Radiology. 229(2):541-4, 2003
5. Lehman CD et al: Position of clip placement after vacuum-assisted breast biopsy: is a unilateral two-view postbiopsy mammogram necessary? Breast J. 9(4):272-6, 2003
6. Rausch D et al: Appearance and artifacts of breast biopsy marking clips. RSNA Educational Exhibit, 2003
7. Rosen EL et al: Accuracy of a collagen-plug biopsy site marking device deployed after stereotactic core needle breast biopsy. AJR Am J Roentgenol. 181(5):1295-9, 2003
8. Philpotts LE et al: Clip migration after 11-gauge vacuum-assisted stereotactic biopsy: case report. Radiology. 222(3):794-6, 2002
9. Burnside ES et al: Movement of a biopsy-site marker clip after completion of stereotactic directional vacuum-assisted breast biopsy: case report. Radiology. 221(2):504-7, 2001

IMAGE GALLERY

Typical

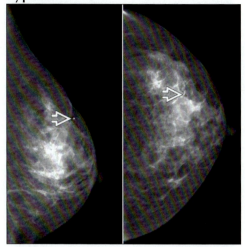
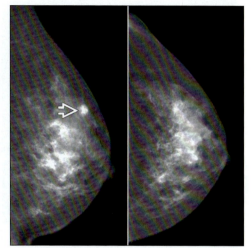

(Left) Mammography (ML, CC) post stereotactic biopsy with benign histology shows clip ➡ near skin surface. Patient phoned 2 months later with complaint of mass at biopsy site. *(Right)* Mammography (ML, CC) 2 months later (same patient as previous), when patient returned complaining of skin lesion and lump, shows a density ➡ on the ML view and no visible clip. US of palpable mass was performed.

Typical

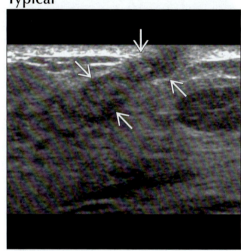
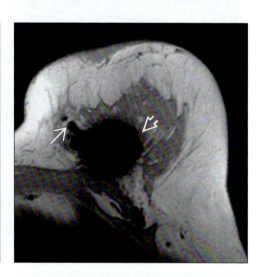

(Left) Ultrasound of palpable mass (same patient as prior 2 images) shows hypoechoic tract ➡ leading to skin. No foreign body was ever visible to patient, but clip was evidently extruded. Physical findings resolved. *(Right)* Axial T1WI MR performed to evaluate chemotherapy treatment response demonstrates large signal void artifact ➡ associated with retained wire fragment and a much smaller adjacent artifact ➡ from a clip.

Typical

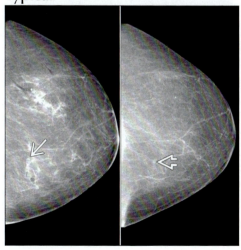
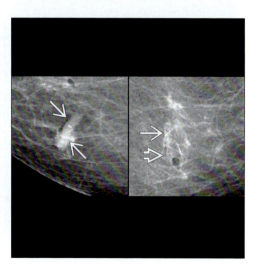

(Left) CC mammography from a case of bilateral 11-gauge stereotactic biopsy procedures shows initial post procedure changes ➡ in medial breast (left) with only the clip ➡ visible 8 months later. *(Right)* CC Photomagnification mammograms of right and left breast (same patient as previous image) show cylindrical outlines of collagen plugs ➡ containing embedded clips. Right image shows a portion of the plug ➡ to be partially radiolucent.

Variant

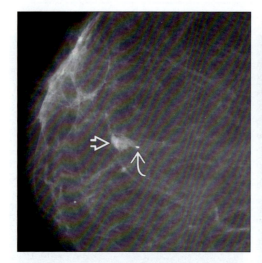 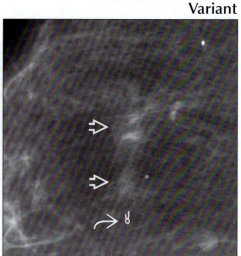

(Left) CC mammography 6 months after stereotactic biopsy (for calcifications = fibrocystic changes) in this 74 year old shows mass ➡ adjacent to clip ➡. *(Right)* MLO mammography spot compression (same patient as previous image) shows mass ➡ elongated toward overlying skin incision from superior biopsy approach. Clip is again seen ➡.

Variant

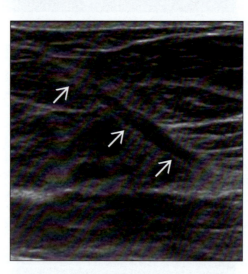 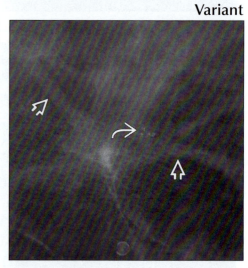

(Left) Radial ultrasound (same patient as prior 2 images) shows oblique hypoechoic track ➡ to overlying skin incision from biopsy. Clip not seen at US. Mass was felt to be scar and moderately decreased at 12 month follow-up. *(Right)* CC mammography magnification in a 57 year old shows cluster of heterogeneous calcifications ➡ adjacent to artery ➡. Stereotactic 11-g biopsy showed sclerosed fibroadenoma with 1 cm hematoma at time of biopsy.

Variant

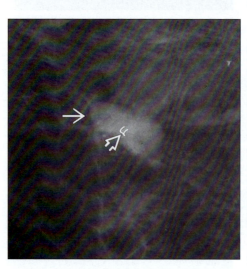 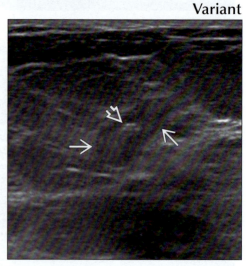

(Left) CC mammography magnification 12 months after biopsy (same patient as previous image) shows an ovoid mass ➡ surrounding clip ➡. *(Right)* Ultrasound (same patient as prior 2 images) shows ovoid, hypoechoic mass ➡ surrounding the echogenic clip ➡. Mass was attributed to scar and decreased at 6 month follow-up.

IV

4

16

Typical

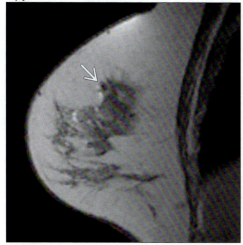
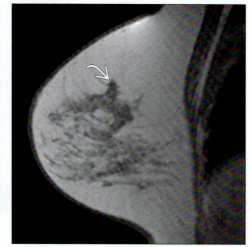

(Left) Sagittal T1WI MR shows signal void and adjacent increased signal ➡ from clip placed at second-look US biopsy of suspicious finding on MR in this 50 year old. US-core biopsy histopathology showed fibrocystic changes and sclerosing adenosis, felt discordant. *(Right)* Sagittal T1WI MR 8 mm more laterally (same patient as previous image) shows persistent spiculated mass ➡ which had been the target of biopsy.

Typical

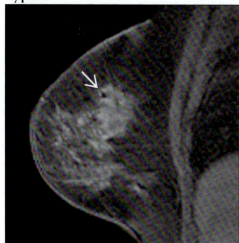
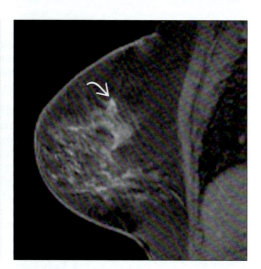

(Left) Sagittal T1 C+ FS MR (same patient as prior 2 images) shows signal void at site of clip ➡. *(Right)* Sagittal T1 C+ FS MR 8 mm more laterally (same patient as prior 3 images) shows enhancing spiculated mass ➡. Needle localization was performed using the clip, deliberately excising tissue lateral to the clip. Findings: Radial scar and micropapillomas.

Typical

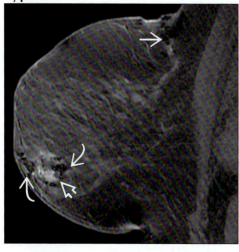
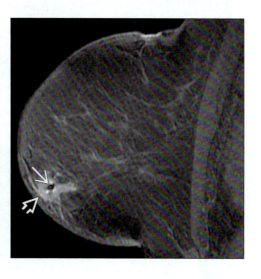

(Left) Sagittal T1 C+ FS MR post-MR-guided biopsy of enhancing lesion 6:00 anteriorly in 63 year old with known DCIS ➡ shows signal voids from air ➡ at target, and increased signal from hematoma ➡, which obscure detection of residual lesion. *(Right)* Sagittal T1 C+ FS MR (same patient as previous) shows signal void from clip ➡ 1.5 cm medial to target, with surrounding hematoma ➡. Air artifacts can mimic clip, and position of clip relative to biopsy target should be reported.

IMPLANT MULTIPLE LUMENS

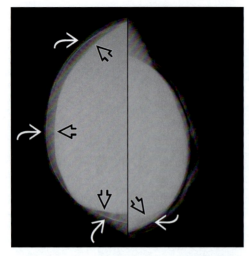

CC mammography in a 49 y/o shows standard double lumen subglandular implants. The more lucent outer saline lumen ⮕ surrounds the dense inner silicone lumen ⮞.

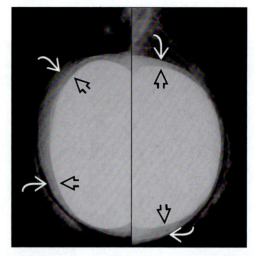

MLO mammography in the same patient confirms intact double lumen implants with both the saline ⮕ and the silicone ⮞ lumina well visualized.

TERMINOLOGY

Definitions
- Multiple lumen implants have > 1 shell; may contain > 1 substance: Usually "bag within a bag"
  - Standard double lumen: Outer lumen saline, inner lumen silicone
    - Outer saline shell can be unfilled or filled to varying degree at time of placement
  - Reverse double lumen: Type of "expander" implant: Outer lumen silicone, inner lumen saline
    - Inner saline lumen gradually filled over months
    - Most often used for reconstruction, gradually stretch chest wall tissue
    - Outer silicone → more natural feel
  - Both lumens silicone: Gel within gel
  - Triple lumen: Variable contents each lumen
- Capsule: Scar tissue that body forms around implant

IMAGING FINDINGS

General Features
- Location
  - Subglandular (retromammary): Implant behind breast tissue, anterior to pectoral muscle
  - Subpectoral (retropectoral): Implant between pectoralis major and minor muscles

Mammographic Findings
- Silicone mammographically denser than saline
  - Thin rim of lucent outer saline lumen in intact double lumen implant
  - May see focal residual lucent saline with failure of inner lumen, mixing of saline and silicone
  - Cannot distinguish types of intracapsular rupture
  - May see extracapsular silicone → implies rupture of both lumens
    - Unless prior ruptured implant with retained extracapsular silicone
- Even with implant displacement, considerable portion of parenchyma obscured

Ultrasonographic Findings
- Difficult to evaluate integrity of double lumen implants on US: Complex internal echoes, folds
- Useful to evaluate breast masses: Distinguish siliconoma from other breast masses

DDx: Mimics of Double Lumen Implants

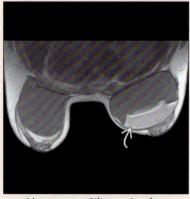

Hematoma, Silicone Implant

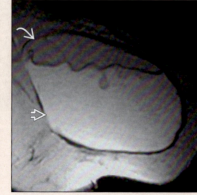

Stacked: Silicone (top), Saline

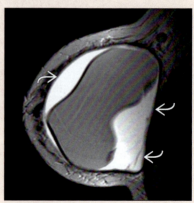

Abscess, Silicone Implant

IMPLANT MULTIPLE LUMENS

Key Facts

Terminology
- Multiple lumen implants have > 1 shell; may contain > 1 substance: Usually "bag within a bag"

Imaging Findings
- Silicone mammographically denser than saline
- Peri-implant fluid hyperintense on T2WI, does not imply rupture of saline lumen
- Isolated failure of outer saline lumen → fluid resorbed, mimics intact single-lumen silicone implant
- Isolated failure of inner lumen results in mixing of contents of inner and outer lumina
- "Salad oil" sign on MR if mixed saline/silicone lumina
- Mammography for screening parenchyma: Routine and implant-displaced views standard
- Routine views include implant: Can prove integrity of double lumen implants when saline lumen well seen

- MR if there is concern for implant rupture

Top Differential Diagnoses
- Moderate fluid around intact single-lumen silicone implant will mimic intact double lumen implant

Pathology
- May have fill valve/tubing, port extending to skin surface

Clinical Issues
- Trend toward reduced sensitivity of mammography in women with implants

Diagnostic Checklist
- Damage to capsule → ↑ risk of rupture
- Capsule alone may be weakened → herniation/contour bulge of intact implant

---

- "Snowstorm" = extracapsular silicone: Echodense noise (due to acoustic scattering)

MR Findings
- T1WI
  - Peri-implant hematoma hyperintense acutely
  - Saline more hypointense than silicone
- T2WI
  - Peri-implant fluid hyperintense on T2WI, does not imply rupture of saline lumen
    - More common with textured-surface implants
  - Capsule hypointense
  - Water signal > silicone signal > fat signal
- T1 C+ FS: Thin rim of enhancement around implant: Capsule
- Assess integrity of each lumen
  - Appearance of outer lumen failure depends on original contents
    - Isolated failure of outer saline lumen → fluid resorbed, mimics intact single-lumen silicone implant
  - Isolated failure of inner lumen results in mixing of contents of inner and outer lumina
    - "Salad oil" sign on MR if mixed saline/silicone lumina
  - Rupture of both lumens
    - Varying degrees of shell collapse: "Subcapsular line sign" of thin rim of silicone external to shell; partial to complete collapse → "linguini sign"
    - May see only one shell or multiple shells collapsing
    - Often see mixing of saline with silicone

Imaging Recommendations
- Best imaging tool
  - Mammography for screening parenchyma: Routine and implant-displaced views standard
    - Routine views include implant: Can prove integrity of double lumen implants when saline lumen well seen
    - Implant-displaced (ID; Eklund) views: Parenchyma pulled forward, implant pushed back: Better visualization of parenchyma

- Protocol advice
  - US to evaluate masses, guide biopsy
  - MR if there is concern for implant rupture
    - T2WI with 3-4 mm slice thickness, breast coil, provide best detail

DIFFERENTIAL DIAGNOSIS

Mimics of Intact Double Lumen Implant
- Moderate fluid around intact single-lumen silicone implant will mimic intact double lumen implant
  - Important to know implant type, particularly if concern for infected fluid
  - Greatest amount of reactive fluid seen around textured-surface implants, esp. polyurethane-covered
  - Hematoma: Recent surgery or trauma, hyperintense on T1WI MR
  - Abscess: Large, growing collection, pain, erythema
- "Stacked" single lumen silicone implant atop a saline implant or vice versa

Mimics of Intact Reverse Double Lumen Implant
- Current saline implant with removal of prior ruptured silicone implant
  - Prior capsule retained, with moderate residual silicone, will mimic outer silicone lumen

Mimics of Double Lumen Rupture
- **Isolated outer lumen failure**
  - Impossible to distinguish from intact single lumen silicone implant except by history or comparison to prior mammograms
  - Outer lumen never filled
- **Isolated inner lumen (internal) failure**
  - Injection of saline, steroids, betadine, antibiotics, or other fluid into a single lumen silicone implant
  - Leakage of internal fill valve → mixing of contents
- **Failure of both lumens**
  - Rupture of a single lumen silicone implant
    - With prior injection of fluids into the implant

IMPLANT MULTIPLE LUMENS

- Or with moderate surrounding reactive fluid prior to rupture
- Only a single layer of collapsing shell will be seen
- Can be difficult to visualize both layers of shell with ruptured double lumen implants

PATHOLOGY

General Features
- Capsule: Dense fibrosis, foreign-body giant cell reaction

Gross Pathologic & Surgical Features
- Configuration
  - Separate patches: Each shell has its own back patch
  - Shared back patch: Complex back patch connects both shells
  - Back patch designed to anchor implant in place
  - May have fill valve/tubing, port extending to skin surface
    - Especially expander type implants

Staging, Grading or Classification Criteria
- Subpectoral or subglandular location
- Implant rupture
  - Isolated outer lumen failure: When saline, no known significance, saline resorbed
    - When silicone outer lumen, explantation (removal) recommended
  - Isolated inner lumen failure (internal failure)
    - Outer lumen still intact: No known clinical significance
  - Failure of both/all lumens
    - May see two layers of shell with varying degrees of collapse as with single lumen implants: Uncollapsed, minimally collapsed, partially to fully collapsed
    - May see mixing of saline and silicone as well, unless earlier failure of outer saline lumen
    - Explantation recommended
- Extracapsular spread of silicone
  - "Snowstorm" appearance on US
  - Silicone-only sequences on MR, typically STIR with water suppression, to map extent

CLINICAL ISSUES

Presentation
- Most common signs/symptoms: Contracture: Hardening of capsule, usually → pain
- Other signs/symptoms: Most ruptures are asymptomatic

Natural History & Prognosis
- Many women with augmentation mammoplasty require additional surgeries
  - Breast implants are not lifetime devices
- No ↑ risk of breast cancer
- Trend toward reduced sensitivity of mammography in women with implants
  - Portion of breast tissue obscured

- Less tissue visualized with subglandular than subpectoral location
- Less tissue visualized with ↑ contracture: Less able to displace implant, breast harder, less able to be compressed
  - Also a function of amount of native breast tissue: If very little, difficult to perform implant-displaced views at all
- Stage of cancers not shown to be different in women with implants
  - Implant may allow cancers to become palpable earlier (controversial)
    - Tissue stretched over implant

Treatment
- Implant complications
  - Capsulotomy for severe contracture
  - Explantation for rupture: Little scientific data on sequelae of leaving ruptured implant in place
- Breast mass: As in women without implants
  - Caution to avoid implant during biopsy

DIAGNOSTIC CHECKLIST

Consider
- Supplemental screening with US and possibly even MR may be appropriate in some patients with implants
  - Very little breast tissue able to be visualized on mammography
  - High risk, dense breast tissue (as with patients without implants): Studies ongoing
- In women with bilateral implants, if one is ruptured, high chance (~ 2/3) that second implant is ruptured

Image Interpretation Pearls
- Important to know type of implant used/history of prior surgery
- Deformity of the implant may be associated with trauma
  - Damage to capsule → ↑ risk of rupture
  - Capsule alone may be weakened → herniation/contour bulge of intact implant

SELECTED REFERENCES

1. Chien CH et al: Spontaneous autoinflation and deflation of double-lumen breast implants. Aesthetic Plast Surg. 30(1):113-7, 2006
2. Middleton MS et al: Breast Implant Imaging. Philadelphia: Lippincott, Williams & Wilkins. 2002
3. Sanger JR et al: False-positive radiographic diagnosis of breast implant rupture because of breast abscess. Ann Plast Surg. 42(5):564-7, 1999
4. Berg WA et al: Single- and double-lumen silicone breast implant integrity: prospective evaluation of MR and US criteria. Radiology. 197(1):45-52, 1995
5. Berg WA et al: MR imaging of the breast in patients with silicone breast implants: normal postoperative variants and diagnostic pitfalls. AJR. 163(3):575-8, 1994
6. Lemperle G et al: Effect of cortisone on capsular contracture in double-lumen breast implants: ten years' experience. Aesthetic Plast Surg. 17(4):317-23, 1993

IMPLANT MULTIPLE LUMENS

IMAGE GALLERY

Typical

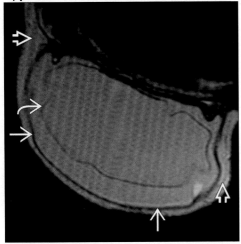 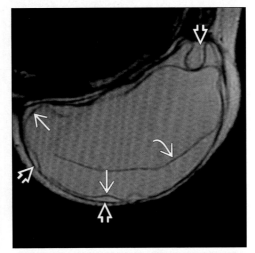

(Left) Axial FSE T2WI of left breast in a 33 y/o shows intact double lumen silicone-silicone implant (inner shell ➡, outer shell ➡). Silicone signal similar to fat ➡ on this sequence. (Right) Axial FSE T2WI (same patient as previous image, right breast) shows intact inner lumen ➡ but rupture of outer lumen with separation of the outer shell ➡ from the capsule with gel between the capsule ➡ and the shell ➡ ("subcapsular line sign" of minimally collapsed rupture).

Typical

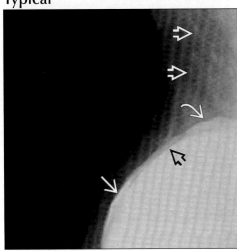 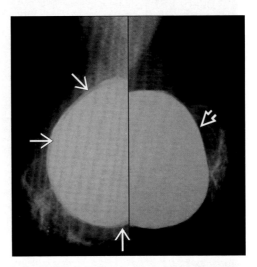

(Left) This 56 y/o had ruptured silicone implant removed. MLO mammogram shows siliconomas in axilla ➡, silicone at edge of implant ➡, calcified capsule ➡, and outer lucent saline lumen of current double lumen implant ➡. (Right) MLO mammography (same as prior image) shows outer lucent saline lumen ➡, confirming current right implant is intact. Left implant ➡ could be a single lumen silicone or double lumen implant with failure of (at least) outer saline lumen.

Typical

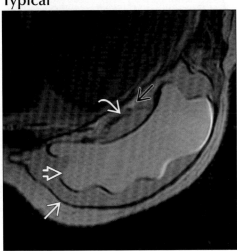 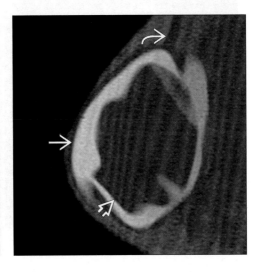

(Left) Axial T2WI MR shows intact expander-type implant with outer silicone ➡ & inner saline ➡ lumina. Minimal saline ➡ is seen near diaphragm ➡ port of entry used to fill inner lumen. (Right) Sagittal STIR WS MR (same as prior image) is "silicone-only": Only outer silicone lumen ➡ is hyperintense. Some infolding of inner saline lumen ➡ is often seen. Subpectoral ➡ location is common for reconstruction as in this 49 y/o status post mastectomy for cancer 4 yrs ago.

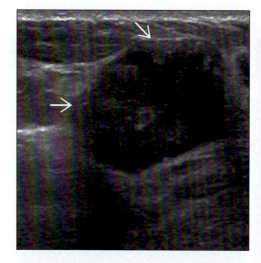
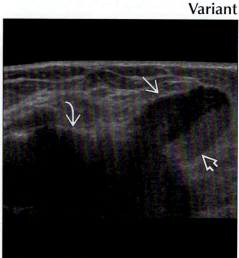

(Left) *This 51 y/o with double lumen implants noted a gradually enlarging lump in her outer breast. US shows what appears to be a complex cystic mass with thick wall ➡. **(Right)** Extended field-of-view US (same as prior image) shows the mass ➡ to be contiguous with a much larger fluid collection ➡. A fluid-debris level is seen within the mass ➡.*

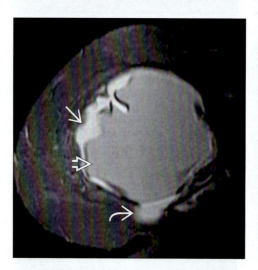
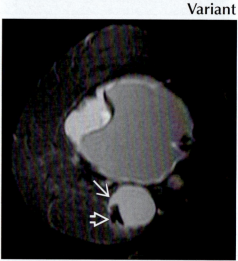

(Left) *Sagittal STIR MR (same case as prior two images) shows subglandular double lumen implant with outer hyperintense saline lumen ➡ and moderately hyperintense inner silicone lumen ➡. Focal herniation of the outer lumen is seen inferiorly ➡. **(Right)** Sagittal STIR MR (adjacent slice, same as prior image) shows rounded palpable mass inferiorly ➡ with internal saline signal. Focal hypointensity ➡ is of uncertain significance.*

IV

4

22

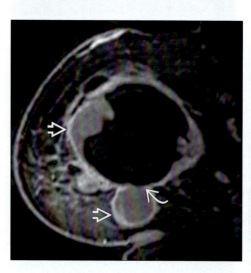
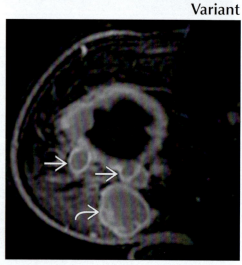

(Left) *Sagittal T1 C+ FS MR (same case as prior 4 images) shows neck of herniation of outer lumen ➡. Rim-enhancement ➡ is noted throughout capsule which has reformed around focal herniation. **(Right)** Sagittal T1 C+ FS MR (same case as left, adjacent slice) shows dominant mass ➡ and smaller outer lumen herniations ➡. Patient stated she always slept this side down. Weakening of capsule can → herniation; does not imply rupture per se. Implant was intact when removed.*

IMPLANT MULTIPLE LUMENS

Typical

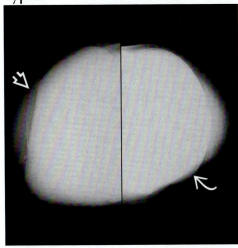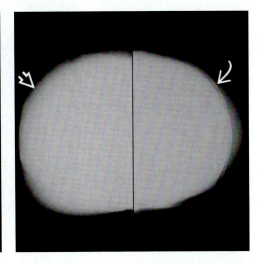

(Left) CC mammography shows intact subglandular double lumen implants with lucent outer saline lumina seen for both right ⮕ and left ⮕ implants in this 49 y/o status post augmentation 9 yrs prior. *(Right)* CC mammography screening the following year (same as left) shows outer lucent saline lumen on left breast ⮕, but only dense silicone on right breast ⮕. There has been interval rupture of one or both lumens since the prior exam. MR is best for further evaluation.

Typical

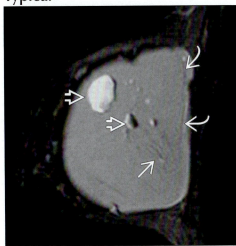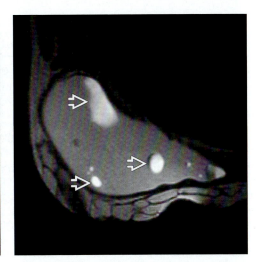

(Left) Sagittal STIR MR (same as prior 2 images) shows mixing of saline and silicone ("salad oil sign") ⮕ due to failed inner lumen. Rupture of outer lumen is confirmed by thin layer of silicone external to shell ⮕ & layers of collapsed slightly hypointense shell ⮕ ("linguine sign"). *(Right)* Axial T2WI MR shows mixing of hyperintense saline ⮕ & silicone lumens ("salad oil sign") without shell collapse (isolated inner lumen failure) in this 27 y/o with 4 y/o double lumen implant.

Typical

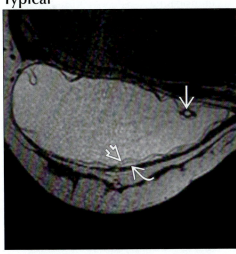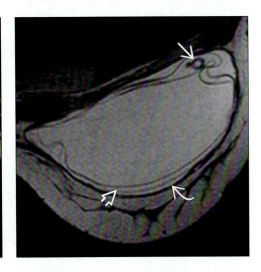

(Left) Axial T2WI MR with water suppression shows ruptured double lumen implant. Note "subcapsular line sign" ⮕, silicone ⮕ between shells, and tubing ⮕ used to instill saline in former outer lumen. Saline had resorbed. *(Right)* Axial T2WI MR of right breast (same patient as left) shows rupture of both lumens, with "subcapsular line sign" ⮕, gel between layers of shells ⮕, and fill tubing ⮕. ~ 2/3 women with one implant rupture will have bilateral rupture.

IMPLANT SALINE

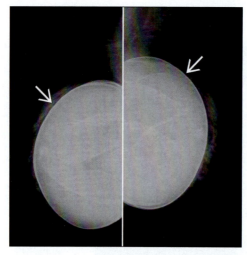

MLO mammography shows intact bilateral subglandular saline implants ➡ in this 41 year old who had them replaced 10 years earlier due to prior rupture.

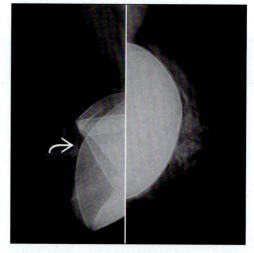

MLO mammography performed two years later (same patient as left-hand image) shows clinically-evident collapse of the right saline implant ➡.

TERMINOLOGY

Abbreviations and Synonyms
- Subglandular = directly behind breast tissue = retroglandular, prepectoral
- Subpectoral = between pectoralis major and minor muscles = retropectoral

Definitions
- Silicone elastomer bags (shell) filled with saline
  - Most have valves through which saline is injected at time of implant operation
    - Optimize cosmetic appearance
  - Some saline implants are prefilled
- Expander type has port at skin, can be gradually inflated or deflated
  - Most often used for reconstruction post mastectomy
  - 50-100 cc instilled each week until reach desired size
  - Tubing to port may be palpable, visible on imaging
- Capsule = scar tissue formed by body around implant
- Contracture = hardening of capsule around implant

IMAGING FINDINGS

General Features
- Best diagnostic clue: Mammography examination includes routine and implant-displaced images
- Location: Distinguish: Subglandular or subpectoral

Mammographic Findings
- Exam can be performed as a screening or diagnostic examination at discretion of facility
- Standard MLO and CC views include implant
- Implant-displaced MLO and CC views (Eklund maneuver) standard to improve tissue visualization
- May be subglandular or subpectoral in location
  - Implant more readily pushed back, breast tissue more completely imaged, with subpectoral placement
- Saline implant semi-opaque
  - Insufficiently lucent to assess overlying breast tissue
- Implant folds and valves often seen
- Smooth or textured surface
- Collapsed implant = silicone elastomer shell only; angular, folded on itself
  - Saline absorbed by body

DDx: Conditions that Mimic Saline Implant

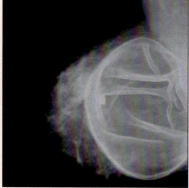

Peanut Oil Implant

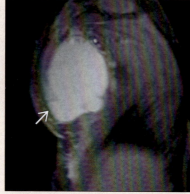

Lymphocele Post Mastectomy, MR

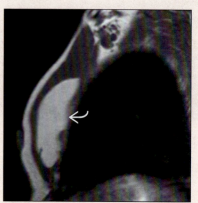

Lipoma, T1WI MR

IMPLANT SALINE

Key Facts

Terminology
- Silicone elastomer bags (shell) filled with saline
- Most have valves through which saline is injected at time of implant operation
- Some saline implants are prefilled
- Expander type has port at skin, can be gradually inflated or deflated

Imaging Findings
- Best diagnostic clue: Mammography examination includes routine and implant-displaced images
- Location: Distinguish: Subglandular or subpectoral
- Reduced sensitivity of mammography: 45 vs. 67% for non-augmented women
- No demonstrated shift in stage distribution or prognosis for cancers in women with implants

- Caution: Even 25-g needle FNA can deflate saline implants

Top Differential Diagnoses
- Silicone Implant
- Peanut oil implant: More radiolucent than saline
- Seroma

Clinical Issues
- Not a lifetime device
- > 20% require revision surgery

Diagnostic Checklist
- Anecdotal reports of implant rupture with mammography
- No need for US or MR to diagnose saline implant rupture

- ○ No residual visible material outside envelope/fibrous capsule
- Capsule can calcify
- Reduced sensitivity of mammography: 45 vs. 67% for non-augmented women
  - ○ No demonstrated shift in stage distribution or prognosis for cancers in women with implants
  - ○ Cancers may be more readily palpable
- No change in specificity compared to women without implants

Ultrasonographic Findings
- Grayscale Ultrasound
  - ○ No need for US to evaluate integrity of saline implants
    - ■ Deflated saline implants will have little or no internal saline
    - ■ Saline is rapidly absorbed
  - ○ Normal findings on US
    - ■ Small amount of fluid at edge of implant, within folds, especially common with textured-surface implants
    - ■ Radial folds in implant surface
    - ■ Shell appears as double parallel echogenic line
    - ■ Very little anterior reverberation artifact
  - ○ US to characterize nonpalpable or palpable masses
    - ■ Edge or folds in implant itself can be palpable when/where implant is superficial
  - ○ "Snowstorm" appearance of residual silicone in patients with prior silicone implant rupture

MR Findings
- T2WI
  - ○ Small amount of fluid at edges of saline implant normal, does not imply leak or rupture
  - ○ Valve, tubing often seen
  - ○ Saline itself hyperintense
- T1 C+ FS
  - ○ Normal: Thin (≤ 4 mm), smooth rim of slow, persistent enhancement around implant = capsule
  - ○ May be helpful in assessing the implanted breast for occult malignancy, disease extent
- No specific role in evaluating saline implant itself

Biopsy
- Path of needle should be parallel to implant surface
- Caution: Even 25-g needle FNA can deflate saline implants

Imaging Recommendations
- Best imaging tool
  - ○ Mammography to screen for breast cancer
    - ■ If most of breast tissue obscured by implant, consider US or MR in high-risk women
    - ■ Digital mammography can be rewindowed to improve tissue or implant visualization
  - ○ US to evaluate masses in women with implants

DIFFERENTIAL DIAGNOSIS

Silicone Implant
- Opaque on mammogram
- Mammogram seldom allows visualization of folds or overlying obscured breast tissue
- Moderately hyperintense on T2WI, hypointense to saline

Other Types of "Implants"
- Peanut oil implant: More radiolucent than saline
  - ○ Complicated by rancidity, infection, no longer being placed
- Other oils, more lucent than saline on mammography
- Fat from liposuction can be instilled into breast: Fat necrosis, infection

Seroma
- Surgical or trauma history
- Large seroma more common in previously irradiated breast/chest wall
- Can form in residual capsule post explantation
  - ○ Often spiculated on mammography
  - ○ US will show fluid collection
  - ○ Should resolve spontaneously

Lymphocele
- Usually post full axillary node dissection

IMPLANT SALINE

Abscess
- Can develop around implant
- Pain, fever, erythema, large fluid collection

PATHOLOGY

General Features
- General path comments
  - As foreign bodies, implants are walled off by body
    - Fibrous capsule
    - May become firm leading to varying degrees of encapsulation, i.e. contracture
  - Deflation rate reports vary greatly
    - 2-76%, increases over time

Gross Pathologic & Surgical Features
- Explanted material includes collapsed envelope
  - With or without fibrous capsule

CLINICAL ISSUES

Presentation
- Most common signs/symptoms
  - Pain is nonspecific
    - Contracture, infection, post-mammogram
- Other signs/symptoms
  - Contracture
    - Increases with increasing duration of implantation
    - More common after reconstruction than augmentation
  - Flattening = rupture = deflation
    - Rate of 0.3-2 per 1000 patient-months
  - Wrinkling or folds in surface of implant can be palpable, may be perceived as a lump by the patient
    - More common with paucity of overlying tissue (e.g. when used for reconstruction)
- Clinical Profile: FDA approved for augmentation and reconstruction
- Physical examination and patient issues are variable
- Frequent history of multiple prior implants of varying types
  - Elicit history of prior ruptured silicone implant in patients with silicone granulomas

Natural History & Prognosis
- Not a lifetime device
- > 20% require revision surgery
- Reported complications
  - Capsular contracture
  - Rupture
    - A clinical diagnosis, "flat tire"
    - Fail more quickly in subpectoral location than subglandular
  - Loss of nipple sensation
  - Asymmetry
  - Wrinkling or puckering of skin at implant sites
  - Edge or folds in implant can mimic breast mass
  - Infection
    - Fever, large peri-implant collection, erythema, warmth
    - 39% positive microbial cultures all implants with fluid vs. 43% without fluid
  - Difficulty with breastfeeding related to implants: 29% rate self-reported
- No known association with breast cancer or collagen vascular disease
  - Careful attention to mammography and clinical examination to avoid missed cancers
    - Implant and implant-displaced views

Treatment
- Ruptured implants are typically surgically removed

DIAGNOSTIC CHECKLIST

Consider
- More breast tissue obscured on mammography with subglandular than subpectoral location
- Anecdotal reports of implant rupture with mammography
- Anecdotal reports of implant rupture during FNA or core biopsy of breast lesions

Image Interpretation Pearls
- Small amount of fluid at surface of implant is normal, does not indicate leakage or rupture
- Large peri-implant collection may suggest infection or hematoma
- No need for US or MR to diagnose saline implant rupture
- US helpful for work-up of suspicious breast lesions
- MR may be used to assess disease extent in women with cancer and implants; MR not recommended for screening women of average risk

SELECTED REFERENCES

1. Handel N et al: A long-term study of outcomes, complications, and patient satisfaction with breast implants. Plast Reconstr Surg. 117:757-67; discussion 768-72, 2006
2. Brown SL et al: Breast implant adverse events during mammography: Reports to the Food and Drug Administration. J Womens Health (Larchmt). 13:371-8, discussion 379-80, 2004
3. Miglioretti DL et al: Effect of breast augmentation on the accuracy of mammography and cancer characteristics. JAMA. 291:442-50, 2004
4. Cunningham BL et al: Saline-filled breast implant safety and efficacy: A multicenter retrospective review. Plast Recon Surg. 105:2143-9, 2000
5. Rohrich RJ: The FDA approves saline-filled breast implants: What does this mean for our patients? Plast Recon Surg. 106:903-5, 2000
6. Strom SS et al: Cosmetic saline breast implants: A survey of satisfaction, breast-feeding experience, cancer screening, and health. Plast Reconstr Surg. 100:1553-7, 1997
7. Ahn CY et al: Clinical significance of intracapsular fluid in patients' breast implants. Ann Plast Surg. 35:455-7, 1995
8. Handel N et al: Factors affecting mammographic visualization of the breast after augmentation mammaplasty. JAMA. 268:1913-7, 1992

IMAGE GALLERY

Variant

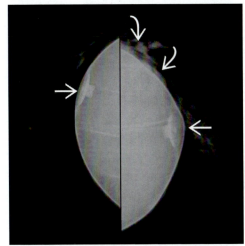

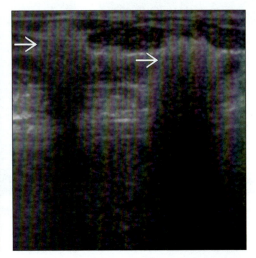

(Left) CC mammography shows dense masses ➔ adjacent to left saline implant in this 55 year old with prior removal of ruptured silicone implant on the left side. Anterior fill valves ➔ are well seen bilaterally. **(Right)** US (same patient as left-hand image) shows "snowstorm" appearance typical for masses due to silicone granulomata ➔ adjacent to the left implant.

Typical

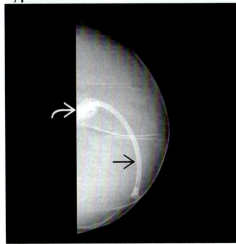

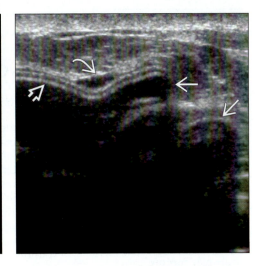

(Left) CC mammography shows normal expander type saline implant with tubing ➔ to port ➔ at chest wall. **(Right)** US in another woman shows lobulated contour ➔ of edge of intact saline implant post mastectomy, perceived as a palpable mass. Note implant shell appears as two parallel echogenic lines ➔. A small amount of fluid ➔ is normally seen adjacent to implant.

Variant

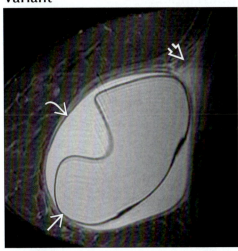

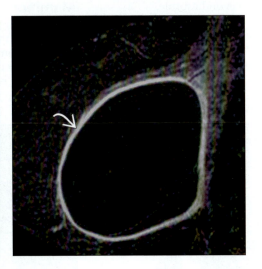

(Left) Sagittal STIR MR shows subpectoral saline implant ➔ placed two months earlier due to prior rupture. A hematoma was noted initially. Now patient has swelling and fever. A large peri-implant collection is noted ➔, with edema in pectoral muscle ➔. **(Right)** Sagittal T1 C+ subtraction MR (same as on left-hand image) shows intense, thick (5 mm) capsular enhancement ➔. Pus was drained from around the implant.

IMPLANT SILICONE

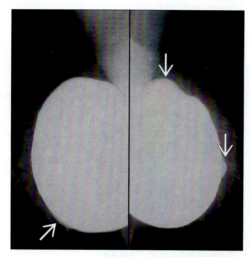

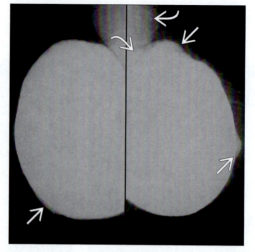

MLO mammography in a 62 y/o shows dense masses of silicone ➡ adjacent to subglandular silicone implants. This was her only set of implants and she had not had silicone injections.

Overexposed MLO views in the same patient better illustrates these masses of silicone ➡. Note extension of free silicone into the left axilla ➡. These findings are diagnostic of extracapsular rupture.

TERMINOLOGY

Definitions

- Silicone implant: Silicone elastomer envelope ("shell") containing silicone gel
- Capsule: Fibrous tissue body forms around an implant
  - Capsulotomy: Procedure to disrupt capsule
    - Closed: Physician twists breast while applying pressure; vs. open (surgical)
    - High risk of causing implant rupture
- Contracture: Hardening of the capsule, often ⇒ pain
- Siliconoma: Mass due to foreign body reaction to silicone gel in tissues, beyond capsule
- Gel bleed: Microscopic diffusion of silicone through shell
- Rupture: Silicone gel macroscopically outside of shell
  - Varying degrees of shell collapse
  - Contained by capsule: "Intracapsular rupture"
  - When silicone gel spreads beyond capsule: "Extracapsular rupture"
- Breast reconstruction: Surgical creation of new breast mound from autologous tissue/implant/combination, typically post mastectomy for cancer

- Breast augmentation: Cosmetic procedure to increase breast size or improve breast contour

IMAGING FINDINGS

General Features

- Location
  - Subglandular (retromammary): Implant behind breast tissue, anterior to pectoral muscle
  - Subpectoral (retropectoral): Implant between pectoralis major and minor muscles
- Features often determined by implant type
  - Envelope may be smooth or textured (including polyurethane covered)
  - Shape variable: Round, oval, teardrop
  - Profile variable: Flat profile for augmentation, rounded profile for reconstruction

Mammographic Findings

- Calcifications (Ca++) in fibrous capsule in ~ 25%
  - Parallel to implant surface, sheet-like dystrophic
  - More common in subglandular than subpectoral
- Implant becomes more rounded with contracture
- Shell may be wrinkled, especially if underfilled

DDx: Large Mammographic Opacities

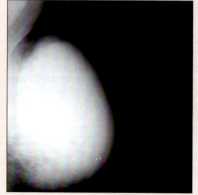

Giant Fibroadenoma

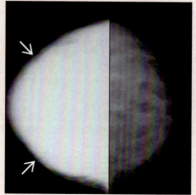

Large Phyllodes

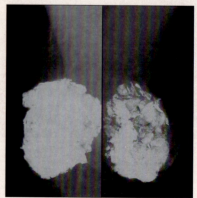

Residual Calcified Capsule

IMPLANT SILICONE

Key Facts

Terminology
- Silicone implant: Silicone elastomer envelope ("shell") containing silicone gel
- Capsule: Fibrous tissue body forms around an implant

Imaging Findings
- Features often determined by implant type
- Calcifications (Ca++) in fibrous capsule in ~ 25%
- Implant becomes more rounded with contracture
- Shell may be wrinkled, especially if underfilled
- Standard screening: Routine and implant-displaced ("ID", "Eklund") mammographic views
- MR most accurate for implant integrity

Top Differential Diagnoses
- Intracapsular Rupture

- Extracapsular Silicone

Clinical Issues
- ↑ Likelihood of rupture: Change in implant shape, recent trauma to breast
- Most implant ruptures are asymptomatic
- ↑ Rupture over time: Median time to rupture = 8-11 yrs all implants; faster if subpectoral
- Majority of patients will require future breast surgery
- No ↑ risk of breast cancer
- Standard recommendation from manufacturers is for removal of known ruptured implant(s)

Diagnostic Checklist
- Trend toward reduced mammographic sensitivity in women with implants
- Peri-implant fluid usually normal

- Dense, oval or round masses due to extracapsular silicone
  - Implies rupture of current implant unless retained from prior implant rupture
  - May develop rim Ca++
- Parenchyma: Implant obscures a portion of breast despite implant-displaced views

Ultrasonographic Findings
- Intact implant is anechoic
  - Appears taller than it is due to slower speed of sound in silicone than in tissue (1,066 vs. ~ 1,540 m/sec)
  - Reverberation artifacts parallel anterior surface
  - Shell is seen as echogenic double parallel lines
- Implant rupture
  - Subtle separation of shell from capsule, gel outside shell along folds
  - Diffuse echoes in lumen
  - "Stepladder" sign: Layers of collapsed shell
- Extracapsular spread of silicone
  - "Snowstorm": Echogenic noise due to scattering
  - Rare: "Silicone cyst(s)": Anechoic collections of gel

MR Findings
- T2WI: May see hyperintense fluid around implant
- STIR
  - Water-suppressed STIR: Only silicone is bright
  - Depict extracapsular silicone, extent
    - Due to fibrotic reaction incited, extracapsular silicone is typically slightly hypointense to gel remaining within capsule
- Folds or wrinkles in implant shell are common
- Positioning on breast coil may thin medial implant: "Rat-tail" appearance, normal
- Implant rupture
  - Uncollapsed rupture: Silicone external to shell, within folds: "Keyhole", "teardrop" or "noose" sign
  - Minimally collapsed rupture: Slight separation of shell from capsule: "Subcapsular line" sign
  - Partially or fully collapsed rupture: Varying degrees of collapse of shell into gel
    - Fully collapsed rupture ⇒ "linguine" sign
- Fluid signal in gel

- Reactive fluid mixing with gel due to rupture
  - Less common: Injected into implant at time of placement: Steroids, betadine, antibiotics
- Extracapsular spread of silicone
  - Silicone seen in breast tissue or lymph nodes

Biopsy
- Not usually a contraindication to needle core biopsy
- Aim to keep implant out of needle trajectory
- Displace implant for stereotactic biopsy: Often possible in at least one view
- Consent patient for specific risk of implant rupture

Imaging Recommendations
- Best imaging tool
  - Standard screening: Routine and implant-displaced ("ID", "Eklund") mammographic views
    - ID views: Parenchyma pulled forward, implant pushed back, off film
    - Improves compression of parenchyma
    - Routine mammography in patients with implants can be a screening or diagnostic exam at discretion of facility/insurance
  - Digital mammography allows windowing/leveling and post-processing, may improve detail
- Protocol advice
  - US to evaluate breast masses, guide biopsy
  - MR most accurate for implant integrity
    - Dedicated breast coil, T2WI, 3-4 mm slice thickness: Best detail for subtle rupture
    - Silicone-only sequence, STIR with water suppression: Best for extracapsular silicone
    - Phase should not be antero-posterior: Minimize respiratory motion artifacts
  - Contrast-enhanced MR can be used for parenchymal evaluation when indicated
    - Not a substitute for mammography, not routine

DIFFERENTIAL DIAGNOSIS

Intracapsular Rupture
- Usually appears intact on mammography

IMPLANT SILICONE

- US: Findings of rupture can be quite subtle
  - Folds of intact implant can → complex echotexture, difficult to distinguish from collapsing shell
- MR: Motion artifacts can mimic
  - Complex radial folds extend to implant surface, more hypointense than collapsing shell as folds represent double layer of shell

Extracapsular Silicone

- Herniation (bulge) of gel through focally weakened capsule, implant intact
  - Mammographically can resemble extracapsular rupture
- Extracapsular rupture
  - Silicone extruded through both implant shell and fibrous capsule
- Residual silicone from prior implant rupture
- Direct injections of silicone oil
- Extremely rare: Gel bleed alone, without rupture

PATHOLOGY

General Features

- General path comments
  - Fibrous capsule
    - Immune system sees implant as foreign body → fibrous tissue encases implant → capsule
- Epidemiology
  - 2/3 of implants placed for augmentation: 225,000 women in 2002 in USA
    - Outside of protocols, only saline implants available for augmentation in USA
  - 1/3 for reconstruction, usually subpectoral
    - Silicone or saline or multiple lumen implants approved

CLINICAL ISSUES

Presentation

- Most common signs/symptoms
  - Discomfort: Common if intact or ruptured
    - ↑ With increasing contracture
    - Siliconomas can be hard, tender
- Other signs/symptoms
  - ↑ Likelihood of rupture: Change in implant shape, recent trauma to breast
    - Includes capsulotomy
  - Most implant ruptures are asymptomatic

Natural History & Prognosis

- FDA restricted silicone implant use in 1992
  - Concerns: Unproven safety
  - Allowed for post mastectomy reconstruction
- Implants are not lifetime medical devices
  - ↑ Rupture over time: Median time to rupture = 8-11 yrs all implants; faster if subpectoral
  - More rapid failure if placed for reconstruction
    - Due to ↓ overlying tissue or subpectoral location
  - Majority of patients will require future breast surgery
- Complications: Infection, loss of nipple sensation, deformity, contracture, rupture
  - Some contracture in nearly all women with implants

- Possible systemic complications: No clear risk or recognizable syndromes
- No ↑ risk of breast cancer

Treatment

- Breast cancer treated in standard manner
  - Subpectoral implant may be left in situ at time of mastectomy or replaced with subpectoral expander
- Standard recommendation from manufacturers is for removal of known ruptured implant(s)
  - Mastopexy, replacement as desired

DIAGNOSTIC CHECKLIST

Consider

- 30-50% ↓ in visualized breast tissue on mammography
  - Worse with less native breast tissue
  - Worse with ↑ capsular contracture
    - More difficult to displace implant
    - Patient less tolerant of compression, "rock hard"
  - Worse with subglandular than subpectoral location
- Trend toward reduced mammographic sensitivity in women with implants
  - No studies to date have shown significantly different breast cancer stage distribution or effect on survival
  - Small cancers may be easier to palpate
- No known clinical significance to implant rupture
  - ~ 80% of implant ruptures are intracapsular
  - Extracapsular silicone ⇒ ↑ incidence of fibromyalgia
  - Natural history of silicone migration not well established

Image Interpretation Pearls

- Peri-implant fluid usually normal
  - Extensive peri-implant fluid may suggest infection
  - More common with textured-surface implants
- Bulge/herniation in implant contour is due to focal weakening of capsule: Does not = rupture
  - May correlate with trauma, ↑ risk of rupture
- Back patch may be visualized on MR (if present)
- Surgical history helpful: Type of implant, prior implant(s), prior rupture if known

SELECTED REFERENCES

1. Lipworth L et al: Silicone breast implants and connective tissue disease: an updated review of the epidemiologic evidence. Ann Plast Surg. 52:598-601, 2004
2. Miglioretti DL et al: Effect of breast augmentation on the accuracy of mammography and cancer characteristics. JAMA. 291:442-50, 2004
3. Scaranelo AM: Evaluation of the rupture of silicone breast implants by mammography, ultrasonography and magnetic resonance imaging in asymptomatic patients: correlation with surgical findings. Sao Paulo Med J. 122:41-7, 2004
4. Middleton MS et al: Breast Implant Imaging. Philadelphia, Lippincott, Williams & Wilkins. 2002
5. Brown SL et al: Prevalence of rupture of silicone gel breast implants revealed on MR imaging in a population of women in Birmingham, Alabama. AJR. 175:1057-64, 2000
6. Soo MS et al: Intracapsular implant rupture: MR findings of incomplete shell collapse. J Magn Reson Imaging. 7:724-30, 1997

IMAGE GALLERY

Typical

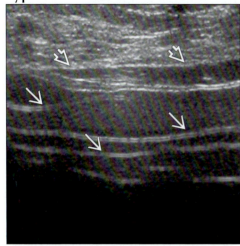
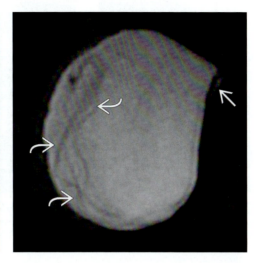

(Left) Radial ultrasound in a 53 y/o shows multiple layers of collapsed implant shell ➡, i.e., the "stepladder sign" of implant rupture. The capsule ➡ is very subtle on US. Shell ➡ is seen as double parallel lines on US. *(Right)* Axial STIR MR with water suppression (same implant as left) shows "linguine" sign of collapsed shell ➡. Note sliver of extracapsular silicone medially ➡. STIR with water suppression is a "silicone only" sequence as only silicone appears bright.

Typical

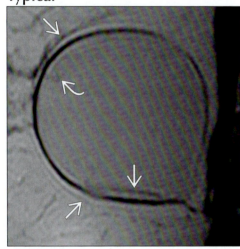
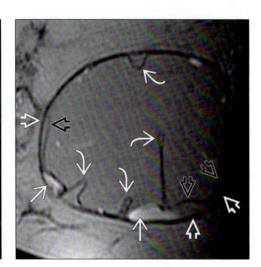

(Left) Sagittal T2WI MR in a 49 y/o shows a subtle collection of silicone gel trapped in a fold ➡ implying rupture. Motion artifacts ➡ are present in the parenchyma and implant. *(Right)* Sagittal T2WI MR (same as left) confirms subtle findings of rupture; the "noose" or "inverted keyhole" sign ➡ of gel trapped within folds and "subcapsular line sign" (separation of shell ➡ from capsule ➡). Fluid ➡ in gel can be unrelated to rupture.

Typical

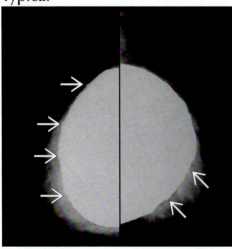
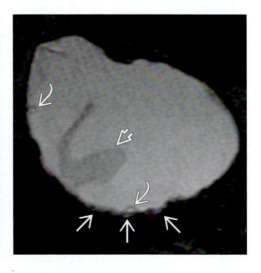

(Left) MLO mammography in a 59 y/o shows subglandular silicone implants with extensive capsular calcification ➡. The mammographic findings are unrevealing as to implant integrity. The patient desired explanation. *(Right)* Axial FSE STIR WS MR (same as left) shows the "noose" sign ➡ as well as tiny amounts of silicone in breast tissue ➡. This "silicone only" sequence proves extracapsular rupture. A normal fold ➡ is incidentally noted.

REDUCTION MAMMOPLASTY

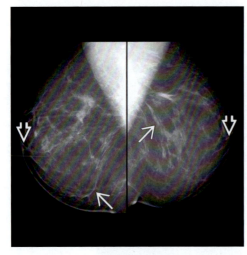

MLO mammography shows reorganization of the breast tissue, elevated nipples ⇨, and the inferior "swirled" pattern of architectural distortion ⇨.

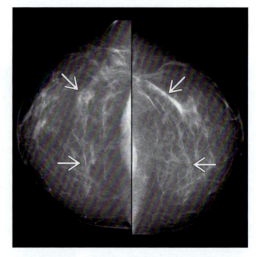

CC mammography shows band-like densities overlying the posterior breasts ⇨ consistent with the areas of the inferior incision sites.

TERMINOLOGY

Abbreviations and Synonyms

- Reduction mammaplasty, breast reduction

Definitions

- Plastic surgery of the breast to reduce its size in the setting of macromastia, contralateral mastectomy or breast conserving surgery, or congenital asymmetry

IMAGING FINDINGS

General Features

- Best diagnostic clue
  - Fibroglandular tissue redistributed from upper outer breast to inferior and inner breast
  - Elevation of nipple
    - More skin inferior to the nipple than superiorly
  - Architectural distortion
    - Inferior and inner breast swirled pattern of fibroglandular tissue

Mammographic Findings

- Parenchymal redistribution as residual breast tissue shifted to a lower position
  - Best seen on MLO or ML views
- Nipple elevation
  - Best seen on MLO or ML views
- Architectural distortion seen as swirling of the fibroglandular tissue
- Fat necrosis
  - Oil cysts which may calcify
  - Calcifications, typically coarse; tend to appear later than other changes (50% of patients by 2 years)
  - Calcifications may begin as fine curvilinear microcalcifications which will eventually coarsen
  - Skin calcifications in periareolar and inferior incision sites
  - Spiculated density
  - Focal mass, usually has lucent fatty center
- Skin thickening
  - Along surgical anastomoses: Periareolar, inferior breast, and inframammary fold
- Retroareolar fibrotic band
  - Parallels skin contour

DDx: Findings Associated with Reduction Mammoplasty

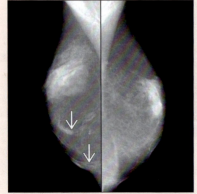

Swirl Distortion

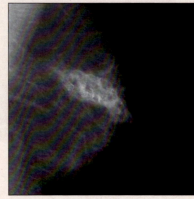

Fat Necrosis

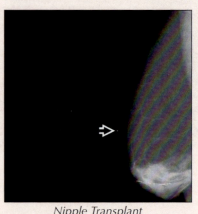

Nipple Transplant

REDUCTION MAMMOPLASTY

Key Facts

Terminology
- Plastic surgery of the breast to reduce its size in the setting of macromastia, contralateral mastectomy or breast conserving surgery, or congenital asymmetry

Imaging Findings
- Parenchymal redistribution as residual breast tissue shifted to a lower position
- Nipple elevation
- Architectural distortion seen as swirling of the fibroglandular tissue
- Fat necrosis
- Skin thickening
- Retroareolar fibrotic band
- Best imaging tool: Mammography

Top Differential Diagnoses
- Carcinoma
- Post-Surgical Changes from Mastopexy

Pathology
- Occult carcinoma detection rates of 0.06-0.4%, or up to 0.8% if ductal carcinoma in situ is included

Diagnostic Checklist
- Post-operative mammographic changes follow a predictable time course
- Distribution of changes should be along the surgical anastomosis sites: Periareolar, inferior breast and inframammary fold (most commonly)
- Nipple elevation and tissue redistribution to inferior breast are the most characteristic changes of the procedure

---

- ○ ≤ 5 mm thick
- Disruption of subareolar ducts
  - ○ Only seen with nipple transplantation type procedures
  - ○ Duct continuity should be preserved with transposition type procedures
- Epidermal inclusion cyst
  - ○ Entire dermoglandular pedicle needs to be carefully deepithelialized prior to nipple-areolar repositioning
  - ○ Cyst may form if there is any retained epithelial element during infolding of the vascularized tissue pedicle
- These findings are variable with none or all of the above being present in any one patient

Imaging Recommendations
- Best imaging tool: Mammography
- Baseline mammogram generally performed prior to procedure in women over 35
  - ○ To detect lesions that need to be evaluated at the time of reduction surgery
- Post-operative mammogram recommended at 3-6 months for new baseline

DIFFERENTIAL DIAGNOSIS

Carcinoma
- Initial findings of fat necrosis may be pleomorphic microcalcifications
- Spiculated density or focal mass of fat necrosis can also be indistinguishable from carcinoma
- Epidermal inclusion cyst may present as a new suspicious post-operative mass
- Atypical post-operative calcifications or masses may require biopsy to exclude carcinoma
- Architectural distortion secondary to surgery may be difficult to distinguish from carcinoma

Post-Surgical Changes from Mastopexy
- Mastopexy differs from reduction mammoplasty in that it is surgery to reduce breast ptosis only with no significant reduction of breast mass or volume

- Performed to restore aesthetic appearance of breasts after volume loss and skin stretching due to natural aging, weight loss, pregnancy, lactation, or menopause
- Many of the post-operative changes are similar to those seen in reduction mammoplasty with the same scar distribution patterns
- Should not exhibit the parenchymal distortion that is often seen with reduction mammoplasty

PATHOLOGY

General Features
- General path comments
  - ○ Reduction tissue should be sent for pathologic analysis
  - ○ Occult carcinoma detection rates of 0.06-0.4%, or up to 0.8% if ductal carcinoma in situ is included
    - ■ Rates are higher in patients having reduction surgery as part of a symmetry procedure for a contralateral carcinoma surgery than for patients with macromastia
- Etiology: Changes after breast reduction are a direct result of iatrogenic trauma to the breast and subsequent healing
- Epidemiology: Patients having reduction for macromastia or congenital asymmetry have the same risk of developing breast cancer as age-matched cohorts who have not had reduction, necessitating tissue biopsy for atypical post-operative findings even if in typical locations

CLINICAL ISSUES

Presentation
- Indications for reduction mammoplasty
  - ○ Macromastia
    - ■ Resulting in physical disability
    - ■ Cosmesis/self image
  - ○ Symmetry procedure following contralateral breast conserving surgery or mastectomy with reconstruction

REDUCTION MAMMOPLASTY

○ Congenital asymmetry
○ Gigantomastia of pregnancy (rare)
- Reimbursement for reduction mammoplasty
  ○ Requirements vary among insurance carriers, but include any or all of the following
    - Long term documentation of multiple symptoms such as back, neck or shoulder pain, submammary intertrigo, shoulder grooving, arm/hand paresthesias and breast pain
    - Documentation that conservative treatments such as an appropriate support bra, nonsteroidal anti-inflammatory drugs, exercise or heat/cold application have failed
    - Documentation of attempted weight loss through a nutritionist, weight loss program or exercise program
    - Estimated minimum weight removal plans of 400-500g per breast
    - Age minimums
- Two general types of reduction surgery are performed
  ○ Nipple transposition on a vascularized parenchymal pedicle
    - Most common technique
    - Inverted-T scar and newer variations on this technique
  ○ Free nipple graft transplantation
    - Easier in large women
    - Operation shorter so may be preferred in older patients or those with systemic disease

Natural History & Prognosis

- Patient satisfaction is high after procedure in vast majority of cases with early improvement in both physical and psychosocial impairment
- Patients may present with palpable abnormality after reduction from various etiologies
  ○ Hematoma
  ○ Fat necrosis
  ○ Scar
- Any palpable mass following reduction should be evaluated in usual manner
  ○ Tissue sampling may be warranted

DIAGNOSTIC CHECKLIST

Consider

- Post-operative mammographic changes follow a predictable time course
- Distribution of changes should be along the surgical anastomosis sites: Periareolar, inferior breast and inframammary fold (most commonly)
- Calcifications and masses are usually typical of fat necrosis
- Atypical calcifications or masses require standard work-up and possibly needle biopsy to exclude carcinoma

Image Interpretation Pearls

- Nipple elevation and tissue redistribution to inferior breast are the most characteristic changes of the procedure

SELECTED REFERENCES

1. Becker H: Breast reduction insurance denials. Plast Reconstr Surg. 114(6):1687, 2004
2. Colwell AS et al: Occult breast carcinoma in reduction mammaplasty specimens: 14-year experience. Plast Reconstr Surg. 113(7):1984-8, 2004
3. Keleher AJ et al: Breast cancer in reduction mammaplasty specimens: case reports and guidelines. Breast J. 9(2):120-5, 2003
4. Yalin CT et al: Breast changes after reduction mammaplasty: a case report with mammographic and ultrasonographic findings and a literature review. Breast J. 9(2):133-7, 2003
5. Chadbourne EB et al: Clinical outcomes in reduction mammaplasty. Mayo Clinic Proceedings. 76(5):503-10, 2001
6. Danikas D et al: Mammographic findings following reduction mammoplasty. Aesthetic Plast Surg. 25(4):283-5, 2001
7. Hidalgo DA et al: Current trends in breast reduction. Plast Reconstr Surg. 104(3):806-15, 1999
8. Miller JA et al: Benign fat necrosis simulating bilateral breast malignancy after reduction mammoplasty. South Med J. 91(8):765-7, 1998
9. Aston SJ et al: Grabb and Smith's Plastic Surgery. 5th Ed. Philadelphia, Lippincott-Raven. Chapter 59, 725, 1997
10. Bassett LW et al: Diagnosis of diseases of the breast. Philadelphia, WB Saunders Co. Chapter 32, 581, 1997
11. Beer GM et al: Diagnosis of breast tumors after breast reduction. Aesthetic Plast Surg. 20(5):391-7, 1996
12. Hogge JP et al: The mammographic spectrum of fat necrosis of the breast. Radiographics. 15(6):1347-56, 1995
13. Mandrekas AD et al: Fat necrosis following breast reduction. Br J Plast Surg. 47(8):560-2, 1994
14. Fajardo LL et al: Epidermal inclusion cyst after reduction mammoplasty. Radiology. 186(1):103-6, 1993
15. Mendelson EB: Evaluation of the postoperative breast. Radiol Clin North Am. 30(1):107-38, 1992
16. Clugston PA et al: Detecting breast cancer after reduction mammoplasty. Can J Surg. 34(1):37-40, 1991
17. Mitnick JS et al: Calcifications of the breast after reduction mammoplasty. Surg Gynecol Obstet. 171(5):409-12, 1990
18. Brown FE et al: Mammographic changes following reduction mammaplasty. Plast Reconstr Surg. 80(5):691-8, 1987
19. Miller CL et al: Mammographic changes after reduction mammoplasty. AJR Am J Roentgenol. 149(1):35-8, 1987
20. Stavrides S et al: Gigantomastia in pregnancy. Br J Surg. 74(7):585-6, 1987

IMAGE GALLERY

Typical

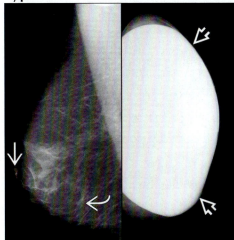 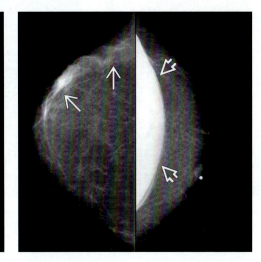

(Left) MLO mammography shows left post mastectomy silicone implant ➡ reconstruction and right reduction with nipple elevation ➡ and inferior swirl distortion ➡. *(Right)* CC mammography (same as on left) shows post left mastectomy reconstruction with visualization of the silicone implant ➡; right breast shows only a small amount of outer quadrant tissue ➡.

Typical

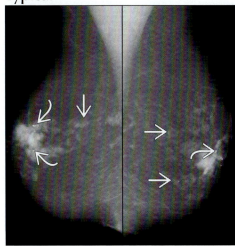 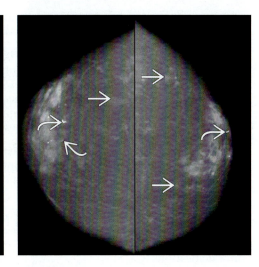

(Left) MLO mammography shows reorganization of breast tissue ➡ and retroareolar coarse calcifications of fat necrosis ➡. *(Right)* CC mammography (same as on left) shows coarse calcifications of fat necrosis ➡ and displaced tissue ➡. Scattered areas of asymmetry are noted, right more than left.

Typical

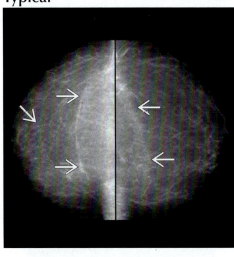 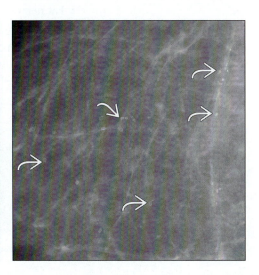

(Left) CC mammography shows band-like areas of density ➡ along the scars corresponding to the sites of incision for the reduction mammoplasty procedure. *(Right)* CC mammography close-up of left breast (same as left) shows numerous small lucent-centered skin calcifications ➡ located within the incisions.

IV

4

35

SILICONE GRANULOMA

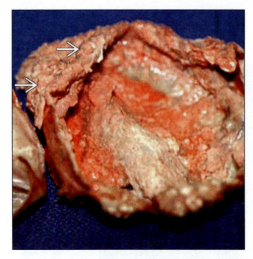

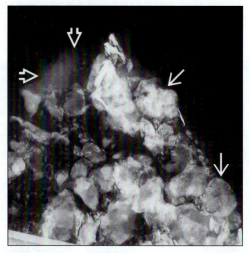

Gross pathology shows an implant capsule after explantation. Chunky Ca++ ➡ seen mammographically are sometimes evident at gross pathology. Extensive Ca++ compromise breast imaging.

Mammography spot compression post explantation in a 73 y/o shows dense mass ➡ with background chunky Ca++ ➡ in retained capsule. Stereotactic biopsy showed silicone granuloma.

TERMINOLOGY

Definitions
- Silicone granuloma = siliconoma: Inflammatory mass caused by foreign body reaction to silicone gel in tissue

IMAGING FINDINGS

General Features
- Best diagnostic clue: Dense, circumscribed mass on mammogram, and/or "snowstorm" on US, in woman with current or prior silicone implants
- Location: Most often at edge of implant or in axilla

Mammographic Findings
- Dense, circumscribed mass ± rim calcifications (Ca++)

Ultrasonographic Findings
- "Snowstorm": Mass of echogenic noise on US
  - Distal border not visible
  - Due to acoustic scattering
  - Shadowing when densely calcified
- Uncommon: "Silicone cyst", anechoic, due to focal collection of gel

MR Findings
- Silicone only sequence
  - Usually FS (inversion recovery) with water suppression
  - Only high signal comes from silicone
- T2WI: Assess bilateral implant integrity or rupture

Imaging Recommendations
- Best imaging tool: Ultrasound demonstration of "snowstorm" highly specific for extracapsular silicone

DIFFERENTIAL DIAGNOSIS

Mass Adjacent to Implant
- Carcinoma
- Fat necrosis/scar
- Fibroadenoma or other benign mass

Fluid Adjacent to Implant
- Cyst: Simple or complicated
- Hematoma/seroma

DDx: Mass or Fluid Adjacent to Implant

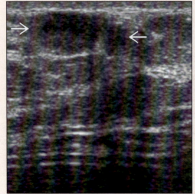

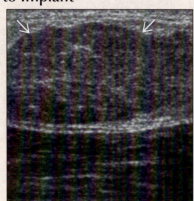

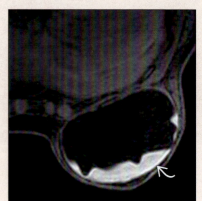

Invasive Cancer

Ductal Carcinoma in Situ

Hematoma (T1WI FS, Silicone Sat)

SILICONE GRANULOMA

Key Facts

Terminology
- Silicone granuloma = siliconoma: Inflammatory mass caused by foreign body reaction to silicone gel in tissue

Imaging Findings
- Location: Most often at edge of implant or in axilla
- Dense, circumscribed mass ± rim calcifications (Ca++)
- "Snowstorm": Mass of echogenic noise on US

Clinical Issues
- Brachial plexus involvement with granulomatous process may cause neuropathy
- Correlates with ↑ incidence fibromyalgia

Diagnostic Checklist
- Siliconoma nearly universally implies "extracapsular" rupture of current or prior silicone implant

---

- Abscess

PATHOLOGY

Microscopic Features
- Foreign body giant cells with asteroid bodies
- Non-specific inflammatory infiltrate and fibrosis
- Silicone itself usually lost in processing

CLINICAL ISSUES

Presentation
- Most common signs/symptoms
  - Asymptomatic, detected mammographically
  - Palpable mass in augmented/reconstructed breast
  - Palpable axillary adenopathy: Biopsy mandatory
    - 25-33% of patients had cancer in addition to silicone granulomata (one series)

Natural History & Prognosis
- If silicone migrates beyond implant it is not biologically inert
  - Granulomatous reaction → tender, hard, inflammatory mass in chest wall musculature, axilla, arm or abdominal wall
  - Brachial plexus involvement with granulomatous process may cause neuropathy
- Correlates with ↑ incidence fibromyalgia
- American College of Rheumatology 1992: No causal relationship to any defined autoimmune syndromes

- No malignant potential

Treatment
- Excision if symptomatic

DIAGNOSTIC CHECKLIST

Consider
- Ask for history of closed capsulotomy
  - May precipitate extracapsular rupture of implant

Image Interpretation Pearls
- Siliconoma nearly universally implies "extracapsular" rupture of current or prior silicone implant
  - Very rare: Microscopic gel bleed through intact implant shell sufficient to cause silicone granuloma

SELECTED REFERENCES

1. Berg WA et al: MR imaging of extracapsular silicone from breast implants: diagnostic pitfalls. AJR. 178:465-72, 2002
2. Brown SL et al: Silicone gel breast implant rupture, extracapsular silicone, and health status in a population of women. J Rheumatol. 28:996-1003, 2001
3. Caskey CI et al: Imaging spectrum of extracapsular silicone: correlation of US, MR imaging, mammographic, and histopathologic findings. Radiographics. 19 Spec No:S39-51; quiz S261-2, 1999
4. Kulber DA et al: Monitoring the axilla in patients with silicone gel implants. Ann Plast Surg. 35:580-4, 1995
5. Harris KM et al: Silicone implant rupture: detection with US. Radiology. 187:761-8, 1993

IMAGE GALLERY

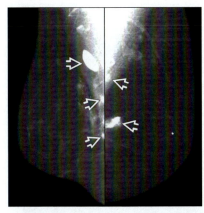
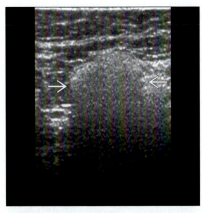
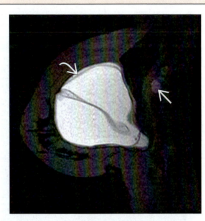

(Left) MLO mammography in a 55 y/o years after removal of ruptured silicone implants demonstrates dense masses ⮞ in both breasts, typical of silicone granulomata. *(Center)* Sagittal ultrasound of left axilla in a 56 y/o shows classic "snowstorm" appearance ⮞ of silicone granuloma, within an axillary node. *(Right)* Sagittal water-suppressed STIR MR (silicone only sequence, same patient as prior image) shows axillary node ⮞ with high signal, confirming silicone. "Subcapsular line sign" ⮞ of minimally collapsed silicone implant rupture is also noted.

ACCELERATED PARTIAL BREAST IRRADIATION

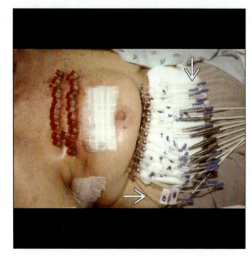

Clinical photograph shows multiple interstitial brachytherapy catheters ➡. Five consecutive days of treatment delivered a total dose of 34 Gy (two 3.4 Gy fractions daily, separated by at least 6 hours).

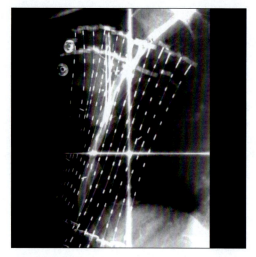

Lateral radiograph oblique (same case as left image) verifies at simulation the proper position of the multiple catheters placed 1 cm apart from each other for brachytherapy.

TERMINOLOGY

Abbreviations and Synonyms
- Accelerated partial breast irradiation (APBI), partial breast irradiation (PBI)
  - Accelerated external beam (3D conformal) radiotherapy (XRT)
  - Interstitial (within tissue) brachytherapy
  - Intracavitary, or, balloon brachytherapy
  - Intra-operative XRT (IORT)

Definitions
- APBI = short course of intra-operative and/or post-operative XRT lasting 1-10 days
- Radiation focused on the lumpectomy cavity plus 1-2 cm margin surrounding the postsurgical cavity
  - Goal is to provide equal tumor cell toxicity as in conventional adjuvant XRT following breast conserving surgery
  - Minimize radiation to normal tissue
  - Rationale: Approximately 95% of tumor recurrences occur at or within 2 cm of the lumpectomy site, 2-7 years after treatment

- Focusing radiation treatment to this vulnerable region may be beneficial
- Brachytherapy: Therapeutic range in mm
  - Radioactive isotope delivers the XRT at a short distance form the source thus limiting dose to normal tissue
- Brachytherapy principles
  - Radioactive materials are placed directly into or near the operated site
    - Radioactive materials may be within needles, seeds, wires, or catheters
  - One or few fractions; variable dose rates, energies, shielding
- Interstitial brachytherapy
  - Multiple catheters placed within tissue 1 cm apart encompassing post-lumpectomy area to be treated
    - Average 16 catheters per treatment site
  - High dose rate therapy for a total dose ~ 34 Gy in 8-10 fractions
  - Treatment given in two daily fractions separated by at least 6 hours for a total of 5 days
- Intracavitary, balloon brachytherapy

DDx: Changes Associated with Whole Breast Irradiation (WBI)

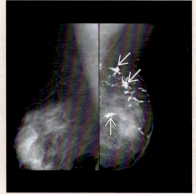

Dystrophic Ca++

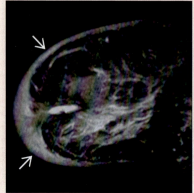

Skin Thickening

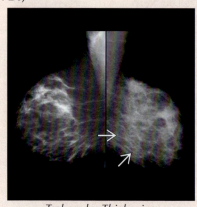

Trabecular Thickening

ACCELERATED PARTIAL BREAST IRRADIATION

Key Facts

Terminology
- Intra-operative XRT (IORT)
- APBI = short course of intra-operative and/or post-operative XRT lasting 1-10 days
- Radiation focused on the lumpectomy cavity plus 1-2 cm margin surrounding the postsurgical cavity
- Interstitial brachytherapy
- Intracavitary, balloon brachytherapy
- External beam 3D conformal intensive modulated radiation therapy (IMRP)

Imaging Findings
- Post-treatment mammography = skin thickening, trabecular coarsening, increased density
- Similar characteristics to adjuvant XRT following breast conserving surgery, but often conform to geographic treated area

Top Differential Diagnoses
- Breast Conserving Therapy
- Mastitis: Typically in lactating women
- Blunt trauma: As in seat belt injuries, trabecular thickening, increased density in traumatized tissue
- Locally advanced or inflammatory breast cancer: May be confused with mastitis

Clinical Issues
- Inclusion Criteria: NSABP Protocol B-39, Radiation Therapy Oncology Group (RTOG) Protocol 413
- AJCC stage 0, I or II treated with lumpectomy with negative margins eligible
- Lesion size ≤ 3 cm; 0 to 3 positive axillary nodes
- No suspicious Ca++ in ipsilateral or contralateral breast

- Balloon placed intra- or post-operatively within lumpectomy site and inflated with 50-70 cc saline and contrast
- Satisfactory device placement confirmed by ultrasound or computer optimized treatment CT
- High dose radiation (HDR) afterloader used to place an Iridium-192 source at the balloon center
- Dosing is typically twice daily for 5 days = 34 Gy in 10 fractions
- External beam 3D conformal intensive modulated radiation therapy (IMRP)
  - External beam restricted to lumpectomy site and immediate surrounding tissue
  - Breast and skin can tolerate a higher focal dose over a shortened period of time
- IORT
  - Single fraction ≈ 21 Gy delivered in operating room immediately following lumpectomy
  - Requires careful lesion selection and no evidence of multifocal or multicentric disease
  - Treatment delivered before final pathologic assessment of margins is available; if margins positive, need whole breast XRT in addition

IMAGING FINDINGS

General Features
- Best diagnostic clue
  - Post-treatment mammography = skin thickening, trabecular coarsening, increased density
    - Similar characteristics to adjuvant XRT following breast conserving surgery, but often conform to geographic treated area

Mammographic Findings
- Pre-treatment imaging essential for lesion selection
- Post-treatment surveillance mammography
  - Post-treatment mammogram standard MLO and CC views with or without ML
  - Post interstitial brachytherapy, 41% abnormal mammograms: Architectural distortion or suspicious Ca++ (single study)

- 17% underwent biopsy with all showing fat necrosis or post XRT changes
  - Post IORT, early appearance of round and punctate Ca++ at site, likely related to directed radiation treatment

Ultrasonographic Findings
- Post-lumpectomy site visible for months to years
- Seroma: Cystic or complex cystic (mixed fluid and solid components)
  - Irregular, hypoechoic margin typical; track visible to overlying incision

MR Findings
- T1WI
  - Post-operative changes may be apparent
    - Architectural distortion, skin thickening and retraction, hemosiderin deposits, signal voids in areas of surgical staples, post-biopsy clips
- T2WI FS: Postsurgical seromas typically hyperintense
- T1 C+ FS
  - Pre-treatment MR to optimize lesion selection
    - Size, exclude additional foci
  - Post-treatment MR findings
    - Benign skin enhancement from recent lumpectomy and XRT
    - Post XRT lumpectomy site (scar) enhancement may be seen for ≥ 18 months
    - Smooth, persistent enhancement of thin rim (≤ 4 mm) around seroma
    - 54% of 14 women treated with pre-operative chemotherapy and brachytherapy demonstrated diffuse but transient (< 3 months) parenchymal enhancement following radiation therapy (single study)

Imaging Recommendations
- Best imaging tool: Post-treatment diagnostic mammography
- Protocol advice
  - Prior to surgery and APBI
    - Bilateral diagnostic mammography, including magnification views of any suspicious findings

ACCELERATED PARTIAL BREAST IRRADIATION

- Targeted or whole breast US as needed
- Optional: Contrast-enhanced MR to evaluate disease extent
- Biopsy of any suspicious areas, establish cancer is unifocal
  - Following APBI
    - Protocols vary; baseline mammogram then q 6 months x 2 years
    - Lumpectomy site may require magnification views (CC and ML or LM) to characterize Ca++
    - MR can be used to aid differentiation of postsurgical scar from residual or recurrent carcinoma

DIFFERENTIAL DIAGNOSIS

Breast Conserving Therapy

- "Gold standard" for conservation of the breast
- Surgical excision (lumpectomy or quadrantectomy) with tumor-free margins
  - Followed by 45 Gy whole breast irradiation (WBI) ± 16 Gy electron boost to cavity site and small margin
- Post-treatment mammogram shows entire breast affected by generic findings of edema
  - Skin and trabecular thickening, diffuse increase in breast density
  - Dystrophic Ca++ (fat necrosis) may develop over 2-5 years typically in lumpectomy site

Other Causes of Unilateral Breast Edema

- Mastitis: Typically in lactating women
- Blunt trauma: As in seat belt injuries, trabecular thickening, increased density in traumatized tissue
  - Fat necrosis may be seen as sequela of the trauma
- Locally advanced or inflammatory breast cancer: May be confused with mastitis
  - Imaging may not demonstrate a dominant mass or focal suspicious finding
- Unilateral vascular or lymphatic obstruction: Axillary adenopathy; venous occlusive disease
- Asymmetric edema: Congestive heart failure

Recurrence or New Primary Carcinoma

- Increase in density, trabecular thickening, skin changes
- Development of suspicious Ca++ (fine pleomorphic, fine linear) ± suspicious mass

PATHOLOGY

General Features

- Epidemiology: Tissue changes are related primarily to the radiation

Microscopic Features

- Findings in the normal irradiated tissue similar to physiologic atrophy but may contain cytologic atypia
- Atypia of stromal fibroblasts and fat necrosis more common in the areas where XRT boosts are given following whole breast XRT and may be more common in APBI-treated tissue

CLINICAL ISSUES

Presentation

- Most common signs/symptoms: Skin thickening and discoloration secondary to radiation

Natural History & Prognosis

- Findings worst at initial 6 month mammogram; should stabilize after 18 months to 2 years

Treatment

- Inclusion Criteria: NSABP Protocol B-39, Radiation Therapy Oncology Group (RTOG) Protocol 413
  - AJCC stage 0, I or II treated with lumpectomy with negative margins eligible
  - Lesion size ≤ 3 cm; 0 to 3 positive axillary nodes
  - No suspicious Ca++ in ipsilateral or contralateral breast
- Exclusion criteria
  - Multicentric carcinoma (disease in more than one quadrant or separated by ≥ 4 cm)
  - Distant metastases, pregnancy or lactation
  - Skin involvement, Paget disease, previously treated breast carcinoma
  - Co-morbid disease with life expectancy < 2 years
  - Collagen vascular disease (specifically dermatomyositis); active skin rash
- Recurrence following APBI is treated in a similar fashion to recurrence following breast conserving surgery and adjuvant XRT
  - Mastectomy typical as XRT cannot be given again

DIAGNOSTIC CHECKLIST

Consider

- Possible exclusion criteria for APBI
  - Positive margins, diffuse disease, positive nodes, lymphovascular invasion, pure DCIS, extensive intraductal component (EIC), pure invasive lobular carcinoma, age ≤ 40
- Unknown risk of low-level radiation at edges of the treated field possibly inducing cancer

SELECTED REFERENCES

1. Dirbas FM et al: The evolution of accelerated partial breast irradiation as a potential treatment option for women with newly diagnosed breast cancer considering breast conservation. Cancer Biotherapy & Radiopharmaceuticals. 19:673-705, 2004
2. Lawenda B et al: Dose-volume analysis of radiotherapy for T1N0 invasive breast cancer treated by local excision and partial breast irradiation by low-dose-rate interstitial implant. Int J Radiat Oncol Biol Phys. 56:671-80, 2003
3. Hlawatsch A et al: MR mammography of response-control in primary chemo-brachytherapy in BCT-inoperable breast cancer. Rofo. 173:31-7, 2001

IMAGE GALLERY

Typical

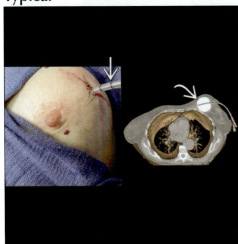

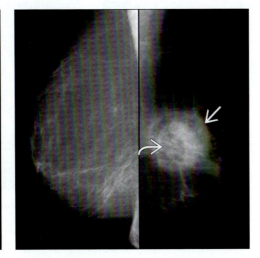

(Left) Clinical photograph (left) shows the external catheter ➡ of an intra-operatively-placed MammoSite™ brachytherapy balloon. Schematic 3D reconstructed CT (right) of the balloon placement ➡ (Courtesy Cytyc Corp). *(Right)* MLO mammography in a 62 y/o woman post intracavitary balloon brachytherapy shows a round fat-containing (fat necrosis) ➡ post-operative site ➡ representing the irradiated region. BI-RADS 2, benign.

Typical

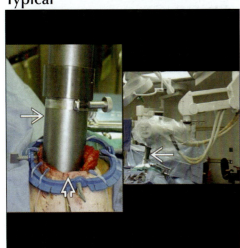

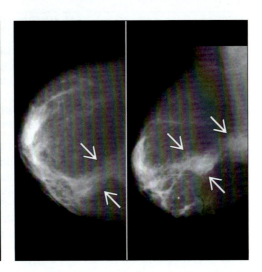

(Left) Intra-operative photographs show linear accelerator collimator ➡ within operative site ➡. Single fraction 21 Gy IORT was administered. Mammograms are shown (same case, right images). (Courtesy FMD). *(Right)* Mammography (CC and MLO) 6 months after IORT shows band of trabecular thickening and increased density ➡ extending anteroposteriorly similar in distribution to the original cylindrical collimator position. BI-RADS 2, benign.

Typical

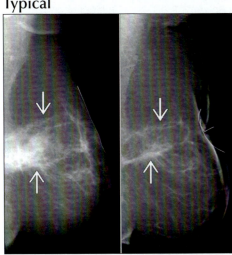

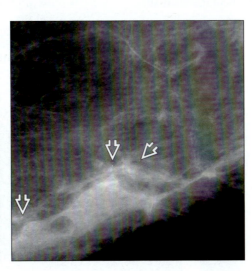

(Left) MLO views (left side) 6 months post treatment for 1.2 cm IDC with IORT shows cylindrical shaped increased density ➡ & trabecular thickening conforming to collimator position. Right side shows diminution of findings ➡ at 1 yr. *(Right)* CC magnification (IORT treated, different case) shows early appearance of punctate calcifications ➡ within treated area likely related to tissue response to single fraction radiation dose. BI-RADS 2, benign.

MYOCUTANEOUS FLAP RECONSTRUCTION

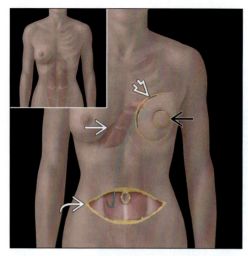

Graphic of TRAM flap reconstruction. Elliptical skin/subcutaneous tissue ➔ on contralateral rectus muscle pedicle ➔ is tunneled (green arrow) to form neobreast ➔. Nipple/areola ➔ are tattooed later.

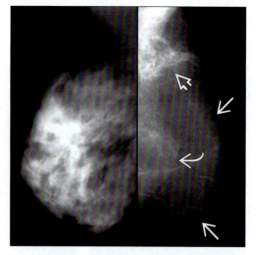

MLO mammography shows the transposed abdominal wall fat ➔ and muscle pedicle ➔ of the TRAM flap. Focal asymmetry and peripheral calcifications ➔ are typical of fat necrosis.

TERMINOLOGY

Abbreviations and Synonyms

- Autologous tissue breast reconstruction
  - Transverse rectus abdominus myocutaneous (TRAM) pedicle and free flaps
  - Deep inferior epigastric perforator (DIEP) flap
  - Latissimus dorsi myocutaneous (LDM) flap
  - Gluteal free flap, inferior gluteal flap, superior gluteal artery perforator (S-GAP) flap
  - Others: Lateral transverse thigh flap; Rubens or periiliac flap
- Neobreast

Definitions

- Autologous breast tissue reconstruction
  - Includes overlying fat and tissue as well as muscle pedicle
  - DIEP flap: Only skin and subcutaneous tissue transferred
  - Flaps may be used alone or in combination with breast implant (usually silicone)

IMAGING FINDINGS

General Features

- Best diagnostic clue
  - Predominantly fatty tissue in neobreast (± implant if used)
    - No normal glandular tissue (unless LDM flap used with partial mastectomy)

Mammographic Findings

- Anatomy differs from normal breast
  - Predominantly fatty neobreast
    - Absence of normal glandular tissue and architecture
  - No nipple-areolar complex
  - Underlying muscle pedicle may be visible posteriorly on mammogram
    - Underlying muscle pedicle absent in DIEP flap
- Common post-flap mammographic findings
  - Fat necrosis
    - Centrally lucent mass, peripheral density
    - Curvilinear and dystrophic calcifications (Ca++) typically develop 2-5 years after surgery

IV

4

42

DDx: Other "Altered Breast" Post-Operative Appearances

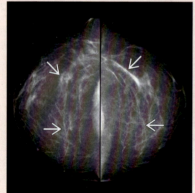

Breast Reduction

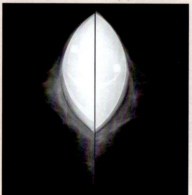

Augmentation

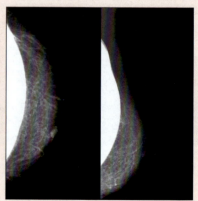

Mastectomy, Silicone Implantation

MYOCUTANEOUS FLAP RECONSTRUCTION

Key Facts

Terminology
- Autologous breast tissue reconstruction

Imaging Findings
- Predominantly fatty tissue in neobreast (± implant if used)
- Absence of normal glandular tissue and architecture
- Underlying muscle pedicle may be visible posteriorly on mammogram

Top Differential Diagnoses
- TRAM flaps
- LDM flap
- Gluteal free flap
- Reduction Mammoplasty
- Predominantly Fatty Breast Parenchyma
- Implant Reconstruction

Pathology
- Epidemiology: 4-11% TRAM flap patients develop recurrence
- Lack of lymphatic anastomoses predisposes to edema

Clinical Issues
- Possible increased risk recurrence with immediate flap reconstruction: Positive margins more common
- Generally XRT prior to reconstruction is preferred
- Avoid traversing flap vascular supply

Diagnostic Checklist
- Annual mammographic surveillance routinely performed at some centers, not in others
- Recurrence in post-TRAM breast has appearance similar to primary breast carcinoma

---

- Often upper outer quadrant with TRAM flaps: Farthest from vascular pedicle
  - Skin thickening early secondary to post-operative edema
- Recurrent malignancy typically at chest wall
  - Appearance similar to primary breast carcinoma
    - New density, mass, suspicious Ca++

Ultrasonographic Findings
- Grayscale Ultrasound
  - Diffuse fatty tissue throughout neobreast
  - Lack of normal glandular tissue and architecture
  - May demonstrate fluid collections post-op
- Color Doppler: May demonstrate flow through vascular pedicle

MR Findings
- T1WI
  - Ipsi- or contralateral muscle absence/atrophy
    - Seen on large field-of-view images (i.e. localizer sequence, abdominal/pelvic MR)
  - Fatty tissue of neobreast hyperintense
  - Hypointense underlying muscle pedicle may be visualized inferoposteriorly
  - De-epithelialized portion of flap surface may be visible deep to native breast skin surface
    - Thin hypointense line
- T2WI FS: Edema hyperintense
- T1 C+ FS: Vascular pedicle will enhance
- Post-operative findings
  - Post-surgical hematoma
    - Early finding: Hyperintense on T1WI & T2WI
    - Late finding: May have hypointense hemosiderin rim
  - Seroma
    - Hyperintense collection on T2WI
    - Smooth rim-enhancement around seroma
  - Skin thickening, edema
    - Diffusely hyperintense on T2WI
  - Fat necrosis
    - Hyperintense on precontrast T1WI
    - Peripherally hypointense on STIR
    - Persistent enhancement

- Correlate with mammogram
  - Scarring, fibrosis
    - Hypointense on all sequences
- Findings suspicious for recurrence
  - Early, rapid enhancement; delayed washout
  - Chest wall enhancement concerning for recurrence
- Findings favoring inflammatory carcinoma over skin edema
  - Both are T2-hyperintense and T1-hypointense
  - Enhancement key to differentiation
    - Diffuse enhancement prominent finding in inflammatory carcinoma
    - Post-surgical enhancement decreases over time

CT Findings
- NECT
  - Predominantly fatty neobreast
  - Underlying muscle pedicle traceable to origin on sequential images
  - Absence/atrophy of ipsi- or contralateral muscle
    - Rectus abdominus, latissimus dorsi, gluteus
    - Ventral hernia may occur

Imaging Recommendations
- Best imaging tool
  - Mammography may detect non-palpable findings including Ca++
  - Time course of MR findings may distinguish post-surgical changes from recurrence
    - US useful to investigate new palpable finding
  - Mammography, US, and MR imaging each may help detect recurrence in reconstruction bed
    - MR enables visualization of chest wall recurrence more readily than mammography

---

DIFFERENTIAL DIAGNOSIS

Myocutaneous Flaps
- TRAM flaps
  - TRAM pedicle flap
    - Uses the entire rectus muscle from one side

MYOCUTANEOUS FLAP RECONSTRUCTION

- Blood flow provided by the superior epigastric vessels
  - Free TRAM pedicle flap
    - Based on the deep inferior epigastric vessels
    - Created to improve blood supply and limit the extensive dissection of a full TRAM pedicle flap procedure
  - DIEP flap: Skin/subcutaneous tissue only
- LDM flap
  - May require implant in addition to flap to achieve adequate volume
- Gluteal free flap
  - Technically most challenging, often staged procedure if bilateral

Reduction Mammoplasty

- Architectural distortion and inferior scar position may mimic flap
- Breast tissue and nipple present

Predominantly Fatty Breast Parenchyma

- Normal pectoralis, lack of surgical changes, normal vascular supply

Implant Reconstruction

- Saline and silicone density higher than that of transposed muscle

PATHOLOGY

General Features

- Etiology
  - Recurrence due to multiple mechanisms
    - Incomplete resection, positive margins
    - Lack of external beam radiation therapy (XRT)
    - Systemic disease spread
    - Residual breast tissue (new primary neoplasm)
- Epidemiology: 4-11% TRAM flap patients develop recurrence

Gross Pathologic & Surgical Features

- Lack of lymphatic anastomoses predisposes to edema
  - Exacerbated by XRT
    - Arterial vasodilatation
    - Tissue friability

Microscopic Features

- Findings in recurrent carcinoma similar to those of primary breast carcinoma
  - Recurrence may have predominantly invasive component
  - Recurrence in patient after hormonal therapy may be estrogen and/or progesterone receptor negative

CLINICAL ISSUES

Natural History & Prognosis

- Possible increased risk recurrence with immediate flap reconstruction: Positive margins more common
- No evidence that reconstruction compromises adjuvant chemotherapy
- XRT not necessarily contraindicated post-flap
  - Generally XRT prior to reconstruction is preferred

- Helps restore woman's self image
- Tactile difference compared with mastectomy and implant reconstruction
  - Provides more tissue bulk and a breast mound more akin to an unaltered breast
- Relative contraindications
  - Older age, infirmity
    - Operations are lengthy, invasive, and costly
  - Smoking, obesity, diabetes, hypertension, prior abdominal surgeries

Treatment

- Biopsy warranted for suspicious findings
  - Fat necrosis can mimic cancer recurrence
  - Obtain surgical history prior to biopsy of possible recurrence
    - Avoid traversing flap vascular supply

DIAGNOSTIC CHECKLIST

Consider

- Post-TRAM flap mammographic surveillance is controversial
  - Annual mammographic surveillance routinely performed at some centers, not in others
  - Chest wall lesion detection difficult except by MR

Image Interpretation Pearls

- Recurrence in post-TRAM breast has appearance similar to primary breast carcinoma

SELECTED REFERENCES

1. Bassett LW et al: Diagnosis of Diseases of the Breast. 2nd ed. Philadelphia, Elsevier Saunders. Chapter 30, 574-5, 2005
2. Morris EA et al: Breast MR Diagnosis and Intervention. Springer, New York. Chapter 26, 486-7, 2005
3. Devon RK et al: Breast reconstruction with a transverse rectus abdominis myocutaneous flap: spectrum of normal and abnormal MR imaging findings. Radiographics. 24(5):1287-99, 2004
4. Mehta VK et al: Postmastectomy radiation therapy after TRAM flap breast reconstruction. Breast J. 10(2):118-22, 2004
5. Helvie MA et al: Mammographic screening of TRAM flap breast reconstructions for detection of nonpalpable recurrent cancer. Radiology. 224(1):211-6, 2002
6. Harris JR et al: Diseases of the Breast. 2nd ed. Philadelphia, Lippincott Williams & Wilkins. Chapter 34, 562-73, 2000

MYOCUTANEOUS FLAP RECONSTRUCTION

IMAGE GALLERY

Typical

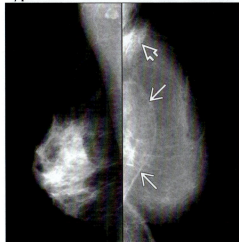 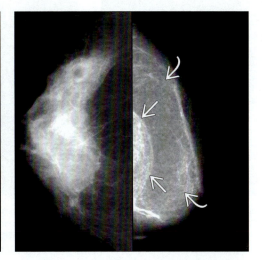

(Left) MLO mammography demonstrates an unaltered right breast and a TRAM reconstructed left breast. The rectus muscle pedicle ➡ is visible. A healing benign biopsy site ➡ is seen superiorly. *(Right)* CC mammography (same patient as left) again shows the neobreast of the TRAM flap reconstruction characterized by anterior fat ➡ and the posterior rectus pedicle ➡.

Typical

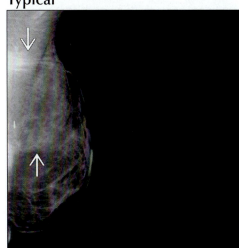 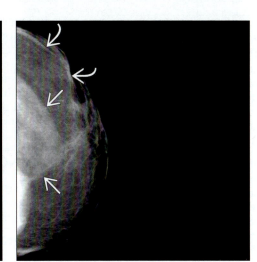

(Left) MLO mammography demonstrates a portion of a lower latissimus dorsi muscle ➡ used to reconstruct the lateral aspect of this partial mastectomy. *(Right)* CC mammography (same patient as left) again demonstrates findings of latissimus dorsi reconstruction, including a portion of the lower latissimus dorsi muscle ➡ and skin and subcutaneous tissue ➡.

Typical

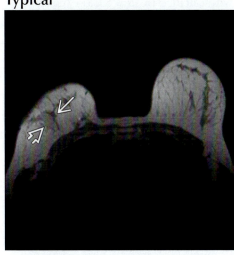 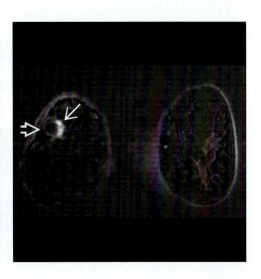

(Left) Axial T1WI MR shows a hyperintense mass ➡ consistent with fat necrosis adjacent to a palpable area of soft tissue ➡ in a TRAM reconstruction. Palpable area = recurrent IDC. (C+ scan, right image). *(Right)* Coronal T1 C+ subtraction MR at the level of the palpable mass shows the known invasive ductal carcinoma (IDC) as a crescentic enhancing mass ➡ along the medial aspect of the rounded nonenhancing mass due to fat necrosis ➡.

POSITIVE MARGINS

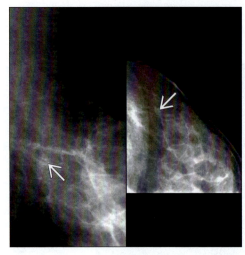

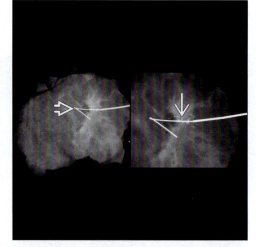

MLO and CC mammography shows a small cluster of residual calcifications ➡ following a bracket wire localization excision for percutaneously proven invasive carcinoma with DCIS.

Specimen mammography magnification (of the same case as previous image) following re-excision shows the distal hookwire ➡ and the targeted Ca++ ➡ shown at pathology to be DCIS with negative margins.

TERMINOLOGY

Abbreviations and Synonyms
- Breast-conserving treatment (BCT) = Breast-conserving surgery (BCS) followed by radiation therapy (XRT)
- Ductal carcinoma in situ (DCIS) = Intraductal carcinoma
- Infiltrating lobular carcinoma (ILC)

Definitions
- Positive margin: Presence of invasive carcinoma or DCIS directly at the inked surface of resection
- Focally positive margin: Cancer at the margin in ≤ 3 low-power microscopic fields
- True margin: Edge of resected tissue which directly faces the tissue remaining in the patient
- Close margins: Variably defined as cancer < 1, 2, or 3 mm from inked surface
  - May not be relevant for invasive carcinoma where any negative margin is negative
- Cavity margin: Additional tissue taken from the edges of the lumpectomy cavity
  - If true margin of cavity margins is negative for cancer, then margins are negative
- Shaved margin: Specimen edge is shaved, allowing examination of large portion of margin
  - Tumor cells in any piece considered positive margin
  - May overestimate positive margins as tumor cells in shaved piece may not be at true margin
- EIC: Intraductal carcinoma represents at least 25% of an at least microscopically invasive main tumor mass, with satellite foci of DCIS in adjacent tissue

IMAGING FINDINGS

General Features
- Best diagnostic clue: Residual suspicious calcifications (Ca++) ± mass at the lumpectomy site

Mammographic Findings
- If original malignancy manifest as Ca++, residual Ca++ highly predictive of residual tumor: PPV 69%
  - In women with calcified DCIS, > 5 Ca++ highly predictive of residual DCIS with PPV 90%
- Difficult to distinguish residual mass from post-surgical changes/seroma

DDx: Post-Lumpectomy Seromas

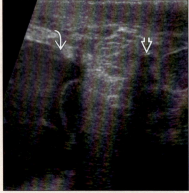

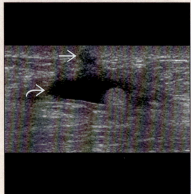

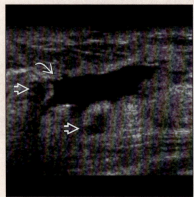

Residual Tubular Carcinoma

Benign

Residual Foci ILC

POSITIVE MARGINS

Key Facts

Terminology
- Positive margin: Presence of invasive carcinoma or DCIS directly at the inked surface of resection
- Close margins: Variably defined as cancer < 1, 2, or 3 mm from inked surface

Imaging Findings
- Intra-operative US ↓ risk of positive margins
- CC and 90° lateral magnification mammographic views: Determine extent of residual Ca++ if any
- MRI can help determine need for mastectomy vs. re-excision for margins

Pathology
- Highly variable reports of initial prevalence at lumpectomy: 15-35%
- ↑ Positive margins with: EIC, DCIS, ILC

- ↑ With larger primary tumor, > 2 cm and esp. > 5 cm

Clinical Issues
- Residual tumor at re-excision in 35-75%
- 7% recurrence at 8 yrs when margins negative
- 14% recurrence rate with focally positive margins
- Local recurrence: ↑ Risk systemic recurrence & death
- Lumpectomy with positive margins → re-excision of margins or mastectomy
- Positive margins at mastectomy: Indication for post-mastectomy XRT

Diagnostic Checklist
- Goal of imaging patients with positive margins is to exclude large and/or remote residual tumor
- Reexcision of margins needed even if imaging negative

Ultrasonographic Findings
- Grayscale Ultrasound
  - Normal lumpectomy site: Simple or complex collection, with track to overlying skin incision
  - Abnormal, suspicious findings: Focal convex mass along cavity; suspicious mass elsewhere in breast

MR Findings
- T1WI
  - Hematoma typically hyperintense
  - Skin thickening, distortion, clip artifacts
- T2WI FS: Fluid-filled lumpectomy site is bright on T2
- Inaccurate in assessing lumpectomy site margins per se: 61% sensitivity overall
  - Thin, smooth ≤ 4 mm rim of enhancement around seroma is a normal finding, does not exclude microscopic residual tumor
    - Granulation tissue can enhance up to 18 months post-op, longer if fat necrosis
  - Irregular mass or clumped, focal nodular enhancement along margin favors residual tumor
- Emphasis is on remainder of breast to exclude multifocal/multicentric disease
  - One series: 23% of breasts had remote suspicious area on MRI: 33% of those malignant, for prevalence of remote cancer = 7%

Nuclear Medicine Findings
- PET: Whole body FDG PET used for staging, may detect unknown metastatic disease, alter treatment

Imaging Recommendations
- Best imaging tool
  - Workup prior to initial surgery to assess extent, including magnification views of Ca++
    - Pre-operative MRI may ↓ risk of positive margins
  - Intra-operative US ↓ risk of positive margins
  - Mammogram as soon after surgery as patient able to tolerate (usually ~ 4 weeks)
  - CC and 90° lateral magnification mammographic views: Determine extent of residual Ca++ if any
- Protocol advice

- If not performed prior to initial surgery, MR can help define extent of residual bulk tumor and detect additional remote tumor foci
  - MRI can help determine need for mastectomy vs. re-excision for margins
  - Due to substantial risk of false positives on MRI, biopsy of remote suspicious area generally necessary prior to mastectomy
  - ↓ False positives if MR performed 28-35 days post-op, but can image as soon as patient can tolerate
  - Contralateral breast US or MRI: 4-6% rate of mammographically & clinically occult cancer

DIFFERENTIAL DIAGNOSIS

Post-Operative Hematoma/Seroma
- Spiculated mass with distortion
- US: Cystic or complex cystic mass connecting to skin

Trauma
- Ill-defined mass/asymmetry, edema
- In the right clinical setting, close interval imaging surveillance rather than biopsy is appropriate

Fat Necrosis
- Ca++ typically not seen until 2-5 yrs post-op or post-trauma

PATHOLOGY

General Features
- Etiology
  - Underestimate extent on pre-operative (± intra-operative) clinical and imaging evaluation
    - Some cases of DCIS lack Ca++ or partially calcified
    - Esp. low-grade and micropapillary DCIS, high frequency of small skip areas (multifocality)
    - ILC extent often underestimated, more often multifocal than invasive ductal carcinoma
- Epidemiology

POSITIVE MARGINS

- ○ Highly variable reports of initial prevalence at lumpectomy: 15-35%
- ○ ↑ Positive margins with: EIC, DCIS, ILC
- ○ ↑ With larger primary tumor, > 2 cm and esp. > 5 cm
- ○ Young age predictive of positive margins, ↑ risk residual tumor at re-excision, and ↑ risk recurrence

Gross Pathologic & Surgical Features

- Specimen is oriented by surgeon at excision
  - ○ Intact specimen is inked by surgeon or pathologist and sections are prepared perpendicular to inked surface (i.e., margin)
    - ■ Can use different color inks on each surface
  - ○ Distance from cancer to margin is measured
  - ○ Pathologist reports which margin(s) show cancer
- Intraoperative frozen section may be used to determine margin status
  - ○ False negative rates to distinguish malignant cells range from 0.1-4.4%
  - ○ Sensitivity = 83-91%; specificity 86-100%

Microscopic Features

- Cancer cells at inked surface of excision

Staging, Grading or Classification Criteria

- Finding additional tumor at or away from initial lumpectomy site may alter tumor grade and/or stage and affect treatment

CLINICAL ISSUES

Presentation

- Most common signs/symptoms: Large primary tumor predicts positive margins

Natural History & Prognosis

- Residual tumor at re-excision in 35-75%
  - ○ ↑ If EIC, more than focally positive, young age
- Obtaining cavity margins greatly ↓ need for re-excision
- ↑ Local recurrence after XRT if positive margins, particularly true or marginal recurrence at original site, usually in first 5 yrs
  - ○ 7% recurrence at 8 yrs when margins negative
  - ○ 7% recurrence rate with margins < 1 mm
  - ○ 14% recurrence rate with focally positive margins
  - ○ 27% recurrence rate with more than focally positive margins
- ↓ Recurrence rates by ≥ 50% if adjuvant chemo- and/or hormonal therapy given in addition to XRT, even with positive margins
- Local recurrence: ↑ Risk systemic recurrence & death

Treatment

- Lumpectomy with positive margins → re-excision of margins or mastectomy
  - ○ Positive deep margin may not be re-excised if initial resection carried down to pectoral fascia
- Re-excision with or without imaging direction
- Multicentric disease is best treated with mastectomy
- Neoadjuvant chemotherapy may shrink tumor and ↑ rate of clear margins with T3 and larger T2 tumors
- Positive margins at mastectomy: Indication for post-mastectomy XRT

DIAGNOSTIC CHECKLIST

Consider

- Ink can penetrate crevices of specimen/tumor → false positive margins
- Pre-operative MR when core biopsy shows ILC or suggests EIC
- Image-guided bracketing of areas of Ca++ > 2 cm using > 1 localization wire may assist in removal of all Ca++
  - ○ Does not assure negative margins: Only 44% clear

Image Interpretation Pearls

- Goal of imaging patients with positive margins is to exclude large and/or remote residual tumor
- Reexcision of margins needed even if imaging negative

SELECTED REFERENCES

1. Morris EA et al: Breast MRI: Diagnosis and Intervention. Springer, New York. 166, 214-26, 2005
2. Chagpar AB et al: Lumpectomy margins are affected by tumor size and histologic subtype but not by biopsy technique. Am J Surg. 188:399-402, 2004
3. Keskek M et al: Factors predisposing to cavity margin positivity following conservation surgery for breast cancer. Eur J Surg Oncol. 30:1058-64, 2004
4. Lee JM et al: MRI before reexcision surgery in patients with breast cancer. AJR. 182:473-80, 2004
5. Dizendorf EV et al: Impact of whole-body 18F-FDG PET on staging and managing patients for radiation therapy. J Nucl Med. 44:24-29, 2003
6. Meric F: Positive surgical margins and ipsilateral breast tumor recurrence predict disease-specific survival after breast-conserving therapy. Cancer. 97:926-33, 2003
7. Singletary SE et al: Surgical margins in patients with early-stage breast cancer treated with breast conservation therapy. Am J Surg. 184:383-93, 2002
8. Liberman L et al: Bracketing wires for preoperative breast needle localization. AJR. 177:565-72, 2001
9. Frei KA et al: MR imaging of the breast in patients with positive margins after lumpectomy: influence of the time interval between lumpectomy and MR imaging. AJR. 175:1577-84, 2000
10. Moore MM et al: Association of infiltrating lobular carcinoma with positive surgical margins after breast-conservation therapy. Ann Surg. 231:877-82, 2000
11. Park CC et al: Outcome at 8 years after breast-conserving surgery and radiation therapy for invasive breast cancer: influence of margin status and systemic therapy on local recurrence. J Clin Oncol. 18:1668-75, 2000
12. Waddell BE et al: Postexcision mammography is indicated after resection of ductal carcinoma-in-situ of the breast. Ann Surg Oncol. 7:665-68, 2000
13. Jardines L et al: Factors associated with a positive reexcision after excisional biopsy for invasive breast cancer. Surgery. 18:803-9, 1995
14. Graham RA et al: The efficacy of specimen radiography in evaluating the surgical margins of impalpable breast carcinoma. AJR. 162:33-6, 1994
15. Schnitt SJ et al: The relationship between microscopic margins of resection and the risk of local recurrence in patients with breast cancer treated with breast-conserving surgery and radiation therapy. Cancer. 74:1746-51, 1994
16. Gluck BS et al: Microcalcifications on postoperative mammograms as an indicator of adequacy of tumor excision. Radiology. 188:469-72, 1993

POSITIVE MARGINS

IMAGE GALLERY

Typical

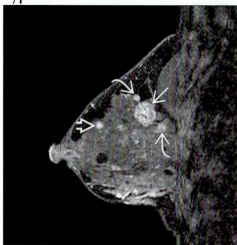
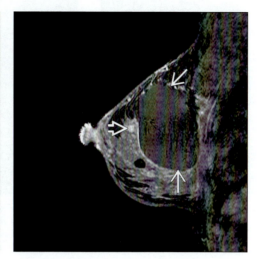

(Left) Sagittal T1 C+ FS MR shows an enhancing mass ➡ with two satellite lesions ⬈. A fourth lesion ⬄ was not included in the surgery. Margins were positive. A pre re-excision MR (right image) was performed. *(Right)* Sagittal T1 C+ FS MR shows the anterior lesion ⬄ adjacent to the lumpectomy site ➡. Pathology confirmed a fourth site of invasive carcinoma anterior to the lumpectomy site.

Typical

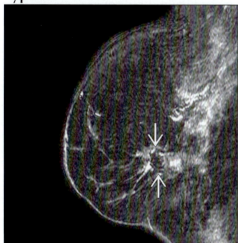
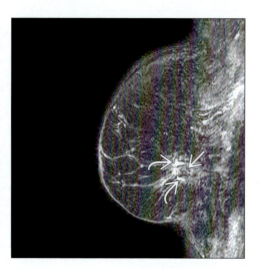

(Left) Sagittal T1 C+ FS MR shows an irregular partially enhancing recent lumpectomy site ➡ in a woman with biopsy proven invasive carcinoma and DCIS. Margins were positive for DCIS. *(Right)* Sagittal T1 C+ FS MR (same case as left image) shows clumped enhancement ⬄ along the anterior margin of the lumpectomy site ➡. Re-excision of lumpectomy site = residual DCIS with negative margins.

Typical

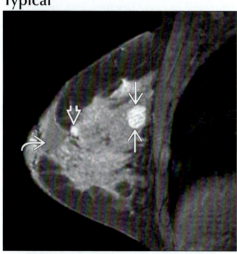
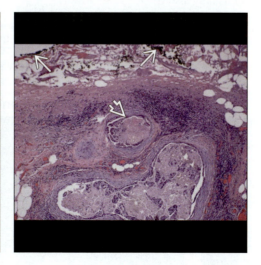

(Left) Sagittal T1 C+ FS MR demonstrates a lumpectomy site ➡ (positive margins) with adjacent enhancing mass ⬄. Both this mass and a mammographically occult enhancing mass ⬄ were carcinoma. (Courtesy DNS). *(Right)* Micropathology, low power, H&E shows high grade DCIS ⬄ < 1 mm away from inked margins ⬄ in a 65 y/o woman s/p biopsy for pleomorphic Ca++ = close margins, usually an indication for reexcision of DCIS.

POST-TREATMENT CHANGES

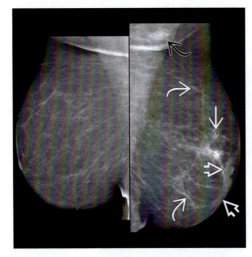

MLO mammography shows early post BCT left breast findings including architectural distortion ➡, trabecular thickening ➡, skin thickening ➡, and axillary scar ➡.

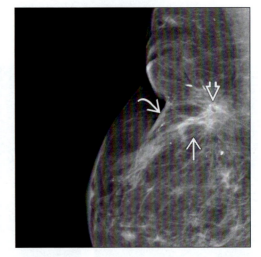

MLO mammography in 82 y/o woman (same patient as previous image) 10 years after BCT shows distortion ➡, focal skin thickening and retraction ➡ at the incision site, and coarse Ca++ ➡ in the upper breast.

TERMINOLOGY

Definitions

- Imaging findings following breast cancer treatment or prophylaxis
- Breast-conserving treatment (BCT), i.e., breast conserving surgery and radiation therapy (XRT)
- Whole breast irradiation (WBI); treatment time course typically 5 days per week over 5-6 weeks
  - Skin tattoos to outline region undergoing treatment
- Boost: Additional radiation treatment to high-risk area, typically the lumpectomy site
- Accelerated partial breast irradiation (APBI)
  - Treatment limited to one to few fractions given over 1-10 days
- Mastectomy: Removal of breast tissue
  - Modified radical mastectomy (MRM), total mastectomy, and skin-sparing mastectomy all remove the breast tissue and usually also the nipple-areolar complex
- Mastectomy with reconstruction: Immediate or delayed reconstructive surgery with implant or autologous tissue, or both

- Expander/implant (saline or silicone or combination) most common method of reconstruction
- Autologous tissue using muscle flap reconstruction; availability and techniques improving
  - Most common: Transverse rectus abdominus myocutaneous (TRAM) flap or latissimus dorsi flap ± implant
  - Nipple reconstruction from autologous tissue; areola tattoo created ~ 2 months later as an outpatient procedure
- Neoadjuvant chemotherapy (NAT)
  - Primary systemic treatment prior to definitive breast surgery (BCT or mastectomy)
- Tamoxifen (TAM): Drug to block estrogen receptors (ER)
  - Most commonly prescribed drug for treatment of breast cancer
    - Both estrogen antagonist and agonist properties
  - ↓ Risk of recurrence of node-negative ER+ breast cancer
    - Node-negative ER+ breast cancer treated with BCT: 3-4% 10 year recurrence with TAM vs. 12-14% 10 year recurrence without TAM

DDx: Calcifications Related to Prior Treatment or Reconstructive Procedures

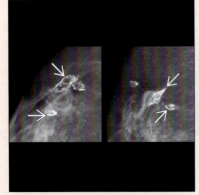

BCT, Coarse Dystrophic Ca++

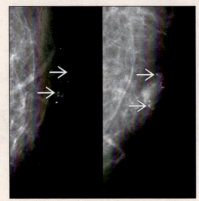

Reconstructed Areola Tattoo

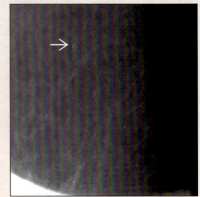

Radiation Port Tattoo

POST-TREATMENT CHANGES

Key Facts

Terminology
- Imaging findings following breast cancer treatment or prophylaxis
- Breast-conserving treatment (BCT), i.e., breast conserving surgery and radiation therapy (XRT)
- Mastectomy: Removal of breast tissue
- Neoadjuvant chemotherapy (NAT)
- Tamoxifen (TAM): Drug to block estrogen receptors (ER)

Imaging Findings
- Breast density may decrease while on TAM
- Mammographic imaging post BCT: Variable protocols
- No standard mammographic follow-up recommended for post-mastectomy or reconstructed breasts

- Monitor NAT-treatment response with mammography ± MR

Top Differential Diagnoses
- Benign Breast Biopsy
- Breast Edema, Unilateral
- Fat Necrosis
- Recurrent Carcinoma

Diagnostic Checklist
- Asymmetry at scar should ↓ over time
- Enlarging, denser scar suspicious
- MR can help distinguish scar from recurrence
- Treated tumor often shows ↓ MR enhancement with or without residual viable tumor; false negative rates up to 67%; false positive overestimates of residual tumor up to 56%

- Breast cancer prevention ("high risk": ≥ 60 years old or risk = 60 years by Gail model)
  - TAM ↓ rates of invasive cancer by 47% and noninvasive cancer by 50%

IMAGING FINDINGS

Mammographic Findings
- Breast conserving treatment
  - Early (immediate-2 years): Trabecular thickening, skin thickening, ↑ density
  - Findings ↓ over time; stable at 2-3 years
  - APBI: Geographic ↑ density in treated area, skin thickening
  - Single fraction intra-operative APBI: Early (< 1 year) punctate Ca++ in treated area
- Myocutaneous flap reconstructed breasts may be imaged with mammography
  - Predominantly fatty neobreast without nipple-areolar complex
  - Underlying muscle pedicle may be visible posteriorly
  - Punctate ± dermal Ca++ at nipple/areolar tattoo
- Curvilinear and dystrophic Ca++ due to fat necrosis typically develop 2-5 years after surgery
  - Often in upper outer quadrant with TRAM flaps (farthest from the vascular pedicle)
- NAT used in locally advanced breast cancer (LABC)
  - Pre-treatment: Mass ± Ca++, skin changes, axillary adenopathy
    - Accuracy in pre-operative size: Correlation coefficients (r^2) with pathology only 0.46-0.72
  - Post-treatment: No change, decrease in tumor size, no visible tumor
    - Treatment-related necrosis and fibrosis may mimic residual tumor
    - Ca++ may remain despite complete treatment response and no residual viable tumor
- Breast density may decrease while on TAM

Ultrasonographic Findings
- Grayscale Ultrasound
  - Limited benefit in evaluation of lumpectomy site

- Architectural distortion, extends to overlying skin scar
- Any new palpable or mammographic mass should be further evaluated; US to guide biopsy
- Breast recurrences are similar to primary tumors
  - Worrisome findings: Hypoechoic, spiculated, irregular, taller-than-wide, posterior shadowing separate from the scar site

MR Findings
- T1WI
  - Post BCT
    - Acute hematoma usually hyperintense; chronic seroma hypointense
    - Distortion, skin thickening
  - NAT
    - Axial bilateral images demonstrate breast size asymmetry, skin changes and axillary and internal mammary node sizes and configurations
    - May show signal void if post-biopsy clip present
- T2WI: Used to evaluate silicone implant integrity
- T2WI FS
  - Post BCT
    - Acute hematoma usually hypointense
    - Chronic seroma typically hyperintense
- T1 C+
  - Surveillance post BCT, contralateral breast, mastectomy site
    - Post-operative lumpectomy site: Seroma with smooth peripheral ≤ 4 mm enhancement normal
    - Enhancement typically resolves by ~ 18 months; may persist for years in some cases
  - Recurrence similar to primary: New enhancing mass, chest wall musculature enhancement when involved
    - Recurrence post-mastectomy can be depicted
  - Serial evaluation of NAT-treated tumors
    - Pre-treatment: 81-94% of known or unsuspected additional ipsilateral tumor reported
    - Chest wall invasion suspected only when muscle(s) enhance
    - Post-treatment: Enhancement may ↓ with or without residual viable tumor

POST-TREATMENT CHANGES

- Non-tumor related enhancement may ↑ secondary to reactive changes (fibrosis, necrosis, inflammation)
- MR spectroscopy: Monitor ↓ choline peak in cancer as measure of treatment response

Nuclear Medicine Findings
- PET
  - Serial evaluation of NAT-treated lesions
    - FDG PET: ↓ Uptake within 8 days of treatment, earlier than ↓ tumor size
    - 75-90% sensitivity to residual tumor
    - 74% specificity (one series)

Imaging Recommendations
- Protocol advice
  - Mammographic imaging post BCT: Variable protocols
    - Mammography of incident breast pre- and post-XRT followed by every 6 months for 2 years
    - Surveillance with MR may be considered
  - No standard mammographic follow-up recommended for post-mastectomy or reconstructed breasts
  - Monitor NAT-treatment response with mammography ± MR
    - Approved indication for FDG PET imaging
  - Surveillance mammography for women treated prophylactically with TAM

DIFFERENTIAL DIAGNOSIS

Benign Breast Biopsy
- Follow-up mammography reported to show a focal finding in ~ 50%
  - Most common findings: Distortion (46%), skin thickening (17%), focal asymmetry (15%)
  - Findings stable or ↓ over 5 years

Breast Edema, Unilateral
- Generic findings of trabecular thickening, ↑ overall density and skin thickening
  - Mastitis, superior vena cava or subclavian vessel thrombosis, trauma, inflammatory breast cancer, lymphatic obstruction due to axillary adenopathy

Fat Necrosis
- Curvilinear Ca++ at edge of lucent mass(es) at scar(s), usually develop 2-5 years post treatment, coarsen over time
- Noncalcified lucent mass(es)

Recurrent Carcinoma
- ↑ Density at scar, new mass(es) ± suspicious Ca++
- Most often near lumpectomy site in first 5 years
- More often remote > 5 years post treatment

PATHOLOGY

General Features
- Pathologic stages of wound healing
  - Inflammatory phase: Immediate to 5 days
    - Hematoma and seroma; fat and tissue necrosis

- Proliferative phase: 2 days to 3 weeks
  - Angiogenesis, granulation tissue
- Remodeling phase: 3 weeks to ≥ 2 years
  - Late fat necrosis: Ca++ and oil cysts
  - Scar: Poorly vascularized dense fibrosis
- Response to NAT
  - Tumor bed: Variable cellularity; residual tumor may be found in scattered nests

Microscopic Features
- Post radiation
  - Atypical fibroblasts and fat necrosis

CLINICAL ISSUES

Presentation
- Most common signs/symptoms: Imaging findings related to post-treatment fat necrosis or NAT-treatment response

DIAGNOSTIC CHECKLIST

Consider
- Post-treatment Ca++ may be related to areolar or radiation planning tattoos, fat necrosis; attentiveness to history and physical examination may avoid unnecessary biopsy
- Core biopsy post XRT may show cellular atypia in benign areas

Image Interpretation Pearls
- Asymmetry at scar should ↓ over time
- As scar contracts, may become denser
- Enlarging, denser scar suspicious
  - MR can help distinguish scar from recurrence
- Fat necrosis Ca++ typically curvilinear at edges of lucent mass at scar site(s), usually develop 2-5 years post-treatment
- Other new Ca++ should be viewed with suspicion
- Treated tumor often shows ↓ MR enhancement with or without residual viable tumor; false negative rates up to 67%; false positive overestimates of residual tumor up to 56%

SELECTED REFERENCES

1. Rosen EL et al: Accuracy of MRI in the detection of residual breast cancer after neoadjuvant chemotherapy. AJR. 181:1275-82, 2003
2. Zenn MR et al: TRAM flap reconstruction: the single pedicle, whole muscle technique. Spear SL, ed. Surgery of the Breast: Principles and Art. Philadelphia, Lippincott. 511-9, 1998
3. Brenner RJ et al: Mammographic changes after excisional breast biopsy for benign disease. AJR. 167:1047-52, 1996
4. Dershaw DD: Mammography in patients with breast cancer treated by breast conservation (lumpectomy with or without radiation therapy). AJR. 164:309-16, 1995
5. Mendelson EB. Evaluation of the postoperative breast. Radiol Clin North Am. 30:107-38, 1992
6. Sickles EA et al: Mammography of the postsurgical breast. AJR. 136:585-8, 1981

POST-TREATMENT CHANGES

IMAGE GALLERY

Typical

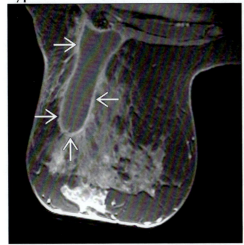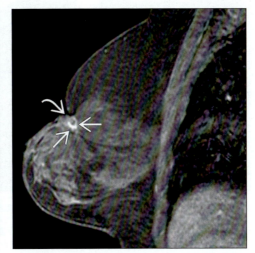

(Left) Axial T1 C+ FS MR shows normal parenchymal enhancement and thin rim of expected enhancement around the lumpectomy seroma (surgical bed) ➡, 4 months after completion of whole breast adjuvant XRT. *(Right)* Sagittal T1 C+ FS MR shows delayed enhancement ➡ 3 years after BCT. The breast is distorted, with skin retraction ➡ at the incision site. The lumpectomy site had shown decreasing enhancement on interval surveillance MRs.

Typical

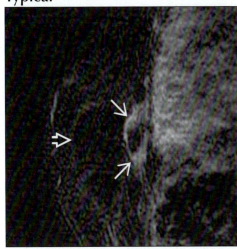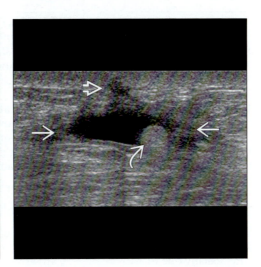

(Left) Sagittal T1 C+ subtraction MR shows enhancement of intercostal muscles ➡ due to recurrent invasive ductal carcinoma post-mastectomy and implant ➡ reconstruction 3 years earlier in this 47 y/o. Mammography is of little value post-mastectomy; MR can be helpful. *(Right)* US shows a pre-boost seroma ➡, track to skin ➡, and an echogenic "mass" ➡, a finding not uncommonly seen. Echogenic "mass" = fibrin & granulation tissue.

Typical

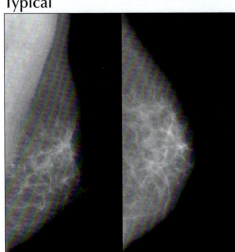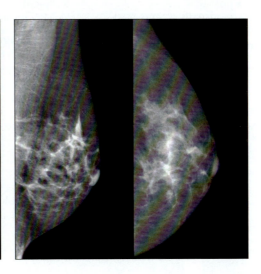

(Left) Unilateral left mammogram shows scattered fibroglandular densities without worrisome focal finding in a pre-menopausal woman taking TAM. *(Right)* Unilateral mammogram 15 months later (same patient as previous image) shows slight increase in diffuse tissue density. The patient had stopped TAM and the increase in density is likely secondary to the removal of the ER antagonist.

RECURRENT BREAST CARCINOMA

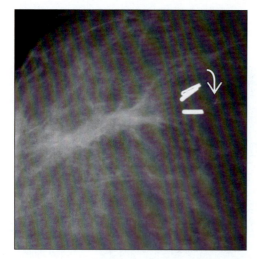

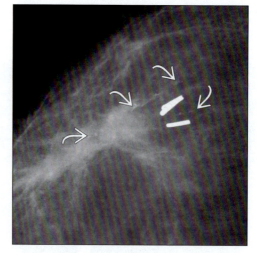

MLO mammography magnification in a 51 y/o woman with prior DCIS and BCT, shows a single fine linear branching calcification ➡ at the lumpectomy site, adjacent to clips. Ca++ was only seen in retrospect.

Lateral mammography magnification 6 months later shows marked interval increase in fine linear and branching Ca++ ➡ in a linear distribution. Stereotactic biopsy showed recurrent DCIS with Ca++.

TERMINOLOGY

Abbreviations and Synonyms

- Local recurrence, locoregional recurrence, local failure
- Ductal carcinoma in situ (DCIS)
- Breast-conserving surgery (BCS), i.e. lumpectomy
- Breast-conserving treatment (BCT) = BCS followed by radiation therapy (XRT)
- Extensive intraductal component (EIC)
  - ≥ 25% of main tumor mass = DCIS, with separate foci of DCIS outside main tumor mass
- TRAM flap: Transverse rectus abdominus myocutaneous flap

Definitions

- Appearance of invasive or noninvasive malignancy in the breast previously treated for cancer
- True recurrence: At original site, usually due to residual tumor, usually < 5 yrs post BCT
- Marginal miss: Near primary site, usually < 5 yrs post
- Elsewhere recurrence: Ipsilateral breast, remote from primary site, usually presumed to be new primary
- Contralateral breast cancer: Typically considered second primary

IMAGING FINDINGS

General Features

- Best diagnostic clue: New suspicious calcifications (Ca++) and/or ↑ density or mass in the treated breast
- Location
  - Usually at or near surgical site in first 5 years
  - Within overlying skin at incision
  - May be quite remote from original primary
- Size: Typically 5-20 mm at diagnosis; larger without regular mammography

Mammographic Findings

- 35-50% of recurrences mammographically detected after BCT
  - DCIS: New suspicious Ca++, esp. fine linear, linear distribution, pleomorphic
  - Invasive carcinoma: Ill-defined, ↑ density/mass or spiculated mass, ↑ distortion
  - May be stable for months or years before enlarging

Ultrasonographic Findings

- Grayscale Ultrasound
  - Benign scar commonly causes posterior shadowing

DDx: Benign Post-Treatment Abnormalities

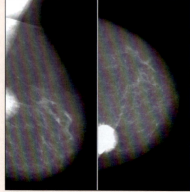

Persistent Seroma

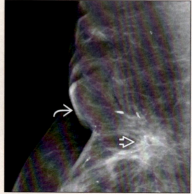

Benign Scarring

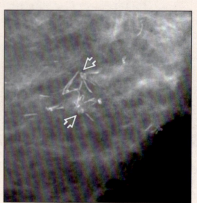

Suture Calcifications, Knots

RECURRENT BREAST CARCINOMA

Key Facts

Terminology
- Local recurrence, locoregional recurrence, local failure
- Appearance of invasive or noninvasive malignancy in the breast previously treated for cancer

Imaging Findings
- Best diagnostic clue: New suspicious calcifications (Ca++) and/or ↑ density or mass in the treated breast
- Usually at or near surgical site in first 5 years
- 35-50% of recurrences mammographically detected after BCT
- Low threshold for biopsy: PPV of 61-72% for suspicious findings
- Best imaging tool: Mammographic surveillance post BCS/BCT
- FDG-PET or PET-CT for metastatic work-up

Top Differential Diagnoses
- Benign Ca++ usually develop 2-5 yrs post-BCT
- Fat necrosis can mimic recurrence
- Dystrophic Ca++ common; coarsen over time
- Scars stable or decrease in size and density over time

Pathology
- Etiology: Most often due to incomplete removal of primary disease at surgery (residual tumor)
- ↑ Risk recurrence if BCS and no XRT: 25-36%
- Positive margins: ↑ Risk recurrence

Clinical Issues
- Majority detected as palpable lump (67%)
- Recurrence rate 1-2% per year; 13% over 7.5 years
- Annual mammography improves survival (OR = 0.77) vs. less frequent surveillance

---

- Mass-like to linear; extends to skin scar
  - Hematoma/seroma common 6-12+ months post-op
    - Resolves sooner if no XRT or intra-operative brachytherapy
  - Recurrent invasive carcinoma: Irregular hypoechoic mass, often near scar

MR Findings
- T1WI
  - Mass or distortion, hypointense to parenchyma
  - Fat necrosis, hematoma hyperintense centrally
- T2WI FS: Mass or distortion, hypointense to parenchyma
- T1 C+ FS
  - Benign scar enhances up to 6 months post-BCS, up to 18 months post-BCT; can be longer
    - Thin, smooth rim (≤ 4 mm) around seroma
    - Fat necrosis can enhance even years later
  - ↓ Parenchymal enhancement common post-XRT
  - Enhancing irregular mass suspicious for invasive carcinoma
  - Linear enhancement suspicious for DCIS

Nuclear Medicine Findings
- PET
  - Focal 18-F-fluorodeoxyglucose (FDG) uptake
    - False negative 5%, false positive 7% of cases
  - Local recurrence: Sensitivity 89%, specificity 84%, accuracy 87%
  - Distant metastases: Sensitivity 100%, specificity 97%, accuracy 98%

Biopsy
- Low threshold for biopsy: PPV of 61-72% for suspicious findings
- Core biopsy preferred to excision: Allows planning of surgical treatment
  - Cytologic atypia may be present due to XRT

Imaging Recommendations
- Best imaging tool: Mammographic surveillance post BCS/BCT
- Protocol advice

- Baseline mammography at 6-12 months post-treatment
- Annual clinical examination and mammography
- Mammography protocol varies across centers
  - After BCT: MLO and CC views for both breasts; lateral view added in some centers
  - After mastectomy: Usually no imaging (clinical evaluation); can do MLO of residual tissue
  - TRAM and other myocutaneous flaps: Consider routine CC + MLO of flap reconstruction (varies)
- T1WI C+ FS MR: Especially if ↑ density at BCS/BCT site, diagnostic uncertainty, too vague to biopsy by mammography or US
- FDG-PET or PET-CT for metastatic work-up

DIFFERENTIAL DIAGNOSIS

Post-Operative Calcifications
- Benign Ca++ usually develop 2-5 yrs post-BCT
- Fat necrosis can mimic recurrence
  - Oil cysts round, lucent; peripheral Ca++
- Dystrophic Ca++ common; coarsen over time
- Coarse linear and curvilinear suture Ca++

Scar
- Commonly produces adjacent parenchymal distortion
- Differs in shape, less dense between views
- Scars stable or decrease in size and density over time
  - May become denser as contract

Seroma
- Dense oval or round mass immediately after surgery
- Usually resolves in 6-12 months; may persist
- May have adjacent irregular scarring

New Primary Cancer (Second Primary)
- Rare; most ipsilateral neoplasia is due to recurrence of original pathology
- Some define according to time of recurrence (e.g., > 5 years post-BCT = new primary)
- More likely new when remote from primary site ± histology differs from original lesion

RECURRENT BREAST CARCINOMA

PATHOLOGY

General Features
- General path comments: Completeness of excision affects risk of recurrence
- Genetics
  - BRCA gene carriers have similar likelihood of recurrence to normal risk women
    - BRCA carriers have higher risk of second primary
- Etiology: Most often due to incomplete removal of primary disease at surgery (residual tumor)
- Epidemiology
  - ↑ Risk recurrence if BCS and no XRT: 25-36%
    - Odds ratio (OR) = 0.64 for recurrence overall & 0.4 for invasive recurrence if XRT given vs. BCS alone
  - ↑ Risk recurrence even with XRT: Young age (< 40 years); estrogen receptor negative tumor; lymphovascular invasion; multifocal tumor
    - DCIS: Close margins (< 2 mm), original lesion > 2.5 cm (more likely multifocal, multicentric)
  - Positive margins: ↑ Risk recurrence
    - 7% recurrence at 8 yrs if negative or < 1 mm margins vs. 14% if margins focally positive vs. 27% if more than focally positive
  - ↓ Recurrence by ≥ 50% if adjuvant chemo- ± hormonal therapy given in addition to XRT
  - Controversial: Preoperative MR ↓ recurrence rate 1.2% vs. 6.8% without MR (one study)
  - EIC does not ↑ risk of recurrence if margins clear

Gross Pathologic & Surgical Features
- Scarring typically dominant macroscopic feature

Microscopic Features
- Usually similar architecture, nuclear grade and receptor status to original primary

CLINICAL ISSUES

Presentation
- Most common signs/symptoms
  - Majority detected as palpable lump (67%)
  - Mammographic surveillance may detect before clinically palpable, esp. DCIS
- Other signs/symptoms
  - Cutaneous nodule or ulceration
  - Cancer en cuirasse: Multiple cutaneous nodules and thickened skin ± ulceration and fixation
  - Axillary or supraclavicular lymphadenopathy
  - Paget disease of the nipple (2% of all recurrences)
  - Distant metastases may present first
- Post-mastectomy recurrence nearly all clinically detected, usually near scar

Natural History & Prognosis
- Local recurrence: ↑ Risk systemic recurrence and death
- Recurrence rate 1-2% per year; 13% over 7.5 years
  - Recurrence < 18 months rare if optimal treatment
- Improved prognosis
  - Annual mammography improves survival (OR = 0.77) vs. less frequent surveillance
- Worse prognosis
  - Concurrent metastatic disease (5-10% of cases)

- Early recurrence, < 5 yrs post BCT, 5 yr survival 41% vs. 68% if later
- Tumors > 2 cm at recurrence, diffuse dermal involvement (5-10% of cases)
- Post-mastectomy recurrence: Poor prognosis, harbinger of systemic disease

Treatment
- "Salvage" mastectomy for recurrence if prior BCT
- Consideration for BCT if no prior XRT
  - Worse local control rate than salvage mastectomy (50 vs. 89%; p = 0.004)
- XRT for post-mastectomy recurrence
  - Nearly all still develop distant metastases
  - Consider resection, chemo- ± hormonal therapy
- "Salvage" axillary node dissection for axillary recurrence after sentinel node biopsy alone

DIAGNOSTIC CHECKLIST

Consider
- Benign conditions mimicking recurrence
- Progressive new densities ± Ca++ are suspicious

SELECTED REFERENCES
1. Lash TL et al: Reduced mortality rate associated with annual mammograms after breast cancer therapy. Breast J. 12:2-6, 2006
2. van der Sangen MJ et al: The prognosis of patients with local recurrence more than five years after breast conservation therapy for invasive breast carcinoma. Eur J Surg Oncol. 32:34-8, 2006
3. Immonen-Räihä P et al: Mammographic screening reduces risk of breast carcinoma recurrence. Cancer. 103:474-82, 2005
4. Warren JL et al: The frequency of ipsilateral second tumors after breast-conserving surgery for DCIS: a population based analysis. Cancer. 104:1840-8, 2005
5. Fischer U et al: The influence of preoperative MRI of the breasts on recurrence rate in patients with breast cancer. Eur Radiol. 14:1725-31, 2004
6. Harris JR et al: Diseases of the Breast, 3rd ed. Philadelphia, Lippincott, Williams & Wilkins. 1067-87, 2004
7. Mollick JA et al: Rational surveillance programs for early stage breast cancer patients after primary treatment. Breast Dis. 21:47-54, 2004
8. Kamel EM et al: [18F]-Fluorodeoxyglucose positron emission tomography in patients with suspected recurrence of breast cancer. J Cancer Res Clin Oncol. 129:147-53, 2003
9. Dershaw DD: Breast imaging and the conservative treatment of breast cancer. Radiol Clin North Am. 40:501-16, 2002
10. Rodrigues N et al: Correlation of clinical and pathologic features with outcome in patients with ductal carcinoma in situ of the breast treated with breast-conserving surgery and radiotherapy. Int J Radiat Oncol Biol Phys. 54:1331-5, 2002
11. Weight SC et al: Optimizing surveillance mammography following breast conservation surgery. Eur J Surg Oncol. 28:11-3, 2002
12. Brenner RJ et al: Mammographic features after conservation therapy for malignant breast disease: serial findings standardized by regression analysis. AJR. 167:171-8, 1996

RECURRENT BREAST CARCINOMA

IMAGE GALLERY

Typical

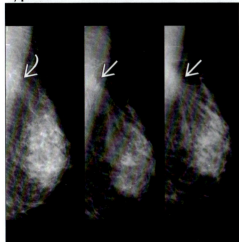

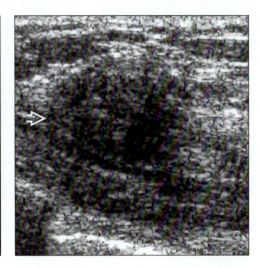

(Left) MLO mammography composite image in this 50 y/o woman shows progressive appearance of spiculated mass ➡ at lumpectomy site ➡ 6 months (left), one year (middle) and 18 months (right) after breast conservation therapy. *(Right)* Sagittal ultrasound (same as left) shows irregular hypoechoic mass ➡ with poorly defined margins. US-guided biopsy showed invasive ductal carcinoma, of same grade and receptor profile as the original cancer.

Typical

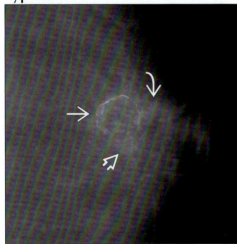

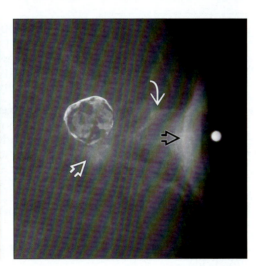

(Left) CC mammography 2 years after breast conservation therapy in a 50 y/o woman shows an oil cyst ➡ with focal density anteriorly ➡ and focal asymmetry ➡, all attributed to post-surgical scarring. *(Right)* CC mammography spot compression 3 years later (same patient as left) shows persistent scarring ➡ and chronic nipple retraction ➡, and a definite ill-defined mass medially ➡, which proved to be recurrent invasive ductal carcinoma at biopsy.

Typical

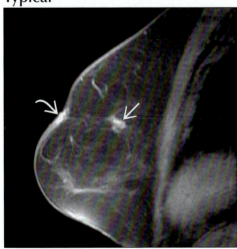

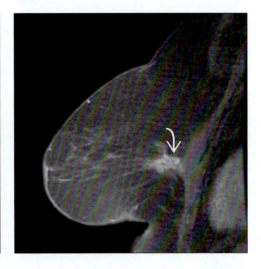

(Left) Sagittal T1 C+ FS MR of the left breast in a 63 y/o woman 5 years after BCT shows abnormal enhancement at the lumpectomy site ➡ and in the skin ➡, both confirmed as invasive carcinoma by mastectomy. (Courtesy DNS). *(Right)* Sagittal T1 C+ FS MR in a 67 y/o woman 10 years after BCT shows abnormal enhancement in the lumpectomy scar ➡. Recurrent invasive ductal carcinoma at excision. (Courtesy DNS).

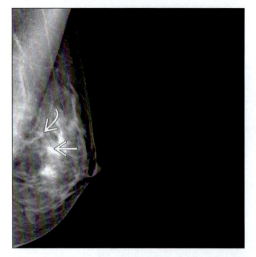

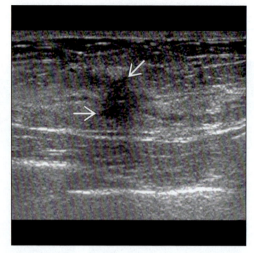

MLO mammography shows architectural distortion ➡ *and calcifications* ➡ *in the left breast in this woman treated with mantle radiation for Hodgkin disease 17 years earlier. This was a screening exam.*

Sagittal ultrasound (same patient as previous image) reveals a spiculated hypoechoic mass ➡. *At mastectomy, high-grade DCIS was found.*

TERMINOLOGY

Definitions
- High risk of secondary breast cancer after treatment for Hodgkin disease (HD)
  - Sequelae of mantle radiation to thorax (lungs shielded): Axillae, medial breasts; no longer standard

IMAGING FINDINGS

General Features
- Best diagnostic clue: History of treatment before age 30
- Location
  - High incidence of medial breast cancer: 39-50%
  - Axillary tail region also vulnerable
    - At edges of mantle radiation fields
  - Frequently bilateral: 21-29%

Mammographic Findings
- Same appearance as in sporadic breast cancer
- Younger age at diagnosis, when breast tissue often dense → decreased sensitivity

Ultrasonographic Findings
- Grayscale Ultrasound
  - Same appearance as in sporadic breast cancer
  - High sensitivity for invasive carcinoma; decreased sensitivity for DCIS

Imaging Recommendations
- Best imaging tool: Initial mammography
- Protocol advice
  - Annual screening mammography
    - Begin 8 years after radiation exposure, if treated before age 30
  - Consider supplemental screening with US or MR for dense breasts

DIFFERENTIAL DIAGNOSIS

New Breast Mass in Hodgkin Survivor
- Intraductal ± infiltrating ductal carcinoma
  - May show suspicious Ca++
- Infiltrating lobular carcinoma
- Fibroadenoma, fibrosis, PASH, other benign
- Rare: Sarcoma of breast

DDx: Infiltrating Cancer

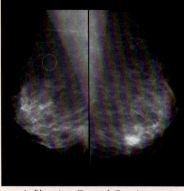

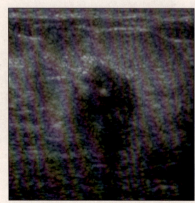

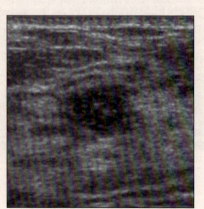

Infiltrating Ductal Carcinoma

Infiltrating Ductal Carcinoma

Infiltrating Lobular Carcinoma

TREATED HODGKIN SURVIVOR SURVEILLANCE

Key Facts

Terminology
- Sequelae of mantle radiation to thorax (lungs shielded): Axillae, medial breasts; no longer standard

Imaging Findings
- Same appearance as in sporadic breast cancer

Pathology
- Younger the patient when treated, the higher the risk of breast cancer

- No significant increased risk if treated after age 30
- Secondary breast cancers rarely seen less than 8 years after treatment
- Peak incidence 15 years after treatment

Clinical Issues
- Mastectomy preferred treatment in conjunction with chemotherapy
- Radiation usually contraindicated

PATHOLOGY

General Features
- Etiology
  - Radiation exposure to developing breast tissue
    - Maximum radiation sensitivity when breast tissue most sensitive to ovarian hormones
    - Chromosomal damage → reduced tumor suppressor activity
  - Linear relationship of dose to breast cancer risk
    - Greatest risk with doses averaging > 40 Gy
- Epidemiology
  - Younger the patient when treated, the higher the risk of breast cancer
    - No significant increased risk if treated after age 30
  - Secondary breast cancers rarely seen less than 8 years after treatment
  - Peak incidence 15 years after treatment
  - Chemotherapy and pelvic radiation decrease risk, secondary to diminished ovarian function

Staging, Grading or Classification Criteria
- Staging and prognosis no different from sporadic breast cancer
- Histopathology same as sporadic breast cancer

CLINICAL ISSUES

Presentation
- Most common signs/symptoms: Asymptomatic
- Other signs/symptoms: Palpable mass in axillary tail or parasternal region

Demographics
- Age: Average age at diagnosis 41 years
- Gender: No reported cases in males

Natural History & Prognosis
- Prognosis determined by stage at diagnosis

Treatment
- Mastectomy preferred treatment in conjunction with chemotherapy
- Breast preservation in selected cases
  - May be indicated in patients treated with radiation to affected areas only
- Radiation usually contraindicated
  - Partial breast irradiation investigational

SELECTED REFERENCES

1. Horwich A et al: Second primary breast cancer after Hodgkin's disease. Brit J Cancer. 90:294-8, 2004
2. Diller L et al: Breast cancer screening in women previously treated for Hodgkin's disease: a prospective cohort study. J Clin Oncol. 20:2085-91, 2002
3. Dershaw D et al: Breast carcinoma in women previously treated for Hodgkin disease: Mammographic evaluation. Radiology. 184:421-23, 1992
4. Meis J et al: Hodgkin's disease involving the breast and chest wall. Cancer. 57:1859-65, 1985

IMAGE GALLERY

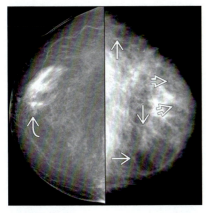 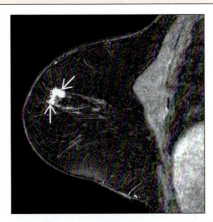 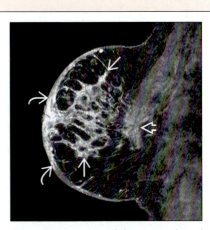

(Left) CC mammography shows left trabecular thickening ➡ and Ca++ ➡ 30 years after mantle radiation for HD. Note subtle mass on the right ➡. *(Center)* Sagittal T1 C+ FS MR right breast (same case as left image) shows irregular enhancing mass ➡. Biopsy showed grade II infiltrating ductal carcinoma (IDC). *(Right)* Sagittal T1 C+ FS MR left breast (same case as prior 2 images) shows diffuse parenchymal ➡, pectoralis muscle ➡ enhancement, & skin thickening & enhancement ➡. Biopsy showed grade III IDC, high-grade DCIS & dermal lymphatic involvement.

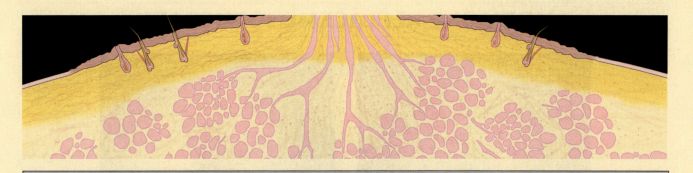

SECTION 5: Special Topics

HORMONE REPLACEMENT THERAPY

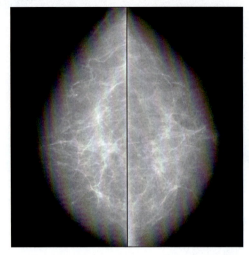

CC mammography shows minimal scattered fibroglandular density in this 70 year old woman.

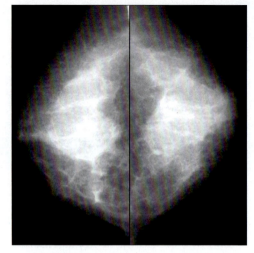

CC mammography (same patient as left-hand image) shows diffuse bilateral increase in parenchymal density one year after beginning combined estrogen and progesterone HRT.

TERMINOLOGY

Abbreviations and Synonyms
- Hormone replacement therapy (HRT)

Definitions
- Exogenous hormonal supplementation to offset declining levels of estrogen and/or progesterone in postmenopausal women
- Combination HRT: Both estrogen and progesterone

IMAGING FINDINGS

General Features
- Best diagnostic clue
  - Bilateral, symmetric increase in breast density after initiating HRT
  - Can occur weeks to years after HRT initiated

Mammographic Findings
- Generalized increase in mammographic density
  - Usually bilateral and symmetrical
  - May be asymmetric and/or patchy
- Most pronounced in patients with lower baseline density
- Density changes more common with combination HRT than estrogen alone
- Focal increase in density (developing asymmetry)
  - Should recapitulate appearance on earlier mammograms: I.e., a focal asymmetry should have been present previously, perhaps involuting near menopause, then more prominent after HRT
  - Merits further evaluation to distinguish from developing mass: Spot compression; US
- Density measured by two methods
  - Qualitative breast density assessment: Upward shift 24% of HRT patients
  - Quantitative density measurement: Increase in 73% of HRT patients
- Increase in breast size
- Proliferation of cysts and fibroadenomas in postmenopausal women
  - More common with estrogen alone
- Slight to no decrease in mammographic sensitivity in women on HRT
  - Reduced sensitivity likely limited to women who show increasing density due to HRT

DDx: Causes of Diffuse Increase in Parenchymal Density

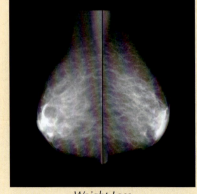

Weight Loss

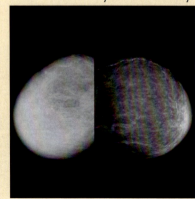

Edema, CHF

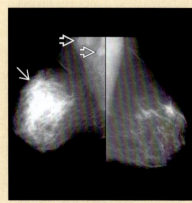

Inflammatory Cancer

HORMONE REPLACEMENT THERAPY

Key Facts

Terminology
- Exogenous hormonal supplementation to offset declining levels of estrogen and/or progesterone in postmenopausal women

Imaging Findings
- Bilateral, symmetric increase in breast density after initiating HRT
- Can occur weeks to years after HRT initiated
- May be asymmetric and/or patchy
- Increase in diffuse or regional parenchymal enhancement on MR, usually symmetric, bilateral, can be focal

Top Differential Diagnoses
- Bilateral edema
- Weight loss

- Normal variant asymmetry
- Indistinctly marginated mass
- 20% of developing focal asymmetries malignant

Clinical Issues
- Greatest risk of breast cancer among users on HRT ten or more years
- Increased risk invasive breast cancer 29%
- Increased risk coronary artery disease, stroke and pulmonary emboli

Diagnostic Checklist
- Focal developing asymmetry merits further evaluation: Spot compression and usually US
- Discontinue HRT and repeat mammogram or MR 6 weeks later to exclude HRT as cause of finding

---

- Slight decrease in specificity

Ultrasonographic Findings
- Grayscale Ultrasound
  - Dense tissue stimulated by HRT can be homogeneously hyperechoic
  - Often normal
  - Helpful in cystic-solid differentiation of masses suspected to be caused by hormonal stimulation

MR Findings
- T1WI: Increase in proportion of glandular tissue to fat
- T2WI: Increase in water content of parenchyma, relatively hyperintense
- T1 C+
  - Increase in diffuse or regional parenchymal enhancement on MR, usually symmetric, bilateral, can be focal
    - Usually slow initial uptake, persistent delayed kinetics
    - 23% showed > 60% initial enhancement on HRT vs. 4% of postmenopausal women not on HRT or 1-3 months after discontinuing HRT (single series)
    - May obscure detection of slowly enhancing masses
  - May increase uptake in benign lesions: Fibrocystic changes, fibroadenomas

Imaging Recommendations
- May recommend interval mammogram 6 weeks following cessation of HRT to evaluate problem cases: If finding due to HRT, it should decrease
- MR may be used at some institutions for problem cases

DIFFERENTIAL DIAGNOSIS

Generalized Increase in Parenchymal Density
- Bilateral edema
  - Trabecular thickening, overall increase in density, skin thickening (may be difficult to perceive on analog mammogram)

- Fluid overload conditions: Congestive heart failure (CHF), hepatic failure, anasarca
  - Superior vena caval obstruction
- Unilateral edema; not typically confused with the expected bilateral increase in breast tissue associated with HRT
  - Post-surgical, usually post-radiation therapy (affected breast)
  - CHF can be asymmetric if patient lies preferentially on one side
  - Lymphatic obstruction in axilla; venous obstruction/thrombosis
- Weight loss
  - Clinical history
  - Loss of subcutaneous fat
  - "Grayness" to mammogram, little soft tissue contrast due to loss of fat
- Pregnancy/lactation
  - Clinical history
  - Changes will persist for several months after discontinuing lactation
  - Can cause focal masses also: Lactating adenoma, focal lobular hyperplasia
- Bilateral inflammatory breast cancer (extremely rare)
  - Associated with edema, erythema and peau d'orange

Focal Increase in Parenchymal Density
- Normal variant asymmetry
  - Spot compression should show thinning of focal asymmetry
  - Interspersed fat
  - Can be seen in perimenopausal women due to native hormonal changes
  - Normal or focal increased echogenicity on US
- Indistinctly marginated mass
  - 20% of developing focal asymmetries malignant
  - Spot compression usually shows persistent mass
  - US will usually reveal hypoechoic mass, guide biopsy
- Trauma
  - Appropriate history
  - Mixed hyper- and hypoechoic mass on US (fat necrosis)

○ Surrounding edema

Multiple Bilateral Rounded Masses
- Cysts
- Fibroadenomas

PATHOLOGY

General Features
- General path comments
  ○ Estrogen effects
    - Normal breast epithelium stimulated to proliferate: Elongation of small terminal ducts; lobule formation
    - Proliferation of stromal elements, interlobular connective tissue
  ○ Progesterone effects
    - Increase in epithelial mitotic activity
    - Increased lobule size
    - Stromal edema

CLINICAL ISSUES

Presentation
- Most common signs/symptoms
  ○ Combined estrogen-progesterone therapy
    - 21-43% of patients will show increase in breast density, can be focal or diffuse
    - Breast tenderness
  ○ Estrogen alone
    - 4-10% of patients show increase in density, not significantly different from no treatment
    - Stimulates growth of cysts and fibroadenomas
    - Breast tenderness
- Clinical Profile
  ○ Route of administration: Oral most common; skin patch; intramuscular injection; vaginal estrogen
  ○ HRT reverses normal postmenopausal involutional processes
    - Proliferation of glandular and stromal elements
    - Cessation or reversal of progressive fatty replacement
  ○ Useful for control of menopause symptoms: Hot flashes; vaginal dryness; insomnia; night sweats
  ○ Health benefits
    - Osteoporosis prevention: 33% decrease in hip fractures; 22% decrease other osseous fractures
    - Colorectal cancer: 37% decrease
  ○ Breast pain
    - Occurs in 25% of women on HRT
    - Dose dependent
    - Associated with increase in mammographic density

Natural History & Prognosis
- Risks of combination HRT: Results of Women's Health Initiative (WHI) controlled, prospective randomized trial
  ○ Greatest risk of breast cancer among users on HRT ten or more years
  ○ Increased risk invasive breast cancer 29%
  ○ Increased frequency of T1, node negative tumors

○ More ductal carcinoma in situ among users
○ HRT before cancer diagnosis may increase survival by as much as 13%
○ Increased risk coronary artery disease, stroke and pulmonary emboli
- Million women study
  ○ Increased relative risk invasive breast cancer with all routes of administration
    - Oral, 1.32 (95% confidence intervals, 1.21-1.45)
    - Transdermal, 1.24 (1.11-1.39)
    - Implanted, 1.65 (1.26-2.16)
  ○ Risk increased with total duration of use
- Risk of breast cancer with combination HRT greater than with estrogen alone

DIAGNOSTIC CHECKLIST

Consider
- Benign effects on breast tissue are reversible
- Focal developing asymmetry merits further evaluation: Spot compression and usually US
- Discontinue HRT and repeat mammogram or MR 6 weeks later to exclude HRT as cause of finding

Image Interpretation Pearls
- Increasing tissue density should recapitulate areas of tissue density present prior to menopause

SELECTED REFERENCES

1. Pfleiderer SO et al: Changes in magnetic resonance mammography due to hormone replacement therapy. Breast Cancer Res. 6:R232-8, 2004
2. Beral V et al: Breast cancer and hormone replacement therapy in the Million Women Study. Lancet. 362:419-27, 2003
3. Carney PA: Individual and combined effects of age, breast density, and hormone replacement therapy use on the accuracy of screening mammography. Ann Int Med. 138:168-75, 2003
4. Roussouw JE et al: Risks and benefits of estrogen plus progestin in healthy postmenopausal women: Principal results from the women's health initiative randomized controlled trial. JAMA. 288:321-33, 2002
5. Colacurci N et al: Effects of different types of hormone replacement therapy on mammographic density. Maturitas. 40:159-64, 2001
6. Rutter CM et al: Changes in breast density associated with initiation, discontinuation, and continuing use of hormone replacement therapy. JAMA. 285:171-6, 2001
7. Kavanagh AM et al: Hormone replacement therapy and accuracy of mammographic screening. Lancet. 355(9200):270-4, 2000
8. Schairer C et al: Menopausal estrogen and estrogen-progestin replacement therapy and breast cancer risk. JAMA. 283:485-91, 2000
9. Thurfjell EL et al: Screening mammography: sensitivity and specificity in relation to hormone replacement therapy. Radiology. 203:339-41, 1997
10. Cyrlak D et al: Mammographic changes in postmenopausal women undergoing hormonal replacement therapy. AJR. 161:1177-83, 1993

IMAGE GALLERY

Typical

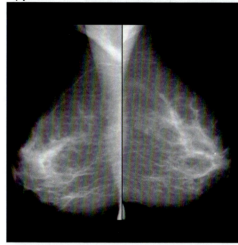
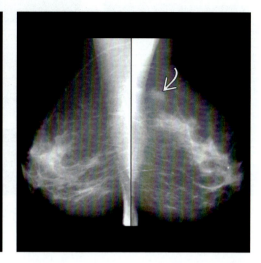

(Left) MLO mammography shows minimal scattered fibroglandular density bilaterally in this 67 year old. MLO views after the initiation of HRT are seen in the next 2 images. **(Right)** MLO mammography one month of HRT shows focal developing asymmetry upper left breast ➡, (where a small amount of tissue was visible prior to HRT) and slight overall increase in parenchymal density bilaterally.

Typical

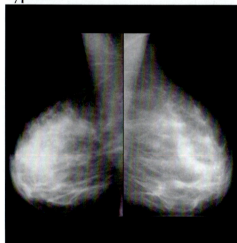
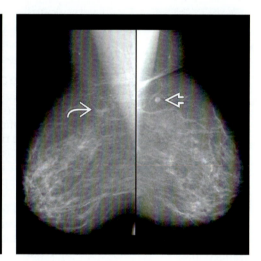

(Left) MLO mammography obtained three years later (same patient as previous 2 images) shows global bilateral increase in parenchymal density due to HRT. **(Right)** MLO mammography shows new focal asymmetry axillary tail right breast ➡ in this 74 year old woman who had been on combined HRT for 12 years. Benign lymph node is noted on the left ➡.

Variant

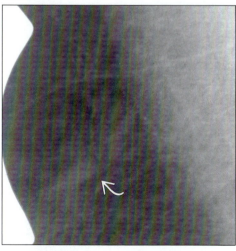
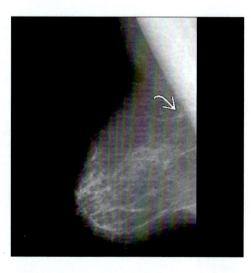

(Left) MLO mammography spot compression (same patient as previous image) shows persistence of the focal asymmetry ➡. US was unrevealing. After discussion with the patient and her physician, HRT was stopped. **(Right)** MLO mammography (same case as previous 2 images) obtained four months after stopping HRT shows near complete resolution of the focal asymmetry ➡. Follow-up over four years showed complete resolution.

GALACTOCELE

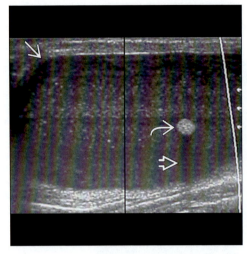

Ultrasound of a palpable mass in an 18 year old pregnant woman shows a complicated cyst ➡ with low level echoes. Hyperechoic focus ➤ with posterior shadowing ▣ is compatible with a fatty plug.

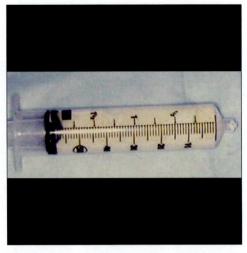

To alleviate patients symptoms, the mass (seen in left image) was aspirated, yielding 60 cc of milk from this galactocele.

TERMINOLOGY

Abbreviations and Synonyms
- Lactocele

Definitions
- A retention cyst that results from occlusion of a lactiferous duct
- Retention of milk-like fluid (fatty material) in areas of cystic duct dilatation appearing usually during or shortly after lactation

IMAGING FINDINGS

General Features
- Best diagnostic clue
  - Fat-containing well-circumscribed mass
    - Cyst with inspissated milk
  - Appearance depends on the amount of fat and protein within the milk
- Location
  - Frequently subareolar but may be anywhere in the breast
  - Solitary or multiple; unilateral or bilateral
- Size
  - Average size: 2 cm
  - Lesions > 5 cm reported

Mammographic Findings
- Circumscribed mass of variable density
  - Pathognomonic finding: Fat-fluid level on upright horizontal beam film
  - May see fluid-calcium level
  - May be associated with fat necrosis, peripheral curvilinear calcifications
- Mottled appearance similar to hamartoma has been described
  - Likened to curdled milk
- Mass is frequently obscured by dense glandular tissue of the lactating patient
- Often indistinguishable from other circumscribed masses

Ultrasonographic Findings
- Grayscale Ultrasound
  - Cyst or complicated cyst appearances
    - Circumscribed, anechoic mass with posterior acoustic enhancement

DDx: Sonographic Appearances of Galactocele

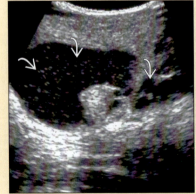

Debris & Loculated Fluid

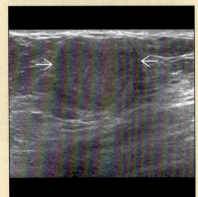

Hyperechoic Fat-Containing

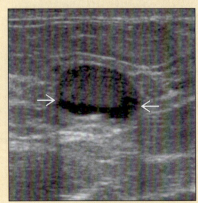

Fluid-Debris Level

GALACTOCELE

Key Facts

Terminology
- Lactocele
- A retention cyst that results from occlusion of a lactiferous duct

Imaging Findings
- Pathognomonic finding: Fat-fluid level on upright horizontal beam film
- Fluid-debris level: Fatty debris nondependent

Top Differential Diagnoses
- Fibroadenoma
- Lactating Adenoma
- Abscess
- Lipoma and variants, fibroadenolipoma (hamartoma), fat necrosis (oil cyst)
- Fat-Containing Skin and Subcutaneous Lesions

- Intracystic papillary cancer
- Invasive ductal carcinoma NOS: Often high grade

Pathology
- General path comments: Single or multi-chambered cysts contain fat and inspissated secretions

Clinical Issues
- Most common signs/symptoms: Palpable, generally painless, firm, freely mobile mass, in pregnant, lactating, or early post-lactational patient
- Most occur in pregnant or lactating women; may be seen up to several years post lactation

Diagnostic Checklist
- Diagnosis established when milky fluid is aspirated or mass with fat-fluid level present on 90° lateral view

---

- Thin septations may be seen
- Low level and bright mobile echoes within fluid
- Fluid-debris level: Fatty debris nondependent
- Thin rim of fluid eccentric to predominantly hypoechoic mass
  - Solid-appearing mass
    - Circumscribed mass; hypo- or hyperechoic; may have posterior enhancement
    - Heterogeneous internal echoes; focal echogenic areas and distal shadowing may be seen
  - Fat hyperechoic relative to protein: Appearance depends on fat content
  - Findings often nonspecific; wide range of US appearances
  - Correlate with mammogram and history
- Color Doppler: No flow within the lesion

MR Findings
- No specific indications

Biopsy
- Only if atypical or suspicious appearance
- Can be drained under US guidance for symptomatic relief: 18-20 g
- Rare reports of milk fistulae after core biopsy or incomplete excision in lactating women

Imaging Recommendations
- Best imaging tool: US in initial evaluation; mammogram if findings suspicious

DIFFERENTIAL DIAGNOSIS

Simple Cyst
- US should be definitive for diagnosis: Anechoic, circumscribed, posterior enhancement
- Small cysts (< 8 mm) can appear slightly hypoechoic due to proteinaceous fluid, especially if deep

Fibroadenoma
- Frequent in women of childbearing age, solid, circumscribed oval or gently lobulated, hypoechoic to isoechoic mass

Lactating Adenoma
- Solid circumscribed oval or gently lobulated mass ± internal flow, in lactating or pregnant women

Abscess
- Associated pain, swelling, tenderness and fever
- Galactocele may become secondarily infected, resulting in abscess
  - US-guided aspiration is diagnostic and therapeutic

Fat-Containing Breast Masses
- Hyperechoic at ultrasound: Encapsulated fat-containing masses are almost always benign
- Do not require further diagnostic imaging or intervention
- Lipoma and variants, fibroadenolipoma (hamartoma), fat necrosis (oil cyst)

Fat-Containing Skin and Subcutaneous Lesions
- Sebaceous and epidermal cysts, severe nodulocystic acne, lipomatosis, xanthomatosis
- Steatocystoma multiplex
  - Malformation of pilosebaceous duct junction: Keratin-filled intradermal cysts containing vellus hair shafts
  - Multiple lesions located on the anterior chest, axillae, groin and neck area
  - Autosomal dominant

Phyllodes Tumor
- Rapidly growing, usually circumscribed mass
- Hypoechoic, may have cystic spaces

Papilloma
- Usually intraductal mass
- May have nipple discharge

Breast Cancer
- Relatively well-circumscribed carcinoma on mammography; most carcinomas have at least one indistinct margin and/or thick wall
  - Intracystic papillary cancer

GALACTOCELE

- Intracystic mass
- Doppler flow within solid areas or vascular stalk
○ Mucinous carcinoma
○ Medullary carcinoma
○ Invasive ductal carcinoma NOS: Often high grade

PATHOLOGY

General Features
- General path comments: Single or multi-chambered cysts contain fat and inspissated secretions
- Etiology
  ○ Causes of galactocele are inferred to include
    - Present or previous stimulation by prolactin
    - Secretory breast epithelium
    - Lactiferous duct dilatation secondary to obstructed duct
  ○ May be related to abrupt suppression of lactation

Gross Pathologic & Surgical Features
- Cyst-like masses containing milk-like fluid and inspissated secretions
- Macroscopically, the milk may appear white and of milk-like viscosity if fresh, or thickened if the liquid is older

Microscopic Features
- Cyst lined by epithelium which exhibits areas of secretory activity (cytoplasmic vacuolization)
- Apocrine metaplasia may be present
- Intact cysts
  ○ Surrounded by fibrous material without inflammation
- Ruptured cysts
  ○ Chronic inflammatory response
  ○ Possible fat necrosis
- Fine needle aspiration
  ○ Cytology of the aspirates show low cellularity and benign epithelial single cells
  ○ Biochemical analysis of the aspirate shows variable proportions of proteins, fat, and lactose

CLINICAL ISSUES

Presentation
- Most common signs/symptoms: Palpable, generally painless, firm, freely mobile mass, in pregnant, lactating, or early post-lactational patient
- Other signs/symptoms: May be seen with chronic galactorrhea
- Clinical Profile
  ○ Stimulated by hyperprolactinemic state
    - At pregnancy and lactation as well as transplacental passage in newborns
    - Prolactin-stimulating pharmaceuticals
    - Pituitary adenoma
- Galactocele formation after augmentation mammoplasty
  ○ In patients under hormonal influence; rare
  ○ Massive painful breast engorgement and inflammation attributable to galactocele formation

○ Post-operative fibrosis and blockage of ducts after augmentation is probable cause

Demographics
- Age
  ○ Most occur in pregnant or lactating women; may be seen up to several years post lactation
  ○ Reported in postmenopausal women
  ○ Reported in newborn infants
- Gender
  ○ Females
  ○ Has been described in males
- Represents 1.1% of breast lesions

Natural History & Prognosis
- Excellent prognosis, mass resolves spontaneously within a few weeks to months
- Infection of galactocele a relatively infrequent complication, requiring antibiotic therapy along with drainage of its contents
  ○ Incision and drainage: Possible milk fistula formation and/or unsatisfactory cosmetic outcome
  ○ If not drained, infection likely to persist and progress into breast abscess
  ○ Repeated aspiration of galactocele suggested as an alternative to incision and drainage

Treatment
- Aspiration for symptomatic relief or diagnosis when uncertain
- Questionable cases may require surgical excision

DIAGNOSTIC CHECKLIST

Consider
- Range of mammographic and US appearances
- Correlate with clinical history

Image Interpretation Pearls
- Diagnosis established when milky fluid is aspirated or mass with fat-fluid level present on 90° lateral view

SELECTED REFERENCES

1. Acarturk S et al: An uncommon complication of secondary augmentation mammoplasty: bilaterally massive engorgement of breasts after pregnancy attributable to postinfection and blockage of mammary ducts. Aesthetic Plast Surg. 29:274-9, 2005
2. Ghosh K et al: Infected galactocele: a perplexing problem. Breast J. 10(2):159, 2004
3. Welch ST et al: Sonography of pediatric male breast masses: gynecomastia and beyond. Pediatr Radiol. 34:952-7, 2004
4. Park KY et al: Steatocystoma multiplex: mammographic and sonographic manifestations. AJR. 180(1):271-4, 2003
5. Sawhney S et al: Sonographic appearances of galactoceles. J Clin Ultrasound. 30:18-22, 2002
6. Rosen PP: Rosen's Breast Pathology. Philadelphia, Lippincott Williams & Wilkins. Chapter 3, 32-3, 2001
7. Kopans D: Breast Imaging. 2nd ed. Philadelphia, Lippincott-Raven. Chapter 19, 557-8, 1998
8. Gomez A et al: Galactocele: three distinctive radiographic appearances. Radiology. 158:43-4, 1986

GALACTOCELE

Typical

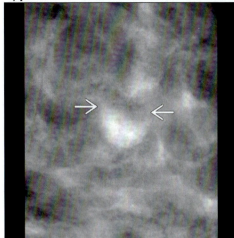
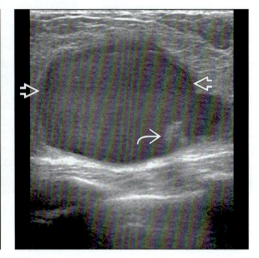

(Left) MLO mammography magnification shows a fat-containing round circumscribed mass ➡ in a 38 year old lactating woman. An US was performed (right-hand image). *(Right)* Transverse ultrasound (same patient as left-hand image) shows a fluid-filled mass ➡ with debris ➡ seen to be mobile with real time imaging. Aspiration was performed (next image).

Typical

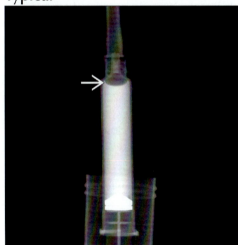
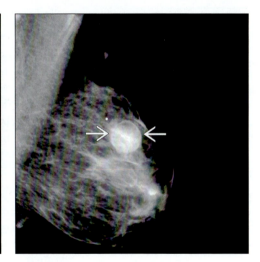

(Left) The aspirated material was white, consistent with milk, with a fat-fluid level ➡ seen on "mammogram" of the syringe. *(Right)* MLO mammogram of a lactating 37 yo with a palpable mass shows a round fat-containing mass ➡. US (not shown) demonstrated a circumscribed mass with fluid-debris level, c/w a galactocele.

Typical

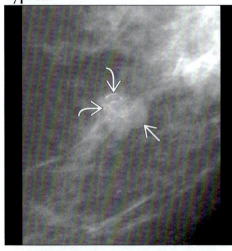
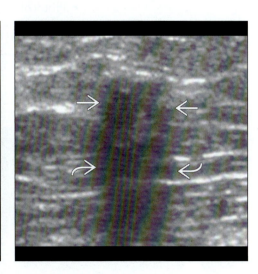

(Left) Left CC magnification mammography in an asymptomatic 50 year old woman shows a lobulated mass ➡ with indistinct borders. Peripheral curvilinear calcifications are present ➡. US (right image) was performed. *(Right)* US shows an irregular hypoechoic mass ➡ with marked posterior shadowing ➡. Surgical biopsy found a ruptured galactocele associated with inflammation and calcifications.

LACTATION

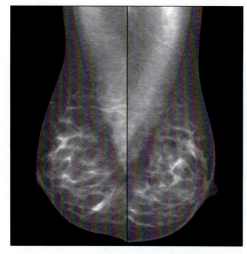

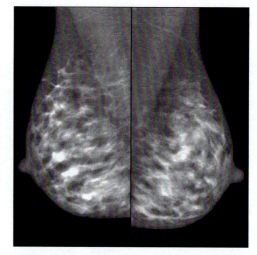

MLO mammography (baseline mammogram) in an asymptomatic 37 yo shows heterogeneously dense breasts. The right image is a screening mammogram 8 months after delivery while lactating.

MLO mammography shows a global increase in breast tissue and breast size consistent with a lactational state. Note that while dense, the breast tissue pattern does not preclude a good mammographic examination.

TERMINOLOGY

Definitions

- Postpartum period when milk produced by mammary glands, secreted through ducts, and actively ejected through stimulation of suckling

IMAGING FINDINGS

General Features

- Best diagnostic clue: Clinical history

Mammographic Findings

- Diffuse increase in size and density typical
- May have little to no change in breast density
- Post lactational benign calcifications (Ca++) reported, including vascular Ca++

Ultrasonographic Findings

- Grayscale Ultrasound: Mild increase in parenchymal echogenicity

MR Findings

- T1WI: Exuberant glandular tissue
- T2WI FS: High signal within tissue, dilated central ducts
- T1 C+
  - Rapid diffuse glandular enhancement; < tumor
  - Nursing infant exposure to gadolinium very small; likely insufficient to warrant 24 h avoidance of breastfeeding

Nuclear Medicine Findings

- PET: High breast uptake of FDG; close infant contact exposure post procedure > GI milk absorption

Biopsy

- Core biopsy, aspiration safe; rare reports of milk fistulae

Imaging Recommendations

- Best imaging tool: US initially for symptomatic women
- Protocol advice
  - Mammography can and should be used when necessary; suspicious findings must be evaluated
  - For screening, ideally wait 2-3 months after discontinuing lactation

DDx: Additional Imaging Examples of Lactating Breasts

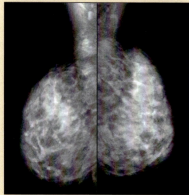

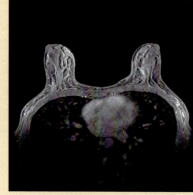

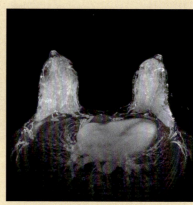

Asymptomatic, Mammogram

Non-Lactating MR C+ MIP

Lactating MR C+ MIP

LACTATION

Key Facts

Terminology
- Postpartum period when milk produced by mammary glands, secreted through ducts, and actively ejected through stimulation of suckling

Imaging Findings
- Best imaging tool: US initially for symptomatic women
- Mammography can and should be used when necessary; suspicious findings must be evaluated

Top Differential Diagnoses
- Hormonal stimulation, exogenous hormone replacement (HRT)
- Bilateral breast edema: Mammo findings = trabecular and skin thickening, overall increase in density

Diagnostic Checklist
- < 3% of breast cancer in pregnant or lactating women; ↓ prognosis; difficulty/delay in diagnosis

DIFFERENTIAL DIAGNOSIS

Normal Variants of Bilateral Breast Density
- Presence of ≥ 50% density varies by decade; 65% 20-30 years of age; 1/2 of 40-50; 30% 70-79 year olds

Bilateral Breast Density Increase
- Hormonal stimulation, exogenous hormone replacement (HRT)
  - Increase in mammographic density ranges from 17-73%; typically diffuse bilateral
- Hormonal stimulation, endogenous: Hormone secreting tumor
- Bilateral breast edema: Mammo findings = trabecular and skin thickening, overall increase in density
- Weight loss: Density increased, decrease in breast size
- Bilateral inflammatory cancer: Very rare

Lump in Lactating Woman
- Abscess: Cracks in nipple/areolar skin → skin organisms; tender, usually near nipple
- Circumscribed oval or gently lobulated mass
  - Lactating adenoma
  - Lobular hyperplasia
  - Fibroadenoma (FA)
- Focally engorged tissue: Usually resolves with breastfeeding
  - Common in axillary tail
- Malignancy: Usually at least partially indistinctly marginated or irregular; suspicious Ca++

PATHOLOGY

General Features
- Etiology: Decrease in prolactin inhibiting factor ⇒ prolactin secretion ⇒ interaction with growth hormone, insulin and cortisol ⇒ secretory state of mammary cells ⇒ suckling ⇒ secretion of oxytocin ⇒ myoepithelial contraction ⇒ milk forced from alveoli into ducts

DIAGNOSTIC CHECKLIST

Consider
- < 3% of breast cancer in pregnant or lactating women; ↓ prognosis; difficulty/delay in diagnosis

SELECTED REFERENCES

1. Espinosa LA et al: The lactating breast: contrast-enhanced MR imaging of normal tissue and cancer. Radiology. 237:429-36, 2005
2. Webb JA et al: The use of iodinated and gadolinium contrast media during pregnancy and lactation. Eur Radiol. 15:1234-40, 2005
3. Giron GL et al: Postlactational microcalcifications. Breast J. 10:247-52, 2004
4. Hicks RJ et al: Pattern of uptake and excretion of ^{18}F-FDG in the lactating breast. J Nucl Med. 42:1238-42, 2001
5. Swinford AE et al: Mammographic appearance of the breasts during pregnancy and lactation: false assumptions. Acad Radiol. 5:467-72, 1998

IMAGE GALLERY

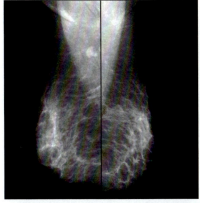 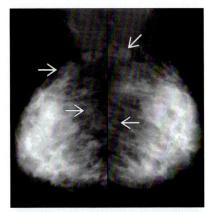 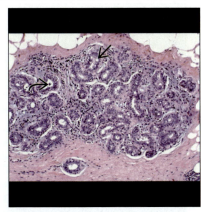

(Left) MLO mammography shows heterogeneously dense breast tissue in this asymptomatic 34 yo woman. *(Center)* One year later she is lactating. MLO mammography shows exuberant breast tissue throughout both enlarged breasts. Bilateral similar oval masses ➡ may represent dilated ducts, cysts or other benign entities. *(Right)* Micropathology shows the histopathological examination typical of lactating tissue: Acinar cells with vacuolated cytoplasm ➜ and occasional luminal cytoplasmic buds ➘ representing benign lactational change (H&E).

LACTATING ADENOMA

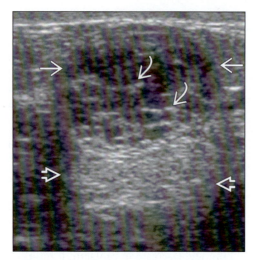

Transverse ultrasound of a palpable lump shows a hypoechoic mass ➡ with echogenic septations ➡ and posterior acoustic enhancement ➡ in a 20 year old pregnant woman. Biopsy was recommended.

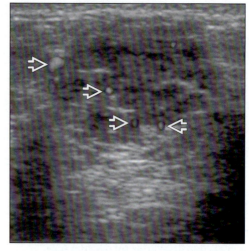

Transverse color Doppler ultrasound (same mass as left image) shows increased vascularity ➡ both within and surrounding the lesion. US-guided biopsy diagnosed lactating adenoma.

TERMINOLOGY

Abbreviations and Synonyms
- Nodular lactational hyperplasia
- Lactating nodule
- Tubular adenoma (outside of United States)

Definitions
- Well-differentiated benign breast tumor in pregnant, lactating or post-partum women

IMAGING FINDINGS

General Features
- Best diagnostic clue
  - Often indistinguishable from fibroadenoma: Circumscribed oval or gently lobulated, slightly hypoechoic mass, parallel to skin, no malignant features
    - Typically palpable
  - Can mimic malignancy
    - Indistinct margins on mammography
      - Presence of any US feature suggesting possible malignancy (margin not circumscribed, marked hypoechogenicity, vertical orientation, echogenic halo, internal mixture of solid and cystic components, posterior acoustic shadowing
- Location
  - Most often occurs in anterior portion of breast
  - May be multiple
- Size: Usually 2-4 cm, up to 21 cm
- Morphology: Well-circumscribed, discrete mass

Mammographic Findings
- Well-circumscribed oval or lobulated mass
- Lower to or equal in density to breast parenchyma
- May be completely obscured by dense surrounding fibroglandular tissue
- Atypical appearances
  - Irregular
  - Ill-defined
  - Spiculated

Ultrasonographic Findings
- Grayscale Ultrasound
  - Oval or gently lobulated, well-circumscribed, homogeneous mass

DDx: Galactocele

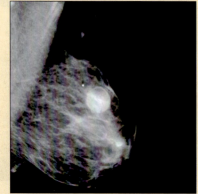

Mixed-Density (Tissue and Fat) Mass

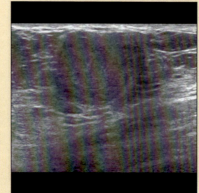

Slightly Hyperechoic Mass

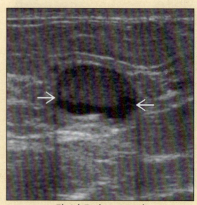

Fluid-Debris Level

LACTATING ADENOMA

Key Facts

Terminology
- Nodular lactational hyperplasia
- Lactating nodule
- Well-differentiated benign breast tumor in pregnant, lactating or post-partum women

Imaging Findings
- Often indistinguishable from fibroadenoma: Circumscribed oval or gently lobulated, slightly hypoechoic mass, parallel to skin, no malignant features
- Can mimic malignancy
- Most often occurs in anterior portion of breast
- May be multiple
- Size: Usually 2-4 cm, up to 21 cm
- Mildly hypoechoic to isoechoic
- Echogenic septations often present

- Best imaging tool: Ultrasound

Top Differential Diagnoses
- Fibroadenoma
- Galactocele
- Complicated Cyst
- Tubular Adenoma
- Well-Circumscribed Carcinoma

Clinical Issues
- Most common signs/symptoms: Soft, palpable, mobile mass occurring during pregnancy or lactation
- Must be distinguished from carcinoma
- Majority of lesions spontaneously regress after completion of breast feeding
- Imaging findings not diagnostic
- Biopsy recommended

- Mildly hypoechoic to isoechoic
- Low level internal echoes
- Posterior acoustic enhancement
  - Large amount of fluid in acinar lumina
- Microlobulated
  - Secretion-distended acini
- Parallel to skin (wider-than-tall)
- Echogenic septations often present
- Echogenic pseudocapsule
- 20-30% Compressibility
  - Most compressible solid lesion except lipoma
- Less common
  - Angulated or ill-defined margins
  - Hyperechoic
  - Posterior acoustic shadowing (occurs with infarction)
- Power Doppler: Hypervascular

Imaging Recommendations
- Best imaging tool: Ultrasound
- Protocol advice
  - Always begin with ultrasound because these are in younger and/or pregnant women
  - Other imaging modalities rarely indicated
- Mammography not routinely recommended during pregnancy
  - Indicated only if malignancy strongly suspected
  - Shield abdomen in pregnant patient

DIFFERENTIAL DIAGNOSIS

Fibroadenoma
- Common in adolescents and women under 30
- Clinically smooth, firm or rubbery and freely movable
- Hypoechoic, solid, circumscribed, oval or gently lobulated mass on ultrasound
- Variable imaging characteristics
- Can enlarge during pregnancy

Galactocele
- Benign breast mass that contains retained milk
- Well-circumscribed mass with thin, echogenic rim

- Presentation may be delayed
  - 6-10 months after cessation of nursing
- Aspiration diagnostic and curative

Complicated Cyst
- Hypoechoic, circumscribed on ultrasound with posterior enhancement
- If equivocal, aspiration diagnostic

Abscess
- Palpable mass or area typically including clinical symptoms of erythema, warmth and tenderness
- Usually of mixed echogenicity: Anechoic, hypoechoic, mixed with isoechoic septations; may be hyperechoic
- Surrounding tissue often with increased echogenicity secondary to edema

Tubular Adenoma
- Uncommon
- Palpable, mobile, firm mass
- Occurs during reproductive years
- Fusiform shape on ultrasound
- Usually smooth, rarely microlobulated

Well-Circumscribed Carcinoma
- Most infiltrating carcinomas have at least some indistinct margins
- May be hypoechoic to isoechoic and difficult to discern from the surrounding breast tissue

Related Pathologic Diagnoses
- Focal lobular hyperplasia of pregnancy: Physiologic, not a discrete lesion, TDLUs expand in all directions
- Focal lactational change (pseudolactational change): Secretory change, not necessarily in pregnant or lactating patient
- Fibroadenoma with lactational change ("lactating fibroadenoma"): Lactational change of epithelial component, fibrous stroma is present
- Secretory carcinoma: Subtype of IDC; microscopically can resemble areas of secretory change, but invasive, myoepithelial layer is absent

LACTATING ADENOMA

PATHOLOGY

General Features
- General path comments: Firm, rubbery circumscribed spherical mass
- Etiology
  - Proposed origins, controversial
    - De novo in hormonally stimulated breast
    - Arises from pre-existing fibroadenoma or tubular adenoma
    - Premature lactational changes, out of phase with surrounding breast tissue
- Cytological Features
  - Moderate cellularity
  - Intact epithelium
  - Foamy to vacuolated cytoplasm
  - Atypia not seen

Gross Pathologic & Surgical Features
- Circumscribed, grayish-white to yellow, firm and rubbery mass
- Lobulated cut surface
- Milky substance may be expressed at surgical excision
- Becomes creamy yellow during lactation
- No true capsule
  - Sharply demarcated from surrounding breast tissue
- Necrosis and hemorrhage uncommon
- 5% undergo infarction

Microscopic Features
- Well-circumscribed lesion with prominent secretory lobules and minimal stromal component
- Large acini surrounded by basement membrane and edematous stroma
- Florid lactational changes
- Tubuloalveolar appearance to glands
- Loosely grouped clusters of epithelial cells with prominent nucleoli

CLINICAL ISSUES

Presentation
- Most common signs/symptoms: Soft, palpable, mobile mass occurring during pregnancy or lactation
- Other signs/symptoms
  - May enlarge rapidly during first two trimesters of pregnancy
  - Infarction
    - Painful, firm mass
- Diagnostic challenge
  - Must be distinguished from carcinoma
    - 3% of breast cancers diagnosed in pregnancy

Demographics
- Age: Reproductive years

Natural History & Prognosis
- Majority of lesions spontaneously regress after completion of breast feeding
- Infarction not uncommon
  - Secondary to relative vascular insufficiency during increased requirements during pregnancy and lactation
- Excellent prognosis
  - No malignant potential
  - No associated increase in future development of malignancy

Treatment
- Imaging findings not diagnostic
  - Biopsy recommended
    - Fine needle aspiration may yield false positive result
    - Core biopsy or excision definitive: Milk fistula reported rare complication
  - Pathologist should be informed that patient is pregnant or lactating
    - Changes may be confused with carcinoma
- Following pregnancy/lactation, bromocriptine may be used to decrease size of lesion
- Surgical excision if mass does not resolve on its own or respond to bromocriptine

SELECTED REFERENCES

1. Saglam A et al: Coexistence of lactating adenoma and invasive ductal adenocarcinoma of the breast in a pregnant woman. J Clin Pathol. 58(1):87-9, 2005
2. Mendelson EB et al: Breast Imaging Reporting and Data System: BI-RADS, Ultrasound, 1st ed. Reston, American College of Radiology, 2003
3. Baker TP et al: Lactating adenoma: a diagnosis of exclusion. Breast J. 7(5):354-7, 2001
4. Choudhury M et al: Lactating adenoma--cytomorphologic study with review of literature. Indian J Pathol Microbiol. 44(4):445-8, 2001
5. Goyal M et al: Palpable breast mass in a lactating woman. Postgrad Med J. 77(909):473, 482-3, 2001
6. Reeves ME et al: Lactating adenoma presenting as a giant breast mass. Surgery. 127(5):586-8, 2000
7. Behrndt VS et al: Infarcted lactating adenoma presenting as a rapidly enlarging breast mass. AJR Am J Roentgenol. 173(4):933-5, 1999
8. Scott-Conner CE: Breast cancer in pregnancy. Rosen Breast Cancer. 30:595-601, 1999
9. Sumkin JH et al: Lactating adenoma: US features and literature review. Radiology. 206(1):271-4, 1998
10. Scott-Conner CEH: Diagnosing and Managing Breast Disease During Pregnancy and Lactation. Medscape Womens Health. 2(5):1, 1997
11. Yang WT et al: Lactating adenoma of the breast: antepartum and postpartum sonographic and color Doppler imaging appearances with histopathologic correlation. J Ultrasound Med. 16(2):145-7, 1997
12. Collins JC et al: Surgical management of breast masses in pregnant women. J Reprod Med. 40(11):785-8, 1995
13. Slavin JL et al: Nodular breast lesions during pregnancy and lactation. Histopathology. 22(5):481-5, 1993
14. Terada S et al: A lactating adenoma of the breast. Gynecol Obstet Invest. 34(2):126-8, 1992
15. Novotny DB et al: Fine needle aspiration of benign and malignant breast masses associated with pregnancy. Acta Cytol. 35(6):676-86, 1991
16. James K et al: Breast tumour of pregnancy ('lactating' adenoma). J Pathol. 156(1):37-44, 1988
17. Bottles K et al: Diagnosis of breast masses in pregnant and lactating women by aspiration cytology. Obstet Gynecol. 66(3 Suppl):76S-78S, 1985
18. O'Hara MF et al: Adenomas of the breast and ectopic breast under lactational influences. Hum Pathol. 16(7):707-12, 1985

LACTATING ADENOMA

IMAGE GALLERY

Typical

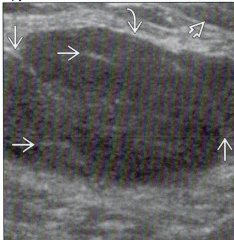 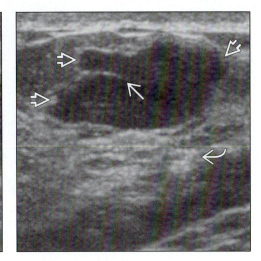

(Left) Radial ultrasound in a lactating woman with two palpable masses, shows gently lobulated mass ➡ which is almost isoechoic to fat ➡. Internal septae ➡ are apparent. *(Right)* Radial ultrasound shows the second mass (same patient as left image) with microlobulation ➡, internal septation ➡, and posterior enhancement ➡. Biopsy of both masses = lactating adenomata. (Courtesy EBM).

Typical

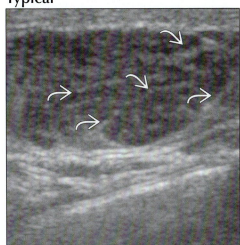 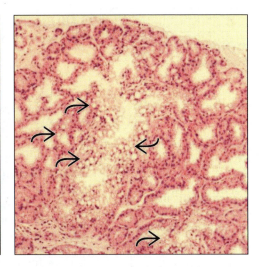

(Left) Radial ultrasound shows circumscribed, slightly hypoechoic mass with multiple echogenic internal septations ➡ in a 20 yo pregnant woman. US 14-gauge core biopsy = lactating adenoma. *(Right)* Specimen micropathology, high power (same patient as left-hand image) shows the mass to be composed of a tight aggregate of lobules with secretory hyperplasia ➡. Such tumors usually do not exhibit true lactational excretion.

Variant

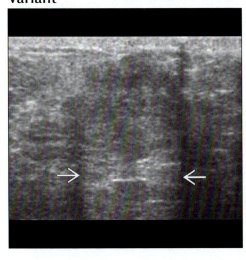 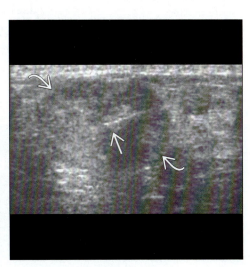

(Left) Transverse ultrasound shows a round irregular isoechoic mass with posterior enhancement ➡ in a lactating woman. Biopsy was recommended (BI-RADS 4). *(Right)* Transverse ultrasound (same patient as left-hand image) shows the mass ➡ with intralesional needle ➡ during core biopsy with a 14-gauge needle. Lactating adenoma was diagnosed.

MALIGNANCY IN PREGNANCY

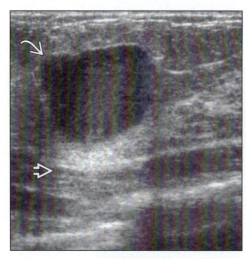

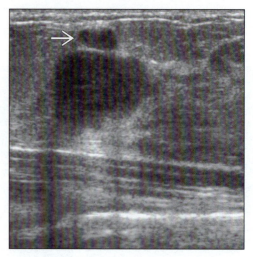

Transverse ultrasound in a pregnant woman shows a well-circumscribed palpable hypoechoic 17 mm mass ➡ with posterior enhancement ⇉. Biopsy revealed infiltrating ductal carcinoma.

Longitudinal ultrasound (same patient as left image) shows a small satellite mass ➡ just below the skin. The well-defined shape, homogeneous texture and acoustic enhancement are typical of pregnancy-related cancers.

TERMINOLOGY

Abbreviations and Synonyms
- Pregnancy-associated breast carcinoma

Definitions
- Breast cancer during pregnancy or within 1 year postpartum

IMAGING FINDINGS

General Features
- Best diagnostic clue: Irregular hypoechoic mass on ultrasound in pregnant or lactating woman
- Size: Typically 2-3 cm diameter at presentation

Mammographic Findings
- Mammography may be falsely negative up to 35%
  - Dense breast tissue may obscure masses
- Two view mammography (0.4 mRad to fetus)
  - Different risks depending on trimester
  - Overall risk to fetus extremely low

Ultrasonographic Findings
- Grayscale Ultrasound
  - Identical to non-pregnancy-related carcinoma
    - Hypoechoic, usually irregular mass, with or without calcifications
  - High grade invasive ductal carcinoma (IDC) can be circumscribed, nearly anechoic
- Power Doppler
  - Hypervascular parenchyma typical
  - Tumors typically hypervascular

MR Findings
- T1 C+
  - Not recommended during first trimester
  - Use of gadolinium in pregnancy guarded
    - Unless potential risk to patient outweighs risk to fetus
    - Increased background parenchymal enhancement due to hormonal stimulation

Nuclear Medicine Findings
- PET: Not recommended in pregnancy

DDx: Other Pregnancy-Related Masses

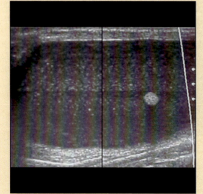

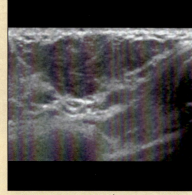

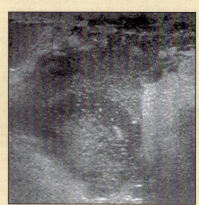

Galactocele

Lactating Adenoma

Breast Abscess

MALIGNANCY IN PREGNANCY

Key Facts

Terminology
- Pregnancy-associated breast carcinoma
- Breast cancer during pregnancy or within 1 year postpartum

Imaging Findings
- Best diagnostic clue: Irregular hypoechoic mass on ultrasound in pregnant or lactating woman
- Mammography may be falsely negative up to 35%
- Different risks depending on trimester
- Use of gadolinium in pregnancy guarded

Top Differential Diagnoses
- Fibroadenoma & Phyllodes Tumour
- Lactating Adenoma
- Lobular Hyperplasia
- Galactocele

Pathology
- BRCA-1 & -2 gene carriers more prone
- ~ 3% of all breast carcinomas
- 1:3,000-10,000 pregnancies
- Grade III carcinomas (80% vs. 33%)
- Usually estrogen- and progesterone-receptor negative

Clinical Issues
- Painless mass or thickening
- ~ 50% have positive axillary nodes
- Age: Typically in mid 30's
- Survival equal stage-for-stage with non-pregnancy-related carcinoma
- Therapeutic abortion not proven to improve survival
- Modified radical mastectomy and lymph node biopsy/dissection
- Breast conservation increasingly common

Biopsy
- Rare reports of milk fistulae after core biopsy in lactating breast; not a reason to avoid biopsy of suspicious findings

Imaging Recommendations
- Best imaging tool: Initial US directed to clinically suspicious findings
- Protocol advice
  - Mammography if clinically and/or US suspicious
    - Shield abdomen with lead apron if pregnant
    - Perform after nursing or pumping, if applicable
  - Investigational: US screening in high risk women while pregnant

DIFFERENTIAL DIAGNOSIS

Fibroadenoma & Phyllodes Tumour
- Usually circumscribed oval or gently lobulated hypoechoic mass
- Small cystic spaces more common in phyllodes
- May enlarge dramatically during pregnancy; biopsy indicated to exclude malignancy

Lactating Adenoma
- Well-differentiated benign tumor of secretory mammary epithelium
- May be variant of pre-existing tubular adenoma or fibroadenoma
- Homogeneous large ovoid or gently lobulated hypoechoic solid mass lesion
- Core biopsy usually necessary to establish diagnosis

Lobular Hyperplasia
- Hormonally induced focal asymmetric hyperplasia
- Typical glandular parenchyma seen on ultrasound

Hamartoma with Hormonal Stimulation
- Fat-containing, mixed echogenicity mass

Galactocele
- Hypoechoic circumscribed mass
  - May show fluid-debris level with nondependent (fatty) debris
- Typically only during lactation

Abscess
- Usually seen during lactation, usually clinically obvious
- Tender, erythematous, palpable mass, usually near nipple

Leukemia, Lymphoma, Sarcoma, and Tuberculosis (Very Rare)
- Lymphoma may be bilateral, readily mistaken for invasive carcinoma on needle biopsy

PATHOLOGY

General Features
- General path comments: Similar to non-pregnancy-related carcinoma
- Genetics
  - BRCA-1 & -2 gene carriers more prone
    - High levels of estrogen may accelerate malignancy
  - Family history of breast cancer more common
- Epidemiology
  - ~ 3% of all breast carcinomas
  - Most common malignancy in pregnancy
    - 1:3,000-10,000 pregnancies
  - Incidence of inflammatory carcinoma similar to non-pregnancy-related carcinoma

Microscopic Features
- Histologically similar to non-pregnancy-related carcinoma, but higher incidence of some findings
  - Grade III carcinomas (80% vs. 33%)
  - Cancerization of lobules (80% vs. 15%)
- If diagnosed during pregnancy
  - Usually estrogen- and progesterone-receptor negative
  - Usually c-erbB-2/HER-2 neu receptor negative
- If diagnosed during lactation
  - Usually c-erbB-2/HER-2 neu receptor positive

MALIGNANCY IN PREGNANCY

○ Many partially or completely mucinous, MUC2 positive

Staging, Grading or Classification Criteria

- Generally present at a later stage than outside pregnancy
  ○ Mostly due to delay in diagnosis
  ○ Aggressive tumor histopathology
- Compared with non-pregnancy-related carcinoma
  ○ Tumors are larger
  ○ More likely to have positive nodes (60-70%)
  ○ More likely to have metastases, and vascular invasion

CLINICAL ISSUES

Presentation

- Most common signs/symptoms
  ○ Painless mass or thickening
  ○ ~ 50% have positive axillary nodes
- Other signs/symptoms
  ○ Nipple discharge
  ○ If breastfeeding, infant may refuse milk from breast
  ○ May have features of remote metastatic disease at diagnosis

Demographics

- Age: Typically in mid 30's

Natural History & Prognosis

- Survival equal stage-for-stage with non-pregnancy-related carcinoma
  ○ Overall worse prognosis due to more advanced presentation
- Recurrence rates high if pregnancy occurs immediately after treatment
  ○ 50% 5 year survival: Pregnancy within 1 year
  ○ 83% 5 year survival: Pregnancy 1-2 years
  ○ 100% 5 year survival: Pregnancy after 2 years
- Future pregnancy not advised if
  ○ Positive nodes (stage II, III) or metastases (stage IV)
  ○ Initial cancer invasive histology (varies)
  ○ < 5 years following diagnosis (varies)

Treatment

- Therapeutic abortion not proven to improve survival
  ○ Usually performed to prevent fetal injury from chemotherapy and radiotherapy
- Modified radical mastectomy and lymph node biopsy/dissection
  ○ Traditional treatment if pregnancy not interrupted
  ○ Reduces need for breast radiation
  ○ For stage I, stage II and some stage III
  ○ Sentinel lymph node requires isotope and/or isosulfan blue dye
    ▪ Safety of isosulfan blue dye not established in pregnant or lactating women
- Breast conservation increasingly common
  ○ Late 2nd or 3rd trimester can perform lumpectomy
    ▪ Chemotherapy can be given after 1st trimester
    ▪ Radiation therapy can be given after delivery
- Radiotherapy usually avoided during pregnancy

○ Absorbed by fetus: Teratogenic or carcinogenic if threshold dose of 0.1-0.2 Gy exceeded
○ This dose is not generally reached with curative radiotherapy during pregnancy
  ▪ Provided suitable shielding and collimation are used to minimize fetal exposure
- Chemotherapy and tamoxifen avoided during first trimester
  ○ Risk of fetal damage is variable
  ○ Successful normal term deliveries possible

DIAGNOSTIC CHECKLIST

Consider

- Lactational mass, e.g., galactocele

Image Interpretation Pearls

- Typical features of carcinoma seen on ultrasound

SELECTED REFERENCES

1. Loibl S et al: Breast carcinoma during pregnancy. International recommendations from an expert meeting. Cancer. 106(2):237-46, 2006
2. Annane K et al: Infiltrative breast cancer during pregnancy and conservative surgery. Fetal Diagn Ther. 20:442-4, 2005
3. Fanale MA et al: Treatment of metastatic breast cancer with trastuzumab and vinorelbine during pregnancy. Clin Breast Cancer. 6(4):354-6, 2005
4. Gentilini O et al: Breast cancer diagnosed during pregnancy and lactation: biological features and treatment options. Eur J Surg Oncol. 31(3):232-6, 2005
5. Kal HB et al: Radiotherapy during pregnancy: fact and fiction. Lancet Oncol. 6(5):328-33, 2005
6. Kerr JR: Neonatal effects of breast cancer chemotherapy administered during pregnancy. Pharmacotherapy. 25(3):438-41, 2005
7. Pavlidis N et al: The pregnant mother with breast cancer: diagnostic and therapeutic management. Cancer Treat Rev. 31(6):439-47, 2005
8. Psyrri A et al: Pregnancy-associated breast cancer. Cancer J. 11(2):83-95, 2005
9. Gentilini O et al: Safety of sentinel node biopsy in pregnant patients with breast cancer. Ann Oncol. 15(9):1348-51, 2004
10. Keleher A et al: The safety of lymphatic mapping in pregnant breast cancer patients using Tc-99m sulfur colloid. Breast J. 10(6):492-5, 2004
11. Bladstrom A et al: Worse survival in breast cancer among women with recent childbirth: results from a Swedish population-based register study. Clin Breast Cancer. 4(4):280-5, 2003
12. Middleton LP et al: Breast carcinoma in pregnant women: assessment of clinicopathologic and immunohistochemical features. Cancer. 98(5):1055-60, 2003
13. Rugo HS: Management of breast cancer diagnosed during pregnancy. Curr Treat Options Oncol. 4(2):165-73, 2003
14. Woo JC et al: Breast cancer in pregnancy: a literature review. Arch Surg. 138(1):91-8; discussion 99, 2003
15. Rosner D et al: Breast cancer and related pregnancy: suggested management according to stages of the disease and gestational stages. J Med. 33(1-4):23-62, 2002
16. Shousha S. Breast carcinoma presenting during or shortly after pregnancy and lactation. Arch Pathol Lab Med. 124: 1053-60, 2000
17. Liberman L et al: Imaging of pregnancy-associated breast cancer. Radiology. 191:245-8, 1994

IMAGE GALLERY

Variant

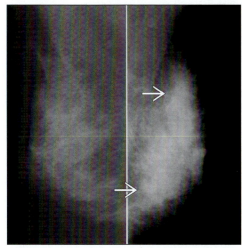 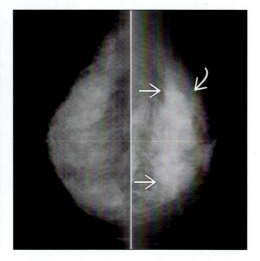

(Left) MLO mammography in a lactating 6 month postpartum woman shows diffuse increase in left breast density ➡ and clinically evident skin and nipple changes. Antibiotics = no change. *(Right)* CC mammography (same patient as left-hand image) shows diffuse increase in glandular density on the left ➡ with hyperdensity of the periglandular fat ➢ due to subcutaneous edema and infiltration. US was performed (next 2 images).

Variant

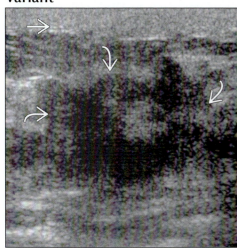 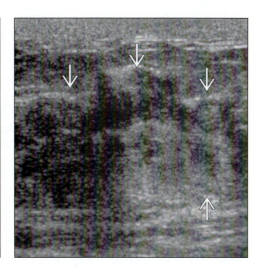

(Left) Transverse ultrasound shows marked skin thickening ➡ and an irregular hypoechoic mass ➢. *(Right)* Longitudinal ultrasound away from main mass shows poorly-defined extensive heterogeneous infiltration ➡. Grade III IDC was confirmed at mastectomy. The patient died from metastatic disease 18 months later.

Typical

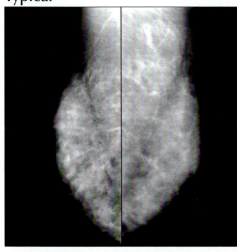 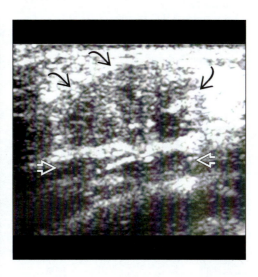

(Left) MLO mammography shows dense glandular parenchyma in this pregnant woman presenting with a palpable lump on the right side (not marked) without visible mass. US (right-hand image) was performed. *(Right)* Transverse ultrasound shows a hypoechoic irregular mass ➤ with posterior acoustic enhancement ➤ in the upper outer quadrant found to be high grade invasive carcinoma.

IV

5

19

TRAUMA

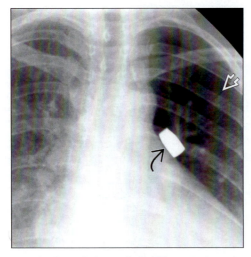
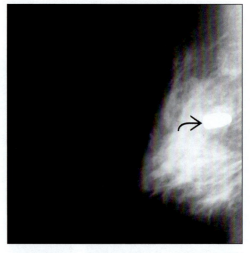

Frontal radiograph shows a bullet ⇗ projected over the right hemithorax. No pneumothorax was present despite the technical hyperlucency ⇒. The bullet was in the left breast (right-hand image).

MLO mammography shows the non-palpable bullet ⇗ lodged in the upper outer quadrant which required needle localization to direct excision.

TERMINOLOGY

Definitions
- Accidental injury to the breast; trauma may be blunt or penetrating

IMAGING FINDINGS

General Features
- Best diagnostic clue
  - Majority of imaging findings attributable to fat necrosis
  - History; elderly in particular may not recall minor trauma

Mammographic Findings
- Early manifestations of blunt trauma may be those of soft tissue mass secondary to hematoma
- Band-like asymmetry may be present on MLO view secondary to edema from seat-belt injury
  - Upper inner quadrant on left when trauma sustained by driver; upper inner right when passenger
- Dystrophic calcifications (Ca++) within areas of fat necrosis may form over time
- Features of post-traumatic fat necrosis/hematomas may mimic carcinoma; mass, irregular margins or even frank spiculation, skin thickening/retraction

Ultrasonographic Findings
- Grayscale Ultrasound
  - Post-traumatic masses may have features identical to carcinoma
    - Margin irregularities, posterior acoustic shadowing or enhancement
  - Increased echogenicity :Edema
  - Fluid collection: Seroma, hematoma, fat necrosis

CT Findings
- CECT: Critical in assessing vascular injuries following severe chest trauma
- NECT: Performed in most cases of severe chest trauma

DIFFERENTIAL DIAGNOSIS

Blunt Trauma
- Seat-belt injuries

DDx: Mammographic and Ultrasound Images of Post Blunt Trauma Fat Necrosis

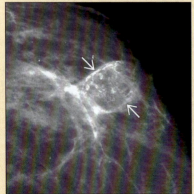
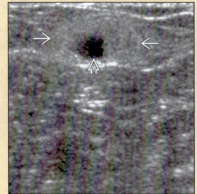
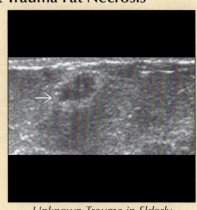

| *Seat-Belt Injury* | *Seat-Belt Injury* | *Unknown Trauma in Elderly* |

TRAUMA

Key Facts

Terminology
- Accidental injury to the breast; trauma may be blunt or penetrating

Imaging Findings
- Majority of imaging findings attributable to fat necrosis
- Post-traumatic masses may have features identical to carcinoma

Top Differential Diagnoses
- Seat-belt injuries
- Direct blows to the chest/breast
- Missiles (metal or plastic bullets, shrapnel), knives, animal and human bites

Diagnostic Checklist
- Without antecedent history, developing densities (particularly in the elderly), suspicious masses, must be further evaluated; often require biopsy

---

- Direct blows to the chest/breast
- Crush injuries
- Complications of blunt trauma
  - Masses, infections, deformities; pressure sores, subcutaneous breast avulsion

Penetrating Trauma
- Missiles (metal or plastic bullets, shrapnel), knives, animal and human bites

PATHOLOGY

General Features
- Etiology
  - Seat-belt injury: Breast tissue compression between belt and bony thorax with deceleration and soft tissue shearing stresses
  - Most common cause of fat necrosis is trauma, either accidental or iatrogenic

Microscopic Features
- Findings are usually typical of fat necrosis, fibrosis; cholesterol granulomas at site of prior hematoma reported
- Focal fat cell damage or destruction → necrotic lipid material filling intracellular cyst-like vacuoles surrounded with fibroblasts, multinucleated giant cells and lipid containing histiocytes (foam cells)
- Area may be replaced by fibrosis or a persistent cavity may remain

CLINICAL ISSUES

Presentation
- Most common signs/symptoms
  - History key; may have to be elicited either due to forgetfulness or passage of time
  - Emergency visits for penetrating trauma should be unambiguous as to breast involvement

Natural History & Prognosis
- Dependent on severity of the trauma

DIAGNOSTIC CHECKLIST

Consider
- Without antecedent history, developing densities (particularly in the elderly), suspicious masses, must be further evaluated; often require biopsy

SELECTED REFERENCES

1. Williams HJ et al: Imaging features of breast trauma: a pictorial review. The Breast. 11:107-15, 2002
2. Hogge JP et al: The mammographic spectrum of fat necrosis of the breast. Radiographics. 15:1247-56, 1995
3. Larsen S et al: Subcutaneous avulsion of the breast caused by a seat belt injury. Report of a case requiring emergency mastectomy. Eur J Surg. 158:131-2, 1992

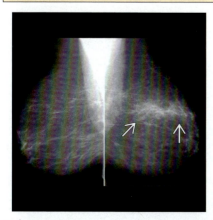 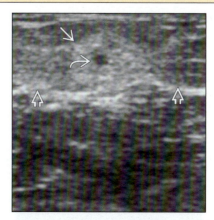 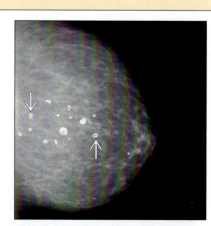

IMAGE GALLERY

(Left) MLO mammography shows a band-like asymmetry in upper (inner) breast ➡ compatible with edema in this woman status post seat-belt injury. Passenger or driver? (Center) US (same patient as left image) shows typical findings of fat necrosis: Diffuse increased echogenicity ➡ = edema + hyperechoic mass ➡ with an anechoic collection ➡. Left inner breast injury = passenger! (Right) CC mammography (different case) shows multiple coarse, round, lucent-centered dystrophic Ca++ ➡ in upper left breast representing sequelae of prior traumatic seat-belt injury.

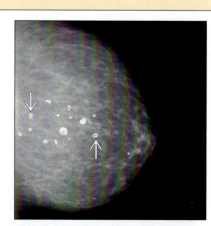

MULTIPLE BILATERAL SIMILAR FINDINGS

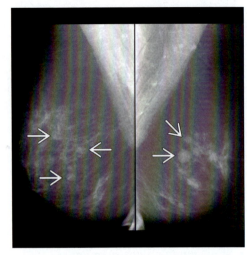
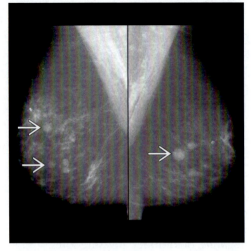

MLO screening mammograms show multiple, bilateral, mostly circumscribed masses ➡ in this 50 year old with a history of cysts and cyst aspirations. BI-RADS 2, benign.

MLO screening mammograms 2 years later show a changing pattern of these circumscribed nodules ➡, with some regressing and some minimally increasing, compatible with cysts, BI-RADS 2.

TERMINOLOGY

Abbreviations and Synonyms
- Multiple rounded densities

Definitions
- Multiple bilateral similar findings: At least 3 total, at least 1 in each breast
  - When applied to masses, refers to multiple bilateral mostly circumscribed, partially obscured masses on mammography
    - Excludes palpable findings
    - Not applicable when there is a dominant mass or suspicious findings
    - Suggests benign etiology
  - Concept that multiplicity and bilaterality favor benign etiology may be relevant to other findings and modalities, but requires further study

IMAGING FINDINGS

General Features
- Best diagnostic clue

- Entity described on screening mammography
  - Fluctuating pattern of bilateral mostly circumscribed masses suggesting cysts
  - May apply to US and MR, but requires further study
- Morphology
  - Oval or gently lobulated, circumscribed masses
  - May apply to other findings

Mammographic Findings
- Multiple, bilateral mostly circumscribed masses
  - Up to 25% of a mass margin may be obscured
  - Carefully evaluate each mass
  - No mass has any indistinct or spiculated margin
  - No associated suspicious calcifications (Ca++)
  - Fluctuating pattern year to year suggests cysts
  - Coarse, popcorn Ca++ suggest fibroadenoma (FA)
  - Can have mixture of cysts and fibroadenoma(s)
- Multiplicity, bilaterality of other similar findings may favor benign etiology
  - Multiple bilateral groupings of coarse, heterogeneous Ca++
  - Multiple bilateral groupings of amorphous and punctate Ca++

DDx: Unilateral Mostly Circumscribed Masses

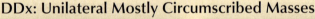

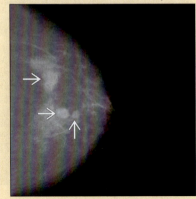
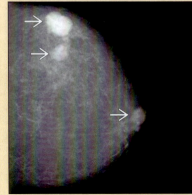
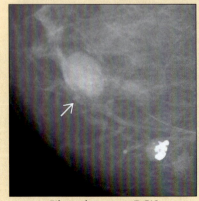

Phyllodes

Medullary Carcinoma

Fibroadenomas, DCIS

MULTIPLE BILATERAL SIMILAR FINDINGS

Key Facts

Terminology
- Multiple bilateral similar findings: At least 3 total, at least 1 in each breast
- When applied to masses, refers to multiple bilateral mostly circumscribed, partially obscured masses on mammography
- Excludes palpable findings
- Not applicable when there is a dominant mass or suspicious findings
- Suggests benign etiology

Imaging Findings
- US indicated in further evaluation of any dominant, palpable, rapidly growing, or other suspicious mass
- Protocol advice: Neither MR nor US indicated for routine evaluation of multiple, bilateral, mostly circumscribed masses absent suspicious findings

Top Differential Diagnoses
- Cysts and complicated cysts
- Fibroadenomas
- Oil cysts
- Papillomas
- Fibrocystic changes (FCC)

Pathology
- 1.7% of screening mammograms show multiple bilateral partially circumscribed masses
- Interval cancer rate with multiple bilateral rounded masses = 0.14% vs. 0.24% in age-matched controls

Diagnostic Checklist
- Avoid satisfaction of search: "Busy" breast may distract from other suspicious findings

---

- Initial full work-up, including CC and true lateral magnification views is recommended

Ultrasonographic Findings
- Grayscale Ultrasound
  - US indicated in further evaluation of any dominant, palpable, rapidly growing, or other suspicious mass
    - Bilateral US if suspicious finding(s) or to assess multiplicity of FA in young women
    - Guide aspiration and/or biopsy if needed
  - If bilateral US performed and multiple bilateral circumscribed oval, gently lobulated masses are identified, consider
    - Evaluate each margin carefully, excluding any thick-walled or indistinctly marginated masses
    - Benign classification for cysts and complicated cysts in the company of simple cysts
    - If solid, likely FA, consider 6 month, 12 month, 24 month follow-up
    - Validation of these approaches in progress
    - Reliable recording of lesion diameters and locations validated: Critical to follow-up

MR Findings
- T1WI
  - Oval or gently lobulated masses isointense to parenchyma
  - Hemorrhagic, proteinaceous cysts hyperintense
  - Fluid-debris levels in complicated cysts
- T2WI FS
  - Simple cysts hyperintense
    - Fluid-debris levels in complicated cysts
    - Proteinaceous fluid intermediate signal
    - Hemorrhagic cysts hypointense
  - Some cellular or myxoid FA hyperintense
- T1 C+
  - FA will enhance; 40-60% will show nonenhancing internal septations
  - Rim-enhancement of ruptured cysts

Imaging Recommendations
- Best imaging tool: Mammography, correlated with prior studies and clinical findings

- Protocol advice: Neither MR nor US indicated for routine evaluation of multiple, bilateral, mostly circumscribed masses absent suspicious findings

DIFFERENTIAL DIAGNOSIS

Multiple, Bilateral Circumscribed Masses
- Cysts and complicated cysts
  - Fluctuating pattern year to year with some developing, others regressing
  - Aspiration of dominant, palpable cysts for symptomatic relief
- Fibroadenomas
  - 15% multiple, bilateral
  - Some may be coarsely calcifying ("popcorn" Ca++)
  - Hypoechoic to isoechoic on US
  - Interval growth > 20% diameter in 6 months may suggest phyllodes tumor
- Fat necrosis
  - Oil cysts
  - May develop peripheral curvilinear Ca++
  - History of trauma or surgery
  - More often bilateral in setting of reduction mammoplasty
    - Associated architectural changes
- Papillomas
  - More often unilateral
  - Can show associated punctate, amorphous Ca++
- Circumscribed malignancy
  - May be in the company of other benign circumscribed masses
  - Most have at least partially indistinct margin
  - Invasive ductal carcinoma (IDC) NOS
    - 16% of high grade IDC is circumscribed
    - Rapid growth
    - May be thick-walled complex cystic lesion at US
  - Intracystic (papillary) carcinoma
    - Special subtype of ductal carcinoma in situ (DCIS)
    - May have associated focal invasive component
  - Mucinous carcinoma
  - Medullary carcinoma

- ○ Metastatic intramammary nodes: Breast, lymphoma
- ○ Metastases to breast: Carcinoid, melanoma, lymphoma
  - ▪ More often unilateral

Multiple, Bilateral Clustered Coarse Heterogeneous Calcifications

- Solitary cluster can be malignant: 7%
- Fibroadenomas
  - ○ Some may show associated circumscribed mass
- Fibrosis
  - ○ Some may actually represent sclerosed FA with loss of epithelial component

Multiple, Bilateral Clustered Punctate and Amorphous Calcifications

- Fibrocystic changes (FCC)
  - ○ Often at least some groupings will show layering on true lateral view, compatible with milk-of-calcium
  - ○ Any new or suspicious (e.g., pleomorphic, fine linear) Ca++ merit further evaluation and possible biopsy
  - ○ Often background of scattered punctate, coarse, and amorphous Ca++
  - ○ May have associated mostly circumscribed nodules due to cysts
- Papillomas
  - ○ Associated circumscribed nodule(s)

PATHOLOGY

General Features

- Epidemiology
  - ○ 1.7% of screening mammograms show multiple bilateral partially circumscribed masses
  - ○ Interval cancer rate with multiple bilateral rounded masses = 0.14% vs. 0.24% in age-matched controls

CLINICAL ISSUES

Presentation

- Most common signs/symptoms: Asymptomatic, screening
- Other signs/symptoms: Palpable lump, may be tender if cyst(s)

Natural History & Prognosis

- Depends on underlying etiology

Treatment

- Multiple, bilateral mostly circumscribed masses can be considered benign
  - ○ Dominant or palpable mass merits US
- Multiple, bilateral similar groupings of Ca++
  - ○ Coarse, heterogeneous Ca++ favors benign: Further study needed, benign or probably benign
    - ▪ Solitary cluster 7% malignancy rate among lesions biopsied
    - ▪ Malignancy rate when multiple, bilateral not established
  - ○ Amorphous, punctate Ca++
    - ▪ Full initial work-up to include magnification views

- ▪ Sampling of dominant grouping may be appropriate
- ▪ Isolated cluster 20% rate of malignancy
- ▪ Follow remaining groupings if dominant grouping benign
- ▪ Approach requires further validation

DIAGNOSTIC CHECKLIST

Consider

- One study suggests even palpable, circumscribed, oval, noncalcified benign appearing solid masses evaluated by both mammography and US may be able to be followed
  - ○ Did not specifically evaluate multiple, bilateral similar masses
  - ○ Not if new or enlarging
- Rapid growth, > 20% in diameter in six months, may be suspicious, merits targeted US and usually rebiopsy

Image Interpretation Pearls

- Carefully evaluate margins of each mass
  - ○ Dominant or palpable mass merits US
  - ○ Any suspicious margins or associated suspicious Ca++ merit work-up
- Avoid satisfaction of search: "Busy" breast may distract from other suspicious findings

SELECTED REFERENCES

1. Berg WA: Screening Breast Ultrasound in High-Risk Women: ACRIN 6666 protocol. www.acrin.org/current protocols/6666
2. Berg WA et al: Operator dependence of physician-performed whole breast sonography: lesion detection and characterization. Radiology (in press), 2006
3. Berg WA: Breast US: Benign and probably benign lesions. In: 2005 Syllabus, Categorical Course in Diagnostic Radiology: Breast Imaging, Ed. SA Feig. Oak Brook, Radiologic Society of North America.115-24, 2005
4. Burnside ES et al: The ability of microcalcification descriptors in the BI-RADS 4th edition to stratify the risk of malignancy. Radiologic Society of North America (abstr). 286, 2005
5. Graf O et al: Follow-up of palpable circumscribed noncalcified solid breast masses with mammography and US: can biopsy be averted? Radiology. 233:850-6, 2004
6. Gordon PB et al: Solid breast masses diagnosed as fibroadenoma at fine-needle aspiration biopsy: acceptable rates of growth at long-term follow-up. Radiology. 229:233-8, 2003
7. Berg WA et al: Biopsy of amorphous breast calcifications: pathologic outcome and yield at stereotactic biopsy. Radiology. 221:495-503, 2001
8. Lamb PM et al: Correlation between ultrasound characteristics, mammographic findings, and histological grade in patients with invasive ductal carcinoma of the breast. Clin Radiol. 55:40-44, 2000
9. Leung JW et al: Multiple bilateral masses detected on screening mammography: Assessment of need for recall imaging. AJR. 175:23-9, 2000

IMAGE GALLERY

Variant

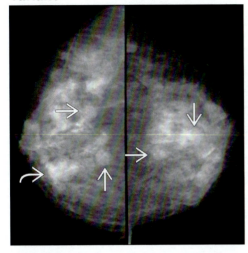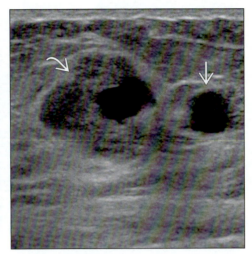

(Left) CC mammography shows multiple, bilateral mostly circumscribed masses ➡ in this 67 year old with a history of cysts. One new dominant circumscribed mass ➡ was noted in the inner right breast, with US performed (right-hand image). *(Right)* Ultrasound shows the dominant mass to be a complex, thick-walled cystic mass ➡, suspicious, BI-RADS 4B. Biopsy showed borderline phyllodes tumor. An adjacent cyst was noted ➡.

Variant

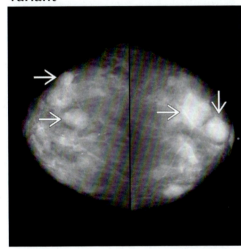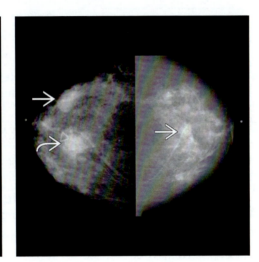

(Left) CC mammography in this 57 year old shows multiple, bilateral, mostly circumscribed masses ➡ compatible with cysts. *(Right)* CC mammography 3 years later (same patient as left-hand image) shows resolution of many of the cysts since the prior study, though a few remain ➡. A palpable mass is also noted ➡, requiring further evaluation (next 2 images).

Variant

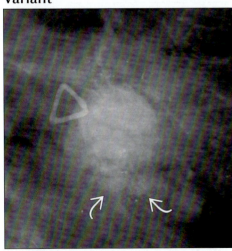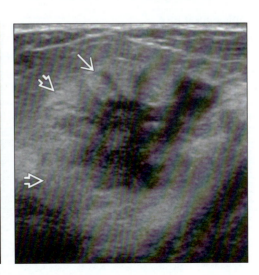

(Left) CC mammography spot compression (same patient as previous 2 images) shows partially spiculated margins ➡ to the palpable mass right breast. US was performed (right-hand image). *(Right)* Ultrasound confirms spiculated, hypoechoic mass ➡ with thick echogenic rim ➡, highly suggestive of malignancy. Initial FNAB was suspicious. Excision showed 3 cm grade III IDC.

IV

5

25

AMYLOID

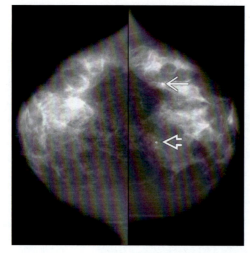 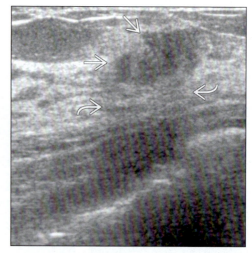

CC mammography shows mammographically-occult, palpable mass marked by BB ➡, in a 49 yo premenopausal woman. Clip ➡ marks an unrelated benign biopsy site.

US (same as on left) shows the 1.5 cm microlobulated, palpable mass ➡. Note subtle posterior acoustic shadowing ➡. US-guided biopsy showed primary amyloid.

TERMINOLOGY

Definitions
- Extracellular deposition of amorphous red Congophilic protein within tissues

IMAGING FINDINGS

General Features
- Best diagnostic clue: Mimics breast carcinoma
- Location: Breast: Right side 3x that of left
- Size: 2-3 cm average; largest reported, 5 cm

Mammographic Findings
- Circumscribed or irregular mass
- Focal asymmetry, architectural distortion reported
- Calcifications, with or without associated mass
- Mimics breast carcinoma
  - No diagnostic mammographic appearance

Ultrasonographic Findings
- Grayscale Ultrasound
  - Well-circumscribed or irregular mass
  - Posterior acoustic shadowing

Biopsy
- Core biopsy preferred; FNA unreliable

Imaging Recommendations
- Best imaging tool: Mammography and ultrasound

DIFFERENTIAL DIAGNOSIS

Infiltrating or Intraductal Carcinoma
- Indistinguishable from amyloid on imaging

Fibrocystic Changes
- Focal asymmetry or mass

Fibroadenoma
- Well-circumscribed mass

PATHOLOGY

General Features
- Etiology

DDx: Lesions that may Mimic Amyloid

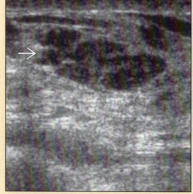 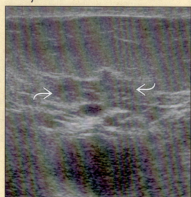 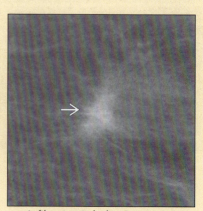

Fibroadenomatoid Changes   *Ductal Carcinoma in Situ*   *Infiltrating Lobular Carcinoma*

AMYLOID

Key Facts

Terminology
- Extracellular deposition of amorphous red Congophilic protein within tissues

Imaging Findings
- Best diagnostic clue: Mimics breast carcinoma

Top Differential Diagnoses
- Infiltrating or Intraductal Carcinoma

Pathology
- Two types of breast amyloid
- Primary: Organ-specific, only involving breast
- Secondary (systemic): Organ involvement elsewhere in body; breast involvement late
- Apple-green birefringence with Congo red stain under polarized light

---

  - Two types of breast amyloid
    - Primary: Organ-specific, only involving breast
    - Secondary (systemic): Organ involvement elsewhere in body; breast involvement late
- Associated abnormalities: Secondary type often associated with underlying diseases like rheumatoid arthritis and multiple myeloma

Gross Pathologic & Surgical Features
- Firm, gray or white and opalescent
- If calcification present, gritty sensation when incised

Microscopic Features
- Eosinophilic, amorphous, homogeneous deposits of amyloid
- Distribution
  - In lobules, fat, fibrocollagenous stroma and blood vessels
  - Around ducts
- Stains red-orange with alkaline Congo red
  - Apple-green birefringence with Congo red stain under polarized light
- Associated multinucleated giant cells, plasma cells and lymphocytes
- Osseous metaplasia reported

CLINICAL ISSUES

Presentation
- Most common signs/symptoms
  - Discrete, firm, palpable mass

- Usually painless
- Skin thickening, peau d'orange reported
- Other signs/symptoms
  - If primary may be asymptomatic, picked up on screening (rare)
  - If secondary, symptoms related to systemic involvement or associated underlying diseases

Demographics
- Age: Range: 45-82; mostly post-menopausal women
- Gender: Only reported in females

Natural History & Prognosis
- Primary amyloid
  - Excellent prognosis
- Systemic
  - Poor prognosis, unrelated to breast involvement

Treatment
- Excisional biopsy

SELECTED REFERENCES

1. Ayers DE et al: Amyloid tumour of the breast mimicking carcinoma. Cytopathology. 13(4):254-6, 2002
2. Gluck BS et al: Amyloid deposition of the breast. AJR Am J Roentgenol. 175(6):1590, 2000
3. Lynch LA et al: Localized primary amyloid tumor associated with osseous metaplasia presenting as bilateral breast masses: cytologic and radiologic features. Diagn Cytopathol. 9(5):570-5, 1993

IMAGE GALLERY

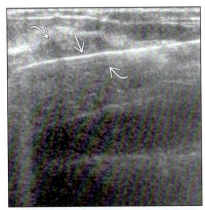
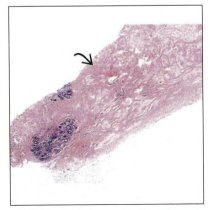
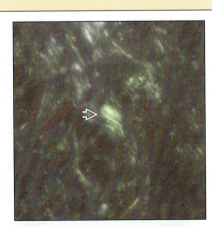

(Left) Transverse ultrasound shows intralesional position of 14-g biopsy needle ➡ at time of US-guided biopsy of palpable mass ➡, establishing diagnosis of primary amyloid of breast. *(Center)* Micropathology, low power, H&E of biopsied lesion shows dense, pink amorphous eosinophilic stroma ➜, suggestive of amyloid. Pathologist ordered Congo red stain (right image). *(Right)* Micropathology, low power shows Congo Red stain, which confirmed diagnosis of amyloid. Note dense stroma ➡ which, with polarization, demonstrates apple-green birefringence.

COLLAGEN VASCULAR DISEASE

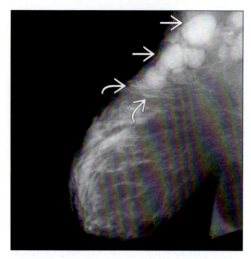

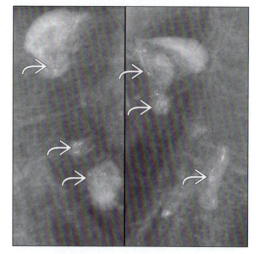

MLO mammography shows findings of mastitis with trabecular thickening ➔. Multiple enlarged nodes without discernible hila ➔, are present, symmetric with the left side in this woman with SLE.

MLO mammography shows radiodensities in several axillary lymph nodes bilaterally ➔, attributable to uptake of gold particles in another woman with a long history of intramuscular gold injections for RA.

TERMINOLOGY

Definitions
- Heterogeneous group of disorders with common features including inflammation of connective tissues, the production of autoantibodies and abnormalities of cell-mediated immunity
- Entities include dermatomyositis, rheumatoid (RA) and psoriatic arthritis, systemic lupus erythematosus (SLE), scleroderma, and mixed connective tissue disorders (MCTD)
- Breast involvement uncommon

IMAGING FINDINGS

General Features
- Best diagnostic clue: Lymphadenopathy, usually bilateral, the most common mammographic abnormality shared by these disorders

Mammographic Findings
- Standard MLO and CC views unless a clinically suspicious finding present

- MLO views may demonstrate axillary adenopathy, typically bilateral
  - Gold deposits within axillary nodes may be seen in some treated cases of RA
- Dermatomyositis may show bizarre subcutaneous dystrophic calcifications (Ca++)
- Skin thickening reported in scleroderma; mass with focal skin thickening reported in SLE

Ultrasonographic Findings
- Grayscale Ultrasound: Used to evaluate clinical and imaging findings

MR Findings
- No specific breast findings, per se

Imaging Recommendations
- Best imaging tool: Screening mammography

DIFFERENTIAL DIAGNOSIS

Axillary Adenopathy of other Causes
- Bilateral

DDx: Other Causes of Findings Reported with Collagen Vascular Diseases

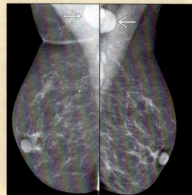

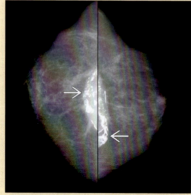

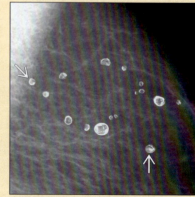

Bilateral Adenopathy, Leukemia

Dystrophic Ca++, Implant Capsule

Coarse Ca++, Seat-Belt Trauma

COLLAGEN VASCULAR DISEASE

Key Facts

Terminology

- Heterogeneous group of disorders with common features including inflammation of connective tissues, the production of autoantibodies and abnormalities of cell-mediated immunity
- Entities include dermatomyositis, rheumatoid (RA) and psoriatic arthritis, systemic lupus erythematosus (SLE), scleroderma, and mixed connective tissue disorders (MCTD)

- Breast involvement uncommon

Imaging Findings

- Dermatomyositis may show bizarre subcutaneous dystrophic calcifications (Ca++)
- Best imaging tool: Screening mammography

Top Differential Diagnoses

- Axillary Adenopathy of other Causes
- Dystrophic Calcifications

- o Lymphoma, leukemia, mononucleosis, HIV, granulomatous diseases (sarcoid, tuberculosis)
- Unilateral or bilateral
  - o Nonspecific benign lymphadenopathy, metastatic disease with or without known primary, mastitis

Dystrophic Calcifications

- Dermatomyositis; reported in SLE
- Post breast conserving treatment (lumpectomy and radiation) for breast cancer
- Fibrous capsule surrounding either silicone or saline implants

Adult Onset Still Disease (AOSD)

- Symptoms of fever, arthritis, and skin rashes reported as first symptoms in patients with breast cancer

PATHOLOGY

General Features

- Epidemiology
  - o No convincing data of association of either typical or atypical connective tissue disease and silicone implants
  - o Mixed reports of breast cancer associated with these disease entities
    - Dermatomyositis; ? RA

CLINICAL ISSUES

Presentation

- Other signs/symptoms: Systemic symptoms include: Arthritides, muscle weakness, skin abnormalities, renal insufficiency

Treatment

- Specific to the systemic disease disorder or any suspicious breast finding
- Active collagen vascular disease a relative contraindication to breast conserving therapy (radiation)

SELECTED REFERENCES

1. Sabate JM et al: Lupus panniculitis involving the breast. Eur Radiol. 16:53-6, 2006
2. Lipworth L et al: Silicone breast implants and connective tissue disease: an updated review of the epidemiologic evidence.Ann Plast Surg. 52:598-601, 2004
3. Von Lilienfeld-Toal M et al: An unusual presentation of a common disease. Ann Rheum DIs. 63:887-8, 2004
4. Opere E et al: Localized scleroderma of the breast. Eur Radiol. 12:1483-5, 2002
5. Feder JM et al: Unusual breast lesions: Radiologic-pathologic correlation. RadioGraphics. 19:811-26, 1999

IMAGE GALLERY

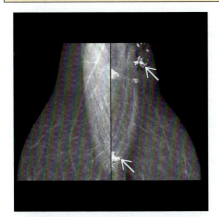 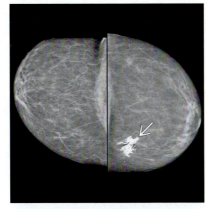 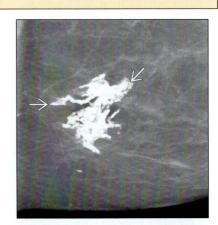

(Left) MLO mammography in a woman with known dermatomyositis demonstrates unilateral left prominent dense dystrophic calcifications ➡ in the upper inner breast and axilla. *(Center)* CC mammography (same case as left image) shows a conglomerate of the dystrophic somewhat bizarrely shaped calcifications ➡. *(Right)* CC photographic close-up (same as previous image) shows to better advantage the coarse nature of this conglomerate of dystrophic calcifications ➡.

DIABETIC MASTOPATHY

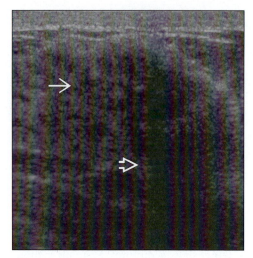

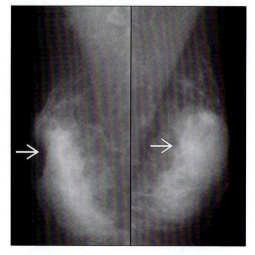

Transverse ultrasound shows a large poorly-defined heterogeneously hypoechoic region ➡ with indistinct margins and posterior shadowing ⇥. This appearance was symmetrical.

MLO mammography shows symmetrical large areas of homogeneous parenchymal density ➡ bilaterally in a patient with long-standing diabetes and stable bilateral hard breast tissue.

TERMINOLOGY

Abbreviations and Synonyms
- Diabetic fibrous breast disease (DFBD)

Definitions
- A variant of stromal fibrosis occurring in diabetics

IMAGING FINDINGS

General Features
- Best diagnostic clue: Bilateral homogeneous marked parenchymal density; clinically hard breasts
- Location: Central glandular cone
- Size: Usually extensive; may be focal 2-6 cm
- Morphology: Indistinct margins

Mammographic Findings
- Symmetric area(s) of homogeneous dense parenchyma

Ultrasonographic Findings
- Grayscale Ultrasound
  - Hypoechoic region or mass with indistinct margins
  - May have marked posterior acoustic shadowing

- Color Doppler: No hypervascularity

MR Findings
- T1 C+
  - Focal slow heterogeneous enhancement
    - Gradual enhancement over time
    - Heterogeneous, regional on delayed imaging

Imaging Recommendations
- Best imaging tool: Ultrasound
- Protocol advice
  - Suspect in patients with longstanding diabetes
  - Clinical palpation important
  - May require biopsy if asymmetric, atypical

DIFFERENTIAL DIAGNOSIS

Carcinoma
- Hypoechoic, indistinct invasive cancers (ductal, lobular)

Focal or Stromal Fibrosis
- Nonspecific imaging findings of dense parenchyma on mammogram

DDx: Dense Breast Tissues

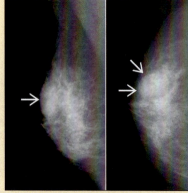

Focal Fibrosis

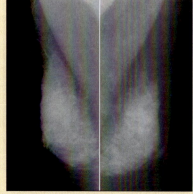

Dense Parenchyma

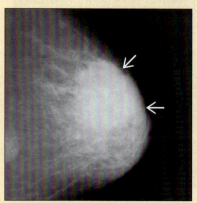

Large Carcinoma

DIABETIC MASTOPATHY

Key Facts

Terminology
- Diabetic fibrous breast disease (DFBD)

Imaging Findings
- Best diagnostic clue: Bilateral homogeneous marked parenchymal density; clinically hard breasts
- Hypoechoic region or mass with indistinct margins
- Suspect in patients with longstanding diabetes

Top Differential Diagnoses
- Carcinoma
- Focal or Stromal Fibrosis

Pathology
- 20 year average interval between diabetes onset and mass

Clinical Issues
- Excellent prognosis, self-limited

Other Palpable Nontender Masses with Nonspecific Imaging Findings
- Dense asymmetric glandular tissue

PATHOLOGY

General Features
- Etiology: Typically seen in type I insulin-dependent diabetics
- Epidemiology
  - 20 year average interval between diabetes onset and mass
  - Mean age of diabetes onset 12-13 years

Gross Pathologic & Surgical Features
- 2-10 cm in size
- Cut surface often indistinguishable from surrounding breast parenchyma

Microscopic Features
- Collagenous stroma
- Increased stromal spindle cells
- Prominent myofibroblasts and perivascular lymphocytic infiltrates

CLINICAL ISSUES

Presentation
- Most common signs/symptoms: Present as palpable, very firm, nontender masses or thickening
- Clinical Profile: Premenopausal woman with long-standing insulin-dependent diabetes

Demographics
- Age: 40-50
- Gender: Most often female; rarely in men

Natural History & Prognosis
- Excellent prognosis, self-limited
- No increased risk for development of invasive cancer

Treatment
- Needle core biopsy suggested to establish diagnosis
- Expectant management, clinical review

SELECTED REFERENCES

1. Goel NB et al: Fibrous lesions of the breast: imaging-pathologic correlation. Radiographics. 25:1547-59, 2005
2. Wong KT et al: Ultrasound and MR imaging of diabetic mastopathy. Clin Radiol. 57:730-5, 2002
3. Rosen PP: Rosen's Breast Pathology. Philadelphia, Lippincott Williams & Wilkins. Chapter 3, 53-6, 2001
4. Bassett LW et al: Diagnosis of Diseases of the Breast. Philadelphia, WB Saunders Co. Chapter 25, 411, 1997

IMAGE GALLERY

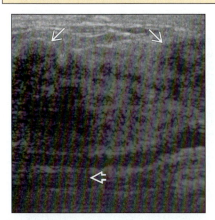 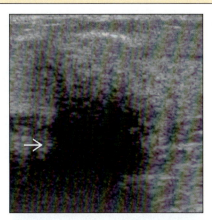 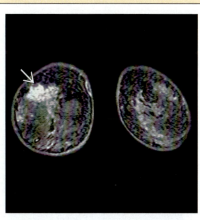

(Left) Anti-radial ultrasound shows two adjacent areas of indistinct hypoechoic change ➡ with some shadowing ➡ and intervening normal parenchyma. Biopsy proven. *(Center)* Transverse ultrasound shows markedly hypoechoic irregular mass ➡ with posterior shadowing at site of palpable lump in this 45 year old with type I diabetes since age 8. *(Right)* Coronal T1 C+ subtraction MR (same patient as previous image) shows heterogeneous, regional enhancement upper right breast ➡ in area of lump. Biopsy proved diabetic mastopathy.

LEUKEMIA

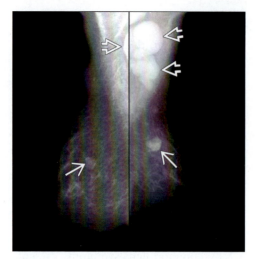

MLO mammography demonstrates a case of chronic lymphocytic leukemia, manifesting as both axillary ➡ and parenchymal masses ➡.

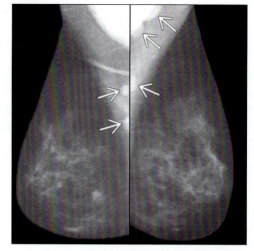

MLO mammography shows an example of recurrent chronic lymphocytic leukemia, manifesting as new axillary adenopathy ➡ on screening mammogram.

IMAGING FINDINGS

General Features
- Best diagnostic clue
  - Systemic disease: Enlarged axillary lymph nodes (LN), usually bilateral
  - Breast disease: Enlarged, hard palpable mass(es) in patient with systemic disease

Mammographic Findings
- Bilateral or unilateral LN enlargement; seen on MLO
  - Hyperdense, round mass(es); often loss of fatty hila
  - Size variable, less important than appearance
- Parenchymal mass
  - May be well-circumscribed or ill-defined; solitary or multiple; often bilateral
  - Can be diffusely infiltrating
- Breast enlargement, edema and skin thickening from lymphatic obstruction

Ultrasonographic Findings
- Grayscale Ultrasound
  - Breast: Irregular, mixed or hypoechoic, echogenic rim
  - Nodes: Nearly anechoic cortex, compressed or absent hila

DIFFERENTIAL DIAGNOSIS

Non-Hodgkin Lymphoma
- Axillary adenopathy most common presentation

Metastatic Disease
- Usually known primary malignancy

Collagen Vascular Disease
- Most common mammographic finding is bilateral axillary adenopathy

HIV-Related Adenopathy
- Incidental finding on screening mammography

PATHOLOGY

General Features
- Genetics: Translocations identified in many leukemias
- Etiology

DDx: Other Causes of Axillary Adenopathy

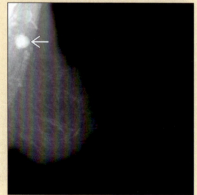

Non-Hodgkin Lymphoma

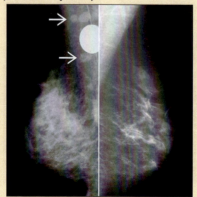

Metastatic Lung Carcinoma

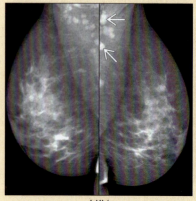

HIV

LEUKEMIA

Key Facts

Imaging Findings
- Systemic disease: Enlarged axillary lymph nodes (LN), usually bilateral

Top Differential Diagnoses
- Non-Hodgkin Lymphoma
- Metastatic Disease
- Collagen Vascular Disease

Pathology
- Usually secondary to known systemic disease
- Acute myelogenous leukemia (AML) most common form to involve breast
- Chloroma: Extramedullary, tumor-forming granulocytic infiltrate in AML

Diagnostic Checklist
- If leukemia suspected → needle biopsy; surgery not necessary

---

- Usually secondary to known systemic disease
  - Occurs by hematogenous spread
  - Breast involvement rarely precedes systemic disease; but if it does, systemic manifestations follow within a year

Gross Pathologic & Surgical Features
- Chronic lymphocytic leukemia (CLL): Adenopathy more common, rarely involves breast
- Acute myelogenous leukemia (AML) most common form to involve breast
- Chloroma: Extramedullary, tumor-forming granulocytic infiltrate in AML
  - Grossly green in color
    - Secondary to enzymatic action of myeloperoxidase in leukemic cells

Microscopic Features
- Small, round leukemic cells within ducts or lobules may simulate infiltrating lobular carcinoma or DCIS
- Chloroma cells: Granular eosinophilic cytoplasm, positive for esterase

CLINICAL ISSUES

Presentation
- Most common signs/symptoms
  - Systemic disease
    - Axillary adenopathy may be detected on screening mammography
    - CLL more common > 50 yrs of age; AML, bimodal

- Clinically evident breast involvement

Treatment
- Systemic disease treated with anti-leukemic drugs
- Chloroma treated with radiation therapy and chemotherapy

DIAGNOSTIC CHECKLIST

Consider
- If leukemia suspected → needle biopsy; surgery not necessary
  - Place tissue cores in saline, not formalin, to allow fluorescence-activated cell sorting

SELECTED REFERENCES

1. Rosen P: Rosen's Breast Pathology. 2nd Ed. Philadelphia, Lippincott Williams & Wilkins. Chapter 42. 881-2, 2001
2. Murray et al: The clinical importance of axillary lymphadenopathy detected on screening mammography. Clin Radiol. 52:458-61, 1997
3. Walsh et al: Axillary lymph nodes: mammographic, pathologic, and clinical correlation. AJR. 168:33-8, 1997

IMAGE GALLERY

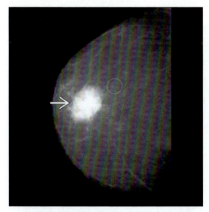 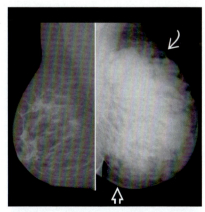 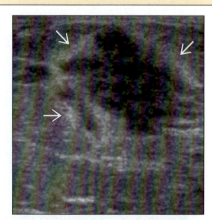

(Left) CC mammography demonstrates a dense, indistinctly marginated mass ➡, corresponding to a palpable lump, known to be a chloroma in this 34 yo with AML. *(Center)* MLO mammography shows enlarged, dense left breast with trabecular thickening ➡ and skin thickening ➡ in a 28 yo with AML. US-guided core biopsy showed chloroma. (Courtesy EBM). *(Right)* US in a 38 yo with AML shows an irregular, hypoechoic (palpable) mass with echogenic halo ➡. US-guided core biopsy showed an esterase positive leukemic infiltrate c/w chloroma.

METASTASES TO BREAST

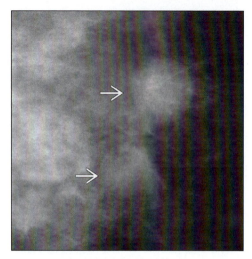

CC mammography shows two partially obscured, partially circumscribed masses ➡. Spot compression views and US (right image) may better define margins & rule out cysts.

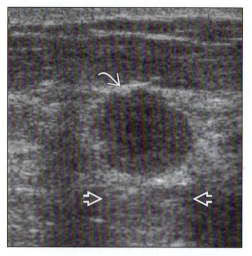

Ultrasound of one of the masses shows it to be hypoechoic ➡ with microlobulated margins and posterior enhancement ➡. US-guided 14-g biopsy revealed metastatic carcinoid.

TERMINOLOGY

Definitions
- Involvement of the breast by metastatic disease
  - From extramammary malignancies
  - Or contralateral breast (rare: Usually second primary)

IMAGING FINDINGS

General Features
- Best diagnostic clue: Circumscribed breast mass(es) in patient with known malignancy
- Location
  - Usually upper outer quadrant, superficial: Parenchymal, or intramammary node
  - Solitary nodule in 75-85%; multiple or bilateral 15-25%, diffuse parenchymal involvement 4%
  - Axillary nodal involvement 25-50%
- Size: Variable, but usually 1-3 cm
- Morphology: Round, circumscribed or slightly irregular mass without spiculations, calcifications, or architectural distortion

Mammographic Findings
- Hematogenous
  - Round, circumscribed, noncalcified mass
  - Multiple & bilateral masses in later stages
  - Spiculations and architectural distortion rare
  - Calcifications rare (some ovarian cancer metastases)
  - Ipsilateral or bilateral axillary adenopathy
- Lymphangitic
  - Breast enlargement, asymmetric density, skin thickening, skin nodules, +/- axillary adenopathy
- Hematologic malignancy such as lymphoma
  - Solitary or multiple, unilateral or bilateral masses, asymmetric density or infiltrative process, +/- axillary adenopathy

Ultrasonographic Findings
- Grayscale Ultrasound
  - Round/ovoid solid, hypoechoic mass(es); sometimes almost anechoic
    - Margins may be indistinct or microlobulated
    - Posterior enhancement more common than shadowing

DDx: Other Well-Defined or Obscured Multiple Masses

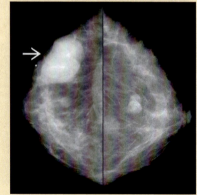

Cancer & FA's

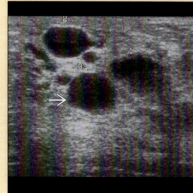

Cysts, Complicated Cysts

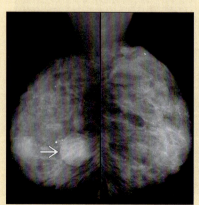

Intracystic Cancer

METASTASES TO BREAST

Key Facts

Terminology
- Involvement of the breast by metastatic disease

Imaging Findings
- Usually upper outer quadrant, superficial: Parenchymal, or intramammary node
- Solitary nodule in 75-85%; multiple or bilateral 15-25%, diffuse parenchymal involvement 4%
- Axillary nodal involvement 25-50%

Top Differential Diagnoses
- Primary Breast Carcinoma
- Cyst
- Benign Breast Tumors
- Intramammary Lymph Node
- Primary or Secondary Lymphoma

Clinical Issues
- Usually indicative of widespread diffuse metastatic disease and very poor prognosis
- Mean survival after diagnosis of metastases within breast less than 1 year

Diagnostic Checklist
- Distinction between primary breast cancer and metastatic disease is critical
- Unnecessary surgery such as radical mastectomy may be avoided
- Appropriate chemotherapy and radiation treatment can be offered
- Solitary palpable, firm, mobile breast mass(es), lacking the typical features of primary breast cancer such as spiculation, calcifications or architectural distortion

MR Findings
- T1 C+: Rapidly enhancing round or ill-defined mass(es); rim-enhancement possible

Nuclear Medicine Findings
- PET: FDG PET-CT moderately high sensitivity for masses > 7-8 mm, whole body scan to determine full extent of metastatic disease

CT Findings
- CECT
  - May detect widespread adenopathy in chest, abdomen, and pelvis
  - Metastatic foci in breast or other organs, soft tissues or skeleton

Imaging Recommendations
- Best imaging tool
  - Mammography and ultrasound
  - Role of PET-CT to be determined
- Protocol advice: Spot compression views and careful scanning for margin details

DIFFERENTIAL DIAGNOSIS

Primary Breast Carcinoma
- Invasive ductal carcinoma (IDC) NOS, medullary, mucinous, papillary

Cyst
- Complicated cyst, ruptured cyst

Benign Breast Tumors
- Fibroadenoma (FA), phyllodes tumor, papilloma

Intramammary Lymph Node
- Normal or pathologic
- Benign reactive or malignant

Primary or Secondary Lymphoma
- Primary lymphoma usually presents as solitary mass
- Secondary lymphoma usually multiple small bilateral nodules, or infiltrative process

PATHOLOGY

General Features
- General path comments
  - Isolated metastasis to breast rare
    - Even when breast is at initial presenting site, other sites usually present
- Etiology
  - Extramammary tumors metastasize to breast via hematogenous spread
    - Melanoma is most common
    - Others in declining order of frequency: Lung, ovarian, soft tissue sarcomas, gastrointestinal, other genitourinary, neuro-endocrine tumors such as carcinoid, and sporadically thyroid, osteosarcoma, cervical, vaginal, and endometrial
  - Hematologic malignancy
    - Lymphoma is second most common non-mammary malignancy of the breast (after melanoma), not always categorized as metastasis
  - Contralateral breast carcinoma via cross lymphatics in anterior chest wall
    - Synchronous or metachronous breast primaries more common than metastases between breasts
- Epidemiology
  - Rare: 0.5-2% of all breast malignancies
  - Median interval from primary cancer diagnosis to appearance of breast metastases 12 months (range: 0-144 months)
  - Incidence of breast as first metastatic site: 25-40%, commonly from small cell lung cancer

Gross Pathologic & Surgical Features
- Circumscribed tumor with multiple satellite foci
- Usually not fixed to adjacent tissues
- Occur in areas of fat rather than parenchymal tissue

Microscopic Features
- Periductal or perilobular malignant cells
- Absence of in situ, ductal or lobular pathology; presence of lymphatic emboli

METASTASES TO BREAST

Staging, Grading or Classification Criteria
- Image guided tissue diagnosis highly accurate
  - Fine needle aspiration cytology or core needle biopsy
- Stage depends on specific primary
  - If primary is contralateral breast: Stage IV

CLINICAL ISSUES

Presentation
- Most common signs/symptoms: Solitary non-tender palpable lump
- Other signs/symptoms
  - Metastatic deposits in intramammary lymph nodes
  - Look for increased density and loss of fatty hilum of nodes
- Hematogenous spread
  - Usually solitary mass; more likely to be multiple and bilateral than primary breast cancer
- Lymphangitic spread
  - Multiple nodules, skin thickening, rarely skin nodules
  - Axillary adenopathy

Demographics
- Age: Median 60 years, range: 20-85
- Gender
  - Females affected 5-6x more commonly than males
  - In males prostate cancer is most common source
    - Important to distinguish breast vs. prostate primary as treatment differs

Natural History & Prognosis
- Usually indicative of widespread diffuse metastatic disease and very poor prognosis
- Mean survival after diagnosis of metastases within breast less than 1 year

Treatment
- Systemic treatment appropriate to primary malignancy
- Mastectomy appropriate for local control of bulky/symptomatic disease
- Lymph node dissection for local control

DIAGNOSTIC CHECKLIST

Consider
- History of previously known non-mammary malignancy
- Distinction between primary breast cancer and metastatic disease is critical
  - Unnecessary surgery such as radical mastectomy may be avoided
  - Appropriate chemotherapy and radiation treatment can be offered

Image Interpretation Pearls
- Solitary palpable, firm, mobile breast mass(es), lacking the typical features of primary breast cancer such as spiculation, calcifications or architectural distortion
- Clinical size of metastatic lesions similar to size on imaging due to lack of desmoplastic reaction

SELECTED REFERENCES

1. Shukla R et al: Fine-needle aspiration cytology of extramammary neoplasms metastatic to the breast. Diagn Cytopathol. 32(4):193-7, 2005
2. Smymiotis V et al: Metastatic disease in the breast from nonmammary neoplasms. Eur J Gynaecol Oncol. 26(5):547-50, 2005
3. Lim ET et al: Pathological axillary lymph nodes detected at mammographic screening. Clin Radiol. 59(1):86-91, 2004
4. Saad RS et al: Diagnostic value of HepPar1, pCEA, CD10, and CD34 expression in separating hepatocellular carcinoma from metastatic carcinoma in fine-needle aspiration cytology. Diagn Cytopathol. 30(1):1-6, 2004
5. Yeh CN et al: Clinical and ultrasonographic characteristics of breast metastases from extramammary malignancies. Am Surg. 70(4):287-90, 2004
6. Bartella L et al: Metastases to the breast revisited: radiological-histopathological correlation. Clin Radiol. 58(7):524-31, 2003
7. Akcay MN: Metastatic disease in the breast. Breast. 11(6):526-8, 2002
8. David O et al: Unusual cases of metastases to the breast. A report of 17 cases diagnosed by fine needle aspiration. Acta Cytol. 46(2):377-85, 2002
9. Fornage BD et al: Interventional breast sonography. Eur J Radiol. 42(1):17-31, 2002
10. Chung SY et al: Imaging findings of metastatic disease to the breast. Yonsei Med J. 42(5):497-502, 2001
11. Vizcaino I et al: Metastasis to the breast from extramammary malignancies: a report of four cases and a review of literature. Eur Radiol. 11(9):1659-65, 2001
12. Deshpande AH et al: Aspiration cytology of extramammary tumors metastatic to the breast. Diagn Cytopathol. 21(5):319-23, 1999
13. Holder WD Jr et al: Effectiveness of positron emission tomography for the detection of melanoma metastases. Ann Surg. 227(5):764-9; discussion 769-71, 1998
14. Rubio IT et al: Carcinoid tumor metastatic to the breast. Arch Surg. 133(10):1117-9, 1998
15. Domanski HA: Metastases to the breast from extramammary neoplasms. A report of six cases with diagnosis by fine needle aspiration cytology. Acta Cytol. 40(6):1293-300, 1996
16. Amichetti M et al: Metastases to the breast from extramammary malignancies. Oncology. 47(3):257-60, 1990
17. Seidelin CM et al: [Breast metastases as the initial symptom of extramammary carcinomas] Ugeskr Laeger. 149(21):1397-8, 1987
18. Bohman LG et al: Breast metastases from extramammary malignancies. Radiology. 144(2):309-12, 1982
19. Paulus DD et al: Metastasis to the breast. Radiol Clin North Am. 20(3):561-8, 1982
20. Nielsen M et al: Metastases to the breast from extramammary carcinomas. Acta Pathol Microbiol Scand [A]. 89(4):251-6, 1981
21. Toombs BD et al: Metastatic disease to the breast: clinical, pathologic, and radiographic features. AJR Am J Roentgenol. 129(4):673-6, 1977

IMAGE GALLERY

Typical

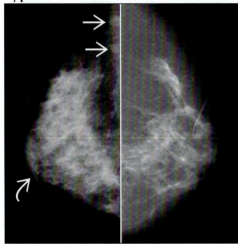

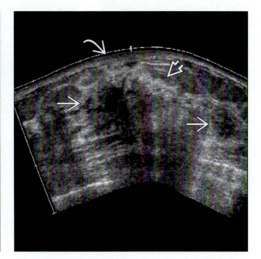

(Left) XCCL mammography shows shrunken right breast with diffuse increased density and skin thickening ➡. Dense nodes are noted in right axilla ➡. This woman had been diagnosed with lung cancer 5 years earlier. *(Right)* US of right breast (same patient as left-hand image) shows multiple irregular hypoechoic masses ➡ and increased echogenicity ➡. Skin thickening is noted ➡. Core biopsy of two masses showed adenocarcinoma metastatic from lung.

Typical

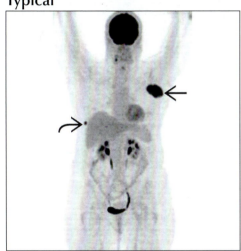

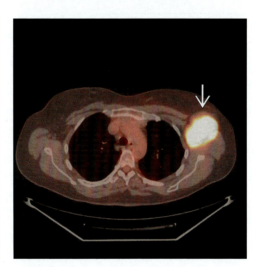

(Left) Coronal PET scan shows intense uptake in left axilla ➡ in this 60 yo woman with axillary mass and a remote history of melanoma over the left scapula. An unsuspected focus in the contralateral right breast ➡ is seen. *(Right)* Axial PET-CT (same case as left) shows the intense uptake in the left axillary mass to better advantage ➡. Biopsy found this to be an 8 cm tumor mass (conglomerate of replaced lymph nodes).

Typical

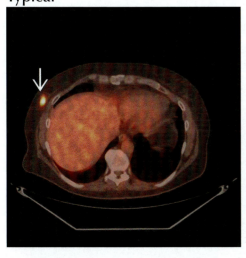

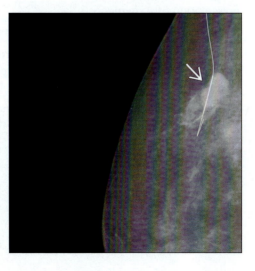

(Left) Axial PET-CT scan (same patient as previous image) better demonstrates the right breast mass ➡. Needle localization and excision of the breast mass (right image) was performed. (Note physiologic heterogeneous hepatic uptake). *(Right)* CC mammography during wire localization shows a lobulated, circumscribed mass in the lateral right breast ➡. Surgical resection and histopathology showed a 1.8 cm metastatic melanoma.

NON-HODGKIN LYMPHOMA

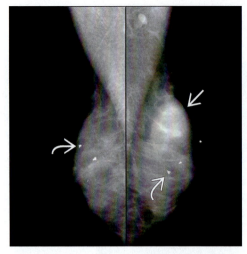
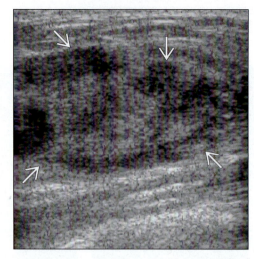

MLO mammography shows dense parenchyma, benign calcifications ⮕ and focal asymmetry ⮕ superiorly on the left, corresponding to palpable lump. US was performed (right-hand image).

Anti-radial ultrasound shows a mixed echogenicity oval mass ⮕, corresponding to the palpable lump. Biopsy, performed due to indeterminate appearance, revealed low grade B-cell lymphoma.

TERMINOLOGY

Abbreviations and Synonyms
- Two distinct entities
  - Primary lymphoma of the breast (PLB)
  - Secondary lymphomatous involvement of the breast (more commonly encountered in breast imaging)

Definitions
- Extra-nodal lymphoma arising from periductal and perilobular lymphoid tissue or from intramammary lymph nodes

IMAGING FINDINGS

General Features
- Best diagnostic clue
  - Uni- or bilateral abnormal axillary nodes most common mammographic presentation of systemic lymphoma
  - Breast mass in patient with history of non-mammary lymphoma
  - Enlarging painless breast lump

- Location: PLB: Most common in upper outer quadrant; right breast more often than left
- Size
  - PLB: 3-12 centimeters
  - Axillary nodes: Variable
- Morphology: Partially circumscribed to indistinct mass

Mammographic Findings
- Solitary or multiple well-circumscribed to ill-defined mass(es) without spiculation or calcifications
- Infiltrative type: Diffuse opacification, trabecular and skin thickening may be present

Ultrasonographic Findings
- Grayscale Ultrasound
  - Partially circumscribed to irregular oval mass
    - Variable posterior acoustic enhancement or shadowing
    - Mixed echogenicity (hyper- and hypoechoic), can be mostly hyperechoic
  - If arising in lymph node, may be almost anechoic, with compressed or absent hilum

MR Findings
- T1WI: Hypointense or isointense; usually well-defined

DDx: Other Circumscribed Breast Masses

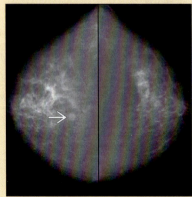
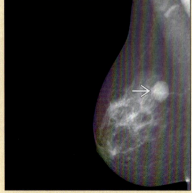
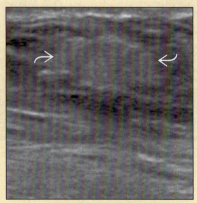

Melanoma Metastasis | Papillary Cancer | Secondary Lymphoma

NON-HODGKIN LYMPHOMA

Key Facts

Terminology
- Two distinct entities
- Primary lymphoma of the breast (PLB)
- Secondary lymphomatous involvement of the breast (more commonly encountered in breast imaging)
- Extra-nodal lymphoma arising from periductal and perilobular lymphoid tissue or from intramammary lymph nodes

Imaging Findings
- Solitary or multiple well-circumscribed to ill-defined mass(es) without spiculation or calcifications
- Infiltrative type: Diffuse opacification, trabecular and skin thickening may be present

Top Differential Diagnoses
- Primary breast cancer
- Benign breast tumors
- Metastatic disease
- Infectious disease
- Inflammatory breast cancer
- Other causes of axillary adenopathy

Pathology
- Represents 0.04-0.5% of all primary malignant breast tumors

Clinical Issues
- Tumor size > 5 cm
- Prognosis better than that of breast carcinoma

Diagnostic Checklist
- Consider in differential of breast masses lacking typical features of breast carcinoma, such as spiculation and microcalcifications

---

- T1 C+: Rapidly enhancing mass

Nuclear Medicine Findings
- PET
  - 18-FDG PET-CT is routinely used for diagnosis, staging and follow-up
    - Gallium scan is the alternative if PET-CT not available

Imaging Recommendations
- Best imaging tool: Mammography and ultrasound, 18-FDG PET-CT

DIFFERENTIAL DIAGNOSIS

Primary Non-Hodgkin Lymphoma of the Breast: Breast Mass
- Primary breast cancer
  - Colloid, mucinous, papillary, tubular or ductal
- Benign breast tumors
  - Fibroadenoma, fibroadenolipoma (hamartoma), phyllodes tumor
- Metastatic disease
  - From extra-mammary lymphoma (e.g., gastro-intestinal)
  - From extramammary primaries
- Infectious disease
  - Chronic abscess
  - Tuberculosis

Primary Lymphoma of Breast Presenting as Infiltrative Process
- Inflammatory breast cancer
- Mastitis
- Venous congestion due to heart failure or venous compromise

Secondary Lymphoma
- Metastases
- Other causes of axillary adenopathy
  - Collagen vascular diseases
  - Lymphoproliferative diseases such as chronic lymphocytic or myeloid leukemia
  - Tuberculosis or other granulomatous disease
  - HIV

PATHOLOGY

General Features
- Genetics: Complex, variable; possible association with t(11;14) translocation
- Epidemiology
  - Represents 0.04-0.5% of all primary malignant breast tumors
  - 0.38-0.7% of all lymphomas
  - 2% of primary extranodal lymphomas
  - Bilateral PLB in puerperal (lactating or peri-lactational) women, usually Burkitt-type

Microscopic Features
- Monotonous round cells with variable nuclear pleomorphism and mitotic activity
- Majority (40-70%) are of B-cell lineage; most common subtype diffuse large cell (40-70%)
- Follicular and MALT (mucosal associated lymphoid tissue) types not uncommon in GI tract, breast
- Immunohistochemical reactivities: CD20, CD45, CD3, CD5, CD10, CD23, CD30, cyclin D1, Ki-67, leukocyte common antigen
- Diagnosis optimally made via fluorescence activated cell sorting, using fresh biopsy specimens in saline

Staging, Grading or Classification Criteria
- Revised European-American Classification of Lymphoid Neoplasms (REAL) based on WHO criteria: Complex family of diseases with four general subtypes
  - Diffuse large B-cell, Anaplastic large cell, Peripheral T-cell, Follicle center lymphoma
- Ann Arbor staging system
  - Stage I: Limited to one lymph node or one extra-nodal site

NON-HODGKIN LYMPHOMA

○ Stage II: Limited to one organ and one or more lymph node groups on the same side of the diaphragm

○ Stage III: NHL in two LN groups +/- extranodal site above and below the diaphragm

○ Stage IV: Extensive or diffuse in one organ site +/- NHL in distant nodes

- Presence or absence of "B symptoms"
  ○ A: Absent or no symptoms
  ○ B: Presence of any of the following: Fever, night sweats, unexplained weight loss (10% within 6 months), severe itching
  ○ E: Involvement of a single extranodal site
  ○ X: "Bulky" disease
  ○ CS: Clinical stage
  ○ PS: Pathological stage
- Staging: Physical eval., complete blood count, blood biochemistry, chest radiography, chest, abdomen & pelvic CT, bilateral bone marrow biopsy

CLINICAL ISSUES

Presentation

- Most common signs/symptoms
  ○ Painless, palpable lump of 2-3 months duration, rapidly enlarging; rarely may present with peau-d'orange, erythema, and diffuse breast swelling
    ▪ Bilateral involvement rare, may be seen in puerperal women
  ○ Secondary lymphoma most commonly presents as axillary adenopathy or with multiple, non-palpable, bilateral breast masses
- Other signs/symptoms
  ○ Axillary adenopathy in 30-50% cases at presentation
  ○ Mycosis fungoides: A rare cutaneous T-cell lymphoma with rash, can involve breasts; lymphadenopathy

Demographics

- Age: Median age at diagnosis 58 years (range 13-90 years); bimodal peaks at 38 and 58
- Gender: Overwhelming female dominance; male PLB reported exceedingly rarely

Natural History & Prognosis

- Five year over-all survival for stage I and IIE 72-85%; disease free survival at 5 years 39-70%
- Survival rates better for low grade lesions & for MALT lymphomas compared to diffuse large B-cell type
- Histologic subtype most important prognostic factor; prognosis worse for younger patients
- Adverse prognostic factors
  ○ Tumor size > 5 cm
  ○ Synchronous bilateral disease
  ○ Axillary nodal metastases
- Prognosis better than that of breast carcinoma
- International Prognostic Index predicts 5 year survival based on age, LDH level, staging, extranodal disease, performance status

Treatment

- Surgical treatment, ranging from biopsy to radical mastectomy, often not indicated

- Chemotherapy regimens vary with histologic type
- Radiation therapy: Effective local control or adjuvant to chemotherapy

DIAGNOSTIC CHECKLIST

Consider

- Diagnosis based on Wiseman and Liao criteria
  ○ 1: Technically adequate pathologic sample
  ○ 2: Close association of mammary tissue with lymphomatous infiltrate
  ○ 3: Exclusion of either systemic lymphoma or previous extramammary lymphoma

Image Interpretation Pearls

- Consider in differential of breast masses lacking typical features of breast carcinoma, such as spiculation and microcalcifications

SELECTED REFERENCES

1. Areia AL et al: Primary breast lymphoma. Eur J Gynaecol Oncol. 26(2):163-4, 2005
2. Baker R et al: Multifocal primary breast lymphoma. South Med J. 98(10):1045-8, 2005
3. Cox J et al: Haematological cancers in the breast and axilla: a drop in an ocean of breast malignancy. Breast. 14(1):51-6, 2005
4. Fruchart C et al: High grade primary breast lymphoma: is it a different clinical entity? Breast Cancer Res Treat. 93(3):191-8, 2005
5. Grubstein A et al: Extranodal primary B-cell non-Hodgkin lymphoma of the breast mimicking acute mastitis. J Clin Ultrasound. 33(3):140-2, 2005
6. Kebudi A et al: Primary T-lymphoma of the breast with bilateral involvement, unusual presentation. Int J Clin Pract Suppl. (147):95-8, 2005
7. Kumar R et al: F-18 FDG positron emission tomography in non-Hodgkin lymphoma of the breast. Clin Nucl Med. 30(4):246-8, 2005
8. Liu MT et al: Primary breast lymphoma: a pooled analysis of prognostic factors and survival in 93 cases. Ann Saudi Med. 25(4):288-93, 2005
9. Maounis N et al: Bilateral primary lymphoma of the breast: a case report initially diagnosed by FNAC. Diagn Cytopathol. 32(2):114-8, 2005
10. Mason HS et al: Primary breast lymphoma: radiologic and pathologic findings. Breast J. 11(6):495-6, 2005
11. Vardar E et al: Primary breast lymphoma cytologic diagnosis. Arch Pathol Lab Med. 129(5):694-6, 2005
12. Venizelos ID et al: Primary non-Hodgkin's lymphoma arising in an intramammary lymph node. Leuk Lymphoma. 46(3):451-5, 2005
13. Vignot S et al: Non-Hodgkin's lymphoma of the breast: a report of 19 cases and a review of the literature. Clin Lymphoma. 6(1):37-42, 2005
14. Carrascosa LA et al: Synchronous primary bilateral breast lymphoma. Am J Clin Oncol. 27(6):635, 2004
15. Loughrey MB et al: WHO reclassification of breast lymphomas. J Clin Pathol. 57(11):1213-4, 2004
16. Mpallas G et al: Primary breast lymphoma in a male patient. Breast. 13(5):436-8, 2004
17. Pruthi S et al: Primary mammary (non-Hodgkin) lymphoma presenting as locally advanced breast cancer. Mayo Clin Proc. 79(10):1310-4, 2004

IMAGE GALLERY

Typical

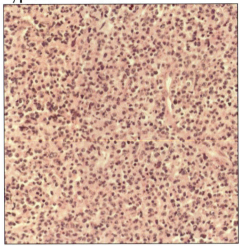 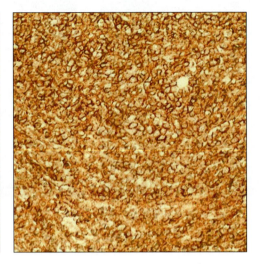

(Left) Micropathology, low power of samples obtained by US-guided 14-g core biopsy of a palpable mass which was of mixed echogenicity by US, shows the typical uniform population of small round cells c/w lymphoma (H&E). *(Right)* Specimen micropathology, low power shows that CD-20 immunostain (same patient as left-hand image) was intensely positive, compatible with a B-cell lymphoma.

Typical

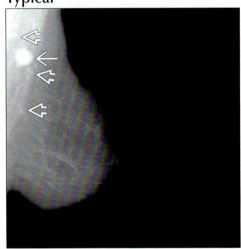 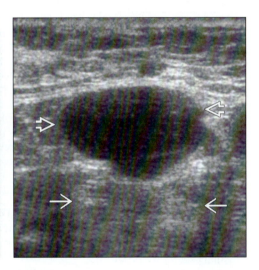

(Left) MLO mammography shows recurrent NHL manifesting as new left axillary mass ➡ seen on routine mammogram in addition to multiple smaller equal-density masses ➡. US of the largest mass (right-hand image) was performed. *(Right)* Anti-radial ultrasound reveals an oval, circumscribed, nearly anechoic mass ➡, without visible fatty hilum and with posterior acoustic enhancement ➡, c/w a lymphomatous node.

Typical

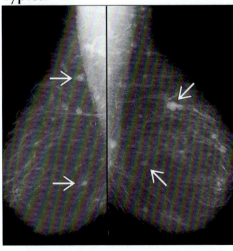 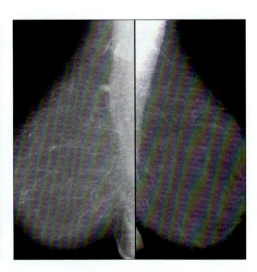

(Left) MLO mammography shows multiple bilateral masses ➡ in a 52 year old woman, later found to have widespread systemic NHL. US-guided core biopsy of the largest mass revealed secondary breast involvement. *(Right)* MLO mammography one year later, after several cycles of chemotherapy, shows resolution of many of the nodules. The patient remains in remission to date, 9 years later.

RENAL DISEASE

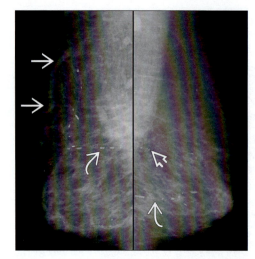

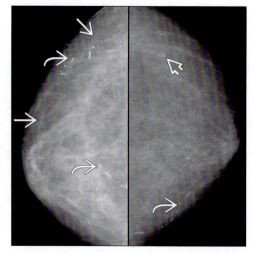

MLO views show superficial varicosities on the right ➡ due to the dialysis graft in the arm. Extensive vascular calcifications ➡ are noted, as is a cluster of coarse calcifications ➡.

CC views (same patient as left-hand image) show again the vascular calcifications ➡ and varicosity ➡. The clustered coarse calcifications ➡ had been stable for 4 years.

TERMINOLOGY

Abbreviations and Synonyms
- Kidney disorder, chronic renal failure (CRF)

Definitions
- Any disorder that affects the function of the kidneys

IMAGING FINDINGS

General Features
- Morphology
  - Anasarca, edema
    - Due to excess fluid ± hypoproteinemia
  - Calcifications: May be extensive
    - Breast calcifications: Up to 68% of CRF patients
    - Stromal, vascular, ductal (usually secretory type), cutaneous
  - Masses
    - Fibroadenomata increase in size under cyclosporine therapy (used for immunosuppression in renal transplant patients)
    - Metastases from renal cell carcinoma (RCC); rare

- Gynecomastia: Frequent in CRF
  - Hormonal abnormalities: Low serum testosterone; raised estradiol, luteinizing hormone and prolactin
- Dilated veins
  - With dialysis arm graft
- Mastitis, abscess
  - Transplant patients with immunosuppression prone to infection
- Calciphylaxis (calcific uremic arteriolopathy)
  - Progressive vascular calcification and ischemic tissue loss in patients with CRF; sepsis, death up to 60% cases

Mammographic Findings
- Edema and anasarca
  - Diffuse increase in density, usually bilateral
  - Diffuse skin and trabecular thickening; may be asymmetric
- Calcifications
  - Stromal, vascular, ductal (usually secretory type), cutaneous
- Masses

DDx: Vascular and Soft Tissue Calcifications Associated with Renal Disease

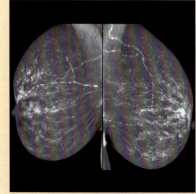

Extensive Calcifications

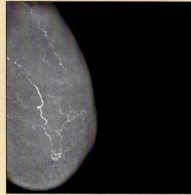

Vascular Calcifications and Edema

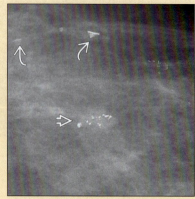

Stromal and Vascular Calcifications

RENAL DISEASE

Key Facts

Terminology
- Any disorder that affects the function of the kidneys

Imaging Findings
- Anasarca, edema
- Breast calcifications: Up to 68% of CRF patients
- Fibroadenomata increase in size under cyclosporine therapy (used for immunosuppression in renal transplant patients)
- Metastases from renal cell carcinoma (RCC); rare

- Gynecomastia: Frequent in CRF
- Dilated veins
- Mastitis, abscess
- Calciphylaxis (calcific uremic arteriolopathy)

Top Differential Diagnoses
- Anasarca
- Diabetes, Type I, Insulin Dependent
- Dermatomyositis

  ○ Well-circumscribed oval (e.g., fibroadenoma) or round (e.g., RCC metastases)

Ultrasonographic Findings
- Grayscale Ultrasound: Mass from fibroadenoma(ta) or intramammary metastases from RCC

MR Findings
- No specific indications

DIFFERENTIAL DIAGNOSIS

Anasarca
- Congestive heart failure, hypoproteinemia in hepatic failure

Diabetes, Type I, Insulin Dependent
- Prominent vascular calcifications; may have secondary renal failure

Dermatomyositis
- May demonstrate extensive subcutaneous skin calcifications

PATHOLOGY

General Features
- Etiology
  ○ Chronic renal failure, most common causes
    ▪ Prolonged medical conditions, such as hypertension or diabetes mellitus

    ▪ Hereditary, such as polycystic kidney disease
  ○ Soft tissue (breast) calcifications
    ▪ Multifactorial mechanism: Secondary hyperparathyroidism ("metastatic calcifications"), metabolic acidosis, adjuvant corticoid medication, hyperoxalemia, calcium deposition in disrupted soft tissue
  ○ Multiple fibroadenomata with cyclosporin (some fibroblasts stimulated with cyclosporin)

CLINICAL ISSUES

Natural History & Prognosis
- Screening for breast cancer among women with CRF is well below the rates of general population
- Patients with renal disease usually have similar incidence of breast cancer as the general population

SELECTED REFERENCES

1. Fleming ST et al: Comorbidity as a predictor of stage of illness for patients with breast cancer. Med Care. 43:132-40, 2005
2. Cowlam TE et al: Cutaneous ectopic breast calcification in a haemodialysis patient. The Breast. 12:342-4, 2003
3. Baildam A et al: Cyclosporin A and multiple fibroadenomas of the breast. Br J Surg. 83:1755-7, 1996
4. Evans SE et al: Extensive calcification in the breast in chronic renal failure. Br J Radiol. 64:757-9, 1991
5. Sommer G et al: Breast calcifications in renal hyperparathyroidism. AJR. 148:855-7, 1987

IMAGE GALLERY

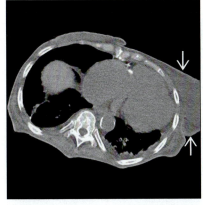 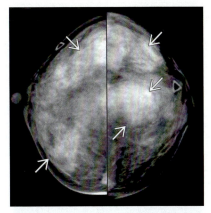 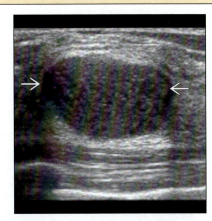

(Left) NECT in a patient with renal failure & pulmonary edema. Infiltration of subcutaneous fat & of incompletely imaged left breast ➡ by soft tissue suggest anasarca. *(Center)* Bilateral fibroadenomata became palpable after 2 month of switching to cyclosporine in this patient with renal transplant. Bilateral CC mammography views show dense & nodular breasts ➡. *(Right)* Bilateral ultrasound (US) (same patient as previous image) revealed four solid masses, largest measuring 4.2 cm. All lesions were fibroadenomata on pathology. US of one of the masses ➡.

SARCOID

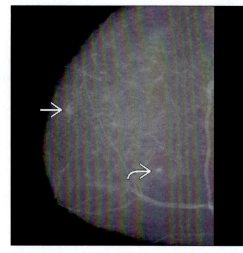

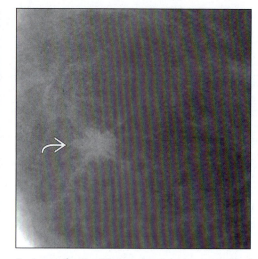

CC mammography shows two ill-defined suspicious right masses in a 47 yo: ⇒ Lateral and ⇒ medial. Spot magnification view (right-hand image) shows margin detail of the medial lesion.

Spot magnification CC view shows the inner spiculated mass ⇒. Biopsy of both masses revealed noncaseating granulomas consistent with sarcoid.

TERMINOLOGY

Abbreviations and Synonyms
- Sarcoidosis, Boeck disease, Hutchinson disease

Definitions
- Chronic inflammatory condition of unknown cause
- Multisystem granulomatous disorder
  ○ Disease first described in 1877 by an English physician, Hutchinson
  ○ Boeck described cutaneous lesions and histology and termed them sarcoid because the lesions resembled sarcoma (sarc-), but were benign (-oid)
  ○ The diagnosis is established when clinical and radiological findings are supported by histological evidence of noncaseating epithelioid granuloma

IMAGING FINDINGS

General Features
- Best diagnostic clue
  ○ Spiculated mass(es)

- Spiculations presumably due to perigranulomatous fibrotic changes in the chronic stage
- Usually < 1 cm
  ○ Circumscribed mass(es)
    ▪ Parenchymal granuloma (no surrounding fibrosis in the early change)
    ▪ Lymph node involvement (intramammary ± axillary lymph nodes)

Radiographic Findings
- Computed tomography
  ○ May show spiculated or less frequently circumscribed nodule(s) in the breast, typically with mediastinal or other sites of lymph node enlargement

Mammographic Findings
- Mass, variable from irregular to circumscribed
  ○ Most commonly irregular, spiculated
- Frequently multiple
- Calcifications are usually absent
  ○ Coarse calcifications within lymph nodes are seen in other specific granulomatous diseases, such as histoplasmosis and tuberculosis

DDx: Other Examples of Sarcoid

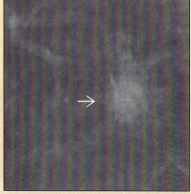

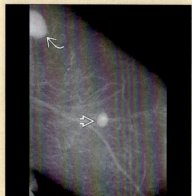

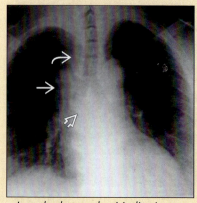

Parenchymal Granuloma, Breast

Lymph Node Involvement

Lymphadenopathy, Mediastinum

SARCOID

Key Facts

Terminology
- Sarcoidosis, Boeck disease, Hutchinson disease

Imaging Findings
- Spiculated mass(es)
- Circumscribed mass(es)
- Lymph node involvement (intramammary ± axillary lymph nodes)
- Calcifications are usually absent

Top Differential Diagnoses
- Invasive cancer
- Post surgical scar
- Radial scar
- Fat necrosis

Pathology
- US prevalence: 10 per 100,000
- Breast involvement in less than 1% of sarcoidosis cases
- Most patients have lesions in areas other than the breast(s) when breast lesions present
- Characteristic lesion is a discrete, compact, noncaseating epithelioid granuloma

Clinical Issues
- Primarily affects the lungs, lymph nodes, skin, spleen, and liver

Diagnostic Checklist
- Sarcoidosis should be included in the differential diagnosis of breast mass lesion in patients with history of sarcoidosis

Ultrasonographic Findings
- Grayscale Ultrasound: Irregular hypoechoic mass or cluster of small masses

MR Findings
- T1WI
  - Inhomogeneous, usually with irregular contours
  - May have a main mass lesion and satellite nodules
- T2WI FS
  - Inhomogeneous, usually with irregular contours
  - May have irregular multinodular appearance
- T1 C+
  - Depending on the inflammatory activity and degree of fibrosis
    - May show rapid enhancement with early washout or gradual enhancement
- Lymphotrophic nanoparticle-enhanced MR
  - May help distinguish nodal metastases from sarcoid
  - Lymph nodes involved by sarcoidosis have preserved contrast uptake by macrophages
  - Metastatic nodes replaced by tumor, no macrophages to take up iron particles

Nuclear Medicine Findings
- PET
  - Sarcoidosis can cause increased 18F-fluorodeoxyglucose (FDG) uptake in lymph nodes and within the breast
    - FDG uptake patterns in sarcoidosis are nonspecific and can be misinterpreted as malignancy
    - FDG uptake correlates well with disease activity
- Ga-67 Scintigraphy: Ga-67 accumulated in sarcoid granulomas (areas of inflammation)
- Tc-99m sestamibi (+ SPECT)
  - Suitable for the diagnosis and follow-up of myocardial sarcoidosis

DIFFERENTIAL DIAGNOSIS

Pathologic Differential Diagnosis
- Granulomatous infection due to specific organism

- Tuberculosis
- Fungal (histoplasmosis)
- Non-necrotizing sarcoid-like granulomatous inflammation accompanying carcinoma
- Foreign body granuloma
- Lymphoma

Imaging Differential Diagnosis
- Spiculated mass
  - Invasive cancer
    - Invasive ductal cancer (IDC): Tubular carcinoma is typically small, stellate mass
    - Invasive lobular cancer (ILC)
  - Post surgical scar
    - Usually larger area, history of treatment
  - Radial scar
    - No central mass
    - Associated calcifications
  - Fat necrosis
    - History of trauma ± dystrophic calcifications
  - Granular cell tumor (GCT)
  - Fibromatosis
- Circumscribed mass
  - Benign mass
    - Cyst, skin cyst, fibroadenoma, lactating adenoma
    - Benign lymph node enlargement
  - Malignancy
    - Carcinoma: IDC, papillary, medullary, mucinous
    - Lymphoma
    - Metastases

PATHOLOGY

General Features
- Genetics
  - Race is an important risk factor
    - Genetic predisposition in people of African descent
- Epidemiology
  - General
    - Worldwide distribution, affecting young and middle-aged adults

SARCOID

- US prevalence: 10 per 100,000
- Highest incidence in African-American women
  - Breast
    - Breast involvement in less than 1% of sarcoidosis cases
    - Most patients have lesions in areas other than the breast(s) when breast lesions present
    - Breast sarcoid can be primary presentation (rare)

Microscopic Features

- Characteristic lesion is a discrete, compact, noncaseating epithelioid granuloma
  - Highly differentiated mononuclear phagocytes (epithelioid cells and giant cells) and lymphocytes
  - Schaumann bodies within Langhans (giant) cells
- Diagnosis requires exclusion of granulomas of known causes and of local sarcoid reactions (sarcoid-like inflammatory response to foreign body or malignancy)

Staging, Grading or Classification Criteria

- Roentgenographic stages in pulmonary disease range from no radiographic abnormalities (stage 0) to advanced fibrosis with honey-combing, hilar retraction, bullae, cysts and emphysema (stage IV)

CLINICAL ISSUES

Presentation

- Most common signs/symptoms
  - Primarily affects the lungs, lymph nodes, skin, spleen, and liver
  - Mammographic or incidental CT finding
  - Palpable breast lump
- Other signs/symptoms
  - Isolated involvement of breast parenchyma by sarcoid exceedingly rare: Evidence of disease in the chest or elsewhere should be obtained
  - General symptoms: Fever, fatigue, malaise, and weight loss in one third of cases
  - Kveim-Siltzbath test may be available and helpful for diagnosis
  - Hypercalcemia in 10% and hypercalcuria in 30%
    - Macrophage/granuloma are sources of 1,25-dihydroxy-vitamin D
  - Angiotensin-converting-enzyme ↑ in 33-90%
    - Produced by macrophage/granuloma
  - Hypergammaglobulinemia

Demographics

- Age: Predilection for adults under 40 years (peak 20-29 years)

Natural History & Prognosis

- The course and prognosis may correlate with the mode or onset and extent of the disease
- Favorable prognosis (≥ 80% spontaneous remission)
  - Acute onset with erythema nodosum
  - Löfgren syndrome: Hilar lymphadenopathy, skin and joint involvement
  - Low stage, self-limited disease
- Poor prognosis
  - Insidious onset, chronic course
  - Lupus pernio (vasculitic skin nodules)
  - Older age at presentation
  - African-American race
- An insidious onset, especially with multiple extrapulmonary lesions, may be followed by relentless, progressive fibrosis of lungs and other organs
  - Mortality range 5-10%
    - Cor pulmonale related to lung fibrosis
    - Cardiac arrhythmia

Treatment

- Corticosteroid therapy, antimalarial agents and cytotoxic agents
- Assessment of disease activity largely determines the type of therapy to be instituted

DIAGNOSTIC CHECKLIST

Consider

- Sarcoidosis should be included in the differential diagnosis of breast mass lesion in patients with history of sarcoidosis

Image Interpretation Pearls

- Imaging is helpful to direct biopsy for histopathological examination, which is usually required to rule out malignancy

SELECTED REFERENCES

1. Harisinghani MG et al: A pilot study of lymphotrophic nanoparticle-enhanced magnetic resonance imaging technique in early stage testicular cancer: a new method for noninvasive lymph node evaluation. Urology. 66:1066-71, 2005
2. Mona el K et al: Quiz case. Breast sarcoidosis presenting as a metastatic breast cancer. Eur J Radiol. 54:2-5, 2005
3. Garcia CA et al: FDG-positron emission tomographic imaging in carcinoma of the breast: interference by massive sarcoidosis. Clin Nucl Med. 28:218-9, 2003
4. Ishimaru K et al: Sarcoidosis of the breast. Eur Radiol. 12 Suppl 3:S105-8, 2002
5. Lower EE et al: Breast disease in sarcoidosis. Sarcoidosis Vasc Diffuse Lung Dis. 18:301-6, 2001
6. Takahashi R et al: Mammary involvement in a patient with sarcoidosis. Intern Med. 40:769-71, 2001
7. Ojeda H et al: Sarcoidosis of the breast: implications for the general surgeon. Am Surg. 66:1144-8, 2000
8. Joint Statement of the American Thoracic Society (ATS), the European Respiratory Society (ERS) and the World Association of Sarcoidosis and Other Granulomatous Disorders (WASOG) adopted by the ATS Board of Directors and by the ERS Executive Committee. Statement on sarcoidosis. Am J Respir Crit Care Med. 160:736-55 1999
9. Kirshy D et al: Sarcoidosis of the breast presenting as a spiculated lesion. AJR. 172:554-5, 1999
10. Yamada Y et al: Fluorine-18-fluorodeoxyglucose and carbon-11-methionine evaluation of lymphadenopathy in sarcoidosis. J Nucl Med. 39:1160-61, 1998
11. Kenzel PP et al: Boeck sarcoidosis of the breast: mammographic, ultrasound, and MR findings. J Comput Assist Tomogr. 21:439-41, 1997
12. Bergkvist L et al: Management of accidentally found pathological lymph nodes on routine screening mammography. Eur J Surg Oncol. 22:250-3, 1996

SARCOID

IMAGE GALLERY

Typical

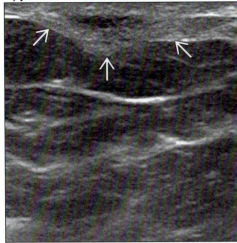

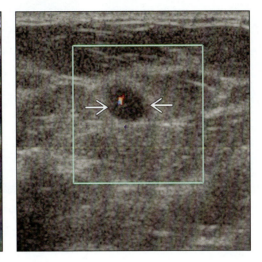

(Left) Ultrasound shows a 36 year old female with right breast tender lesions, possibly associated with her known diagnosis of sarcoid. Ultrasound showed superficial dermal lesions c/w her sarcoid ➡. *(Right)* Ultrasound in the same woman's ipsilateral breast is a 7 mm solid hypoechoic mass ➡, which is not superficial in nature. US-guided core biopsy = non-caseating granulomatous inflammation c/w sarcoidosis.

Typical

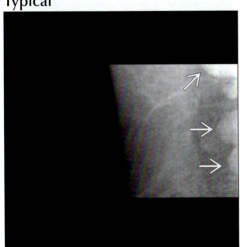

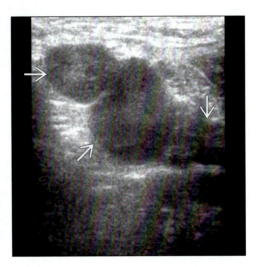

(Left) MLO mammography magnification view in a 50 year old woman with a palpable axillary mass includes partial visualization of multiple round to oval high density, well-circumscribed masses ➡. *(Right)* Transverse ultrasound (same case as on left) reveals multiple, well-circumscribed hypoechoic masses ➡, corresponding to the mammographic findings. Findings of sarcoid were seen at biopsy.

Typical

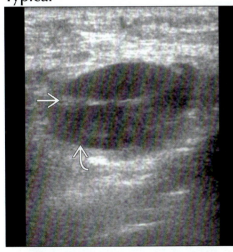

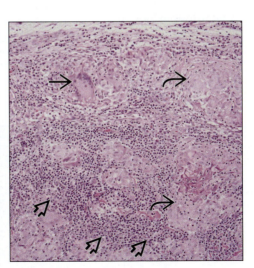

(Left) Longitudinal ultrasound image of a palpable axillary lymph node shows a thin echogenic hilum ➡ and a diffusely, markedly thickened hypoechoic cortex ➡ in this 50 year old. Biopsy showed noncaseating granuloma consistent with sarcoid. *(Right)* Medium power histopathology picture (same patient as left image) shows lymphoid tissue ➡, multinucleated cells ➡ and granulomas ➡, compatible with sarcoid (H&E).

WEIGHT-FLUCTUATIONS

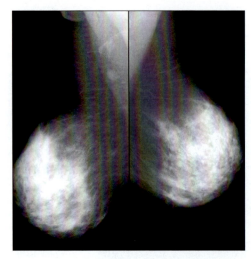

MLO mammography demonstrates moderately large breasts, dense tissue, and no worrisome focal findings in this asymptomatic woman. A marked change in appearance is seen 1 year later (right image).

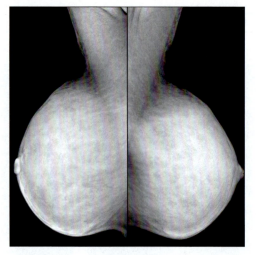

MLO mammography shows decrease in size and markedly dense tissue secondary to a 120 pound loss. (Caution: This remarkable change is unusual; be alert to a possible confusion with a different patient).

TERMINOLOGY

Definitions
- Alteration of breast size attributable to systemic weight changes
- Breast density varies related to weight shift
  - Density increases with weight loss
    - Breast size decreases
  - Density decreases with weight gain
    - Breast size changes often not so apparent as in cases of weight loss

IMAGING FINDINGS

General Features
- Best diagnostic clue: History

Mammographic Findings
- Apparent increase in breast tissue with weight loss
  - Increase in breast density due to fat loss and decreased breast size
  - Loss of subcutaneous fat
  - Poor soft tissue contrast: Increased "grayness"

DIFFERENTIAL DIAGNOSIS

Bilateral Increase in Breast Density
- Hormonal stimulation, exogenous hormone replacement (HRT)
  - Mammographic density increase reported range from 17-73% of cases
  - Findings are typically diffuse and bilateral
    - Breast may be increased (rather than decreased) in size
    - Unilateral and or focal density increases require further evaluation to rule out developing density of cancer
  - Breast cancer risk is increased
    - Multifactorial; HRT regimen, duration of use, tissue density, genetic predisposition
- Hormonal stimulation, endogenous
  - Pregnancy, lactation; hormone secreting tumors
  - Findings diffuse and bilateral; breasts are increased in size
- Bilateral breast edema
  - Mammographic findings bilateral, usually symmetric and may include an increase in breast size

DDx: Changes in Breast Size and/or Density

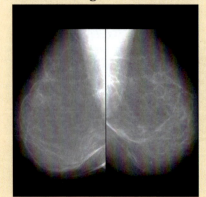

Reduction Mammoplasty

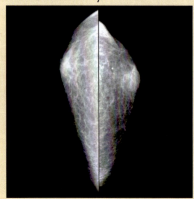

Edema, Heart Failure

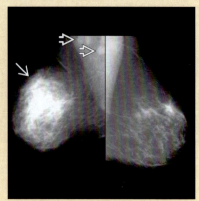

Inflammatory Breast Cancer

WEIGHT-FLUCTUATIONS

Key Facts

Terminology
- Alteration of breast size attributable to systemic weight changes

Top Differential Diagnoses
- Bilateral Increase in Breast Density
- Hormonal stimulation, exogenous hormone replacement (HRT)
- Hormonal stimulation, endogenous
- Bilateral breast edema

- Bilateral Decrease in Breast Density and/or Size
- Normal fatty involution with aging process
- Reduction mammoplasty

Diagnostic Checklist
- Possible inaccurate patient identification when interval mammographic examinations extremely altered

---

- Trabecular thickening, skin thickening, increase in overall density
- Bilateral breast trauma
  - Seat-belt injuries are typically unilateral
- Bilateral inflammatory cancer: Very rare

Bilateral Decrease in Breast Density and/or Size
- Normal fatty involution with aging process
- Reduction mammoplasty
  - Constellation of findings as well as clinical history should differentiate
    - Decrease in breast size, nipple elevation, displacement of residual tissue, swirling fibrotic bands

PATHOLOGY

General Features
- Epidemiology
  - Body mass index is inversely related to risk of pre-menopausal breast cancer
    - Possibly secondary to delayed detection/diagnosis; greater number of irregular menstrual cycles
    - Dense breast tissue itself is a risk factor
  - Body fat only weakly related to postmenopausal breast cancer risk
    - Elevated endogenous estrogen levels
    - Relative risk reduction from being heavy during premenopausal years may persist

CLINICAL ISSUES

Presentation
- Most common signs/symptoms: Asymptomatic screening mammogram

DIAGNOSTIC CHECKLIST

Consider
- Possible inaccurate patient identification when interval mammographic examinations extremely altered
- Digital mammography depicts subcutaneous fat and skin better than film: Breasts may appear larger

SELECTED REFERENCES

1. Patella A et al: Breast density changes associated with hormone replacement therapy in postmenopausal women. Effects on the specificity and sensitivity of mammographic screening. Eur J Gynaecol Oncol. 26:485-90, 2005
2. Ikeda DM: The Requisites: Breast Imaging. Philadelphia, Elsevier Mosby. Chapter 10, 296-7, 2004
3. Swinford AE et al: Mammographic appearance of the breasts during pregnancy and lactation: false assumptions. Acad Radiol. 5:467-72, 1998

IMAGE GALLERY

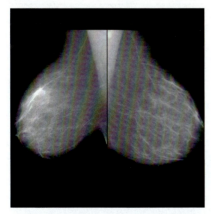 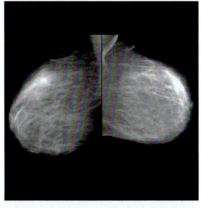 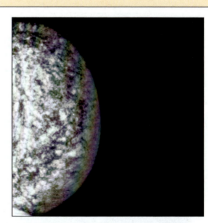

(Left) MLO mammography shows baseline negative examination. Annual screening MLO view obtained the following year, 9 months after gastric bypass surgery, is shown in next image. *(Center)* MLO mammography demonstrates reduction in size of breasts and slight overall increase in apparent fibroglandular density compatible with interval 168 pound weight loss. *(Right)* CC mammography in this transsexual male to female who was taking exogenous hormones shows diffuse densities throughout left breast (right side similar, not shown) from direct oil injections.

GYNECOMASTIA

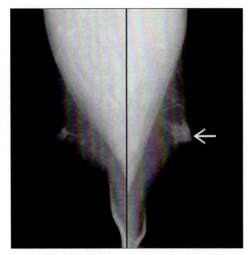

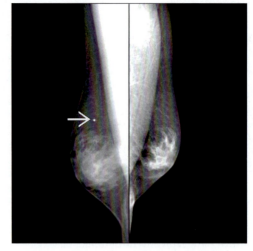

MLO mammography illustrates a case of bilateral, asymmetric gynecomastia in a 29 year old male with a palpable left mass ➡. *Note round-to-conical shape of left subareolar density.*

MLO mammography shows bilateral gynecomastia in a 55 yo male with a palpable right lump ➡ *related to superior breast tissue. Patient gave a history of previous heroin abuse, now on methadone.*

TERMINOLOGY

Definitions
- Enlargement of the male breast, secondary to ductal hyperplasia and stromal proliferation

IMAGING FINDINGS

General Features
- Best diagnostic clue: Fan- or flame-shaped density, emanating from nipple, blends into surrounding fat
- Location
  - Subareolar; usually asymmetric
    - Unilateral in 70% in one series
    - Of bilateral cases, 67% asymmetric in one series
  - May extend into upper outer quadrant
- Size: 2-6 cm; may involve entire breast

Mammographic Findings
- Three patterns
  - Early nodular
    - Less than one year's duration
    - Well-demarcated subareolar mass, extending into posterior tissue in a fan-like configuration (tapering peripherally)
  - Late dendritic
    - Usually occurs after one year
    - Flame-shaped central subareolar mass with prominent linear projections radiating into deep adipose tissue
    - May extend into upper outer quadrant
  - Diffuse glandular
    - Secondary to exogenous estrogen (e.g., treatment for prostate cancer, transsexuals)
    - Dense, nodular parenchyma in enlarged breast
    - Mimics appearance of female breast, except for absence of Cooper ligaments

Ultrasonographic Findings
- Grayscale Ultrasound
  - Early nodular pattern
    - Small, subareolar hypoechoic mass
    - Prominent subareolar ducts
    - Slightly lobulated posterior border
    - May be hyperemic on Doppler interrogation
  - Late dendritic phase

DDx: Gynecomastia

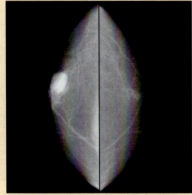

Male Breast Cancer

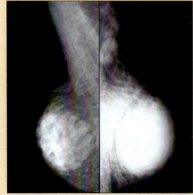

Bilateral Male Breast Cancer

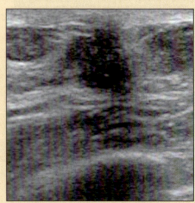

Male Breast Cancer

GYNECOMASTIA

Key Facts

Terminology
- Enlargement of the male breast, secondary to ductal hyperplasia and stromal proliferation

Imaging Findings
- Best diagnostic clue: Fan- or flame-shaped density, emanating from nipple, blends into surrounding fat
- Subareolar; usually asymmetric
- May extend into upper outer quadrant

Top Differential Diagnoses
- Male Breast Cancer
- Pseudogynecomastia
- Lipoma
- Diabetic Mastopathy

Pathology
- Causes of gynecomastia: Hormonal, drug-induced, systemic, idiopathic
- Hormone imbalance: Relative excess of estrogen in relation to testosterone at level of breast tissue
- 85% of breast masses in males

Clinical Issues
- Most common signs/symptoms: Painful, tender subareolar mass
- Prevalence in general population, 32-65%

Diagnostic Checklist
- Thorough physical exam
- Careful drug history

- Hypoechoic mass centered at nipple
  - Stellate, posterior finger-like projections
  - No flow on Doppler
- Diffuse glandular pattern
  - Similar to normal female breast tissue pattern

MR Findings
- T1WI: Appearance similar to normal female breast
- T1 C+: Slow, persistent non-mass-like enhancement of the retroareolar breast tissue

Biopsy
- Core biopsy when diagnostic uncertainty

DIFFERENTIAL DIAGNOSIS

Male Breast Cancer
- Circumscribed or spiculated mass usually evident
- Usually convex posteriorly; often eccentric to nipple

Pseudogynecomastia
- Fatty enlargement; no ductal or stromal proliferation
- Radiolucent on mammography
- Secondary to obesity, especially in older men

Lipoma
- Radiolucent mass on mammography with thin capsule
- Slightly hyperechoic, oval mass on US

Diabetic Mastopathy
- Firm, palpable mass in long-standing type I diabetic males (and females)

Abscess
- Erythema, acute history; heterogeneous mass on US

PATHOLOGY

General Features
- General path comments
  - Abnormal increase in stromal & ductal components
  - Early nodular phase (reversible)

- Dilatation, lengthening, increase in number of ducts
- Epithelial hyperplasia; ↑ stromal vascularity; edema
  - Late dendritic (irreversible)
    - Dense periductal hyalinization; exceeds volume of ductal tissue
    - Extensive fibrosis; ↓ vascularity
  - Unilateral or asymmetric, 72%
- Genetics
  - Most cases not genetically based
  - Familial cases reported (rare): Increased extraglandular aromatization
  - Klinefelter syndrome: Usually 47 XXY
- Etiology
  - Causes of gynecomastia: Hormonal, drug-induced, systemic, idiopathic
  - Hormone imbalance: Relative excess of estrogen in relation to testosterone at level of breast tissue
  - Pharmacologic: Alcohol, alkylating chemotherapeutic agents, amiodarone, amphetamines, anabolic steroids, captopril, cimetidine, cocaine, diazepam, digitalis, haloperidol, heroin, isoniazid, marijuana, metronidazole, nifedipine, omeprazole, phenytoin, spironolactone, tricyclic antidepressants, thiazide diuretics, verapamil
  - Systemic
    - Underlying diseases: Chronic renal failure, cirrhosis, HIV, hypo- and hyperthyroidism, nutritional deprivation → refeeding gynecomastia
    - Testicular tumors: Germ cell, Leydig, Sertoli
    - Non-testicular tumors: Adrenal, liver, lung, renal [ectopic human chorionic gonadotropin (HCG)]
- Epidemiology
  - 85% of breast masses in males
  - Hormonal: Tri-modal age distribution
    - Neonatal: 60-90% newborns transiently develop palpable breast tissue; enlargement may be considerable; "witch's milk" clear or cloudy, colostrum-like discharge; usually resolves spontaneously in few weeks

GYNECOMASTIA

- Pubertal: Transient surge in estrogen in adolescent boys; usually bilateral and asymmetrical; 60% of young males affected to some degree; often resolves in a few months
- Senescent: Men older than 60; age-related decrease in testosterone; increased estradiol from peripheral conversion in adipose tissue, secondary to aromatization of androgens to estrogens

Gross Pathologic & Surgical Features
- Soft, rubbery or firm gray/white mass
- Fat rarely dispersed in fibrous tissue

Microscopic Features
- Increased number and length of ducts
- Proliferation of ductal epithelium
- Periductal edema; fibroblastic stroma

CLINICAL ISSUES

Presentation
- Most common signs/symptoms: Painful, tender subareolar mass
- Other signs/symptoms
  - Breast enlargement
    - May be unilateral, bilateral; sometimes painless
- Clinical Profile
  - Prevalence in general population, 32-65%
    - 40% non-obese men
    - 85% obese men

Demographics
- Age
  - Hormonal: Tri-modal age distribution - neonatal, pubertal, senescent
  - Drug-induced or systemic: Any age

Natural History & Prognosis
- If present less than a year, may spontaneously regress if underlying cause withdrawn
- If present more than one year, often irreversible
  - Ductal proliferation resolves, but fibrosis permanent
- Not causally related to male breast cancer
  - Often coexists due to high prevalence of gynecomastia

Treatment
- Expectant: Reversible cases
- Surgical/interventional: Non-reversible cases
  - Simple excision
  - Subcutaneous mastectomy with concentric skin resection
  - Liposuction
- Medical: Tamoxifen, Danozal
- Prevention in prostate cancer patients treated with estrogen
  - Radiation therapy
  - Tamoxifen, aromatase inhibitors (investigational)

DIAGNOSTIC CHECKLIST

Consider
- Thorough physical exam

  - Meticulous breast exam to differentiate from pseudogynecomastia or cancer
    - Patient supine
    - Examiner's fingers opposite sides of breast
    - Elevate tissue off chest wall by pinching
  - Careful testicular evaluation to rule out tumor
  - Thyroid and liver palpation
- Careful drug history
- Hormonal investigation in selected cases: Serum testosterone, estradiol, HCG, prolactin, luteinizing hormone

Image Interpretation Pearls
- If mass eccentric on physical exam or imaging, think malignancy: Biopsy

SELECTED REFERENCES

1. Di Lorenzo G et al: Management of gynaecomastia in patients with prostate cancer: a systematic review. Lancet Oncol. 6(12):972-9, 2005
2. Prisant LM et al: Gynecomastia and hypertension. J Clin Hypertens (Greenwich). 7(4):245-8, 2005
3. Wise GJ et al: Male breast disease. J Am Coll Surg. 200(2):255-69, 2005
4. Bembo SA et al: Gynecomastia: its features, and when and how to treat it. Cleve Clin J Med. 71(6):511-7, 2004
5. Gabro et al: Gynaecomastia in the adolescent: a surgically relevant condition. Eur J Pediatr Surg. 14(1):3-6, 2004
6. Fruhstorfer BH et al: A systematic approach to the surgical treatment of gynaecomastia. Br J Plast Surg. 56(3):237-46, 2003
7. Lazala C et al: Pubertal gynecomastia. J Pediatr Endocrinol Metab. 15(5):553-60, 2002
8. Gruntmanis U et al: Treatment of gynecomastia. Curr Opin Investig Drugs. 2(5):643-9, 2001
9. Ismail AA et al: Endocrinology of gynaecomastia. Ann Clin Biochem. 38(Pt 6):596-607, 2001
10. McLeod DG et al: Gynecomastia in patients with prostate cancer: a review of treatment options. Urology. 56(5):713-20, 2000
11. Sher ES et al: Evaluation of boys with marked breast development at puberty. Clin Pediatr (Phila). 37(6):367-71, 1998
12. Stewart RA et al: Pictorial review: the imaging features of male breast disease. Clin Radiol. 52(10):739-44, 1997
13. Chantra PK et al: Mammography of the male breast. AJR. 164(4):853-8, 1995
14. Cooper RA et al: Mammography in men. Radiology. 191:651-6, 1994
15. Glass AR: Gynecomastia. Endocrinol Metab Clin North Am. 23(4):825-37, 1994
16. Braunstein GD: Gynecomastia. N Engl J Med. 328(7):490-5, 1993
17. Mladick RA: Gynecomastia. Liposuction and excision. Clin Plast Surg. 18(4):815-22, 1991
18. Mahoney CP: Adolescent gynecomastia. Differential diagnosis and management. Pediatr Clin North Am. 37(6):1389-404, 1990
19. Dershaw DD: Male mammography. AJR. 146(1):127-31, 1986
20. Jackson VP et al: Male breast carcinoma and gynecomastia: comparison of mammography with sonography. Radiology. 149(2):533-6, 1983
21. Michels LG et al: Radiography of gynecomastia and other disorders of the male breast. Radiology. 122(1):117-22, 1977

GYNECOMASTIA

IMAGE GALLERY

Typical

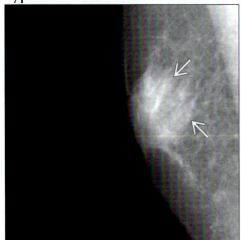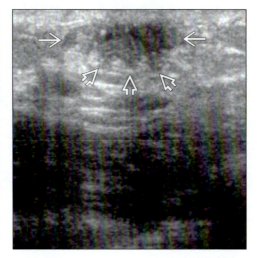

(Left) MLO mammography magnification demonstrates a flame-shaped retroareolar density ➡ in this 46 year old male who presented with a palpable lump. **(Right)** Transverse ultrasound in the immediate retroareolar area of same case as left-hand image demonstrates findings consistent with gynecomastia seen as hypoechoic area ➡ with posterior, finger-like projections ➡.

Typical

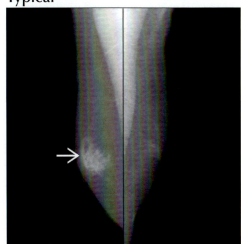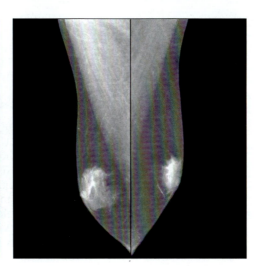

(Left) MLO mammography demonstrates a case of pubertal gynecomastia in a 13 year old boy who presented with a palpable right retroareolar lump ➡. Note: Mammography is not usually indicated in this setting. **(Right)** MLO mammography shows typical appearance of asymmetric gynecomastia in a man with a history of long-standing marijuana abuse.

Typical

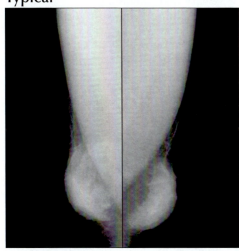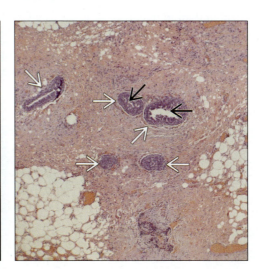

(Left) MLO mammography demonstrates extensive bilateral breast tissue in this male patient, illustrative of the diffuse glandular pattern. This is often seen in men on exogenous estrogen. **(Right)** Micropathology, low power shows typical appearance of gynecomastia. Note proliferation of ducts ➡ with florid hyperplasia ➡. As the male breast lacks lobules, there is no lobular differentiation.

MALE BREAST CANCER

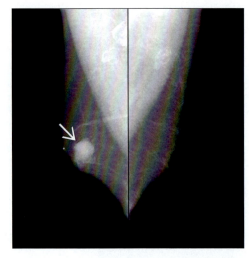

MLO mammography shows a fairly well-circumscribed hyperdense palpable mass ➡ in a 75 year old male. Eccentric location of the mass, just inferior to right nipple, increases suspicion.

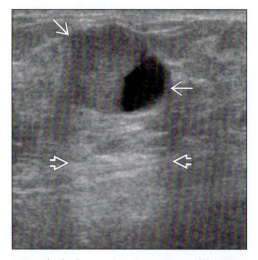

Longitudinal ultrasound (same mass as left image) reveals a complex cystic mass ➡ with posterior acoustic enhancement ⇨. Subsequent excision revealed DCIS, suspected on initial core biopsy.

TERMINOLOGY

Definitions
- Carcinoma of the male breast

IMAGING FINDINGS

General Features
- Best diagnostic clue: Firm, tender, subareolar mass, typically eccentric to nipple
- Location: Most often subareolar, eccentric to nipple
- Size: Mean diameter 2.0-3.5 cm

Mammographic Findings
- Mass 80-90%
  - Shape: Round, oval, irregular or lobulated
  - Margins
    - Spiculated, ill-defined
    - Well-circumscribed: More often than in females, due to higher incidence of intracystic papillary ductal carcinoma in situ (DCIS)
- Calcifications uncommon
  - Tend to be coarser, larger, rounder, less numerous and scattered
  - Pleomorphic morphology less common in men
- Associated findings may be present: Axillary adenopathy, skin thickening, skin and/or nipple retraction
- Florid gynecomastia may mask carcinoma

Ultrasonographic Findings
- Grayscale Ultrasound
  - Usually round-to-oval or irregular hypoechoic mass
    - Margins: Indistinct, angular or circumscribed
    - Posterior acoustic properties: Variable, shadowing common
  - Echogenic halo
  - Complex cystic mass
    - Highly suspicious for malignancy
    - Mural nodule may be present
    - May represent papillary DCIS
  - Evaluate for axillary node metastases
    - Absence of fatty hilum, asymmetric cortical thickening suspicious
    - Fatty hilum may be visible, though often compressed; nonspecific

DDx: Benign Symptomatic Male Breast Complaints

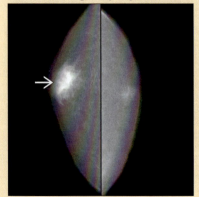

Gynecomastia, Asymmetric

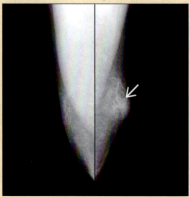

Gynecomastia, Unilateral

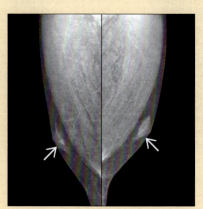

Gynecomastia, Symmetric

MALE BREAST CANCER

Key Facts

Terminology
- Carcinoma of the male breast

Imaging Findings
- Best diagnostic clue: Firm, tender, subareolar mass, typically eccentric to nipple
- Size: Mean diameter 2.0-3.5 cm
- Usually round-to-oval or irregular hypoechoic mass
- Best imaging tool: Mammography and ultrasound

Top Differential Diagnoses
- Gynecomastia
- Fat Necrosis

Pathology
- Majority of male breast cancer infiltrating ductal carcinoma (IDC)

- 85% NOS (not otherwise specified)
- Associated DCIS 35-50%
- Pure DCIS 7-11%
- Bilaterality 1.4%
- High frequency of BRCA-2 gene mutation
- 0.2-0.9% of breast cancers in the United States
- 1,500 new cases annually; 400 deaths per year
- Estrogen receptor positive 65-85%

Clinical Issues
- Overall prognosis worse due to later stage of diagnosis
- Equivalent to female breast cancer stage for stage

Diagnostic Checklist
- Consider genetic counseling, especially if other relatives with breast or ovarian cancer

MR Findings
- T1 C+: Rapid initial contrast-enhancement and washout worrisome for invasive malignancy
- MR not generally indicated unless chest wall invasion suspected

Imaging Recommendations
- Best imaging tool: Mammography and ultrasound
- Protocol advice
  - Begin with CC and MLO mammography
    - Reverse CC (from below) may show more tissue in male breast
    - Supplemental views as needed: Magnification, spot compression or tangential
  - Ultrasound
    - Mandatory if mammographic and clinical findings are not consistent with gynecomastia

DIFFERENTIAL DIAGNOSIS

Gynecomastia
- Fan- or flame-shaped subareolar density extending into upper outer quadrant
- Usually unilateral or asymmetric

Fat Necrosis
- Spiculated or irregular mass; band-like density or oil cyst
- Coarse, dystrophic, lucent-center or eggshell calcifications
- History of trauma

Pseudogynecomastia
- Fatty enlargement
- Absence of glandular tissue

Granular Cell Tumor
- Spiculated mass; majority are benign

Extramammary Metastasis to Breast
- Prostate most common; melanoma, lung

PATHOLOGY

General Features
- General path comments
  - Majority of male breast cancer infiltrating ductal carcinoma (IDC)
    - 85% NOS (not otherwise specified)
  - Associated DCIS 35-50%
    - Paget disease reported, up to 12%
  - Pure DCIS 7-11%
    - Usually low to intermediate grade
    - Intracystic papillary DCIS more common in men
    - High grade usually associated with invasive lesions
  - Infiltrating lobular carcinoma rare
    - Male breast lacks lobules, unless stimulated by exogenous estrogen
    - In prostate cancer patients treated with diethystilbesterol (DES)
    - May occur in transsexuals on long term, high dose estrogen therapy
  - Sarcoma (rare)
    - Arise from vascular, neural, adipose or fibrous elements in fat, skin or chest wall
  - Bilaterality 1.4%
  - Slight predilection for left breast
  - Embryology-anatomy
    - Normal: Subareolar ducts with epithelium
    - Male breast lacks terminal ductal lobular unit (TDLU)
    - Lobule formation rare, except in Klinefelter syndrome or other states of excess estrogen
    - Cyst formation rare: Ductal dilation
- Genetics
  - High frequency of BRCA-2 gene mutation
    - 18-33% of male breast cancer patients
    - Relative risk (RR) breast cancer 1.4; 6% absolute risk by age 70; up to 14% lifetime risk
    - Worse prognosis, younger age at diagnosis
    - Pancreatic cancer, RR 5.9; prostate RR 2.5; pharynx RR 7.3; digestive tract RR 1.5

MALE BREAST CANCER

- ○ Female relatives of men with breast cancer have increased risk
  - ▪ Equivalent to increased risk with female breast cancers
- ○ Positive family history increases risk two to fourfold
- ○ 30% male breast cancer cases have positive family history
- ○ Family history of prostate cancer increases risk 4x
- ○ Klinefelter syndrome (usually XXY): RR 50
- Etiology: Ducts give rise to infiltrating ductal carcinoma
- Epidemiology
  - ○ Less than 1% of all male cancers in the United States
  - ○ 0.2-0.9% of breast cancers in the United States
    - ▪ 1,500 new cases annually; 400 deaths per year
  - ○ Risk factors
    - ▪ Advanced age
    - ▪ Genetic: Klinefelter, BRCA-2
    - ▪ Family history of female or male breast cancer
    - ▪ Testicular disease: Undescended testes, orchiectomy, mumps orchitis, testicular injury
    - ▪ Treatment with estrogen (prostate cancer, male-to-female transsexuals)
    - ▪ Obesity
    - ▪ Excess alcohol consumption
    - ▪ Head trauma, resulting in increased prolactin production
- Associated abnormalities
  - ○ Gynecomastia
    - ▪ Common in general population
    - ▪ Not considered a risk factor by most authorities

Gross Pathologic & Surgical Features
- Similar to female breast cancer

Microscopic Features
- Estrogen receptor positive 65-85%
- Androgen receptor positivity worse prognosis

CLINICAL ISSUES

Presentation
- Most common signs/symptoms: Firm, painless subareolar mass, usually eccentric to the nipple
- Other signs/symptoms
  - ○ Axillary adenopathy; 50% of cases at time of diagnosis
  - ○ Nipple discharge: Serosanguineous more often than bloody
  - ○ Nipple retraction or inversion; Paget disease; ulceration
  - ○ Skin changes present at diagnosis more often than with women
    - ▪ Retraction and thickening, even ulceration

Demographics
- Age
  - ○ Average age of diagnosis, range 60-64 years; later than in women
    - ▪ Males less aware, less concerned about breast cancer
    - ▪ Screening not routinely performed in men
- Ethnicity

- ○ Greater prevalence in some groups
  - ▪ African-American; Native Africans from Western nations; men of Jewish ancestry

Natural History & Prognosis
- Overall prognosis worse due to later stage of diagnosis
  - ○ Depends on size of primary tumor, histologic grade and lymph node status
  - ○ Mucinous, medullary, papillary and tubular subtypes more favorable prognosis than NOS
- Equivalent to female breast cancer stage for stage
- Metastatic spread similar to that observed in females
  - ○ Lung and bone most common sites
  - ○ Hepatic involvement less common
- Second primary cancers in 5-15% cases
  - ○ Prostate, gastrointestinal (primarily colon and rectal), lung and skin

Treatment
- Most treatment regimens similar to those established for female breast cancer
  - ○ Modified radical mastectomy; lumpectomy not appropriate
  - ○ Sentinel node biopsy; full axillary dissection if sentinel lymph node biopsy positive
- Adjuvant chemotherapy: Stage II, III
- Hormonal treatment for metastatic carcinoma
  - ○ Tamoxifen or aromatase inhibitors if ER positive

DIAGNOSTIC CHECKLIST

Consider
- Frequent association with BRCA-2 mutation
  - ○ Consider genetic counseling, especially if other relatives with breast or ovarian cancer
- Annual CBE and mammographic surveillance of contralateral breast if sufficient breast tissue

Image Interpretation Pearls
- Usually eccentric to nipple, often convex margins
- Distinguish from gynecomastia: Centered at nipple, typically tapers peripherally

SELECTED REFERENCES

1. Fentiman IS et al: Male breast cancer. Lancet. 367(9510):595-604, 2006
2. VanAsperen CJ et al: Cancer risks in BRCA2 families: estimates for sites other than breast and ovary. J Med Genet. 42:711-9, 2005
3. Kwiatkowska E et al: BRCA2 mutations and androgen receptor expression as independent predictors of outcome of male breast cancer patients. Clin Cancer Res. 9:4452-4459, 2003
4. Frank TS et al: Clinical characteristics of individuals with germline mutations in BRCA1 and BRCA2: analysis of 10,000 individuals. J Clin Oncol. 20:1480-90, 2002
5. Wang WT et al: Sonographic features of primary breast cancer in men. AJR. 176:413-16, 2001
6. Csokay B et al: High frequency of germ-line BRCA2 mutations among Hungarian male breast cancer patients without family history. Cancer Res. 59:995-8, 1999
7. Dershaw DD et al: Mammographic findings in men with breast cancer. AJR. 160:267-70, 1993

IMAGE GALLERY

Typical

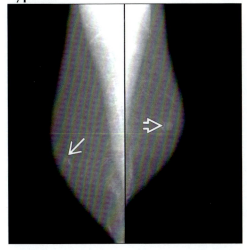
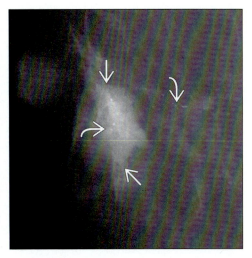

(Left) MLO mammography reveals a small unsuspected right subareolar ➡ mass in an elderly male who presented with a left lipoma, not mammographically evident. The left nipple ⇥, as the right, is not in profile. (Right) CC mammography magnification (same case as left-hand image) reveals indistinct margins ➡ and linear microcalcifications both within and beyond mass ⇥, not seen on standard views. Core biopsy and surgery revealed high grade DCIS without invasion.

Typical

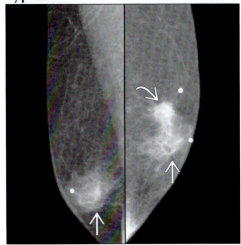
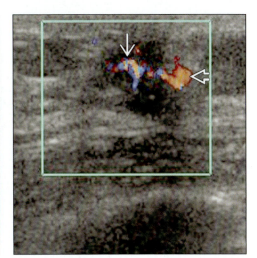

(Left) MLO mammography shows bilateral, palpable gynecomastia ➡ and an eccentric palpable spiculated mass ⇥ on the left. Gynecomastia, though not a risk factor, often coexists with breast cancer. (Right) Anti-radial color Doppler ultrasound (same case as left-hand image) shows marked increased vascularity within ➡ and adjacent ➡ to the mass; biopsy = grade II IDC, NOS.

Typical

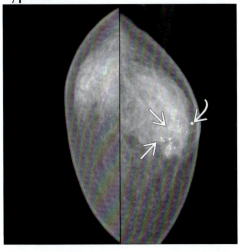
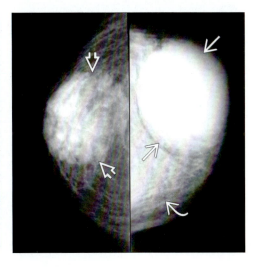

(Left) CC mammography shows bilateral gynecomastia, as well as a palpable, obscured left mass ➡ associated with fine linear and pleomorphic calcifications ➡. Biopsy = IDC and DCIS. (Right) CC mammography (different patient) shows bilateral poorly differentiated adenocarcinoma. The large left mass ➡ is associated with trabecular thickening ➡. The palpable right mass was obscured by extensive tissue ⇥.

IV

5

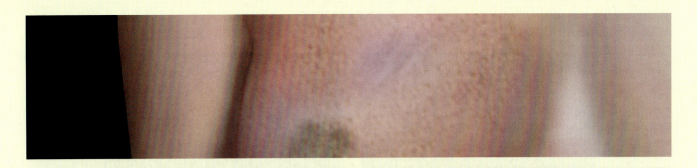

SECTION 6: Infections and Inflammation

ABSCESS

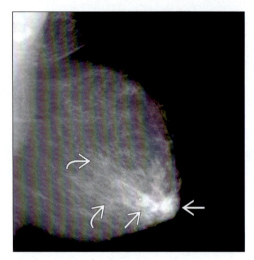

MLO mammography shows lobulated retroareolar mass ➜, corresponding to palpable lump, with associated trabecular thickening ⬏, compatible with edema.

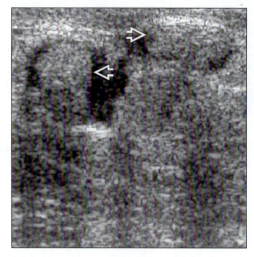

US (same patient as previous) shows lobulated mass is due to duct(s) containing echogenic masses or debris ➜. Limited initial response to antibiotics required aspiration, & change in antibiotics, leading to resolution.

TERMINOLOGY

Abbreviations and Synonyms
- Focal breast infection

Definitions
- Localized pus collection within the breast tissue
- Puerperal abscess = lactational breast abscess

IMAGING FINDINGS

General Features
- Best diagnostic clue: Tender, palpable mass near nipple, complex on US with surrounding edema
- Location: Subareolar common; may be peripheral
- Size: Variable: Often 2-4 cm but can be up to 10-12 cm
- Morphology: Irregular mass with ill-defined margins; focal asymmetry on mammography

Mammographic Findings
- Ill-defined, noncalcified mammographic mass or focal asymmetry
- Adjacent trabecular thickening due to edema
- Often subareolar or periareolar
- Mammography not indicated in lactating or young women (< 30 years) with typical clinical constellation
- Pain limits use of mammography
- Can be spiculated
- Ipsilateral adenopathy may be present

Ultrasonographic Findings
- Grayscale Ultrasound
  - Hypoechoic mass with heterogeneous texture
  - Complex cystic-solid mass ± thick wall or septations
  - May have fluid-debris level, mimic complicated cyst
  - Gentle probe pressure may show movement of thick, echogenic purulent material within cavity
  - Air may be present within abscess cavity
    - Bright specular reflectors
  - Surrounding increased echogenicity due to edema
  - ± Extension toward skin surface: "Pointing"
- Power Doppler
  - Hyperemia in surrounding tissue common
  - Inspissated fluid may be isoechoic; ballottement to show color from sloshing of contents

DDx: Complex Fluid Collections

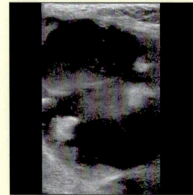

Necrotic Metastasis

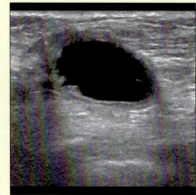

Post-Operative Seroma

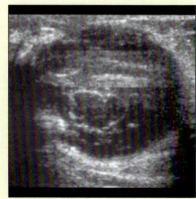

Sub-Acute Hematoma

ABSCESS

Key Facts

Terminology
- Localized pus collection within the breast tissue
- Puerperal abscess = lactational breast abscess

Imaging Findings
- Best diagnostic clue: Tender, palpable mass near nipple, complex on US with surrounding edema
- Location: Subareolar common; may be peripheral
- US-guided aspiration for diagnosis and treatment

Top Differential Diagnoses
- Inflammatory Carcinoma
- Invasive Carcinoma
- Mastitis
- Seroma
- Hematoma

Pathology
- Puerperal abscess: Nipple fissure → sub-areolar inflammation, duct obstruction, milk stasis, infection
- Duct ectasia, stasis, obstruction and inflammation
- Break in skin/nipple while breastfeeding
- Diabetes, HIV, steroids, recent surgery, radiation increase risk
- 90% of women with non-puerperal periductal mastitis are smokers

Clinical Issues
- Age: Most common during reproductive years
- Systemic antibiotics typically directed to skin organisms
- Cavities < 3 cm usually successfully aspirated
- 50-60% require repeat aspiration

MR Findings
- MR not indicated: Conventional imaging usually sufficient
- Edema presents as high signal on T2WI
- Abscess cavity may show intense rim enhancement due to hyperemia
- Adjacent edema and skin thickening can be seen
- Adenopathy may be present

Biopsy
- US-guided aspiration for diagnosis and treatment
  - Thick pus often requires 18-g or larger needle
  - Culture not usually necessary unless refractory to treatment

Imaging Recommendations
- Best imaging tool: US: May require lower frequency transducer for larger abscess

DIFFERENTIAL DIAGNOSIS

Inflammatory Carcinoma
- Can mimic infectious process
  - May appear to respond to antibiotics
  - May lead to delay in diagnosis
- Skin punch biopsy usually diagnostic

Invasive Carcinoma
- Invasive ductal carcinoma (IDC) NOS
- Invasive lobular carcinoma (ILC) or mixed IDC-ILC

Necrotic Tumor
- Poorly differentiated IDC NOS
- Squamous cell metastases

Mastitis
- Diffuse infection with inflammation and edema; may harbor a small focal abscess
- Often associated with lactation

Seroma
- Appropriate clinical history, no signs of infection

Hematoma
- May be echogenic acutely
- Subacute may show fluid-debris level(s), septations

Epidermal Inclusion or Sebaceous Cyst
- Can distinguish clinically

PATHOLOGY

General Features
- General path comments
  - Puerperal abscess: Nipple fissure → sub-areolar inflammation, duct obstruction, milk stasis, infection
    - Lobar or sublobar origin
    - Patterns of involvement: Central, peripheral, or non-specific
    - Central: Rapid lobar spread with hyperemia; infection in dilated central ducts, usually unilocular, parallel to ducts
    - Peripheral: Sublobar ducts or infection in pre-existing galactocele: Abscess forms early, often multi-loculated
    - Non-specific pattern: Ill-defined hyperemia, edema; poorly distinguished ducts; diagnosis difficult until abscess forms
  - Non-puerperal or peri-areolar abscess
    - Underlying duct ectasia, less often cysts
    - Nipple inversion may precede or be caused by periductal inflammation, fibrosis
    - Pathogenesis: Stasis, inflammation, infection
    - Weakened, inflamed duct wall ruptures releasing fatty secretions, causing inflammation
    - Migratory focal abscesses: Different lobar ducts affected
    - Prone to fistula formation
- Etiology
  - Duct ectasia, stasis, obstruction and inflammation
    - Rare: Obstructing intraductal mass with secondary infection
  - Break in skin/nipple while breastfeeding

ABSCESS

- Diabetes, HIV, steroids, recent surgery, radiation increase risk
  - Peripheral location of abscess more common
- Squamous metaplasia of lactiferous ducts (SMOLD)
  - Recurrent mastitis which can result in abscess
  - High association with smoking
- Can occur as a delayed infection in post-lumpectomy seroma cavities
- Various agents
  - Staphylococcus aureus, S. epidermidis most common
  - Streptococcus more diffuse; associated with cellulitis & chronic abscess
  - Anaerobic or microaerophilic organisms
  - Less common causative agents: Fungal, viral, parasitic, mycobacterium (including TB), cat scratch disease
- Epidemiology
  - Puerperal abscess: 4.8-11% incidence in lactating women
  - Non-puerperal abscess: Incidence 5.5-25%
    - Peri-menopausal: Etiology less clear, possibly related to hormonal changes
    - Late teens/early twenties: Associated with underlying congenital nipple inversion and squamous metaplasia
  - 90% of women with non-puerperal periductal mastitis are smokers
- Associated abnormalities: Nipple inversion may be intermittent and recurrent

Gross Pathologic & Surgical Features
- Focal mass
- Inflammation

Microscopic Features
- Mixed acute and chronic inflammation
- May have fat necrosis

CLINICAL ISSUES

Presentation
- Most common signs/symptoms: Erythematous, indurated, painful breast lump near nipple
- Other signs/symptoms: Nipple retraction ± discharge; mammary fistula

Demographics
- Age: Most common during reproductive years

Natural History & Prognosis
- May resolve spontaneously
- Non-puerperal sub-areolar abscesses often indolent, chronic and recurrent
  - Recurrence rate: 10-38%
- Nipple retraction or inversion can become permanent
- If untreated
  - "Pointing" of abscess with subsequent drainage through skin, creating mammary fistula
  - May lead to rupture of multiple ducts

Treatment
- Local and systemic treatment necessary

- Systemic antibiotics typically directed to skin organisms
  - Cephalexin 250-500 mg qid x 10 d or Zithromycin, Z-pak
- Percutaneous US-guided drainage of cavity
  - Cavities < 3 cm usually successfully aspirated
- 50-60% require repeat aspiration
- Cavities > 3-4 cm may require catheter drainage
- Occasionally surgical incision & drainage
- Puerperal abscess
  - Encourage continued breast emptying by breastfeeding or pumping
  - Surgical excision rarely required for refractory cases
- Non-puerperal abscess
  - Recurrent subareolar abscesses may require surgical excision of plugged lactiferous ducts
  - Wedge excision of affected area of nipple in chronic cases
- Exclude malignancy, especially in older women

DIAGNOSTIC CHECKLIST

Consider
- Clinical presentation key to selecting appropriate imaging

Image Interpretation Pearls
- Abscess may be isoechoic due to complex fluid: Ballottement useful to distinguish from solid mass

SELECTED REFERENCES

1. Bassett LW et al: Diagnosis of Diseases of the Breast. Philadelphia, Elsevier Saunders. 421-4, 2005
2. Christensen AF et al: Ultrasound-guided drainage of breast abscesses: results in 151 patients. Br J Radiol. 78(927):186-8, 2005
3. Eryilmaz R et al: Management of lactational breast abscesses. Breast. 14(5):375-9, 2005
4. Varey AH et al: Treatment of loculated lactational breast abscess with a vacuum biopsy system. Br J Surg. 92(10):1225-6, 2005
5. Versluijs-Ossewaarde FN et al: Subareolar breast abscesses: characteristics and results of surgical treatment. Breast J. 11(3):179-82, 2005
6. Lannin DR: Twenty-two year experience with recurring subareolar abscess and lactiferous duct fistula treated by a single breast surgeon. Am J Surg. 188(4):407-10, 2004
7. Ulitzsch D et al: Breast abscess in lactating women: US-guided treatment. Radiology. 232(3):904-9, 2004
8. Berg WA et al: Cystic lesions of the breast: sonographic-pathologic correlation. Radiology. 227(1):183-91, 2003
9. Leborgne F et al: Treatment of breast abscesses with sonographically guided aspiration, irrigation, and instillation of antibiotics. AJR Am J Roentgenol. 181(4):1089-91, 2003
10. Rosen PP: Rosen's Breast Pathology. Philadelphia, Lippincott Williams & Wilkins. Chapter 4, 65-75, 2001
11. Hook GW et al: Treatment of breast abscesses with US-guided percutaneous needle drainage without indwelling catheter placement. Radiology. 213(2):579-82, 1999
12. Berna JD et al: Percutaneous catheter drainage of breast abscesses. Eur J Radiol. 21(3):217-9, 1996

ABSCESS

IMAGE GALLERY

Typical

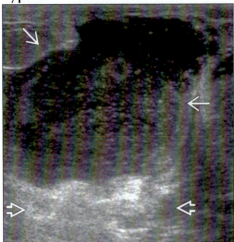
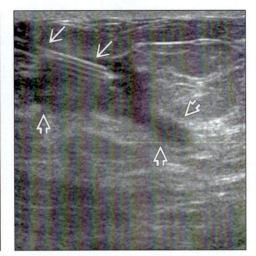

(Left) Ultrasound of a tender swelling in 26 year old with history of trauma and resolving hematoma, shows an irregular fluid collection ➡ with mobile internal echoes & posterior enhancement ➡. (Right) US (same patient as previous image) shows needle ➡ within the fluid and almost complete aspiration, yielding frankly purulent material. Residual hypoechoic area ➡ likely represents surrounding inflammation.

Typical

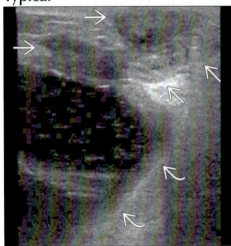
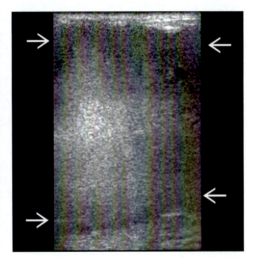

(Left) US of a 41 year old two weeks post breast augmentation shows an irregular, complex fluid collection ➡ extending from the implant ➡ to the skin surface. US-guided aspiration confirmed infection. (Right) US in 31 year old with markedly enlarged, firm, tender breast shows echogenic material ➡, representing pus in an unrecognized abscess with rupture of multiple ducts. Treatment: Surgical incision & drainage.

Typical

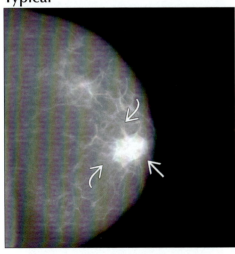
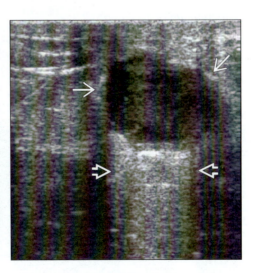

(Left) CC mammography in a 39 year old with tender swelling shows sub-areolar density with slightly spiculated margins ➡ Trabecular thickening ➡ is also seen. US shows typical features of abscess, which resolved with aspiration & antibiotics. (Right) Radial ultrasound shows a thick-walled fluid collection ➡ with posterior enhancement ➡. Culture of aspirated fluid grew staphylococcus aureus. The patient was successfully treated with oral antibiotics.

GRANULOMATOUS MASTITIS

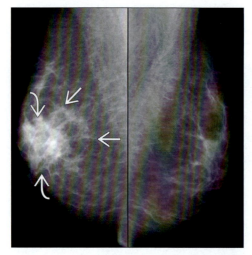

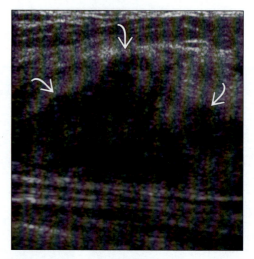

MLO mammography shows retroareolar asymmetry ⮞ & trabecular thickening ⮞ in a woman presenting with periareolar discharging sinuses some months after stopping breastfeeding. US was performed (next).

US shows typical findings of granulomatous mastitis (biopsy-proven) with poorly defined hypoechoic mass ⮞ and no significant distortion or posterior features. This woman responded well to oral steroids.

TERMINOLOGY

Abbreviations and Synonyms
- Idiopathic mastitis, nonspecific mastitis
- Granulomatous lobular mastitis, nonspecific granulomatous mastitis

Definitions
- Noninfective granulomatous inflammation of the breast
- Tuberculosis and other granulomatous infections excluded

IMAGING FINDINGS

General Features
- Location: Breast cone, often retroareolar
- Size: 2-10 cm
- Morphology: Irregular, poorly marginated

Mammographic Findings
- Focal, poorly-defined asymmetry
  - Often retroareolar

- Trabecular thickening due to edema

Ultrasonographic Findings
- Grayscale Ultrasound
  - Multiple, irregular, clustered, often contiguous, tubular hypoechoic lesions
  - Large, irregular hypoechoic mass(es)
    - May be confluent
  - Hypoechoic linear tracks to skin (cutaneous sinuses)
  - Typically without change in posterior acoustic features
  - Surrounding increased echogenicity due to edema
- Color Doppler: Hypervascularity common in surrounding parenchyma

MR Findings
- T1WI: Hypointense or isointense irregular mass(es)
- T2WI FS: Microabscesses: Small pockets of hyperintense pus
- T1 C+ FS
  - Intensely but slowly enhancing irregular geographic region(s) on MR
    - Nonenhancing focal rounded rim-enhancing abscesses

DDx: Asymmetric Irregular Pathology

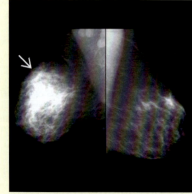

Inflammatory Carcinoma

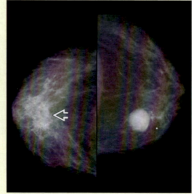

Bacterial Mastitis (Arrow; Left ILC)

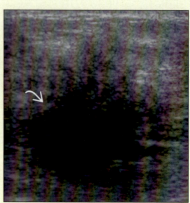

Diabetic Mastopathy

GRANULOMATOUS MASTITIS

Key Facts

Terminology
- Idiopathic mastitis, nonspecific mastitis
- Noninfective granulomatous inflammation of the breast

Imaging Findings
- Focal, poorly-defined asymmetry
- Intensely but slowly enhancing irregular geographic region(s) on MR
- Multiple, irregular, clustered, often contiguous, tubular hypoechoic lesions
- Large, irregular hypoechoic mass(es)

Top Differential Diagnoses
- Bacterial Mastitis
- Diffuse or Inflammatory Breast Carcinoma
- Other Infective Mastitis

Pathology
- Idiopathic, probably autoimmune etiology
- Inflammatory mass with discharging sinuses
- Noncaseating granulomas
- Multinucleated Langhans-type giant cells

Clinical Issues
- Typically postpartum: Breastfeeding history very common
- Resolves on oral steroid therapy in many cases
- Antibiotic, antituberculous therapy are of minimal benefit

Diagnostic Checklist
- Mimics malignancy: Aspiration/biopsy often needed

- Circumscribed lesion with heterogeneous enhancement

Imaging Recommendations
- Best imaging tool: Ultrasound
- Protocol advice
  - Mammography and ultrasound initially
  - MR for mapping of extent and monitoring response to treatment

DIFFERENTIAL DIAGNOSIS

Bacterial Mastitis
- Draining sinuses uncommon
- Staphylococcal and streptococcal infection most common
  - Culture required to differentiate
- Lacks granuloma formation on biopsy

Tuberculosis (TB) of the Breast
- Discharging sinuses may be present
- Typically "cold" abscess presentation
- Caseating granulomas on biopsy
- TB polymerase chain reaction (PCR) positive
- Culture may be negative

Diffuse or Inflammatory Breast Carcinoma
- No discharging sinuses or pus
- Needle biopsy should be performed to confirm

Other Infective Mastitis
- Culture usually required for diagnosis
- Potential organisms
  - Other mycobacterial infections
  - Fungal or worm infection (e.g., sparganosis)
  - Actinomycosis
  - Histoplasmosis
  - Brucellosis

Other Systemic Granulomatous Conditions
- Wegener granulomatosis
  - May present with granulomatous mastitis initially
- Sarcoidosis

  - Very rare presentation

Cholesterol Granulomas of the Breast
- Foreign body reaction to ruptured intraduct material
- Clinical presentation usually as focal tender mass
- Diagnosis usually made incidentally on needle biopsy

Oil Granulomas
- History of cosmetic enhancement injections
- Paraffin oil injections
  - Can produce hypoechoic suspicious irregular masses
  - May be apparent only on biopsy
- Silicone oil granulomas
  - History of prior silicone breast implants
  - History of direct silicone oil breast injections (Asia)
  - Radiographically dense droplets
  - Dense widespread calcifications

Conditions Producing Localized Breast Fibrosis
- Mainly imaging differentials
- Diabetic fibrous mastopathy
- Mass-like focal or stromal fibrosis

PATHOLOGY

General Features
- General path comments: Diagnosis of exclusion; esp. exclude tuberculosis
- Etiology
  - Idiopathic, probably autoimmune etiology
  - Triggering incident often lactation
  - Sometimes spontaneous
  - One report suggests strong association with Corynebacterium infection, esp. C. kroppenstedtii
- Epidemiology
  - Vast majority associated with lactation
    - Usually months after starting lactation
    - May be lactating at presentation
    - May present many years later

GRANULOMATOUS MASTITIS

Gross Pathologic & Surgical Features
- Irregular areas of poorly-defined inflammation
- Inflammatory mass with discharging sinuses
- Thick pus in multiple microabscesses

Microscopic Features
- Cytology suggestive
- Histology characteristic
  - Noncaseating granulomas
  - Epithelioid cells
  - Multinucleated Langhans-type giant cells
  - Neutrophils, lymphocytes, and stromal cells
- No organisms on culture
- No gram positive or acid-fast bacilli, fungi, oil or cholesterol deposits

CLINICAL ISSUES

Presentation
- Most common signs/symptoms
  - Clinical signs of inflammation
    - Tenderness and mass
    - Skin reddening & warmth
    - Pus discharging from skin sinuses & nipple
- Clinical Profile
  - Typically postpartum: Breastfeeding history very common
  - Lactation may have been many years earlier

Demographics
- Age
  - Usually childbearing years
  - May occur in prepubertal and post-menopausal women: Ages 11-60
- Gender
  - Almost exclusively female
  - In men, usually due to an infective cause or Wegener granulomatosis (extremely rare)

Natural History & Prognosis
- Excellent if treated correctly
- 50% of cases may resolve spontaneously with expectant management
- Often relapses intermittently
- May recur metachronously in opposite breast

Treatment
- Resolves on oral steroid therapy in many cases
- Surgical excision often incomplete
  - Some reports show almost 100% cured if surgical excision complete
  - Microscopically disease free margins required
- Methotrexate reported useful for resistant or recurrent cases
- Antibiotic, antituberculous therapy are of minimal benefit
  - Useful only if specific microbial infection likely or proven

DIAGNOSTIC CHECKLIST

Consider
- Bacterial infection
- Tuberculosis of the breast
- Inflammatory breast cancer
- Other unusual infections of the breast

Image Interpretation Pearls
- Mimics malignancy: Aspiration/biopsy often needed
- Large area of poorly defined hypoechoic change on ultrasound in a woman with subacute or relapsing breast inflammation and discharging cutaneous sinuses
- Large irregular enhancing region with rim-enhancing abscesses on contrast-enhanced MR

SELECTED REFERENCES

1. Asoglu O et al: Feasibility of surgical management in patients with granulomatous mastitis. Breast J. 11:108-14, 2005
2. Lai EC et al: The role of conservative treatment in idiopathic granulomatous mastitis. Breast J. 11:454-6, 2005
3. Diesing D et al: Granulomatous mastitis. Arch Gynecol Obstet. 269:233-6, 2004
4. Kocaoglu M et al: Imaging findings in idiopathic granulomatous mastitis: a review with emphasis on magnetic resonance imaging. J Comput Assist Tomogr. 28:635-41, 2004
5. Tse GM et al: Granulomatous mastitis: a clinicopathological review of 26 cases. Pathology. 36:254-7, 2004
6. Kim J et al: Methotrexate in the management of granulomatous mastitis. ANZ J Surg. 73:247-9, 2003
7. Taylor GB et al: A clinicopathological review of 34 cases of inflammatory breast disease showing an association between corynebacteria infection and granulomatous mastitis. Pathology. 35:109-19, 2003
8. Memis A et al: Granulomatous mastitis: imaging findings with histopathologic correlation. Clin Radiol. 57:1001-6, 2002
9. Sakurai T et al: A case of granulomatous mastitis mimicking breast carcinoma. Breast Cancer. 9:265-8, 2002
10. Yilmaz E et al: Mammographic and sonographic findings in the diagnosis of idiopathic granulomatous mastitis. Eur Radiol. 11:2236-40, 2001
11. Engin G et al: Granulomatous mastitis: gray-scale and color Doppler sonographic findings. J Clin Ultrasound. 27:101-6, 1999
12. Martinez-Parra D et al: Utility of fine-needle aspiration in the diagnosis of granulomatous lesions of the breast. Diagn Cytopathol. 17:108, 1997

GRANULOMATOUS MASTITIS

IMAGE GALLERY

Typical

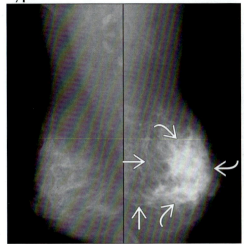

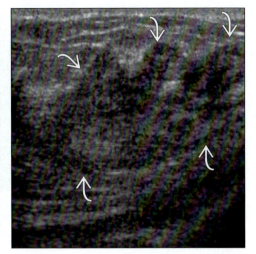

(Left) MLO mammography shows marked asymmetry ⮞ and evidence of parenchymal edema with trabecular thickening ⮞ in a woman presenting with typical signs of inflammation and left breast induration. *(Right)* Radial ultrasound (same as left) in the lateral left breast shows irregular hypoechoic changes corresponding to biopsy proven granulomatous inflammation ⮞.

Typical

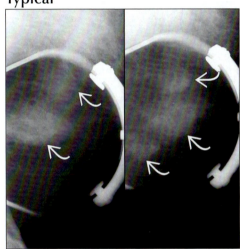

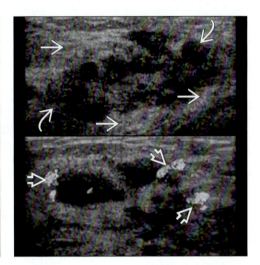

(Left) Mammography spot compression views in the MLO (left) and CC (right) projections show indistinct lobulated mass(es) ⮞ in the lower outer left breast in this woman presenting with tender lumps. *(Right)* Longitudinal ultrasound (same patient as left) (above) shows an irregularly marginated hypoechoic mass ⮞ with thick echogenic rim ⮞. Color Doppler (below) shows prominent marginal hypervascularity ⮞. Biopsy proven granulomatous mastitis.

Variant

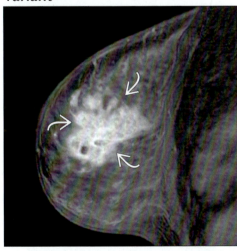

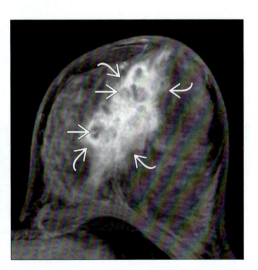

(Left) Sagittal T1 C+ FS MR in a lactating woman with biopsy-proven granulomatous mastitis. Mammograms showed marked diffuse density bilaterally. MR shows the extent of disease ⮞. *(Right)* Axial T1 C+ FS MR (same as left) shows the granulomatous inflammation in the left breast as a large central area of intense irregular enhancement ⮞ with nonenhancing microabscesses ⮞. Excellent response to oral steroid therapy.

MASTITIS

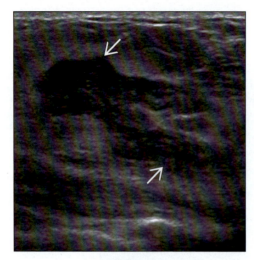
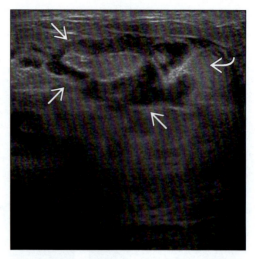

Radial ultrasound over tender, erythematous area in 29 y/o with symptoms for 1 month, shows complex fluid in dilated, thickened ducts ➡. Aspiration yielded minimal thick pus. Intravenous antibiotics required for resolution.

Radial ultrasound of 44 y/o with painful swelling while nursing shows dilated ducts in subareolar region ➡. Echogenicity in adjacent tissue ➡ likely due to edema. Symptoms resolved on oral antibiotics.

TERMINOLOGY

Definitions
- Focal or diffuse breast inflammation, often associated with duct ectasia; includes cellulitis of the breast
  ○ May be infectious or non-infectious
- Several distinct clinical entities
  ○ Puerperal or lactational mastitis: In lactating breast, bacterial, may → abscess
  ○ Nonpuerperal mastitis: Bacterial, not related to pregnancy or lactation
  ○ Granulomatous mastitis: Usually idiopathic
  ○ Unusual infections: Tuberculosis, other
  ○ Lymphocytic mastitis: Intense lymphocytic infiltrate → fibrosis
- Periductal mastitis: Secretory disease: Response to irritative contents of intraluminal lipid in ducts
  ○ Plasma cells accumulate in periductal stroma (formerly "plasma cell mastitis")
  ○ Duct ectasia
  ○ Secretory calcifications (Ca++) accumulate
    ▪ Smooth, rod-like, ≥ 1 mm in diameter
    ▪ In wall of duct or lumen
    ▪ Unusual < age 60

IMAGING FINDINGS

General Features
- Best diagnostic clue: Non-cyclical breast pain, erythema, induration, breast mass, nipple discharge or inversion
- Location: Commonly subareolar, may be peripheral

Mammographic Findings
- Not routinely performed in puerperal mastitis
  ○ Clinical diagnosis
- Dilated subareolar ducts, may extend peripherally
- Findings consistent with inflammation
  ○ Skin and trabecular thickening
  ○ Overall or focal increase in breast density
- Acute, intense mastitis may mimic carcinoma
  ○ Bacterial or granulomatous
  ○ Possible focal mass with abscess formation
- Adenopathy often present

Ultrasonographic Findings
- Grayscale Ultrasound
  ○ Diffuse or focal skin thickening

DDx: Other Causes of Mammographic Asymmetries

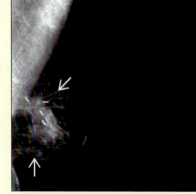
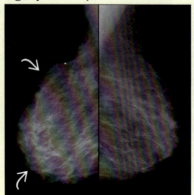
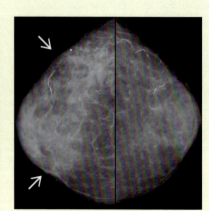

Lumpectomy and Radiation

Inflammatory Cancer

Venous Congestion

MASTITIS

Key Facts

Terminology
- Focal or diffuse breast inflammation, often associated with duct ectasia; includes cellulitis of the breast
- May be infectious or non-infectious
- Puerperal or lactational mastitis: In lactating breast, bacterial, may → abscess
- Nonpuerperal mastitis: Bacterial, not related to pregnancy or lactation
- Periductal mastitis: Secretory disease: Response to irritative contents of intraluminal lipid in ducts

Imaging Findings
- Best diagnostic clue: Non-cyclical breast pain, erythema, induration, breast mass, nipple discharge or inversion
- Location: Commonly subareolar, may be peripheral

- Best imaging tool: Ultrasound: Edema, indistinct dilated ducts, skin thickening, identify and guide drainage of abscess if present

Top Differential Diagnoses
- Inflammatory Carcinoma
- Granulomatous Mastitis
- Lymphocytic Mastitis

Pathology
- Staphylococcus aureus and streptococcal bacteria most common agents

Diagnostic Checklist
- Constellation of clinical symptoms are key to diagnosis
- Punch biopsy to exclude inflammatory carcinoma

- Edema: Diffuse ↑ echogenicity, may see dilated lymphatics
- Irregular hypoechoic mass or no discrete mass
- Mixed echogenicity, often complex cystic mass with thick wall due to abscess
  - May have fluid-debris level
  - Air: Echogenic specular reflectors with "dirty" shadowing
- ± Dilated ducts
- Power Doppler: Hyperemia in inflamed tissues

MR Findings
- T2WI FS
  - High signal in areas of edema
  - Focal hyperintense collection(s) suggest abscess
- T1 C+ FS: Irregular enhancing mass

Imaging Recommendations
- Best imaging tool: Ultrasound: Edema, indistinct dilated ducts, skin thickening, identify and guide drainage of abscess if present
- Protocol advice: Findings of duct wall thickening and edema may be subtle

DIFFERENTIAL DIAGNOSIS

Inflammatory Carcinoma
- Clinical, imaging findings may be indistinguishable
- Both entities may respond to antibiotic treatment
- Often requires punch skin biopsy for diagnosis

Granulomatous Mastitis
- Local granulomatous inflammation

Lymphocytic Mastitis
- Local inflammatory reaction of unknown etiology
- Prominent accumulation of lymphocytes

PATHOLOGY

General Features
- General path comments

- Unclear whether duct ectasia precedes periductal mastitis or inflammation causes obstruction leading to dilatation
  - Bacteria present in nipple discharge of majority of patients with duct ectasia
- Staphylococcus aureus and streptococcal bacteria most common agents
- Leukocyte count > 10^6, bacterial count > 10^3 per ml of breast milk distinguishes from non-infectious milk stasis in lactating patients
- Etiology
  - Puerperal mastitis
    - Pathogens transmitted to breast from infant or through irritated, cracked nipple
    - Milk stasis causing duct dilation and disruption
    - Lipids in periductal tissue incite inflammatory response
  - Non-puerperal mastitis in late teens, early twenties
    - Often associated with congenital nipple inversion (present in 3% of live births)
    - Chronic intermittent nipple discharge common
    - Keratin scales fill duct lumen causing obstruction
    - May be due to squamous metaplasia of lactiferous ducts (SMOLD)
  - Non-puerperal mastitis in peri-menopausal age group
    - Duct ectasia or peri-ductal inflammation
    - Nipple inversion often seen
    - Symptoms last average of 3 years
    - Smoking associated with worse clinical cases and more complications of mastitis
  - Periductal mastitis: Obstructed ducts distend & rupture, extravasation of lipid contents into adjacent tissues causes inflammatory reaction
  - Rarely as complication of percutaneous breast biopsy or surgery
  - Staphylococcus more localized and invasive
  - Streptococcus more diffuse; cellulitis
  - Abscesses may form in untreated or advanced cases
- Epidemiology
  - Incidence: 1-9% of women in puerperal period

MASTITIS

○ 3-12% benign breast lumps in non-lactational women are due to duct ectasia and periductal mastitis
• Associated abnormalities
  ○ Mammary fistula (Zuska disease)
    ▪ Fistula may be lined by squamous epithelium
    ▪ ~ 90% cases in heavy smokers
    ▪ Staphylococci and anaerobes often present in fistula
    ▪ Treatment requires complete excision of affected ducts including terminal portion in the nipple

Gross Pathologic & Surgical Features
• Diffuse or focal breast inflammation, edema, skin thickening, induration
• Focal mass: Abscess or focal duct ectasia

Microscopic Features
• Excised specimens: Mixed acute and chronic inflammation
• Focal accumulation of plasma cells
• Local inflammatory reaction
• Inspissated secretions or immune response
• Rod-like "secretory" calcifications may develop
• May have fat necrosis

CLINICAL ISSUES

Presentation
• Most common signs/symptoms: Diffuse or focal pain, localized tenderness, erythema, edema, warmth
• Other signs/symptoms
  ○ Pain & abscess: Younger women
  ○ Nipple retraction & nontender mass
  ○ May have fever & leukocytosis; focal mass (abscess)
  ○ Periductal mastitis often asymptomatic

Demographics
• Age
  ○ Puerperal mastitis: Reproductive years
  ○ Duct ectasia-periductal mastitis: Peak 40-49 years
  ○ Secretory disease (plasma cell mastitis): > 60 years
• Gender: Rarely in immune compromised males

Natural History & Prognosis
• Puerperal or lactational mastitis
  ○ Usually responsive to conservative local treatment and systemic antibiotics
• Duct ectasia-periductal mastitis complex
  ○ May be chronic, indolent, recurrent; average duration 3 years
  ○ Chronic fibrosis may lead to persistent nipple inversion

Treatment
• Puerperal mastitis
  ○ Broad coverage antibiotics
  ○ Warmth and regular emptying of breast by continued breastfeeding or pumping
  ○ If symptoms do not resolve promptly, US should be performed to detect abscess
  ○ Percutaneous drainage of abscess if present, obtain culture & sensitivity

○ Pathogen-specific antibiotics
○ Repeat aspiration may be necessary
• Peripheral non-puerperal abscess
  ○ May be successfully treated by percutaneous aspiration if abscess present
  ○ Agent-specific antibiotics
• Granulomatous mastitis
  ○ Oral steroids
  ○ Surgical excision may be necessary in some cases
  ○ Methotrexate reported effective for resistant or recurrent cases
• Duct ectasia-periductal mastitis complex
  ○ Depends on presentation
  ○ Focal mass: Biopsy to exclude malignancy
  ○ Persistent nipple discharge: Duct excision
  ○ SMOLD: Complete excision of all diseased ducts, possibly including wedge of nipple

DIAGNOSTIC CHECKLIST

Consider
• Constellation of clinical symptoms are key to diagnosis
• Punch biopsy to exclude inflammatory carcinoma

Image Interpretation Pearls
• US best modality to demonstrate areas of inflammation and focal abscess
  ○ Can guide drainage of abscesses

SELECTED REFERENCES

1. Cerveira I et al: Lupus mastitis. Breast. 2006
2. Lee JH et al: Radiologic and clinical features of idiopathic granulomatous lobular mastitis mimicking advanced breast cancer. Yonsei Med J. 47(1):78-84, 2006
3. Nagpal V et al: Breast lump as a presentation of a hydatid disease. Trop Doct. 36(1):57-8, 2006
4. Stricker T et al: Nonpuerperal mastitis in adolescents. J Pediatr. 148(2):278-81, 2006
5. da Silva BB et al: Primary tuberculosis of the breast mimicking carcinoma. Am J Trop Med Hyg. 73(5):975-6, 2005
6. Edey AJ et al: Ductal breast carcinoma presenting with methicillin-resistant Staphylococcus aureus mastitis. Breast J. 11(6):491-2, 2005
7. Lai EC et al: The role of conservative treatment in idiopathic granulomatous mastitis. Breast J. 11(6):454-6, 2005
8. Rosen PP: Rosen's Breast Pathology. Philadelphia, Lippincott Williams & Wilkins. 65-75, 2001
9. Kopans D: Breast Imaging, 2nd edition. Philadelphia, Lippincott-Raven. 523-4, 1998
10. Bassett LW et al: Diagnosis of Diseases of the Breast. Philadelphia, WB Saunders Co. 382-5, 1997
11. O'Hara RJ et al: Conservative management of infective mastitis and breast abscesses after ultrasonographic assessment. Br J Surg. 83:1413-4, 1996
12. Karstrup S et al: Acute puerperal breast abscesses: US-guided drainage. Radiology. 188:807-9, 1993
13. Watt-Boolsen S et al: Primary periareolar abscess in the nonlactating breast: risk of recurrence. Am J Surg 153:571-3, 1987

IMAGE GALLERY

Typical

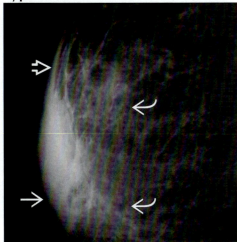 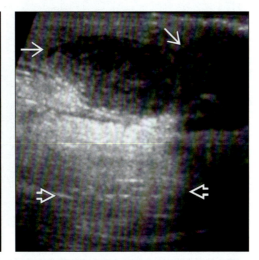

(Left) CC mammography spot compression shows increased density ➡, trabecular thickening ➡, and skin thickening ➡ in this 38 y/o diabetic with painful swelling of the breast. *(Right)* Radial ultrasound (same patient as left) shows a heterogeneous collection ➡ with posterior enhancement ➡, compatible with mastitis & abscess. Aspirated purulent material showed Staphylococcus aureus. Resolved completely on oral antibiotics.

Typical

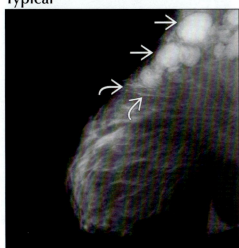 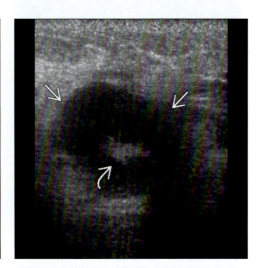

(Left) MLO mammography of a 37 y/o with SLE illustrates typical findings of mastitis: Trabecular thickening ➡ from edema, and multiple large nodes without visible fatty hila ➡; (fatty hila of left axillary nodes preserved). Skin thickening evident clinically. *(Right)* Radial ultrasound of a node (same as left) shows thickened cortex ➡ & compressed hilum ➡. Symptoms resolved after 10 days of antibiotics directed to skin organisms. Lupus itself can also cause mastitis.

Typical

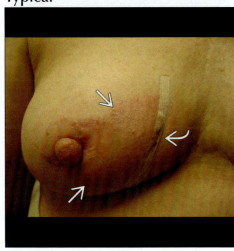 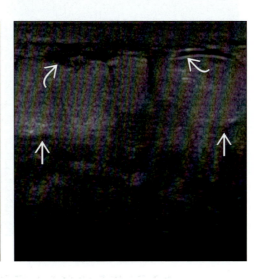

(Left) Frontal clinical photograph of a 45 y/o after core biopsy shows erythema ➡ next to biopsy site ➡, compatible with cellulitis. Infection, occurring in < 1% of percutaneous procedures, usually responds promptly to oral antibiotics (courtesy DNS). *(Right)* Sagittal US of a different patient shows typical sonographic appearance of cellulitis: Diffuse edema manifest as hyperechoic featureless tissue ➡, obscuring normal anatomy. Fluid is seen between tissue planes ➡.

IV

6

13

MASTITIS

(Left) Sagittal T2WI FS MR shows mild increased signal ➡ compatible with edematous tissue in the retroareolar region in this 34 y/o with a nontender lump and strong family history of breast cancer. *(Right)* Sagittal T1 C+ FS MR (same case as left) shows rim-enhancing irregular mass ➡ retroareolar region. Excision showed mastitis without abscess.

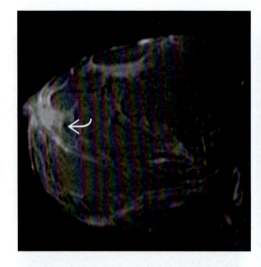 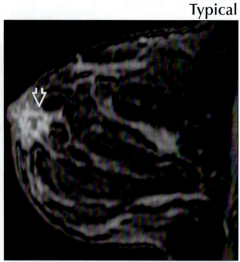

(Left) CC mammography shows dense, round mass ➡ (palpable lump left breast), and palpable global asymmetry with distortion ➡, with associated trabecular thickening ➡, on right side in this 67 y/o. *(Right)* MLO mammography (same as left) again shows left breast mass ➡ and global asymmetry and trabecular thickening right breast ➡. No adenopathy is seen.

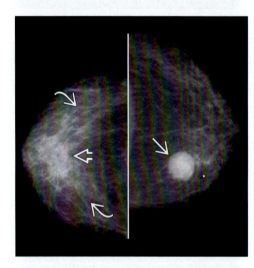 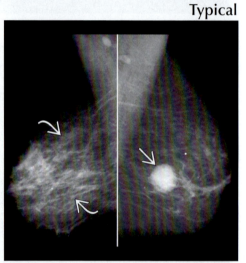

(Left) US of the left breast (same case as prior 2 images) shows microlobulated hypoechoic mass ➡ with echogenic rim/halo ➡. US-guided biopsy showed invasive lobular carcinoma and lobular carcinoma in situ. *(Right)* US of the upper outer right breast 10:00 (same as prior 3 images) shows diffuse increased echogenicity ➡ due to edema, as well as vague areas of decreased echogenicity ➡ (palpable thickening).

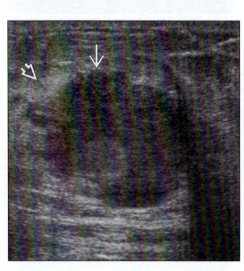 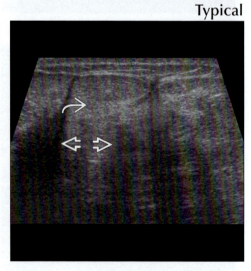

IV

6

MASTITIS

Typical

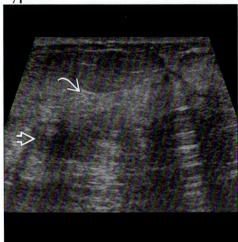 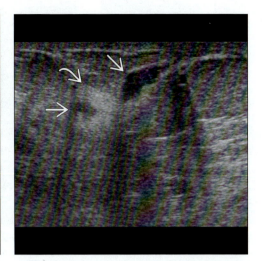

(Left) *US of 12:00 region right breast (this and the next 5 images are a continuation of the same case as the prior 4 images) shows similar findings of diffuse increased echogenicity ➡ and vague hypoechoic mass ⬇. US-guided core biopsy showed moderate acute and chronic inflammation.* **(Right)** *Radial US 12:00 near the nipple shows dilated ducts with debris ➡ and periductal edema ➡.*

Typical

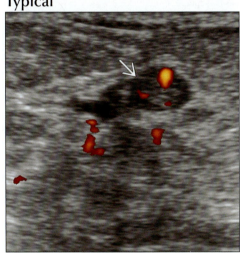 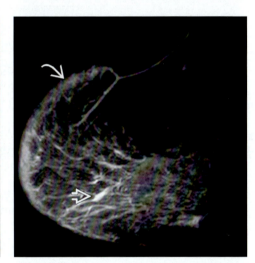

(Left) *US of the 6:00 periareolar region right breast shows unexpected hypervascular intraductal mass ➡. Bloody nipple discharge was also evident on exam. US-guided core biopsy showed papilloma (excised after MR seen in next 3 images).* **(Right)** *Because of her recent diagnosis of contralateral invasive lobular carcinoma, MR was performed. Sagittal T2WI FS of the right breast shows diffuse edema ➡ and skin thickening ➡.*

Typical

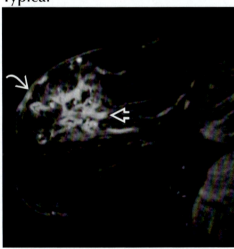 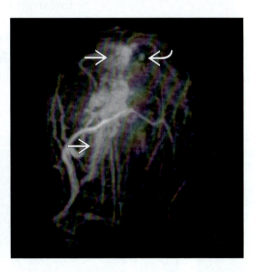

(Left) *Sagittal T1 C+ subtraction MR of the right breast shows irregular reticulated region of enhancement ➡, less discrete than most malignancies, in area of biopsy-proven mastitis. Overlying skin enhancement ➡ is noted.* **(Right)** *Axial MIP of T1 C+ subtraction MR shows distribution of enhancement ➡ is segmental, extending to nipple. Enhancing known papilloma is seen ➡. Symptoms resolved after 3 weeks on cephalexin.*

UNUSUAL INFECTIONS

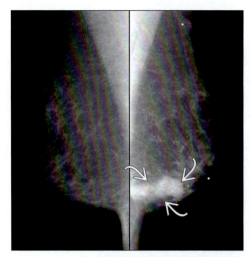

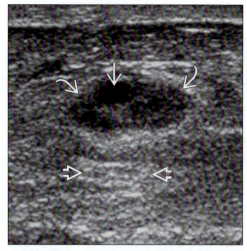

MLO mammography in an 80 y/o woman with a palpable lump shows an elongated asymmetry in the inferior left breast ➨. (Courtesy GT & AP).

Ultrasound (same as left) shows an oval hypoechoic indistinctly-marginated mass ➨ with a focal cystic change ➨ and mild posterior enhancement ➨. Sparganosis was proven at culture.

TERMINOLOGY

Definitions
- Infection by organisms other than pyogenic bacteria
  - Atypical or uncommon infection

IMAGING FINDINGS

General Features
- Best diagnostic clue: Rarely suspected prior to histological diagnosis
- Location: Tendency to be retroareolar
- Size: Wide range: Small calcifications (Ca++) to large palpable mass

Mammographic Findings
- Focal or global asymmetry
  - ± Trabecular thickening due to edema
- Linear or serpiginous Ca++ in filariasis
- Focal Ca++ in axillary nodes in tuberculosis (TB)

Ultrasonographic Findings
- Grayscale Ultrasound

- Granuloma: Hypo- to mixed echogenicity irregular mass
  - May show cystic areas, posterior enhancement
  - ± Surrounding ↑ echogenicity due to edema
  - Nodes may be circumscribed ± Ca++
- Worms: Well-defined, hypoechoic serpiginous tubular masses

MR Findings
- T2WI FS: Hyperintense mass due to internal pus or necrosis
- T1 C+ FS: Variably enhancing mass(es), with or without rim-enhancing abscesses

DIFFERENTIAL DIAGNOSIS

Inflammatory and Pyogenic Infections
- Granulomatous mastitis
- Staphylococcus aureus most common bacterial agent

Necrotic Tumor
- Poorly differentiated infiltrating ductal carcinoma

DDx: Atypical Necrotic Masses

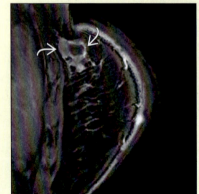

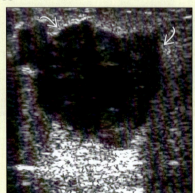

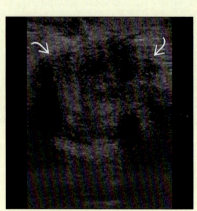

Granulomatous Mastitis *Infiltrating Ductal Carcinoma* *Pyogenic Abscess*

UNUSUAL INFECTIONS

Key Facts

Terminology
- Infection by organisms other than pyogenic bacteria

Imaging Findings
- Best diagnostic clue: Rarely suspected prior to histological diagnosis

Top Differential Diagnoses
- Inflammatory and Pyogenic Infections
- Necrotic Tumor

Pathology
- Travel to or origin from endemic regions
- May be isolated or part of systemic infection
- Following surgical or other intervention, esp. cosmetic oil or gel injections
- Mycobacterial
- Parasitic (esp. in endemic regions)
- Fungal (very rare, usually isolated)

PATHOLOGY

General Features
- Etiology
  - Travel to or origin from endemic regions
  - May be isolated or part of systemic infection
  - Following surgical or other intervention, esp. cosmetic oil or gel injections
  - Culture or serology usually required for diagnosis
  - Mycobacterial
    - TB (Mycobacterium tuberculosis) & atypical mycobacteria
  - Parasitic (esp. in endemic regions)
    - Worms: Filariasis (Wucheria bancrofti), dirofilariasis (D. repens, D. tenuis), loiasis (Dracunculus medinensis)
    - Tapeworms: Cysticercosis (Taenia solium), coenurosis (T. multiceps), sparganosis (Spirometra)
    - Other: Schistosomiasis (S. japonicum), hydatid (Echinococcus granulosus)
  - Fungal (very rare, usually isolated)
    - Histoplasmosis, aspergillosis, cryptococcosis, blastomycosis, coccidioidomycosis
  - Other infections are very rare
    - Granulomatous bacterial infections: Actinomycosis, typhoid mastitis, brucellosis
    - Uncommon bacterial infections (e.g., pseudomonas) in immunocompromised patients

Microscopic Features
- Frequently granulomatous inflammation diagnosed
- Infective organism may be seen microscopically

CLINICAL ISSUES

Presentation
- Most common signs/symptoms: Palpable asymmetric mass ± signs of inflammation
- Other signs/symptoms: Skin nodules, inflammation of nipple, nipple discharge

Treatment
- Specific antimicrobial, antiparasitic or antifungal therapy for microorganism
- Surgical excision may be required

SELECTED REFERENCES

1. Park JH et al: A surgically confirmed case of breast sparganosis showing characteristic mammography and ultrasonography findings. Korean J Parasitol. 44:151-6, 2006
2. Cherubini M et al: Mycobacterium infection directly observed in a surgical outpatient centre. Minerva Chir. 58:77-82, 82-5, 2003
3. Bastarrika G et al: Calcified filariasis of the breast: report of four cases. Eur Radiol. 11:1195-7, 2001
4. Rosen PP. Rosen's Breast Pathology, 2nd Ed. Philadelphia, Lippincott Williams & Wilkins. 65-75, 2001

IMAGE GALLERY

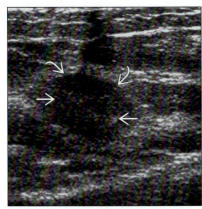 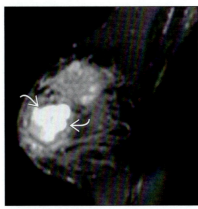 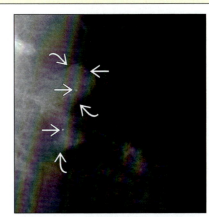

(Left) Ultrasound in an 27 y/o woman with a palpable right breast lump shows a hypoechoic partly circumscribed mass ➡ with heterogeneous internal echoes ➡. *(Center)* Sagittal T2WI FS MR (same as left) shows a hyperintense lobulated irregular cystic mass ➡. Culture and biopsy-proven tuberculous breast abscess (Courtesy GT & AP). *(Right)* MLO mammography magnification of the left axilla in a 46 y/o woman shows lymphadenopathy ➡ with multiple focal dense calcifications ➡. Biopsy-proven TB lymphadenitis.

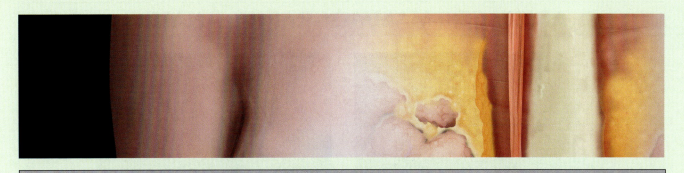

SECTION 7: Artifacts

ARTIFACTS: MAMMOGRAPHY, ANALOG

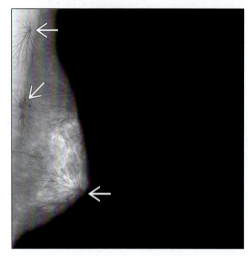

MLO mammography shows plus-density artifacts ➡ due to static electrical discharge at surface of film prior to processing. Light emitted during electrical discharge has exposed film, causing characteristic static pattern.

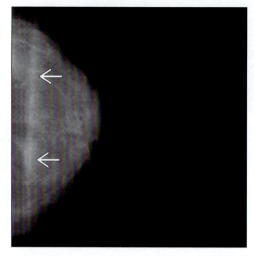

CC mammography shows linear minus density artifact ➡ parallel to chest wall. Could be due to misaligned compression paddle, filter, or mirror in tube (if recurring) or due to crimped film (as an isolated event).

TERMINOLOGY

Abbreviations and Synonyms
- American College of Radiology (ACR)
- US Food and Drug Administration (FDA)
- Mammography Quality Standards Act (MQSA)
- Automatic exposure control (AEC)
- Quality control (QC)

Definitions
- Artifact: Any physical or chemical process that adds structured noise to an image
  - Can obscure normal or pathologic structures; sometimes mimics pathologic structure
- Plus density: Higher optical density (darker)
- Minus density: Lower optical density (lighter)
- Pickoff: Focal removal of emulsion from film, usually due to build up of gelatin on rollers in dryer of processor

IMAGING FINDINGS

General Features
- Best diagnostic clue
  - Appearance or finding that does not correspond to normal anatomy or typical pathology
  - Film processing is the major source of artifacts in analog mammography
  - X-ray imaging chain and film handling are less common sources of analog artifacts
  - ACR phantom simulates a 4.5 cm breast, contains standardized fibers, speck groups, and masses; an excellent tool to analyze artifacts
    - Artifacts can obscure objects in phantom
    - 4 fibers, 3 speck groups, and 3 masses must be seen to meet ACR/FDA requirements
  - Uniform phantom covering the entire x-ray field is also helpful in analyzing artifacts
- Location: Can occur in isolated areas (e.g., foreign matter on screen) or can occur repeatedly across entire image (e.g., pickoff, processor chatter lines or wet pressure)
- Size: Larger in size than the structure of quantum mottle (random noise)

DDx: Calcifications and Artifacts that Mimic Them

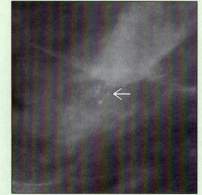

Ductal Carcinoma in Situ

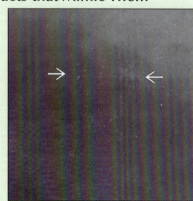

Fingerprint

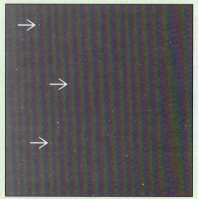

Dust and Underlying Grid Lines

ARTIFACTS: MAMMOGRAPHY, ANALOG

Key Facts

Terminology
- Artifact: Any physical or chemical process that adds structured noise to an image
- Can obscure normal or pathologic structures; sometimes mimics pathologic structure

Imaging Findings
- Appearance or finding that does not correspond to normal anatomy or typical pathology
- Film processing is the major source of artifacts in analog mammography
- Artifacts appear as either minus or plus density and as specks, lines, or blotches
- Poor positioning leads to patient-derived object artifacts: Patient's hair, nose, chin, arm, axillary fold, belly superimposed on film

- Inadequate compression promotes blur due to breast motion

Top Differential Diagnoses
- Point-like minus density artifacts are typically higher contrast (e.g., pickoff, dust, other foreign objects) or more regular (e.g., skin talc) than Ca++ due to ductal carcinoma in situ (DCIS)
- Analog Artifacts: Structured Noise, ↓ Conspicuity of Breast Lesions
- Those occurring on every film due to persistent problem are most bothersome

Pathology
- General path comments: Careful attention is needed to differentiate image artifacts from lesions

---

- Morphology
  - Artifacts appear as either minus or plus density and as specks, lines, or blotches
    - Often obvious, but may mimic or obscure pathology
- Types of analog mammography artifacts
  - Film defects
  - Film handling artifacts
  - Processing artifacts
  - Screen artifacts, including foreign matter on screen
  - X-ray equipment artifacts
  - Motion artifacts
- Identifying source of artifacts often requires investigation with phantoms
  - Film processor is most likely source of artifacts
  - Artifacts constant across different cassettes and processors are likely due to x-ray unit
  - Placing cassette atop breast support tray can test for artifacts due to grid or breast support assembly
  - Isolating artifacts to processor, x-ray unit, or film facilitates appropriate service correction

Radiographic Findings
- Radiography
  - Film defects, film handling, and screen artifacts
    - Can occur on any film, anywhere on film
    - Can be plus density or minus density
    - Dust: Between screen and film prevents light from exposing film → minus artifacts resembling calcifications (Ca++); similar pattern seen on multiple images obtained with same cassette
    - Fingerprints: Can be minus or plus density
    - Minus density fingerprint can resemble Ca++
    - Minus density streaks or mass-like areas on film can be due to foreign matter (fingernail polish, pencil marks, cleaning chemicals) on screen
    - Stains, blotches: Film may be affected before or after exposure and before or during processing (e.g., damp screen when film is placed in cassette)
    - Scratches: Sharply-defined, irregular, linear defects in emulsion
    - Static electricity: Jagged linear or star-like plus density marks

  - Processing artifacts
    - Roller marks: Straight, parallel lines, often in repeating pattern, usually plus density, always perpendicular to direction of film travel
    - Delay streaks: Plus density deposits of developer parallel to the direction of film travel
    - Guide shoe marks: Plus or minus density fine lines parallel to the direction of film travel
    - Wet pressure: Plus density blotches on film due to rollers in developer tank having rough surfaces or uneven buildup of developer
  - Film processing problems
    - Poor contrast, lighter films: Contaminated or exhausted developer, improper developer replenishment
    - Films too light or too dark: Improper developer temperature or replenishment, improper fixer replenishment, recent service to processor
    - Films too dark or too light despite consistent processor QC results & exposure settings: Faulty film batch
    - Tacky films or films turning brown over time: Incomplete wash of fixer from film: Check water supply and filter for wash tank
  - Cassette and film storage problems
    - Recurring plus density areas at edges of film: Light leak due to cracked cassette; use cassette number on film to identify damaged cassettes
    - Plus density areas on film: Improper film or cassette storage, light leaks in darkroom or processor, cracked or improper safelight filter, safelight bulb too bright, new light sources placed in darkroom
    - Fogged films: Loaded cassettes may be improperly stored where x-rays can fog film
    - Film far too light: Film loaded upside down in cassette
    - Rectangular criss-crossed pattern on film: Cassette placed upside down in Bucky

Mammographic Findings
- Procedure-related

- ○ Poor positioning leads to patient-derived object artifacts: Patient's hair, nose, chin, arm, axillary fold, belly superimposed on film
- ○ Inadequate compression promotes blur due to breast motion
- ○ Poor exposure: Incorrect AEC photocell positioning; generator and power supply failures, recent service to x-ray unit that changed AEC performance
- Mammography machine-related
  - ○ Incorrect collimation
  - ○ Grid line artifacts: Parallel lines visible due to incomplete grid motion
  - ○ Grid inhomogeneity, stationary grid lines (Bucky failure)
  - ○ Compression system failure
- Film & screen-related
  - ○ Faulty screens: Variable density across image
  - ○ Quantum mottle: Mottled variation in radiographic density over moderately dense tissues
- Foreign material: Radiodense opacities which are usually recognizable, may mimic suspicious Ca++
  - ○ On screens: Fingerprints, dust, smoke particles, hair
  - ○ On cassettes: Contrast media, metallic particles
  - ○ On patient: Clothing, talc
  - ○ In patient: Pacemaker, tattoos, foreign bodies

Imaging Recommendations

- Best imaging tool
  - ○ Uniform phantom covering entire image receptor is best way to evaluate artifacts
    - ▪ Expose a 2-4 cm thick phantom using AEC to get optical density (OD) between 1.5 and 2.0
    - ▪ Expose same phantom on each film-screen unit
    - ▪ Process an identically exposed phantom on each film processor
    - ▪ This process helps distinguish x-ray equipment artifacts from processing artifacts
    - ▪ On non-daylight processors, rotating direction of film feed can help separate processing artifacts from equipment-caused artifacts
- Protocol advice: Minimizing artifacts improves lesion conspicuity and can minimize spurious lesions
- Recognition and awareness of artifacts are crucial
- Feedback to technologists and medical physicist about identified artifacts is essential
- Quality control (QC) for mammography is required by MQSA and is prescribed in FDA's Final Rules
- Details for QC are specified in the ACR Mammography QC Manual (4th Edition), which is consistent with FDA requirements

DIFFERENTIAL DIAGNOSIS

Suspicious Minus-Density Artifacts on Mammography Mimic DCIS Ca++

- Point-like minus density artifacts are typically higher contrast (e.g., pickoff, dust, other foreign objects) or more regular (e.g., skin talc) than Ca++ due to ductal carcinoma in situ (DCIS)

Suspicious Minus Density Linear or Focal Artifacts

- May mimic neoplasm, focal lesion
- Can be due to finger pressure on film, foreign substance on film or screen, superimposed foreign object at edge of film

Analog Artifacts: Structured Noise, ↓ Conspicuity of Breast Lesions

- Those occurring on every film due to persistent problem are most bothersome
  - ○ Processing artifacts
  - ○ Breast support tray artifacts
  - ○ Grid lines
  - ○ Filtration artifacts

PATHOLOGY

General Features

- General path comments: Careful attention is needed to differentiate image artifacts from lesions

DIAGNOSTIC CHECKLIST

Consider

- Using your QC technologist or medical physicist to identify source of perceived artifacts

Image Interpretation Pearls

- Keep an eye out for persistent artifacts seen on multiple cases, identify source, and correct
- Film processor is the cause of most artifacts
- ACR Mammography QC Manual is an excellent reference for image quality and artifact issues

SELECTED REFERENCES

1. Minigh J: Mammographic film artifacts. Radiol Technol. 77(5):389M-402M, 2006
2. Ikeda D et al: Breast Imaging: The Requisites. Philadelphia, Elsevier Mosby Publishing Co. 1-23, 2004
3. Rothenberg LN et.al: NCRP Report #149. A Guide to Mammography and Other Breast Imaging Procedures, Bethesda, National Council of Radiation Protection and Measurements, 2004
4. Bassett LW et al: Reasons for failure of a mammography unit at clinical image review in the American College of Radiology Mammography Accreditation Program. Radiology. 215(3):698-702, 2000
5. Hendrick RE et. al: ACR Mammography Quality Control Manual, 4th Ed. Reston, American College of Radiology, 1999
6. Hogge JP et al: Quality assurance in mammography: artifact analysis. Radiographics. 19(2):503-22, 1999
7. Hedrick WR et al: Unusual artifact with mammography film. Radiology. 206(3):835-7, 1998
8. Quality Mammography Standards; Final Rule. Federal Register, Volume 62, No. 208, p. 55852-55994, 1997
9. Farria DM et al: Mammography quality assurance from A to Z. Radiographics. 14(2):371-85, 1994

IMAGE GALLERY

Variant

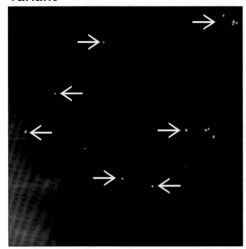 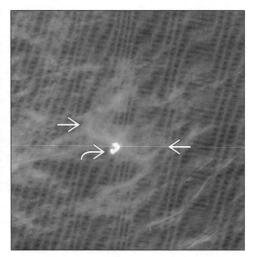

(Left) Mammography shows pickoff artifacts ➡ as minus density points resembling Ca++. Pickoff is usually brighter than calcifications or dust, as film emulsion has been removed locally; pattern often repeats. *(Right)* MLO mammography shows minus density artifact due to a radiodense object ➡. Surrounding structures are blurred ➡ due to poor screen-film contact near object (and resulting scatter), caused by small metal fragment found between screen and film.

Variant

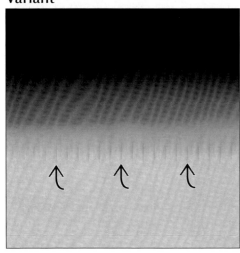 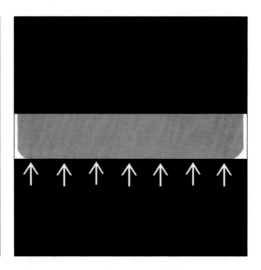

(Left) Mammography shows parallel, evenly spaced plus density artifacts ➡ due to excessive entrance roller pressure or wet rollers. Film traveled vertically through processor, parallel to the dark lines. *(Right)* Mammography shows guide shoe marks ➡ as evenly spaced plus density lines running parallel to the direction of film travel, usually occurring at the leading edge of film. Guide shoe marks can be dark or light and sometimes persist across entire film.

Variant

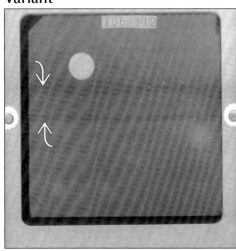 

(Left) Mammography of ACR phantom shows two horizontal plus density bands ➡. Bands running perpendicular to direction of film travel are usually roller marks. Those running parallel to film travel (like these) are delay streaks. Both are due to developer buildup on rollers. *(Right)* Mammography shows criss-crossed minus-density pattern due to incomplete hexagonal grid motion. Incomplete linear grid motion caused horizontal bands in last DDx image.

ARTIFACTS: MAMMOGRAPHY, DIGITAL

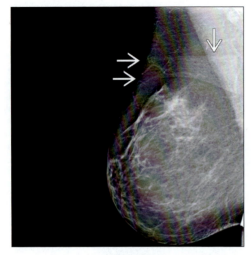

MLO mammography using digital detector shows minus density ghosting artifacts ➡ due to prior x-ray exposures using phantoms, which left remnant image on detector.

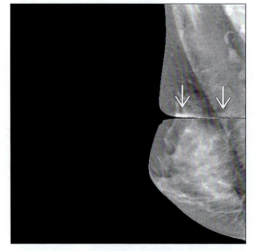

MLO mammography with digital detector shows plus-minus density horizontal line obscuring breast tissue ➡ due to detector dropout or misregistration, enhanced near skin line by thickness compensation.

TERMINOLOGY

Abbreviations and Synonyms
- American Association of Physicists in Medicine (AAPM)
- American College of Radiology (ACR)
- Maximum optical density in film (Dmax)
- Food and Drug Administration (FDA)
- Quality control (QC)
- Society of Motion Picture and Television Engineers (SMPTE)
- Window width (WW)
- Window level (WL)

Definitions
- Artifact: Any physical phenomenon that adds structured noise to the image, degrades image quality, and can mimic pathology or interfere with image interpretation
- Full-field digital mammography (FFDM): Electronic device designed to acquire and store images of the entire breast

- Computed radiography (CR): Digital modality in which latent images are recorded on cassettes with photostimulable phosphor screens
  - These screens are scanned in a reader device using a laser point-by-point, generating stimulated emissions in proportion to x-ray exposure
- Review workstation: Softcopy display device suitable for primary interpretation of digital mammograms
- Ghosting: Remnant image from prior exposures superimposed on current digital image
- Thickness compensation or thickness equalization: Image post-processing algorithm applied to tissue near skin line to yield approximately uniform background density compensating for breast thickness roll-off
- Detector saturation: X-ray flux to detector exceeding dynamic range of detector, causing registration of maximum possible signal and eliminating contrast between pixels
- Digital systems are required to score at least 4 fibers, 3 speck groups, and 3 masses on ACR Phantom, just as for film-screen-film; some digital system manufacturers have set higher requirements
- Minus density: Lower optical density (lighter)
- Plus density: Higher optical density (darker)

DDx: ACR Phantom Images on Digital: The Good, the Bad, and the Ugly

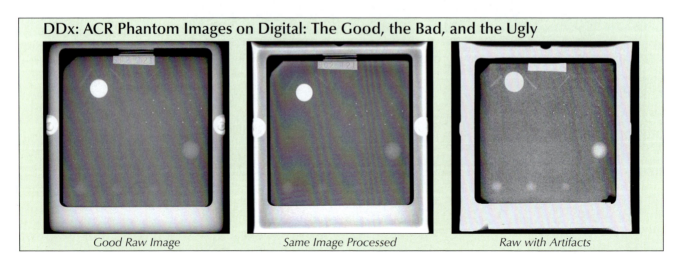

| Good Raw Image | Same Image Processed | Raw with Artifacts |

ARTIFACTS: MAMMOGRAPHY, DIGITAL

Key Facts

Terminology
- Artifact: Any physical phenomenon that adds structured noise to the image, degrades image quality, and can mimic pathology or interfere with image interpretation

Imaging Findings
- Detector miscalibration is the primary source of image artifacts in digital mammography
- X-ray imaging chain is a less-common source of image artifacts
- Same equipment artifacts that occur in analog mammography can occur in digital
- Fixed digital detector systems use calibration or gain correction to remove sensitivity differences and x-ray non-uniformities (e.g., heel effect)

- ACR phantom or uniform phantom imaged with appropriate clinical technique is excellent way to check for artifacts
- Minimizing artifacts in digital mammography requires constant attention to image quality, recognition of digital artifacts when they occur, and feedback to technologists and the medical physicist

Clinical Issues
- Specks, lines, streaks, or blotches due to signal calibration problems
- Most detector failures are catastrophic, causing obvious artifacts or preventing exposure

Diagnostic Checklist
- Beware of assessing lesion sizes from digital hardcopy

IMAGING FINDINGS

General Features
- Best diagnostic clue
  - Detector miscalibration is the primary source of image artifacts in digital mammography
  - X-ray imaging chain is a less-common source of image artifacts
  - Artifacts seen on hardcopy should be checked on softcopy workstation to determine if due to imaging chain or laser printer
- Location
  - Can occur anywhere on image
  - Check carefully for white or black lines at chest wall edge of digital image, indicating excluded tissue
- Size: Can repeat over entire image or occur locally
- Morphology
  - Straight or curved lines not conforming to anatomy are common indicators of digital artifacts
  - Pattern sometimes repeats over entire image (e.g., grid line artifacts)

Radiographic Findings
- Same equipment artifacts that occur in analog mammography can occur in digital
- Fixed digital detector systems use calibration or gain correction to remove sensitivity differences and x-ray non-uniformities (e.g., heel effect)
  - Calibration generally reduce artifacts, but also can introduce persistent artifacts
- Recalibrating the gain correction file can remove persistent artifacts
- Recalibrating too soon after patient or phantom exposures can introduce ghosting artifacts into the calibration file
  - These artifacts will appear on every subsequent image
  - Recalibration is best done in the morning, before any exposures are made

Imaging Recommendations
- Best imaging tool

  - ACR phantom or uniform phantom imaged with appropriate clinical technique is excellent way to check for artifacts
    - To analyze artifacts using ACR phantom, set WW and WL to best reveal objects in phantom, then check for artifacts throughout phantom
    - To analyze artifacts using uniform phantom, set WW at a fixed value similar to that used for clinical image evaluation or ACR phantom (e.g., WW = 200)
    - Too narrow a WW will always show some artifacts, including those not clinically relevant
    - Too wide a WW will obscure clinically relevant artifacts
  - Digital phantoms such as SMPTE pattern or AAPM TG-18 test pattern best for evaluating digital display devices
- Protocol advice
  - Minimizing artifacts in digital mammography requires constant attention to image quality, recognition of digital artifacts when they occur, and feedback to technologists and the medical physicist
  - FDA requirement for QC in digital mammography is to follow the QC manual of the digital equipment manufacturer, including test frequencies and criteria
  - Each digital system type has an equipment-specific QC program

DIFFERENTIAL DIAGNOSIS

Types of Digital Mammography Artifacts
- Gain calibration file non-uniformities
- Filtration artifacts: Mottled background across entire image
- Bad pixel artifacts: Isolated white or black pixels
- Cluster artifacts: Several bad pixels in a group, black or white
- Line artifact: Row or column of defective pixels, black or white

ARTIFACTS: MAMMOGRAPHY, DIGITAL

- Dust artifacts: Dust can accumulate atop digital detector, breast support tray, compression paddle, mirror, or filter, producing a similar pattern of minus density specks in each image
- Grid artifacts: Resemble grid artifacts in screen-film; could be "calibrated" into gain calibration file, resulting in an unwanted grid pattern in every subsequent image
- Improper collimation or detector alignment: Black or white bands at edge of detector
- Damaged detector or detector housing
- Image ghosting: Lighter or darker regions on image due to prior exposure
- Pre- or post-processing algorithm artifacts
- Motion artifacts

Laser Printer Artifacts
- Lines or streaks in horizontal or vertical direction
- Criss-crossed background
- Images too light or too dark
  - Check film type loaded in laser imager
  - Call laser printer service to adjust printed films to match displayed images

Image Display Monitor Artifacts
- Broad area non-uniformities
- Lines, streaks, or dots: Black or white
  - Both are best evaluated with uniform digital phantom
- Monitor background density too bright
  - Have service or medical physicist check and adjust dark level of monitor
- Monitors fail to match
  - Can be evaluated by displaying same clinical image on both monitors at same WW and WL
  - Check that all areas match for brightness and contrast
  - QC on display monitors is often neglected: Make sure it is done regularly

Design-Specific Artifacts
- Scan line artifacts: Slot-scanning or CR systems
  - Check for banding artifacts in direction of slot or laser scanning
- Cassette phosphor or scanning non-uniformities: CR systems
  - Produces broad area background differences
  - Best evaluated with a uniform phantom
- Damaged cassette: CR systems
- Signal dropout: Any digital system, but especially those with multiple detector elements
  - Best evaluated with uniform phantom containing a high-contrast grid pattern

Other Image Quality Problems
- Poor or excessive contrast
  - Could be due to image processing
  - Could be due to too wide or too narrow a WW setting on displayed images
  - Could be due to incorrect look-up table applied to image
  - Low contrast on laser printed images could be due to too low a Dmax

- Laser imager needs service adjustment to raise Dmax and possibly mid-density gray level

CLINICAL ISSUES

Presentation
- Most common signs/symptoms
  - Specks, lines, streaks, or blotches due to signal calibration problems
    - Best evaluated with a uniform phantom
- Other signs/symptoms
  - White or black bands at edges of image receptor (especially chest wall edge)
  - Most detector failures are catastrophic, causing obvious artifacts or preventing exposure

DIAGNOSTIC CHECKLIST

Consider
- Using your QC technologist, medical physicist, and digital service engineer to resolve artifact issues
- As interpreting physician, you are responsible for the quality of interpreted images, even if it is not your imaging equipment
- When submitting phantom images for ACR accreditation, submit "raw" or "for processing" images, so that thickness equalization does not introduce spurious artifacts in phantom (see DDx images)

Image Interpretation Pearls
- Compare hardcopy and softcopy output to see if artifact occurs in both
  - This can eliminate the laser imager or review workstation as cause of artifact
- Beware of assessing lesion sizes from digital hardcopy
  - Sizes on printed digital do not necessarily reflect true sizes
  - Can affect assessment of lesion stability or growth between film and digital

SELECTED REFERENCES

1. Bloomquist AK et.al: Quality control for digital mammography in the ACRIN DMIST trial: part I. Medical Physics. 33:719-36, 2006
2. Yaffe MJ et.al: Quality control for digital mammography: part II. Recommendations from the ACRIN DMIST trial. Medical Physics. 33:737-52, 2006
3. Ikeda D et al: Breast Imaging: the Requisites. Philadelphia, Elsevier Mosby Publishing Co. 1-23, 2004
4. Lewin JM et al: Digital mammography. Radiol Clin North Am. 42:871-84, 2004
5. Pisano ED et al: Digital mammography. Philadelphia, Lippincott, Williams & Wilkins. 2004
6. Boyle ER et al: Motion artifact seen on slot-scanning direct digital mammography. AJR. 172:697-701, 1999
7. Hendrick RE et.al: ACR Mammography QC Manual, 4th Edition. Reston, American College of Radiology. 1999
8. Chotas HG et al: Memory artifact related to selenium-based digital radiography systems. Radiology. 203:881-3, 1997
9. Bick U et al: Density correction of peripheral breast tissue on digital mammograms. RadioGraphics. 16:1403-11, 1996

IMAGE GALLERY

Variant

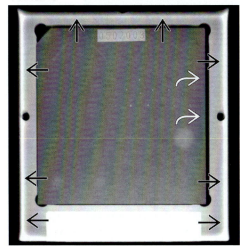

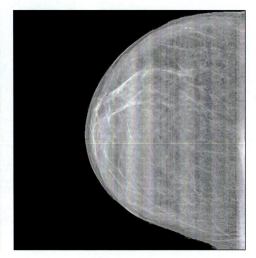

(Left) Mammography with full-field digital detector shows phantom image with thickness-equalization algorithm applied, causing white bands around edge of phantom ➡ and edge of insert ➡. Algorithm causes artifacts on sharp-edged phantoms. Insert area has mottled appearance due to poor detector calibration. *(Right)* CC mammography shows vertical banding along direction of slot motion in a poorly calibrated slot-scanning full-field digital mammography system.

Variant

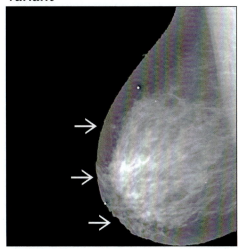

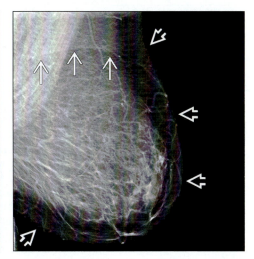

(Left) MLO mammography with full-field digital detector shows jagged edges at skin line ➡ due to detector saturation into breast tissue. Usually can be corrected with better compression. *(Right)* MLO mammography shows ghost artifact ➡ due to miscalibrated detector (if recurring) or ghost from prior exposure (if on isolated images or differs from image to image). This and prior image (left) both show dark rim between center of breast and skin line ➡ due to thickness compensation.

Variant

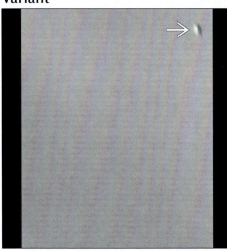

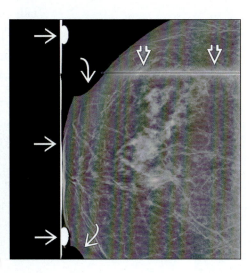

(Left) Mammography of uniform phantom with full-field digital detector shows plus-minus density artifact ➡ due to metallic fleck on mirror that was calibrated into detector response, then shifted position slightly between calibration and exposure. *(Right)* CC mammography shows detector misregistration artifact ➡, thickness compensation defects ➡, and extra metallic object ➡ in image.

ARTIFACTS: OBJECTS

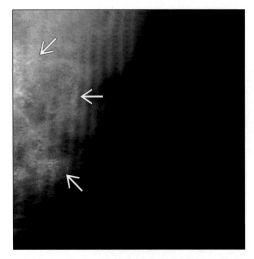

CC mammography shows curvilinear densities due to the patient's hair ➡ projecting over the posteromedial breast, mimicking calcifications.

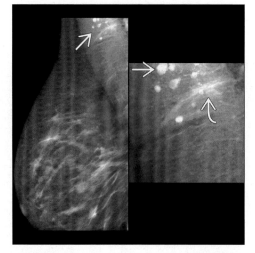

MLO mammography (left image) shows densities due to deodorant ➡ in the right axilla, mimicking calcifications. Photomagnification better illustrates the clumped ➡ and fine ➡ particles within skin folds.

TERMINOLOGY

Definitions
- Any object that interferes with image interpretation
  - Mimics or obscures normal or pathologic structures
- May be inside or outside the patient

IMAGING FINDINGS

General Features
- Best diagnostic clue
  - Appearance or finding that does not correspond to anatomy or range of pathology
    - Some appearances are pathognomonic
    - Others require history and/or physical exam
- Location
  - Some locations typical for certain artifacts
    - Deodorant: Axilla
    - Hair: Inner breast, seen on CC view
    - Vascular catheters, pacemakers: Close to chest wall
- Morphology
  - Appearance may vary according to imaging modality

- Due to physics of modality, positioning, technique, anatomy of patient

Mammographic Findings
- Procedure-related
  - Poor positioning
    - Hair, nose, chin, axillary fold
- Foreign material: Radiodense opacities, usually recognizable, may mimic suspicious Ca++
  - On analog screens
    - Fingerprints, dust, smoke particles, hair
    - Large dust → blur due to poor film-screen contact
    - Pick-off of emulsion during processing
  - On analog cassettes
    - Contrast media, metallic particles
  - On patient
    - Talc (magnesium silicate): Radiopaque
    - Ointment: Density due to mineral content (or other additives), sticky surface to which radiopaque material may adhere
    - Bandages: May trap air within
    - Transdermal patches: May contain thin metallic stiffener filaments

DDx: Foreign Bodies Within the Breast

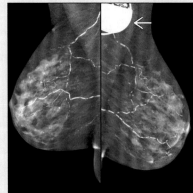

Pacemaker

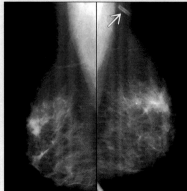

Catheter Cuff

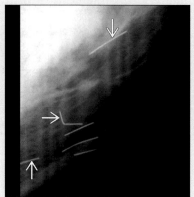

Needles

ARTIFACTS: OBJECTS

Key Facts

Terminology
- Any object that interferes with image interpretation
- Mimics or obscures normal or pathologic structures
- May be inside or outside the patient

Imaging Findings
- Some appearances are pathognomonic
- Others require history and/or physical exam

Top Differential Diagnoses
- Suspicious Calcifications
- Suspicious Shadowing on Ultrasound

Diagnostic Checklist
- Perform careful imaging work-up to accurately distinguish mimics of Ca++ (talc, deodorant) and dermal Ca++ before biopsy

---

- In patient: Pacemaker, tattoos, foreign bodies (iatrogenic and traumatic, implants)

Ultrasonographic Findings
- Grayscale Ultrasound
  - Echogenic clips, air introduced by biopsy
  - Siliconoma → "snowstorm" appearance

MR Findings
- T1WI
  - Multiple substances T1-hypointense
    - DDx: Calcium, gas, metal
- T2* GRE
  - "Blooming" artifact on gradient echo sequences
    - Magnetic susceptibility artifact
    - Biopsy markers, surgical clips, sutures, ports
    - Also seen with chunky Ca++ as in fibroadenomas
- T1 C+ FS
  - Misregistration on subtraction → bands of alternating bright signal (especially at skin) and dark signal, mimics enhancement
  - Inhomogeneous fat suppression → bright signal

Imaging Recommendations
- Recognition, awareness, history are crucial
- Change imaging parameters or plane
- Correct presumed problems and repeat imaging

DIFFERENTIAL DIAGNOSIS

Suspicious Calcifications
- Small particulate, fingerprints can mimic DCIS

Suspicious Shadowing on Ultrasound
- Confirm in multiple planes, compare to mammography (if available)
  - Correlate with known scars, foreign bodies

DIAGNOSTIC CHECKLIST

Consider
- Perform careful imaging work-up to accurately distinguish mimics of Ca++ (talc, deodorant) and dermal Ca++ before biopsy

Image Interpretation Pearls
- Skin localization, repeat views can be helpful

SELECTED REFERENCES

1. Coulthard A et al: Pitfalls of breast MRI. Br J Radiol. 73:665-71, 2000
2. Hogge JP et al: Quality assurance in mammography: artifact analysis. Radiographics. 19:503-22, 1999

IMAGE GALLERY

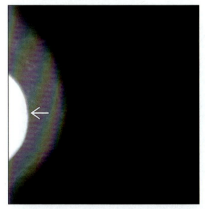 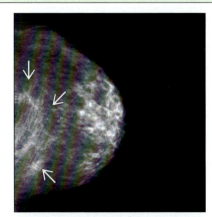 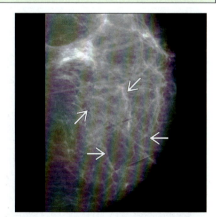

(Left) CC mammography shows a crescentic dense object superimposed on the posterior breast ➡, mimicking an implant. This was the patient's chin. *(Center)* CC mammography shows linear densities with intervening lucencies ➡, superimposed on the medial breast, corresponding to the patient's wig. *(Right)* CC mammography magnification shows artifact ➡ from an adhesive bandage applied to the skin. This and medication patches may occasionally demonstrate bubbles of air beneath the adhesive.

ARTIFACTS: ULTRASOUND

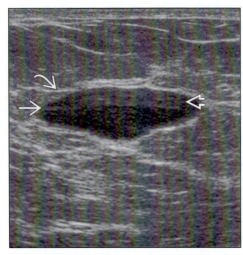

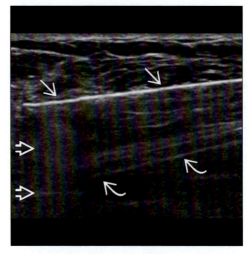

US shows reverberation artifact in anterior aspect of cyst, most of which parallels the anterior wall of the cyst ➡. Focally ➡, the reverberation is due to the adjacent echogenic Cooper ligament ➡.

US shows reverberation artifacts ➡ paralleling the 14-g core needle ➡ as well as echogenic band of ring-down artifact ➡ from the needle tip.

TERMINOLOGY

Definitions
- Artifact: Physical, electronic, or technical phenomenon → abnormal echogenicity or shadowing on ultrasound (US)
- Dynamic range: Ratio of highest and lowest amplitudes that can be displayed, in decibels (dB)
  - Typically 55-60 dB optimal for breast imaging
- Spatial compounding: Use of multiple off-angle beams (or splitting the beam to insonate only a part of the image at a time) to create an image
  - Averages signal from the multiple beams: Noise cancels out
  - ↓ Specular reflection, reverberation artifacts
  - ↑ Detail within masses and along side and posterior margins
  - ↓ Posterior enhancement and shadowing
    - Turn off this feature to ascertain posterior features
- Tissue harmonic imaging: Insonate tissue with one frequency (usually 5-6 MHz) and receive at a multiple of that frequency (e.g., 10-12 MHz)
  - Reduces artifactual internal echoes in cysts

  - ↑ Soft tissue contrast: ↑ Conspicuity of nearly isoechoic masses
  - Posterior features are retained
  - Less effective beyond ~ 3 cm depth

IMAGING FINDINGS

Mammographic Findings
- Correlate echogenic findings with clips, calcifications (Ca++), air

Ultrasonographic Findings
- Grayscale Ultrasound
  - Crystal dropout
    - Focal signal dropout in one part of the image
    - Extends from skin surface down
    - Minimized when spatial compounding used
  - Dynamic range inappropriate
    - ↓ Dynamic range → ↑ contrast: Fewer shades of grey
    - Too wide a dynamic range: Cysts often appear hypoechoic due to slight protein content
  - Gain improper
    - Gain too high → artifactual internal echoes

DDx: US Artifacts Due to Foreign Matter

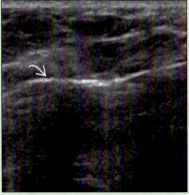

Air Along Biopsy Track

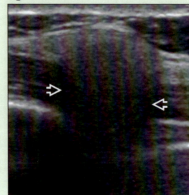

Snowstorm from Siliconoma

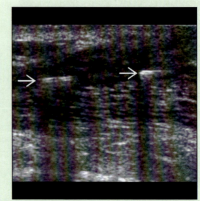

Surgical Clips in Lumpectomy Bed

ARTIFACTS: ULTRASOUND

Key Facts

Terminology
- Artifact: Physical, electronic, or technical phenomenon → abnormal echogenicity or shadowing on ultrasound (US)

Imaging Findings
- Gain too high → artifactual internal echoes
- Gain too low → solid masses can appear cystic
- Refractive edge shadowing: US beam is refracted around the curved edge of a mass
- Reverberation: Series of echoes deep to and paralleling an interface with large differences in acoustic impedance
- High-frequency linear array transducer with center frequency of 10 MHz preferred
- Field of view to reach chest wall but not beyond
- Appropriate positioning of patient is critical
- Gradually increasing time-gain-compensation (TGC) curve with increasing depth
- Gentle pressure while scanning
- Change angle of insonation: ↓ Artifactual shadowing
- Glob of gel or standoff pad for superficial structures
- Most transducers are not optimally focused in the most superficial 7 mm of tissue

Diagnostic Checklist
- Minimizing depth needed to penetrate is most effective method to improve image quality
- Real-time adjustment of gain, focal zones, depth of scanning, scanning pressure, angle of insonation all necessary to produce optimal image
- Spatial compounding → ↓ posterior features: May hamper lesion characterization

---

- Gain too low → solid masses can appear cystic
  - Posterior enhancement
    - ↓ Absorption of sound by the structure
    - More sound penetrates deep to lesion than surrounding tissue
    - Most pronounced in cysts
    - Can be seen in malignancies: Invasive ductal carcinoma (IDC), metastatic nodes, lymphoma, intracystic ductal carcinoma in situ (DCIS)
  - Posterior shadowing
    - ↑ Absorption of sound by the structure
    - Less sound penetrates deep to the lesion than surrounding tissue
    - Nipple itself can cause shadowing: Change angle of insonation, pressure
  - Refractive edge shadowing: US beam is refracted around the curved edge of a mass
    - Less of the insonating beam proceeds directly along edge of mass → shadowing
    - Not true shadowing for purposes of lesion description
    - Can cause apparent mass at interface of fat lobules: ↑ Pressure or change angle of insonation
  - Reverberation: Series of echoes deep to and paralleling an interface with large differences in acoustic impedance
    - On its way back to transducer, beam is instead reflected off wall of structure to then insonate the tissue a second time
    - Sound waves take longer to return to transducer as they make a longer net trip
    - Reflected sound waves (and structure) are mapped deeper in tissue than they really are
    - Reverberation parallels structure which causes it, usually parallel to insonating beam
    - Common with needles, anterior wall of cysts, silicone implants
  - Ring-down
    - Echogenic bands perpendicular to transducer
    - Typically from air collections
    - At tip of needle during biopsy
  - Specular reflection
    - Bright linear echoes due to sound bouncing back to transducer off edge of structure
    - Ligaments
    - Edges of circumscribed solid masses → pseudocapsule
  - Volume averaging
    - Finite slice thickness (typically 1-1.5 mm): Adjacent structures superimpose
    - Long-axis of biopsy needle appears to be within mass when it is only near it
    - Confirm needle within mass on short-axis (perpendicular) view
- Color Doppler
  - Any movement will be mapped as "color"
  - Respiratory motion
  - Speech
    - Vocal fremitus can be used to distinguish a true mass from normal tissue
    - Filling in of tissue with color or power Doppler "flow" when patient hums, sings, talks
    - Masses vibrate less than normal tissue, resulting in "defect" against otherwise color filled-in background
    - Can be used to distinguish fat lobules from isoechoic masses
- Silicone implant artifacts
  - Snowstorm: Extracapsular silicone
    - Acoustic scattering
    - Multiple interfaces due to fibrotic reaction to small silicone foci
  - Artificially increased thickness
    - Sound travels slower in silicone (1066 m/sec) than in tissue (~ 1540 m/sec)
    - Implant appears taller than it really is
  - Echogenic noise in silicone implants
    - Mixing of fluids with gel due to rupture or injection of saline, iodine, antibiotics, other
    - Reverberation artifacts off of invaginated folds of redundant implant shell

Imaging Recommendations
- Best imaging tool

ARTIFACTS: ULTRASOUND

- ○ High-frequency linear array transducer with center frequency of 10 MHz preferred
- ○ Field of view to reach chest wall but not beyond
  - ▪ Improves detail within the breast
- Protocol advice
  - ○ Intermittent use of spatial compounding for lesion characterization
  - ○ Appropriate positioning of patient is critical
    - ▪ "Modeling pose" for outer breast: Ipsilateral arm raised, elevate that side
    - ▪ Supine for inner breast
    - ▪ Inferior portion very large breasts: Patient can help support upper breast with opposite hand
  - ○ Gradually increasing time-gain-compensation (TGC) curve with increasing depth
    - ▪ Compensates for absorption of sound by tissue: Equivalent shades of gray throughout image
  - ○ Set focal zone at lesion
    - ▪ Most current transducers have broad focal range, allow real-time scanning with multiple focal zones
    - ▪ Adjustment is most critical for superficial lesions
    - ▪ Horizontal band-like artifact at interface of focal zones
  - ○ Gentle pressure while scanning
    - ▪ ↓ Artifactual shadowing
    - ▪ ↓ Depth of tissue to penetrate, improve detail
    - ▪ Can artificially reduce flow in lesions
  - ○ Change angle of insonation: ↓ Artifactual shadowing
    - ▪ Angle behind nipple
    - ▪ "Rolled nipple" technique: Roll nipple over finger and elongate duct(s)
  - ○ Glob of gel or standoff pad for superficial structures
    - ▪ Most transducers are not optimally focused in the most superficial 7 mm of tissue
    - ▪ Artificially ↑ depth of the lesion to match focal zone: Improve detail
    - ▪ Very high frequency transducers (e.g., 13-14 MHz), 1.5D array, improve detail in extreme near field

DIFFERENTIAL DIAGNOSIS

Posterior Shadowing
- Invasive ductal (IDC) ± lobular carcinoma (ILC)
  - ○ Difficult to assess for possible chest wall invasion
- Fibrosis
- Scar
  - ○ Hypoechoic track to overlying skin incision
- Artifact
  - ○ Refractive edge shadowing: Often at edge/interface of fat lobules, can create pseudomass

Echogenic Findings
- Large calcifications (Ca++): > 0.5 mm
  - ○ When > 1-2 mm, may also shadow
- Cooper ligaments: Horizontal linear or curvilinear brightly echogenic lines at edges of fat lobules
- Air: Mobile on real-time scanning
  - ○ Can cause minimal shadowing
- Clips, needles, other hardware
- Edema: Diffuse increased echogenicity
  - ○ ± Dilated anechoic lymphatic channels

- Special fat-containing lesions
  - ○ Oil cysts, lipomas, hilar fat in lymph nodes, galactoceles: Slightly hyperechoic
- Snowstorm: Extracapsular silicone
  - ○ Usually incites extensive fibrotic reaction: Silicone granuloma ("siliconoma")
  - ○ May also have silicone "cysts" (rare)

Complicated Cyst
- Proteinaceous debris in an otherwise simple cyst
  - ○ May be visibly mobile in cyst
  - ○ Power Doppler can impart energy and cause particulate to move
  - ○ Fluid-debris level pathognomonic
- Hypoechoic solid mass
- Complex cystic and solid lesion
  - ○ Mural mass vs. debris: Debris will typically move on changing patient position
  - ○ Internal vascularity → at least partially solid
  - ○ Thick wall (> 0.5 mm) or septations (> 0.5 mm)

"Flow" on Color or Power Doppler
- Motion of any kind
  - ○ Vascular flow: Compressible
    - ▪ Can help distinguish intraductal debris from papilloma(s): Fibrovascular stalk in papillomas
    - ▪ Malignancies can appear anechoic: Internal vessels can confirm solid nature and need for biopsy
  - ○ Mobile echoes within complicated cysts

DIAGNOSTIC CHECKLIST

Consider
- Minimizing depth needed to penetrate is most effective method to improve image quality
  - ○ Position appropriately, gentle scan pressure
  - ○ Allows use of higher frequency transducers → improved resolution

Image Interpretation Pearls
- Real-time adjustment of gain, focal zones, depth of scanning, scanning pressure, angle of insonation all necessary to produce optimal image
- Spatial compounding → ↓ posterior features: May hamper lesion characterization

SELECTED REFERENCES

1. Cha JH et al: Differentiation of benign from malignant solid breast masses: conventional US versus spatial compound imaging. Radiology. 237:841-6, 2005
2. Szopinski KT et al: Tissue harmonic imaging: utility in breast sonography. J Ultrasound Med. 22:479-87; quiz 488-9, 2003
3. Rosen EL et al: Tissue harmonic imaging sonography of breast lesions: improved margin analysis, conspicuity, and image quality compared to conventional ultrasound. Clin Imaging. 25:379-84, 2001
4. Lopez H et al: Ultrasound interactions with free silicone in a tissue-mimicking phantom. J Ultrasound Med. 17:163-70, 1998
5. Kremkau FW et al: Artifacts in ultrasound imaging. J Ultrasound Med. 5:227-37, 1986

IMAGE GALLERY

Variant

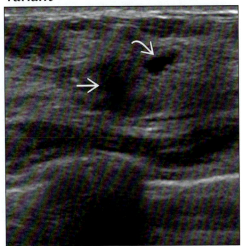
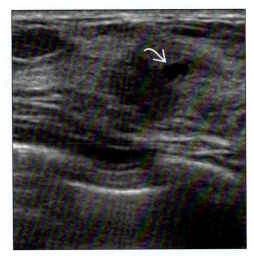

(Left) Ultrasound shows vague hypoechoic area ➡ adjacent to a cyst ➡ on screening US in this 51 y/o with dense breasts. *(Right)* US (same patient as previous image) with slight change in pressure and angle of insonation shows apparently normal tissue with the cyst ➡ again noted. Six-month follow-up was recommended.

Variant

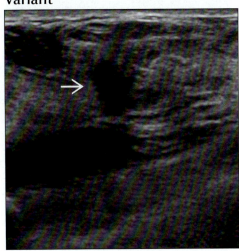
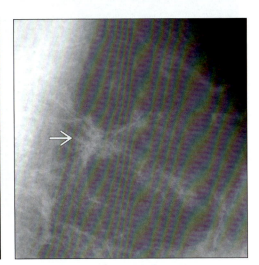

(Left) US seven months later (same as prior 2 images) shows irregular, vertical, spiculated, nearly anechoic mass ➡. US-guided biopsy and excision showed 7 mm invasive lobular carcinoma. It can be difficult to distinguish subtle tissue shadowing due to artifact from a true mass. *(Right)* Lateral mammography magnification shows spiculated mass with subtle amorphous Ca++ ➡ in this asymptomatic 50 y/o.

Typical

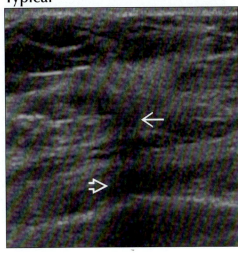
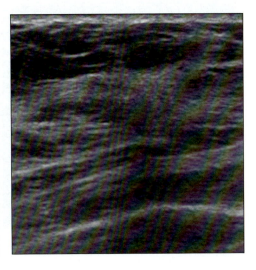

(Left) US targeted to mammographic mass (see prior image) shows subtle decreased echogenicity ➡ and posterior shadowing ➡. US-guided core biopsy showed grade I IDC and DCIS from mammographic finding (confirmed by clip placed at biopsy). *(Right)* Spatial compounding US (same field as prior image) shows slightly heterogeneous echotexture, but no definite abnormality. Spatial compounding reduces artifactual as well as true shadowing.

Typical

(Left) US shows hypoechoic area ⮕ at the interface of adjacent fat lobules ⮕. This was questioned as a mass vs. artifact. *(Right)* US (same field as on left) with greater scanning pressure applied shows the fat lobules ⮕, with the intervening hypoechoic area nearly gone, and likely due to converging areas of refractive edge shadowing. This patient remains cancer free three years later.

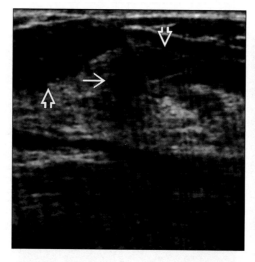

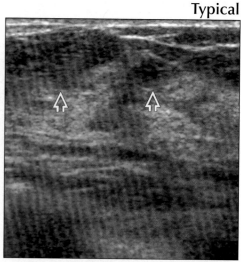

Typical

(Left) Ultrasound shows refractive edge shadowing ⮕ from both a known fibroadenoma ⮕ and an adjacent fat lobule ⮕ in this 42 y/o. *(Right)* Ultrasound shows subtle vertical band of decreased echogenicity ⮕ due to crystal dropout in this uniformity test using Model 50 Near-Field US phantom (Computerized Imaging Reference Systems, Norfolk, VA). Likely the transducer had been dropped and a crystal cracked.

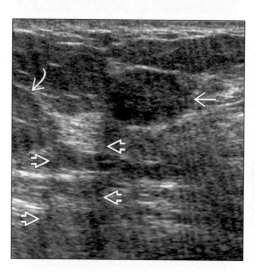

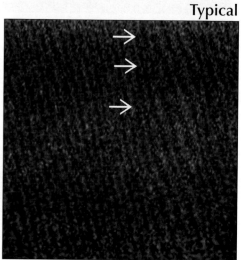

Typical

(Left) US images obtained during 14-g core biopsy show needle tip ⮕ just adjacent to hypoechoic mass ⮕ prior to firing (upper image). On post-fire image (below), needle ⮕ appears to have speared mass. *(Right)* Short-axis US image post-fire shows echogenic needle ⮕ adjacent to mass ⮕, a proven fibroadenoma. Volume averaging can produce a long-axis image (prior image) with needle appearing to be within the targeted mass when it is actually adjacent to it.

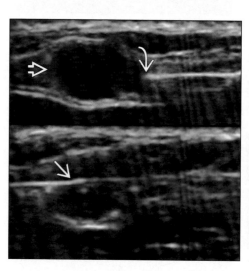

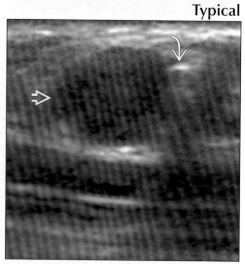

Typical

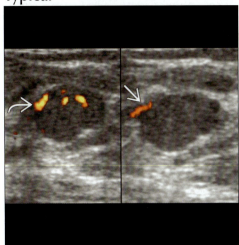

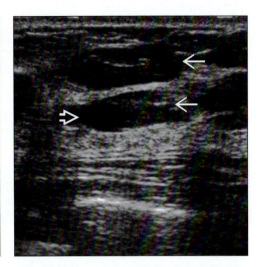

(Left) Power Doppler US shows moderate internal vascularity ➡ within this fibroadenoma, greatly reduced ➡ when usual scanning pressure is applied (right-hand image). *(Right)* Antiradial US shows fat lobules ➡ with possible hypoechoic mass ➡.

Typical

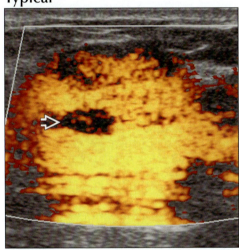

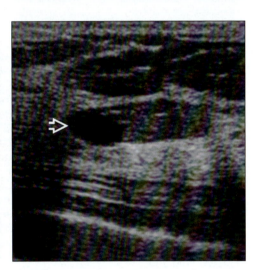

(Left) Power Doppler US (same as prior image) shows use of "vocal fremitus" (patient hummed) to create motion (color), with the mass now more conspicuous as a defect ➡ because it vibrates less than normal tissue. *(Right)* Radial US with tissue harmonic imaging (same as prior two images) better shows the hypoechoic mass ➡, stable for years, in this 37 y/o with known fibroadenomas.

Typical

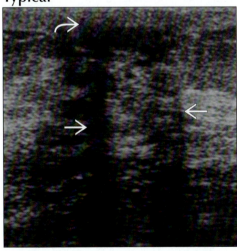

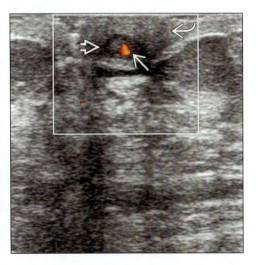

(Left) US shows shadowing ➡ from the nipple ➡, a common problem. This was initially interpreted as normal in this 80 y/o with bloody nipple discharge. *(Right)* Power Doppler US (same patient as previous image) with the gain adjusted shows oval hypoechoic mass ➡ within the nipple ➡. Flow is seen in the vascular stalk ➡ of this large-duct papilloma.

ARTIFACTS: MRI

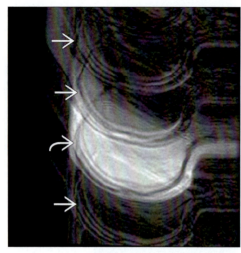

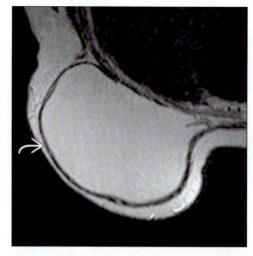

Axial FSE T2WI FS MR image shows extensive respiratory motion artifact ➡ causing "ghosting" of implant ➤, mimicking rupture. Phase encoding was inadvertently set AP, exacerbating motion artifacts.

Repeat axial FSE T2WI FS MR (same patient as previous image), with frequency encoding now set AP and phase encoding now right to left, shows intact subpectoral silicone implant ➤.

TERMINOLOGY

Definitions
- Any physical, electronic, or technical phenomenon that causes abnormal signal intensity
- Most MR artifacts interfere with image quality and potentially interpretation; some mimic pathology

IMAGING FINDINGS

Mammographic Findings
- Clip artifacts can be correlated with biopsy history and mammography → signal void, signal flare (localized ↑ signal) or both, on MR
- Coarse calcifications (Ca++) → signal void and magnetic susceptibility artifacts
- Air can be well seen as dark area(s) on mammography → signal void on MR

Ultrasonographic Findings
- Not usually helpful in distinguishing sources of MR artifacts

MR Findings
- Ghosting: Replication of bright areas or interfaces propagating in phase encoding direction
  - Respiratory motion: Adds extra noise pattern across breasts if phase encoding is in anteroposterior (AP) direction
  - Cardiac: Adds motion artifacts across left breast if phase encoding is AP; set frequency encoding AP
  - Vascular pulsation can cause spurious bright ghost "vessels" at evenly spaced intervals
  - Patient motion during scanning causes ghosting of bright areas and interfaces
- Motion: Causes blur in primary images and misregistration on subtracted images
  - Typically bright at skin surface, with adjacent parallel bands of decreased signal
  - Can obscure lesions on subtracted images and MIP reconstructions
  - Can mimic linear/ductal enhancement
  - Correlate with raw, unsubtracted post-contrast T1WI
    - Fat suppression → ↑ perceptibility of enhancing structures against now darkened fat background; reduces motion artifacts

DDx: Motion Artifacts

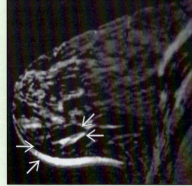

Misregistration on Subtraction

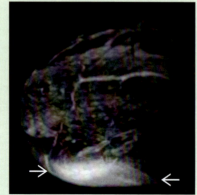

MIP: Skin Bright, Vessels Poorly Seen

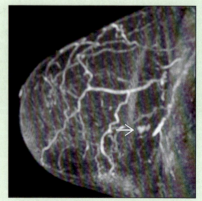

MIP: Repeat Scan, Benign Node

ARTIFACTS: MRI

Key Facts

Terminology
- Any physical, electronic, or technical phenomenon that causes abnormal signal intensity
- Most MR artifacts interfere with image quality and potentially interpretation; some mimic pathology

Imaging Findings
- Inhomogeneous or failed fat suppression
- Partial volume: Thicker slices (> 3 mm) can blur interfaces and reduce visibility of small structures
- Poor in-plane spatial resolution: Pixels > 1 mm x 1 mm blur image details
- Poor temporal resolution → erroneous kinetics
- Schedule at days 7-14 of menstrual cycle to minimize background parenchymal enhancement
- Patient history and questionnaire prior to imaging
- Gentle breast compression to minimize motion
- Manual fine tuning of fat suppression often necessary
- Recognition of artifacts at time of imaging → change parameters or scan plane, repeat scan

Top Differential Diagnoses
- Clips show signal void or void plus flare due to magnetic susceptibility artifact
- Subtle magnetic susceptibility artifacts can cause signal voids in areas of prior surgery
- Large calcifications → signal void
- Breast abutting coil: Void and flare at surface of breast
- Motion and misregistration on subtraction can mimic DCIS or enhancing lesion

Diagnostic Checklist
- Attention to careful positioning and contrast bolus injection critical

---

- ○ Minimize by applying gentle compression around breast, discussing need for shallow breathing with patient
- ○ Claustrophobia and discomfort can exacerbate: Premedicate (e.g., benzodiazepines) as needed
- ○ Post-processing can correct for minimal motion
- Wrap artifact: Improperly small field of view → bright structures outside of field of view "wrap" into image
  - ○ Usually at edges of field of view, recognizable structures from opposite side of body wrap in phase encoding direction
  - ○ Most often arms, especially if patient unable to raise arms for axial scans
  - ○ In 3D imaging, slices can wrap in slice-select direction if bright tissue is outside selected volume
- Magnetic susceptibility: Focal distortion of magnetic field → usually bright at edge of focal signal void, "directional blurring"
  - ○ Metallic hardware: Usually ferromagnetic clips
- Signal void: Focal absence of signal (e.g., air)
- Inhomogeneous or failed fat suppression
  - ○ Fat is hyperintense on T1WI and T2WI without fat suppression
    - ▪ Fat suppression → fat becomes hypointense
  - ○ Poor magnetic field shimming causes non-uniform fat suppression; if non-uniform fat suppression observed, reshim magnet
  - ○ Can be inconsistent over time → subtraction images can show artificial "enhancement" in areas of inconsistent fat suppression
  - ○ In fatty breasts, tuning on fat peak instead of water peak misplaces fat saturation pulse, causing fat saturation to fail
- Magnetic field inhomogeneity → regional, heterogeneous patchy signal loss across all sequences
  - ○ Usually due to metallic objects in bore of scanner
  - ○ Can be due to poor coil design or loss of input from one or more receiver coil channels
- Inhomogeneous gradients → distortion of image
  - ○ Worse at field strengths < 1.5 T
- Partial volume: Thicker slices (> 3 mm) can blur interfaces and reduce visibility of small structures

- ○ Artificially smoothes mass margins and reduces conspicuity of subtle spiculations
- Poor in-plane spatial resolution: Pixels > 1 mm x 1 mm blur image details
  - ○ Blurs mass margins and low-contrast structures such as subtle spiculations
- Chemical shift artifact: Results in black or white band at fat-water interface
  - ○ Resonant frequency of fat, water, and silicone all differ (silicone > fat > water)
  - ○ Fat image, water image, and silicone image are shifted relative to one another in frequency-encoding direction, causing chemical shift artifact
  - ○ When frequency shift causes fat and water to overlap, bright band occurs at fat-water interface
  - ○ When frequency shift causes fat and water to separate, dark band occurs at fat-water interface
  - ○ Fat-water chemical shift artifact reduced by using fat suppression
  - ○ Often seen at edges of silicone implants
- Poor temporal resolution → erroneous kinetics
  - ○ Must have adequate temporal resolution to see peak contrast within lesion
  - ○ Typically entire breast must be imaged within 2.5 minutes of contrast injection
  - ○ Follow-up imaging for at least 5 minutes post injection
  - ○ Longer time intervals → averaging of signal over time, miss peak
    - ▪ Washout kinetics can appear to be persistent
- Failed injection: Evaluate cardiac and great vessel contrast uptake
  - ○ Can be difficult to recognize clinically due to small volume (10-20 cc) of contrast used
  - ○ May still see vascular and nipple enhancement if only part of bolus intravascular
- Other patient-related artifacts
  - ○ Lesion outside field of view
    - ▪ Most common with large breast/body habitus and posterior ± axillary lesion
  - ○ Intense background parenchymal enhancement

- Cyclical dependency: Least in days 7-14 of menstrual cycle
  - Breast abutting coil
    - Usually large breast, at edge of tissue → signal void and magnetic susceptibility artifacts
    - Focally inhomogeneous fat suppression
  - Positioning: May hamper interpretation and correlation with other imaging modalities
    - Nipple quite medial or lateral
    - Large breast "stuffed" into coil

Imaging Recommendations
- Protocol advice
  - Schedule at days 7-14 of menstrual cycle to minimize background parenchymal enhancement
  - Patient history and questionnaire prior to imaging
    - History of surgery, foreign objects in breast
    - History of claustrophobia → risk for motion
  - Gentle breast compression to minimize motion
  - Manual fine tuning of fat suppression often necessary
  - Recognition of artifacts at time of imaging → change parameters or scan plane, repeat scan
  - Recognition of artifacts at time of reporting → correct protocol if needed and recommend repeat scan at no charge if interpretation adversely affected

DIFFERENTIAL DIAGNOSIS

Signal Void
- Clips
  - Clips show signal void or void plus flare due to magnetic susceptibility artifact
- Post-surgical changes
  - Subtle magnetic susceptibility artifacts can cause signal voids in areas of prior surgery
  - Often extend to skin surface
  - May show associated distortion
  - Correlate with clinical history
  - Typically no clips or Ca++ visible on mammography
- Other metallic objects
  - Catheter ports
  - Implant valve
- Large calcifications → signal void
  - Correlate with mammogram
- Air
  - Correlate with mammogram, history
  - Recent biopsy most common
- Plastic obturator or localization wires introduced for biopsy
  - Tip: Distal image showing discrete signal void
- Breast abutting coil: Void and flare at surface of breast
  - Can deform contour of breast
  - More problematic for larger breasts

Bright on C+ Subtraction Images
- Ductal carcinoma in situ (DCIS)
  - Often linear or ductal, clumped
- Invasive ductal or lobular carcinoma
- Benign breast masses
  - Fibroadenoma (FA), fibrocystic changes (FCC), fibrosis, papillomas, other

- High risk lesions: E.g., atypical hyperplasias, lobular carcinoma in situ, radial sclerosing lesions
- Motion and misregistration on subtraction can mimic DCIS or enhancing lesion
- Normal variant parenchymal enhancement
  - Usually patchy, regional, slow, persistent enhancement
  - Typically relatively symmetric bilaterally
  - Most common in upper outer quadrant and at edges of parenchyma
    - Inflow phenomenon, ↑ vascularity these areas
  - Worst on days 1-6 and 15-28 of menstrual cycle
    - ↓ By scanning at days 7-14 after onset of menses
  - Can be problematic in post-menopausal women on hormone replacement therapy (HRT)
    - Consider discontinuing HRT for 6 weeks and repeating scan

Bright on T1 C+ FS
- Enhancing breast lesion: Malignant, high risk, benign
- Normal variant parenchymal enhancement
- Acute blood: Will not be bright on subtraction images unless motion occurs
- Areas of failed fat suppression: Will be less prominent on subtraction images, unless motion occurs

Lack of Enhancement of Malignancy
- Outside field of view
- Poor contrast bolus
- Excessive breast compression
  - Most often occurs at time of planned MR-guided biopsy: Obtain follow-up scan
- Intrinsic features of tumor
  - Very small size, usually < 5 mm
  - Poor vascularity
  - More common with DCIS

DIAGNOSTIC CHECKLIST

Consider
- Attention to careful positioning and contrast bolus injection critical

SELECTED REFERENCES

1. Rausch DR et al: How to optimize clinical breast MR imaging practices and techniques on your 1.5-T system. RadioGraphics. 26:1469-84, 2006
2. Murphy TJ et al: Correlation of single-lumen silicone implant integrity with chemical shift artifact on T2-weighted magnetic resonance images. J Magn Reson Imaging 15:159-64, 2002
3. Teifke A et al: Undetected malignancies of the breast: dynamic contrast-enhanced MR imaging at 1.0 T. Radiology 224:881-8, 2002
4. Shellock FG: Metallic marking clips used after stereotactic breast biopsy: ex vivo testing of ferromagnetism, heating, and artifacts associated with MR imaging. AJR 172:1417-9, 1999
5. Kuhl CK et al: Healthy premenopausal breast parenchyma in dynamic contrast-enhanced MR imaging of the breast: normal contrast medium enhancement and cyclical-phase dependency. Radiology 203:137-44, 1997

IMAGE GALLERY

Typical

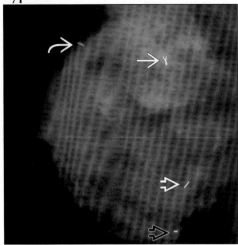

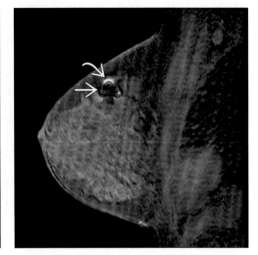

(Left) Lateral mammography magnification shows multiple clips at sites of prior biopsies in this 54 year old: FCC on US-guided biopsy ➡; ALH on stereotactic biopsy ➡; DCIS on MR-guided vacuum-biopsy ➡; and FCC on MR-guided vacuum biopsy ➡. *(Right)* Sagittal T1 C+ FS MR (same patient as previous image) shows artifact from ferromagnetic clip with signal void ➡ and flare ➡ at site of remote US-guided biopsy showing fibrocystic changes.

Typical

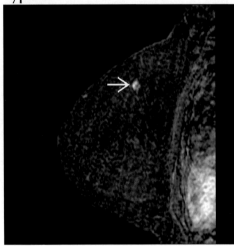

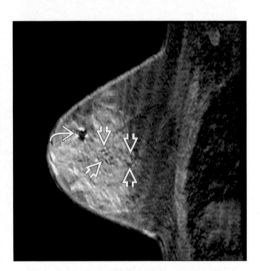

(Left) Sagittal T1 C+ subtraction MR (same as prior two images) shows apparent enhancement at site of ferromagnetic clip ➡. This is due to artifact. *(Right)* (Same patient as prior 3 images) shows artifact from Micromark II clip ➡ at site of biopsy showing atypical lobular hyperplasia (ALH). Subtle signal voids ➡ at site of excision of MR-detected DCIS are also noted.

Typical

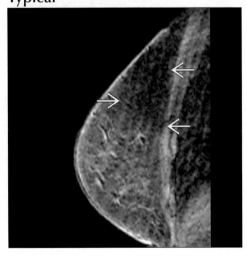

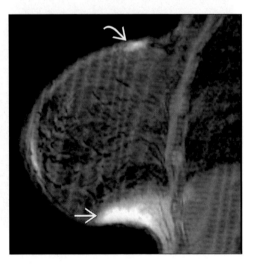

(Left) Sagittal T1 C+ FS MR shows global loss of signal from upper breast ➡. A hairpin had lodged in bore of the magnet causing magnetic field inhomogeneity. *(Right)* Sagittal T1 C+ FS MR shows bright areas at edges of field/breast due to flaring close to the coil ➡ where the coil is more sensitive, as well as inhomogeneous fat suppression ➡. Both can obscure detection of bright enhancing lesions; subtraction will correct most of this.

Typical

(Left) MLO mammography shows diffuse coarse, linear, secretory Ca++ ➡ in this 82 year old s/p left mastectomy for cancer. *(Right)* Sagittal T2WI FS MR (same patient as previous image) shows signal voids in ductal pattern ➡ due to the large Ca++. Signal voids due to Ca++ are most evident on T2WI FS images.

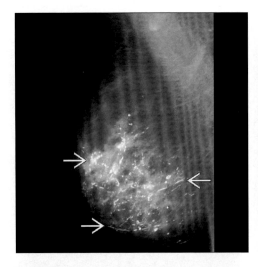
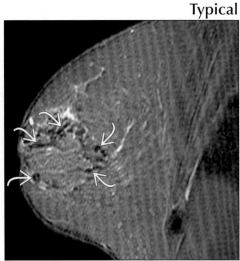

Typical

(Left) Sagittal STIR image with water suppression (WS) shows intact subpectoral expander-type implant with hyperintense outer silicone ➡ & hypointense inner saline ⮞ lumens in this 49 y/o s/p prophylactic mastectomy. *(Right)* Sagittal STIR WS MR, more medial image (same as left) shows failed water suppression in inferior half of the implant, with saline remaining hyperintense ⮞ & silicone becoming focally hypointense ➡. Minimal ghosting is also seen ➡.

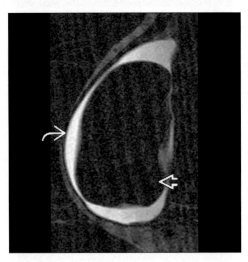
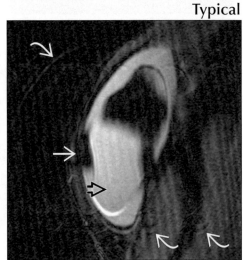

Typical

(Left) Sagittal T1 C+ FS MR (same as prior 2 images) shows extensive artifacts ➡ along the inferior half of the image. *(Right)* Axial T1WI scout (same as prior 3 images) shows the source of the artifacts ➡ to be centered at waist level. This proved to be due to a metal snap on her clothing. Repeat scan was unremarkable.

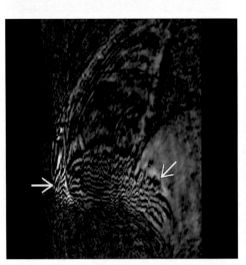
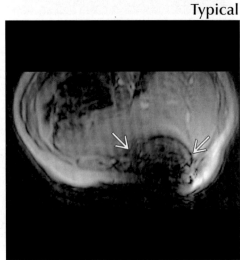

Typical

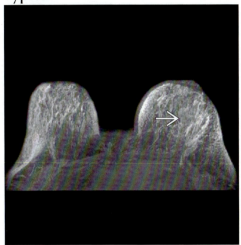 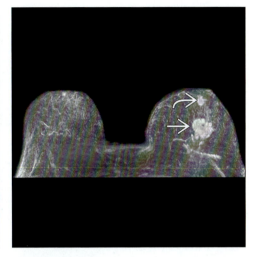

(Left) Axial MIP of T1 C+ subtraction MR shows patchy background enhancement with no discrete lesion in the area of known left breast cancer ➡. *(Right)* Axial MIP of T1 C+ subtraction MR (same dataset as left), after applying computer-assisted motion correction, demonstrates intense rim-enhancement in known cancer ➡, as well as satellite malignancy more anteriorly ➡, and virtually no background enhancement. (Courtesy DynaCad, Inc.)

Typical

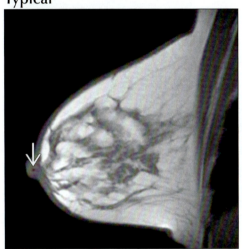 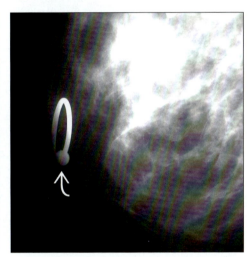

(Left) Sagittal T1WI MR shows signal void ➡ in nipple in this 36 year old. *(Right)* MLO mammography (same patient as previous image) shows nipple ring ➡ which had been removed for the MR scan, resulting in air artifact on the MR images.

Typical

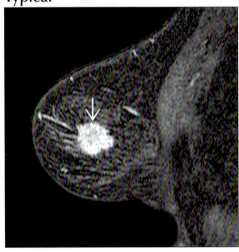 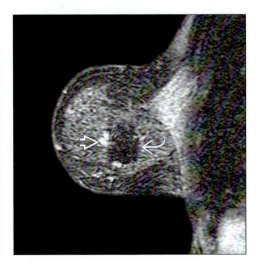

(Left) Sagittal T1 C+ FS MR in 65 y/o shows irregular enhancing mass ➡. Clip was placed at US-guided biopsy which showed invasive ductal cancer; neoadjuvant chemotherapy (NAT) given. *(Right)* Sagittal T1 C+ FS MR (same as left) after 4 cycles NAT shows marked artifact from clip placed at US biopsy ➡. Minimal enhancement anterior to clip ➡ was due to residual tumor. Treatment response could not be assessed due to clip artifacts. This clip is off market.

PART V

Management and Procedures

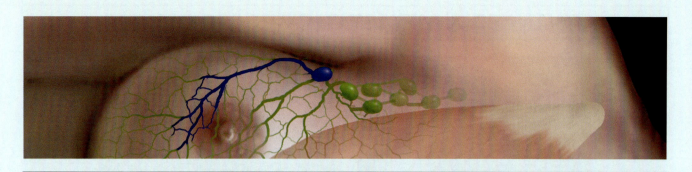

SECTION 1: Treatment Planning Issues

ADVANCED & METASTATIC BREAST CANCER

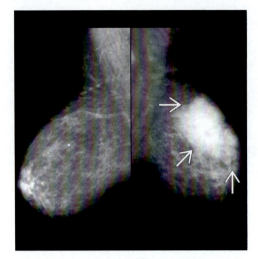

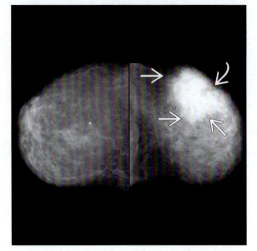

MLO mammography shows a large, dense, poorly circumscribed mass ➡ in the left breast. This is the typical appearance of a locally advanced breast cancer.

CC mammography (same case as left) shows the large mass ➡ and associated skin retraction ➘. Note the retraction of the breast parenchyma causing reduction in size compared to the right breast.

TERMINOLOGY

Abbreviations and Synonyms
- Locally advanced breast cancer (LABC)
- Axillary lymph node dissection (ALND)
- Sentinel node biopsy (SNB)

Definitions
- Metastatic breast cancer (MBC): Stage IV, distant metastases, spread beyond the breast and ipsilateral nodes
  - TNM (tumor-node-metastasis) classification used for description
- LABC: Stage III breast cancer, excluding inflammatory cancer
  - T3: Primary invasive tumor > 5 cm
  - T4: Skin/chest wall involvement
  - N2: Fixed axillary nodes
  - N3: Ipsilateral metastatic infra- or supraclavicular nodes or clinically apparent (* includes imaging) internal mammary nodes with clinically apparent* axillary nodes
  - Stage IIIa: T0-2 N2 M0 or T3 N1-2 M0
  - Stage IIIb: T4 N0-2 M0
  - Stage IIIc: Any T N3 M0
- Inflammatory breast cancer reported separately from LABC due to distinct clinical presentation/behavior

IMAGING FINDINGS

Radiographic Findings
- Radiography
  - Chest X-ray: MBC
    - Lung nodules, pleural effusion, rib/spine metastases
  - Bone Films: MBC
    - Mixed lytic/sclerotic bone lesions may be presenting feature of breast cancer

Mammographic Findings
- LABC
  - Large dominant mass
  - Large area of suspicious calcifications
  - Diffuse increased density
  - Large area of architectural distortion
  - Skin thickening/ulceration
  - Nipple retraction
  - "Shrinking" breast

DDx: Clinical Presentation Similar to LABC

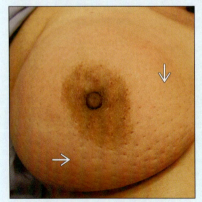

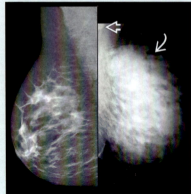

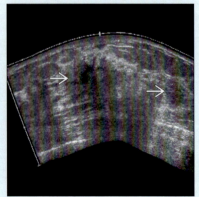

Inflammatory Breast Cancer

Leukemic Infiltration

Metastatic Lung Cancer

ADVANCED & METASTATIC BREAST CANCER

Key Facts

Terminology
- Metastatic breast cancer (MBC): Stage IV, distant metastases, spread beyond the breast and ipsilateral nodes
- LABC: Stage III breast cancer, excluding inflammatory cancer

Imaging Findings
- PET/CT whole body imaging → metastatic disease identified earlier → treatment decisions influenced

Top Differential Diagnoses
- Inflammatory Breast Cancer
- Metastases to Breast
- Lymphoma (1° or 2°), leukemia
- Post-Radiation/Post-Surgical Change
- Mastitis/Abscess

Clinical Issues
- Clinical findings may be more prominent than mammographic findings
- May present with diffuse infiltration of breast without dominant mass
- Complete pathologic response (no residual tumor at surgery) → improved long-term survival
- Disease progression → extremely poor prognosis
- Evaluation of response can be difficult due to fibrosis or small volume of residual disease
- Multimodality therapy most effective

Diagnostic Checklist
- Node positive LABC most common presentation of breast cancer in low resource countries
- Axillary nodal involvement in LABC impacts long-term prognosis but not treatment plan

---

- - May be only manifestation of diffuse invasive lobular carcinoma
- Metastatic disease
  - May see involved axillary lymph nodes
  - May see intramammary nodal metastases

Ultrasonographic Findings
- Grayscale Ultrasound
  - Breast
    - Large solid irregular mass
    - Diffuse shadowing without discernible mass
  - Lymph nodes
    - Loss of normal hilar fat and "bean" shape
- Color Doppler: In palpable nodes, peripheral vascularity increases suspicion for malignancy

MR Findings
- T1 C+
  - Define tumor extent
    - Pectoralis major, chest wall involvement
    - Skin/nipple involvement (usually direct extension)
  - Evaluate response to chemotherapy
    - Good response → tumor necrosis → ↓ enhancement
    - MR may be most helpful to confirm response in the face of tumor necrosis → edema/erythema/↑ size palpable mass

Nuclear Medicine Findings
- PET
  - PET/CT whole body imaging → metastatic disease identified earlier → treatment decisions influenced
    - Allows anatomic localization of sites of 18F fluoro-2-deoxy-D-glucose (FDG) uptake
    - Improved accuracy over PET alone
  - More accurate than bone scan for skeletal metastases
  - Predict/monitor response to chemotherapy
- Bone Scan: May see tracer uptake in breast primary on bone scan

CT Findings
- CECT: Useful for mediastinal & liver metastases

- NECT
  - Useful for lung & pleural metastases
  - Lymphangitic spread

Biopsy
- US-guided core biopsy of breast mass → establish diagnosis, receptor studies
- US-guided FNAB or core biopsy & axillary node(s)

Imaging Recommendations
- Best imaging tool
  - FDG PET CT for whole body staging
  - MR or PET to assess response to treatment

DIFFERENTIAL DIAGNOSIS

Inflammatory Breast Cancer
- Tumor cells in dermal lymphatics
- Erythema/edema, often no discrete primary tumor
- Dismal prognosis: 5 yr survival < 5% without multimodality therapy

Metastases to Breast
- Primary tumor usually known: Melanoma, lung, ovarian, soft tissue sarcoma
- Lymphoma (1° or 2°), leukemia
- May require biopsy to exclude breast as second primary

Post-Radiation/Post-Surgical Change
- Appropriate history
- May be difficult to distinguish residual/recurrent tumor from scar

Mastitis/Abscess
- Typically seen in nursing mothers
- Confined to breast, usually responds dramatically to antibiotics

Diabetic Mastopathy
- Florid fibrotic masses → architectural distortion and dense acoustic shadowing
- Insulin-dependent diabetics often > 20 yr duration

ADVANCED & METASTATIC BREAST CANCER

PATHOLOGY

General Features
- Genetics
  - Microarray analysis
    - Individual tumor gene profiles (ongoing studies)
    - May identify more aggressive tumor → potentially individualized treatment plan
- Epidemiology
  - > 1,000,000 new cases breast cancer annually worldwide
  - 370,000 deaths annually worldwide
  - LABC at presentation
    - 5% cases in industrialized countries with screening programs
    - 50% in developing countries without screening

Staging, Grading or Classification Criteria
- Tumor-node-metastasis (TNM) system developed in 1942 by Denoix
- American Joint Committee on Cancer staging manual 6th edition published in 2002 reflects
  - New information on immunohistochemical staining
  - Clinical outcomes associated with various nodal metastatic patterns
  - Clinical importance of total number of axillary nodes involved

CLINICAL ISSUES

Presentation
- Clinical findings may be more prominent than mammographic findings
- Easily palpable
- May present with diffuse infiltration of breast without dominant mass
- Clinical features for inoperable breast cancer
  - Extensive skin edema
  - Satellite nodules in skin
  - Parasternal tumor
  - Arm edema
  - Supraclavicular metastases
  - 2 or more of the following
    - Skin ulceration
    - Tumor fixed to chest wall
    - Fixed axillary lymph nodes
    - Axillary nodes > 2.5 cm on palpation

Natural History & Prognosis
- 10 yr survival
  - 10% with stage IV
  - 40% with stage III
- Depends on response to chemotherapy
  - Complete pathologic response (no residual tumor at surgery) → improved long-term survival
  - Disease progression → extremely poor prognosis
- Evaluation of response can be difficult due to fibrosis or small volume of residual disease

Treatment
- Multimodality therapy most effective
  - Chemotherapy
    - Neoadjuvant: First-line treatment
    - Adjuvant: After surgery
    - Taxane based regimes → better clinical response than standard regimen in neoadjuvant setting
  - Surgery
    - Modified radical mastectomy
    - Axillary nodal excision for palpable nodes
    - Neoadjuvant chemotherapy may → ↓ tumor size → breast conservation possible
    - If neoadjuvant chemotherapy → ALND preferred over SNB (↑ risk false negatives on SNB)
    - Consider pre-treatment SNB if neoadjuvant chemotherapy planned
  - Radiation therapy (XRT)
    - Chest wall/regional nodes post-operatively
    - LABC may be treated with XRT prior to surgery
    - May be mainstay of therapy in inoperable LABC if poor response to chemotherapy
- Hormonal therapy
  - Used with estrogen receptor (ER) positive tumors
    - Post-menopausal: Tamoxifen for 5 yrs
    - Pre-menopausal: Tamoxifen +/- ovarian ablation
    - Aromatase inhibitors very effective in post-menopausal population, limited side effects

DIAGNOSTIC CHECKLIST

Consider
- Node positive LABC most common presentation of breast cancer in low resource countries
  - Case fatality rates highest in low resource countries
  - Breast cancer most common cause of cancer deaths in women worldwide
- Axillary nodal involvement in LABC impacts long-term prognosis but not treatment plan
  - Patients may benefit from minimally invasive approach to axilla: Fewer side effects with no change in treatment outcome
- If palpable adenopathy: Full axillary dissection is therapeutic/important for local control
- No imaging modality reliably predicts complete pathologic response

Image Interpretation Pearls
- Beware the shrinking breast
  - Weight loss → symmetric decrease in breast size
  - In absence of surgery, unilateral ↓ breast size is very suspicious for diffuse tumor infiltration particularly invasive lobular carcinoma

SELECTED REFERENCES

1. Singletary SE et al: Breast cancer staging: working with the sixth edition of the AJCC Cancer Staging Manual. CA Cancer J Clin. 56(1):37-47; quiz 50-1, 2006
2. Moon YW et al: Neoadjuvant chemotherapy with infusional 5-fluorouracil, adriamycin and cyclophosphamide (iFAC) in locally advanced breast cancer: an early response predicts good prognosis. Ann Oncol. 16(11):1778-85, 2005
3. Thor A: A revised staging system for breast cancer. Breast J. 10 Suppl 1:S15-8, 2004
4. Zangheri B et al: PET/CT and breast cancer. Eur J Nucl Med Mol Imaging. 31 Suppl 1:S135-42, 2004

ADVANCED & METASTATIC BREAST CANCER

IMAGE GALLERY

Typical

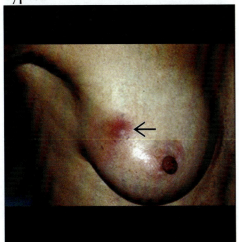
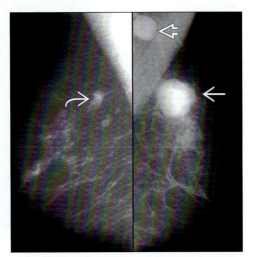

(Left) Clinical photograph shows a clinically visible locally advanced breast cancer ➡ with erythema and infiltration of the overlying skin. *(Right)* MLO mammography (different patient) shows a dense, irregular 3 cm mass ➡ in the upper outer left breast with a dense, round node ➡ in the left axilla. A dense, irregular mass is also noted in the upper outer right breast ➡.

Typical

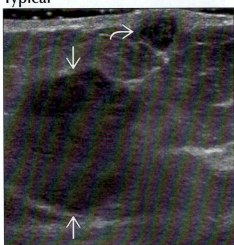
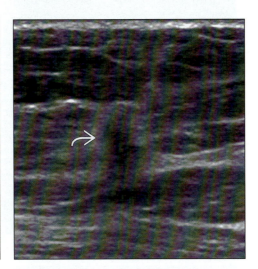

(Left) Sagittal ultrasound of the left breast (same patient as prior image) confirms a solid mass ➡ with an associated solid skin nodule ➡. Core biopsy of the mass showed invasive ductal cancer and FNAB of skin nodule showed metastasis. *(Right)* Sagittal ultrasound of the upper right breast (same patient as previous image) shows an irregular mass ➡ with posterior acoustic shadowing at site of the mammographic abnormality. Biopsy confirmed invasive ductal cancer.

Typical

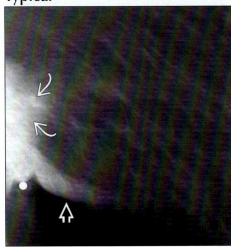
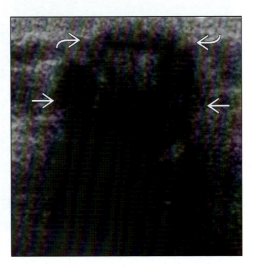

(Left) MLO mammography spot compression shows only a portion of a palpable indistinctly marginated mass with amorphous calcifications ➡, skin retraction and skin thickening ➡. This posteroinferior mass could not be included on the CC view. *(Right)* Ultrasound (same patient as previous image) shows a mass ➡ with posterior shadowing & probable skin invasion ➡. MR performed to evaluate full tumor size and extent confirmed skin invasion.

(Left) MLO mammography shows multiple foci of left breast cancer ➡ with lymph node metastases ➡. The 6:00 left breast mass shows extension to involve the overlying skin ➡, also seen on US (see next image).
(Right) Transverse ultrasound (same patient as left) of the largest left breast lesion at 6:00 shows skin ulceration ➡ associated with an irregular hypoechoic mass ➡.

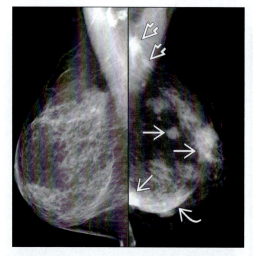
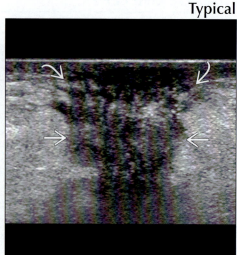

(Left) Axial CECT for staging (same patient as prior two images) shows metastatic disease to bone with sclerotic foci ➡ seen in the T11 vertebral body. Patient had no complaints of pain.
(Right) Axial CECT of the abdomen (same patient as previous image) shows extensive ascites ➡ secondary to widespread tumor dissemination. Bone metastases ➡ are less apparent on soft tissue windows.

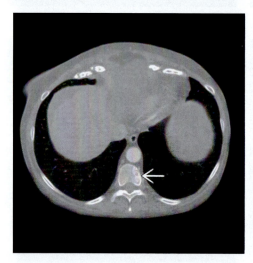
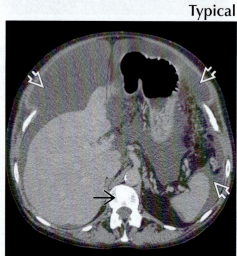

(Left) Sagittal breast US shows almost complete replacement by tumor ➡ in 28 y/o pregnant woman whose mother died of breast cancer at age 26. She was successfully treated with neoadjuvant chemotherapy and delivered a healthy infant at 36 weeks gestation.
(Right) Coronal PET in a 36 y/o with a poorly differentiated invasive ductal cancer shows extensive metastatic infraclavicular ➡, paratracheal ➡, mediastinal ➡ and left hilar ➡ adenopathy.

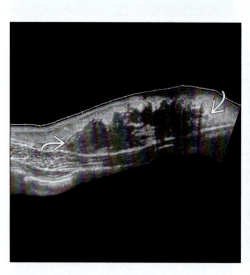
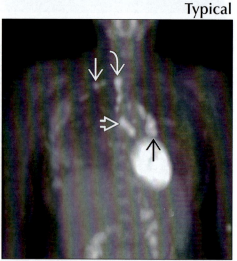

Typical

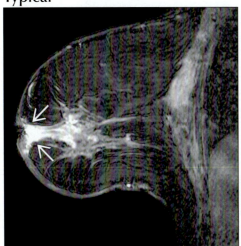 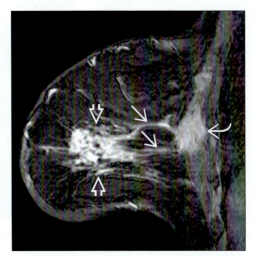

(Left) Sagittal T1 C+ FS MR in a patient with locally advanced breast cancer shows extensive involvement of most of the central breast. There is enhancement extending to involve the nipple-areolar complex ➡. *(Right)* Sagittal T1 C+ FS MR at a different plane (same paitent as left) shows more of the central tumor ➡ with enhancing tumor ➡ extending through the breast with enhancement of the pectoral muscle ➡ consistent with tumor involvement.

Typical

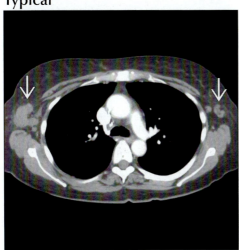 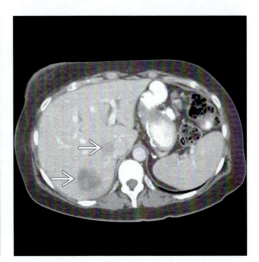

(Left) Axial CECT in a 41 y/o presenting with palpable axillary adenopathy ➡. Several of the right nodes were necrotic. At biopsy, the right axilla was positive, but the left was negative; size alone cannot be used as a determinant of nodal involvement. *(Right)* Axial CECT through the abdomen (same patient as previous image) shows multiple liver metastases ➡ confirming widespread metastatic disease.

Typical

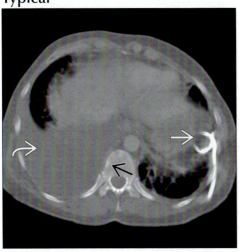 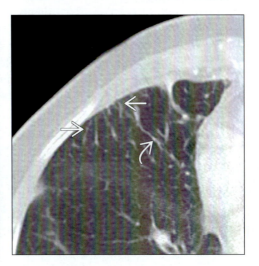

(Left) Axial NECT in a 42 year old Bosnian refugee presenting with disseminated disease shows skeletal metastases ➡, a large right pleural effusion ➡ and a pigtail catheter ➡ in the left pleural space placed to drain a malignant effusion prior to pleurodesis. She had never had a mammogram. *(Right)* Axial NECT (same patient as prior image) shows interlobular septal thickening ➡ which is nodular in places ➡. This is the typical appearance of lymphangitic tumor spread.

AXILLARY ADENOPATHY, OCCULT PRIMARY

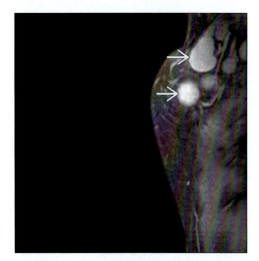

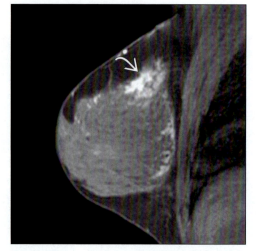

Sagittal T1 C+ FS MR shows multiple round and oval enhancing axillary nodes ➡ *in this 44 yo presenting with palpable right axillary nodes. Breast physical examination and mammography were negative.*

Sagittal T1 C+ FS MR (from the same MR as left image) shows an irregular enhancing mass ➡ *in the upper breast found at biopsy to represent the otherwise occult infiltrating ductal carcinoma.*

TERMINOLOGY

Definitions

- Axillary nodal metastatic adenocarcinoma consistent with breast origin, with no clinical or mammographic depiction of the breast cancer

IMAGING FINDINGS

General Features

- Best diagnostic clue
  - Enlarged axillary nodes may be visible on MLO mammogram
    - Finding may initiate work-up of previously unknown metastatic or systemic disease
    - Enlarged or dense round nodes (abnormal appearances) seen in 0.3% of screening mammograms (varying etiologies including hyperplastic, infectious, manifestations of systemic disease)

Mammographic Findings

- Bilateral mammogram should be performed with additional images as needed

Ultrasonographic Findings

- Grayscale Ultrasound
  - Abnormal lymph nodes may demonstrate asymmetrically thick hypoechoic cortex with absent or compressed echogenic fatty hila
  - May reveal breast primary initially or on targeted examination after MR

MR Findings

- T2WI FS: Lymph node cortex hyperintense; fatty hilum hypointense
- T1 C+ FS
  - Any enhancing morphologically suspicious lesion deserves further evaluation
    - Targeted US often beneficial for lesion assessment, direct biopsy

Imaging Recommendations

- Best imaging tool: MR test of choice with identification of breast primary in 50-86%

DDx: Axillary Masses with Positive Mammographic or Clinical Findings

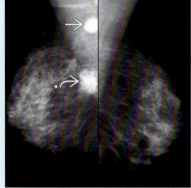

Breast Cancer, Nodal Metastasis

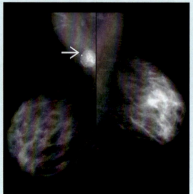

Epidermal Inclusion Cyst

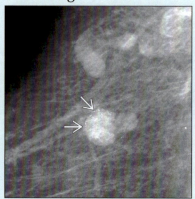

Metastatic Ovarian Cancer

AXILLARY ADENOPATHY, OCCULT PRIMARY

Key Facts

Terminology

- Axillary nodal metastatic adenocarcinoma consistent with breast origin, with no clinical or mammographic depiction of the breast cancer

Imaging Findings

- Enlarged axillary nodes may be visible on MLO mammogram
- Best imaging tool: MR test of choice with identification of breast primary in 50-86%

Top Differential Diagnoses

- Axillary Metastases with Known Primary

Pathology

- 0.3-1.0% of cases of operable breast cancer at presentation

Clinical Issues

- Mastectomy with axillary node dissection historically most common treatment

---

DIFFERENTIAL DIAGNOSIS

Axillary Metastases with Known Primary

- Metastatic breast cancer, ovarian, melanoma, lung

Systemic Disease Manifestations

- Benign: Collagen vascular disease, sarcoid, tuberculosis, HIV
- Malignant: Lymphoma, leukemia

PATHOLOGY

General Features

- Etiology
  - 0.3-1.0% of cases of operable breast cancer at presentation
  - Underlying invasive ductal carcinoma (IDC) most common; less often invasive lobular cancer

CLINICAL ISSUES

Presentation

- Most common signs/symptoms: Axillary mass(es)

Demographics

- Age: Range 36-79 years (single series)

Natural History & Prognosis

- Prognosis intermediate between stage I and stage II breast cancer

Treatment

- Mastectomy with axillary node dissection historically most common treatment
  - Breast cancer not found even at mastectomy in 1/3
- If no primary detected, whole breast irradiation with 50-55 Gy an alternative to mastectomy
- If MR depicts primary, 37-58% eligible for breast-conserving treatment (BCT)
- Chemo- ± hormonal therapy

DIAGNOSTIC CHECKLIST

Consider

- Adenocarcinomas from sites other than breast uncommonly present as isolated axillary metastases
  - Extensive search for disease other than breast usually not indicated

SELECTED REFERENCES

1. Buchanan CL et al: Utility of breast magnetic resonance imaging in patients with occult primary breast cancer. Ann Surg Oncol. 12:1045-53, 2005
2. Fourquet A et al: Occult primary cancer with axillary metastases. In: Harris JR, et al, eds. Diseases of the Breast. 2nd ed. Philadelphia, Lippincott. 703-07, 2000
3. Orel SG et al: Breast MR imaging in patients with axillary node metastases and unknown primary malignancy. Radiology. 212:543-9, 1999

IMAGE GALLERY

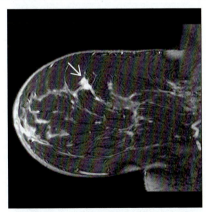 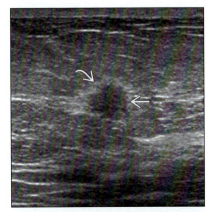 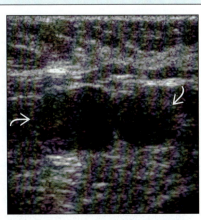

(Left) Sagittal T1 C+ FS MR in a woman with axillary metastases, negative mammogram and clinical exam depicts a left breast spiculated 1.1 x 0.7 x 0.5 cm enhancing mass ➡. Targeted look US (next image) was performed. (Center) Ultrasound shows a spiculated hypoechoic mass ➡ with an irregular echogenic rim ➡. US-guided core biopsy yielded IDC. BCT was carried out. (Right) Ultrasound of metastatic axillary lymph nodes ➡ demonstrates marked hypoechogenicity. Metastatic nodes, when fully replaced by tumor, can appear nearly anechoic.

CONTRALATERAL BREAST CANCER

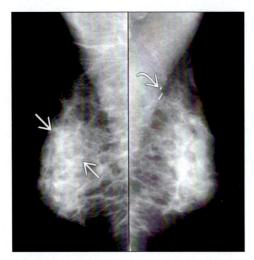

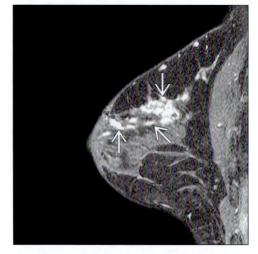

MLO mammography in a 23 y/o shows findings of recent left lumpectomy ➡ for self-discovered cancer. No mammogram was performed. Now has second self-discovered right breast mass with Ca++ ➡ on right.

Sagittal T1 C+ FS MR (same patient as previous image) demonstrates extensive clumped enhancement ➡, due to high-grade DCIS. The patient underwent bilateral mastectomies with TRAM reconstruction.

TERMINOLOGY

Abbreviations and Synonyms
- Synchronous bilateral breast cancer (SBBC)
- Metachronous bilateral breast cancer (MBBC)
- Clinical breast examination (CBE)
- Unilateral breast cancer (UBC)

Definitions
- Breast cancer (BC): Invasive ductal carcinoma (IDC), invasive lobular carcinoma (ILC), ductal carcinoma in situ (DCIS)
- Simultaneous bilateral primary breast cancer (SBBC)
  - Defined variably as simultaneous, within 3 months, or within one year of incident tumor diagnosis
    - Historical incidence ~ 2%
    - Some reports indicate these cases may be more advanced at time of presentation
- Contralateral breast second primary cancer (MBBC) diagnosed after incident tumor treatment
  - Range of timing from > 3 months to years following initial breast cancer diagnosis/treatment
  - Risk 0.5-1%/year; cumulative risk = 15%: Risk differs based on age at time of diagnosis

- < 45 years at diagnosis of initial BC, annual rate ~ 1%: Lifetime risk as high as 40%
- > 50 years at initial diagnosis of BC, annual rate ~ 0.5%
  - More likely to be younger at initial diagnosis compared to UBC or SBBC
- Breast-conserving treatment (BCT) followed by adjuvant radiation therapy (XRT)
- Tamoxifen (TAM): Nonsteroidal agent that binds to estrogen receptors (ER)

IMAGING FINDINGS

General Features
- Best diagnostic clue
  - Palpable or suspicious imaging finding in contralateral breast either at time of initial BC diagnosis (SBBC) or following BC treatment (MBBC)
  - ↑ Frequency of multicentricity in one or both breasts compared to those with UBC
- Location: Mirror image mammographic location: 53%
- Morphology: Mammographic findings similar in index and contralateral BC in 33-36%

DDx: Age 37 Left BC, Had BCT; Age 47 Right IDC, Had BCT

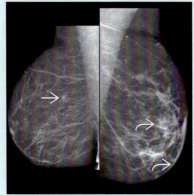

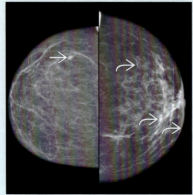

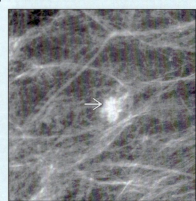

Mass Right, XRT Changes Left

Mass Right, XRT Changes Left

Microlobulated Grade III IDC

CONTRALATERAL BREAST CANCER

Key Facts

Terminology
- Simultaneous bilateral primary breast cancer (SBBC)
- Historical incidence ~ 2%
- Contralateral breast second primary cancer (MBBC) diagnosed after incident tumor treatment
- Risk 0.5-1%/year; cumulative risk = 15%: Risk differs based on age at time of diagnosis
- More likely to be younger at initial diagnosis compared to UBC or SBBC

Imaging Findings
- MR: SBBC occult on mammography, CBE in 4-6%
- US: SBBC occult on mammography, CBE in 3-6%
- Vigilant surveillance credited for increased detection and earlier stage detection of contralateral cancers
- Consider MR for supplemental surveillance of known high-risk populations

Top Differential Diagnoses
- Benign Contralateral Imaging Findings
- Suspicious contralateral findings deserve biopsy: ~ Double rate of malignacy compared to women without BC

Pathology
- ↑ Contralateral BC with family history of breast cancer, multicentric index disease, invasive lobular histology

Diagnostic Checklist
- Contralateral findings with history of BC should be evaluated with a lower threshold for further work-up and/or biopsy

Mammographic Findings
- Suspicious masses, calcifications (Ca++), architectural distortion in contralateral breast must be further evaluated
  - Lower threshold for work-up including biopsy than in those women without known BC

Ultrasonographic Findings
- Direct biopsy of suspicious masses
- US: SBBC occult on mammography, CBE in 3-6%
- Targeted US following a suspicious finding on MR
  - On average 55% (23-89%) of MR-detected lesions referred for biopsy seen with US
  - MR more sensitive than US for DCIS

MR Findings
- T1 C+ FS
  - MR: SBBC occult on mammography, CBE in 4-6%
  - Mammographically and clinically occult suspicious lesions in contralateral breast needing biopsy in 8-32% of women with BC
  - Cancer in 20-84% of MR-prompted biopsies of contralateral breast

Biopsy
- Compared to women without BC, contralateral biopsy in women with BC more likely to show cancer: 58% vs. 30% one series (mammographically prompted biopsies)
- Blind contralateral upper outer quadrant surgical biopsy malignant in 3%

Imaging Recommendations
- Best imaging tool
  - Bilateral mammography
    - Vigilant surveillance credited for increased detection and earlier stage detection of contralateral cancers
    - Screened group: 41% DCIS, 23% stage II or III compared with 22% DCIS and 50% stage II or III in non-screened
- Protocol advice

  - Consider MR for supplemental surveillance of known high-risk populations
    - Recurrence following BCT
    - BRCA mutation carriers: BRCA-1 risk of contralateral BC up to 65%
    - Hodgkin disease survivors (prior mantle radiation including chest and axillae): Bilateral BC 21-29%
    - Prior biopsy demonstrating infiltrating lobular carcinoma (ILC), lobular carcinoma in situ (LCIS)

DIFFERENTIAL DIAGNOSIS

Benign Contralateral Imaging Findings
- Suspicious contralateral findings deserve biopsy to direct management decisions
- High-risk lesions common: 12% of biopsies one series

Benign Surveillance Incident Findings
- Suspicious contralateral findings deserve biopsy: ~ Double rate of malignacy compared to women without BC

Metastatic Cancer
- Breast cancer usually second primary
- Melanoma, lymphoma, lung, ovarian most common

PATHOLOGY

General Features
- Genetics
  - Tumor phenotype similarities higher in SBBC than MBBC
  - Family history twice as common in MBBC than SBBC
- Etiology
  - Environmental influences, both internal and external, more likely related to SBBC
  - ↑ Contralateral BC with family history of breast cancer, multicentric index disease, invasive lobular histology

CONTRALATERAL BREAST CANCER

Microscopic Features

- Histologic characteristics of SBBC similar in 57-67%
- SBBC as compared with UBC may have higher rate of ER and PR positivity

CLINICAL ISSUES

Presentation

- Palpable mass one side, mammographic finding contralateral side
- Post-BCT surveillance mammographic finding
- MR-detected clinically, mammographically occult contralateral suspicious finding

Demographics

- Gender: Male BC: < 1% of all BC cases; bilateral male BC ~ 2% of all male BC

Natural History & Prognosis

- Trend toward ↓ overall survival compared to UBC

Treatment

- Breast-conserving treatment (BCT)
  ○ Malignancy confined to one quadrant, negative margins possible with acceptable cosmesis, patient willing and has no contraindications to XRT
    ▪ Contraindications to XRT: Collagen vascular diseases, prior breast or chest XRT; cancer presenting in 1st or 2nd trimester of pregnancy
  ○ Feasible for both SBBC and MBBC
- Modified radical mastectomy (MRM)
  ○ Post-mastectomy XRT
    ▪ Close or positive margins, advanced primary disease, ≥ 4 axillary nodal metastases
    ▪ Decreases local-regional recurrence by 66%
- Prophylactic mastectomy
  ○ Procedure should be advocated only when risk is moderate to high and patient desires
  ○ Significant reduction in BC incidence, 80-90%
  ○ Counseling should include consultation with a reconstructive surgeon
  ○ Total (simple) mastectomy most effective procedure
- Tamoxifen
  ○ Used both to ↓ risk recurrent BC and as prophylaxis against contralateral BC
  ○ National Surgical Adjuvant Breast and Bowel Project (NSABP) breast cancer prevention trial P-1
    ▪ 13,388 women: Age ≥ 60 or risk considered = 60 years of age per Gail model
    ▪ TAM or placebo
    ▪ Women taking TAM: ↓ Risk invasive cancer by 47% and DCIS by 50%
    ▪ Subset of women at risk due to prior diagnosis of LCIS: 56% ↓ risk

DIAGNOSTIC CHECKLIST

Consider

- Candidates for BCT who test positive for BRCA-1, -2 mutation choose bilateral mastectomies over surveillance (recent study)

- Risk of patient request for prophylactic contralateral mastectomy when MR suspicious lesion(s) lead to biopsy recommendation (even if proven benign)

Image Interpretation Pearls

- Contralateral findings with history of BC should be evaluated with a lower threshold for further work-up and/or biopsy

SELECTED REFERENCES

1. Gilroy JS et al: Breast-conserving therapy in patients with bilateral breast cancer: do today's treatment choices burn bridges for tomorrow? Int J Radiat Oncol Biol Phys. 62(2):379-85, 2005
2. Kahla PB et al: Bilateral synchronous breast cancer in a male. Mt Sinai J Med. 72(2):120-3, 2005
3. Lehman CD et al: Added cancer yield of MRI in screening the contralateral breast of women recently diagnosed with breast cancer: results from the International Breast Magnetic Resonance Consortium (IBMC) trial. J Surg Oncol. 92(1):9-15; discussion 15-6, 2005
4. Pediconi F et al: CE-Magnetic Resonance Mammography for the evaluation of the contralateral breast in patients with diagnosed breast cancer. Radiol Med (Torino). 110(1-2):61-8, 2005
5. Stolier AJ et al: Newly diagnosed breast cancer patients choose bilateral mastectomy over breast-conserving surgery when testing positive for a BRCA1/2 mutation. Am Surg. 71(12):1031-3, 2005
6. Yamauchi C et al: Bilateral breast-conserving therapy for bilateral breast cancer: results and consideration of radiation technique. Breast Cancer. 12(2):135-9, 2005
7. Berg WA et al: Diagnostic accuracy of mammography, clinical examination, US, and MR imaging in preoperative assessment of breast cancer. Radiology. 233:830-49, 2004
8. Horwich A et al: Second primary breast cancer after Hodgkin's disease. Br J Cancer. 90(2):294-8, 2004
9. Intra M et al: Clinicopathologic characteristics of 143 patients with synchronous bilateral invasive breast carcinomas treated in a single institution. Cancer. 101(5):905-12, 2004
10. Lee SG et al: MR imaging screening of the contralateral breast in patients with newly diagnosed breast cancer: preliminary results. Radiology. 226(3):773-8, 2003
11. Liberman L et al: MR imaging findings in the contralateral breast of women with recently diagnosed breast cancer. AJR Am J Roentgenol. 180(2):333-41, 2003
12. Moon WK et al: Multifocal, multicentric, and contralateral breast cancers: bilateral whole-breast US in the preoperative evaluation of patients. Radiology. 224(2):569-76, 2002
13. Brown H et al: Histopathologic features of bilateral and unilateral breast carcinoma: a comparative study. Mod Pathol 13:18A, 2000
14. Fisher B et al: Tamoxifen for prevention of breast cancer: report of the National Surgical Adjuvant Breast and Bowel Project P-1 Study. J Natl Cancer Inst. 90(18):1371-88, 1998
15. Fischer U et al: Prognostic value of contrast-enhanced MR mammography in patients with breast cancer. Eur Radiol. 7(7):1002-5, 1997
16. Roubidoux MA et al: Women with breast cancer: histologic findings in the contralateral breast. Radiology. 203(3):691-4, 1997
17. Murphy TJ et al: Bilateral breast carcinoma: mammographic and histologic correlation. Radiology. 195(3):617-21, 1995
18. Roubidoux MA et al: Bilateral breast cancer: early detection with mammography. Radiology. 196(2):427-31, 1995

IMAGE GALLERY

Typical

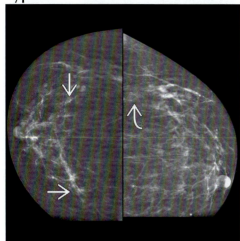

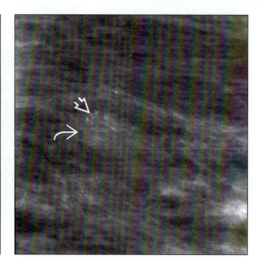

(Left) CC mammography in a 65 y/o patient shows extensive linear Ca++ on the right ➡ and vague soft tissue density ➡ on the left. Right biopsy showed small invasive focus (2 mm) and extensive intermediate grade DCIS. (Right) MLO mammography magnification of the left breast (same patient as previous image) shows mass ➡ with pleomorphic Ca++ ➡. Biopsy showed grade II IDC and DCIS. Patient had bilateral mastectomies.

Typical

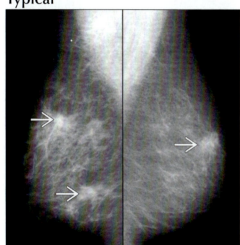

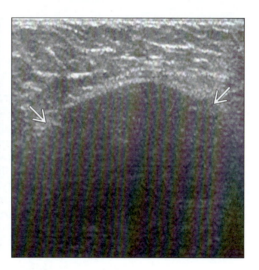

(Left) MLO mammography in a 45 y/o presenting with a right axillary mass (not seen) shows bilateral ill-defined masses ➡. Right breast edema is likely due to lymphatic obstruction by the axillary mass. (Right) US of the right axilla (same patient as previous image) shows clinically matted lymph node conglomerate ➡ measuring at least 3.3 cm.

Typical

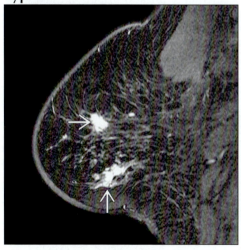

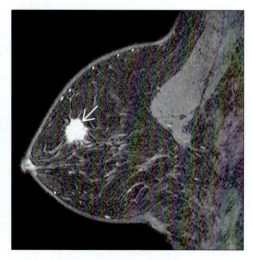

(Left) Sagittal T1 C+ FS MR (same patient as prior 2 images) of the right breast shows two of the numerous spiculated masses ➡ present in multiple quadrants. (Right) Sagittal T1 C+ FS MR of left breast (same patient as prior 3 images) found only one spiculated mass ➡. The patient had right mastectomy for multicentric grade II IDC and left BCT for grade II IDC. Synchronous bilateral breast cancer is commonly multicentric in at least one breast.

EXTENSIVE INTRADUCTAL COMPONENT (EIC)

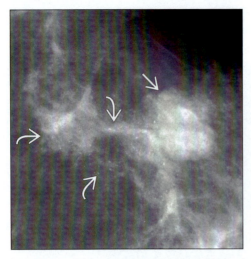

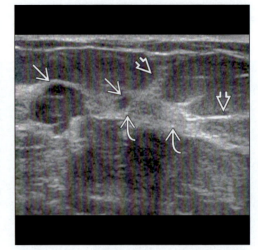

Magnification CC mammogram shows 1 cm lobulated mass ➡ with adjacent pleomorphic calcifications and asymmetry ➡, highly suggestive of malignancy. US was performed (see next image).

US: 1 cm and 2 mm masses ➡, Ca++ ➡ & tethered Cooper ligaments ➡. Excision: 3 cm cancer (60% DCIS), adjacent 2 mm IDC, & separate foci DCIS. US better depicts invasive component than DCIS.

TERMINOLOGY

Abbreviations and Synonyms

- American Joint Committee on Cancer (AJCC), generates Cancer Staging Manual

Definitions

- Invasive carcinoma with associated ductal carcinoma in situ (DCIS)
  - DCIS represents at least 25% of main tumor mass
  - Satellite foci of DCIS beyond main tumor mass
- Includes DCIS with microinvasion (T1 mic)
  - Variable definitions of microinvasion in literature:
    AJCC = ≤ 1 mm invasive carcinoma
  - Multifocal invasive carcinomas each ≤ 1 mm still qualify as microinvasion
- Distinguish from invasive ductal carcinoma (IDC) only with adjacent extensive DCIS

IMAGING FINDINGS

General Features

- Best diagnostic clue

  - Malignant-appearing mass with associated & adjacent fine linear or pleomorphic calcifications (Ca++)
  - Malignant-appearing mass with adjacent linear or segmental enhancement on MR

Mammographic Findings

- Appearances overlap with pure DCIS
  - Particularly for cases of DCIS with microinvasion
    - More often associated suspicious mass (63% of those with microinvasion vs. 33% without)
    - More likely multicentric than pure DCIS
- Malignant-appearing mass or asymmetry usually invasive component (invasive ductal carcinoma [IDC] or mixed invasive ductal-lobular)
  - DCIS can be manifest as mass or asymmetry
- EIC+ more likely to have Ca++ ± mass than EIC- IDC (65-83% vs. 17-27%)
  - Pleomorphic or fine linear Ca++ radiating toward nipple in segmental or linear distribution usually = DCIS component
  - Ca++ may also be within IDC
- Noncalcified DCIS may be mammographically occult

DDx: Findings that Mimic EIC

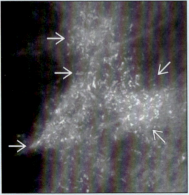

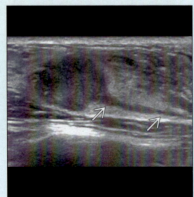

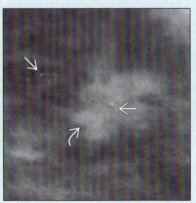

Extensive DCIS + 1.3 cm IDC

IDC, Adjacent DCIS

ILC (mass) + DCIS (Ca++)

EXTENSIVE INTRADUCTAL COMPONENT (EIC)

Key Facts

Terminology
- Invasive carcinoma with associated ductal carcinoma in situ (DCIS)
- DCIS represents at least 25% of main tumor mass
- Satellite foci of DCIS beyond main tumor mass
- Includes DCIS with microinvasion (T1 mic)

Imaging Findings
- Malignant-appearing mass with associated & adjacent fine linear or pleomorphic calcifications (Ca++)
- Malignant-appearing mass with adjacent linear or segmental enhancement on MR

Top Differential Diagnoses
- Pleomorphic and/or fine linear Ca++ without a mass most common in pure DCIS

- Ca++ often seen with IDC, does not necessarily imply associated DCIS
- IDC + DCIS Without EIC
- The larger the area of DCIS, the more likely an associated invasive component
- Fibrocystic Changes (FCC)

Clinical Issues
- EIC ↑ frequency positive margins at lumpectomy
- No greater risk of recurrence if clear margins

Diagnostic Checklist
- Disease extent often underestimated with mammography (especially if DCIS noncalcified)
- EIC likely when core biopsy shows mixed IDC + DCIS
- Pre-operative MR more accurate than mammography, US at depicting full extent of EIC

Ultrasonographic Findings
- Grayscale Ultrasound
  - Irregular mass ± echogenic Ca++
  - Duct extension of mass suggests DCIS component
  - ~ 50% of DCIS is occult on US
    - Subtle intraductal echogenic Ca++ ± mass
    - Tubular, hypoechoic structures with increased vascularity
    - Subtle indistinctly-marginated mass
  - US can identify invasive component in large areas of DCIS
    - When Ca++ in malignancies are visualized on US, 72% are invasive
- Color Doppler: Increased vascularity typical

MR Findings
- T1 C+ FS
  - Most common: Clumped linear or segmental enhancement in DCIS component
    - Morphology more helpful than kinetics (can be slow, persistent in DCIS)
  - May or may not appreciate discrete irregular mass due to invasive component
- EIC depicted only on MR in 6/19 (32%) [one series] with mammography, US, clinical exam, MR

Nuclear Medicine Findings
- PET: Dedicated breast FDG-PET (positron emission mammography) may depict EIC

Biopsy
- Presence of both DCIS and IDC on core biopsy predictive of EIC at surgery
  - 30-45% have EIC vs. 0% with invasive carcinoma alone
  - Quantify amount of DCIS (one series) in cores
    - At least 3 cores show low-grade DCIS
    - At least 2 cores show high-grade DCIS
    - 87% had EIC at excision
    - 60% of lumpectomies with EIC: Positive margins

Imaging Recommendations
- Best imaging tool: MR most accurate at depicting full extent of EIC
- Protocol advice
  - Large (> 2.5 cm²) area of malignant-appearing Ca++ on mammography
    - Magnification CC and 90° lateral views to depict extent
    - US targeted to any associated mass or asymmetry
    - US-guided biopsy of associated mass: Helps identify invasive component

DIFFERENTIAL DIAGNOSIS

Ductal Carcinoma in Situ (DCIS)
- No associated invasive component
- Pleomorphic and/or fine linear Ca++ without a mass most common in pure DCIS
- Associated mass or asymmetry favors invasive component

Invasive Ductal Carcinoma (IDC)
- Duct extension can be purely invasive
- Ca++ often seen with IDC, does not necessarily imply associated DCIS

IDC + DCIS Without EIC
- Adjacent DCIS not admixed with primary tumor mass, not an EIC per se
- The larger the area of DCIS, the more likely an associated invasive component
- 30-35% chance of invasive component when DCIS area is > 2.5 cm² in size
  - Invasive tumor mass has < 25% DCIS within it

Invasive Lobular Carcinoma (ILC)
- Ca++ infrequent
- Can have associated DCIS with Ca++
- ILC with duct extension of associated lobular carcinoma in situ (LCIS)

EXTENSIVE INTRADUCTAL COMPONENT (EIC)

Fibrocystic Changes (FCC)

- Masses: Cysts, complicated cysts, apocrine metaplasia, ruptured cysts, sclerosing adenosis
- Associated Ca++ can be pleomorphic, rarely linear in morphology or distribution

PATHOLOGY

General Features

- Epidemiology
  - 18-20% of breasts with IDC have associated EIC
  - DCIS with microinvasion
    - More often high grade DCIS
    - 20% of high grade DCIS has microinvasion
- Associated abnormalities: Axillary nodal metastases in 4-5% of cases of DCIS with microinvasion
- Grade of DCIS usually parallels grade of invasive carcinoma
- High likelihood of large extent of cancer
  - 30-64% of EIC+ cases have tumor extension ≥ 2 cm beyond edge of primary cancer vs. 2-26% if EIC-
  - Risk of large residual tumor burden
  - Possible to have "clear" margins and residual tumor
    - Skip areas usually < 1 mm: Wider clear margins favored
- More likely to have multicentric carcinoma

Microscopic Features

- DCIS with microinvasion: Basement membrane breached by tumor cells
  - Laminin stain can help confirm
  - More reliable than loss of myoepithelial cell layer which can appear focally discontinuous

CLINICAL ISSUES

Presentation

- Most common signs/symptoms: Asymptomatic: Abnormal mammogram
- Other signs/symptoms
  - Palpable mass
  - Rarely nipple discharge, Paget disease

Demographics

- Age
  - > 50% of EIC in women < 50 years of age
    - 7% of cases are in women ≥ age 70

Natural History & Prognosis

- EIC not a prognostic factor
- EIC ↑ frequency positive margins at lumpectomy
- Increased risk of recurrence if incompletely resected
  - No greater risk of recurrence if clear margins
- Worse pathologic response to neoadjuvant chemotherapy: ↑ Likelihood of residual tumor

Treatment

- Lumpectomy surgery with negative cavity margins
- Sentinel node biopsy even for T1(mic)
- Re-excise close margins (≤ 2 mm) for DCIS if EIC+
  - EIC increases yield of + reexcision: 38-74% vs. 11-42% without EIC

- Residual carcinoma is typically DCIS
- Consider post-lumpectomy mammogram to verify complete excision of suspicious Ca++
- Mastectomy may be needed due to large size of involved area, poor cosmesis if conserved
- Radiation therapy (XRT) if breast conserved
  - EIC is contraindication to partial breast irradiation
- Adjuvant chemotherapy when appropriate

DIAGNOSTIC CHECKLIST

Consider

- Disease extent often underestimated with mammography (especially if DCIS noncalcified)
- EIC likely when core biopsy shows mixed IDC + DCIS
- Pre-operative MR more accurate than mammography, US at depicting full extent of EIC
  - MR frequently alters surgical planning in breasts with EIC when conservation planned

Image Interpretation Pearls

- Magnification views help depict extent of malignant Ca++ on mammography

SELECTED REFERENCES

1. Dzierzanowski M et al: Ductal carcinoma in situ in core biopsies containing invasive breast cancer: Correlation with extensive intraductal component and lumpectomy margins. J Surg Oncol. 90:71-6, 2005
2. Berg WA et al: Diagnostic accuracy of mammography, clinical examination, US, and MR imaging in preoperative assessment of breast cancer. Radiology. 233:830-49, 2004
3. Ikeda O et al: Magnetic resonance evaluation of the presence of an extensive intraductal component in breast cancer. Acta Radiol. 45:721-5, 2004
4. Ishida T et al: Pathological assessment of intraductal spread of carcinoma in relation to surgical margin state in breast-conserving surgery. Jpn J Clin Oncol. 33(4):161-6, 2003
5. Smitt MC et al: Predictors of reexcision findings and recurrence after breast conservation. Int J Radiat Oncol Biol Phys. 57(4):979-85, 2003
6. Nishimura R et al: An evaluation of predictive factors involved in clinical or pathological response to primary chemotherapy in advanced breast cancer. Breast Cancer. 9(2):145-52, 2002
7. Ferranti C et al: Relationships between age, mammographic features and pathological tumour characteristics in non-palpable breast cancer. Br J Radiol. 73(871):698-705, 2000
8. Mai KT et al: Predictive value of extent and grade of ductal carcinoma in situ in radiologically guided core biopsy for the status of margins in lumpectomy specimens. Eur J Surg Oncol. 26(7):646-51, 2000
9. Wazer DE et al: The influence of age and extensive intraductal component histology upon breast lumpectomy margin assessment as a predictor of residual tumor. Int J Radiat Oncol Biol Phys. 45(4):885-91, 1999
10. Hurd TC et al: Impact of extensive intraductal component on recurrence and survival in patients with stage I or II breast cancer treated with breast conservation therapy. Ann Surg Oncol. 4:119-24, 1997
11. Holland R et al: The presence of an extensive intraductal component following a limited excision correlates with prominent residual disease in the remainder of the breast. J Clin Oncol. 8(1):113-8, 1990

IMAGE GALLERY

Typical

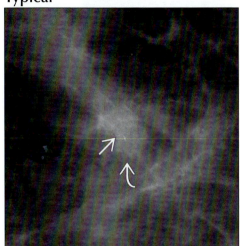

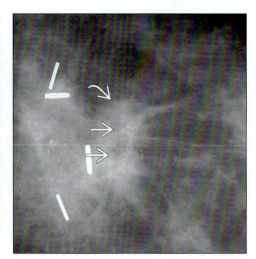

(Left) Magnification CC mammogram shows indistinctly marginated mass ➔ with associated fine linear Ca++ ➔. Excision showed 1 cm grade III IDC with EIC, with 7 positive lymph nodes, and clear margins. *(Right)* Magnification CC mammogram 19 months later, post lumpectomy and XRT shows new pleomorphic and fine linear Ca++ ➔ at lumpectomy site, with associated mass ➔ = recurrent grade III IDC + EIC.

Variant

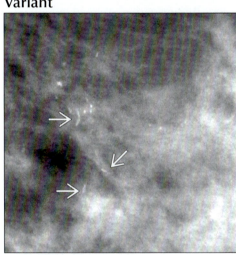

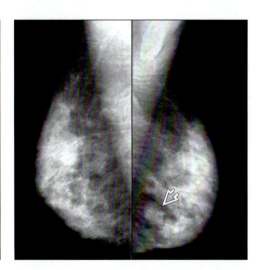

(Left) Lateral mammography magnification in this 65 year old shows fine linear Ca++ ➔, highly suggestive of malignancy. Core biopsy showed DCIS. At excision, a < 1 mm IDC was found, together with DCIS, i.e. DCIS with microinvasion. *(Right)* MLO mammography shows 2 cm oval mass ➔ in this 43 year old. This was new and solid on US, and underwent direct excision showing a 1.8 cm mucinous carcinoma with margins positive for both DCIS and IDC. MR was performed.

Typical

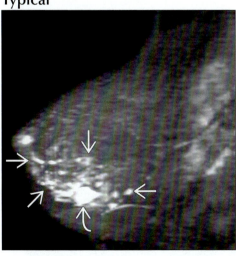

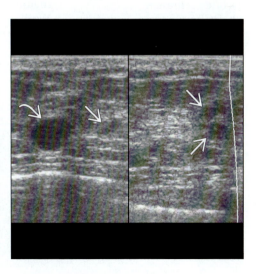

(Left) Postoperative sagittal MIP of T1C+ subtraction MR (same patient as prior image) shows a dominant 15 mm mass ➔ as well as segmental clumped enhancement throughout the lower left breast ➔. *(Right)* Radial US targeted to the areas on MR (same patient as prior 2 images) shows multiple small hypoechoic masses ➔ and one larger 15 mm mass ➔. Mastectomy confirmed residual mucinous carcinoma and EIC.

MULTIFOCAL BREAST CANCER

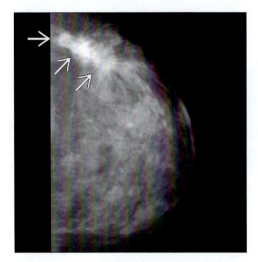

CC mammography shows large spiculated mass or masses ➡ in a 36 year old with a lump.

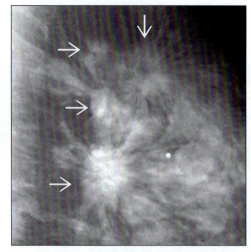

MLO mammography (same patient as previous) shows multiple adjacent spiculated masses ➡. These proved to be multifocal mixed invasive ductal and lobular carcinoma at initial core biopsy and mastectomy.

TERMINOLOGY

Definitions

- Breast cancer: Invasive ductal (IDC) or lobular carcinoma (ILC) or ductal carcinoma in situ (DCIS) or a combination of these entities
- Multiple (≥ 2) separate foci of breast cancer within 4 or sometimes 5 cm of each other
  - Typically within the same quadrant
  - Usually along the same ductal system

IMAGING FINDINGS

General Features

- Best diagnostic clue
  - Multiple suspicious masses ± suspicious calcifications (Ca++) within 4-5 cm span
    - "Separate" clusters of Ca++ often represent contiguous disease (usually DCIS)

Mammographic Findings

- Multiple suspicious masses ± suspicious Ca++ in one quadrant

- Solitary suspicious finding with additional lesion(s) mammographically occult

Ultrasonographic Findings

- Grayscale Ultrasound
  - Multiple suspicious hypoechoic masses
  - US to guide biopsy of multiple lesions

MR Findings

- T1 C+ FS
  - Two or more suspicious findings within 4-5 cm span
  - 64-75% of suspicious findings seen only on MR in same quadrant as known cancer → malignant
- Performed at initial diagnosis or with positive or close (< 2 mm) margins at initial excision

Nuclear Medicine Findings

- PET
  - Dedicated breast [18]FDG-PET (positron emission mammography, PEM) performance similar to MR: Work in progress
  - Higher risk of false negatives with ILC, low tumor grade

DDx: Mimics of Multifocal Carcinoma

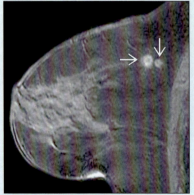

Contiguous IDC + DCIS

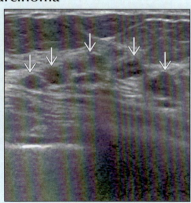

Papillomas, Focal DCIS

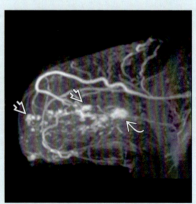

Multicentric ILC

MULTIFOCAL BREAST CANCER

Key Facts

Terminology
- Multiple (≥ 2) separate foci of breast cancer within 4 or sometimes 5 cm of each other
- Typically within the same quadrant
- Usually along the same ductal system

Imaging Findings
- MR most sensitive in depicting tumor extent
- Magnification CC and 90° lateral mammographic views to assess extent of suspicious Ca++
- When performing US for biopsy of highly suspicious masses, evaluate that quadrant carefully

Top Differential Diagnoses
- Multiple papillomas
- Atypical/High-Risk Lesions
- Multicentric breast cancer

Pathology
- 48% of cancers thought to be unifocal clinically and mammographically have additional tumor foci
- 75% of additional foci are multifocal; 25% are multicentric

Clinical Issues
- Bracket needle localization

Diagnostic Checklist
- MR particularly indicated in certain situations
- ILC
- DCIS > 2.5 cm in size
- Extensive intraductal component suspected
- Young woman, < 45 years of age
- Sample by core biopsy sufficient to prove extent for appropriate surgical planning

---

Biopsy
- Sample suspicious lesions farthest apart to prove extent pre-operatively: US-guidance helpful
- Suspicious Ca++: Sample differing morphologies, widely separated clusters when possible
- Needle localization of malignancies farthest apart, i.e. bracket localization

Imaging Recommendations
- Best imaging tool
  - MR most sensitive in depicting tumor extent
    - Risk of false positives: Sample additional suspicious lesions before recommending change in surgical management
- Protocol advice
  - Magnification CC and 90° lateral mammographic views to assess extent of suspicious Ca++
    - Post-lumpectomy mammogram to assure complete removal of Ca++ prior to radiation therapy (XRT)
  - When performing US for biopsy of highly suspicious masses, evaluate that quadrant carefully

DIFFERENTIAL DIAGNOSIS

Benign Lesions: Alone or with Breast Cancer
- Multiple fibroadenomas
  - Mostly circumscribed masses ± Ca++
- Multiple papillomas
  - Multiple intraductal masses ± Ca++
  - Associated DCIS or atypia common

Atypical/High-Risk Lesions
- Atypical ductal (ADH) or lobular hyperplasia (ALH)
  - Frequent association with amorphous Ca++: Within (ADH) or adjacent to (ALH)
  - ADH on core biopsy requires excision, recommended for ALH
- Lobular carcinoma in situ (LCIS)
  - Usually mammographically occult
  - Irregular mass on US or MR

  - Frequent association with ILC

Malignancies
- Systemic metastases to breast
  - Can be mostly circumscribed, especially when in intramammary node(s)
  - Melanoma, lymphoma, lung, ovarian, soft tissue sarcomas, carcinoid most common
  - Rarely have Ca++ (except ovarian)
  - Late in course of disease; poor prognosis
- Multicentric breast cancer
  - Multiple cancers separated by at least 4-5 cm
  - Cancers in different quadrants
- Metastatic intramammary lymph node and breast cancer

PATHOLOGY

General Features
- General path comments
  - Multifocality more common with low grade DCIS than high grade DCIS
    - High grade DCIS tends to have continuous growth pattern
    - Low grade DCIS tends to have small skip areas, typically < 1 cm separating foci
    - Particularly common with micropapillary DCIS
    - More common with DCIS > 2.5 cm in diameter
  - 48% of cancers thought to be unifocal clinically and mammographically have additional tumor foci
    - 75% of additional foci are multifocal; 25% are multicentric
  - More common with ILC than invasive ductal carcinoma (IDC)
    - More common with tubular carcinoma and mixed IDC-ILC than IDC NOS
- Etiology
  - Field effect: Vast majority of multifocal carcinomas are of same histology
    - Chromosomal studies show variable monoclonal or polyclonal origin

MULTIFOCAL BREAST CANCER

CLINICAL ISSUES

Presentation
- Most common signs/symptoms: Solitary breast cancer clinically ± mammographically; additional foci on US and/or MR

Demographics
- Age: Multifocal tumor more common in younger women, < age 45

Natural History & Prognosis
- Absent XRT, risk of local recurrence parallels frequency of additional occult tumor foci: 25-36% at five years
- Increased risk of local recurrence even with XRT
  - 11% local failure with unifocal cancer
  - 16% with bifocal cancer
  - 35% with 3 or more tumor foci (one series)
  - May be confounded by positive or close margins
- ↑ Risk recurrence after lumpectomy in young women (< 40-45 years), even with boost to lumpectomy site
  - May be related to increased frequency of mammographically and clinically occult multifocal tumor

Treatment
- Goal of surgical management is complete excision of all tumor foci with clear margins and good cosmesis
  - Farthest apart foci dictate size of area to be excised: Wide excision usually sufficient
  - Tumor: Breast size needs to be considered
  - Bracket needle localization
- Sentinel node biopsy for invasive cancer
  - Inject Tc-99m sulfur colloid subareolar or double peritumoral or subdermally
  - Equivalent accuracy to unifocal cancers
- Radiation with boost to lumpectomy site
  - Boost decreases recurrence rate by half

DIAGNOSTIC CHECKLIST

Consider
- Increased risk of local recurrence and positive margins
  - Pre-operative MR may reduce risk of recurrence (controversial)
  - Low risk of recurrence with clear margins and post-lumpectomy radiation in absence of MR
- Apparently separate groups of Ca++ on mammography due to DCIS may prove to be contiguous disease
  - MR can help map extent of DCIS, more accurate than mammography
- MR particularly indicated in certain situations
  - ILC
  - DCIS > 2.5 cm in size
  - Extensive intraductal component suspected
    - Mixed IDC and DCIS on core biopsy
  - Young woman, < 45 years of age
- US accurate in mapping extent of IDC
  - Limited value of US with DCIS except to identify invasive component
  - Size of ILC often underestimated

Image Interpretation Pearls
- Sample by core biopsy sufficient to prove extent for appropriate surgical planning
- MR can be helpful in mapping full extent of tumor
  - Risk of false positives, overestimation of extent
- Identification of DCIS on MR relies on morphology more than kinetics
  - Enhancement can be slow, persistent
  - Segmental, linear distribution, clumped morphology favor DCIS

SELECTED REFERENCES

1. Menell JH et al: Determination of the presence and extent of pure ductal carcinoma in situ by mammography and magnetic resonance imaging. Breast J. 11(6):382-90, 2005
2. Tafra L et al: Pilot clinical trial of 18F-fluorodeoxyglucose positron-emission mammography in the surgical management of breast cancer. Am J Surg. 190:628-32, 2005
3. Wallace AM et al: Rates of reexcision for breast cancer after magnetic resonance imaging-guided bracket wire localization. J Am Coll Surg. 200(4):527-37, 2005
4. Berg WA et al: Diagnostic accuracy of mammography, clinical examination, US, and MR imaging in preoperative assessment of breast cancer. Radiology. 233:830-49, 2004
5. Fischer U et al: The influence of preoperative MRI of the breasts on recurrence rate in patients with breast cancer. Eur Radiol. 14(10):1725-31, 2004
6. Lee JM et al: MRI before reexcision surgery in patients with breast cancer. AJR Am J Roentgenol. 182(2):473-80, 2004
7. Morrow M: Magnetic resonance imaging in breast cancer: one step forward, two steps back? JAMA. 292:2779-80, 2004
8. Liberman L et al: MR imaging of the ipsilateral breast in women with percutaneously proven breast cancer. AJR Am J Roentgenol. 180(4):901-10, 2003
9. Hlawatsch A et al: Preoperative assessment of breast cancer: sonography versus MR imaging. AJR. 179:1493-501, 2002
10. Bartelink H et al: Recurrence rates after treatment of breast cancer with standard radiotherapy with or without additional radiation. N Engl J Med. 345(19):1378-87, 2001
11. Fisher ER et al: Fifteen-year prognostic discriminants for invasive breast carcinoma. Cancer. 91(8 Suppl):1679-87, 2001
12. Orel SG et al: MR imaging of the breast for the detection, diagnosis, and staging of breast cancer. Radiology. 220(1):13-30, 2001
13. Fischer U et al: Breast carcinoma: effect of preoperative contrast-enhanced MR imaging on the therapeutic approach. Radiology. 213(3):881-8, 1999
14. Faverly DR et al: Three dimensional imaging of mammary ductal carcinoma in situ: clinical implications. Semin Diagn Pathol. 11(3):193-8, 1994
15. Harms SE et al: MR imaging of the breast with rotating delivery of excitation off resonance: clinical experience with pathologic correlation. Radiology. 187:493-501, 1993
16. Holland R et al: Extent, distribution, and mammographic/histological correlations of breast ductal carcinoma in situ. Lancet. 335(8688):519-22, 1990
17. Kurtz JM et al: Breast-conserving therapy for macroscopically multiple cancers. Ann Surg. 212:38-44, 1990
18. Leopold KA et al: Results of conservative surgery and radiation therapy for multiple synchronous cancers of one breast. Int J Radiat Oncol Biol Phys. 16:11-6, 1989
19. Holland R et al: Histologic multifocality of Tis, T1-2 breast carcinomas. Implications for clinical trials of breast-conserving surgery. Cancer. 56(5):979-90, 1985

IMAGE GALLERY

Typical

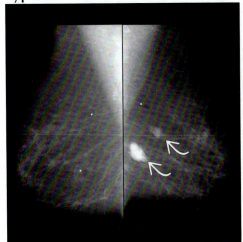 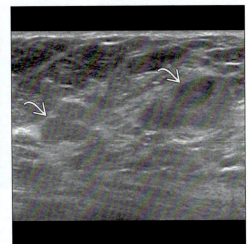

(Left) MLO mammography shows two dense, indistinctly marginated masses ➡ left breast in this 66 year old woman. *(Right)* Anti-radial ultrasound (same patient as prior image) shows two adjacent nearly isoechoic, lobulated masses ➡, quite subtle on US. US-guided core biopsy and excision confirmed multifocal mucinous carcinoma.

Typical

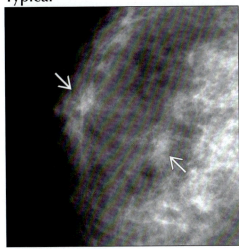 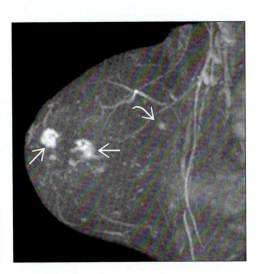

(Left) CC mammography spot compression in this 44 year old with nipple retraction shows two spiculated masses ➡. US-guided core biopsy of both showed infiltrating and in situ carcinoma, predominantly lobular type. *(Right)* Sagittal MIP of T1 C+ subtraction MR (same patient as previous image) confirms the multifocal carcinoma ➡. A faintly enhancing mass in the posterior breast ➡ proved to be a fibroadenoma.

Variant

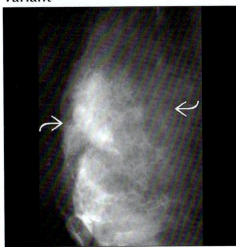 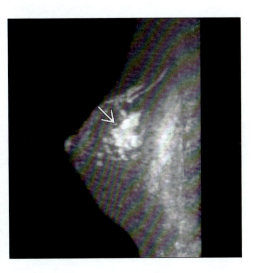

(Left) Lateral mammography magnification in this 51 year old shows two subtle clusters of pleomorphic calcifications ➡, each proven to be intermediate grade DCIS on 11-g biopsy, thought to be multifocal disease. *(Right)* Sagittal MIP of T1 C+ subtraction MR (same patient as previous image) shows contiguous regional enhancement ➡ in the area between the groups of calcifications. This proved to be contiguous DCIS at mastectomy.

MULTICENTRIC BREAST CANCER

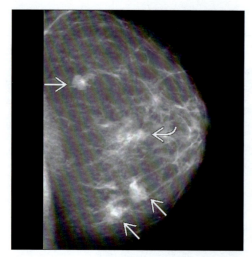
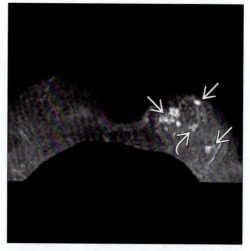

CC mammography shows multiple irregular masses ➡ *in different quadrants in this 28 y/o with lump inner left breast. Central asymmetry* ➡ *was also suspicious. US-guided biopsies: Multicentric IDC, grade I.*

Axial MIP of T1 C+ FS subtraction MR confirms extent of disease as on mammography (see previous image), with multiple irregular enhancing masses ➡ *. Central ill-defined mass* ➡ *proved malignant at mastectomy.*

TERMINOLOGY

Definitions

- Breast cancer: Invasive ductal (IDC) or invasive lobular carcinoma (ILC) or ductal carcinoma in situ (DCIS) or a combination of these entities
- Multiple (≥ 2) separate foci of breast cancer where the greatest distance between two foci is > 4 cm or sometimes defined as > 5 cm
  - Typically in different quadrants of the breast
  - Usually in different duct systems

IMAGING FINDINGS

General Features

- Best diagnostic clue: Multiple suspicious masses ± suspicious calcifications (Ca++) in different quadrants

Mammographic Findings

- Multiple suspicious masses ± Ca++ in different quadrants
- Solitary suspicious finding with additional malignancy(ies) mammographically occult

Ultrasonographic Findings

- Grayscale Ultrasound
  - ≥ 2 suspicious masses ± Ca++ in different quadrants and/or > 4-5 cm apart
  - Guide biopsy of suspicious breast masses
  - US highly accurate in depicting extent of invasive carcinoma
  - Less helpful in assessing extent of DCIS
    - Can help target associated invasive component (usually a mass) for core biopsy
  - Evaluate ipsilateral axillary nodes
    - Guide FNAB or core biopsy of suspicious node(s)
  - Screen contralateral breast if dense (optional)
    - 3-6% rate of mammographically and clinically occult carcinoma

MR Findings

- T1 C+ FS
  - ≥ 2 suspicious findings separated by at least 4-5 cm
  - Evaluate ipsilateral lymph nodes and contralateral breast
  - 6-34% of breasts anticipating conservation have additional malignant foci ipsilateral breast on MR (3-24% in different quadrants)

DDx: Mimics of Multicentric Carcinoma

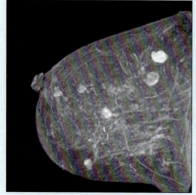
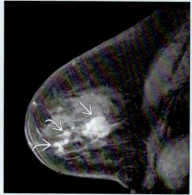
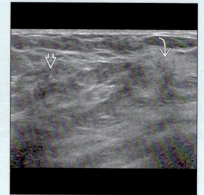

Multiple Fibroadenomas

Dominant IDC and Fibrosis

Multifocal Disease (DCIS, IDC)

MULTICENTRIC BREAST CANCER

Key Facts

Terminology
- Multiple (≥ 2) separate foci of breast cancer where the greatest distance between two foci is > 4 cm or sometimes defined as > 5 cm
- Typically in different quadrants of the breast

Imaging Findings
- Multiple suspicious masses ± Ca++ in different quadrants
- > 50% of suspicious findings seen only on MR ipsilateral to a known cancer → malignant
- Sample by core biopsy suspicious lesions farthest apart to prove extent preoperatively
- MR highly sensitive to disease extent, with substantial risk of false positives
- Mammography with magnification views of suspicious Ca++

- ↑ Risk synchronous bilateral breast cancer

Top Differential Diagnoses
- Benign or Atypical Lesions ± Breast Cancer
- Metastases to breast

Pathology
- Multicentric more common with DCIS ≥ 2.5 cm
- If suspect breast has single cancer by mammography and clinical breast examination
- 7-10% will have occult multicentric foci

Diagnostic Checklist
- ~ 25% of additional unsuspected tumor foci are multicentric
- ~ 25% of recurrences are in different quadrant from index cancer

---

- > 50% of suspicious findings seen only on MR ipsilateral to a known cancer → malignant
  - ↑ Malignant in same quadrant as index lesion: 64-75% vs. 31-47% in different quadrants

Nuclear Medicine Findings
- PET
  - FDG-PET with dedicated high resolution dedicated positron emission mammography (PEM): Can depict local extent of disease
    - 91% of DCIS and 89% of invasive cancer depicted, median size 21 mm (one series)
    - Potential false negatives with ILC

Biopsy
- Sample by core biopsy suspicious lesions farthest apart to prove extent preoperatively

Imaging Recommendations
- Best imaging tool
  - MR highly sensitive to disease extent, with substantial risk of false positives
    - Sample additional suspicious lesions before recommending change in surgical management
  - US for biopsy guidance of breast masses, FNAB or core biopsy of axillary node if needed
- Protocol advice
  - Mammography with magnification views of suspicious Ca++
  - When performing initial US of highly suspicious masses, evaluate that quadrant as well as the remainder of that breast carefully
  - Evaluation should include the contralateral breast
    - ↑ Risk synchronous bilateral breast cancer
  - MR performed at initial diagnosis or when lumpectomy margins positive or close

DIFFERENTIAL DIAGNOSIS

Benign or Atypical Lesions ± Breast Cancer
- Lobular carcinoma in situ (LCIS) frequently associated with ILC

  - Suspicious mass on US ± MR; occult on mammography
- Atypical ductal hyperplasia (ADH) often coexists with malignancies: Most often amorphous Ca++
- Fibroadenomas, papillomas, fibrocystic changes

Malignancies
- Multifocal breast cancer
  - Multiple malignant foci within 4-5 cm span; same quadrant
- Metastases to breast
  - Melanoma, lymphoma, lung, ovarian most common

PATHOLOGY

General Features
- Genetics
  - Loss of heterogosity (LOH) studies: Independent origin of vast majority multicentric tumors
  - Biologic definition: Tumors of clonal origin termed multifocal even if geographically widely separated
- Associated abnormalities
  - Multifocal breast cancer also present in > half
  - ↑ Contralateral breast cancer
  - Increased risk of axillary node metastases compared to unifocal cancer
    - Consider largest or aggregate tumor volume with multicentric cases to predict risk nodal spread
    - Odds ratios 2.2-2.34 of axillary metastases compared to similar sized unifocal cancer
- 20-47% of all breasts undergoing mastectomy will have cancer in more than one quadrant
- In breasts with DCIS undergoing mastectomy, 23-47% involve more than one quadrant
  - High-grade DCIS tends to contiguous spread
  - Low-grade DCIS more frequent skip areas
  - Gaps > 1 cm in 8% of DCIS
  - Multifocal, multicentric DCIS most common with micropapillary subtype
  - Multicentric more common with DCIS ≥ 2.5 cm
- If suspect breast has single cancer by mammography and clinical breast examination

MULTICENTRIC BREAST CANCER

○ Average 48% have additional occult tumor foci (either multifocal or multicentric) at detailed histopathology
○ 7-10% will have occult multicentric foci

Microscopic Features

• ILC more likely multicentric than IDC
• More common with DCIS component than with pure invasive carcinomas: 17% vs. 5% one series

Staging, Grading or Classification Criteria

• T stage determined by largest individual tumor, with invasive cancer taking precedence to DCIS
  ○ Tis: DCIS
  ○ T1: Invasive component ≤ 2 cm in greatest dimension
  ○ T2: Invasive tumor > 2 cm and ≤ 5 cm
  ○ T3: Invasive tumor > 5 cm
  ○ T4: Tumor of any size with direct extension to skin or chest wall
• In TNM staging system, designate T stage with parentheses indicating multiple foci (m) [e.g., T1(m)] or number of "grossly recognizable" multiple foci, e.g., T1(3): Largest invasive tumor 2 cm or smaller, with 3 tumor foci known

CLINICAL ISSUES

Natural History & Prognosis

• Increased risk of recurrence if breast conserved compared to unifocal cancer

Treatment

• Mastectomy usually recommended
  ○ No higher risk of locoregional recurrence than unifocal disease stage for stage
• Double lumpectomy with needle localization if nonpalpable (controversial) in select patients
  ○ Strong patient preference, agrees to post-operative radiation (XRT)
  ○ Large breast, small tumors, clear margins required
    ■ No extensive intraductal component
  ○ Contraindication to partial breast irradiation
• Sentinel node biopsy for invasive cancer
  ○ Subareolar or double peritumoral or subdermal injection of Tc-99m sulfur colloid
  ○ Inject blue dye around both (invasive) tumors
  ○ 96% sensitivity to axillary metastases in multicentric breast cancer: No different than performance with unifocal breast cancer

DIAGNOSTIC CHECKLIST

Consider

• ~ 25% of additional unsuspected tumor foci are multicentric
• ~ 25% of recurrences are in different quadrant from index cancer
• More common with family history of breast cancer
  ○ Younger age at diagnosis
  ○ More likely to have dense breast tissue
  ○ ↑ Detection potential from pre-operative MR

• Pre-operative MR identification of all tumor foci → change in management in 8-15% of breasts anticipating conservation
  ○ May decrease risk of local recurrence (one study)

Image Interpretation Pearls

• Avoid satisfaction of search

SELECTED REFERENCES

1. Berg WA et al: High-Resolution Fluorodeoxyglucose Positron Emission Tomography with Compression ("Positron Emission Mammography") is Highly Accurate in Depicting Primary Breast Cancer. Breast J. 12:309-23, 2006
2. Gentilini O et al: Sentinel lymph node biopsy in multicentric breast cancer. The experience of the European Institute of Oncology. Eur J Surg Oncol. 32(5):507-10, 2006
3. Andea AA et al: Correlation of tumor volume and surface area with lymph node status in patients with multifocal/multicentric breast carcinoma. Cancer. 100(1):20-7, 2004
4. Berg WA et al: Diagnostic accuracy of mammography, clinical examination, US, and MR imaging in preoperative assessment of breast cancer. Radiology. 233:830-49, 2004
5. Fischer U et al: The influence of preoperative MRI of the breasts on recurrence rate in patients with breast cancer. Eur Radiol. 14(10):1725-31, 2004
6. Bedrosian I et al: Changes in the surgical management of patients with breast carcinoma based on preoperative magnetic resonance imaging. Cancer. 98(3):468-73, 2003
7. Liberman L et al: MR imaging of the ipsilateral breast in women with percutaneously proven breast cancer. AJR Am J Roentgenol. 180(4):901-10, 2003
8. Tousimis E et al: The accuracy of sentinel lymph node biopsy in multicentric and multifocal invasive breast cancers. J Am Coll Surg. 197(4):529-35, 2003
9. Hlawatsch A et al: Preoperative assessment of breast cancer: sonography versus MR imaging. AJR Am J Roentgenol. 179(6):1493-501, 2002
10. Moon WK et al: Multifocal, multicentric, and contralateral breast cancers: bilateral whole-breast US in the preoperative evaluation of patients. Radiology. 224(2):569-76, 2002
11. Elling D et al: Intraductal component in invasive breast cancer: analysis of 250 resected surgical specimens. Breast. 10(5):405-10, 2001
12. Fukutomi T et al: Multicentricity and histopathological background features of familial breast cancers stratified by menopausal status. Int J Clin Oncol. 6(2):80-3, 2001
13. Berg WA et al: Multicentric and multifocal cancer: whole-breast US in preoperative evaluation. Radiology. 214(1):59-66, 2000
14. Fischer U et al: Breast carcinoma: effect of preoperative contrast-enhanced MR imaging on the therapeutic approach. Radiology. 213(3):881-8, 1999
15. Lagios MD et al: Ductal carcinoma in situ. The success of breast conservation therapy: a shared experience of two single institutional nonrandomized prospective studies. Surg Oncol Clin N Am. 6(2):385-92, 1997
16. Hartsell WF et al: Should multicentric disease be an absolute contraindication to the use of breast-conserving therapy? Int J Radiat Oncol Biol Phys. 30(1):49-53, 1994
17. Harms SE et al: MR imaging of the breast with rotating delivery of excitation off resonance: clinical experience with pathologic correlation. Radiology. 187:493-501, 1993
18. Holland R et al: Histologic multifocality of Tis, T1-2 breast carcinomas. Implications for clinical trials of breast-conserving surgery. Cancer. 56(5):979-90, 1985
19. Lesser ML et al: Multicentricity and bilaterality in invasive breast carcinoma. Surgery. 91(2):234-40, 1982

Variant

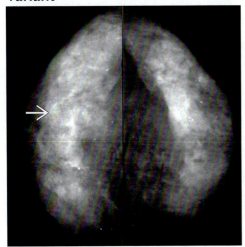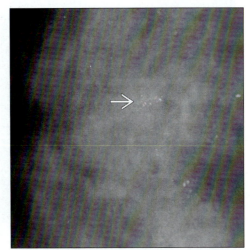

(Left) CC mammography shows dense breast tissue with multiple bilateral groupings of coarse heterogeneous Ca++ in this 57 y/o with a lump inner right breast. A cluster of pleomorphic Ca++ in outer retroareolar right breast was new ➡. *(Right)* CC mammography magnification (same patient as previous image) shows new clustered pleomorphic Ca++ to better advantage ➡. Stereotactic 11-g biopsy showed high grade DCIS with microinvasion.

Variant

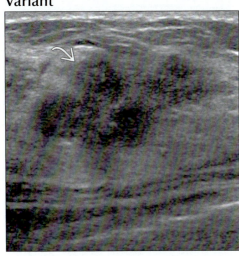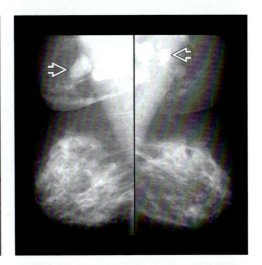

(Left) US of the palpable medial right breast mass (same patient as prior two images) shows an irregular, lobulated hypoechoic mass ➡. Initial US-guided biopsy showed fibrosis, discordant. Rebiopsy under US showed ILC. With proven multicentric disease, patient had mastectomy. *(Right)* MLO mammography shows bilateral axillary adenopathy ➡ in this 57 y/o who presented with palpable right supraclavicular lymph node compatible with metastatic ILC.

Variant

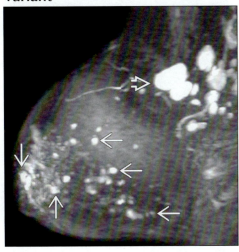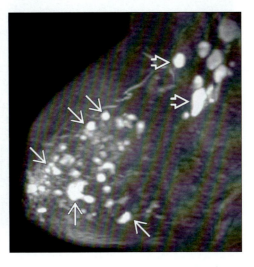

(Left) Sagittal MIP of T1 C+ FS subtraction MR (same as prior image) shows multiple enhancing masses ➡ right breast, as well as extensive enhancing adenopathy ➡. *(Right)* Sagittal MIP of T1 C+ subtraction MR of contralateral breast (same as previous image) shows diffuse irregular masses ➡ & axillary adenopathy ➡. A representative mass was biopsied bilaterally under US → ILC. Mastectomies confirmed bilateral diffuse multifocal & multicentric ILC & metastatic nodes.

MULTICENTRIC BREAST CANCER

Typical

(Left) MLO mammography shows dense, palpable mass lower inner right breast ➡. A second, subtle mass was noted in the upper inner right breast ➡. *(Right)* MLO mammography spot compression (same patient as previous image) shows circumscribed margins to the palpable mass inferiorly ➡, and indistinct margins to the superior mass ➡.

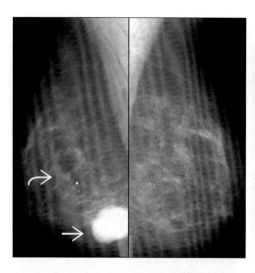
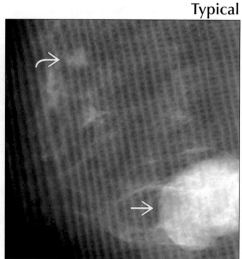

Typical

(Left) Ultrasound of the palpable lower inner mass (same as prior 2 images) shows intracystic mass ➡ and fluid-debris level ➡. US-guided aspiration then immediate 14-g core biopsy showed papillary DCIS. *(Right)* US directed to the mammographic mass upper inner right breast (same as prior 3 images) shows spiculated, hypoechoic mass ➡. US-guided core biopsy: Grade II IDC. Patient had double lumpectomy and XRT, and remains disease free over 5 years later.

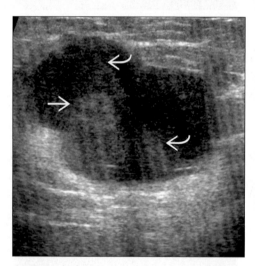
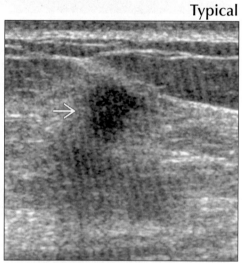

Typical

(Left) MLO mammography shows subtle spiculated mass upper outer left breast ➡ adjacent to multiple large, palpable cysts in this 56 y/o. US-guided biopsy: Mixed IDC-ILC. Ca++ in lower inner left breast ➡ were initially overlooked. *(Right)* CC mammography magnification (same patient as previous image) shows fine linear and pleomorphic Ca++ ➡. Stereotactic biopsy: High-grade DCIS. Patient had double lumpectomy with clear margins and XRT.

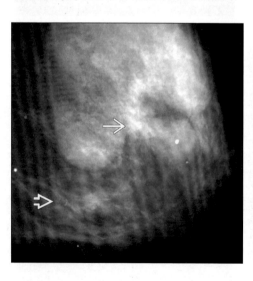
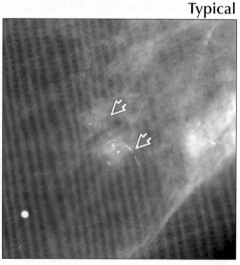

Typical

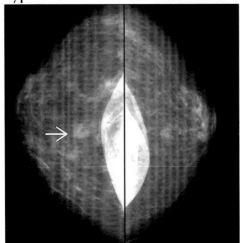 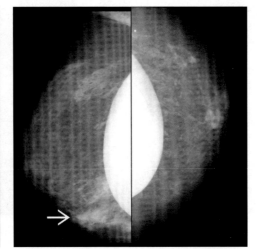

(Left) Implant-displaced CC mammograms in this 52 y/o with a palpable mass 6:00 right breast show ill-defined mass ➡ adjacent to subglandular saline implant. (Right) Implant-displaced MLO mammograms (same patient as previous image) confirm ill-defined mass 6:30 position right breast ➡.

Typical

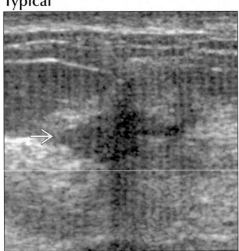 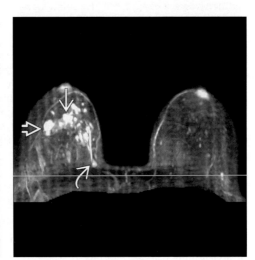

(Left) US of the palpable mass (same patient as prior 2 images) shows spiculated hypoechoic mass ➡ with posterior shadowing. US-guided core biopsy: Grade I IDC. (Right) Axial MIP of T1 C+ FS subtraction MR (same as prior 3 images) shows enhancement of the known cancer ➡. Additional suspicious masses were noted medially ➡ and laterally ➡.

Typical

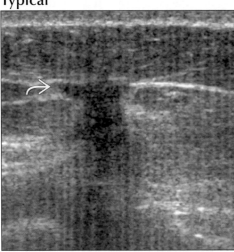 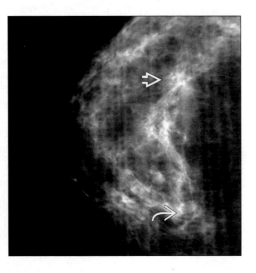

(Left) US of inner right breast (same patient as previous) shows second spiculated, shadowing, hypoechoic mass ➡. US-guided core biopsy confirmed multicentric grade I IDC. Mastectomy was performed. (Right) CC mammography spot compression shows subtle spiculated masses upper outer right breast ➡ and lower inner right breast ➡ first noted on screening in this 52 y/o. US-guided biopsy, showed both = grade II IDC, confirmed at mastectomy.

NEOADJUVANT CHEMOTHERAPY

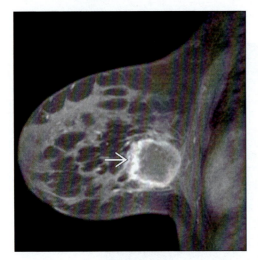

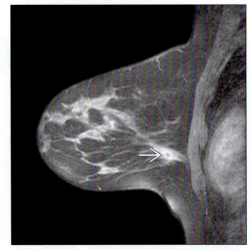

Sagittal T1 C+ FS MR in this 40 y/o woman shows irregular, rim-enhancing mass ➡. US-guided biopsy showed poorly differentiated IDC. NAT was given & a follow-up MR performed (next image). (Courtesy DNS).

Sagittal T1 C+ FS MR shows marked decrease in tumor size with minimal residual enhancement ➡. Lumpectomy showed no residual tumor. Complete pathologic response with false positive enhancement.

TERMINOLOGY

Abbreviations and Synonyms
- Neoadjuvant chemotherapy (NAT)

Definitions
- NAT: Systemic chemotherapy ± hormonal treatment of breast cancer prior to definitive breast surgery
- Major use in primary inoperable locally advanced breast cancer (LABC)
  - Primary goal: Facilitate clear margins at surgery by clearing skin, chest wall invasion
  - Secondary goal: Shrink tumor → potential for breast conservation surgery and adjuvant radiation therapy (XRT)
  - Assess treatment response if measurable lesion present
    - Responders and nonresponders can be identified
  - Carcinoma gene expression and proteins as well as treatment-related changes can be studied
    - Understanding tumor characteristics allows possible tailoring of individual treatment
  - Earlier treatment may decrease appearance of resistant tumor clones

  - Treat occult micrometastases
- NAT used to reduce tumor burden in operable breast cancer (controversial)
- Assessment of response: CR = complete (no residual tumor), PR = partial (≥ 50% tumor reduction), NR = stable (no) response
  - Clinical, imaging, pathologic assessments
- Adjuvant therapy: Chemotherapy or hormonal treatment following definitive breast surgery

IMAGING FINDINGS

General Features
- Best diagnostic clue
  - LABC imaging abnormalities (some or all)
    - Mass(es), extensive calcifications (Ca++), skin thickening or retraction, nipple retraction, axillary adenopathy

Mammographic Findings
- Pre-treatment: Mass ± Ca++, skin changes, axillary adenopathy
  - Accuracy in pre-operative size: Correlation coefficients (r^2) with pathology only 0.46-0.72

DDx: LABC in 47 Yr Old with Little Clinical Response to 4 Cycles NAT

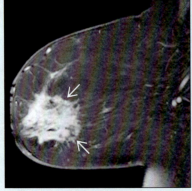

MR Pre-NAT

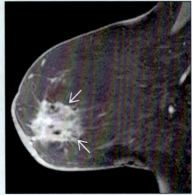

MR Post (Decreased Enhancement)

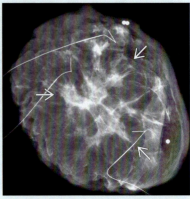

Specimen, Extensive Tumor

NEOADJUVANT CHEMOTHERAPY

Key Facts

Terminology

- NAT: Systemic chemotherapy ± hormonal treatment of breast cancer prior to definitive breast surgery
- Major use in primary inoperable locally advanced breast cancer (LABC)
- Assessment of response: CR = complete (no residual tumor), PR = partial (≥ 50% tumor reduction), NR = stable (no) response

Imaging Findings

- Post-treatment: Tumor size may decrease yet still be viable secondary to focal therapy-induced changes
- Place clip at time of initial biopsy of LABC
- Size of tumor most accurately determined by MR
- MR during and/or at conclusion of treatment to assess response

Top Differential Diagnoses

- Post NAT Fibrosis, Scar
- Post NAT Residual Viable Tumor

Pathology

- Metastases to axillary lymph nodes (LN) most important prognostic factor before and after NAT
- Response to treatment is an additional strong prognostic feature

Clinical Issues

- Randomized trials demonstrate equivalent survival for neoadjuvant and adjuvant chemotherapy in women with primary operable breast cancer

Diagnostic Checklist

- Potential to tailor treatment if no response

- ○ Particularly inaccurate for invasive lobular carcinoma (ILC), noncalcified tumor in dense breast tissue
- Post-treatment: No change, decrease in tumor size, no visible tumor
  - ○ Treatment-related necrosis and fibrosis may mimic residual tumor
  - ○ Ca++ may remain despite complete treatment response and no residual viable tumor

Ultrasonographic Findings

- Evaluate ipsilateral breast and axilla, guide biopsy of both pre-treatment
- US relatively inaccurate in sizing tumor: r^2 with pathology 0.45-0.72
  - ○ More inaccurate with tumors > 2 cm
  - ○ Fibrosis can mimic residual cancer

MR Findings

- T1WI: Axial bilateral images demonstrate breast size asymmetry, skin changes and axillary and internal mammary nodes
- T1 C+ FS
  - ○ Pre-treatment: Size and focality of primary tumor, nodes
    - Size accuracy vs. pathology, r^2 = 0.82-0.98
  - ○ Chest wall invasion: Enhancement of pectoral or intercostal muscles
  - ○ Evaluate contralateral breast
  - ○ Post-treatment: Tumor size may decrease yet still be viable secondary to focal therapy-induced changes
    - Non-tumor related enhancement may increase secondary to reactive changes (fibrosis, necrosis, inflammation)
    - False negative rates as high as 67%; false positive overestimates of residual tumor as high as 56%
  - ○ MR imaging may accurately determine response to NAT
- MR spectroscopy
  - ○ Choline present in malignancies >> normal tissue
  - ○ Monitor response to treatment: ↓ Choline peak within days, precedes ↓ size of tumor

- ○ Technique limited to one lesion, minimum of 1 cm³ voxel
- ○ Benefit to higher field strength, ↑ signal: 3-4 T

Nuclear Medicine Findings

- PET
  - ○ Serial evaluation of NAT-treated lesions
    - FDG PET: ↓ Uptake within 8 days of treatment, earlier than ↓ size of tumor
    - 75-90% sensitivity to residual tumor
    - 74% specificity (one series)

Biopsy

- US-guided core biopsy to establish diagnosis
- Place clip at time of initial biopsy of LABC
  - ○ Clip facilitates excision and identification of tumor bed with CR
    - Response may result in ambiguity as to original tumor site by palpation, mammography, US, MR
- US-guided FNAB or core biopsy suspicious axillary node(s)
- Biopsy suspicious findings in contralateral breast

Imaging Recommendations

- Best imaging tool
  - ○ Imaging prior to initiation of treatment
    - 81-94% of known or unsuspected additional ipsilateral tumor depicted with MR; 48-84% with mammography; 63-91% with mammography + US
    - Size of tumor most accurately determined by MR
    - Tumor extent assessment with MR vulnerable to both over (12%) and underestimation (6%)
    - Contralateral synchronous breast cancer in 6-10% of patients: MR or US can help depict
  - ○ Core biopsy with clip placement to establish diagnosis, receptor studies
  - ○ FNAB or core biopsy of suspicious axillary node
  - ○ MR during and/or at conclusion of treatment to assess response

NEOADJUVANT CHEMOTHERAPY

DIFFERENTIAL DIAGNOSIS

Post NAT Fibrosis, Scar
- May be misinterpreted as residual tumor by palpation
- May enhance on MR

Post NAT Residual Viable Tumor
- Treated tumors may demonstrate a decrease in enhancement on MR despite viable tumor cells
- Residual tumor often found at pathology in scattered nests within tumor bed

PATHOLOGY

General Features
- Metastases to axillary lymph nodes (LN) most important prognostic factor before and after NAT
  - Known LN positivity prior to treatment is only setting where a complete LN response can be accurately assigned
  - High false negative sentinel lymph node (SLN) rates reported after treatment
- Response to treatment is an additional strong prognostic feature
- Presently 8 pathologic evaluation systems for breast cancer treatment response
  - B-18 (Fisher), Chevallier, Sataloff, Miller-Payne (Ogston), RCB (Symmans), AJCC (Carey), Rouzier, MNPI (Abrial)
    - Most of these systems define complete pathologic response (pCR) as the absence of invasive breast cancer in the breast; tumor bed must be identified
    - Systems differ as to number of response categories
    - All but one evaluation system includes LN evaluation

Gross Pathologic & Surgical Features
- Tumors may not show significant change in size despite marked decrease in cellularity
- Treated tumors typically softer

Microscopic Features
- Tumor bed does not have the appearance of normal breast tissue
  - Variable amount of residual tumor cellularity
    - Residual tumor may be present in scattered nests
  - Typically has loose fibrous stroma, histiocytes, and lymphocytes
  - May have hemosiderin-laden macrophages, giant cells
- Treated tumor is unlikely to change in tumor grade

CLINICAL ISSUES

Presentation
- Most common signs/symptoms
  - Mass, either palpable or image-detected
  - Locally advanced breast cancer changes may include skin retraction, skin thickening, axillary adenopathy
  - Inflammatory breast cancer less likely to include a frank mass: Tumor throughout the breast and skin

- Symptoms may dramatically improve or even resolve following systemic treatment prior to definitive surgery
  - High false positive rates due to fibrosis and tumor cell death
  - High false negative results possibly due to tumor changes related to decreased cellularity, vascularity

Natural History & Prognosis
- Including inflammatory and NAT (often lumped in reported statistics), systemic treatment +/- radiation therapy prior to lumpectomy or mastectomy 5 year survival = 35-50%
  - Surgery or radiation therapy alone 5 year survival < 10%
  - Surgery and radiation therapy 5 year survival = 20%
- Overall LABC response rates vary between 60-100%
  - Complete clinical responses range 10-50%
  - Clinical responders have a better prognosis than nonresponders
  - Pathologic responders: Those with complete response or minimal residual disease have longer disease-free and overall survival than those with residual gross disease

Treatment
- Randomized trials demonstrate equivalent survival for neoadjuvant and adjuvant chemotherapy in women with primary operable breast cancer
- Invasive carcinomas of higher grade are more likely to respond to chemotherapy

DIAGNOSTIC CHECKLIST

Consider
- Potential to tailor treatment if no response
- Tumor response, allowing the option of breast conservation and adjuvant radiation, may be problematic: One study suggests tumors > 2 cm after NAT treated with breast conservation and radiation are more likely to recur

SELECTED REFERENCES

1. Padhani AR et al: Reduction of clinicopathologic response of breast cancer to primary chemotherapy at contrast-enhanced MR imaging: initial clinical results. Radiology. 239:361-74, 2006
2. Yeh E et al: Prospective comparison of mammography, sonography, and MRI in patients undergoing neoadjuvant chemotherapy for palpable breast cancer. AJR. 184:868-77, 2005
3. Tseng J, et al: ^{18}F-FDG kinetics in locally advanced breast cancer: correlation with tumor blood flow and changes in response to neoadjuvant chemotherapy. J Nucl Med. 45:1829-1837, 2004
4. Rosen EL et al: Accuracy of MRI in the detection of residual breast cancer after neoadjuvant chemotherapy. AJR. 181:1275-82, 2003
5. Rouzier R et al: Primary chemotherapy for operable breast cancer: incidence and prognostic significance of ipsilateral breast tumor recurrence after breast-conserving surgery. J Clin Oncol. 19:3823-35, 2001

IMAGE GALLERY

Typical

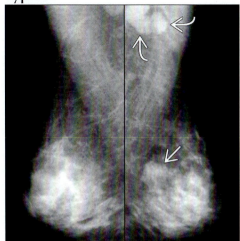
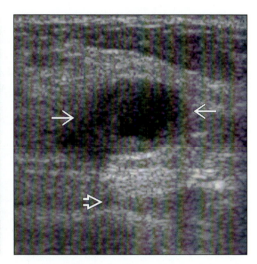

(Left) MLO mammography in a 43 yr old woman shows an indistinct mass in the upper left breast ➡ and dense enlarged axillary nodes ➡. US-guided FNA confirmed metastatic adenopathy. (Right) Radial ultrasound (same patient as previous image, breast mass) shows an indistinctly marginated complex cystic mass ➡ with posterior enhancement ➡. US-guided core bx showed IDC, NOS, grade III. NAT was initiated.

Typical

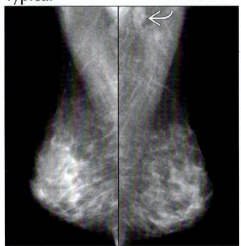
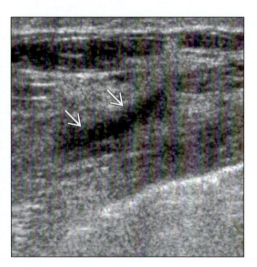

(Left) MLO mammography (same patient as previous 2 images) four months later shows resolution of breast mass and adenopathy ➡. Post-NAT US was also performed (next image). (Right) Radial ultrasound shows an oval hypoechoic residual "mass" ➡. Needle localization was performed with US-guidance, fluid obtained. Mammography and US complete response. At surgery, no residual tumor in the breast or axilla.

Typical

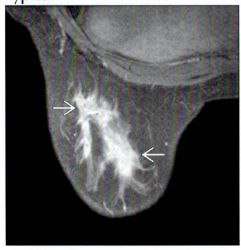
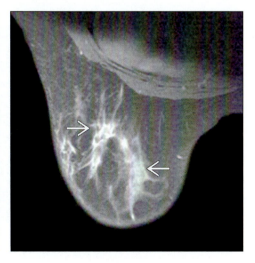

(Left) Axial T1 C+ FS MR in a 29 yr old woman shows 6 cm irregular enhancing mass ➡ found at core biopsy to represent IDC. NAT was initiated and post-NAT MR (next image) performed. (Right) Axial T1 C+ FS MR shows partial response with the lesion ➡ now 4 cm in size. Note the decrease in avidity of enhancement. Mastectomy showed 4 cm of residual IDC and extensive DCIS (case courtesy DNS).

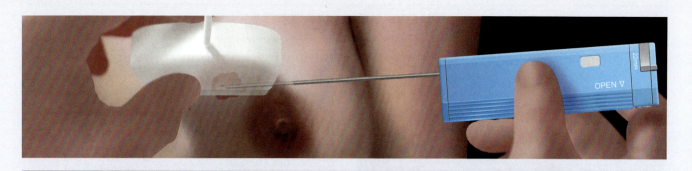

SECTION 2: Procedures, Image-Guided

CYST ASPIRATION

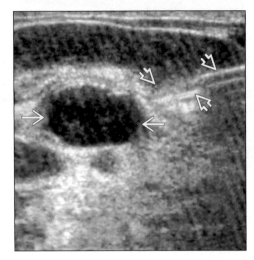

Longitudinal ultrasound demonstrates aspiration of a complicated cyst ➡ with internal echoes in a 44 year old woman. Because thick fluid was suspected, a 16-g needle ➡ was used.

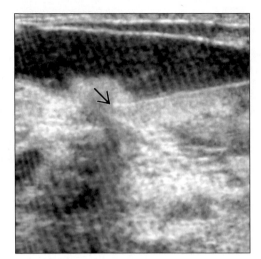

Post-aspiration US (same as left) shows complete resolution of cyst. Tip of needle ➡ indicates location of aspirated cyst. 0.5 cc of thick amber fluid (typical of benign cyst contents) was obtained and discarded.

TERMINOLOGY

Definitions
- Percutaneous aspiration of fluid from breast cyst
  - Most efficiently performed with real-time ultrasound (US) guidance, usually by radiologist
  - Alternatively, may be performed by clinician using palpation

PRE-PROCEDURE

Indications
- Painful or tender cysts
  - Improved tolerance of mammographic compression
- Patient anxiety or request
- Improved sensitivity of clinical exam
- Cyst recurrence after previous aspiration
- Diagnostic uncertainty: Hypoechoic, complicated cyst vs. solid mass, which would need biopsy if solid: e.g. Irregular wall, new on mammography, or palpable

Contraindications
- Asymptomatic simple cysts
- Complex cystic and solid lesion: Intracystic mass, mural nodule(s), thick wall, or thick septation(s), predominantly solid with cystic component(s)
  - Biopsy: US-guided core or vacuum-assisted biopsy or excision

Getting Started
- Things to Check
  - Document size, location and number of cysts to be aspirated
  - Informed, written consent
- Medications
  - 1% lidocaine ± buffered with sodium bicarbonate, 25-g needle, for local anesthesia

- - Can be done without anesthesia
- Equipment List
  - Syringe for aspiration (some radiologists prefer red-topped vacuum tube)
  - Needle
    - 21 or 22-gauge adequate for most cysts
    - 16, 18 or 19-gauge for viscous fluid
  - Betadine or other skin disinfectant
  - Sterile drape and gel ± probe cover

PROCEDURE

Patient Position/Location
- Best procedure approach
  - Patient supine on exam table; ipsilateral arm raised, hand resting behind head
  - Slight contralateral decubitus position for outer hemispheric cysts
- Long-axis approach (preferred)
  - Needle pierces skin adjacent to short end of transducer
  - Needle advanced toward lesion along plane of ultrasound beam
  - Good needle visualization, relatively short needle travel
    - Visualization of needle improves the closer the needle is to perpendicular to US beam
    - Spatial compounding can help depict needle
- Short-axis approach
  - Needle pierces skin alongside the middle of the transducer; more direct route
  - Shows needle only in cross section; entire length not seen; difficult to identify tip per se

Equipment Preparation
- If sterile probe cover not used, must sterilize probe
  - Avoid any Betadine contact with probe surface

CYST ASPIRATION

Key Facts

Terminology
- Percutaneous aspiration of fluid from breast cyst
- Most efficiently performed with real-time ultrasound (US) guidance, usually by radiologist

Pre-procedure
- 1% lidocaine ± buffered with sodium bicarbonate, 25-g needle, for local anesthesia
- 21 or 22-gauge adequate for most cysts
- 16, 18 or 19-gauge for viscous fluid

Procedure
- Long-axis approach (preferred)
- Aspirate cyst to completion
- Document lesion gone
- Usually discard fluid; if bloody or mucoid, send to cytology
- Document number and location of cysts aspirated, amount of fluid withdrawn and any complications

Procedure Steps
- Area of interest cleansed with disinfectant
- Fenestrated drape or towels to define sterile field
- Using sterile technique, apply local anesthesia
- Needle, with attached syringe, advanced toward cyst under long axis of transducer
  - Radiologist holds transducer in nondominant hand and needle/syringe in other
- Puncture cyst wall
  - If fibrous tissue present, quick jabbing motion helpful to pass through wall
- Aspirate cyst to completion
  - Document lesion gone
  - Optional: Remove fluid-filled syringe and use fresh syringe to instill equal volume of air (↓ recurrence)
- Usually discard fluid; if bloody or mucoid, send to cytology
- If lesion solid or partially solid → convert to US-guided core biopsy
- If grossly bloody fluid encountered → stop
  - May lose US landmark of possibly malignant lesion
  - Consider vacuum-bx/clip placement or excision

Findings and Reporting
- Document number and location of cysts aspirated, amount of fluid withdrawn and any complications

Alternative Procedures/Therapies
- Surgical
  - For recurrent cysts, excision may be considered
    - Rarely necessary for simple cysts

POST-PROCEDURE

Expected Outcome
- Complete clinical and imaging resolution of cyst

PROBLEMS & COMPLICATIONS

Complications
- Most feared complication(s): Pneumothorax (rare)
- Other complications: Bleeding and infection

SELECTED REFERENCES

1. Bassett LW et al: Diagnosis of Diseases of the Breast. 2nd edition. Philadelphia, Elsevier Saunders. Chapter 20, 323-8, 2005
2. Stavros AT: Breast Ultrasound. Philadelphia, Lippincott Williams and Wilkins. Chapter 17, 742-8, 2004
3. Gizienski TA et al: Breast cyst recurrence after postaspiration injection of air. Breast J. 8:34-7, 2002
4. Smith DN et al: Impalpable breast cysts: utility of cytologic examination of fluid obtained with radiologically guided aspiration. Radiology. 204:149-51, 1997
5. Ciatto S et al: The value of routine cytologic examination of breast cyst fluids. Acta Cytol. 31:301-4, 1987

IMAGE GALLERY

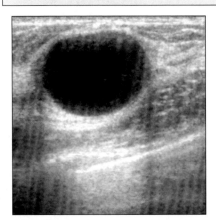 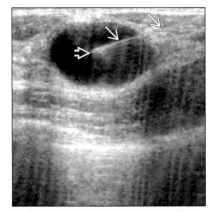 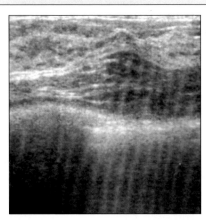

(Left) Transverse ultrasound shows a palpable simple left upper outer quadrant cyst in a 53 year old woman. Because it was symptomatic, the patient requested aspiration. (Center) Transverse ultrasound (same as prior image) demonstrates tip ⇨ of 21-gauge needle ➡ in cyst, just prior to evacuation of contents. (Right) Ultrasound post-aspiration (same as prior image) confirms resolution of cyst. 2.5 ccs of clear yellow fluid were obtained, then discarded.

DUCTOGRAPHY

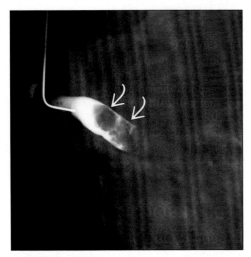

Lateral galactography demonstrates intraductal filling defects ➡ in a patient who presented with bloody nipple discharge. Excision revealed multiple benign papillomas.

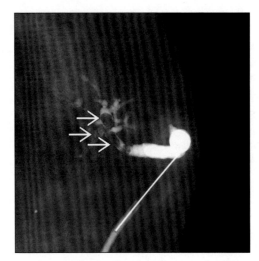

CC galactography shows multiple filling defects ➡ in a 46 year old woman with bloody nipple discharge. Excision confirmed intraductal papilloma, duct ectasia, debris and fibrosis.

TERMINOLOGY

Synonyms
- Galactography

Definitions
- Contrast examination of mammary ducts performed to identify intraductal lesions
  - Once identified → image-guided biopsy or pre-operative localization

PRE-PROCEDURE

Indications
- Unilateral, single-duct spontaneous nipple discharge
  - Bloody, serosanguineous, clear or colorless
- Bloody nipple discharge with stimulation

Contraindications
- Multiple discharging ducts, physiologic discharge, pregnancy or lactation
- Active mastitis
- Previous nipple/areolar surgery (disrupts ducts)
- History of severe allergy to iodinated contrast material

Getting Started
- Things to Check
  - Recent pre-procedure subareolar magnification views
  - Active nipple discharge
  - US unrevealing
- Equipment List
  - 27 or 30-gauge blunt cannula, straight or right-angled, attached to extension tubing
  - 1-3 cc syringe (attached to cannula system)
  - Contrast material, lidocaine gel
  - High-intensity light source; headset magnification device
  - Sterile alcohol swabs, paper tape, warm compresses and latex or non-latex gloves

PROCEDURE

Patient Position/Location
- Best procedure approach: Patient supine or seated

Equipment Preparation
- Eliminate air bubbles from cannula, syringe, extension tubing

Procedure Steps
- Sterilize nipple with alcohol swab, removing dried secretions
- Localize discharging duct
  - Express small drop of discharge onto nipple surface, applying gentle pressure to trigger point
- Stabilize nipple between thumb and forefinger → guide cannula into duct
  - Gentle twirling and angling of cannula helpful
- If cannulation unsuccessful, apply warm compresses to nipple and reattempt procedure
- If second attempt unsuccessful → another radiologist
  - If unsuccessful after three attempts, reschedule procedure in 7-14 days
- Once cannula in place, slowly inject 0.2-0.3 cc contrast material
  - Inject until meet resistance, patient feels fullness; pain or burning → stop
  - If reflux occurs at beginning → consider distal obstructing lesion near nipple
  - Intense pain/unimpeded flow may indicate duct rupture → stop injection, obtain film
- Secure cannula in place with paper tape; tape syringe to ipsilateral shoulder

DUCTOGRAPHY

Key Facts

Terminology
- Galactography
- Contrast examination of mammary ducts performed to identify intraductal lesions

Pre-procedure
- Unilateral, single-duct spontaneous nipple discharge
- 27 or 30-gauge blunt cannula, straight or right-angled, attached to extension tubing

Procedure
- Localize discharging duct
- Once cannula in place, slowly inject 0.2-0.3 cc contrast material

Problems & Complications
- Duct rupture
- Mastitis, vasovagal reaction

- Obtain craniocaudal and 90° lateral magnification mammograms
  - Nonmagnified views may be needed if process extensive
  - Mild to moderate compression
- If opacification of duct system incomplete → re-inject small amount of contrast and re-image
  - Total contrast volume rarely exceeds 1 cc
- Obtain supplemental views as needed
- Untape breast, remove cannula
- Give patient sterile gauze pad to place in bra

Findings and Reporting
- Lesion location, size and distance from nipple should be reported

Alternative Procedures/Therapies
- Radiologic
  - Ultrasound
    - Less invasive, sensitive to lesions near nipple
    - If intraductal mass identified → US-guided biopsy
  - Contrast-enhanced MR
- Surgical
  - Intraoperative duct exploration ± ductoscopy, excision of abnormal duct system
    - Possible incomplete removal of causative lesion(s)
- Other
  - Percutaneous ultrasound-guided ductography
    - Consider when ductography fails and dilated ducts are visualized with ultrasound
  - Nipple fluid cytology: Frequent atypia problematic
  - Duct lavage: Frequent atypia problematic

POST-PROCEDURE

Expected Outcome
- Identification of intraductal abnormality(ies) to account for nipple discharge
- Increased discharge may occur for a few days

PROBLEMS & COMPLICATIONS

Complications
- Most feared complication(s)
  - Duct rupture
    - Due to forceful contrast administration or duct perforation by cannula insertion
    - Treat with mild analgesics; reschedule in 7-14 days
- Other complications: Mastitis, vasovagal reaction

SELECTED REFERENCES

1. Bhattarai N et al: Intraductal papilloma: features on MR ductography using a microscopic coil. AJR Am J Roentgenol. 186:44-7, 2006
2. Slawson SH et al: Ductography: How to and what if? Radiographics. 21:133-50, 2001
3. Hild F et al: Ductal orientated sonography improves the diagnosis of pathological nipple discharge of the female breast compared with galactography. Eur J Cancer Prev. 7 Suppl 1:S57-62, 1998
4. Cardenosa G et al: Ductography of the breast: technique and findings. AJR Am J Roentgenol. 162:1081-7, 1994

IMAGE GALLERY

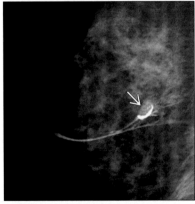 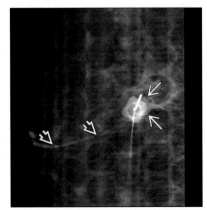 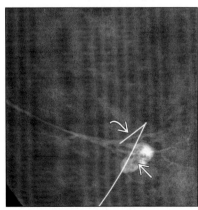

(Left) Lateral galactography shows filling defect ➡ remote from nipple in 53 year old woman with brownish-colored discharge. This was not apparent on US. (Center) Lateral mammography shows galactographic needle localization (same patient as previous image). After contrast was injected, filling defect ➡ was localized from a medial approach. Note contrast in duct leading to lesion ➡. (Right) CC mammography (same patient as previous image) confirms hookwire ➡ is appropriately positioned near filling defect ➡. Pathology: Benign intraductal papilloma.

FINE NEEDLE ASPIRATION BIOPSY

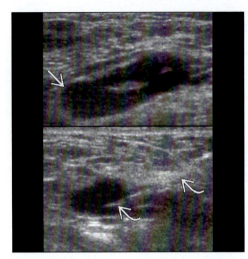

US shows enlarged axillary node with thickened cortex ➡. 21-g needle ➜ was used to perform FNAB under US-guidance using suction technique. Smears were prepared and material was sent for cell block.

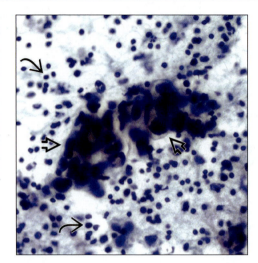

Cytology, high power, shows clump of large, irregular epithelial cells ⟡ in background of small blue lymphocytes ➜. The diagnosis of lymph node metastasis from breast cancer is easily made on FNAB.

TERMINOLOGY

Abbreviations
- Fine needle aspiration (FNA) biopsy (FNAB)

Definitions
- Percutaneous sampling of a suspicious lesion using a small, 22 to 25-gauge needle for cytologic diagnosis
- "Aspiration" if only fluid, FNAB if for solid mass

PRE-PROCEDURE

Indications
- Suspected axillary nodal metastasis
- Suspicious palpable mass; core biopsy problematic or not available
  - Anticoagulation therapy cannot be safely discontinued (note: Core biopsy can be performed , varies by center)
- Probable complicated cyst
  - Contents: Thick fluid or solid
    - Most commonly small mass, ≤ 8 mm, aspirated under US guidance

Contraindications
- Lack of adequately trained cytopathologist
- Calcifications without a mass

Getting Started
- Things to Check
  - Usually done with imaging guidance
    - Ultrasound (most common)
    - Mammography (stereotactic guidance)
- Equipment List
  - When possible, US is guidance method of choice
    - > 7 MHz linear transducer
    - Sterile probe, usually covered

  - Stereotactic prone table or add-on upright unit
  - 22 to 25-g needles, 5-10 cc syringes
  - Slides or liquid-based ThinPrep specimen
  - Betadine or other method to sterilize skin
  - 1% lidocaine ± buffered with sodium bicarbonate

PROCEDURE

Patient Position/Location
- Patient supine for US-guided approach; prone or upright for stereotactic approach

Procedure Steps
- Skin overlying lesion cleansed in standard fashion
- Application of local anesthetic
- Image-guided needle placement
  - Real-time US monitoring during needle placement
  - Confirmation of needle placement with +15 and -15 stereotactic views
- Meticulous technique essential
  - Once needle in lesion, confirmed on imaging guidance, apply continuous suction via syringe
  - Capillary technique (without suction) can be used
  - To-and-fro shearing or jabbing motion, collect cells in needle/syringe
    - 5-10 excursions usually sufficient
    - Needle angle varied between excursions → broad region of lesion sampled
    - Stop if/when blood obtained
- Suction released before needle removed from lesion
- Needle detached from syringe, air sucked into syringe, then needle reattached
- Two options for specimen preparation
  - Conventional smears
    - Immediate on-site preparation by radiologist, cytopathologist or assistant

FINE NEEDLE ASPIRATION BIOPSY

Key Facts

Terminology
- Percutaneous sampling of a suspicious lesion using a small, 22 to 25-gauge needle for cytologic diagnosis

Pre-procedure
- When possible, US is guidance method of choice

Problems & Complications
- Limited usefulness for breast lesions

- Unacceptably high insufficient sampling rate for breast masses: 10% (US-guided) to 40% (stereotactic)
- Worse for calcifications: 49% insufficient samples
- Bloody aspirates may limit sampling and diagnosis
- Small, blood-filled lesions may disappear
- Consider post-procedure clip placement
- Non-diagnostic procedure, need for repeat biopsy

- ■ Material in needle gently pushed onto slides: Air-dried or wet-fixed
- ○ Liquid-based ThinPrep (cytological preservative)
  - ■ Aspirate from syringe submitted in preservative for automated processing of cell block
- ○ Papanicolaou stain, Giemsa, or modified Giemsa (e.g., Diff-Quik) for smears, H&E for cell block

Alternative Procedures/Therapies
- Radiologic
  - ○ Core needle biopsy (CNB) with image guidance
    - ■ More accurate than FNAB
    - ■ Provides specific histopathologic diagnosis
    - ■ Usually distinguish invasive from noninvasive cancer → appropriate surgical management
- Surgical: Needle-localized excision; FNAB or CNB without image guidance if palpable (higher miss rate)

POST-PROCEDURE

Expected Outcome
- Lymph nodes
  - ○ Epithelial cells imply metastasis
  - ○ Monomorphic lymphocytes suspicious for lymphoma: Recommend core biopsy or excision
  - ○ Heterogeneous population of lymphocytes in reactive nodes
- Insufficient, atypical, suspicious results → rebiopsy or excision
- Cyst contents: Proteinaceous debris, macrophages, old blood, may be acellular

PROBLEMS & COMPLICATIONS

Problems
- Limited usefulness for breast lesions
  - ○ Unacceptably high insufficient sampling rate for breast masses: 10% (US-guided) to 40% (stereotactic)
  - ○ Worse for calcifications: 49% insufficient samples
  - ○ Less accurate than core biopsy
- Bloody aspirates may limit sampling and diagnosis
- Small, blood-filled lesions may disappear
  - ○ Consider post-procedure clip placement

Complications
- Most feared complication(s)
  - ○ Non-diagnostic procedure, need for repeat biopsy
    - ■ Bleeding, infection rare
- Other complications
  - ○ Vasovagal reaction (uncommon)
    - ■ Possible when patient upright (e.g., add-on stereotactic mammography unit)

SELECTED REFERENCES

1. Pisano ED et al: Fine-needle aspiration biopsy of nonpalpable breast lesions in a multicenter clinical trial: results from the radiologic diagnostic oncology group V. Radiology. 219(3):785-92, 2001
2. Dowlatshahi K et al: Nonpalpable breast lesions: findings of stereotaxic needle-core biopsy and fine-needle aspiration cytology. Radiology. 181(3):745-50, 1991
3. Schmidt R et al: Benefits of stereotactic aspiration cytology. Adm Radiol. 9(10):35-6, 39, 41-2, 1990

IMAGE GALLERY

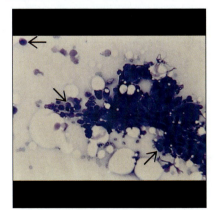 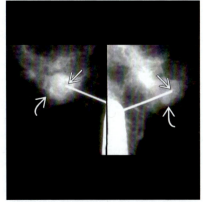 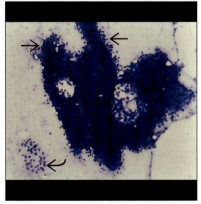

(Left) Diff-Quik stained aspirate (160x) shows loose aggregates of atypical epithelial cells w/large nuclei ➡, consistent w/ductal carcinoma. *(Center)* Stereotactic images show 22-g needle ➡ in center of mass ➡ in 38 year old asymptomatic woman. Rapid passes were made through mass w/suction technique, & smears prepared. *(Right)* Cytology specimen (same patient as previous image), stained w/Diff Quik (40x), shows cohesive epithelial cells w/small nuclei ➡ in "antler-horn" configuration ➡ characteristic of fibroadenoma, & concordant w/imaging findings.

MR-GUIDED VACUUM-ASSISTED BIOPSY

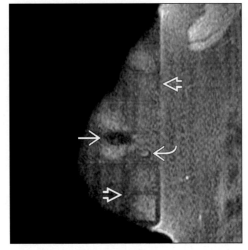

Sagittal T1WI FS MR shows grid ➡ compressing breast, with artifact from obturator ➡ and localizing fiducial ➡ in place.

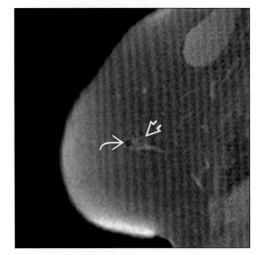

Sagittal T1WI FS MR image (same as left) shows obturator artifact ➡ confirming location within enhancing target lesion ➡. Pathology: Grade I invasive ductal cancer.

TERMINOLOGY

Definitions
- Percutaneous MR-guided core breast biopsy using vacuum-assisted devices
  - Biopsy itself typically performed outside the magnet (unless open bore)
  - MR used to identify lesion, confirm plastic cannula tip at edge of lesion, and confirm clip at biopsy site
- Important component to facility offering breast MR
- May be performed either with a grid or free-hand
- Obturator: MR-compatible plastic stylet used while imaging to confirm proper placement of coaxial cannula
- Trocar: Metallic stylet to aid insertion of plastic cannula
- Targeted US: US directed to MR abnormality
- Fiducial marker: T1-hyperintense marker on skin surface (vitamin E or fish oil capsule, Gd-impregnated marker)
- Grid: Fenestrated compression paddle
- Template: Paper, clear sheet of film, or software to record location of lesion with respect to fiducial
  - Facilitates 90° translation of images as viewed on scanner to prone position of patient

PRE-PROCEDURE

Indications
- Suspicious lesion detected on MR
- Lesion seen only on MR: Unable to biopsy lesion using US or stereotactic guidance

Contraindications
- Same as for general MR examinations (e.g., pacemaker, other metallic implants, etc.)

- Breast implants: Relative contraindication; possible if lesion far enough removed from implant surface
- Extreme posterior lesions: If unable to include in grid
- Very large breasts may demonstrate anterior "puddling" as breast rests on gantry top; may limit access to anterior lesions
- Very thin breast (< 3 cm): Can use reverse compression paddle with open grids on both sides of breast
  - "Build up" breast thickness with positioning maneuvers as in stereotactic biopsy
- Very small lesion (< 5 mm): Very low rate of malignancy (3%), technical success may be reduced

Getting Started
- Things to Check
  - MR safety questionnaire
  - Staff must ensure safety within MR environment
    - Remove metallic objects, cards with magnetic stripe, etc.
  - Establish need for biopsy using MR
    - Review of current mammography, US (targeted US often helpful)
    - Limit hormonal influence by scheduling MR at days 7-14 after onset of menses
  - Discontinue anticoagulants; variable per facility
- Medications
  - Pre-medication for claustrophobic patient
    - Typically benzodiazepine
  - Pre-medication if history of known Gd-contrast reaction
    - Oral steroids, diphenhydramine
- Equipment List
  - Closed-bore magnet, high field strength (≥ 1.5 T)
  - Open-bore magnets
    - Disadvantage: < 1.5 T generally considered insufficient for quality breast imaging; may be acceptable for interventional procedures
  - Dedicated breast coil

MR-GUIDED VACUUM-ASSISTED BIOPSY

Key Facts

Pre-procedure
- Suspicious lesion detected on MR
- Staff must ensure safety within MR environment
- Closed-bore magnet, high field strength (≥ 1.5 T)
- Dedicated breast coil
- MR-compatible equipment

Procedure
- Prone positioning within dedicated breast coil, grid with compression
- Review all appropriate imaging: Assure lesion persists on immediate pre-biopsy diagnostic MR
- Image: Verify tip of plastic obturator (signal void) at target
- Obtain 6-12 samples with 11-g or larger biopsy device
- Place clip at biopsy site

- Significant rate of malignancy among lesions occult at targeted US: 6-14% → need for MR-guided biopsy

Post-procedure
- 96-97% of lesions successfully biopsied, 95% successful clip deployment
- 25-37% malignant: Most series > 50% DCIS
- Radiologic-pathologic concordance critical
- Consider post-biopsy MR to verify lesion removal
- Atypical or high-risk lesion should prompt excision

Problems & Complications
- Lesion non-visualization at time of biopsy
- Up to 13% of biopsies canceled due to nonvisualization: 10% malignant on follow-up
- No MR sequence for specimen imaging

- Required for diagnostic/screening breast MR
- Used in conjunction with grid or free-hand technique
- Allows for lateral and medial approaches
○ MR-compatible equipment
  - Fiducial marker, biopsy clip
  - 10-14 cm long open plastic cannula, obturator
  - Light: MR-compatible, or (standard) flashlight held away from magnet
○ Biopsy equipment used outside the magnet bore
  - Standard syringe/needle(s) for local anesthesia; scalpel
  - Coaxial metal stylet/trocar to advance plastic cannula
  - Vacuum-assisted biopsy device and probe: Hand-held, designed for MR-biopsy
  - Many devices have lengthy tubing connecting to vacuum canister outside of scanning room
○ Grid compression paddle, needle guide (optional)

PROCEDURE

Patient Position/Location
- Best procedure approach
  ○ Prone positioning within dedicated breast coil, grid with compression
    - Compression minimizes breast motion and breast thickness; consistent lesion location
    - Avoid overly tight compression (vascular compression hinders enhancement)
  ○ Lateral approach
    - Technically easier for operator
  ○ Medial approach when required, more technically challenging
    - Patient obliquely positioned with right breast in left breast coil (for example)
    - Non-imaged breast (and left side of patient) must be accommodated on upper coil surface
    - Due to oblique position, access to posteromedial lesions may be problematic

- Alternatively, right breast can be positioned in right breast coil with left coil opening covered
- Here, the operator must lean further under the coil to reach exposed medial breast surface

Procedure Steps
- Review all appropriate imaging: Assure lesion persists on immediate pre-biopsy diagnostic MR
- Position patient in breast coil with grid in place
- Imaging performed in magnet bore; all other steps outside magnet bore
- Place fiducial marker on skin near expected lesion location
- Perform T1WI scout sequence
  ○ Ensure inclusion of breast tissue, grid, fiducial
  ○ Note coordinate location of fiducial marker on template
- Inject intravenous Gd-contrast
- Image with T1WI FS technique
  ○ Subtraction may be necessary to visualize lesion
  ○ If lesion no longer seen, biopsy canceled
    - Ensure successful injection of Gd-contrast; follow-up
  ○ Compare fiducial and enhancing target lesion locations, recording each on template
  ○ Alternative: Proprietary integrated lesion localization software (e.g. on computer-assisted detection software)
- Mark skin entry site relative to known position of fiducial marker
- Prepare area in usual sterile fashion
- Instill lidocaine into marked entry site
- Perform dermatotomy through skin wheal
- Use needle guide electively
  ○ Advance trocar through guide: Secure guide in grid box before or after placing trocar in skin incision
- Advance plastic cannula/coaxial metal trocar to calculated depth
- Remove metal trocar, insert plastic obturator
- Image: Verify tip of plastic obturator (signal void) at target
  ○ At superficial edge or center of lesion (varies by device)

- ○ Require additional ~ 2 cm depth from imaged stylet tip to projected full extension of biopsy probe
- Remove obturator, insert biopsy probe into plastic cannula
- Obtain 6-12 samples with 11-g or larger biopsy device
  - ○ Can sample circumferentially if centered in lesion or eccentrically, e.g. anteriorly, if cannula/probe are e.g. along posterior aspect of lesion
- Place clip at biopsy site
- Post-biopsy MR images of entire breast, sagittal only or sagittal and axial
  - ○ Demonstrate post-biopsy findings, removal of lesion
  - ○ Post-biopsy hematoma hyperintense on T1WI, may obscure site
    - ■ Non-visualization may not = lesion removal
  - ○ Demonstrate clip position relative to location of abnormality
- Post-biopsy CC and 90° lateral mammogram to document clip position

Findings and Reporting

- Convey to pathologist size of lesion & expected result
- Report from procedure
  - ○ Lesion size, location, morphology, kinetics
  - ○ # Specimens, gauge, clip placement, complications
  - ○ Specimen radiography if performed (optional); post-biopsy mammogram
- Addend with pathology findings, concordance (or not), management recommendations

Alternative Procedures/Therapies

- Radiologic
  - ○ MR-guided core biopsy: Usually 14-g
    - ■ Approach similar to vacuum-assisted biopsy
  - ○ Targeted US (rarely stereotactic) biopsy
    - ■ Highly variable success with targeted US, 23-89% success (averaging 55% across 3 series)
    - ■ Significant rate of malignancy among lesions occult at targeted US: 6-14% → need for MR-guided biopsy
- Surgical: MR-guided needle localization and excision
- Other: Short-interval MR follow-up

POST-PROCEDURE

Expected Outcome

- 30-45 minute procedure
- Technical success rates: 87-96% lesions visualized at time of biopsy
  - ○ 96-97% of lesions successfully biopsied, 95% successful clip deployment
  - ○ 25-37% malignant: Most series > 50% DCIS
    - ■ DCIS over-represented in lesions seen only at MR

Things To Do

- Radiologic-pathologic concordance critical
  - ○ If discordant, action depends on clinical judgment
    - ■ Mammography-guided localization of clip or relative to clip
  - ○ Consider post-biopsy MR to verify lesion removal
- Atypical or high-risk lesion should prompt excision
  - ○ ~ 25-29% upgraded to malignancy

PROBLEMS & COMPLICATIONS

Problems

- Lesion non-visualization at time of biopsy
  - ○ Extravasation of contrast, failed contrast injection
  - ○ Ensure compression not overly tight
  - ○ Obtain follow-up MR to verify resolution of finding
  - ○ Up to 13% of biopsies canceled due to nonvisualization: 10% malignant on follow-up
- Rapid washout of lesion during biopsy
  - ○ "Vanishing target": Proceed quickly; may re-bolus
- Bilateral/multi-site biopsy
  - ○ Position cannulae/obturators at both sites initially
    - ■ Verify position with one imaging sequence
    - ■ Proceed with biopsy and clip placement both sites
  - ○ Allow 20 minutes between sites if re-bolus Gd-contrast
- Cost
- No MR sequence for specimen imaging
  - ○ MR enhancement does not persist ex vivo

Complications

- Most feared complication(s)
  - ○ Adverse reaction to Gd-contrast
    - ■ Idiosyncratic; variable severity
    - ■ Less common than with iodinated contrast
- Clip migration along track when compression released ("accordion effect")
- Patient inability to complete procedure
  - ○ Pre-medication if needed

SELECTED REFERENCES

1. Ghate SV et al: MRI-guided vacuum-assisted breast biopsy with a handheld portable biopsy system. AJR. 186:1733-6, 2006
2. Liberman L et al: Does size matter? Positive predictive value of MRI-detected breast lesions as a function of lesion size. AJR. 186:426-30, 2006
3. Orel SG et al: MR imaging-guided 9-gauge vacuum-assisted core-needle breast biopsy: initial experience. Radiology. 238:54-61, 2006
4. Perlet C et al: Magnetic resonance-guided, vacuum-assisted breast biopsy: results from a European multicenter study of 538 lesions. Cancer. 106:982-90, 2006
5. Beran L et al: Correlation of targeted ultrasound with magnetic resonance imaging abnormalities of the breast. Am J Surg. 190:592-4, 2005
6. Lehman CD et al: Clinical experience with MRI-guided vacuum-assisted breast biopsy. AJR. 184:1782-7, 2005
7. Liberman L et al: MRI-guided 9-gauge vacuum-assisted breast biopsy: initial clinical experience. AJR. 185:183-93, 2005
8. Morris EA et al: Breast MRI: Diagnosis and Intervention. 1st ed. Springer, New York. 297-315, 2005
9. Sim LS et al: US correlation for MRI-detected breast lesions in women with familial risk of breast cancer. Clin Radiol. 60:801-6, 2005
10. Hefler L et al: Follow-up of breast lesions detected by MRI not biopsied due to absent enhancement of contrast medium. Eur Radiol. 13:344-6, 2003
11. LaTrenta LR et al: Breast lesions detected with MR imaging: utility and histopathologic importance of identification with US. Radiology. 227:856-61, 2003

MR-GUIDED VACUUM-ASSISTED BIOPSY

IMAGE GALLERY

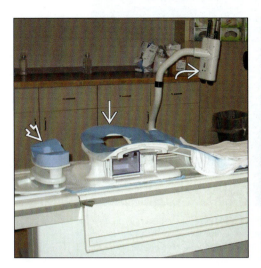

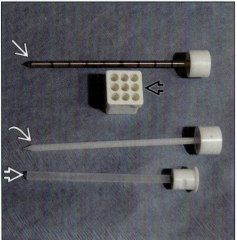

(Left) The bilateral breast coil ➡ may be accessed from a lateral or medial approach, with the patient in a prone position (head support ➡). Contrast injection is via power injector ➡. (Right) Photograph shows coaxial metal trocar ➡ used to initially advance hollow plastic cannula ➡ through optional needle guide ➡ to the desired depth. The metal stylet is then removed and replaced by plastic obturator stylet ➡ for MR imaging.

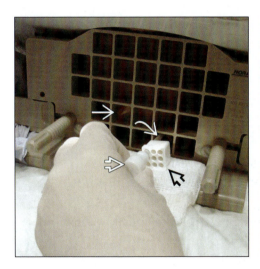

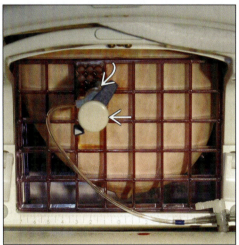

(Left) Metal trocar ➡ in plastic cannula ➡ is inserted in skin incision first, then needle guide ➡ is moved into position in grid box. Note nearby fish oil fiducial ➡ and (typically) poor lighting conditions. (Right) After removing metal trocar, a plastic stylet (obturator) ➡ is introduced in cannula ➡ allowing post-placement imaging. Neither the metal trocar nor biopsy needle can be imaged because of large artifacts.

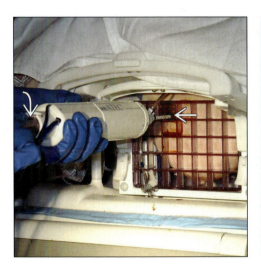

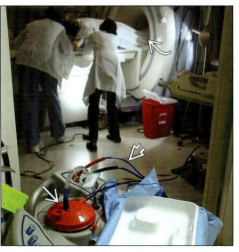

(Left) Following verification of alignment with enhancing target lesion, probe ➡ is placed through the plastic sheath & rotated to obtain samples which, in this device, are collected in a posterior enclosed chamber ➡. (Right) The procedure is performed with the patient lying prone within the dedicated breast coil on the gantry outside the bore ➡. Vacuum canister ➡ remains outside the immediate magnet area attached to the needle via tubing ➡.

PRE-OP LESION LOCALIZATION, BRACKETING

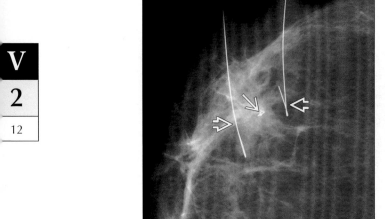

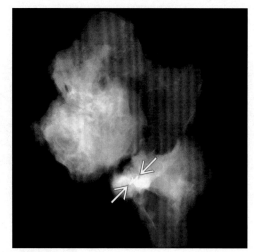

CC mammography shows clip ➡ from prior US guided vacuum-assisted biopsy, flanked by localizing wires ➡ in right upper outer quadrant of a 46 year-old woman. Radial scar diagnosis prompted excision.

Specimen radiograph of preceding case confirms that clip ➡ was excised. Final pathology revealed radial scar, florid ductal epithelial hyperplasia and fibroadenoma.

TERMINOLOGY

Definitions
- Image-guided localization of breast lesion, using two or more wires, prior to surgical excision
  - Assists surgeon in excising entire lesion by delineating extent of abnormality
  - Mammographic, US, or MR guidance

PRE-PROCEDURE

Indications
- Known cancer(s), at least some of which is nonpalpable, ≈ > 2 and < 5 cm in diameter
- Most often performed for malignant Ca++
- > 2 cm area of Ca++ highly suggestive of malignancy for which direct excision is performed
- Nonpalpable high-risk or locally aggressive lesion for which wide excision desired, e.g., phyllodes tumor

Contraindications
- Lesion(s) not appropriate for lumpectomy, e.g., small breast size relative to size of cancer
- Small lesion(s) which could be adequately localized and excised with a single wire
- Low suspicion lesion(s) for which excision would yield cosmetic defect: Initial core biopsy preferred

Getting Started
- Things to Check
  - Initial diagnosis by percutaneous core biopsy recommended
  - Surgeon's approval: Essential in balancing potential competing interests of good cosmesis & adequate excision
- Medications: 1% lidocaine ± sodium bicarbonate (buffering agent)

- Localization needles and wires
- Betadine or other skin disinfectant
- Rigid, fenestrated mammographic localizing paddle
  - Alpha-numeric grid for precise placement of needles
  - Open window or perforated hole plate
- Ruler to measure skin-to-lesion distance

PROCEDURE

Patient Position/Location
- Choose shortest distance from skin to lesion over largest diameter of lesion
  - Parallel to chest wall
- Best if entire lesion to be localized fits within window of localization paddle

Procedure Steps
- Informed, written consent
  - Explain that more than one wire will be used
- Patient positioned upright in mammography unit, breast in compression, paddle open at skin entry sites
- Ink marks placed on skin to detect patient movement
  - At corners of open window device
  - Around inner perimeter of perforated holes
- Scout film obtained with patient in compression
  - Coordinates of each point to be localized determined
    - Two wires usually adequate to define longest dimension of lesion: Anterior-posterior, superior-inferior or medial-lateral
- Skin disinfected
- Local anesthesia: 1-3 cc lidocaine per site
- Needles advanced to appropriate depth, following path of X-ray beam
  - Most posterior needle placed first → maximizes unobstructed access for subsequent needle placement

PRE-OP LESION LOCALIZATION, BRACKETING

Key Facts

Terminology
- Image-guided localization of breast lesion, using two or more wires, prior to surgical excision
- Assists surgeon in excising entire lesion by delineating extent of abnormality
- Mammographic, US, or MR guidance

Pre-procedure
- Initial diagnosis by percutaneous core biopsy recommended

Procedure
- Choose shortest distance from skin to lesion over largest diameter of lesion
- Best if entire lesion to be localized fits within window of localization paddle

Post-procedure
- Complete removal of imaging finding(s): 81% one series
- High risk of positive margins: 56% in one series

- ○ Field localizing light used for guidance
  - ▪ Shadows of needle hubs should superimpose on skin entry sites
- Radiograph obtained to verify that needle tips project over targeted areas
- Compression paddle removed
  - ○ May be most challenging part of procedure
    - ▪ All needles must be individually secured to prevent inadvertent removal by advancing paddle
- Patient repositioned for orthogonal projection
- Radiograph obtained to assess depth of needles
  - ○ Needles adjusted to desired positions
    - ▪ Rigid needle systems: Curved J-wires deployed, needles left in place
    - ▪ Hookwire systems: Wires deployed, needles removed
- Final radiograph obtained
  - ○ Wires should be within 5 mm of lesion(s) with tips through and < 1 cm deep to lesion(s)
- Final radiograph and film of wires passing through lesion(s) on orthogonal view sent to OR
  - ○ Individual wire positions should be clearly marked on films: e.g., anterior, posterior, superior
  - ○ Distance from skin entry site to lesion and wire tip should be documented for each wire
- May need to annotate wires themselves with tape markers e.g., "A", "B"
- Specimen radiograph required
  - ○ Must account for all wires used in procedure
  - ○ Call findings to surgeon while patient still in OR

- ▪ Verify lesion(s) included, location relative to margins, hookwires included ± intact
- ○ Annotate specimen in container or by placing needles for pathologist as needed

Alternative Procedures/Therapies
- Stereotactic placement of needles
  - ○ Less accurate in depth determination

POST-PROCEDURE

Expected Outcome
- Complete removal of imaging finding(s): 81% one series
- High risk of positive margins: 56% in one series

PROBLEMS & COMPLICATIONS

Complications
- Most feared complication(s): Vasovagal reaction, missed localization
- Other complications: Infection, bleeding, retained wire fragments and wire migration

SELECTED REFERENCES
1. Bassett LW et al: Diseases of the Breast, 2nd Ed. Philadelphia, Elsevier Saunders. Chapter 15, 266, 2005
2. Liberman L et al: Bracketing wires for preoperative breast needle localization. Am J Roentgenol. 177(3):565-72, 2001

IMAGE GALLERY

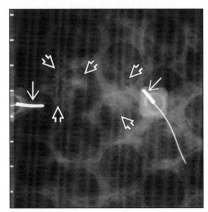 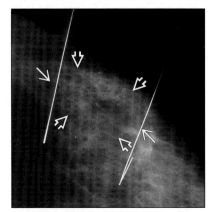 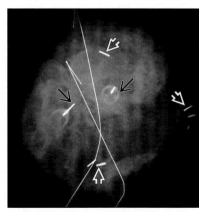

(Left) Lateral mammography with localization grid demonstrates ➡ two needles bracketing widespread pleomorphic Ca++ ➡ in a 46 year old asymptomatic woman. *(Center)* CC mammography (same as previous) shows successful deployment of hookwires ➡ which surround the Ca++ ➡. *(Right)* Specimen radiograph (same as prior 2 images) confirms that the Ca++, marked for pathologist with hypodermic needles ➡, were excised. Pathology revealed high-grade DCIS with comedonecrosis. Clips ➡ placed by surgeon. Initial margins very close, negative at reexcision.

PRE-OP LESION LOCALIZATION, MAMMO

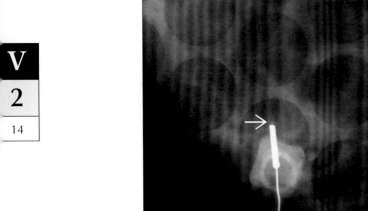

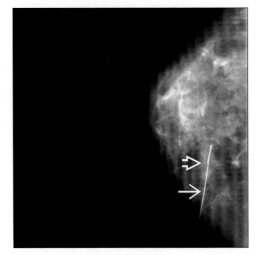

Lateral mammography shows grid in place over medial aspect of left breast after needle placement for localization of calcifications ➡. *The tissue was too thin for stereotactic biopsy.*

CC mammography of prior case after needle removal shows hookwire ➡ *in place. The tip of the wire is just distal to the calcifications* ➡. *Pathology revealed benign breast tissue with calcifications.*

TERMINOLOGY

Synonyms
- Pre-operative needle/wire placement

Definitions
- Mammographically-guided localization of non-palpable breast lesion(s) prior to surgical excision

PRE-PROCEDURE

Indications
- Known non-palpable malignancy or high-risk lesion
  - Prior percutaneous biopsy (± clip placement)
- Diagnostic surgical biopsy of non-palpable lesion(s) not amenable to image-guided biopsy
  - Architectural distortion on mammogram (no underlying mass detected by US) e.g., radial scar
  - Widely distributed suspicious calcifications
    - Possible insufficient sampling stereotactically
  - Lesion not amenable to stereotactic biopsy
    - Breast tissue too thin (< 3 cm), not able to be "thickened" by foam support
    - Extreme posterior or immediate subareolar location

Contraindications
- Lesion(s) not clearly visible by mammography
  - Localize by modality where depicted: e.g., US, MR
- Clearly benign finding, biopsy not warranted

Getting Started
- Things to Check
  - Pre-operative mammograms
    - Lesion should be visualized in two orthogonal views: CC and 90° lateral
- Medications: 1% lidocaine ± sodium bicarbonate

- Equipment List
  - Mammographic unit
    - X-ray tube and image receptor must rotate 180° allowing inferior approach when needed
  - Localizing device
    - Rigid-needle system (needle and J-wire): Needle left in place, curved J-wire advanced into tissue
    - Hook-wire system (needle and barb-type wire): Needle removed after wire deployed
    - Various needle lengths available (choose based on skin-to-lesion distance)
  - Fenestrated mammographic localizing paddle
    - Alpha-numeric grid for precise needle placement
    - Open window or holes
  - Ruler to measure skin to wire tip (lesion) distance
  - Localizing dye (optional, not widely used, causes discomfort)
    - Methylene blue dye (interferes with estrogen/progesterone receptor (ER/PR) assay); isosulfan blue, no interference

PROCEDURE

Patient Position/Location
- Best procedure approach: Shortest distance from skin to lesion (parallel to chest wall)

Procedure Steps
- Informed, written consent
- Patient positioned upright in mammography unit, breast in compression, paddle against skin entry site
  - Ink marks placed on skin to detect patient movement
    - At corners of open window device
    - Around inner perimeter of holes with hole plate
- Scout film obtained with patient in compression
  - Magnification can be used if needed: Patient stands

PRE-OP LESION LOCALIZATION, MAMMO

Key Facts

Terminology
- Mammographically-guided localization of non-palpable breast lesion(s) prior to surgical excision

Pre-procedure
- Lesion should be visualized in two orthogonal views: CC and 90° lateral

Procedure
- Coordinates of lesion determined from scout image

- Needle advanced to appropriate depth, following path of X-ray beam
- Orthogonal view obtained to assess depth of needle
- Wire should be within 5 mm of lesion, tip through and < 1 cm deep to lesion
- Specimen radiograph required

Problems & Complications
- Vasovagal reaction, lesion not excised (3%)

- ○ Patient left in compression while image developed
- ○ Coordinates of lesion determined from scout image
- Skin cleansed with Betadine or sterile soap
- Local anesthesia obtained: 1-3 ml of 1% lidocaine and sodium bicarbonate
- Needle advanced to appropriate depth, following path of X-ray beam
  - ○ Field localizing light used for guidance
    - ■ Shadow of needle hub should superimpose on skin entry site
- Radiograph to verify needle tip projects over lesion
- Compression paddle removed → patient repositioned
- Orthogonal view obtained to assess depth of needle
  - ○ Needle adjusted to desired position
    - ■ Rigid needle system: Curved J-wire deployed, needle left in place
    - ■ Hookwire system: Hookwire deployed, needle removed
- Final radiograph obtained, skin entry in target or marked with BB
  - ○ Wire should be within 5 mm of lesion, tip through and < 1 cm deep to lesion
- Final radiograph and film of wire passing through lesion on orthogonal view sent to OR
  - ○ Radiologist should indicate on film distance from skin entry site to lesion and wire tip
- Specimen radiograph required
  - ○ Call findings to surgeon while patient still in OR
    - ■ Verify lesion inclusion, location relative to margins and +/- intact wire
  - ○ Mark lesion location(s) for pathologist

- Note: Digital technique reduces procedure time 50%

POST-PROCEDURE

Expected Outcome
- Accurate localization and excision of lesion

Things To Avoid
- Excessive compression
- Stereotactic placement (less accurate for depth determination due to accordion effect)

PROBLEMS & COMPLICATIONS

Complications
- Most feared complication(s): Vasovagal reaction, lesion not excised (3%)
- Other complications: Bleeding, infection, retained wire fragments and wire migration

SELECTED REFERENCES

1. Bassett LW et al: Diagnosis of Diseases of the Breast. 2nd Edition. Philadelphia, Elsevier & Saunders. Chapter 16, 263-72, 2005
2. Jackman RJ et al: Needle-localized breast biopsy: why do we fail? Radiology. 204(3):677-84, 1997
3. Homer MJ: Localization of nonpalpable breast lesions with the curved-end, retractable wire: leaving the needle in vivo. AJR Am J Roentgenol. 151(5):919-20, 1988

IMAGE GALLERY

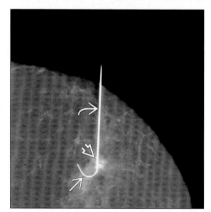 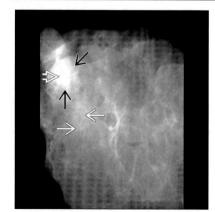 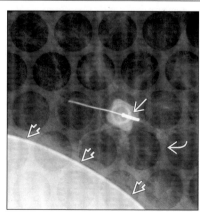

(Left) CC mammography shows rigid needle ➡ and J-wire ➡ in place after localization of clip ➡ placed at stereotactic biopsy of low-grade DCIS in a 79 year old woman. *(Center)* Specimen mammography (same patient as previous image) shows clip ➡, post-stereo hematoma ➡ and residual Ca++ ➡. Pathology: Invasive ductal carcinoma and low-grade DCIS. *(Right)* Lateral mammography demonstrates localizing needle ➡, grid ➡, and implant ➡ in a 65 year old woman. A spiculated lesion was successfully localized. Pathology: Invasive ductal carcinoma.

PRE-OP LESION LOCALIZATION, MRI

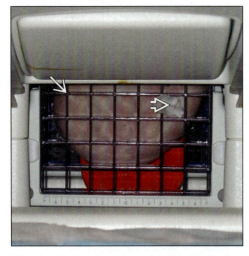

Clinical photograph shows left breast in light compression within grid ➡️ (medial approach shown, patient's head to right). Fiducial marker ⇥ is secured with tape near expected location of the abnormality.

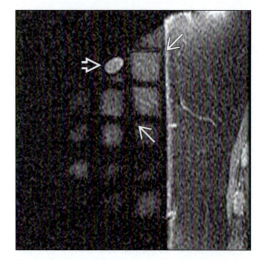

The patient is moved back into bore of the magnet and sagittal T1 FS images are obtained to confirm the area of interest is included in the grid ➡️, expected to be near the fiducial marker ⇥ (same as left).

TERMINOLOGY

Definitions
- MR-guided pre-operative needle localization with wire placement prior to surgical excision
- Targeted US: US directed to MR abnormality
- Fiducial marker: T1-hyperintense marker to place on skin surface (vitamin E or fish oil capsule, Gd-impregnated marker)
- Grid: Fenestrated compression paddle
- Template: Paper, clear sheet of film, or software system to record location of lesion with respect to fiducial
  - Facilitates 90° translation of images as viewed on scanner to prone position of patient

PRE-PROCEDURE

Indications
- Suspicious lesion seen best or only on MR
  - Unable to confidently localize using mammographic, stereotactic, or US guidance
  - Patient prefers excision to initial MR-guided vacuum-assisted biopsy (MRVAB)
  - Initial MRVAB missed lesion or additional MR-only lesions
  - MR demonstrated wider extent of disease than either mammography or US
    - Initial MRVAB preferred over surgery due to false positives on MR imaging

Contraindications
- Same as for general MR examinations (e.g., pacemaker, other metallic implants, etc.)
- Breast implants: Relative contraindication; possible if lesion far enough removed from implant surface
- Extreme posterior lesions: If unable to include in grid

- Very large breasts may demonstrate anterior "puddling" as breast rests on gantry top; may limit access to anterior lesions
- Very thin breast (< 3 cm): Can use reverse compression paddle with open grids on both sides of breast
  - "Build up" breast thickness with positioning maneuvers as in stereotactic biopsy
- Very small lesion(s): < 5 mm very low rate of malignancy (3%), consider follow-up

Getting Started
- Things to Check
  - MR safety questionnaire
  - Staff must ensure safety within MR environment
    - Remove metallic objects, cards with magnetic stripe
  - Establish need for biopsy using MR
    - Review of current mammography, US (targeted US often helpful)
    - Limit hormonal influence by scheduling MR at days 7-14 after onset of menses
  - Discontinue anticoagulants
- Medications
  - Pre-medication for claustrophobic patient
    - Typically benzodiazepine
  - Pre-medication if history of known Gd-contrast reaction
    - Oral steroids, diphenhydramine
- Equipment List
  - Closed-bore magnet, high field strength ≥1.5 Tesla
  - Open-bore magnets
    - Minimize patient claustrophobia
    - Disadvantage: < 1.5 T generally considered insufficient for quality breast imaging; may be acceptable for interventional procedures
  - Dedicated breast coil: Grid or free-hand
  - MR-compatible equipment
    - Fiducial marker

PRE-OP LESION LOCALIZATION, MRI

Key Facts

Terminology
- MR-guided pre-operative needle localization with wire placement prior to surgical excision

Pre-procedure
- Suspicious lesion seen best or only on MR
- Review of current mammography, US (targeted US often helpful)
- Closed-bore magnet, high field strength ≥1.5 Tesla
- Dedicated breast coil: Grid or free-hand
- MR-compatible hookwire needle system

Procedure
- Prone positioning within dedicated breast coil, grid with compression
- Place the fiducial marker on skin near expected lesion location

- Perform T1WI scout sequence
- Inject intravenous Gd-contrast
- Compare fiducial and enhancing target lesion locations
- Insert MR-compatible hollow needle to calculated depth
- Deploy hookwire through hollow needle, desiring hook to be within 1 cm deep to lesion

Post-procedure
- Technical success rates 93-100%
- Positive predictive value for cancer 31-73%

Problems & Complications
- Lesion non-visualization at time of localization
- No MR sequence for specimen imaging
- Inaccurate hookwire placement relative to lesion

- MR-compatible hookwire needle system
- Light: MR-compatible, or (standard) flashlight held away from magnet
  - Biopsy equipment used outside magnet bore
    - Standard syringe/needle(s) for local anesthesia
  - Grid compression paddle, needle guide (optional)

PROCEDURE

Patient Position/Location
- Best procedure approach
  - Prone positioning within dedicated breast coil, grid with compression
    - Compression minimizes motion; consistent lesion location
    - Avoid overly tight compression (vascular compression hinders enhancement)
  - Lateral approach: Technically easier for operator
  - Medial approach when required, more technically challenging
    - Patient obliquely positioned with right breast in left breast coil (for example)
    - Non-imaged breast (and left side of patient) must be accommodated on upper coil surface
    - Due to oblique position, access to posteromedial lesions may be problematic
    - Alternatively, the right breast can be positioned in right breast coil with left breast coil opening covered
    - Operator must lean further under the coil to reach exposed medial breast surface

Procedure Steps
- Review all appropriate imaging: Ensure lesion persists on immediate pre-biopsy diagnostic MR
- Position patient in breast coil with grid in place
- Place the fiducial marker on skin near expected lesion location
- Perform T1WI scout sequence
  - Ensure inclusion of breast tissue, grid, fiducial
  - Note coordinate location of fiducial marker on template

- Inject intravenous Gd-contrast
- Image with T1WI FS technique
  - Subtraction may be necessary to visualize lesion
  - If lesion no longer seen, procedure canceled
    - Ensure successful injection of Gd-contrast
  - Compare fiducial and enhancing target lesion locations
    - Record coordinate location of lesion in three planes
    - Determine depth of lesion from skin entry site
  - Alternative: Proprietary integrated lesion localization software (e.g., on computer-assisted detection software)
- Patient brought out of bore of magnet
- Mark skin entry site relative to known position of fiducial marker
- Prepare area in usual sterile fashion
- Instill lidocaine into marked entry site
- Use needle guide electively
- Insert MR-compatible hollow needle to calculated depth
- Reposition patient in magnet bore
- Image (axial and sagittal) to verify needle spears lesion or within < 1 cm
  - Aim to be through lesion, not shallow
  - Adjust needle position and re-image if necessary
- Patient brought out of bore of magnet
- Deploy hookwire through hollow needle, desiring hook to be within 1 cm deep to lesion
  - Remove hollow needle
- Verify wire position on post-procedure MR sagittal and axial images
- Secure wire prior to patient transport
- CC and 90° lateral mammograms
  - Annotate depth of hook from skin entry site
  - Annotate relative positions of hookwire and lesion, lesion size
  - Films to operating room with the patient

Findings and Reporting
- Report includes
  - Size, location, morphology and enhancement characteristics of targeted lesion

PRE-OP LESION LOCALIZATION, MRI

○ Opinion of success in targeting, any complications
- Radiologic-pathologic concordance critical
  ○ If discordant, action depends on clinical judgment
  ○ Consider post-excision MR to verify lesion removal

Alternative Procedures/Therapies
- Radiologic
  ○ Targeted US after MR
    - Highly variable success: 23-89% success (averaging 55% across 3 series)
    - Significant rate of malignancy among lesions occult at targeted US: 6-14% → need for MR-guided biopsy or localization
  ○ MR-guided vacuum-assisted biopsy with clip placement
    - Technical success rates: 87-96% lesions visualized at time of biopsy
    - 96-97% of lesions successfully biopsied, 95% successful clip deployment
    - Clip localized for excision using standard mammographic approaches
  ○ MR-guided clip placement only, with needle localization of clip using mammography
    - May facilitate scheduling magnet time relative to day of surgery
- Surgical
  ○ Use of adjacent landmarks, other known adjacent lesion(s), to include MR-suspicious findings in excised area
  ○ Mastectomy not recommended without confirmation that MR-only findings are malignant
    - High rate of false positives on MR imaging
- Other: MR follow-up may be reasonable for some lesions, work in progress

POST-PROCEDURE

Expected Outcome
- Technical success rates 93-100%
- Positive predictive value for cancer 31-73%

Things To Do
- Prompt review of specimen image, if obtained
  ○ Ensure hook-wire included
- In cases of equivocal imaging-pathologic concordance
  ○ Entire specimen should be processed and examined
  ○ Post-procedure follow-up MR to verify lesion removal if findings ambiguous

Things To Avoid
- Non-ferromagnetic MR-compatible wire properties impact surgical technique
  ○ Use caution with electrocautery
    - Lower resistance metal may conduct heat more readily and cause burns
  ○ Weaker metal may break
    - Avoid excessive traction on wire while removing specimen from breast
    - Examine specimen radiograph carefully for all wire components, including hook
- Wire displaced between procedure and arrival in OR

PROBLEMS & COMPLICATIONS

Problems
- Lesion non-visualization at time of localization
  ○ Extravasation of contrast, failed contrast injection
  ○ Ensure compression not overly tight
  ○ Obtain follow-up MR to verify resolution of finding if procedure canceled
- Rapid washout of lesion during localization
  ○ "Vanishing target"; proceed quickly
  ○ Utilize anatomic landmarks, coordinate location of lesion
  ○ Consider re-bolus Gd-contrast
- Inability to access lesion
  ○ Posterior location
  ○ Large breast size may limit anterior tissue visualization
- Bilateral/multi-site localization
  ○ Position both (all) hollow needles initially
    - Verify position with one imaging sequence
    - If staff/equipment permit, localize both simultaneously
  ○ Allow 20 minutes between sites if Gd-contrast re-bolused
- Cost
- No MR sequence for specimen imaging
  ○ Lesion visualization on MR relies on vascularity
  ○ MR enhancement does not persist ex vivo
  ○ Entire specimen should be processed and examined
- Impact on surgical technique
  ○ Route to lesion may not be as direct as with conventional needle localization

Complications
- Most feared complication(s)
  ○ Adverse reaction to Gd-contrast
    - Idiosyncratic; variable severity
    - Less common than with iodinated contrast
- Other complications
  ○ Patient inability to complete procedure
    - Pre-medication if needed
  ○ Hookwire breakage
    - Occurred in 3% of one series of 101 patients
  ○ Inaccurate hookwire placement relative to lesion
    - Single-institution series: 53% within 1 cm of lesion, 46% within 1.1-2.0 cm, 1% > 2 cm

SELECTED REFERENCES

1. Morris EA et al: Breast MRI: Diagnosis and Intervention. 1st ed. Springer, New York. 280-96, 2005
2. Lampe D et al: The clinical value of preoperative wire localization of breast lesions by magnetic resonance imaging--a multicenter study. Breast Cancer Res Treat. 75:175-9, 2002
3. Morris EA et al: Preoperative MR imaging-guided needle localization of breast lesions. AJR. 178:1211-20, 2002
4. Orel SG et al: MR imaging of the breast for the detection, diagnosis, and staging of breast cancer. Radiology. 220:13-30, 2001
5. Smith LF et al: Magnetic resonance imaging-guided core needle biopsy and needle localized excision of occult breast lesions. Am J Surg. 182:414-8, 2001

IMAGE GALLERY

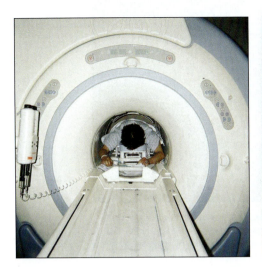

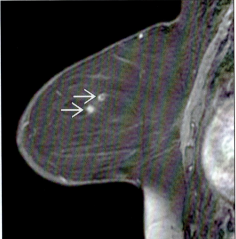

(Left) The patient is imaged prone, and pre- and post-gadolinium images are used to guide placement of the wire into the lesion. Patient is moved into the bore for imaging and out for the procedural elements. *(Right)* Three almost contiguous enhancing masses ➡ (two of which are visible on this image) are identified and their location/depth is compared to location of the fiducial marker. Note: Next 4 images are from same case.

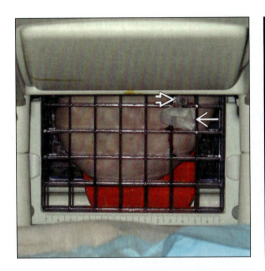

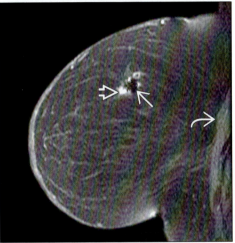

(Left) The fiducial marker ➡ (obscured by tape) and the adjacent hollow localization needle ➡ are seen. Differences in patient position (head right, feet left and back superior) from the sagittal image (right) are apparent. *(Right)* Sagittal T1WI FS post-contrast shows needle in place ➡ within enhancing targeted abnormality ➡ upper breast, approximately midway between the anterior breast and chest wall ➡.

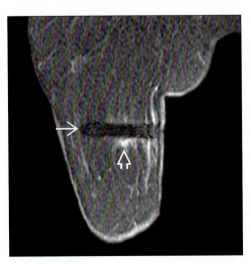

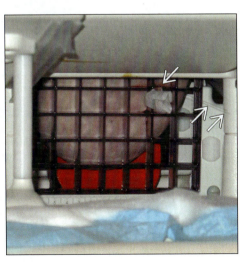

(Left) Axial T1WI post-contrast MR verifies needle position/depth ➡ with respect to the target ➡. Note prominent 21-g needle artifact. The needle is deep to the lesion and was withdrawn slightly prior to placing hookwire. *(Right)* Hookwire ➡ has been placed through the needle (which was subsequently removed) and final position verified on post-placement MR and mammographic images. Pathology: Benign tissue with fat necrosis.

PRE-OP LESION LOCALIZATION, US

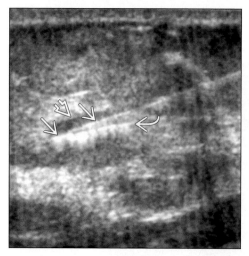

Transverse ultrasound shows a localizing wire ⇨ and hook ➡ within mass ⇨ known to be mucinous carcinoma by prior core biopsy in a 68 year old woman.

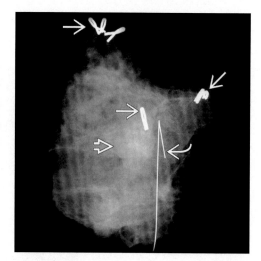

Specimen radiograph (same patient as previous image) confirms excision of known malignant mass ⇨ & hookwire ➡. Clips ➡ placed by surgeon to orient specimen. Margins were free of tumor.

TERMINOLOGY

Synonyms
- Pre-operative US needle/wire localization

Definitions
- US-guided localization of non-palpable or vaguely palpable breast lesion prior to surgical excision

PRE-PROCEDURE

Indications
- Any nonpalpable or vaguely palpable breast lesion, requiring surgical excision, that can be seen on US
  - Usually known malignant or high-risk lesion by prior core biopsy (± clip placed)

Contraindications
- Obviously palpable lesions
- Small, subtle lesions seen better on mammography

Getting Started
- Things to Check
  - Initial core biopsy preferred to excision
  - Verify lesion location and depth from skin surface
  - Compare US and mammographic images: Concordance of suspicious findings essential
  - Informed, written consent
- Medications: 1% lidocaine ± buffered with sodium bicarbonate
- Equipment List
  - High-resolution ultrasound unit
    - 10-13 MHz transducer
  - Localizing device
    - Rigid-needle system (needle and J-wire); needle left in place → curved J-wire advanced into tissue
    - Hook-wire system (needle and barb-type wire); needle removed after wire deployment
  - 25-gauge needle for local anesthesia
  - Betadine or other surgical-cleansing soap
  - Sterile drape, gel, optional probe cover

PROCEDURE

Patient Position/Location
- Best procedure approach
  - Patient supine on exam table; ipsilateral arm raised, hand resting behind head
  - Contralateral decubitus position for lateral lesions
- Long-axis approach
  - Needle enters skin near narrow end of transducer, parallel to long axis
    - Needle oblique to skin for most lesions
    - Horizontal orientation (paralleling chest wall) for deep lesions
- Short-axis (vertical) approach
  - Needle enters skin adjacent to mid-portion of long-axis of transducer
  - Shortest distance to lesion
  - Technically challenging: Hard to see needle and tip

Procedure Steps
- Breast cleansed with disinfectant
- If sterile probe cover not used, must disinfect probe
- Fenestrated drape or towels placed to define sterile field
- Local anesthesia given
- Choose length of needle = measured distance from distal end of lesion to estimated skin entry + 2 cm
- Using free-hand technique, advance needle under real-time US guidance through lesion
  - Transducer in non-dominant hand, needle in other
- Once needle placed through lesion, wire is deployed

Key Facts

Terminology
- US-guided localization of non-palpable or vaguely palpable breast lesion prior to surgical excision

Pre-procedure
- Verify lesion location and depth from skin surface
- Compare US and mammographic images: Concordance of suspicious findings essential

Procedure
- Using free-hand technique, advance needle under real-time US guidance through lesion
- Once needle placed through lesion, wire is deployed
- "X" marked on overlying skin with permanent marker, directly over lesion
- If lesion not seen on mammography → specimen US lesion scanned in saline bath

- o Wire tip should be just beyond lesion
- "X" marked on overlying skin with permanent marker, directly over lesion
  - o Depth from mark to lesion should be noted for surgeon
- Hard-copy US image, documenting wire placement, sent to OR with patient
  - o If possible, image should demonstrate lesion and full length of wire
  - o Distance from skin entry site to lesion should be documented and noted on film
    - ▪ Attached schematic drawing of wire, skin, lesion, and distances, helpful to orient surgeon
- Orthogonal mammograms (not necessary if appropriate wire placement unequivocally documented with US)
  - o Surgeon preference
    - ▪ Some more comfortable with mammographic orientation
- Specimen imaging required
  - o If lesion not seen on mammography → specimen US lesion scanned in saline bath
    - ▪ Lesion scanned in saline bath

Alternative Procedures/Therapies
- Radiologic
  - o Mark skin over lesion without placing needle/wire
    - ▪ Acceptable for superficial lesions, especially if vaguely palpable
  - o Mammographic localization if seen better on mammography

- Surgical: Intraoperative US localization (by surgeon)

POST-PROCEDURE

Expected Outcome
- Accurate localization and excision of lesion

PROBLEMS & COMPLICATIONS

Complications
- Most feared complication(s)
  - o Failed excision of lesion
  - o Wire in pectoralis muscle
  - o Pneumothorax
- Other complications
  - o Wire tip more distal than expected due to poor conspicuity
  - o Infection, bleeding

SELECTED REFERENCES

1. Bassett LW et al: Diagnoses of Diseases of the Breast. 2nd Ed. Philadelphia, Elsevier Saunders. Chapter 20, 328-30, 2005
2. Harlow SP et al: Intraoperative ultrasound localization to guide surgical excision of nonpalpable breast carcinoma. J Am Coll Surg. 189(3):241-6, 1999
3. Kopans DB et al: Breast sonography to guide cyst aspiration and wire localization of occult solid lesions. AJR Am J Roentgenol. 143(3):489-92, 1984

IMAGE GALLERY

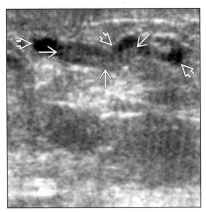
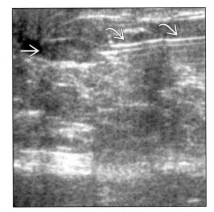
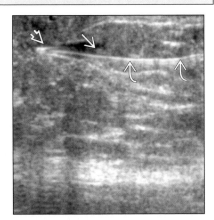

(Left) US depicts a dilated right retroareolar duct ⧨ with an elongated intraductal mass ➡. The patient is a 54 year old woman with clear nipple discharge. *(Center)* US during needle localization (same patient as previous image) shows Kopans needle ➡ being advanced toward the intraductal mass ➡. *(Right)* US (same patient as prior 2 images) confirms deployment of hookwire ➡ through mass ➡, with hook ➡ optimally positioned distally within the duct. Pathology revealed an intraductal papilloma with a well-defined vascular stalk.

SKIN LOCALIZATION

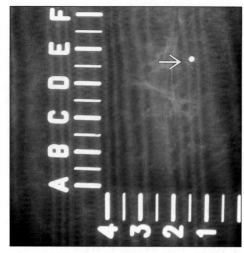

Lateral skin localization was performed for linearly distributed rather superficial Ca++ considered somewhat suspicious. A BB was placed over the calcifications and position of the BB confirmed ➡.

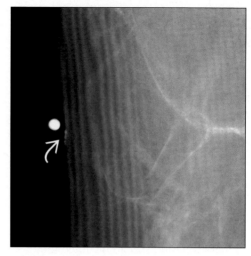

CC Spot magnification tangential view confirms the calcifications to be within the skin ➡, and therefore benign, BI-RADS 2.

TERMINOLOGY

Synonyms
- Skin calcification (Ca++) localization
- Dermal Ca++ localization
- Skin or dermal Ca++ work-up

Definitions
- Most common: Determination of dermal location of Ca++ by tangential imaging
  - Dermal Ca++ are benign and can be dismissed without further evaluation
  - Grid localization technique performed in a fashion similar to parenchymal needle localization but with skin marking rather than needle insertion
- Mammography ± ultrasound (US) for skin masses
  - BB skin marker and confirmatory mammogram
  - US may be needed to confirm intradermal location
- Pre-surgical excision may be directed by US-guided skin BB placement approximating a superficial underlying lesion
  - Include depth of lesion from skin in report

PRE-PROCEDURE

Indications
- Distinguish dermal vs. parenchymal Ca++ location
  - Some skin Ca++ morphology quite distinctive
    - Geometric in shape with umbilicated or lucent centers, often grouped together
  - Other morphologies may be similar to and worrisome for suspicious parenchymal Ca++
    - Most of breast skin projects over breast parenchyma on the MLO and CC views
    - Ambiguous Ca++ forms may be close to a skin surface on one view but may or may not lie within the skin

Contraindications
- None

Getting Started
- Things to Check
  - Possible image artifacts simulating Ca++
    - Skin talc, powder, deodorant
    - Analog film artifacts such as incomplete fingerprint
    - Thorough skin cleansing may be helpful
- Equipment List
  - Standard mammographic unit
    - Analog or digital

PROCEDURE

Patient Position/Location
- Best procedure approach: Grid localization technique using mammography

Equipment Preparation
- Use modified compression paddle with the fenestrated portion outlined by an alpha-numeric grid
- Magnification should be used for tangential view

Procedure Steps
- Place breast in compression in fenestrated grid localization paddle
- Expose the skin surface closest to the Ca++ in question, centering over area of interest
- Acquire a mammogram
- Determine the Ca++ location on image
- Find the intersecting X and Y coordinates and create a mark on the skin
- Place a skin BB directly on the skin mark indicated by the intersecting X and Y coordinates

SKIN LOCALIZATION

Key Facts

Terminology
- Skin calcification (Ca++) localization
- Dermal Ca++ localization
- Most common: Determination of dermal location of Ca++ by tangential imaging

Procedure
- Place breast in compression in fenestrated grid localization paddle

- Place a skin BB directly on the skin mark indicated by the intersecting X and Y coordinates
- Obtain an image to verify that the radiopaque marker is directly over the Ca++
- Obtain a magnified tangential view of the skin directly beneath the skin BB
- Digital imaging may demonstrate dermal location of Ca++ on standard images

---

- Obtain an image to verify that the radiopaque marker is directly over the Ca++
- Remove the breast from compression and replace grid compression paddle with a spot compression paddle
- Obtain a magnified tangential view of the skin directly beneath the skin BB
- Assess the tangential view for the presence (or absence) of the targeted Ca++ within the skin
- Evaluate surrounding area closely for presence of the targeted Ca++ near, but not within the skin

Findings and Reporting
- Determination of dermal Ca++ is reassuring as these are a benign finding
- Further evaluation with orthogonal spot magnification views of any suspicious non-dermal Ca++ must be carried out if the skin localization fails to demonstrate the Ca++ to be dermal in location

Alternative Procedures/Therapies
- Radiologic
  - Digital imaging enhances visibility of the skin
    - Digital imaging may demonstrate dermal location of Ca++ on standard images
- Surgical: Suspicious Ca++ found to lie within the parenchyma require biopsy, either stereotactic or surgical excision

POST-PROCEDURE

Expected Outcome
- Determination of Ca++ within the skin
- If not within the skin, further evaluation required

Things To Do
- Be certain the skin is cleansed of any possible radiopaque confounding elements such as talc, deodorant

PROBLEMS & COMPLICATIONS

Complications
- Most feared complication(s): Misinterpretation of suspicious ductal Ca++ as dermal in location

SELECTED REFERENCES

1. Bassett LW et al: Diagnosis of Diseases of the Breast. 2nd ed. Philadelphia, Elsevier. 402-4, 2005
2. Cardenosa G: Breast Imaging. Philadelphia, Lippincott Williams & Wilkins. 141-4, 2004
3. Diekmann F et al: Reduced-dose digital mammography of skin calcifications. AJR. 178:473-4, 2002
4. Berkowitz JE et al: Dermal breast calcifications: localization with template-guided placement of skin marker. Radiology. 163:282, 1987

IMAGE GALLERY

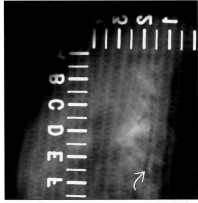 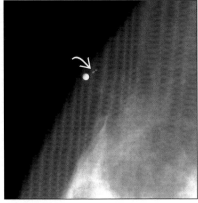 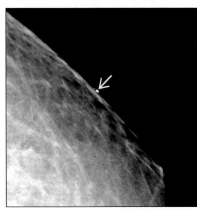

(Left) CC skin localization of a superior superficial cluster of round Ca++ was performed to determine their location. The area with Ca++ was placed within grid, the Ca++ located ➡ and a BB placed on skin. *(Center)* Spot tangential magnification view was obtained (same as on left) with BB in tangent, confirming Ca++ to be within the skin ➡. Benign, BI-RADS 2. *(Right)* CC digital mammogram shows a small group of round smooth Ca++ ➡, easily seen on tangential skin surface because of increased conspicuity of the skin on digital mammograms.

SPECIMEN IMAGING

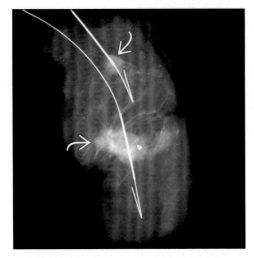

Magnification specimen radiograph shows inclusion of two wire-localized spiculated masses ➡ within this lumpectomy specimen; both masses were invasive ductal carcinoma (IDC).

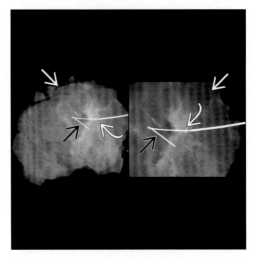

Magnification specimen radiographs show irregular mass with Ca++ ➡ (better seen on higher magnification image on right) adjacent to hookwire ➡ within lumpectomy specimen ➡. Pathology = IDC.

TERMINOLOGY

Definitions
- Imaging of tissue specimen to identify imaging abnormalities

PRE-PROCEDURE

Indications
- Confirm successful retrieval of imaging abnormality
  - Mass, architectural distortion, ± calcifications (Ca++)
- Communicate location of finding to pathologist
- Assure retrieval of post-core biopsy clip(s)
  - Clip may be at a distance from the biopsy site
    - When at a distance, clip removal not mandatory
- Assure retrieval of hookwire(s)
  - Hook rarely transected, not in specimen
    - Communicate to surgeon, may require retrieval
- Helps predict involvement of surgical margins
  - Requires immediate evaluation during operation
    - Guides resection of additional marginal specimens
    - Requires attention to specimen orientation
  - Can also be used for clinical/palpable findings
  - Potential for false negatives and false positives

Getting Started
- Things to Check: Correlate with pre-procedure imaging
- Equipment List
  - Standard mammogram unit
    - Dedicated specimen imaging unit optional
  - Standard ultrasound unit
  - Appropriate specimen containers
    - Should allow orientation of specimen
    - Facilitates annotation for pathologist, e.g. grid box

PROCEDURE

Patient Position/Location
- Best procedure approach: Magnification specimen radiograph standard when targeting Ca++

Equipment Preparation
- Utilize standard precautions when handling specimen

Procedure Steps
- Stereotactic or US-guided core biopsy samples
  - Magnification mammography: 16-22 kVp, 8 mAs
  - Orient core samples on receptacle
  - Separate & label samples with and without Ca++ and send in formalin to pathology
  - Immediate post-biopsy imaging of breast
    - Ca++ missing; air/density at proper site
    - Clip in proper position
- Surgically excised specimen
  - Surgeon inks margins and/or affixes suture ties ± clips for orientation
  - Magnification mammography
    - 25-26 kVp, 40-60 mAs, 0.1 mm focal spot
    - Compression may not be needed
  - Single view generally accepted as adequate
    - Orthogonal view may better demonstrate lesion distance to specimen edges
- Mastectomy specimen
  - Radiologist can place needle in lesion(s) to direct pathologist to area(s) of greatest concern
  - Need to image entire specimen: Usually no magnification used
- Paraffin blocks: If targeted lesion not found at initial histologic assessment
  - 22 kVp, 5 mAs (10 mAs for upright orthogonal view)

Findings and Reporting
- Prompt examination of sample imperative

SPECIMEN IMAGING

Key Facts

Procedure
- Magnification specimen radiograph standard when targeting Ca++
- Single view generally accepted as adequate
- Prompt examination of sample imperative
- Compare to pre-procedure imaging
- For excisional tissue, communicate findings to operating surgeon

Post-procedure
- Specimen image should demonstrate target
- Ca++ on core biopsy specimen radiograph, present on pathology: Specific diagnosis made in 81%
- Follow-up imaging important in some circumstances
- Resection of large (roughly > 2.5 cm) area of malignant Ca++ or when specimen radiograph equivocal

- MR-guided core biopsy or needle localization with equivocal concordance of histologic findings
- "Negative" margin on specimen does not guarantee negative pathologic margin
- "Positive" margin on specimen imaging may prompt surgeon to obtain additional tissue

Problems & Complications
- Nonvisualization of Ca++ on specimen imaging
- Nonvisualization of mass on specimen imaging
- Nonvisualization of Ca++ at histologic examination
- Undertreatment of cancer (false negative)
- Incomplete sampling of target area
- Incomplete sectioning of specimen at pathology

- ○ Compare to pre-procedure imaging
- ○ For excisional tissue, communicate findings to operating surgeon
  - Do Ca++ extend to margin of specimen?
  - Does suspicious mass appear transected?
  - Surgeon may opt to resect additional tissue if margin(s) appear close or lesion incompletely or not excised: Communicate which margin(s) appear positive
- Trend towards smaller tumor size at diagnosis
  - ○ Increased reliance on specimen imaging to guide pathologic sectioning
    - 15% invasive carcinoma, 80% DCIS cannot be seen on gross pathology
    - Proper localization increases diagnostic yield of pathologic analysis
- Key findings to include in report to pathologist
  - ○ Type of lesion: Mass ± Ca++, architectural distortion
  - ○ Location, size, characteristics of lesion(s)
    - Especially critical for lesions < 1 cm in size

Alternative Procedures/Therapies
- Radiologic
  - ○ Post-procedure specimen imaging standard for needle-localized surgical excision and core biopsy of Ca++
  - ○ If specimen imaging not performed or does not clearly contain target
    - Document in report; recommend post-procedure mammogram (when patient able) to confirm lesion excised
    - Post-procedure mammogram may be difficult to interpret due to edema, hematoma, patient unable to tolerate adequate compression
- Specimen US
  - ○ Scan specimen within receptacle, cover transducer
  - ○ Limited by reverberation artifacts from receptacles
- MR-guided localization or biopsy
  - ○ No ability as yet to perform specimen MR
  - ○ Clip placement post MR-guided core biopsy valuable
    - Separates task of MR guidance from day of surgery
    - Facilitates needle localization using mammographic guidance

- May enable surgeon to resect smaller area
- ○ Post-procedural follow-up breast MR
  - Helps confirm target lesion sampling/removal
  - Recommended for any nonspecific or equivocal result at MR-guided biopsy

POST-PROCEDURE

Expected Outcome
- Specimen image should demonstrate target
- Proven high efficacy in visualizing target on specimen imaging
- Core biopsy
  - ○ Ca++ targeted
    - Ca++ on core biopsy specimen radiograph, present on pathology: Specific diagnosis made in 81%
    - Ca++ not seen on specimen radiograph: 13% still seen on pathology: Diagnosis made in 38%
  - ○ Mass targeted
    - 91% of dense core specimens diagnostic
    - 18% of low density specimens diagnostic
    - Less helpful when background parenchyma dense
- Surgically excised specimen
  - ○ 84% masses seen as well as or better than on pre-procedure mammogram; 98% of noncalcified masses visualized
    - Usually unaffected by dense breast parenchyma
    - Irrespective of mass shape/margin
    - If mass not seen on image, likely not included in specimen
  - ○ Similar results expected for mastectomy specimen
- Paraffin blocks
  - ○ Single institution data: Ca++ nonvisualized after block preparation in 13.6% and after slide preparation in 12.6%
    - X-ray blocks and prepare additional levels from appropriate block(s) → diagnosis
- Post-procedure mammogram may demonstrate removal of the previously seen abnormality
  - ○ Area may be obscured immediately post-procedure (hematoma, seroma)

SPECIMEN IMAGING

Things To Do

- Implement department policy for specimen radiography
  - Ensure prompt direct communication with surgeon and pathologist
  - Maintain high quality standards
  - Report specimen imaging findings as separate paragraph in procedure report
- Radiologic-pathologic correlation particularly important for percutaneous core biopsy results
  - Interdisciplinary conference to discuss cases
    - Facilitates management decisions for discordant or unusual findings
    - Increases radiologist and pathologist familiarity with imaging-pathologic correlation
    - Improves communication among departments
  - Maintain proper records for internal audit
- Follow-up imaging important in some circumstances
  - Resection of large (roughly > 2.5 cm) area of malignant Ca++ or when specimen radiograph equivocal
    - Obtain follow-up mammogram to assure all Ca++ resected prior to radiation treatment
  - MR-guided core biopsy or needle localization with equivocal concordance of histologic findings
    - Result of fibrosis particularly problematic

Things To Avoid

- Displacement of localizing wire before excision
- Over-reliance on specimen appearance as predictor of surgical margins
  - "Negative" margin on specimen does not guarantee negative pathologic margin
    - Margins may appear falsely clear with multifocal disease, seen in 32% of cases with Ca++
    - Reflects non-masslike DCIS in ductal distribution
  - "Positive" margin on specimen imaging may prompt surgeon to obtain additional tissue
- Delay in specimen handling with drying of tissue → artifacts
- If lymphoma or leukemia suspected, place specimen in saline rather than formalin

PROBLEMS & COMPLICATIONS

Problems

- Nonvisualization of Ca++ on specimen imaging
  - Ca++ may not be present
  - Ca++ may be below radiographic resolution
    - Ca++ oxalate in microcysts may be difficult to visualize
    - More Ca++ visible on pathology than imaging
    - Magnification, low kVp technique to optimize visualization
- Nonvisualization of mass on specimen imaging
  - Repeat specimen image at higher mAs
  - Consider orthogonal specimen radiograph, US of specimen
  - Surgeon may attempt further excision
  - Post-procedure mammogram
  - Cysts may be decompressed at surgery/biopsy

- Nonvisualization of architectural distortion on specimen imaging
  - May be due to different orientation
- Nonvisualization of Ca++ at histologic examination
  - Ca++ phosphate most common type in breast
    - Readily visible on standard hematoxylin-eosin (H&E) stain
  - Ca++ oxalate form less common in breast
    - Not visible on standard H&E stain
    - Birefringency: Examine under polarized light
  - Ca++ may fall out during sectioning
    - More common with Ca++ oxalate
  - Sections analyzed may not contain Ca++
    - Not every portion of specimen is examined
    - Radiograph paraffin blocks to guide re-sectioning
- Size discrepancy between pathology and imaging
  - Lesion may not be well seen
  - Lesion not sectioned along longer axis
  - Lesion may shrink in formalin
  - Original lesion may have been transected during biopsy
    - Fibrosis may occur between mass areas
    - May appear as two masses
    - May appear smaller in size than original imaging

Complications

- Most feared complication(s): Loss of specimen, mislabeling or inadequate labeling or orientation of specimen
- Other complications: Specimen compression may "push" edge of lesion closer to margin, yielding potential false + surgical margin
- Undertreatment of cancer (false negative)
  - Incomplete sampling of target area
  - Incomplete sectioning of specimen at pathology

SELECTED REFERENCES

1. Mendez JE et al: Tissue compression is not necessary for needle-localized lesion identification. Am J Surg. 190:580-2, 2005
2. Liberman L et al: To excise or sample the mammographic target: what is the goal of stereotactic 11-gauge vacuum-assisted biopsy? AJR. 179:679-83, 2002
3. Berg WA et al: Predictive value of specimen radiography for core needle biopsy of noncalcified breast masses. AJR. 171:1671-8, 1998
4. Homer MJ et al: Radiography of the surgical breast biopsy specimen. AJR. 171:1197-9, 1998
5. D'Orsi CJ: Management of the breast specimen. Radiology. 194:297-302, 1995
6. Lee CH et al: Detecting residual tumor after excisional biopsy of impalpable breast carcinoma: efficacy of comparing preoperative mammograms with radiographs of the biopsy specimen. AJR. 164:81-6, 1995
7. Liberman L et al: Radiography of microcalcifications in stereotaxic mammary core biopsy specimens. Radiology. 190:223-5, 1994
8. D'Orsi CJ et al: Breast specimen microcalcifications: radiographic validation and pathologic-radiologic correlation. Radiology. 180:397-401, 1991
9. Stomper PC et al: Efficacy of specimen radiography of clinically occult noncalcified breast lesions. AJR. 151:43-7, 1988

SPECIMEN IMAGING

IMAGE GALLERY

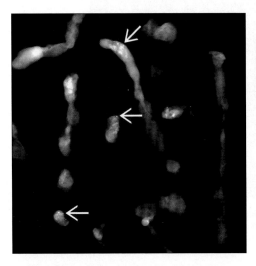

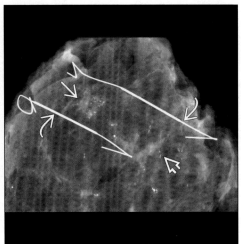

(Left) Magnification specimen radiograph of material obtained at stereotactic 11-g vacuum-assisted core needle biopsy shows calcifications ➡ in some samples. Pathology showed invasive ductal carcinoma. *(Right)* Magnification specimen radiograph shows 2 wires from a bracket localization ➡ and fine linear ➡ and pleomorphic Ca++ ➡ where a core had shown ADH. Excision = DCIS, intermediate grade.

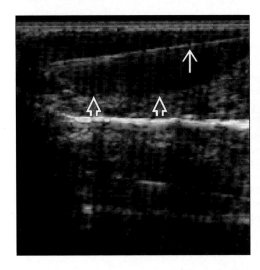

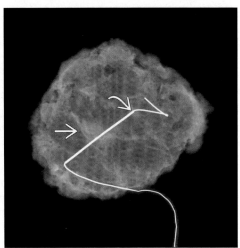

(Left) Specimen ultrasound demonstrates a targeted oval, hypoechoic mass ➡ with localization hookwire ➡ traversing the lesion. Pathology was fibroadenoma. *(Right)* Magnification specimen radiograph after MR-guided localization shows wire ➡ through focal asymmetry ➡. MR finding prompting biopsy = irregular area of persistent enhancement in a high-risk 42 year old. Pathology = benign tissue.

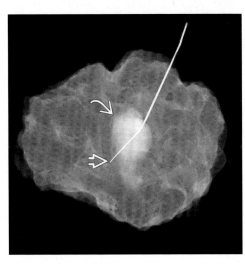

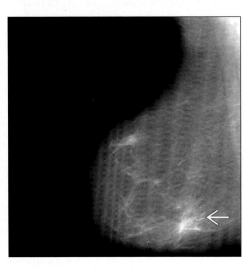

(Left) Magnification specimen radiography of excisional biopsy specimen after needle localization shows oval mass ➡, proven fibroadenoma. Note the hookwire tip is absent ➡, a finding not noted prospectively. *(Right)* Lateral mammography (same case as left, later date) shows the retained hookwire tip ➡. The patient underwent successful needle localization and excision of the fragment; pathology = normal breast tissue.

STEREOTACTIC BIOPSY, PRONE

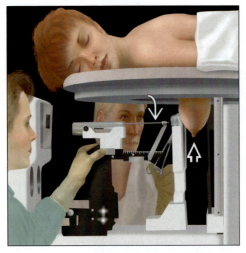

Drawing shows prone dependent position of compressed breast ➡ about to be biopsied using vacuum-assisted probe ➡. Suction tubing not shown.

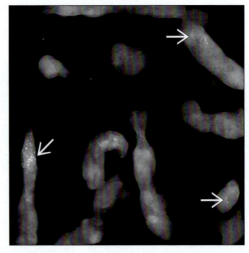

Specimen radiograph shows successful retrieval of numerous pleomorphic Ca++ ➡ at 11-g SVAB. Histopathology showed high grade DCIS with Ca++.

TERMINOLOGY

Synonyms
- Stereotaxic biopsy, stereotactic vacuum-assisted biopsy (SVAB), stereotactic core needle biopsy (SCNB), typically automated 14-g core device

Definitions
- Use of mammographic images, taken at +15° and -15° angles, to calculate three-dimensional target(s) for percutaneous biopsy of suspicious breast lesions

PRE-PROCEDURE

Indications
- Nonpalpable, mammographically-detected BI-RADS 4 or 5 lesions, not amenable to percutaneous ultrasound-guided biopsy
  - Calcifications (Ca++)
    - Underlying mass on ultrasound → US-guided biopsy may be more appropriate
  - Desirable to sample extremes of suspicious area to confirm need for wide excision and/or mastectomy
    - E.g., most anterior and most posterior Ca++
    - Sample differing suspicious Ca++ morphologies
  - Masses not seen on ultrasound

Contraindications
- Patient inability to lie prone for at least 30 minutes
- Thin breast: Breast thickness < aperture size of biopsy device
  - < 3 cm thick may require tricks in positioning
  - Breast thickness can be artificially increased by surrounding breast by flexible cushioning
  - Deep lesion: Use open compression paddle on both sides of breast to allow some "give" when firing probe

- Superficial lesion: Advance probe to target with portion of aperture protruding from skin; devices available to partially cover probe aperture
- Lesion unable to be targeted: Subtle asymmetry
  - Large breast: Central lesion may be beyond reach of biopsy device
  - Extreme posterior location
    - Can attempt positioning arm through table opening
- Sub-areolar lesions (relative): ↓ Breast thickness
- Architectural distortion (relative): ↓ Accuracy, 62% one series
  - Reasonable to excise possible radial scars directly
    - High rate of associated malignancy or atypical hyperplasias, but often microscopic malignancy
- Large area of suspicious Ca++ (relative): Difficult to target specific Ca++

Getting Started
- Things to Check
  - Complete imaging workup prior to procedure
    - CC and 90° lateral magnification mammograms
    - Milk of calcium may only layer when patient prone on stereotactic table
  - American College of Radiology accreditation
    - 3 hours continuing education credit every 3 years
    - Perform ≥ 12 per year; initial can be 3 under supervision of one who has performed ≥ 24
    - Qualify as mammography interpreting physician (MQSA, Mammography Quality Standards Act, if radiologist, USA)
- Medications
  - Anticoagulants should be discontinued before procedure; aspirin typically held one week prior
    - If need for biopsy urgent or therapy cannot be stopped → may proceed with caution
- Equipment List
  - Dedicated prone stereotactic biopsy table

STEREOTACTIC BIOPSY, PRONE

Key Facts

Terminology
- Use of mammographic images, taken at +15° and -15° angles, to calculate three-dimensional target(s) for percutaneous biopsy of suspicious breast lesions

Pre-procedure
- Complete imaging workup prior to procedure
- Anticoagulants should be discontinued before procedure; aspirin typically held one week prior
- If need for biopsy urgent or therapy cannot be stopped → may proceed with caution

Procedure
- Breast suspended through table opening, positioned against image receptor plate
- Scout image obtained; goal = lesion in center of field

- Lesion targeted on stereotactic images at digital monitor → numerical coordinates calculated to localize lesion in three dimensions: Adjusted depth: "z"
- Specimen radiograph to verify Ca++ lesion retrieval
- Stainless steel or titanium clip placed via hollow probe
- Communicate specifics of imaging findings and level of suspicion to pathologist; multidisciplinary review can be helpful

Post-procedure
- No proven benefit to devices larger than 11-g
- Sensitivity to malignancy: 94-95% including immediate rebiopsy
- 89-92% with SCNB; 95-96% with SVAB
- Discordant results: 3% of biopsies

- Vacuum-assisted biopsy system with various probe-size options, 14- to 8-gauge (g)
  - Tru-cut needle (rarely used, small samples)
- Lidocaine ± sodium bicarbonate 10:1 (superficial)
- Lidocaine with 1:100,000 epinephrine (deep)
- Betadine or surgical cleansing soap to disinfect skin
- Specimen radiography system: Dedicated unit or standard mammography equipment

PROCEDURE

Procedure Steps
- Informed, written consent obtained
- Breast suspended through table opening, positioned against image receptor plate
  - Scout image obtained; goal = lesion in center of field
- Stereotactic images obtained
- Lesion targeted on stereotactic images at digital monitor → numerical coordinates calculated to localize lesion in three dimensions: Adjusted depth: "z"
  - Negative stroke margin may require repositioning patient, changing approach
- Skin thoroughly cleansed, local anesthesia → skin wheal
- Small, 2-3 mm, skin incision made with scalpel
- Probe/needle advanced to pre-fire position
  - Stereotactic images obtained to verify position
  - Slight retargeting may be needed: Withdraw probe so just inside skin and adjust, reconfirm with stereotactic paired images
- Probe/needle "fired" into breast
  - Position verified with stereotactic images (optional)
- Samples retrieved
  - Vacuum-assisted: Tissue drawn into open aperture with vacuum suction → severed by cutting sheath → transported to collection chamber
  - Tru-cut: Multiple passes, repositioning required
  - 10-12 samples recommended (varies with size of probe or needle)
- Specimen radiograph to verify Ca++ lesion retrieval
  - Standard for Ca++; optional for noncalcified masses

- Specimens containing Ca++ placed in a separate container (optional)
- Stainless steel or titanium clip placed via hollow probe
  - Verifies biopsy location if entire lesion removed
  - Preloaded clips can be placed after Tru-cut sampling
- Post-procedure orthogonal-view mammograms obtained (not typically billable)
  - Document location of clip relative to biopsy site
- If doing two lesions, ideally center both in template
  - Widely separated lesions: Perform more posterior biopsy first

Findings and Reporting
- Document lesion retrieval
  - Number of specimens containing calcifications
- Location of clip on post-biopsy mammograms
- Communicate specifics of imaging findings and level of suspicion to pathologist; multidisciplinary review can be helpful
  - Addend biopsy procedure report stating histopathology results, concordance, management recommendation(s), including need for rebiopsy
- Telephone or fax referring physician if malignant or otherwise needs excision or rebiopsy
  - Radiologist or referring physician contacts patient directly; document communication of results

Alternative Procedures/Therapies
- Radiologic
  - US-guided when visible sonographically
  - MR-guided biopsy for lesions seen best/only on MR
- Surgical
  - Needle localization and excisional biopsy
    - Widespread calcifications: May ↓ sampling error

POST-PROCEDURE

Expected Outcome
- Technical success sampling targeted lesion: 98%
  - Most failures related to poor lesion visualization
  - 5 specimens, 14-g SCNB diagnostic for 99% of masses

- ≥ 10 specimens with 11-g SVAB ↑ diagnostic accuracy for Ca++
- No proven benefit to devices larger than 11-g
- Sensitivity to malignancy: 94-95% including immediate rebiopsy
  - 89-92% with SCNB; 95-96% with SVAB
- Underestimation of disease
  - Common with biopsies for Ca++
    - 37% with 14-g SCNB; 23% with 11-g SVAB
  - Atypical ductal hyperplasia upgrade to malignancy
    - 45% after 14-g SCNB; 25% after 14-g SVAB; 18% after 11-g SVAB
  - Ductal carcinoma in situ (DCIS) upgraded to invasive carcinoma
    - 11% after 11-g SVAB across multiple series
- Discordant results: 3% of biopsies
  - Absence of Ca++ retrieval
  - Benign histology when lesion highly suspicious
  - Average 24% malignancy rate at rebiopsy

Things To Do

- Vacuum around biopsy site prior to placing clip
  - Evacuates small post-biopsy hematomas
- Pathologist fails to identify Ca++ which were retrieved
  - Assure slides reviewed with polarized light: Ca++ oxalate will be clear, translucent on standard H&E
  - Prepare additional levels; ± magnification mammogram of tissue blocks
  - Ca++ may be lost in processing
- Needle-localized excision of all malignancies
  - Even if all imaging evidence of lesion removed: Residual cancer in 79%
- Needle-localized excision of high-risk lesions
  - Atypical ductal hyperplasia, atypical papilloma
  - Lobular carcinoma in situ and atypical lobular hyperplasia
  - Radial scar
    - May not require excision if incidental finding when target is Ca++, well sampled
  - Possible phyllodes
    - Result of "cellular fibroadenoma" in woman ≥ 50: Consider excision
  - Columnar cell lesions with atypia
- Needle-localized excision: Other lesions
  - Benign papilloma
    - 12-14% malignancy rate at excision, ↑ if peripheral, multiple
  - Mucocele-like lesions
- Mammographic follow-up
  - Variable protocols: Usually treated as diagnostic examination
    - Magnification views if residual suspicious Ca++
    - 12 month follow-up if benign, concordant result and lesion well-sampled (e.g., fibroadenoma)
    - Initial 6 month follow-up of non-specific benign results [e.g., fibrocystic changes (FCC) and residual Ca++], then 12 month, usually 24 month
    - Suspicious change at any follow-up should prompt rebiopsy: e.g., ↑ suspicious Ca++

Things To Avoid

- Targeting clip for subsequent excision when clip is at a distance from the biopsy site

PROBLEMS & COMPLICATIONS

Complications

- Most feared complication(s): Uncontrolled bleeding → surgical intervention
- Other complications
  - Infection, clip migration
  - 2% of follow-up mammograms show density along track

SELECTED REFERENCES

1. Ciatto S et al: Accuracy and Underestimation of Malignancy of Breast Core Needle Biopsy: the Florence Experience of Over 4000 Consecutive Biopsies. Breast Cancer Res Treat. 2006
2. Liberman L et al: Is surgical excision warranted after benign, concordant diagnosis of papilloma at percutaneous breast biopsy? AJR Am J Roentgenol. 186(5):1328-34, 2006
3. Berg WA: Image-guided breast biopsy and management of high-risk lesions. Radiol Clin North Am. 42(5):935-46, vii, 2004
4. Fajardo LL et al: Stereotactic and sonographic large-core biopsy of nonpalpable breast lesions: results of the Radiologic Diagnostic Oncology Group V study. Acad Radiol. 11(3):293-308, 2004
5. Jackman RJ et al: Stereotactic histologic biopsy with patients prone: technical feasibility in 98% of mammographically detected lesions. AJR Am J Roentgenol. 180(3):785-94, 2003
6. Jacobs TW et al: Nonmalignant lesions in breast core needle biopsies: to excise or not to excise? Am J Surg Pathol. 26(9):1095-110, 2002
7. Liberman L et al: To excise or to sample the mammographic target: what is the goal of stereotactic 11-gauge vacuum-assisted breast biopsy? AJR Am J Roentgenol. 179(3):679-83, 2002
8. Liberman L: Percutaneous image-guided core breast biopsy. Radiol Clin North Am. 40(3):483-500, vi, 2002
9. Brenner RJ et al: Stereotactic core-needle breast biopsy: a multi-institutional prospective trial. Radiology. 218(3):866-72, 2001
10. Jackman RJ et al: Stereotactic breast biopsy of nonpalpable lesions: determinants of ductal carcinoma in situ underestimation rates. Radiology. 218(2):497-502, 2001
11. Darling ML et al: Atypical ductal hyperplasia and ductal carcinoma in situ as revealed by large-core needle breast biopsy: results of surgical excision. AJR Am J Roentgenol. 175(5):1341-6, 2000
12. Lamm RL et al: Mammographic abnormalities caused by percutaneous stereotactic biopsy of histologically benign lesions evident on follow-up mammograms. AJR Am J Roentgenol. 174(3):753-6, 2000
13. Liberman L: Clinical management issues in percutaneous core breast biopsy. Radiol Clin North Am. 38(4):791-807, 2000
14. Melotti MK et al: Core needle breast biopsy in patients undergoing anticoagulation therapy: preliminary results. AJR Am J Roentgenol. 174(1):245-9, 2000
15. Jackman RJ et al: Atypical ductal hyperplasia diagnosed at stereotactic breast biopsy: improved reliability with 14-gauge, directional, vacuum-assisted biopsy. Radiology. 204(2):485-8, 1997
16. Liberman L et al: Stereotaxic 14-gauge breast biopsy: how many core biopsy specimens are needed? Radiology. 192(3):793-5, 1994
17. Parker SH et al: Percutaneous large-core breast biopsy: a multi-institutional study. Radiology. 193(2):359-64, 1994

IMAGE GALLERY

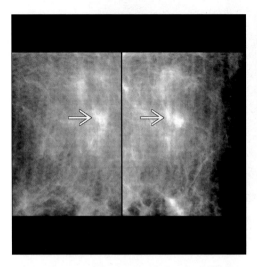
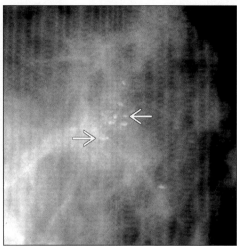

(Left) CC stereotactic mammography confirms visualization of subtle spiculated mass ➡ on ± 15° images. Although US-guidance is preferred for masses, stereotactic biopsy is appropriate for lesions occult on US. Biopsy showed tubular carcinoma. *(Right)* Stereotactic scout image shows layering ➡ of some Ca++ in this 51 y/o, compatible with milk of calcium. Because some did not layer, 11-g biopsy was performed → intermediate grade DCIS and FCC.

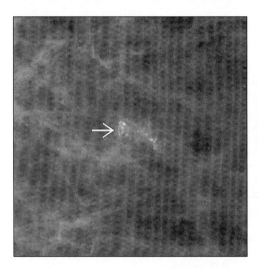
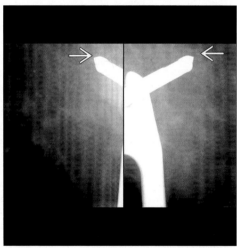

(Left) CC mammography magnification demonstrates a cluster of coarse heterogeneous Ca++ in the left upper inner quadrant ➡ of a fatty breast. *(Right)* CC stereotactic mammography (same as left) obtained in pre-fire position, shows tip of 11-g probe adjacent to targeted Ca++ ➡. After appropriate positioning of the probe is verified, it is "fired" and deep anesthesia given. The vacuum is activated; tissue is excised and transported through probe to collection chamber.

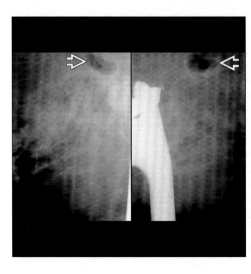
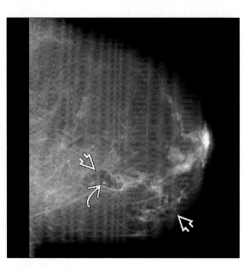

(Left) CC stereotactic mammography after 12 samples obtained (same as prior 2 images) shows removal of targeted Ca++ (confirmed on specimen radiograph) with small air collection ➡ at biopsy site. Clip was placed. *(Right)* Post-biopsy mammogram (same as left image) confirms accurate deployment of radiopaque marker ➡. Post-biopsy air is noted along course of probe ➡ and more diffusely. Histopathology: Sclerosed fibroadenoma with Ca++.

STEREOTACTIC BIOPSY, UPRIGHT

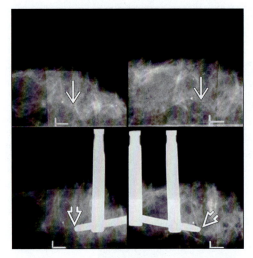

Targeting paired stereotactic images with a calcification in the lesion visible ➡ on computer screen in the upper pair. In the lower pair, inserted core needle tip ➡ is confirmed to be correctly positioned.

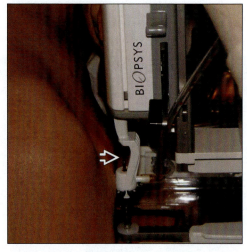

Clinical photograph during vertical upright vacuum-assisted biopsy shows the specimen ➡ in the specimen trough ready for retrieval.

TERMINOLOGY

Synonyms
- Stereotactic biopsy, conventional

Definitions
- Mammographically guided needle biopsy using conventional mammogram unit and stereotactic attachment
- Core needle biopsy (CNB) or vacuum-assisted biopsy (VAB) in most centers

PRE-PROCEDURE

Indications
- Suspicious lesion on mammography, not able to be targeted for biopsy under US guidance
  - Most commonly calcifications (Ca++) ± associated asymmetry
    - Sample Ca++ and adjacent tissue
    - 14-g minimum; 11-g or larger biopsy device preferable
  - Rarely, suspicious mass, most often in large, fatty breast
    - 14-g or larger device, VAB optional

Contraindications
- Relative: Clearly visible corresponding lesion on ultrasound
- Extremely posterior lesions
  - Can be performed with lateral arm needle holder
  - Consider prone biopsy system if available
  - Consider hookwire localization and excision

Getting Started
- Things to Check
  - Lesion clearly visible on relevant workup views
  - Stereotactic equipment accuracy and calibration
  - Biopsy system (gun, vacuum device) functioning
- Medications
  - 1% lidocaine (± sodium bicarbonate) local anesthetic
  - Atropine for iV injection if vasovagal episode
- Equipment List
  - Stereotactic system
    - Analog (slow, film-based)
    - Digital (rapid, with integrated computer targeting)
  - Stereotactic needle holder (vertical or horizontal attachment)
  - Dedicated mammographic stereotactic biopsy chair
  - Biopsy system
    - Core biopsy: 14-g core cut needle and disposable or reusable gun
    - Vacuum assisted: 11 to 8-g needle, holders and vacuum biopsy device
  - Biopsy cart
    - Skin preparation solutions
    - Local anesthetic injection
    - Scalpel blade
    - Appropriate needle guides (sterilized)
    - Glass slides if cytology performed
    - Filter paper or petri dish for core biopsies
    - Fine tweezers for core specimen handling
    - Specimen bottle with fixative solution for core samples
  - Styrofoam pad 2-4 cm thick
    - For women with small breasts, < 3 cm thick on compression

PROCEDURE

Patient Position/Location
- Best procedure approach

STEREOTACTIC BIOPSY, UPRIGHT

Key Facts

Terminology
- Mammographically guided needle biopsy using conventional mammogram unit and stereotactic attachment
- Core needle biopsy (CNB) or vacuum-assisted biopsy (VAB) in most centers

Pre-procedure
- Sample Ca++ and adjacent tissue
- Lesion clearly visible on relevant workup views

Procedure
- Craniocaudal approach may be uncomfortable
- Lateromedial approach most practical
- Decide if more than one lesion to be biopsied
- Insert needle at targeted position
- Pre-fire stereotactic images to confirm targeting

- Perform initial biopsy in center of lesion, followed by radial pattern 2-4 mm from center
- > 10 cores for high diagnostic accuracy for Ca++
- Core specimen cytology (optional)
- Deploy marker clip or coil
- Post-biopsy CC and 90° lateral mammograms ideally
- Specimen X-ray of cores to ensure Ca++ are present

Post-procedure
- 80-90% presurgical diagnostic accuracy
- Adequate specimen in 90-95% CNB
- Adequate specimen in 99% VAB

Problems & Complications
- Inability to position patient/lesion for biopsy (< 5%)

- ○ Patient seated at front of imaging platform, tube and plate rotated to appropriate approach position
- ○ Craniocaudal approach may be uncomfortable
    - ■ Tube shield may be in patient's face (depends on machine design)
    - ■ Suitable for superior lesions
- ○ Mediolateral oblique approach usually very uncomfortable
- ○ Lateromedial approach most practical
    - ■ Requires adequate and accurate initial workup
    - ■ May be performed upright or reclining
    - ■ Less suitable for very medial lesions
    - ■ Vacuum-assisted specimen notch well-positioned for sample removal (Mammotome)
- ○ Mediolateral and inferior approaches rarely practical
    - ■ Contralateral breast, torso or legs may interfere

Equipment Preparation
- Test exposure and targeting calibration (usually weekly QA procedure)
- Replace standard compression paddle with biopsy paddle, attach stereotactic needle holder and targeting system
- Check targeting computer and stereotactic system are correctly installed and functioning
- Familiarize staff with targeting system, biopsy system and precise needle positioning
    - ○ May require practice with biopsy phantom

Procedure Steps
- Decide if more than one lesion to be biopsied
- Determine most practical approach(es)
    - ○ Ideally same approach if more than one lesion
- Compress breast in selected position
- Perform test exposure to check lesion is in biopsy window
    - ○ Adjust position and compression as needed
    - ○ With digital, zoom, window and invert to optimize targeting
- Perform paired stereotactic exposures
- Target lesion and compute depth
    - ○ Target same point near lesion center on both images (e.g., specific microcalcification)

- ■ Ensure correct needle length and type selected
- ■ Transmit computed location and depth to stereotactic system
- ○ Ensure depth adequate for needle throw
    - ■ May require foam block padding to lift breast away from bucky
- Insert needle holders & mark skin at targeted puncture site
- Insert needle at targeted position
    - ○ Prep skin, inject 2-5 cc local anesthetic (too much may obscure lesion)
    - ○ Nick skin with scalpel blade
- Pre-fire stereotactic images to confirm targeting
    - ○ Needle tip at proximal edge short of lesion
        - ■ May require needle retraction of 5-10 mm for small (< 5 mm) lesions
        - ■ Fire vacuum-assisted gun prior to commencing biopsy
        - ■ Additional deep anesthesia: 1% lidocaine ± epinephrine
- Perform initial biopsy in center of lesion, followed by radial pattern 2-4 mm from center
- Core needle (non-vacuum)
    - ○ After firing, remove needle and open notch
    - ○ Five-core approach (central plus 4-corner) useful routine
        - ■ Minimum of 3 cores for high diagnostic accuracy for masses
        - ■ Rarely additional diagnostic benefit for > 12 cores
    - ○ Rotate biopsy notch to face outer aspect of lesion for each position
- Vacuum-assisted core biopsy
    - ○ Perform rotational vacuum biopsy
    - ○ Remove cores with tweezers from specimen trough (Mammotome)
    - ○ > 10 cores for high diagnostic accuracy for Ca++
- Core specimen cytology (optional)
    - ○ Permits rapid processing and diagnosis (< 1 hour)
    - ○ Core needle wash or touch imprint onto glass slides
    - ○ > 80% sensitivity to malignancy if suspicious results are classified as malignant

- Perform post-biopsy stereotactic images of site after completion
  - Deploy marker clip or coil
    - May not be needed if discrete lesion with clearly visible residual Ca++
  - Post-biopsy CC and 90° lateral mammograms ideally
- Specimen X-ray of cores to ensure Ca++ are present
  - Place each core onto filter paper or petri dish in serial positions
  - If inadequate, re-target, obtain additional cores
  - If adequate, end procedure and place cores in specimen jar with fixative
    - Place cores with and without Ca++ into separate specimen containers
- If patient has vasovagal episode
  - Minimize by performing procedure rapidly (ideally with digital system)
  - May require procedure to be paused, iV atropine administered and supine positioning to recover
  - May have to terminate and reschedule, or consider alternative methods

Findings and Reporting

- Whether procedure was completed satisfactorily
- Approach used and lesion(s) biopsied including side and location
- Needle biopsy type and number of passes for each lesion
- Number of core specimens containing Ca++ (if applicable)
- Accuracy of marker clip or coil placement relative to biopsy site

Alternative Procedures/Therapies

- Radiologic
  - US-guided CNB if lesion visible on US
    - 95-97% accurate management
  - Stereotactically-guided fine needle aspiration biopsy (FNAB): Limited utility in most centers
    - 40% insufficient samples for masses
    - 49% insufficient samples for Ca++
    - Limited for indeterminate lesions especially
    - Best with onsite cytotechnician
- Surgical: Hookwire localization and excision biopsy

POST-PROCEDURE

Expected Outcome

- 80-90% presurgical diagnostic accuracy
  - Appropriate triage to excision for high-risk lesions
    - ~ 18% of atypical ductal hyperplasia upgraded to malignancy
- ~ 11% of ductal carcinoma in situ upgraded to invasive cancer
- Adequate specimen in 90-95% CNB
- Adequate specimen in 99% VAB

Things To Do

- Informed consent includes risk of inadequate biopsy

Things To Avoid

- Lesions very close to chest wall or skin surface
- Patients with known bleeding diathesis

  - Cease warfarin or antiplatelet medications 1-2 weeks before procedure
  - Cover clotting deficiencies or thrombocytopenia with appropriate infusions
- Beware biopsying arterial wall microcalcifications

PROBLEMS & COMPLICATIONS

Problems

- Inability to position patient/lesion for biopsy (< 5%)
- Inadequate specimen or poor radiologic-pathologic correlation
  - Careful radiologic-pathologic review of all biopsies
  - Re-biopsy or consider excision if inconclusive result

Complications

- Most feared complication(s)
  - Hematoma at biopsy site (< 1% delayed)
  - Infection (rare)
- Other complications
  - May biopsy skin beyond lesion
    - Particularly if thin breast needing foam block padding for targeting
  - Intramammary scarring after 11-g vacuum-assisted biopsy (rare)
  - Skin entry site tumor seeding (rare)

SELECTED REFERENCES

1. Fahrbach K et al: A comparison of the accuracy of two minimally invasive breast biopsy methods: a systematic literature review and meta-analysis. Arch Gynecol Obstet. 274(2):63-73, 2006
2. Uriburu JL et al: Local recurrence of breast cancer after skin-sparing mastectomy following core needle biopsy: case reports and review of the literature. Breast J. 12(3):194-8, 2006
3. Yazici B et al: Scar formation after stereotactic vacuum-assisted core biopsy of benign breast lesions. Clin Radiol. 61(7):619-24, 2006
4. Koskela AK et al: Add-on device for stereotactic core-needle breast biopsy: how many biopsy specimens are needed for a reliable diagnosis? Radiology. 236(3):801-9, 2005
5. Lomoschitz FM et al: Stereotactic 11-gauge vacuum-assisted breast biopsy: influence of number of specimens on diagnostic accuracy. Radiology. 232(3):897-903, 2004
6. Pisano ED et al: Fine-needle aspiration biopsy of nonpalpable breast lesions in a multicenter clinical trial: results from the radiologic diagnostic oncology group V. Radiology. 219(3):785-92, 2001
7. Sneige N et al: Accuracy of cytologic diagnoses made from touch imprints of image-guided needle biopsy specimens of nonpalpable breast abnormalities. Diagn Cytopathol. 23(1):29-34, 2000
8. Lankford KV et al: Utilization of core wash material in the diagnosis of breast lesions by stereotactic needle biopsy. Cancer. 84(2):98-100, 1998
9. Parker SH et al: Nonpalpable breast lesions: stereotactic automated large-core biopsies. Radiology. 180(2):403-7, 1991
10. Lofgren M et al: Stereotactic fine-needle aspiration for cytologic diagnosis of nonpalpable breast lesions. AJR Am J Roentgenol. 154(6):1191-5, 1990
11. Parker SH et al: Stereotactic breast biopsy with a biopsy gun. Radiology. 176(3):741-7, 1990

STEREOTACTIC BIOPSY, UPRIGHT

IMAGE GALLERY

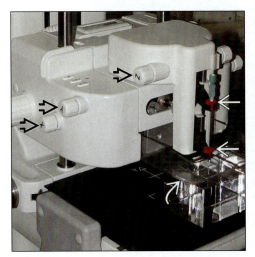

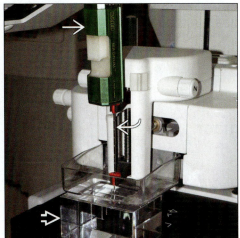

(Left) Clinical photograph of biopsy device set up for fine needle biopsy with a Perspex calibration phantom ➡, shows tridirectional (X,Y,Z) control knobs ➡. Fine needle is held in sterile red plastic needle guides ➡. *(Right)* Clinical photograph shows automated core biopsy gun ➡ and needle ➡ mounted using a calibration Perspex phantom ➡. This digital stereotactic device is remotely targeted from a stereotactic computer.

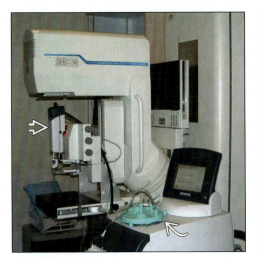

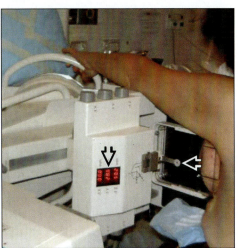

(Left) Clinical photograph shows vacuum-assisted biopsy device ➡ mounted in a stereotactic biopsy holder. The vacuum pump and controller is seen nearby ➡. *(Right)* Clinical photograph during stereotactic positioning shows the lateromedial approach prior to needle biopsy. The vacuum-assisted biopsy needle guide ➡ is in place. This device has direct feedback ➡ for X, Y, & Z directions.

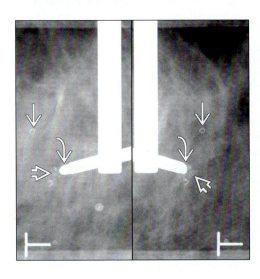

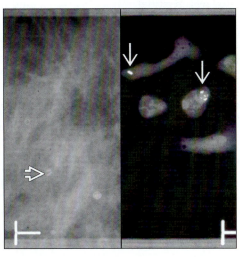

(Left) Stereotactic image pair (pre-fire) shows the core needle tip ➡ positioned just short of a cluster of casting calcifications ➡ in a patient with DCIS. Note the relative shift in position of the oil cyst in the two images ➡. *(Right)* Mammography magnification (same patient as previous) shows biopsy site after CNB completion (left), with residual calcifications ➡. The specimen core radiograph (right) shows Ca++ in some cores ➡.

IMAGE-GUIDED THERMAL ABLATION

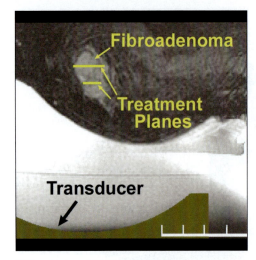

FUS treatment. T2WI FS MR of a fibroadenoma. The patient is prone, with the breast positioned on the water pillow. The transducer is outlined at the bottom.

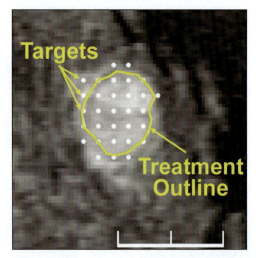

Corresponding MR image of planned treatment volume and foci positions. (Courtesy Nathan J McDanold PhD. Both images reproduced from Radiology 2001;219:176-185, © 2001. All rights reserved.)

TERMINOLOGY

Abbreviations
- Focused ultrasound surgery (FUS)
- Radiofrequency ablation (RFA)
- Laser interstitial thermal therapy (LITT)

Definitions
- FUS: Focal heating of target tissue achieved by deposition of acoustic energy (1-2 MHz) generated by curved piezoelectric transducer array
  - Transducer is acoustically coupled with water bath to breast of prone patient
  - Completely noninvasive, trackless ablation method
- Interstitial ablative therapies
  - Interstitial probe(s) can be pulled back after initial energy delivery, in order to treat larger targets
  - RFA: Destruction of tissue by application of electromagnetic fields, created by interstitial electrode delivery of RF energy (0.4-8 MHz)
    - Current density is induced in tissue, causing resistive heating
  - Cryoablation: Destruction of tissue using rapid cooling, typically to -40°C and held for at least 10 minutes
  - LITT: Light energy delivered by percutaneous optical fiber directly to tissue and creates zone of thermal ablation
  - Microwave ablation: Destruction of tissue by energy on order of 1GHz with interstitial antennae

PRE-PROCEDURE

Requirements
- Ability to localize tumor and its surrounding anatomic structure, define targeted tissue volume

- Ability to target tumor with interstitial probe or focused ultrasound array
- Ability to monitor temperature or thermal effects during energy deposition in real time
- Ability to control amount of energy deposited and spatial extent of ablation
- Core biopsy to establish histology prior to procedure

Patient Preparation for Interstitial Image-Guided Therapy
- Similar requirements as for image-guided diagnostic procedures (e.g., core needle biopsy, FNAB) regarding imaging, patient preparation, anesthesia and analgesia, and approach
  - Deeper planes of anesthesia (e.g., conscious sedation) may be used in ablative procedures
    - Local anesthetic typically used in biopsy due to potential pain from more invasive intervention and longer procedure duration

PROCEDURE

Guidance Modalities
- X-ray, Ultrasound, CT, MR

Temperature Monitoring
- Temperature sensors
  - Fiber optic temperature sensors or thermocouples may be inserted through cannula into breast
- MR thermal monitoring
  - MR enables visualization of targeted lesion before, during, and after ablation
  - Delivery of energy can be quantitatively monitored using temperature sensitive sequences (T1WI or proton resonant frequency images)
  - Effect can qualitatively be seen with T2WI during or immediately after ablation

IMAGE-GUIDED THERMAL ABLATION

Key Facts

Terminology

- FUS: Focal heating of target tissue achieved by deposition of acoustic energy (1–2 MHz) generated by curved piezoelectric transducer array
- Transducer is acoustically coupled with water bath to breast of prone patient
- Completely noninvasive, trackless ablation method
- RFA: Destruction of tissue by application of electromagnetic fields, created by interstitial electrode delivery of RF energy (0.4–8 MHz)
- Cryoablation: Destruction of tissue using rapid cooling, typically to -40°C and held for at least 10 minutes
- LITT: Light energy delivered by percutaneous optical fiber directly to tissue and creates zone of thermal ablation

Procedure

- Fiber optic temperature sensors or thermocouples may be inserted through cannula into breast

Problems & Complications

- Major argument against ablative therapies: Margin status cannot be assessed due to lack of pathologic specimen
- Radiologic assessment must replace histopathology
- Advantage: Greater cosmesis, patient comfort and reduced hospital stays and cost savings
- Advantage: No or greatly reduced risks of anesthesia-related complications and of hemorrhage, infection, scarring and disfigurement

○ Changes seen on MR broadly correlate with areas of tumor necrosis

Focused Ultrasound Surgery (FUS)

- Trackless (non-invasive) ablative therapy
- Ultrasound array embedded into MR table
  ○ Patient lies prone with breast in water pillow
- For 10 second sonication, treated zone can have dimensions of 1-5 mm in diameter and 0.5-3 cm long
- Many focal points within treatment zone are individually heated to sculpt ablation zone
- Heat builds and dissipates quickly; rapid temperature elevation to 50-90°C is produced
- Treatment times are about 45 minutes for 1 cm treated zone and 2 hours for 2 cm treated zone

Radiofrequency Ablation (RFA)

- US or MR guidance is provided for insertion of needle electrode connected to radiofrequency (RF) generator
- Larger electrode pads placed on patient's anterior thighs to return current to generator
  ○ MR may cause heating of conductive materials: Return electrode pad is potential site for skin burn induced by energies used in MR imaging
- RF power deposition is function of tissue conductivity and difficult to predict or control
  ○ Effect and treated zone formation may be inhomogeneous
- Ablation zone of 3-6 cm
- Tissue heating is in vicinity of electrode
- Duration of treatment based on time to achieve optimal heating, resistance measurements, and/or temperature measurements

Cryoablation

- Cooling is achieved by liquid nitrogen flowing through probe
  ○ More recently via Joule-Thompson effect cooling: High pressure gas is expanded through nozzle inside probe
- Probe diameter correlates to maximum iceball diameter (2 mm probe creates 2 cm iceball)

- Single/few large probes or multiple small diameter probes can be used to sculpt zone of freezing
- Cryonecrosis correlates with zone slightly inside leading edge of iceball (-40°C isotherm)
- Iceball is easily appreciated on MR
- Acoustic shadow created by iceball on US which limits monitoring of leading edge of zone of freezing to that which is closest to US probe

Laser Interstitial Thermal Therapy (LITT)

- LITT can be direct extension of biopsy procedure
  ○ Optical fiber introduced through outer cannula of biopsy needle
- Optical laser fibers are inherently MR compatible; extension fibers can be used to position laser outside MR room
- Beam splitters and diffusion tips can be used to treat larger targets
- Treated area expands with continued delivery of energy
  ○ Expansion of region on T1WI plateaus after 270-400 seconds of treatment
- Negative margins were reported to be achieved in one study with 2500 Joule/mL of tissue or when thermal sensor adjacent to fiber read 60°C

Microwave Ablation Therapy

- Approach for microwave ablation is similar to RFA, except
  ○ Treatment areas are typically smaller
  ○ Duration of energy delivery to create treated zone is shorter
  ○ Multiple tracks must be used to treat larger targets
- Percutaneous temperatures probes can also serve as antennae to guide microwave energy
- Procedure is well established for liver tumors but has yet to be applied in breast

IMAGE-GUIDED THERMAL ABLATION

PROBLEMS & COMPLICATIONS

Problems

- Short term studies are needed to prove total ablation of dominant target with negative margins
- Long-term studies to prove that equivalent or even greater efficacy is achieved as with surgery
- Extensive DCIS away from ablated zone: Not appropriate for thermal ablation
- Large vessels may act as heat source or heat sink and islands of cells in their vicinity may survive
- MR thermal monitoring
  - Proton resonance frequency shift techniques work in aqueous tissue, but not in fatty tissue
  - Low field open scanners (< 1.5T) have limited signal-to-noise ratio and limited temperature resolution; best done at high field (≥ 1.5T)
  - In subtraction-based temperature sensitive sequences, misregistration due to breathing or bulk patient movement may be problematic
- Concerns specifically about FUS
  - Analgesic injectate has been reported to cavitate
  - Limited patient access when using MR-guidance/monitoring
  - Risk for skin burn for superficial targets
- Concerns specifically about RFA
  - Concern about margin assessment/status
    - Less than perfect correlation between core biopsy and surgical tumor grading
  - Residual tumor reported in ablated zone
    - Necrotic cells with normal-appearing cells interspersed reported with H&E staining
    - Thermally treated zone close to probe has appearance different from remainder of ablation zone: Pitfall for pathologists new to RFA
  - No commercially available solution for performing simultaneous RFA and MR
    - Electromagnetic emissions from RF generator appear as noise in MR image
  - Pre/post treatment image subtraction of limited use because treated tissue shrivels
  - RF electrode with tines reported to not deploy well into hard fibrous tissue
  - Very lengthy procedure
  - Can be painful, especially with superficial targets near skin (less painful with cryoablation)
- Concerns specifically about cryoablation
  - Can be difficult to obtain high pressure, high purity gases in many parts of the world
- Concerns specifically about LITT
  - Expensive capital equipment compared to RFA
  - Accreditation with lasers required
  - Multiple pull backs (time) or multiple fibers (cost) necessary to treat larger targets
- Concerns specifically about microwave ablation
  - Limited ablation size; requires multiple tracks

Complications

- The same complications that apply to breast biopsy are also concerns in ablation procedures using interstitial techniques: Infection, bleeding, pneumothorax
- Complications specific to ablation include damage to skin, chest wall, or pleura due to ablative energy

Summary of Limitations and Disadvantages

- Major argument against ablative therapies: Margin status cannot be assessed due to lack of pathologic specimen
  - Radiologic assessment must replace histopathology

Advantages

- Advantage: Greater cosmesis, patient comfort and reduced hospital stays and cost savings
- Advantage: No or greatly reduced risks of anesthesia-related complications and of hemorrhage, infection, scarring and disfigurement

SELECTED REFERENCES

1. Agnese DM et al: Ablative approaches to the minimally invasive treatment of breast cancer. Cancer J. 11(1):77-82, 2005
2. Kaufman CS et al: Office-based cryoablation of breast fibroadenomas with long-term follow-up. Breast J. 11(5):344-50, 2005
3. Copeland EM 3rd et al: Are minimally invasive techniques for ablation of breast cancer ready for "Prime Time"? Ann Surg Oncol. 11(2):115-6, 2004
4. Kacher DF et al: MR imaging--guided breast ablative therapy. Radiol Clin North Am. 42(5):947-62, vii, 2004
5. Morin J et al: Magnetic resonance-guided percutaneous cryosurgery of breast carcinoma: technique and early clinical results. Can J Surg. 47(5):347-51, 2004
6. Sabel MS et al. Cryoablation of early-stage breast cancer: work-in-progress report of a multi-institutional trial. Ann Surg Oncol. 11;5:542-9, 2004
7. Gianfelice D et al: MR imaging-guided focused US ablation of breast cancer: histopathologic assessment of effectiveness-- initial experience. Radiology. 227(3):849-55, 2003
8. Singletary ES: Feasibility of radiofrequency ablation for primary breast cancer. Breast Cancer. 10(1):4-9, 2003
9. Dowlatshahi K et al: Laser therapy for small breast cancers. Am J Surg. 184(4):359-63, 2002
10. Pfleiderer SO et al: Cryotherapy of breast cancer under ultrasound guidance: initial results and limitations. Eur Radiol. 12:3009– 14, 2002
11. Huber PE et al: A new noninvasive approach in breast cancer therapy using magnetic resonance imaging-guided focused ultrasound surgery. Cancer Res. 61(23):8441-7, 2001
12. Hynynen K et al: MR imaging-guided focused ultrasound surgery of fibroadenomas in the breast: a feasibility study. Radiology. 219(1):176-85, 2001
13. Hynynen K et al: Temperature monitoring in fat with MRI. Magn Reson Med. 43(6):901-4, 2000
14. Jeffrey SS et al: Radiofrequency ablation of breast cancer: first report of an emerging technology. Arch Surg. 134(10):1064-8, 1999
15. Mumtaz H et al: Biopsy and Intervention Working Group report. J Magn Reson Imaging. 10(6):1010-5, 1999
16. Ablin RJ: The use of cryosurgery for breast cancer. Arch Surg. 133(1):106, 1998
17. Kuroda K et al: Temperature mapping using the water proton chemical shift: a chemical shift selective phase mapping method. Magn Reson Med. 38(5):845-51, 1997
18. Mumtaz H et al: Laser therapy for breast cancer: MR imaging and histopathologic correlation. Radiology. 200(3):651-8, 1996

IMAGE-GUIDED THERMAL ABLATION

IMAGE GALLERY

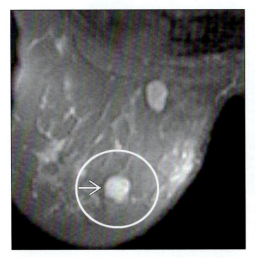
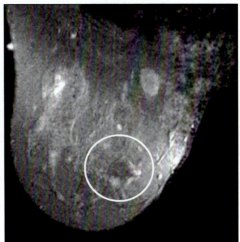

(Left) T1 C+ FS MR of a fibroadenoma ⇨ 2 months prior to FUS. *(Right)* 6 months after FUS (same patient as previous image). (Both images reproduced from Radiology 2001; 219:176-185, copyright © 2001. All rights reserved.)

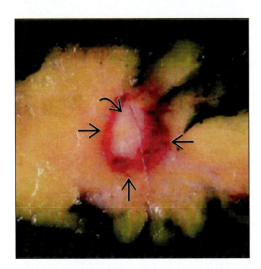
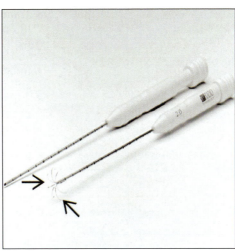

(Left) Macroscopic specimen 5 days after FUS shows the treated target as white area ⇨ with a hyperemic rim ⇨. (Cancer Res.1;61:8441-7, 2001, Copyright © 2001. All rights reserved.) *(Right)* Photograph of MR-compatible RF electrode with secondary electrodes that are deployed in a star-like array (15 cm, 15-gauge, 10 tine) ⇨. (Arch. Surg 134:1064-8; 1999, Copyright © 1999 AMA. All rights reserved.)

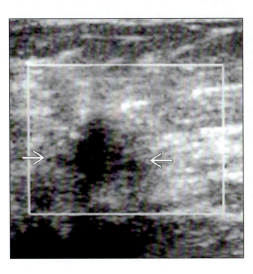
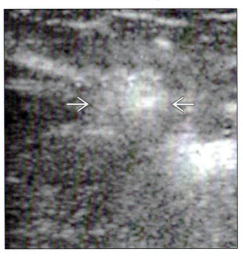

(Left) Intra-operative breast US showing irregular, hypoechoic cancer ⇨ before RFA. *(Right)* Intra-operative US immediately after RFA (same as prior image), demonstrates increased echogenicity of the treated cancer ⇨. (Arch Surg 134:1064−8; 1999, Copyright © 1999 AMA. All rights reserved.)

US-GUIDED CORE BIOPSY

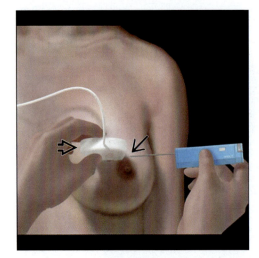

Drawing shows positioning of 14-g spring-loaded biopsy device and needle ➔ for core needle biopsy of a left upper inner quadrant lesion. Note alignment of the needle shaft along long axis of the transducer ➔.

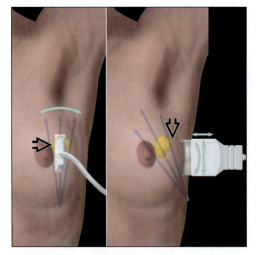

Graphic shows the multiple degrees of freedom of motion of the probe and the needle (blue arrows) relative to the lesion ➔.

TERMINOLOGY

Abbreviations
- Ultrasound-guided core needle biopsy (USCNB)
- Fine needle aspiration biopsy (FNAB)

Synonyms
- Sonographically-guided core needle biopsy

Definitions
- Use of US to guide core needle biopsy of a lesion
- Needle removed between passes
- Can use coaxial trocar

PRE-PROCEDURE

Indications
- Ultrasound-visible mass needing needle biopsy
- Confirmation of axillary node metastasis
- Confirmation of clinically evident malignancy
  - Prior to surgery
  - Prior to neoadjuvant chemotherapy or radiotherapy

Contraindications
- Lesion poorly seen on ultrasound
  - Ca++ without a mass: Larger device, esp. vacuum-assisted preferred
- Extremely deep lesion
- Very small lesion in very large breast
- Anticoagulants: (Relative) may proceed if area can be compressed, risk to discontinuing anticoagulation

Getting Started
- Things to Check
  - Appropriate training and practice prior to procedure
    - Accuracy and needle visualization greatly improved by training
    - Training on phantoms ideal, e.g., turkey breast phantom with olives/pimientos as "targets"
  - American College of Radiology accreditation requirements
    - Images documenting lesion, needle position pre- and post-fire
    - 3 hours continuing education credit; ≥ 12 biopsies per year
  - Multiple degrees of motional freedom for needle and probe relative to lesion
    - Needle tip and shaft: Forward, back, superficial, deep, above & below or lateral & medial
    - Probe: Translation forward, back, up, down; rotation clockwise and counter-clockwise
  - Check for bleeding diathesis, warfarin
- Medications
  - Lidocaine 1%, 5-10 cc
    - Can buffer with 0.5-1.0 cc sodium bicarbonate
- Equipment List
  - High resolution ultrasound system
    - Real-time 3D can improve biopsy accuracy, esp. for less well-trained operators
    - Spatial compounding improves needle visualization
  - High frequency linear array probe
  - Skin preparation kit and solution
  - Coupling media
    - Alcohol or saline effective as coupling media
    - Coupling gel can be used if no cytology to be performed
    - Avoid gel if touch prep cytopathology performed (mimics mucin)
  - Probe cover (optional, sterile or nonsterile)
  - Local anesthetic syringe and needle (21-25 gauge spinal needle if deep lesion)
  - Scalpel blade
  - 14-g (or 12-g) core needles
    - Needles smaller than 14-g → less diagnostic

US-GUIDED CORE BIOPSY

Key Facts

Terminology
- Use of US to guide core needle biopsy of a lesion

Pre-procedure
- Ultrasound-visible mass needing needle biopsy
- Confirmation of axillary node metastasis
- Confirmation of clinically evident malignancy
- Prior to neoadjuvant chemotherapy or radiotherapy
- Appropriate training and practice prior to procedure

Procedure
- Patient supine or rolled, ipsilateral arm raised
- Mark skin at planned puncture site location
- Keep needle shaft angle < 30° relative to probe face
- Direct visual check of needle and probe alignment
- Semi-automated biopsy system ("fire-in-place" type)
- Automated biopsy gun system ("fire-forward" type)

- Mobile mass: Can anchor tip of needle in edge of mass prior to firing
- 3 cores diagnostic in vast majority of masses
- ↑ # Cores for small lesion (< 7-10 mm), target = Ca++, uncertainty in targeting and/or needle gauge (e.g., 12-g)
- Consider insertion of marker, clip or coil

Post-procedure
- Sensitivity & specificity 92-99%, average 98%, including immediate rebiopsies
- Rebiopsy rates 4-11%, average 7%
- Tumor grade accuracy 75-80%
- Receptor status accuracy 70%
- Her-2/neu status 60%
- Touch imprint cytology sensitivity and specificity 90-95%

- ○ Automated high performance metal biopsy gun with single-use needles
  - Multiple springs, very rapid sampling (0.1 second)
  - Consistently high quality cores
  - Heavy, expensive, need maintenance, gun not sterile
- ○ Single-use, spring-loaded plastic biopsy gun with integrated needle
  - Single spring usually weaker than metal guns
  - Semi-automatic and automatic designs
  - Performance, yield vary with device
  - Light, consistent, sterile-packed, cost-effective
- ○ Specimen jar(s) with 10% formalin or alcohol
- ○ If touch imprint cytology: Slides, fixative, etc., as for FNAB
- ○ Outer coaxial trocar/cannula (optional): Facilitates repeated needle placement
- ○ Marker clip or coil may be required
  - Needle-mounted automatic release spring clip or gel marker
  - Angiographic embolization coils can be used

PROCEDURE

Patient Position/Location
- Best procedure approach
  - ○ Patient supine or rolled, ipsilateral arm raised
    - Usually operator on right side of patient; may need left-sided approach or swap hands
    - Needle path ideally near-horizontal, lesion directly in front of operator
    - Minimize operator stretching or angulation

Equipment Preparation
- Arrange couch, US machine & monitor according to approach
- Ensure appropriate probe and tissue presets selected

Procedure Steps
- Informed consent signed
- Ensure proper lesion being targeted
- Mark skin at planned puncture site location

- ○ Farther from probe for deeper lesions
- ○ Needle path preferably along probe face
- Inject local anesthetic into skin subcutaneously
  - ○ Raise wheal by injecting just deep to skin first then withdrawing slightly
  - ○ Inject to edge of lesion, deep to lesion, and beyond lesion along expected path of core needle
  - ○ For posterior lesions, can "elevate" lesion off chest wall by injecting anesthetic posterior to mass
- Make small skin nick (2-3 mm) with scalpel blade
- Insert (optional) 12-13 gauge coaxial trocar/cannula to edge of lesion
- Probe-needle-lesion alignment
  - ○ Keep needle shaft angle < 30° relative to probe face
  - ○ Gentle compression over lesion to stabilize
  - ○ Alternately move needle and probe to confirm needle position
  - ○ Needle tip has specular reflection, especially with bevel facing downwards
  - ○ Direct visual check of needle and probe alignment
  - ○ Document needle position before ("pre") and after ("post") firing gun
    - Can confirm needle through lesion with short-axis perpendicular view
- Semi-automated biopsy system ("fire-in-place" type)
  - ○ Push inner needle through lesion
  - ○ Ensure trough is across lesion, then fire
- Automated biopsy gun system ("fire-forward" type)
  - ○ Desirable to sample edge of lesion: Avoid necrotic center
  - ○ Mobile mass: Can anchor tip of needle in edge of mass prior to firing
  - ○ Double check alignment & depth of needle throw (15 mm or 22 mm typical)
  - ○ Compress lesion with probe to stabilize, then fire
- Remove needle, open notch and place core into specimen jar
  - ○ If touch imprint cytology, first touch core in trough onto clean slide
  - ○ Smear, fix and stain slides as for fine needle biopsy
- 3 cores diagnostic in vast majority of masses
  - ○ ~ 70% accuracy with 1 core, ~ 95% with 3 cores

US-GUIDED CORE BIOPSY

○ ↑ # Cores for small lesion (< 7-10 mm), target = Ca++, uncertainty in targeting and/or needle gauge (e.g., 12-g)
• Consider insertion of marker, clip or coil
  ○ Through coaxial cannula, or independently if needle-mounted
• Apply dressing: Sterile tape over skin incision
• For multiple lesions, check numbering and consistency

Findings and Reporting
• Confirm lesion numbering, location and sequence, especially if multiple lesions
• Describe approach(es), puncture site(s), biopsy type, # passes
• Report any problems or complications
• Addend report with histopathology results, statement of concordance, final management recommendation, to whom results were communicated

Alternative Procedures/Therapies
• Radiologic
  ○ Stereotactic core or vacuum-assisted biopsy (if mammographically visible)
  ○ US-guided vacuum-assisted biopsy (esp. if lesion is very small or target is Ca++ without a mass)
  ○ US-guided FNAB of axillary lymph nodes
  ○ US-guided FNAB of highly suspicious masses
    ▪ 10% insufficient samples with nonpalpable lesions
• Surgical
  ○ Freehand core biopsy for palpable lesions
    ▪ Higher miss rate (13% vs. < 2% for US CNB in one series)
  ○ Diagnostic surgical biopsy, needle-localized if nonpalpable

POST-PROCEDURE

Expected Outcome
• Minimal sequelae
• US-guided 14-g CNB efficacy
  ○ Sensitivity & specificity 92-99%, average 98%, including immediate rebiopsies
  ○ Rebiopsy rates 4-11%, average 7%
    ▪ High risk lesions → excision
    ▪ Imaging-histopathologic discordance → excision
  ○ Tumor grade accuracy 75-80%
  ○ Upgrades at excision
    ▪ Nearly half of atypical ductal hyperplasia upgraded to malignancy
    ▪ ~ 20% of DCIS upgraded to invasive carcinoma
  ○ Receptor status accuracy 70%
  ○ Her-2/neu status 60%
  ○ Touch imprint cytology sensitivity and specificity 90-95%

Things To Do
• Place clip if any question of difficulty identifying lesion in future
  ○ Subtle finding
  ○ Neoadjuvant therapy planned: Mass may shrink or resolve
  ○ Facilitate correlation with mammography

○ Post-clip CC and 90° lateral mammograms
• Compress over lesion for 5-10 minutes
• Explain pressure and management if delayed hematoma develops

Things To Avoid
• Lack of visualization of needle tip

PROBLEMS & COMPLICATIONS

Complications
• Most feared complication(s)
  ○ Pneumothorax (< 0.1%)
  ○ Large delayed hematoma (< 1%)
• Other complications
  ○ Local pain (common, mild, transient)
  ○ Acute significant hematoma (< 1%)
  ○ Inadequate or inconclusive biopsy (depends on biopsy type), < 5%
  ○ Discordant needle and surgical biopsy histology
    ▪ Occurs in < 1% of cases
  ○ Infection (rare)

SELECTED REFERENCES

1. Cahill RA et al: Preoperative profiling of symptomatic breast cancer by diagnostic core biopsy. Ann Surg Oncol. 13(1):45-51, 2006
2. Crystal P et al: Accuracy of sonographically guided 14-gauge core-needle biopsy: results of 715 consecutive breast biopsies with at least two-year follow-up of benign lesions. J Clin Ultrasound. 33(2):47-52, 2005
3. Dillon MF et al: The accuracy of ultrasound, stereotactic, and clinical core biopsies in the diagnosis of breast cancer, with an analysis of false-negative cases. Ann Surg. 242(5):701-7, 2005
4. Klevesath MB et al: Touch imprint cytology of core needle biopsy specimens: a useful method for immediate reporting of symptomatic breast lesions. Eur J Surg Oncol. 31(5):490-4, 2005
5. Topal U et al: Role of ultrasound-guided core needle biopsy of axillary lymph nodes in the initial staging of breast carcinoma. Eur J Radiol. 56(3):382-5, 2005
6. Pijnappel RM et al: Diagnostic accuracy for different strategies of image-guided breast intervention in cases of nonpalpable breast lesions. Br J Cancer. 90(3):595-600, 2004
7. Smith WL et al: Comparison of core needle breast biopsy techniques: freehand versus three-dimensional US guidance. Acad Radiol. 9(5):541-50, 2002
8. Pisano ED et al: Fine-needle aspiration biopsy of nonpalpable breast lesions in a multicenter clinical trial: results from the radiologic diagnostic oncology group V. Radiology. 219(3):785-92, 2001
9. White RR et al: Impact of core-needle breast biopsy on the surgical management of mammographic abnormalities. Ann Surg. 233(6):769-77, 2001
10. Hatada T et al: Diagnostic value of ultrasound-guided fine-needle aspiration biopsy, core-needle biopsy, and evaluation of combined use in the diagnosis of breast lesions. J Am Coll Surg. 190(3):299-303, 2000
11. Jacobs TW et al: Accuracy of touch imprint cytology of image-directed breast core needle biopsies. Acta Cytol. 43(2):169-74, 1999
12. Harvey JA et al: Evaluation of a turkey-breast phantom for teaching freehand, US-guided core-needle breast biopsy. Acad Radiol. 4(8):565-9, 1997

IMAGE GALLERY

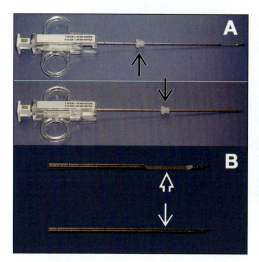

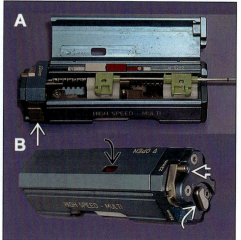

(Left) (A) Disposable plastic biopsy gun of "fire-in-place" type. Position of needle tip does not change when outer needle moves forward ➡. (B) Typical core notch opened ➡ and closed ➡. **(Right)** (A) Metal automated biopsy gun of "fire-forward" type with needle mounted in fired position. Note trigger ➡. (B) Indicator window ➡ shows gun is cocked. Note trigger throw length switch ➡ and safety catch ➡.

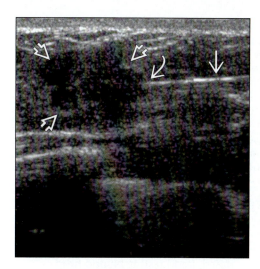

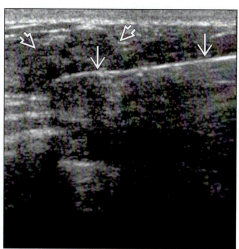

(Left) Transverse ultrasound during CNB shows pre-fire position with needle tip ➡ at leading edge of a hypoechoic irregular mass ➡. Note the needle shaft ➡ parallels the transducer face. **(Right)** Transverse ultrasound (same patient as previous image) post-fire. The needle ➡ has advanced into the lesion ➡. Note relative position of probe, lesion and needle. Histology showed grade II invasive ductal carcinoma (IDC).

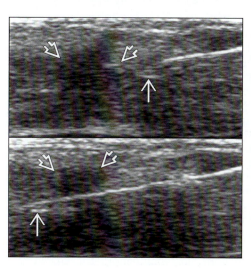

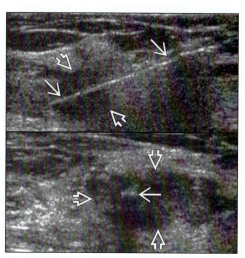

(Left) Ultrasound shows CNB needle tip ➡ and a hypoechoic 12 mm lesion ➡ pre-fire (upper) and post-fire (lower). Note the needle tip pre-fire is short of this grade II IDC. The 22 mm throw carries the tip through the lesion. **(Right)** Ultrasound shows a core needle ➡ fired into an irregular hypoechoic lesion ➡. Upper image is parallel to needle shaft; lower image perpendicular to needle shaft, showing needle ➡ near the center of this invasive carcinoma.

US-GUIDED VACUUM-ASSISTED BIOPSY

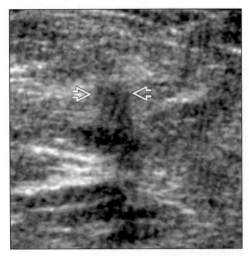

US shows a nonpalpable 5 mm mass ⊳ upper outer right breast in an 89 year old woman. US-guided vacuum-assisted biopsy was recommended.

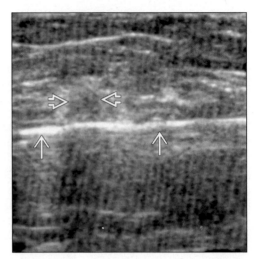

US (same patient as previous image) shows probe ⊳ well positioned, just posterior to lesion ⊳ prior to biopsy. Aperture is still closed. Pathology revealed infiltrating ductal carcinoma.

TERMINOLOGY

Synonyms
- Ultrasound-guided directional vacuum-assisted breast biopsy (US-VAB or US-DVB)

Definitions
- US-guided biopsy technique, using vacuum suction to remove significantly more tissue than standard automated core biopsy

PRE-PROCEDURE

Indications
- Lesions which benefit from greater tissue retrieval
  - Suspicious calcifications (Ca++) visible on US
  - Very small, subtle, or insinuating lesions
    - Practices vary from lesions ≤ 1.5 cm to only those smaller than 5 mm
    - **No proven diagnostic benefit for masses compared to 14-g core**
- Complete excision of probably benign palpable lesions: Controversial, not standard of care
  - Fibroadenoma, gynecomastia

Contraindications
- Anticoagulants or other medications which promote bleeding: May proceed if medication can be temporarily discontinued or effects reversed
- Bleeding disorders
- Lesions ≥ 1.5 cm diameter
- Subcutaneous lesions
- Lesions immediately adjacent to implants

Getting Started
- Things to Check: Verify lesion can be seen on US
- Medications

- 1% lidocaine ± buffered with sodium bicarbonate
- 1% lidocaine & epinephrine (deep anesthesia)
- Equipment List
  - High-resolution ultrasound unit (10-13 MHz transducer)
  - Vacuum-assisted biopsy device: 11-, 10-, 9-, or 8-gauge probe
  - Scalpel, hemostat, 25-gauge needle (local anesthetic)
  - Betadine or other surgical-cleansing soap for skin
  - Sterile drape, gel, (optional) probe cover
  - Radiopaque clip/marker

PROCEDURE

Patient Position/Location
- Best procedure approach: Patient supine with ipsilateral arm raised, hand resting behind head

Procedure Steps
- Breast cleansed with disinfectant
- Fenestrated drape or towels to define sterile field
- Sterile probe, usually covered
- Administration of local anesthetic
  - Should be given along desired route as well as anterior, posterior & distal to lesion
- Small skin incision made with scalpel
  - Hemostat to spread tissue → facilitates probe entry
    - Additional local anesthetic with large gauge needle also "breaks up" dense tissue
- Probe advanced manually under US guidance posterior to lesion with aperture toward lesion
  - If anterior → "shadows out" lesion
  - Posterior position prevents chest wall/implant harm
- Cutter retracted to expose aperture; ring down artifact
- Vacuum activated → tissue cut → excised → transported to collection chamber or retrieved
- Aperture rotated

US-GUIDED VACUUM-ASSISTED BIOPSY

Key Facts

Terminology
- US-guided biopsy technique, using vacuum suction to remove significantly more tissue than standard automated core biopsy

Procedure
- Probe advanced manually under US guidance posterior to lesion with aperture toward lesion
- Vacuum activated → tissue cut → excised → transported to collection chamber or retrieved

- Disappearance of lesion monitored under realtime US guidance
- Marking clip placed through probe
- Post-procedure CC & 90° lateral mammograms

Post-procedure
- Average 7.5% re-biopsy rate, 23% malignant

Problems & Complications
- Bleeding (hematoma), infection

- Samples acquired between 9:00 & 3:00, traveling through 12:00
- Unless lesion posterior to aperture, no need to acquire tissue at other positions
- Disappearance of lesion monitored under realtime US guidance
- Marking clip placed through probe
- Specimen radiograph for Ca++
  - May help direct pathologist's attention
  - Place specimens with Ca++ in separate container
- Post-procedure CC & 90° lateral mammograms
  - Clip position documented for follow-up mammograms or needle localization

Findings and Reporting
- Document clip location in relation to lesion
- Document if lesion removed using imaging criteria
  - Disappearance of lesion on imaging does not usually indicate complete pathologic removal

Alternative Procedures/Therapies
- Radiologic
  - Ultrasound-guided multipass 14-g core biopsy
    - Much cheaper, less invasive
    - 7.4% re-biopsy rate; 21% malignant

POST-PROCEDURE

Expected Outcome
- Complete or near-complete removal of imaging finding; target obscured during procedure

- Average 7.5% re-biopsy rate, 23% malignant
  - Atypical or high-risk lesions need excision

PROBLEMS & COMPLICATIONS

Complications
- Most feared complication(s): Bleeding (hematoma), infection
- Other complications: Pneumothorax: Avoid by parallel position of probe tip to chest wall

SELECTED REFERENCES

1. Cho N et al: Sonographically guided core biopsy of the breast: comparison of 14-gauge automated gun and 11-gauge directional vacuum-assisted biopsy methods. Korean J Radiol. 6(2):102-9, 2005
2. March DE et al: Breast masses: removal of all US evidence during biopsy by using a handheld vacuum-assisted device--initial experience. Radiology. 227(2):549-55, 2003
3. Parker SH et al: Sonographically guided directional vacuum-assisted breast biopsy using a handheld device. AJR Am J Roentgenol. 177(2):405-8, 2001
4. Simon JR et al: Accuracy and complication rates of US-guided vacuum-assisted core breast biopsy: initial results. Radiology. 215(3):694-7, 2000
5. Parker SH et al: Performing a breast biopsy with a directional, vacuum-assisted biopsy instrument. Radiographics. 17(5):1233-52, 1997

IMAGE GALLERY

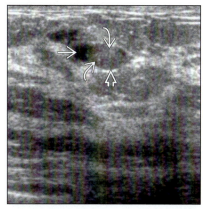 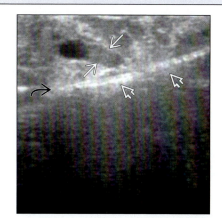 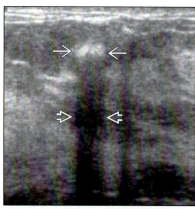

(Left) Transverse US shows a dilated duct ➡ with an intraductal mass ➡ containing Ca++ ➡, just superior to the right nipple, in a 41 year old woman. (Center) US shows intraductal mass ➡ (same patient as previous image) at time of vacuum-assisted biopsy. Probe ➡ is posterior to mass ➡, its tip ➡ distal to lesion. (Right) Sagittal US (same patient as prior 2 images) confirms lesion removal. A metallic clip ➡ with its associated shadowing ➡ has been placed at biopsy site. Pathology revealed a benign papilloma. The lesion was not excised.

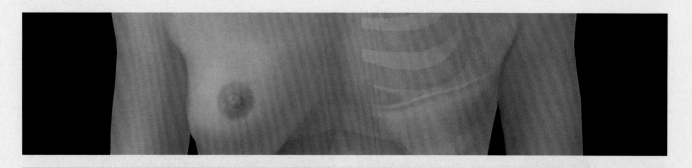

SECTION 3: Procedures, Surgical

AXILLARY DISSECTION

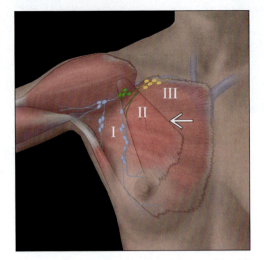

Graphic shows lymphatic channels (light blue). Most drainage leads to axillary nodes ➔. The locations of the internal mammary ➔, intramammary ➔, and infraclavicular nodes ➔ are also illustrated.

In ALND, level I nodes lateral to (blue), and level II nodes posterior to (green) the pectoralis minor muscle ➔ are typically removed. Medial level III nodes (yellow) are not typically removed.

TERMINOLOGY

Abbreviations
- Axillary lymph node dissection (ALND)
- Sentinel lymph node (SLN) biopsy (SNB)

Synonyms
- Axillary lymphadenectomy

Definitions
- Surgical removal of axillary contents (fat and lymph nodes) for the purposes of staging breast cancer and control of local disease
- Traditional approach to ALND includes dissection of the level I and level II axillary nodes
  - Level I axillary nodes: Nodes that lie inferior and lateral to the pectoralis minor muscle
  - Level II axillary nodes: Nodes that lie posterior to the pectoralis minor muscle and below the axillary vein
  - Level III axillary nodes: Nodes that lie medial to the pectoralis minor muscle and below the clavicle
- Dissection of level III nodes generally reserved for gross disease in an effort to maximize local control
- Completion ALND: Performed after initial SNB

PRE-PROCEDURE

Indications
- ALND performed for staging invasive breast cancer
- When SNB contraindicated
  - Clinically suspicious axillary nodes
    - 10-50% of clinically suspicious axillary nodes do not contain tumor by H&E staining
    - 15-40% of clinically negative axillary nodes reveal metastatic disease on histologic evaluation

- Pregnancy: Reluctance to use radiocolloid; methylene blue can be used
- Prior axillary surgery or cosmetic breast surgery
  - Lymphatic channels may be disrupted
  - Area of ongoing investigation
- Following neoadjuvant chemotherapy
  - Higher rate of false negative SNB (ongoing studies)
- Axillary nodal metastasis known by prior fine needle aspiration biopsy (FNAB) or core biopsy (CNB)
- SLN known to have metastasis
  - Result of isolated tumor cells (ITC, typically by immunohistochemistry, IHC) in SLN controversial
    - Likely does not merit ALND; ongoing studies
  - Metastasis (more than ITC) in SLN on intraoperative frozen section, touch prep, or final sectioning
- Failure to identify SLN
- Previous mastectomy: Lymphatic channels disrupted, SNB not an option
- Local control: Elderly patient with suspicious axillary nodes, not a candidate for chemotherapy

Contraindications
- In clinically node-negative disease, SNB used alone for axillary staging
  - Reduced mortality
  - Completion ALND if SNB shows metastasis
- Ductal carcinoma in situ (DCIS)
  - SNB may be performed for large area of DCIS (> 2.5 cm) or when mastectomy planned

Getting Started
- Things to Check
  - In the patient with newly diagnosed breast cancer, physical examination by the surgeon is critical
    - Review of imaging studies and clinical findings: Confirm extent of disease (plan lumpectomy vs. mastectomy)

AXILLARY DISSECTION

Key Facts

Terminology

- Axillary lymph node dissection (ALND)
- Sentinel lymph node (SLN) biopsy (SNB)
- Surgical removal of axillary contents (fat and lymph nodes) for the purposes of staging breast cancer and control of local disease

Pre-procedure

- ALND performed for staging invasive breast cancer
- Clinically suspicious axillary nodes
- Axillary nodal metastasis known by prior fine needle aspiration biopsy (FNAB) or core biopsy (CNB)
- Metastasis (more than ITC) in SLN on intraoperative frozen section, touch prep, or final sectioning
- In clinically node-negative disease, SNB used alone for axillary staging
- Completion ALND if SNB shows metastasis

Procedure

- Multiple anatomic structures must be identified and preserved to minimize morbidity of ALND

Post-procedure

- 5-year disease-free survival (DFS) for node-negative patients: ~ 80%
- 5-year DFS ≥ 16 involved axillary nodes: ~ 20%

Problems & Complications

- Upper extremity lymphedema
- May take several years to manifest: 13% initially; up to 25% on delayed follow-up
- Hematoma/seromas requiring drainage
- Axillary recurrence in 0.25-3.0% of node-negative patients
- Post-operative infection: 8-19% of patients

- Clinical examination of axilla: Suspicious nodes prompt ALND rather than SNB
- Medications: Generally performed under general anesthesia unless precluded by severity of comorbid conditions

PROCEDURE

Patient Position/Location

- Best procedure approach
  - Patient supine on operating room table with ipsilateral arm abducted 90 degrees on an armboard
  - Pre-operative single dose intravenous antibiotics (optional)
  - Dissection follows anatomic boundaries of axilla
    - Lateral extent of dissection: Border of latissimus dorsi muscle
    - Medial extent of dissection: Three levels of axillary nodes as defined by their relationship to pectoralis minor muscle
    - Superior extent of dissection: Axillary vein
    - Inferior extent of dissection: Where thoracodorsal bundle courses inferiorly and enters latissimus dorsi muscle on its deep surface
  - Multiple anatomic structures must be identified and preserved to minimize morbidity of ALND
    - At lateral border of pectoralis minor muscle, the medial pectoral neurovascular bundle is preserved
    - Along the anterior border of latissimus dorsi muscle, preserve intercostobrachial nerves
    - Along the axillary vein, a cuff of adjacent fat is preserved; stripping all fat from the axillary vein increases risk of subsequent arm lymphedema
    - Thoracodorsal nerve (within the thoracodorsal bundle) preserved
    - Long thoracic nerve is identified as it courses along the chest wall and is preserved
  - A closed-suction drain may be placed as wound is closed to minimize hematoma/seroma formation

Findings and Reporting

- Generally, an adequate ALND specimen will contain 10 or more lymph nodes for histologic analysis
  - Average of 16 nodes obtained (averages range from 11-23 across series)
- Histologic analysis usually consists of bivalving the nodes and examining H&E stained sections
  - IHC not typically performed except on SLN
- Pathologist to report number and size of nodes, category (single cells or clusters, micro- or macrometastases), maximal size of largest metastatic deposit, presence of extranodal extension
- p Staging = Pathologic staging: pN0 = No regional lymph node metastasis histologically
  - pN1mi: Micrometastasis = 0.2 mm < tumor deposit ≤ 2 mm
  - pN1a: Metastasis in 1-3 axillary lymph nodes
  - pN2a: Metastasis in 4-9 axillary lymph nodes (at least one tumor deposit > 2.0 mm)
  - pN3a: Metastasis in 10 or more axillary lymph nodes (at least one tumor deposit > 2.0 mm) or infraclavicular nodal metastasis

Alternative Procedures/Therapies

- Radiologic
  - No imaging test sufficiently accurate to preclude need for surgical axillary node sampling by SNB or ALND
  - Initial US-guided FNAB or CNB of node to confirm metastasis: Skip SNB proceed directly to ALND
- Surgical
  - In appropriate candidates, SNB can be substituted for ALND for axillary staging
    - If SLN negative, ALND usually not performed
    - 7% false negative rate of SNB
- Other
  - Therapeutic radiation of the axilla
    - In clinically node-negative patients, primary axillary radiation without ALND has low rate of loco-regional recurrence comparable to ALND (0.8-3.0%) (ongoing studies)
    - Does not allow for pathologic nodal staging

■ Salvage ALND for axillary recurrence

POST-PROCEDURE

Expected Outcome
- Presence or absence of metastasis in axillary nodes is the single most important prognostic indicator in predicting survival from breast cancer
  - 5-year disease-free survival (DFS) for node-negative patients: ~ 80%
  - 5-year DFS ≥ 16 involved axillary nodes: ~ 20%
- Direct relationship exists between number of axillary nodes involved with metastases & DFS
- Predictive value of nodal involvement in overall survival is independent of tumor size
- Axillary recurrence rates range from 0.25-3.0% in clinically node-negative patients undergoing ALND
  - ↑ Axillary recurrence rates with ↑ # nodes found metastatic at initial ALND and fewer nodes resected
  - Surgical removal of axillary nodes containing metastatic disease decreases risk of axillary recurrence

Things To Do
- Treatment decisions for adjunctive chemotherapy and radiotherapy are based, in part, on axillary node status
  - Post-mastectomy radiation therapy (XRT) typically given when 4 or more nodes show metastases
  - Adjuvant chemotherapy typically given when any metastatic node(s) identified
    - Significance of ITC in SLN unknown

PROBLEMS & COMPLICATIONS

Complications
- Most feared complication(s)
  - Upper extremity lymphedema
    - May take several years to manifest: 13% initially; up to 25% on delayed follow-up
    - Risk is related to extent of surgical dissection
    - Risk increases with increasing patient age
    - Adjunctive axillary radiotherapy after ALND doubles risk of lymphedema
    - Treatment includes manual lymphatic drainage, pneumatic compression devices, compressive bandaging, therapeutic exercise, use of elastic compression garments
- Other complications
  - Hematoma/seromas requiring drainage
    - 8% of patients in whom closed-suction axillary drain was used vs. 50% of patients without
  - Axillary recurrence in 0.25-3.0% of node-negative patients
  - Nerve injury (frequent)
    - Pectoral neurovascular bundle: Atrophy of portion of pectoralis muscle
    - Intercostobrachial nerves: Numbness of upper inner arm, paresthesias, ↓ arm strength

- Thoracodorsal nerve: Atrophy of latissimus dorsi muscle and loss of shoulder abduction (transection of thoracodorsal vessels precludes use of latissimus dorsi muscle in breast reconstruction)
- Long thoracic nerve: Atrophy of serratus anterior muscle and winged scapula
  - Post-operative infection: 8-19% of patients
    - May be reduced with administration of single-dose, intravenous, pre-operative antibiotics
  - Post-operative shoulder immobility, cording
    - Usually resolves within 6 months with physical therapy
  - Axillary vein thrombosis

SELECTED REFERENCES

1. Kim T et al: Lymphatic mapping and sentinel lymph node biopsy in early-stage breast carcinoma: a metaanalysis. Cancer. 106(1):4-16, 2006
2. Lyman GH et al: American Society of Clinical Oncology guideline recommendations for sentinel lymph node biopsy in early-stage breast cancer. J Clin Oncol. 23(30):7703-20, 2005
3. Coen JJ et al: Risk of lymphedema after regional nodal irradiation with breast conservation therapy. Int J Radiat Oncol Biol Phys. 55(5):1209-15, 2003
4. Singletary SE et al: Revision of the American Joint Committee on Cancer staging system for breast cancer. J Clin Oncol. 20(17):3628-36, 2002
5. Petrek JA et al: Lymphedema in a cohort of breast carcinoma survivors 20 years after diagnosis. Cancer. 92(6):1368-77, 2001
6. Martin J: Axillary Dissection. Operative Techniques Gen Surg. 2:152-60, 2000
7. Nason KS et al: Increased false negative sentinel node biopsy rates after preoperative chemotherapy for invasive breast carcinoma. Cancer. 89(11):2187-94, 2000
8. Newman LA et al: Presentation, management and outcome of axillary recurrence from breast cancer. Am J Surg. 180(4):252-6, 2000
9. Bold RJ et al: Prospective, randomized, double-blind study of prophylactic antibiotics in axillary lymph node dissection. Am J Surg. 176(3):239-43, 1998
10. Hilsenbeck SG et al: Time-dependence of hazard ratios for prognostic factors in primary breast cancer. Breast Cancer Res Treat. 52(1-3):227-37, 1998
11. Zavotsky J et al: Evaluation of axillary lymphadenectomy without axillary drainage for patients undergoing breast-conserving therapy. Ann Surg Oncol. 5(3):227-31, 1998
12. Carter CL et al: Relation of tumor size, lymph node status, and survival in 24,740 breast cancer cases. Cancer. 63(1):181-7, 1989
13. Pezner RD et al: Arm lymphedema in patients treated conservatively for breast cancer: relationship to patient age and axillary node dissection technique. Int J Radiat Oncol Biol Phys. 12(12):2079-83, 1986
14. Fisher B et al: The accuracy of clinical nodal staging and of limited axillary dissection as a determinant of histologic nodal status in carcinoma of the breast. Surg Gynecol Obstet. 152(6):765-72, 1981
15. Berg JW: The significance of axillary node levels in the study of breast carcinoma. Cancer. 8(4):776-8, 1955

IMAGE GALLERY

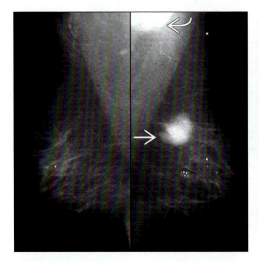

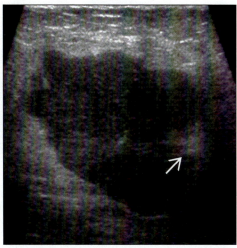

(Left) MLO mammography shows lobulated dense mass upper left breast ➡ and large, palpable mass left axilla ➡ in this 62 year old woman. Core biopsy of breast mass: Grade III IDC. *(Right)* US of left axillary mass (same patient as previous image) shows lobulated hypoechoic mass & small echogenic hilum ➡. US-guided FNAB: Metastatic node. She underwent lumpectomy + ALND. ALND is appropriate when nodal metastases are known preoperatively.

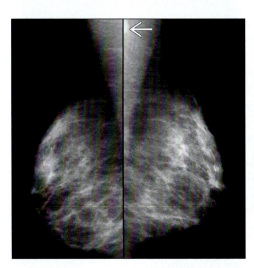

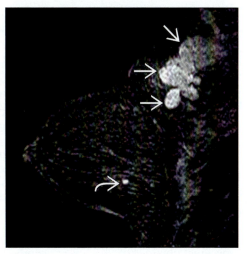

(Left) MLO mammography shows portion of palpable dense mass left axilla ➡ in this 41 year old. US-guided FNAB showed metastatic node. *(Right)* Sagittal T1 C+ FS MR (same patient as previous image) shows multiple, confluent proven metastatic nodes left axilla ➡. The primary cancer was not identified. An incidental enhancing mass on MR ➡ showed fibrocystic change. Neoadjuvant chemotherapy was given followed by ALND and breast XRT.

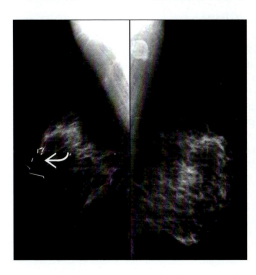

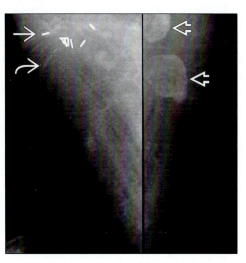

(Left) MLO mammography in this 59 year old shows post-surgical changes s/p right lumpectomy 4 years earlier, with right breast smaller than left and clips at surgical site ➡. *(Right)* Close-up of axillae (same patient as previous image) shows clips ➡ and minimal linear scarring ➡ right axilla following ALND. Several normal nodes remain on the left ➡.

LUMPECTOMY

The target is localized using imaging guidance (here, mammography was utilized), and a wire is placed through the lesion.

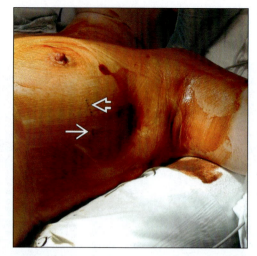

With the wire ➡ now in place, (same as on left) the patient is positioned supine with the arm abducted. The entire area has been prepped with an iodine-based antiseptic. The planned incision site is marked ➡.

TERMINOLOGY

Abbreviations
- Breast-conserving treatment (BCT); i.e., breast-conserving surgery followed by adjuvant radiation therapy (XRT)
- Accelerated partial breast irradiation (APBI)

Synonyms
- Partial mastectomy

Definitions
- Lumpectomy: Breast-conserving surgery with goal of removing breast malignancy and surrounding margin of histologically benign breast parenchyma
  - Connotes removal of a cancer with intention to treat
  - Term also used to describe specimen obtained at re-excision for margins
- Cavity margins: Additional tissue taken at edges of lumpectomy to aid in assuring clear margins
- Sentinel lymph node (SLN) biopsy (SNB)
  - Full axillary lymph node dissection (ALND) performed when SLN shows metastasis
- Quadrantectomy: Resection of triangular sector of breast (apex toward nipple) including skin and pectoralis fascia
  - Based on segmental growth of cancer
  - Includes wide margin of normal breast tissue; ↑ deformity
- Excisional biopsy: Surgical tissue removal for diagnosis, connotes benign result
- Incisional biopsy: Surgical tissue sampling of a large lesion for diagnosis, not intended to treat
- Oncoplastic resection surgery
  - Surgical techniques emphasizing cosmetic outcome
    - Malignant breast tissue removed with wide surgical margins
    - Remaining glandular tissue transposed to achieve best possible cosmetic outcome

PRE-PROCEDURE

Indications
- Radiologic evidence and physical examination suggests malignancy is confined to one quadrant of the breast
- Size and location of tumor in context of breast size suggests cosmetically acceptable outcome will be achieved with lumpectomy
- Patients with locally advanced breast cancer undergoing neoadjuvant chemotherapy (NAT) with good response
  - Those with significant tumor response may become candidates for BCT rather than mastectomy

Contraindications
- Presence of two or more primary tumors in separate quadrants of the breast or association with diffuse malignant-appearing calcifications (Ca++)
- Inability to obtain negative histologic margins after reasonable attempts at surgical excision/re-excision
- 4-5 cm or larger tumor in small breast
- History of prior therapeutic XRT to the involved breast
- First or second trimester pregnancy: XRT contraindicated
  - In third trimester, BCT with deferral of XRT until after delivery is often feasible
- History of collagen vascular disease: Relative contraindication to XRT, may be poorly tolerated
- Known BRCA-1, -2 carrier (relative): High risk of second primary breast cancer

LUMPECTOMY

Key Facts

Terminology
- Lumpectomy: Breast-conserving surgery with goal of removing breast malignancy and surrounding margin of histologically benign breast parenchyma

Pre-procedure
- Radiologic evidence and physical examination suggests malignancy is confined to one quadrant of the breast
- Patient willing and able to have XRT
- Percutaneous biopsy: ↓ Rates positive margins, ↓ number of surgeries, ↓ costs

Procedure
- Outpatient procedure

- Pre-operative needle localization for nonpalpable lesions and/or to define radiologic extent of disease, may require bracketing
- Surgeon orients specimen
- Intra-operative specimen imaging if needle localized
- Additional marginal tissue often resected

Post-procedure
- When combined with XRT in appropriate candidates, survival rate equivalent to mastectomy
- Local recurrence rates of 5-19% 10 years after BCT with clear margins
- Local recurrence ↓ with hormonal therapy in patients with ER+ cancer(s): 2-7% at 10 years
- Post-operative mammography prior to XRT when margins close or positive & original tumor had Ca++

- When genetic testing results unknown, delay in procedure may occur (patient choice) until testing results available (~ 5 weeks); patient may elect bilateral mastectomies if results are positive

Getting Started
- Things to Check
  - Careful patient selection and multidisciplinary approach critical to success
  - Patient willing and able to have XRT
  - Physical examination by surgeon, extensive imaging assessment as to size and location of lesion(s)
    - Mammographic evaluation (within 2 months) to assess extent of disease
    - Extent of malignant-appearing Ca++ should be documented; magnification CC and 90° lateral views
  - Percutaneous biopsy: ↓ Rates positive margins, ↓ number of surgeries, ↓ costs
    - Facilitates patient counseling in preparation for cancer-related surgery(ies)
    - When > one finding, biopsy lesions farthest apart to confirm extent of disease; mastectomy may be indicated
    - If core biopsy with clip placement determined the malignancy, pre- and post-biopsy mammogram assessment critical to avoid pitfall of localizing a misplaced clip rather than the targeted lesion(s)
  - Evaluate contralateral breast: 2-3% rates synchronous bilateral cancer historically
  - Consider supplementing mammography with US or MR to assess disease extent if BCT contemplated
    - ↑ Tumor size ± foci occult on mammography ± CBE common: Especially young patients (< 40-45 years), dense breast parenchyma, strong family history of breast cancer, known gene mutation, invasive lobular histology, extensive intraductal component (EIC, best seen on MR)
    - Detection of synchronous contralateral breast cancer (CBC) on US and/or MR in another 3-6% of patients
  - Contralateral breast may need reduction surgery for symmetry

PROCEDURE

Patient Position/Location
- Best procedure approach
  - Outpatient procedure
  - Local anesthesia ± supplemental sedation
    - General anesthesia may be used in some cases
  - Patient positioned supine in the operating suite with ipsilateral arm abducted
  - Pre-operative needle localization for nonpalpable lesions and/or to define radiologic extent of disease, may require bracketing
  - Ideal wire placements
    - Wire through or close to (< 1 cm from) lesion
    - Hook or J-tip ~ 1 cm deep to lesion, not superficial
    - Thickened part of internal wire stiffener (when present) straddles lesion
    - Wire entry site, lesion and nipple all included on same annotated image
  - New localization techniques being used or tested
    - Intraoperative US
    - Radioisotope seeds for lesion marking
    - Pre-operative placement of lesion tethering devices: Grasp ± surround lesion, facilitating its identification and removal

Procedure Steps
- Incision often made over tumor or circumareolar, with minimal tunneling
- Not necessary to remove skin or to excise needle track(s) from percutaneous biopsy
- Attention to hemostasis: ↓ Post-operative hematoma
  - Hematomas: ↑ Scarring, distortion on mammography
- Tissue of excisional cavity is not approximated
  - Cavity fills in with serum → more natural post-operative breast
- Surgeon orients specimen
  - Margins inked and/or affixed with suture ties
  - Specimen sent for imaging in a specimen container
- Intra-operative specimen imaging if needle localized
  - Assess removal of radiologic evidence of malignancy

LUMPECTOMY

- ○ Mammography and/or ultrasound may be used
- ○ No practical MR specimen imaging sequence to date
- ○ Intra-operative report to surgeon as to presence of lesion and intact wire within specimen
  - ■ May advise operating surgeon as to location of lesion(s) in relationship to specimen edges, may prompt additional tissue removal
- ○ Specimen image annotated to direct pathologist
- • Additional marginal tissue often resected
- • Axillary lymph node sampling
  - ○ If pre-operative FNAB or core biopsy of axillary node is positive, ALND performed
  - ○ SNB for invasive tumor with unknown node status; consider for high-grade DCIS > 2.5 cm
  - ○ If frozen section or touch prep of SNB positive → completion ALND
- • Oncoplastic resections performed with increasing frequency
  - ○ Smaller lesions removed through incisions along relaxed skin tension lines
  - ○ Internal defect may or may not be closed
  - ○ Consideration given to specialized incisions with skin resection
    - ■ "Batwing" or "donut" skin incisions
    - ■ Volume displacement closure techniques
- • Lumpectomy cavity marking clips placed to orient radiation oncologist for "boost"
- • Lumpectomy cavity may be maintained (no clips) for APBI balloon catheter brachytherapy

Findings and Reporting

- • Pathology report includes size and type of invasive tumor, grade of tumor, margin status, presence or absence of DCIS, grade of DCIS, % DCIS in tumor
- • EIC + tumors ⇒ ↑ likelihood of positive margins and ↑ residual malignancy at re-excision

Alternative Procedures/Therapies

- • Radiologic: Image-guided ablation undergoing study; tumor size and margin assessment limited
- • Surgical: Mastectomy → equivalent survival rates
- • Other: If patient not a candidate for surgery due to other (severe) comorbid conditions, consider tamoxifen for estrogen-receptor (ER) positive tumors

POST-PROCEDURE

Expected Outcome

- • When combined with XRT in appropriate candidates, survival rate equivalent to mastectomy
- • Local recurrence rates of 5-19% 10 years after BCT with clear margins
  - ○ Local recurrence ↓ with hormonal therapy in patients with ER+ cancer(s): 2-7% at 10 years
- • Acceptable cosmetic results in most patients

Things To Do

- • Post-operative mammography prior to XRT when margins close or positive & original tumor had Ca++
- • Consider MR if margins positive
  - ○ Sensitivity and specificity for residual disease = 61-70%; MR changes original treatment plan ~ 30%
- • Ongoing imaging surveillance is essential

- ○ Variable mammographic imaging protocols: q 6 months for 1-5 years, annual for contralateral breast

Things To Avoid

- • Over-reliance on specimen imaging to predict surgical margin status
  - ○ Apparent clear margins on specimen imaging no guarantee of negative pathologic margins
    - ■ Margins falsely negative with multifocal disease
- • Loss of orientation of specimen or marginal tissue
- • Intraoperative frozen section for diagnosis
  - ○ 3% false positive rate

PROBLEMS & COMPLICATIONS

Complications

- • Most feared complication(s)
  - ○ Positive margins → re-excision
    - ■ ↑ With EIC, large area (> 2.5 cm) malignant Ca++
  - ○ Poor cosmesis
  - ○ Wound infection uncommon ~ 1%
    - ■ Delayed breast abscess appearance median time = 5 months
    - ■ Infection risk increased with re-excision, XRT
  - ○ Failed excision of target following needle localization procedure ~ 3%
  - ○ Long term: Persistent seroma; fat necrosis

SELECTED REFERENCES

1. Choi JY et al: Aesthetic and reconstruction considerations in oncologic breast surgery. J Am Coll Surg. 202(6):943-52, 2006
2. Anderson BO et al: Oncoplastic approaches to partial mastectomy: an overview of volume-displacement techniques. Lancet Oncol. 6(3):145-57, 2005
3. Newman LA et al: Advances in breast conservation therapy. J Clin Oncol. 23(8):1685-97, 2005
4. Dirbas FM et al: The evolution of accelerated, partial breast irradiation as a potential treatment option for women with newly diagnosed breast cancer considering breast conservation. Cancer Biother Radiopharm. 19(6):673-705, 2004
5. Kepple J et al: Minimally invasive breast surgery. J Am Coll Surg. 199(6):961-75, 2004
6. Lee JM et al: MRI before reexcision surgery in patients with breast cancer. AJR Am J Roentgenol. 182(2):473-80, 2004
7. Rampaul RS et al: Randomized clinical trial comparing radioisotope occult lesion localization and wire-guided excision for biopsy of occult breast lesions. Br J Surg. 91(12):1575-7, 2004
8. Fisher B et al: Twenty-year follow-up of a randomized trial comparing total mastectomy, lumpectomy, and lumpectomy plus irradiation for the treatment of invasive breast cancer. N Engl J Med. 347(16):1233-41, 2002
9. Liberman L et al: One operation after percutaneous diagnosis of nonpalpable breast cancer: frequency and associated factors. AJR Am J Roentgenol. 178(3):673-9, 2002
10. Morrow M et al: Standard for breast conservation therapy in the management of invasive breast carcinoma. CA Cancer J Clin. 52(5):277-300, 2002
11. Veronesi U et al: Twenty-year follow-up of a randomized study comparing breast-conserving surgery with radical mastectomy for early breast cancer. N Engl J Med. 347(16):1227-32, 2002

LUMPECTOMY

IMAGE GALLERY

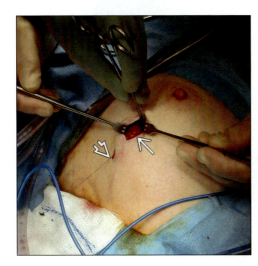
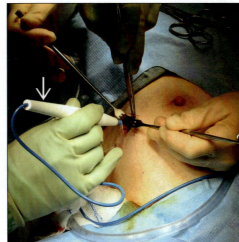

(Left) Intraoperative photographs demonstrate procedural steps of lumpectomy (same case as prior 2 and next 5 images). An incision ➡ is made medial to the entrance site ➡ of the localization wire. *(Right)* Electrocautery ➡ is used to dissect down along the expected path to the target lesion. Localizing the target is facilitated by intraoperative availability of post-localization mammograms.

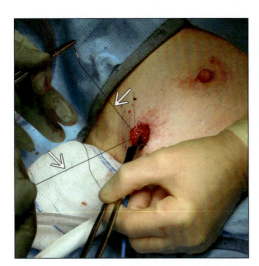
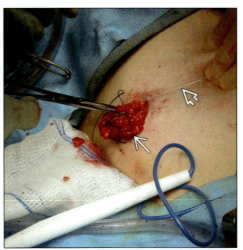

(Left) Prior to removal, the specimen orientation is marked with suture ties ➡ to facilitate margin examination by the pathologist. *(Right)* The specimen ➡ is delivered, along with the wire ➡, from the incision site.

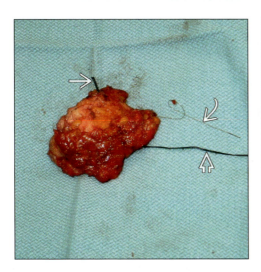
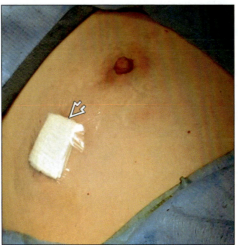

(Left) Specimen shows the single short stitch superiorly ➡ and a long stitch laterally ➡ both placed by the surgeon before tissue removal. The localization wire ➡ is seen exiting the specimen. *(Right)* Post-operatively, the incision is sutured closed and covered with a sterile dressing ➡.

MASTECTOMY

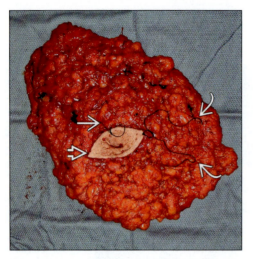

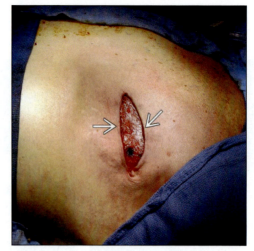

Skin-sparing mastectomy specimen including the nipple-areolar complex ➡️ *is marked with sutures to indicate orientation (short suture* ➡️ *= superior, long sutures* ➡️ *= lateral).*

Immediate post-mastectomy incision site ➡️ *(same as on left). Care is taken to assure smoothly tapering fat planes beneath the subcutaneous tissues to assure a good cosmetic result.*

TERMINOLOGY

Definitions

- Mastectomies
  - Total mastectomy (or simple): Complete excision of breast tissue without inclusion of axillary lymph nodes
    - Nipple-areolar complex traditionally removed
    - New areolar sparing techniques
  - Subcutaneous mastectomy: Removal of breast tissue, with preservation of the nipple-areolar complex
    - No intentional lymph node removal
  - Modified radical mastectomy (MRM): Complete excision of breast tissue and underlying fascia of the pectoralis major muscle
  - "Skin-sparing" mastectomy of any type focuses on minimal unnecessary skin removal; performed when immediate reconstruction is planned
  - Radical mastectomy: Complete excision of breast tissue, pectoralis major and minor muscles and level I, II, and III axillary lymph nodes; frequently requires skin graft
  - Extended radical mastectomy: Radical mastectomy plus excision of ipsilateral internal mammary nodal chain
  - Prophylactic mastectomy: Removal of a normal breast to prevent future development of malignancy
    - Total mastectomy most common; consider sentinel node biopsy (SNB)
- Sentinel lymph node (SLN) biopsy (SNB)
  - SNB often performed at time of mastectomy; cannot be done after mastectomy
  - When axillary nodes known to be positive for tumor (e.g., prior FNAB or core biopsy, positive SLN at frozen section or touch prep), full axillary lymph node dissection (ALND) performed
- Axillary lymph node dissection (ALND)

  - Performed when axillary nodes known to be positive for tumor
    - Prior FNAB or core biopsy
    - Positive SLN at frozen section or touch prep → "completion" ALND
  - May be performed when SLN cannot be identified
- Generic patient consent form: Mastectomy, SNB, completion ALND if SLN+
- Reconstructions
  - Prostheses
    - Saline or silicone gel-filled implants
    - Tissue expander: Inflatable, temporary implant
  - Tissue transfers: Vascular pedicle flaps
    - TRAM (transverse rectus abdominus myocutaneous)
    - Latissimus dorsi (generally need additional prosthesis)
  - Tissue transfers: Free flaps, defined by vascular supply
    - Deep inferior epigastric perforator (DIEP)
    - Superficial inferior epigastric artery (SIEA)
    - Superior gluteal artery perforator (S-GAP)
    - Inferior gluteal artery perforator (I-GAP)
- Breast-conserving treatment (BCT): Lumpectomy or quadrantectomy, followed by adjuvant radiation therapy (XRT)

PRE-PROCEDURE

Indications

- Presence of two or more primary cancers in separate quadrants of the breast
- Multifocal carcinoma in young woman (< 40-45 years): High risk of local recurrence, especially if ≥ 3 foci
- Association of cancer with diffuse malignant-appearing calcifications (Ca++)
- Cancer recurrence in a therapeutically irradiated breast

MASTECTOMY

Key Facts

Terminology
- Modified radical mastectomy (MRM): Complete excision of breast tissue and underlying fascia of the pectoralis major muscle
- Sentinel lymph node (SLN) biopsy (SNB)
- SNB often performed at time of mastectomy; cannot be done after mastectomy

Pre-procedure
- Presence of two or more primary cancers in separate quadrants of the breast
- Cancer recurrence in a therapeutically irradiated breast
- Chest wall invasion, diffuse skin involvement may preclude mastectomy
- Immediate reconstruction possible if potential need for XRT is low

Procedure
- Resection performed through an elliptical transverse incision encompassing the nipple-areolar complex (total mastectomy or MRM)
- Plane is developed between breast tissue and subcutaneous fat

Post-procedure
- Consider post-mastectomy XRT: Close or positive margins, advanced primary disease (T3, T4), ≥ 4 axillary lymph nodes positive for metastasis

Problems & Complications
- Local recurrence
- Seroma (most common), easily aspirated or drained
- Necrosis of skin flaps

- Patient unable or unwilling to undergo adjuvant XRT in conjunction with BCT
  - Cancer presenting in the first or second trimester of pregnancy
  - Other contraindications to XRT
    - Collagen vascular diseases
    - Prior breast and/or chest XRT
- Presence of extensive intraductal component (EIC) may ↑ recommendation for mastectomy
  - Variable: No higher risk of recurrence if clear margins achieved with good cosmesis
- Size and location of cancer in context of size of the breast suggest that lumpectomy (with clear margins) would fail to achieve a cosmetically acceptable result
  - General rule: Tumor > 5 cm in total extent prompts mastectomy
- Inability to achieve histologically negative margins after reasonable attempts at surgical excision ± re-excision lumpectomy
- Locally advanced breast cancer (LABC) in most cases
  - Neoadjuvant chemotherapy (NAT) fails to achieve tumor downsizing or cannot be tolerated
  - Even if cancer shrinks, high risk of recurrence with BCT
- Prevent development of malignancy in patients at high risk of breast cancer
  - Documented BRCA-1 or BRCA-2 genetic mutation
    - Lifetime risk of breast cancer: 50%-85%
  - Contralateral normal breast in patients presenting with breast cancer
    - Annual rate of contralateral breast cancer in women < 45 yrs of age diagnosed with breast cancer ~ 1% per year
    - Often chosen by patients when index cancer was mammographically occult
    - Invasive lobular cancer histology: ↑ Contralateral cancer
  - Lobular carcinoma in situ (LCIS): 18-37% lifetime risk in either breast

Contraindications
- Chest wall invasion, diffuse skin involvement may preclude mastectomy

- Inflammatory breast cancer without adequate NAT response
- Known distant metastases (relative): May be performed for local control
- Patient not able to tolerate major surgery

Getting Started
- Things to Check
  - Physical examination by the surgeon
    - Breasts, axillae, and supraclavicular regions
  - Mammographic evaluation within 2 months of treatment
    - Size and location of masses ± malignant-appearing Ca++
    - CC and 90° lateral magnification views of suspicious Ca++
    - Assess for possible disease in contralateral breast: Synchronous bilateral cancer 2-3% historically
    - Particular attention should be given to assessment for the presence of multicentric disease
  - Consider supplemental ultrasound or MR
    - Assess extent of disease in ipsilateral breast if otherwise a candidate for BCT
    - Attention to contralateral breast: Synchronous bilateral cancer seen only by MR, US: 3-6%
    - May be of particular benefit: Young women, dense parenchyma on mammogram, strong family history ± known BRCA-1, -2 carrier
    - ~ 50% of additional suspicious findings are malignant: Additional suspicious findings should be proven by core biopsy
- Medications: Generally performed under general anesthesia after single dose of preoperative antibiotics
- Decide on immediate or delayed or no reconstruction
- Immediate reconstruction possible if potential need for XRT is low
  - When XRT is likely, preferable to delay reconstruction until after XRT
  - XRT can be given following immediate reconstruction
    - Reported ~ 40% risk of complications
  - Type planned by patient and reconstructive surgeon pre-operatively

MASTECTOMY

- ○ Tissue expander may be needed prior to implant
- ○ Acellular dermal matrix (new) may be used as "sling" to improve contour of neobreast
- ○ Rates of local recurrence and development of distant metastases are equivalent with immediate or delayed reconstruction

PROCEDURE

Patient Position/Location
- Best procedure approach: Patient positioned supine on operating room table with ipsilateral arm abducted

Procedure Steps
- Resection performed through an elliptical transverse incision encompassing the nipple-areolar complex (total mastectomy or MRM)
- If incisional biopsy was performed for diagnosis, that incision should be incorporated in the specimen
- Boundaries of resection
  - ○ Laterally to the latissimus dorsi muscle
  - ○ Medially to the lateral border of the sternum
  - ○ Superiorly to the inferior margin of the clavicle
  - ○ Inferiorly to inframammary crease
- Plane is developed between breast tissue and subcutaneous fat
  - ○ Purpose is to completely excise breast tissue
- Breast tissue is dissected off the pectoralis muscle, taking its fascia
  - ○ May include part of muscle if it appears infiltrated by tumor
- Specimen is delivered from the incision, margins are marked with sutures for orientation
- Skin is closed over drain(s) to minimize hematoma/seroma formation

Alternative Procedures/Therapies
- Surgical
  - ○ BCT may be an acceptable alternative if
    - Malignancy confined to one quadrant of the breast
    - Histologically negative margins can be achieved
    - Size and location of tumor suggest that a cosmetically acceptable result will be obtained
    - Patient able and willing to undergo whole breast XRT or accelerated partial breast irradiation (APBI)

POST-PROCEDURE

Things To Do
- Consider post-mastectomy XRT: Close or positive margins, advanced primary disease (T3, T4), ≥ 4 axillary lymph nodes positive for metastasis
  - ○ ↓ Risk local-regional recurrence by ~ 66%; ↑ survival benefit ~ 10%
  - ○ Controversial when 1-3 nodes positive, large T2 tumors

Things To Avoid
- Incising skin involved by tumor

PROBLEMS & COMPLICATIONS

Complications
- Most feared complication(s)
  - ○ Local recurrence
    - Closely associated with larger primary tumor size and higher numbers of axillary lymph nodes positive for metastasis
    - 5% recurrence without axillary nodal metastasis
    - 25% in patients presenting with axillary nodal metastasis
    - Minimized through use of adjuvant XRT in patients at high risk for local recurrence
- Other complications
  - ○ Seroma (most common), easily aspirated or drained
  - ○ Necrosis of skin flaps
    - Occurs in up to 18% of cases, but often minor in degree
    - Associated with closure of flaps under tension ± perioperative infection
    - May require closure by secondary intention
  - ○ Wound infection
    - Reported incidence ranges from 6% to 14%
    - ~ 40% reduction can be achieved with single-dose peri-operative intravenous antibiotics

SELECTED REFERENCES

1. Choi JY et al: Aesthetic and reconstruction considerations in oncologic breast surgery. J Am Coll Surg. 202(6):943-52, 2006
2. Salhab M et al: Skin-sparing mastectomy and immediate breast reconstruction: patient satisfaction and clinical outcome. Int J Clin Oncol. 11(1):51-4, 2006
3. Stolier AJ et al: Areola-sparing mastectomy: defining the risks. J Am Coll Surg. 201(1):118-24, 2005
4. Staradub VL et al: Factors influencing outcomes for breast conservation therapy of mammographically detected malignancies. J Am Coll Surg. 196(4):518-24, 2003
5. Buchholz TA et al: Controversies regarding the use of radiation after mastectomy in breast cancer. Oncologist. 7(6):539-46, 2002
6. Medina-Franco H et al: Factors associated with local recurrence after skin-sparing mastectomy and immediate breast reconstruction for invasive breast cancer. Ann Surg. 235(6):814-9, 2002
7. Chilson TR et al: Seroma prevention after modified radical mastectomy. Am Surg. 58(12):750-4, 1992
8. Rosen PP et al: Contralateral breast carcinoma: an assessment of risk and prognosis in stage I (T1N0M0) and stage II (T1N1M0) patients with 20-year follow-up. Surgery. 106(5):904-10, 1989
9. Valagussa P et al: Patterns of relapse and survival following radical mastectomy. Analysis of 716 consecutive patients. Cancer. 41(3):1170-8, 1978
10. Auchincloss H: Modified radical mastectomy: why not? Am J Surg. 119(5):506-9, 1970

MASTECTOMY

IMAGE GALLERY

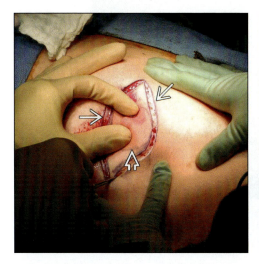
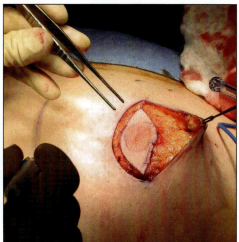

(Left) Intraoperative photographs from total left mastectomy with planned saline implant reconstruction demonstrate the procedural steps (same case as prior 2 and next 5 images). An elliptical incision ➡ is made to include the nipple-areolar complex ⇒. *(Right)* Using blunt dissection and an electrocautery, a plane is created between the breast tissue and the dermis/subcutaneous tissues.

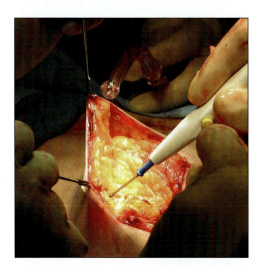
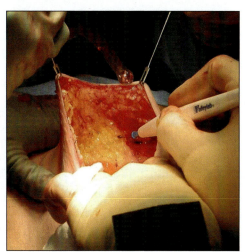

(Left) With careful attention to the thickness of the skin, dissection continues, balancing the need to remove breast tissue while retaining enough skin thickness to retain blood supply and remain viable. *(Right)* The dissection plane is continued to the clavicle superiorly, sternum medially, inframammary fold inferiorly, and latissimus dorsi laterally.

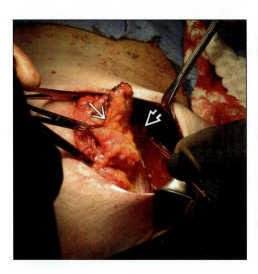
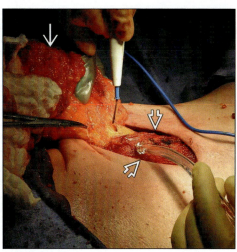

(Left) The breast tissue ➡ is subsequently dissected off the pectoralis muscle ⇒. *(Right)* The tissue ➡ is delivered from the elliptical incision ⇒, marked with sutures to indicate orientation, then removed from the field.

REDUCTION MAMMOPLASTY, PROCEDURE

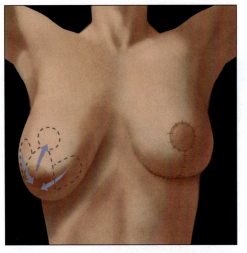

Graphic shows typical keyhole pattern of excision for reduction mammoplasty with nipple transposition on the right breast. The post-operative scar pattern is depicted on the left breast.

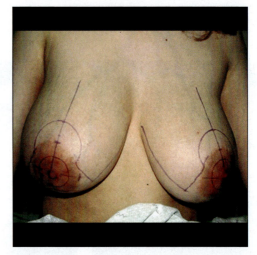

Clinical photograph shows pre-operative skin marking for a traditional "keyhole" inverted T-scar reduction mammoplasty. (All clinical photos courtesy of JJP).

TERMINOLOGY

Synonyms
- Reduction mammaplasty, breast reduction surgery

Definitions
- Plastic surgery to reduce breast size
- Mastopexy is surgery to reduce breast ptosis, but does not alter breast mass or volume

PRE-PROCEDURE

Indications
- Macromastia: Causing physical disability or poor self-image
  - Physical disability
    - Neck pain
    - Back pain
    - Shoulder pain
    - Shoulder grooving from pressure of brassiere straps
    - Chronic breast pain
    - Inframammary skin maceration and dermatoses
    - Hand/arm paresthesias
  - Psychological disability
    - Distorted body image
    - Interference with daily activities
    - Difficulty in participating in recreational activities
- Symmetry procedure following or concurrent with contralateral breast conservation surgery or mastectomy and reconstruction
- Congenital asymmetry
- Primary breast cancer prevention
  - In women with a high-risk profile (e.g., gene mutations) who find prophylactic mastectomy unacceptable
  - Breast cancer risk decreases proportional to amount of tissue resected

Getting Started
- Things to Check
  - Pre-operative patient assessment
    - Medical history: Comorbidities may affect the type of reduction performed
    - Preoperative mammography: Generally performed in all patients 35 years and older
    - Physical exam: Both to assess for any worrisome masses or skin changes as well as to assess skin type for surgical planning
  - Pre-operative patient counseling
    - Expectations of surgical scars
    - Possible nipple loss
    - Possible skin necrosis
    - Possible loss of nipple sensation
    - Possible impairment of normal lactation
    - Various techniques for reduction that may alter operative time, recovery period, scar pattern, and complication rates
  - Surgical planning
    - Measurements of the degree of nipple and breast ptosis with respect to the inframammary fold
    - Estimates of any size and shape disparity between the breasts
    - Skin tone
  - Reduction mammoplasty technique chosen based on
    - Surgeon experience
    - Breast size
    - Degree of breast ptosis
    - Patient age
    - Patient comorbidities
  - Variability in reimbursement by third-party payers
    - Variability exists as to what constitutes "medical necessity"

REDUCTION MAMMOPLASTY, PROCEDURE

Key Facts

Terminology
- Plastic surgery to reduce breast size
- Mastopexy is surgery to reduce breast ptosis, but does not alter breast mass or volume

Pre-procedure
- Macromastia: Causing physical disability or poor self-image
- Pre-operative patient counseling
- Various techniques for reduction that may alter operative time, recovery period, scar pattern, and complication rates
- Variability in reimbursement by third-party payers

Procedure
- Skin resection pattern and resultant scars distinguish various methods of reduction

- Most common techniques involve nipple-areolar complex transposition on a dermoglandular flap
- Less common techniques: Breast amputation with free nipple graft and suction mammoplasty

Post-procedure
- Multiple reviews and meta-analyses show procedure is associated with a statistically significant improvement in physical disability and quality of life
- Resected breast tissue should be sent for pathology review
- Occult breast carcinomas in 0.06-0.4% of reduction specimens; up to 0.8% if DCIS is included

Problems & Complications
- Post-operative scarring

- Documentation of the severity and duration of symptoms
- Documentation that conservative measures such as weight loss, exercise, dietary counseling, anti-inflammatory medications, muscle relaxants, support bras, and heat/cold treatments have failed to relieve symptoms
- Most insurers require estimates of the amount of breast tissue to be removed with minimums set around 400-500 g per side
- Some insurers have body mass index requirements
- The position of the American Society of Plastic Surgeons is that the definition of macromastia should focus on the degree of symptomology rather than the degree of hypertrophy
- Studies have shown that symptomatic macromastia is related to breast size and chest circumference independent of body weight

PROCEDURE

Procedure Steps
- For conventional reduction mammoplasties
  - Skin marking performed with the patient seated upright or standing
  - New site for nipple-areolar complex marked with varying techniques; approximately at the level of the submammary fold along a line from the mid clavicle projecting out to the nipple
  - Traditional keyhole incision pattern; new variations described
  - Skin flap is deepithelialized
  - Designated amount of parenchymal tissue is removed from the inferior portion of the breast
  - Dermoglandular pedicle with attached nipple-areolar complex is repositioned superiorly
  - Skin anastomoses sutured

Reduction Mammoplasty Techniques
- Skin resection pattern and resultant scars distinguish various methods of reduction

- Most common techniques involve nipple-areolar complex transposition on a dermoglandular flap
  - Inverted T-scar reduction
    - Variations based on the dermoglandular pedicle with inferior, superior, central, and medial pedicle techniques performed
    - Modifications of technique to increase survival of the transposed nipple-areola and skin flaps, improve aesthetic shape, and preserve nipple sensation and lactation function
  - Vertical-scar reduction
    - Reduced scar length as it eliminates the traditional scar along the inframammary fold
    - More technically challenging surgery, especially with larger breast sizes
  - No vertical-scar reduction
    - Another variation on the inverted T pattern which maintains the periareolar and inframammary anastomoses, but eliminates the visible vertical scar line
    - Ideal patients are those with a lot of ptosis, ≥ 5 cm of skin between the areola and the new areolar site
  - Pattern of skin de-epithelialization and glandular resection based on which technique is chosen
- Less common techniques: Breast amputation with free nipple graft and suction mammoplasty
  - Breast amputation with free nipple graft
    - Better results in very large breasts (2,500g or more per breast)
    - Surgery is faster; older patients or those with comorbidities may benefit
    - Disadvantages = loss of nipple sensation, loss of nipple projection, and loss of lactation function
  - Suction mammoplasty = liposuction reduction
    - Ideal for individuals with good skin quality and tone, predominantly fatty breast tissue, normal areola size and location, and small to moderate volume reduction desired
    - Less predictable results than with conventional reduction mammoplasty

- Alternative for those patients who find traditional scarring unacceptable
- Preserves nipple sensation and lactation function
- Faster recovery time to return to daily activities and exercise
- Mastopexy
  - Similar procedure to reduction mammoplasty, however only entails skin removal and nipple-areola repositioning without the parenchymal resection

POST-PROCEDURE

Expected Outcome
- Multiple reviews and meta-analyses show procedure is associated with a statistically significant improvement in physical disability and quality of life
- Symptom relief and improved body image are independent of pre-operative body weight
- Most patients would have the surgery again and would recommend it to others

Things To Do
- Resected breast tissue should be sent for pathology review
- Occult breast carcinomas in 0.06-0.4% of reduction specimens; up to 0.8% if DCIS is included

Post-Procedure Care
- Use of post-surgical drains is variable, with removal usually by 24 hours if used
- Bandage wrap similar to a brassiere
- Bandages and skin sutures usually removed by post-operative day 3
- Patients usually instructed to wear a sports bra for the first 2-3 weeks
- Bruising in the inferior breasts is expected post-operatively with gradual resolution
- Heavy exercise should be avoided for about 2 months with traditional reduction surgery
- Recommendations for post-operative mammography
  - Usually only in patients over age 35
  - Some recommend new baseline imaging as early as 3-6 months, others at 1 year
  - Patients having reduction for macromastia or congenital asymmetry have the same breast cancer risk as age-matched cohorts who have not had reduction, necessitating biopsy of any atypical post-operative findings
  - Changes from reduction as a symmetry procedure for contralateral mastectomy or breast conservation surgery do not delay the diagnosis of a subsequent primary cancer in the reduced breast

PROBLEMS & COMPLICATIONS

Problems
- Post-operative scarring

Complications
- Placing the nipple too high: Should be at or near the level of the inframammary fold

- Misplacing the nipple either too medially or too laterally: Breast meridian defined as line from mid clavicle through nipple to inframammary fold
- Inadequate skin or glandular resection at periphery of the breast may produce an unaesthetic-appearing breast
- Scar hypertrophy: Can be accentuated by excess skin resection or increased skin tension
- Dog ears (skin excess) at the end of the vertical wound: Usually occurs in elderly patients or those with poor skin elasticity, requires surgical correction
- Breast asymmetry
- Overly narrowed pedicle may lead to nipple-areola ischemia resulting in areolar depigmentation, scar hypertrophy or even total nipple-areola loss
- Loss of nipple sensation: May be prevented by maintaining a lateralized dermoglandular pedicle as innervation is thought to arise from the lateral cutaneous branch of the fourth intercostal nerve

SELECTED REFERENCES

1. Abramson DL et al: Improving long-term breast shape with the medial pedicle Wise pattern breast reduction. Plast Reconstr Surg. 115(7):1937-1943, 2005
2. Colwell AS et al: Occult breast carcinoma in reduction mammaplasty specimens: 14-year experience. Plast Reconstr Surg. 113(7):1984-8, 2004
3. Moskovitz MJ et al: Outcome study in liposuction breast reduction. Plast Reconstr Surg. 114(1):55-60, 2004
4. Poell JG: Vertical reduction mammaplasty. Aesth Plast Surg. 28:59-69, 2004
5. Tarone RE et al: Breast reduction surgery and breast cancer risk: does reduction mammaplasty have a role in primary prevention strategies for women at high risk of breast cancer? Plast Reconstr Surg. 113(7):2104-10, 2004
6. Lalonde DH et al: The no vertical scar breast reduction: a minor variation that allows you to remove vertical scar portion of the inferior pedicle Wise pattern T scar. Aesth Plast Surg. 27:335-44, 2003
7. Matarasso A: Suction mammaplasty: the use of suction lipectomy alone to reduce large breasts. Clin Plastic Surg. 29:433-443, 2002
8. Chadbourne EB et al: Clinical outcomes in reduction mammaplasty: a systematic review and meta-analysis of published studies. Mayo Clin Proceed. 76(5):503-10, 2001
9. Netscher DT et al: Physical and psychological symptoms among 88 volunteer subjects compared with patients seeking plastic surgery procedures to the breast. Plast Reconstr Surg. 105(7):2366-73, 2000
10. Glatt BS et al: A retrospective study of changes in physical symptoms and body image after reduction mammaplasty. Plast Reconstr Surg. 103(1):76-82, 1999
11. Hidalgo DA et al: Current trends in breast reduction. Plast Reconstr Surg. 104(3):806-15, 1999
12. Spear SL: Surgery of the Breast: Principles and Art. Philadelphia, Lippincott-Raven. Chapter 49, 673, 1998
13. Aston SJ et al: Grabb and Smith's Plastic Surgery, 5th ed. Philadelphia, Lippincott-Raven. Chapter 59, 725, 1997
14. Burk RW et al: Conceptual considerations in breast reconstruction. Clin Plast Surg. 22(1):141-152, 1995

IMAGE GALLERY

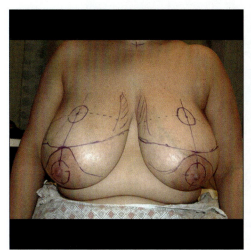

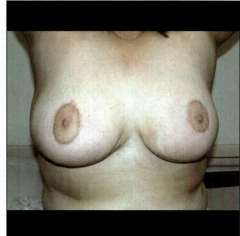

(Left) Clinical photograph shows pre-operative skin marking for new nipple-areola site, new inframammary fold line, and area for de-epithelialization. *(Right)* Clinical photograph shows post-operative appearance (same patient as on left) after 1290 g and 1095 g of breast tissue were removed from the right and left breasts, respectively, using the "no vertical scar" technique.

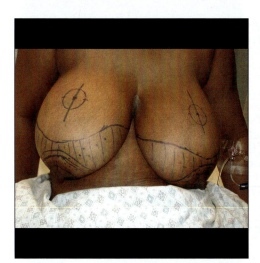

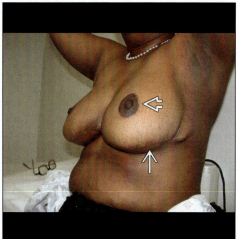

(Left) Clinical photograph shows pre-operative skin marking for a "no vertical scar" reduction. New site of nipple-areola complex and cross-hatched area for de-epithelialization marked. *(Right)* Clinical photograph 4 months post-op (same patient as on left). Breast tissue removed was 1100 g (R) and 1020 g (L). Periareolar ➾ and inframammary ➡ scars visible.

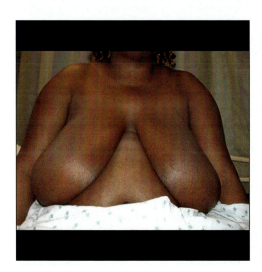

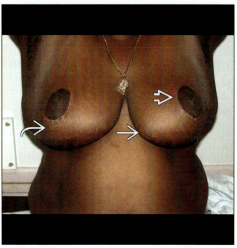

(Left) Clinical photograph shows pre-operative appearance of large breasts with extensive ptosis, making this patient a good candidate for the traditional inverted T scar reduction. *(Right)* Clinical photograph 6 weeks post-op (same patient as on left). 2325 g (R) and 2355 g (L) of breast tissue removed. Inverted T with periareolar ➾, vertical ➘, and inframammary ➡ scars.

SENTINEL NODE BIOPSY

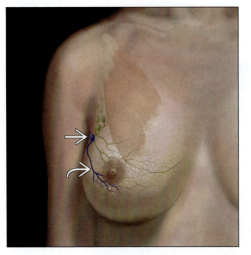

Graphic shows uptake of blue dye by lymphatic channels ➤ and level I axillary lymph node ➤. A few minutes following peritumoral injection, an axillary incision is made, and the blue node is resected.

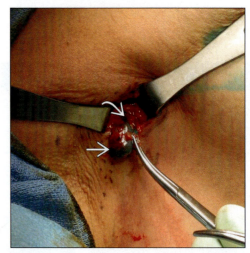

Blue axillary SLN ➤ and lymphatic channels ➤ are identified. A gamma probe is used intraoperatively to confirm identity of the "hot" sentinel node(s) containing radiocolloid (which may or may not also be "blue").

TERMINOLOGY

Abbreviations
- Sentinel lymph node (SLN) biopsy (SNB)

Synonyms
- Sentinel lymphadenectomy

Definitions
- Surgical removal of first draining node(s) for histologic nodal staging in patients with breast cancer
  - Premise: Breast cancer will spread to one or a few "sentinel" nodes in regional nodal basin before spreading to any other nodes
  - Hypothesis: If sentinel node(s) are negative, no need for full ALND
- SLN(s): Node(s) identified by uptake of Tc-99m sulfur colloid ± blue dye ± intraoperative palpation
- Axillary lymph node dissection (ALND); typically level I and II nodes
- Immunohistochemistry (IHC): Using antibody to cytokeratin (present in epithelial cells) to identify isolated tumor cells (ITC)
- Lymphoscintigraphy: Preoperative gamma camera imaging following injection of Tc-99m sulfur colloid into breast with cancer
- Staging: pN0: No regional lymph node metastasis by H&E; IHC not performed
  - pN0(i-): No regional lymph node metastasis by H&E; IHC negative
  - pN0(i+): No regional lymph node metastasis by H&E; positive IHC, no IHC cluster (ITC) > 0.2 mm
  - pN1mi = Micrometastasis (> 0.2 mm, none > 2.0 mm)
  - pN1 = Macrometastasis: Tumor deposit > 2.0 mm
- Nonsentinel node (NSN): Lymph node not identified by SNB

- False negative SNB: NSN shows metastatic disease when SLN negative

Location
- When SLN identified, ipsilateral axillary location in ~ 92-97% of patients
- Internal mammary node (IMN) as well as axillary SLNs in ~ 14-20%
- Isolated IMN drainage in 3-8%
  - Isolated IMN metastasis in 1-3% of all patients (10% of patients with negative axilla)
- Isolated contralateral axillary, and supraclavicular sentinel node(s) rare

PRE-PROCEDURE

Indications
- Patients with invasive breast cancer who are operative candidates
  - Unifocal, multifocal, and multicentric carcinoma all appropriate
  - Prior fine needle aspiration biopsy (FNAB), core, incisional, or excisional biopsy of primary cancer
- DCIS with microinvasion
- DCIS when mastectomy is planned
- High-grade DCIS > 2.5 cm in size (variable)
- Prior to neoadjuvant chemotherapy
- At time of prophylactic mastectomy (variable)

Contraindications
- Note: ALND recommended when SNB contraindicated
- Clinically suspicious axillary nodes
  - May be completely replaced by tumor, source of false negative SNBs
- Known lymph node metastasis(es) by prior imaging-directed FNAB
- Prior mastectomy (no way to identify SLN)

SENTINEL NODE BIOPSY

Key Facts

Terminology
- Surgical removal of first draining node(s) for histologic nodal staging in patients with breast cancer
- Premise: Breast cancer will spread to one or a few "sentinel" nodes in regional nodal basin before spreading to any other nodes
- SLN(s): Node(s) identified by uptake of Tc-99m sulfur colloid ± blue dye ± intraoperative palpation

Pre-procedure
- Lymphoscintigraphy optional
- Pre-operative radiocolloid injection: Intratumoral or peritumoral, subdermal, or subareolar routes all successful

Procedure
- Failure to identify SLN → perform ALND

- Mean of 1.9 (median of 2) SLNs identified (range 1-4)
- IHC to identify ITC if H&E negative: Use and significance are controversial

Post-procedure
- Metastasis in axillary node(s): Most important adverse prognostic indicator of breast cancer survival
- SNB results in significantly less morbidity than ALND
- Combined radiotracer + blue dye: ~ 93% sensitivity; ~ 97% NPV; and > 95% accuracy of SNB for axillary staging
- Successful identification of SLN: Blue dye alone = 83%; radiocolloid alone = 89%; combined radiocolloid and blue dye = 92%
- Half of false negatives are clinically suspicious
- Completion ALND if SLN + on touch prep, H&E

- Patients with DCIS (< 2.5 cm or not high grade) undergoing lumpectomy
- Prior axillary surgery
- Prior cosmetic breast surgery other than implants
- Prior neoadjuvant chemotherapy (NAT)
  - Higher false negative rate (treated metastasis)
  - SNB may be of benefit prior to NAT
- Inflammatory, T3 (> 5 cm) or T4 (involving skin or chest wall) carcinomas: Higher false negative rate
- Pregnancy: Reluctance to use radioisotope; safety of isosulfan blue dye not established; methylene blue ok

Getting Started
- Things to Check
  - Clinical examination of axilla
    - Clinically suspicious nodes → ALND
  - Lymphoscintigraphy optional
    - Can depict non-axillary SLN: Significance controversial
- Medications
  - SNB generally performed under general anesthesia
    - Unless precluded by severity of comorbid conditions
  - Tc-99m sulfur colloid ± Isosulfan or methylene blue dye injection
    - Radiocolloid: Varying volumes (0.1-5 cc), preparations (filtered or not), doses (0.1-10 mCi, divided or not)
    - Smaller particles may migrate more rapidly
  - Pre-operative radiocolloid injection: Intratumoral or peritumoral, subdermal, or subareolar routes all successful
    - Intra- or peritumoral: Upper outer quadrant cancer/injection may obscure detection of axillary SLN due to "shine through"
    - Slower uptake with intra- or peritumoral route (hours): Massage breast to facilitate uptake
    - Subdermal, subareolar routes: Rapid uptake in axilla, may fail to identify non-axillary sentinel nodes (not thought to be clinically relevant)
    - Subareolar route preferred with multifocal or multicentric carcinomas
  - Blue dye injected intra-operatively around tumor

  - Pre-operative, single dose, intravenous antibiotics to minimize risk of wound infection (optional)
- Equipment List: Hand-held gamma probe

PROCEDURE

Patient Position/Location
- Best procedure approach: Patient supine with ipsilateral arm abducted 90° on armboard

Procedure Steps
- Inject radiocolloid 2-24 hours (intra- or peritumoral) or less (subareolar or periareolar) prior to surgery
- Optional: Inject blue dye (1-5 cc) around tumor intraoperatively, followed by 5 minutes manual breast massage to facilitate lymphatic uptake
- 2-3 cm low axillary incision (same as for ALND)
  - No separate incision if in conjunction with mastectomy
- If radiocolloid was injected, use gamma probe to identify area of high counts, indicating location of SLN(s) (guides removal)
  - Confirm high counts in resected node ex vivo
- If blue dye utilized, visually inspect to trace blue lymphatic channels to SLN
- Palpate axillary contents intraoperatively to identify any grossly positive nodes
- Intra-operative inspection of cut faces, frozen section or touch prep (= imprint cytology) of SLN(s)
  - Particularly if clinically suspicious
- Immediate conversion to ALND recommended if
  - SLN shows metastasis on intraoperative frozen section or touch prep
    - Touch prep: 81% sensitivity for macrometastases; 22% for micrometastases
  - Failure to identify SLN → perform ALND
- Once SLNs have been removed, wound is closed without a drain if no ALND

Findings and Reporting
- Mean of 1.9 (median of 2) SLNs identified (range 1-4)
- Serial longitudinal paraffin sections SLN(s), H&E

○ #, size of nodes blue and/or hot intra-operatively
○ Report micro- and macrometastases
  ▪ Maximal diameter of largest tumor cell deposit
○ Micrometastases seen in 10-12% of nodes negative by conventional bivalve examination
• IHC to identify ITC if H&E negative: Use and significance are controversial

Alternative Procedures/Therapies

• Radiologic
  ○ Suspicious node(s) on imaging (e.g., mammography, US, MR) → FNAB or core biopsy
    ▪ If known positive node(s) preoperatively, then ALND performed
• Surgical
  ○ ALND: Mean of 16 nodes identified (range of means 11-23)
  ○ Trend to broader sampling of level I nodes only without full ALND if SLN not identified
• Other
  ○ Axillary XRT in lieu of completion ALND if SLN positive (controversial, ongoing studies)
    ▪ Good local control (together with chemotherapy); salvage ALND for axillary recurrence
    ▪ Reduced lymphedema, pain, numbness

V

3

20

POST-PROCEDURE

Expected Outcome

• Metastasis in axillary node(s): Most important adverse prognostic indicator of breast cancer survival
  ○ Guides treatment planning
  ○ Micrometastasis significant in T1 disease, may not be with T2 tumor (NSABP B-32)
  ○ N0(i+) disease may not affect overall survival
• SNB results in significantly less morbidity than ALND
• Combined radiotracer + blue dye: ~ 93% sensitivity; ~ 97% NPV; and > 95% accuracy of SNB for axillary staging
• Successful identification of SLN: Blue dye alone = 83%; radiocolloid alone = 89%; combined radiocolloid and blue dye = 92%
• If SNB negative, axillary staging is complete
  ○ Half of false negatives are clinically suspicious
• Significance of pN0(i+) debated, may not merit ALND
• If SNB shows metastatic disease by H&E, "completion" ALND recommended
  ○ Completion ALND shows additional positive nodes in 48% (95% confidence interval, 35-62)
  ○ Positive NSN more common in certain situations
    ▪ Larger primary tumor size
    ▪ Increasing number of positive SLN(s)
    ▪ Fewer SLN(s) examined
    ▪ Tumor not in upper outer quadrant
    ▪ Tumor shows lymphovascular invasion

Things To Do

• Completion ALND if SLN + on touch prep, H&E
• Recognized learning curve: Surgeon should perform 20 cases of SNB followed by immediate completion ALND
  ○ Goals: Identify SLN ≥ 85%, false negative rate ≤ 5%
• Adjuvant treatment influenced by SNB ± ALND results

○ Positive lymph nodes generally an indication for adjuvant chemotherapy
○ ≥ 4 positive nodes prompts post-mastectomy radiation

PROBLEMS & COMPLICATIONS

Complications

• Most feared complication(s)
  ○ Upper extremity lymphedema: ~ 5-7% for SNB vs. 13% for ALND
  ○ 7% seroma, 1% hematoma, 1% wound infection
• Other complications
  ○ Injury to nerves, arm numbness, rare
  ○ Axillary web syndrome: Tender lymphatic cords upper inner arm
  ○ Allergic reaction to isosulfan blue dye: 1-2%, mostly hives; 0.25-0.5% anaphylactic
• Insignificant radiation exposure from radiocolloid to patient, staff, pathologist, others

SELECTED REFERENCES

1. Cox CE et al: Sentinel node biopsy before neoadjuvant chemotherapy for determining axillary status and treatment prognosis in locally advanced breast cancer. Ann Surg Oncol. 13(4):483-90, 2006
2. Kim T et al: Lymphatic mapping and sentinel lymph node biopsy in early-stage breast carcinoma: a metaanalysis. Cancer. 106(1):4-16, 2006
3. Mansel RE et al: Randomized multicenter trial of sentinel node biopsy versus standard axillary treatment in operable breast cancer: the ALMANAC Trial. J Natl Cancer Inst. 98(9):599-609, 2006
4. Wilke LG et al: Surgical complications associated with sentinel lymph node biopsy: results from a prospective international cooperative group trial. Ann Surg Oncol. 13(4):491-500, 2006
5. Hong J et al: Extra-axillary sentinel node biopsy in the management of early breast cancer. Eur J Surg Oncol. 31(9):942-8, 2005
6. Lyman GH et al: American Society of Clinical Oncology guideline recommendations for sentinel lymph node biopsy in early-stage breast cancer. J Clin Oncol. 23(30):7703-20, 2005
7. Tew K et al: Meta-analysis of sentinel node imprint cytology in breast cancer. Br J Surg. 92(9):1068-80, 2005
8. Singletary SE et al: Revision of the American Joint Committee on Cancer staging system for breast cancer. J Clin Oncol. 20(17):3628-36, 2002
9. Cody HS 3rd et al: Complementarity of blue dye and isotope in sentinel node localization for breast cancer: univariate and multivariate analysis of 966 procedures. Ann Surg Oncol. 8(1):13-9, 2001
10. Haigh PI et al: Biopsy method and excision volume do not affect success rate of subsequent sentinel lymph node dissection in breast cancer. Ann Surg Oncol. 7(1):21-7, 2000
11. McMasters KM et al: Preoperative lymphoscintigraphy for breast cancer does not improve the ability to identify axillary sentinel lymph nodes. Ann Surg. 231:724-31, 2000
12. Veronesi U et al: Sentinel-node biopsy to avoid axillary dissection in breast cancer with clinically negative lymph-nodes. Lancet. 349(9069):1864-7, 1997

IMAGE GALLERY

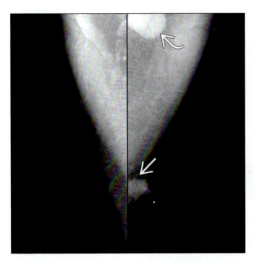
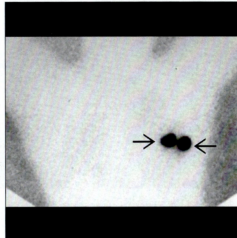

(Left) MLO mammography shows irregular palpable mass ➡ in a 59 y/o male. Core biopsy showed grade III IDC. Large, dense left axillary node is noted ⮧. FNAB or core biopsy can confirm metastatic node preoperatively, and SNB can be falsely negative with clinically suspicious nodes. *(Right)* Frontal scintigram (same patient as previous image) obtained immediately after injection of 576 μCi Tc-99m sulfur colloid shows hot spots ➡ corresponding to peritumoral injection sites.

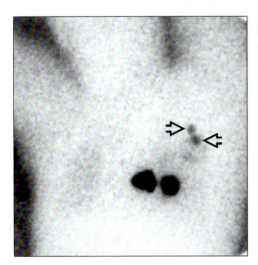
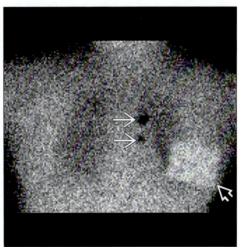

(Left) LAO scintigram at 2 hours (same as prior two images) shows tracer in two SLNs ⮧ left axilla. Intraoperative frozen section = metastatic nodes. Full ALND showed 18 metastatic lymph nodes. *(Right)* Scintigram (different case) shows two internal mammary SLNs ➡ without axillary uptake (peritumoral injection site shielded ⮧). 14-18% of internal mammary (IM) SLNs are malignant; isolated IM SLN are seen in ~ 3-8% of cases, but are often not resected.

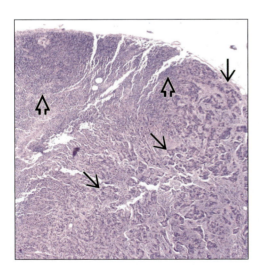
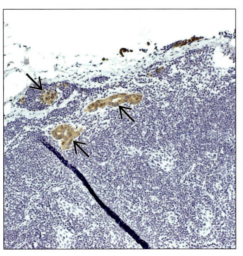

(Left) Micropathology, low power, H&E shows metastatic carcinoma ➡ in SLN, with minimal residual lymphatic tissue ⮧. Completion ALND is typically performed when SLN shows metastatic disease on frozen or permanent section. *(Right)* Micropathology, low power, shows several < 2 mm groups of keratin-positive metastatic epithelial cells ➡ in subcapsular sinus of SLN, i.e., micrometastasis. Completion ALND is usually recommended.

TRAM AND OTHER FLAP PROCEDURES

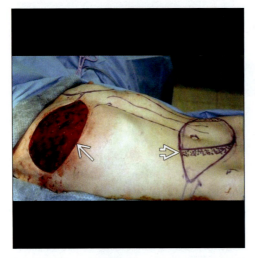

Intra-operative photograph demonstrates right mastectomy site ➡ with planned construction of pedicle TRAM flap ➡. (All clinical photos courtesy of JJP).

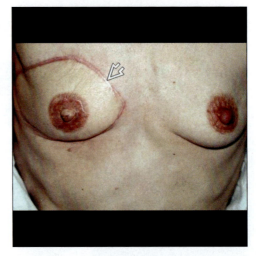

Post-operative photograph of the same patient as previous image demonstrates appearance of right pedicle TRAM flap ➡ with post-operative nipple reconstruction.

TERMINOLOGY

Abbreviations
- Transverse rectus abdominus myocutaneous (TRAM) pedicle and free flap
- Deep inferior epigastric perforator (DIEP) flap
- Latissimus dorsi myocutaneous (LDM) flap
- Gluteal free flap, inferior gluteal artery perforator (I-GAP), superior gluteal artery perforator (S-GAP) flap
- Others: Lateral transverse thigh flap; Rubens or periiliac flap

Synonyms
- Neobreast

Definitions
- Autologous breast tissue reconstruction
  - Flaps may be used alone or in combination with breast implant (usually silicone)

PRE-PROCEDURE

Indications
- Following mastectomy for breast cancer
  - Patient desires cosmetic approximation of pre-surgical breast appearance
    - Current trend towards immediate flap reconstruction at time of mastectomy
    - May provide a more natural feel than implants
- Following prophylactic mastectomy
  - Unilateral or bilateral
  - BRCA-1, -2 carrier or other high risk patient
- Following partial mastectomy
  - LDM flap to bulk up lateral resection site
- Reconstruction after implant removal

Contraindications
- Relative contraindications
  - Poor overall health increases risk of complications
  - Obesity
    - Too much abdominal tissue relative to contralateral native breast (for TRAM flaps)
  - Extreme underweight
    - Too little abdominal tissue to achieve breast symmetry
  - Extensive abdominal scarring, prior surgery (for TRAM flaps)
    - Including prior unilateral TRAM flap: Cannot do second TRAM later
  - Young patient desiring potential future childbirth
    - Relative abdominal wall weakness (for TRAM flaps)
  - Vascular disease
    - History of smoking, atherosclerosis, collagen vascular disease, diabetes
  - High cost of procedure: Usually covered by insurance
- Locally advanced primary breast malignancy
  - Extensive skin/subcutaneous tissue involvement may complicate flap placement
  - Neoadjuvant chemotherapy prior to surgery may shrink tumor, even allow breast conservation

Getting Started
- Complete pre-mastectomy preoperative work-up
  - Breast biopsy +/- axillary node FNAB or core biopsy
  - Comprehensive imaging evaluation
    - Extent of ipsilateral and/or contralateral disease
    - Nipple-areolar complex involvement
    - Clear margins anticipated at skin and chest wall
- Consultation with oncologist, radiation oncologist
  - Plan for neoadjuvant and/or adjuvant chemotherapy

TRAM AND OTHER FLAP PROCEDURES

Key Facts

Terminology
- Transverse rectus abdominus myocutaneous (TRAM) pedicle and free flap
- Latissimus dorsi myocutaneous (LDM) flap

Pre-procedure
- Following mastectomy for breast cancer
- Following prophylactic mastectomy
- Reconstruction after implant removal
- Complete pre-mastectomy preoperative work-up
- Consultation with oncologist, radiation oncologist
- Delayed reconstruction if post-mastectomy XRT anticipated
- Consultation with surgeon and plastic surgeon
- Assessment of patient emotional readiness

Procedure
- Skin ellipse and underlying subcutaneous tissue with rectus muscle tunneled through abdominal subcutaneous tissues to mastectomy site
- Skin of flap used to appose edges of oblique mastectomy incision

Post-procedure
- Lengthy post-procedure hospitalization, recovery
- No increased risk of recurrence
- Possible improved psychological adjustment to mastectomy(ies)
- More natural feel compared to implants

Problems & Complications
- Post-surgical imaging follow-up controversial

- ○ Delayed reconstruction if post-mastectomy XRT anticipated
  - ■ Close or positive margins likely
  - ■ Large primary cancer (T3 or T4)
  - ■ ≥ 4 axillary lymph nodes metastatic
- • Consultation with surgeon and plastic surgeon
  - ○ Pre-operative surgical planning
    - ■ Type of flap, choice of donor site, +/- skin-sparing technique
    - ■ Need for ipsilateral implant
    - ■ Need for contralateral mastopexy, reduction, augmentation to achieve symmetry with neobreast
    - ■ History of prior TRAM
  - ○ Assessment of patient emotional readiness
    - ■ Provision of educational materials
    - ■ Patient meeting with others who have had similar procedure
- • Preoperative or intraoperative color Doppler can help map vascular supply of planned flap

PROCEDURE

Patient Position/Location
- Best procedure approach: Patient supine, arm abducted 90 degrees

Procedure Steps
- Mastectomy ± SNB and/or ALND
  - ○ Total (simple) mastectomy: Complete excision of breast tissue and usually nipple-areolar complex
  - ○ Modified radical mastectomy
- TRAM pedicle flap technique
  - ○ Skin ellipse and underlying subcutaneous tissue with rectus muscle tunneled through abdominal subcutaneous tissues to mastectomy site
  - ○ Rectus muscle (and associated vascular pedicle) to contralateral mastectomy generally used
    - ■ Bilateral TRAM flaps are derived from ipsilateral side to avoid crossing pedicles, kinked vessels
  - ○ Skin of flap used to appose edges of oblique mastectomy incision

- ■ Alternative in nipple/areolar complex-sparing procedure: De-epithelialize flap, position beneath native skin
- ○ Mesh occasionally used to strengthen abdominal wall
  - ■ Present emphasis on "minimal muscle plug" (adipomyocutaneous flap) to minimize risk of abdominal hernia
- ○ Traditional approach: Superior epigastric artery (SEA) blood supply to pedicle
- ○ Generally does not require additional implant
  - ■ Two pedicles (bilateral rectus muscle flaps) may be used on the same side to match size of large contralateral breast
  - ■ Contralateral breast reduction may improve symmetry
- ○ Advantages
  - ■ Least technically complicated flap procedure
  - ■ Lower likelihood necrosis compared to free flap
  - ■ Shorter procedure time and hospital stay than free flap
- • Free TRAM flap technique: Inferior epigastric artery (IEA) supply
  - ○ Smaller portion of rectus muscle is removed from abdominal wall compared to pedicle flap technique
  - ○ Overlying skin and subcutaneous fat transferred to mastectomy site
  - ○ Artery transected and anastomosed to thoracodorsal artery, subscapular artery, or internal mammary artery (IMA)
    - ■ Vascular anastomosis enters from upper outer quadrant of flap
    - ■ Thoracodorsal artery most accessible if axillary node dissection performed
  - ○ Advantages over pedicle TRAM flap
    - ■ Robust vascular supply
    - ■ Less extensive abdominal dissection
  - ○ Disadvantages over pedicle TRAM flap
    - ■ Requires meticulous technique, experience
    - ■ Longer procedure and hospital stay, higher cost
- • Deep inferior epigastric perforator (DIEP) flap technique

- ○ Skin and subcutaneous tissues only are transferred
  - May preserve abdominal wall strength
  - ○ Blood supply: Perforating branches of deep inferior epigastric vessels
  - ○ Additional technical challenges, requires experienced surgeon
- Latissimus dorsi flap (LDM)
  - ○ Muscle, fat, skin transferred similar to TRAM
  - ○ Blood supply: Thoracodorsal artery
  - ○ Requires intra-operative patient repositioning
  - ○ Generally requires implant beneath flap
  - ○ Smaller size may better approximate contralateral breast size in small-breasted patient
    - May not need additional implant
  - ○ Larger scar, less obscured by some clothing
  - ○ Alternative site in patient with prior TRAM flap and cancer recurrence, or flap failure
- Gluteal free flap
  - ○ Portion of buttock including skin, fat, muscle
  - ○ S-GAP: Superior gluteal artery to internal mammary artery
  - ○ I-GAP: Inferior gluteal artery to thoracodorsal artery
  - ○ Requires flipping patient intraoperatively
  - ○ Advantage: Alternative if cannot use abdominal donor site
  - ○ Disadvantage: Possible discomfort while sitting
- Post-reconstruction nipple-areola reconstruction
  - ○ May be performed in office under local anesthesia then tattoo

Alternative Procedures/Therapies
- Surgical
  - ○ Total mastectomy with implant reconstruction
    - Expander often placed initially, then delayed silicone or saline implant, usually subpectoral
    - Technically easier than flap construction
    - Wider availability for patients far from secondary/tertiary care hospital center
    - Less expensive
    - Alterable (implant may be explanted/augmented if needed)
    - Shorter recovery time than for flap
    - Preserves abdominal musculature (i.e., singer, athlete)
    - Expected implant lifetime 10-13 years, may need re-operation
  - ○ Total mastectomy without flap construction or implant placement: Use external prosthesis
  - ○ Lumpectomy with radiation therapy (XRT) if clear margins can be achieved
  - ○ Delayed breast reconstruction
    - When need for post-mastectomy XRT
    - Lack of necessary specialized staff or facility at time of initial mastectomy
    - Patient preference

POST-PROCEDURE

Expected Outcome
- Compared to uncomplicated total mastectomy
  - ○ Lengthy post-procedure hospitalization, recovery
  - ○ No increased risk of recurrence

- Possible improved psychological adjustment to mastectomy(ies)
- Immediate reconstruction more cost-effective than delayed
- More natural feel compared to implants
- TRAM, DIEP flaps → relocate fat of abdomen ("tummy tuck")
  - ○ Secondary cosmetic benefit in some patients
- Possible XRT after flap reconstruction
  - ○ May be needed if immediate reconstruction performed, pending margin and lymph node status
  - ○ Higher complication rates observed
  - ○ External XRT favored before reconstruction when possible

Post-Flap Imaging Surveillance
- Controversial, institution-dependent
- Requires familiarity with expected post-operative appearance

PROBLEMS & COMPLICATIONS

Problems
- Size discrepancy with contralateral breast

Complications
- Most feared complication(s): Partial or complete loss of flap: Vascular compromise → tissue/skin necrosis
- Other complications
  - ○ Abdominal muscle weakness
    - Smaller free flap: Greater preservation of abdominal wall strength
  - ○ Ventral hernia (5-9%)
  - ○ Fat necrosis (2-14%)
    - Often upper outer quadrant of TRAM flap (reduced vascularity)
    - May present as calcified mass
    - Mammography usually definitive
  - ○ Disease recurrence: Usually in skin, subcutaneous tissues
    - Mammography, US, MR: Can depict recurrent disease in flap
    - Mammography best to distinguish from fat necrosis
    - Post-surgical imaging follow-up controversial
  - ○ Post-reconstruction XRT complications
    - Flap shrinkage, change in color/texture
    - Vascular insufficiency causing necrosis
    - Possibly less effective treatment due to wider apposition of surgical margins around flap tissues

SELECTED REFERENCES
1. Devon RK et al: Breast reconstruction with a transverse rectus abdominis myocutaneous flap: spectrum of normal and abnormal MR imaging findings. Radiographics. 24:1287-99, 2004
2. Helvie MA et al: Mammographic screening of TRAM flap breast reconstructions for detection of nonpalpable recurrent cancer. Radiology. 224:211-6, 2002
3. Shaikh N et al: Detection of recurrent breast cancer after TRAM flap reconstruction. Ann Plast Surg. 47:602-7, 2001

IMAGE GALLERY

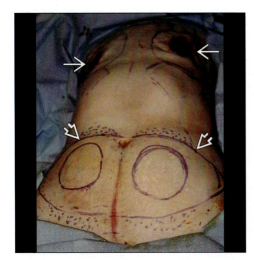 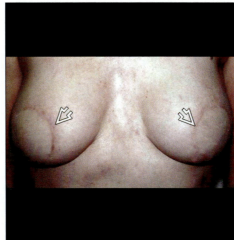

(Left) Intra-operative photograph of a patient status post bilateral skin-sparing mastectomies ➡, with planned bilateral pedicle TRAM flap ➡ reconstruction. **(Right)** Post-operative photograph of the same patient as previous image demonstrates appearance of bilateral TRAM flaps ➡ without post-operative nipple reconstruction.

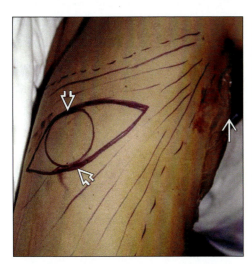 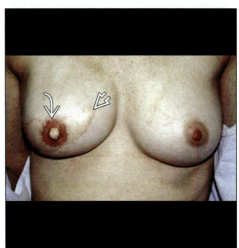

(Left) Intra-operative photograph of a patient undergoing right mastectomy ➡ with ipsilateral latissimus dorsi flap reconstruction ➡. **(Right)** Post-operative photograph of the same patient as previous image status post latissimus dorsi flap reconstruction ➡ with implant placement, and post-operative nipple reconstruction ➡.

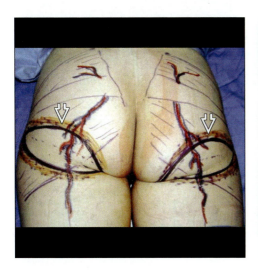 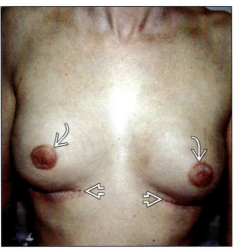

(Left) Intra-operative photograph demonstrates planned approach for bilateral inferior gluteal flap reconstruction ➡ in a patient status post explantation of bilateral ruptured silicone implants. **(Right)** Post-operative photograph of the same patient as previous image demonstrates bilateral gluteal flaps ➡ with post-operative nipple reconstruction ➡.

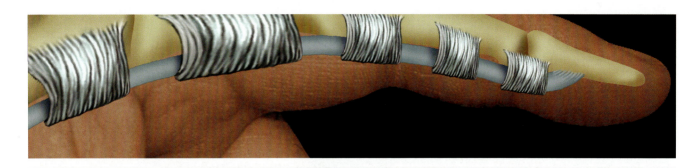

INDEX

INDEX

INDEX

INDEX

INDEX

i

v

INDEX

INDEX

INDEX

i

ix

INDEX

INDEX

INDEX

INDEX

INDEX

INDEX

INDEX

xx

i

INDEX

INDEX